Operative
Orthopaedics
Volume 2

Operative Orthopaedics

Volume 2

Edited by

Michael W. Chapman, M.D.

Professor and Chair
Department of Orthopaedics
University of California, Davis
Davis, California

Michael Madison, Ph.D.

Managing Editor

196 Contributors

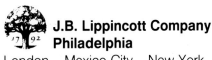

J.B. Lippincott Company
Philadelphia
London   Mexico City   New York
St. Louis   São Paulo   Sydney

Acquisitions Editor: Darlene Barela Cooke
Developmental Editor: Richard Winters
Manuscript Editor: Patrick O'Kane
Indexer: Barbara Littlewood
Developmental Designer: Susan Blaker
Design Coordinator: Michelle Gerdes
Production Manager: Carol Florence
Production Coordinator: Barney Fernandes
Compositor: TAPSCO Inc.
Printer/Binder: Halliday Lithograph Corp.

1   3   5   6   4   2

LIBRARY OF CONGRESS
Library of Congress Cataloging-in-Publication Data

Operative orthopaedics/edited by Michael W. Chapman;
Michael Madison, managing editor.
    p.   cm.
    Includes bibliographies and index.
    1. Orthopedic surgery.   I. Chapman, Michael W.
II. Madison, Michael,
[DNLM: 1. Orthopedics.   WE 168 061]
RD731.064 1988
617'.3—dc19
DNLM/DLC
for Library of Congress   87-34225
                             CIP
ISBN 0-397-50919-7 (vol. 1)
ISBN 0-397-50920-0 (vol. 2)
ISBN 0-397-50921-9 (vol. 3)

ISBN 0-397-50772-0 (3 vol. set)

The authors and publisher have exerted every effort to ensure
that drug selection and dosage set forth in this text are in
accord with current recommendations and practice at the time
of publication. However, in view of ongoing research, changes
in government regulations, and the constant flow of information relating to drug therapy and drug reactions, the reader is
urged to check the package insert for each drug for any change
in indications and dosage and for added warnings and precautions. This is particularly important when the recommended
agent is a new or infrequently employed drug.

Associate Editors

LEWIS D. ANDERSON, M.D.
Professor and Chairman
Department of Orthopaedics
University of South Alabama
College of Medicine
Mobile, Alabama
Infections

WILLIAM L. BARGAR, M.D.
Assistant Clinical Professor
Department of Orthopaedics
University of California, Davis
Davis, California
Department of Surgery, Orthopaedic Section
Sutter General Hospital
Sacramento, California
Joint Reconstruction

DANIEL R. BENSON, M.D.
Professor of Orthopaedics
University of California, Davis
Davis, California
Chief, Spinal Deformity Service
University of California, Davis Medical Center
Sacramento, California
The Spine

TIMOTHY J. BRAY, M.D.
Assistant Clinical Professor of Orthopaedics
University of California, Davis
Davis, California
Reno Orthopaedic Clinic
Reno, Nevada
Fractures and Dislocations

MICHAEL W. CHAPMAN, M.D.
Professor and Chairman
Department of Orthopaedics
University of California, Davis
Davis, California
Surgical Principles and Techniques
Amputations

DAVID B. COWARD, M.D.
Assistant Clinical Professor of Orthopaedic Surgery
University of California, Davis
Davis, California
Department of Surgery, Orthopaedic Section
Sutter General Hospital
Sacramento, California
Arthroscopic Surgery

JAMES O. JOHNSTON, M.D.
Clinical Professor of Orthopaedics
University of California, San Francisco
Chief, Department of Orthopaedics
Kaiser Foundation Hospital
Oakland, California
Tumors

ROGER A. MANN, M.D.
Associate Clinical Professor of Orthopaedic Surgery
University of California, San Francisco
Chief of Foot Surgery
Samuel Merritt Hospital
Oakland, California
The Foot

GEORGE T. RAB, M.D.
Associate Professor of Orthopaedic Surgery
University of California, Davis
Davis, California
Chief, Section of Children's Orthopaedics
University of California, Davis Medical Center
Sacramento, California
Pediatric Disorders

RICHARD S. RIGGINS, M.D.
Professor of Orthopaedics
Emory University School of Medicine
Atlanta, Georgia
Arthrodesis

JUAN J. RODRIGO, M.D.
Associate Professor of Orthopaedics
University of California, Davis
Chief, Adult Reconstructive Service
University of California, Davis Medical Center
Sacramento, California
The Knee

PHILLIP G. SPIEGEL, M.D.
Professor and Chairman
Department of Orthopaedic Surgery
University of South Florida
Tampa, Florida
Malunions and Nonunions

ROBERT M. SZABO, M.D.
Assistant Professor of Orthopaedics
University of California, Davis,
Davis, California
Chief, Hand & Microvascular Service
University of California, Davis Medical Center
Sacramento, California
The Hand

ANDREW J. WEILAND, M.D.
Professor, Department of Orthopaedic Surgery
Division of Plastic Surgery and
Department of Emergency Medicine
Chief, Division of Upper Extremity Surgery
Johns Hopkins University School of Medicine
Baltimore, Maryland
Microvascular Surgery

Contributors

PAUL J. ABBOTT, JR., M.D.
Virginia Beach Sports Medicine
Virginia Beach, Virginia

BEHROOZ A. AKBARNIA, M.D.
Professor and Vice Chairman
Department of Orthopedic Surgery
St. Louis University School of Medicine
Director of Orthopedics
Cardinal Glennon Children's Hospital
St. Louis, Missouri

A. HERBERT ALEXANDER, M.D.
Captain, Medical Corps, United States Navy
Clinical Associate Professor
Uniformed Services University of the Health Sciences
Bethesda, Maryland
Chairman, Department of Orthopaedic Surgery
Naval Hospital
Oakland, California

DANIEL D. ANDERSON, M.D.
Resident in Orthopaedic Surgery
University of California, Davis Medical Center
Sacramento, California

LEWIS D. ANDERSON, M.D.
Professor and Chairman
Department of Orthopaedics
University of South Alabama
College of Medicine
Mobile, Alabama

T. A. ANDREW, M.Sc., M.B.B.S.(Hons.), F.R.C.S.,
    F.R.C.S.(Ed.)
Consultant Orthopaedic Surgeon
Corbett Hospital
Stourbridge, West Midlands
England

JAMES R. ANDREWS, M.D.
Clinical Professor
Department of Orthopaedics
Section of Sports Medicine
Tulane University School of Medicine
Orthopaedic Surgeon
South Highlands Hospital
Birmingham, Alabama

WILLIAM L. BARGAR, M.D.
Assistant Clinical Professor
University of California, Davis
Davis, California
Department of Surgery, Orthopaedic Section
Sutter General Hospital
Sacramento, California

JAMES E. BATEMAN, M.D., F.R.C.S.(C)
Associate Professor of Surgery
University of Toronto
Surgeon-in-Chief (Emeritus)
Orthopaedic & Arthritic Hospital
Toronto, Ontario
Canada

LOUI G. BAYNE, M.D.
Clinical Associate Professor of Orthopedics
Emory University
Director Hand Clinic
Scottish Rite Children's Hospital
Atlanta, Georgia

ALFRED BEHRENS, M.D., F.R.C.S.(C)
Associate Professor of Orthopaedic Surgery
University of Minnesota
St. Paul Ramsey Medical Center
St. Paul, Minnesota

DEBORAH BELL, M.D., F.R.C.S.(C)
Lecturer, Division of Orthopaedic Surgery
University of Toronto
Orthopaedic Surgeon, Hospital for Sick Children
Toronto, Ontario
Canada

DANIEL R. BENSON, M.D.
Professor of Orthopaedics
University of California, Davis
Davis, California
Chief, Spinal Deformity Service
University of California,
Davis Medical Center
Sacramento, California

MARVIN H. BLOOM, M.D.
Associate Clinical Professor of Orthopaedic Surgery
University of California, San Francisco
Director, Sports Medicine Clinic
San Francisco General Hospital
San Francisco, California

DR. RENATO BOMBELLI
Specialist in Orthopaedics and Radiology
L. D. Clinica Ortopedica
University of Milano
Consultant in Orthopaedics and Traumatology
Hospital of Busto Arsizio
Legnano, Italy

LAWRENCE B. BONE, M.D.
Assistant Professor of Orthopaedic Surgery
State University of New York at Buffalo
Director, Musculoskeletal Trauma Service
Erie County Medical Center
Buffalo, New York

F. WILLIAM BORA, JR., M.D.
Professor of Orthopaedic Surgery
University of Pennsylvania
School of Medicine
Chief of Hand Surgery
Hospital of the University of Pennsylvania
Philadelphia, Pennsylvania

MICHAEL J. BOTTE, M.D.
Assistant Professor of Surgery
Chief, Foot and Ankle Surgery
University of California, San Diego
Chief of Hand Surgery
Veterans Administration Hospital
San Diego, California

J. RICHARD BOWEN, M.D.
Pediatric Orthopedic Surgeon
Alfred I. DuPont Institute
Wilmington, Delaware

PAUL W. BRAND, C.B.E., M.B., F.R.C.S.
Clinical Professor of Orthopaedics and Surgery
Louisiana State University Medical School
Senior Consultant
Gillis W. Long Hansen's Disease Center
Carville, Louisiana

TIMOTHY J. BRAY, M.D.
Assistant Clinical Professor of Orthopaedics
University of California, Davis
Davis, California
Reno Orthopaedic Clinic
Reno, Nevada

HUGH P. BROWN, M.D.
Clinical Assistant Professor of Orthopaedic Surgery
University of Tennessee College of Medicine
Chattanooga, Tennessee

WILTON H. BUNCH, M.D., PH.D.
Professor, Department of Surgery
University of Chicago Pritzker School of Medicine
Dean of Medical Affairs
University of Chicago Hospitals & Clinics
Chicago, Illinois

B. D. BURDEAUX, JR., M.D.
Assistant Clinical Professor of Orthopaedic Surgery
Baylor College of Medicine
Associate Clinical Professor
Department of Surgery
University of Texas
Health Science Center at Houston
Houston, Texas

WILLIAM E. BURKHALTER, M.D.
Professor and Vice-Chairman
Department of Orthopaedics and Rehabilitation
Chief, Division of Hand Surgery
University of Miami
Jackson Memorial Medical Center
Miami, Florida

J. KENNETH BURKUS, M.D.
Assistant Clinical Professor
Department of Orthopaedic Surgery
University of California, Davis Medical Center
Sacramento, California
Director, Spine Clinic
Department of Orthopaedic Surgery
Naval Hospital
Oakland, California

CHARLES CARROLL IV, M.D.
Instructor of Orthopaedic Surgery
Northwestern University Medical School
Chicago, Illinois

RICHARD B. CASPARI, M.D.
Clinical Associate Professor of Orthopaedics
Medical College of Virginia
Richmond, Virginia

JOSEPH R. CASS, M.D., M.S.
Orthopaedic Surgeon
Midwest Orthopaedic Center
Sioux Falls, South Dakota

MICHAEL W. CHAPMAN, M.D.
Professor and Chairman of Orthopaedics
University of California, Davis
Davis, California

LARRY K. CHIDGEY, M.D.
Department of Orthopaedic Surgery
University of California, Davis Medical Center
Sacramento, California

WILLIAM G. CLANCY, JR., M.D.
Professor and Head
Section of Sports Medicine
Division of Orthopaedic Surgery
University of Wisconsin
Madison, Wisconsin

THOMAS H. COMFORT, M.D.
Associate Professor of Orthopaedics
University of Minnesota
Chief, Orthopaedic Surgery
St. Paul-Ramsey Hospital
St. Paul, Minnesota

MICHAEL J. COUGHLIN, M.D.
Clinical Assistant Professor
Division of Orthopaedics and Rehabilitation
Oregon Health Sciences University
Portland, Oregon
Chief of Orthopaedic Surgery
St. Alphonsus Regional Medical Center
Boise, Idaho

MARK B. COVENTRY, M.D., M.S.
Emeritus Professor
Mayo Medical School
Emeritus Orthopaedic Consultant
Mayo Clinic
Rochester, Minnesota

DAVID B. COWARD, M.D.
Assistant Clinical Professor, Orthopaedic Surgery
University of California, Davis
Davis, California
Department of Surgery, Orthopaedic Section
Sutter General Hospital
Sacramento, California

EDWARD V. CRAIG, M.D.
Assistant Professor, Orthopaedics
University of Minnesota
Minneapolis, Minnesota

JAMES J. CREIGHTON, JR., M.D.
Assistant Chief, Hand Surgery Service
Maricopa Medical Center
Phoenix, Arizona

JOHN CSONGRADI, M.D.
Assistant Professor of Surgery (Orthopaedics)
Stanford University School of Medicine
Stanford, California

R. RAYMOND CUNNINGHAM, M.D.
Orthopaedic Surgeon
St. John's Hospital
Jackson, Wyoming

AVRON DANILLER, M.D., F.R.C.S.
Professor and Chief
Division of Plastic Surgery
University of California, Davis Medical Center
Sacramento, California

LAWRENCE D. DORR, M.D.
Consultant Orthopaedics, Rancho Los Amigos Medical Center
Assistant Clinical Professor
University of California, Irvine
Associate, Kerlan-Jobe Orthopaedic Clinic
Centinela Hospital
Inglewood, California

KAREN DUANE, M.D.
Instructor in Orthopaedic Surgery
New York Medical College
Valhalla, New York

DR. H. G. ENDER
University of Vienna
Oberarzt at the Unfallkrankenhaus Lorenz Bohler
Vienna, Austria

JOHN A. FEAGIN, JR., M.D.
Orthopaedic Surgeon
St. John's Hospital
Jackson, Wyoming

HARRY E. FIGGIE III, M.D.
Assistant Professor of Orthopaedic Surgery
Case Western Reserve University
School of Medicine
Cleveland, Ohio

HENRY A. FINN, M.D.
Assistant Professor, Department of Surgery
Section of Orthopaedics and Rehabilitation Medicine
The University of Chicago
Pritzker School of Medicine
Attending Physician, Department of Surgery
Section of Orthopaedics and Rehabilitation Medicine
Adult Reconstruction and Orthopaedic Oncology
The University of Chicago Medical Center
Chicago, Illinois

J. P. FLANAGAN, F.R.C.S., F.R.C.S.(Ed.)
Consultant Orthopaedic Surgeon
Black Notley Hospital
Braintree—Bloomfield Hospital
Chelmsford, Essex
England

JOSEPH C. FLYNN, M.D.
Clinical Teaching Staff
Post Graduate Orthopaedic Education
Clinical Instructor of Orthopaedics
Emeritus Chairman
Department of Orthopaedic Surgery
Orlando Regional Medical Center
Medical Director
Florida Elks Children's Hospital
Orlando, Florida

ALVIN A. FREEHAFER, M.D.
Professor of Orthopaedics
Case Western Reserve University
School of Medicine
Director of Orthopaedics
Chief of Spinal Cord Injury Center
Cuyahoga County Hospital
Cleveland, Ohio

ALAN E. FREELAND, M.D.
Professor, Department of Orthopaedic Surgery
University of Mississippi Medical Center
Chief, Hand and Upper Extremity Surgery
Department of Orthopaedic Surgery
Jackson, Mississippi

ROBERT W. GAINES, JR., M.D.
Associate Professor of Orthopaedics
University of Missouri School of Medicine
Columbia, Missouri

RICHARD H. GELBERMAN, M.D.
Professor of Orthopaedic Surgery
Harvard Medical Center
Chief of Hand and Upper Extremity Surgery
Massachusetts General Hospital
Boston, Massachusetts

DAVID H. GERSHUNI, M.D., F.R.C.S.(ENG)
    F.R.C.S.(EDIN)
Associate Professor of Orthopaedic Surgery
University of California, San Diego
Co-Chief, Fracture Service
University of California Medical Center, San Diego
Chief, Orthopaedic Surgery
VA Medical Center
San Diego, California

DALE B. GLASSER, M.S.
Research Coordinator
Orthopaedics
Memorial Sloan-Kettering Cancer Center
New York, New York

J. LEONARD GOLDNER, M.D.
James B. Duke Professor and Chief Emeritus
Department of Orthopaedics
Duke University Medical Center
Durham, North Carolina

STUART B. GOODMAN, M.D., MSc., F.R.C.S.C.
Assistant Professor of Surgery
Stanford University Medical Center
Stanford, California

JOHN S. GOULD, M.D.
Professor and Chairman
Department of Orthopaedic Surgery
Medical College of Wisconsin
Milwaukee, Wisconsin

JAMES A. GOULET, M.D.
Clinical Instructor
Section of Orthopaedic Surgery
The University of Michigan Medical Center
Ann Arbor, Michigan

STEVEN M. GREEN, M.D.
Clinical Associate Professor of Orthopaedic Surgery
Mt. Sinai Medical School
Assistant Chief of Hand Services
Mt. Sinai Hospital and Orthopaedic Institute
Hospital of Joint Diseases
New York, New York

WILLIAM L. GREEN, M.D.
Assistant Clinical Professor
University of California, San Francisco
School of Medicine
Children's Hospital
San Francisco, California

SIGVARD T. HANSEN, JR., M.D.
Professor, Department of Orthopaedics
University of Washington School of Medicine
Orthopaedist-in-Chief, Harborview Medical Center
Seattle, Washington

KEVIN D. HARRINGTON, M.D.
Clinical Associate Professor of Orthopaedic Surgery
University of California, San Francisco
San Francisco, California

LELAND G. HAWKINS, M.D.
Orthopaedic Surgeon
Mercy Hospital and St. Lukes Hospital
Cedar Rapids, Iowa

KINGSBURY G. HEIPLE, M.D.
C. H. Herndon Professor and Chairman
Department of Orthopaedics
Case Western Reserve University
School of Medicine
Director, Department of Orthopaedics
University Hospitals of Cleveland
Cleveland, Ohio

AARON A. HOFMANN, M.D.
Associate Professor of Orthopaedic Surgery
University of Utah School of Medicine
Staff Physician, Orthopaedic Surgery
University of Utah Medical Center
Salt Lake City, Utah

JACK C. HUGHSTON, M.D.
Clinical Professor, Department of Orthopaedics
Division of Sports Medicine
Tulane University School of Medicine
Hughston Sports Medicine Hospital
Columbus, Georgia

WILLIAM G. HUMPHREYS, M.D.
Resident Physician
University of Missouri, Columbia
Resident Physician
University of Missouri Hospital and Clinics
Columbia, Missouri

ALLAN E. INGLIS, M.D.
Professor of Clinical Surgery
Professor of Anatomy in Cell Biology and Anatomy
Cornell University Medical College
Director, Comprehensive Arthritis Service
The Hospital for Special Surgery
New York, New York

MICHAEL E. JABALEY, M.D.
Clinical Professor of Surgery (Plastic)
University of Mississippi Medical Center
Jackson, Mississippi

DOUGLAS W. JACKSON, M.D.
Director
Southern California Center for Sports Medicine
Medical Director
Memorial Bone and Tissue Bank
Long Beach, California

RAE R. JACOBS, M.D.
Professor of Surgery (Orthopaedic)
University of Kansas
Chief, Problem Spine Clinic
Kansas University Medical Center
Chief, Orthopaedic Section
VA Medical Center
Kansas City, Kansas

KURT E. JACOBSON, M.D.
Staff Surgeon, Hughston Orthopaedic Clinic
Hughston Sports Medicine Hospital
Columbus, Georgia

ROBERT J. JOHNSON, M.D.
Professor of Orthopaedic Surgery
Head, Division of Sports Medicine
University of Vermont
Attending Physician
Medical Center Hospital of Vermont
Burlington, Vermont

JAMES O. JOHNSTON, M.D.
Clinical Professor of Orthopaedics
University of California, San Francisco
Chief, Department of Orthopaedics
Kaiser Foundation Hospital
Oakland, California

JESSE B. JUPITER, M.D.
Assistant Professor of Orthopaedic Surgery
Harvard Medical School
Assistant Orthopaedic Surgeon
Massachusetts General Hospital
Boston, Massachusetts

WILLIAM J. KANE, M.D., PH.D.
Professor of Orthopaedic Surgery
Northwestern University Medical School
Attending in Orthopaedic Surgery
Northwestern Memorial Hospital
Attending in Orthopaedic Surgery
Children's Memorial Hospital
Chicago, Illinois

MARY ANN E. KEENAN, M.D.
Assistant Clinical Professor of Orthopaedic Surgery
University of Southern California
School of Medicine
Director of Neuromuscular Research
The Adult Head Trauma Service
Rancho Los Amigos Medical Center
Downey, California

MICHAEL W. KEITH, M.D.
Assistant Professor of Orthopedics
Hand Surgeon
University Hospital
Cleveland, Ohio

JAMES F. KELLAM, M.D., F.R.C.S.(C)
Assistant Professor
University of Toronto
Clinical Director
Sunnybrook Hospital
and Regional Trauma Unit
Toronto, Ontario
Canada

HOWARD A. KING, M.D.
Clinical Associate Professor of Orthopaedic Surgery
University of Washington
Chief Spine Section
Children's Hospital and Medical Center
Seattle, Washington

HOWARD W. KLEIN, M.D., F.R.C.S.(C)
Assistant Professor of Surgery
Division of Plastic and Reconstructive Surgery
University of California, Davis
Davis, California

L. ANDREW KOMAN, M.D.
Associate Professor, Section on Orthopaedic Surgery
Wake Forest University Medical Center
North Carolina Baptist Hospital
Winston-Salem, North Carolina

RICHARD F. KYLE, M.D.
Assistant Chairman, Department of Orthopaedics
Hennepin County Medical Center
Clinical Assistant Professor
Department of Orthopaedic Surgery
University of Minnesota
Minneapolis, Minnesota

KENNETH L. LAMBERT, M.D.
Orthopaedic Surgeon
St. John's Hospital
Jackson, Wyoming

JOSEPH M. LANE, M.D.
Professor of Orthopaedic Surgery
Cornell University Medical College
Chief, Metabolic Bone Disease Unit
The Hospital for Special Surgery
Chief, Orthopaedic Division
Memorial Sloan-Kettering Cancer Center
New York, New York

ROBERT L. LARSON, M.D.
Orthopaedic Consultant
University of Oregon Athletic Department
Clinical Associate Professor of Orthopaedics
University of Oregon Medical School
Eugene, Oregon

ROBERT D. LEFFERT, M.D.
Associate Professor of Orthopaedic Surgery
Harvard Medical School
Chief, Department of Rehabilitation Medicine
and the Surgical Upper Extremity Rehabilitation Unit
Massachusetts General Hospital
Visiting Orthopaedic Surgeon
Massachusetts General Hospital
Boston, Massachusetts

ROSS K. LEIGHTON, M.D., F.R.C.S.(C)
Lecturer, Dalhousie University
Orthopaedic Surgeon, The Moncton Hospital
Moncton, New Brunswick
Canada

DAVID W. LHOWE, M.D.
Instructor in Orthopaedic Surgery
Harvard Medical School
Staff Physician
Massachusetts General Hospital
Boston, Massachusetts

TERRY R. LIGHT, M.D.
Associate Professor of Orthopaedics and Rehabilitation
Loyola University School of Medicine
Attending Surgeon
Loyola University Medical Center
Shriners Hospital for Crippled Children
Chicago, Illinois

JAMES A. LILLA, M.D.
Assistant Clinical Professor of Plastic Surgery
University of California, Davis
Davis, California

PAUL R. LIPSCOMB, M.D.
Professor Emeritus, Mayo Foundation and Clinic
Professor Emeritus, University of California, Davis
Davis, California

WILLIAM LONON, M.D.
Department of Orthopaedic Surgery
Naval Hospital
Oakland, California

G. DEAN MacEWEN, M.D.
Professor and Chief, Department of Orthopaedics
Section of Pediatric Orthopaedics
Louisiana State University Medical Center
Chairman, Department of Pediatric Orthopaedics
Children's Hospital
New Orleans, Louisiana

MICHAEL MADISON, PH.D.
Orthopaedic Research Laboratories
University of California, Davis
Davis, California

BRUCE A. MALLIN, M.D.
Associate in Surgery
The University of Arizona
Chief of the Medical Staff
Phoenix Memorial Hospital
Phoenix, Arizona

ROGER A. MANN, M.D.
Associate Clinical Professor of Orthopaedic Surgery
University of California, San Francisco
School of Medicine
Chief of Foot Surgery
Samuel Merritt Hospital
Oakland, California

PAUL R. MANSKE, M.D.
Fred C. Reynolds Professor and Chairman
Orthopaedic Surgery
Washington University School of Medicine
St. Louis, Missouri

RANDALL E. MARCUS, M.D.
Assistant Professor of Orthopaedics
Case Western Reserve University
School of Medicine
Attending Surgeon
University Hospitals of Cleveland
Cleveland, Ohio

RICHARD A. MARDER, M.D.
Assistant Professor of Orthopaedics
University of California, Davis
Davis, California

JOEL M. MATTA, M.D.
Associate Professor of Orthopaedic Surgery
University of Southern California School of Medicine
Director of Orthopaedic Reconstruction Service
Los Angeles County/University of Southern California
    Medical Center
Los Angeles, California

PETER MATTER, M.D.
Professor Dr. med.
University of Basle
Chief of Surgery
Hospital of Davos
Davos, Switzerland

RICHARD C. MAURER, M.D.
Clinical Professor of Orthopaedic Surgery
Vice Chairman, Department of Orthopaedic Surgery
University of California, San Francisco
Chief of Orthopaedic Surgery
Veterans Administration Medical Center
San Francisco, California

JACK K. MAYFIELD, M.D., M.S.
Chairman, Section of Orthopaedic Surgery
Phoenix Children's Hospital
Phoenix, Arizona

PAUL C. McAFEE, M.D.
Assistant Professor of Orthopaedic Surgery
Assistant Professor of Neurological Surgery
Chief of Spinal Reconstructive Surgery
The Johns Hopkins Hospital
Baltimore, Maryland

DOUGLAS J. McDONALD, M.D.
Mayo Graduate School
Department of Orthopaedics
Rochester, Minnesota

DANA C. MEARS, M.D., PH.D.
Associate Professor
Department of Orthopaedic Surgery
University of Pittsburgh School of Medicine
Pittsburgh, Pennsylvania

ALAN C. MERCHANT, M.D., M.S.
Clinical Professor of Surgery (Orthopaedic Division)
Stanford University School of Medicine
Stanford, California
Active Staff Surgeon
Department of Orthopaedic Surgery
El Camino Hospital
Mountain View, California

FREDERICK N. MEYER, M.D.
Assistant Professor, Orthopaedic Surgery
Chief, Division of Hand Surgery
University of South Alabama Medical Center
Mobile, Alabama

GARY MILLER, M.D.
Hand Fellow
Department of Orthopaedic Surgery
University of Pennsylvania School of Medicine
Philadelphia, Pennsylvania

ROBERT H. MILLER III, M.D.
Clinical Instructor
University of Tennessee Center for Health Sciences
Baptist Memorial Hospital, Regional Medical Center
Memphis, Tennessee

H. MILLESI, M.D.
Professor of Plastic Surgery
University of Vienna Medical Faculty
Chief of Plastic Surgery
I. Chirurgische Universitatsklinik Wien
Director of the Ludwig-Boltzmann-Institute of
Experimental Plastic Surgery
Vienna, Austria

ROBY MIZE, M.D.
Assistant Clinical Professor of Orthopaedic Surgery
University of Texas Southwestern Medical School
Staff Orthopaedic Surgeon
Presbyterian Medical Center of Dallas
Dallas, Texas

PASQUALE X. MONTESANO, M.D.
Instructor of Orthopaedics
University of California, Davis
Orthopaedic Surgeon
University of California, Davis Medical Center
Sacramento, California

J. RUSSELL MOORE, M.D.
Associate Professor
Department of Orthopaedic Surgery
Johns Hopkins University School of Medicine
Baltimore, Maryland

THOMAS J. MOORE, M.D.
Medical Director
Charlotte Rehabilitation Hospital
Miller Orthopaedic Clinic
Charlotte, North Carolina

JOHN R. MORELAND, M.D.
Assistant Clinical Professor of Orthopaedics
UCLA School of Medicine
Los Angeles, California

BERNARD F. MORREY, M.D.
Associate Professor of Orthopedic Surgery
Mayo Medical School
St. Mary's Hospital
Rochester, Minnesota

JAMES M. MORRIS, M.D.
Associate Professor of Orthopaedic Surgery
University of California, San Francisco
San Francisco, California

DAVID S. MORRISON, M.D.
Clinical Instructor in Orthopaedic Surgery
University of California, Irvine
Director of Shoulder and Elbow Surgery
Southern California Center for Sports Medicine
Long Beach, California

VINCENT S. MOSCA, M.D.
Assistant Clinical Professor of Orthopaedics
University of Washington
Head, Orthopaedic Clinical Services
Children's Hospital and Medical Center
Seattle, Washington

SCOTT J. MUBARAK, M.D.
Associate Clinical Professor of Orthopaedic Surgery
University of California, San Diego
Pediatric Orthopaedic Surgeon
Children's Hospital & Health Center
San Diego, California

MICHAEL J. MURPHY, M.D.
Assistant Clinical Professor of Orthopaedic Surgery
Yale University School of Medicine
Attending Spine Surgeon
Yale New Haven Hospital
New Haven, Connecticut

ROBERT J. NEVIASER, M.D.
Professor and Chairman, Department of Orthopaedic Surgery
Director, Hand and Upper Extremity Service
George Washington University Medical Center
Washington, DC

BETH NICHOLSON, OTR
Clinical Instructor,
School of Community and Allied Health
University of Alabama
Birmingham, Alabama

JOHN J. NIEBAUER, M.D.
Clinical Professor of Orthopaedic Surgery
University of California, San Francisco
Former Chief, Department of Hand Surgery
Pacific Presbyterian Hospital
Kentfield, California

TOM R. NORRIS, M.D.
Pacific Presbyterian Medical Center
San Francisco, California

RICHARD D. PARKER, M.D.
Sports Medicine Clinical Research Fellow
Latter Day Saints Hospital
Salt Lake City, Utah

SIR DENNIS PATERSON, M.D., F.R.C.S., F.R.A.C.S.
Clinical Senior Lecturer
University of Adelaide
Director & Chief Orthopaedic Surgeon
The Adelaide Children's Hospital
Adelaide, Australia

MICHAEL J. PATZAKIS, M.D.
Associate Professor of Orthopedic Surgery
University of Southern California
School of Medicine
Los Angeles County-University of Southern California
    Medical Center
Los Angeles, California

LONNIE E. PAULOS, M.D.
Clinical Assistant Professor
Division of Orthopedic Surgery
University of Utah School of Medicine
Salt Lake City, Utah

P. HUNTER PECKHAM, PH.D.
Associate Professor of Biomedical Engineering
Case Western Reserve University
Director, Rehabilitation Engineering
Cleveland Metropolitan General/Highland View Hospital
Cleveland, Ohio

CLAYTON A. PEIMER, M.D.
Associate Professor of Orthopaedic Surgery
Clinical Assistant Professor of Anatomical Sciences
Clinical Assistant Professor of Rehabilitation Medicine
School of Medicine
State University of New York at Buffalo
Chief of Hand Surgery
Department of Orthopaedics
Millard Fillmore Hospitals and
Erie County Medical Center
Buffalo, New York

LANDRUS L. PFEFFINGER, M.D.
Assistant Clinical Professor
University of California, San Francisco
Chief of Foot Clinic
Children's Hospital of Northern California
Attending Physician, Samuel Merritt Hospital
Oakland, California

NORMAN K. POPPEN, M.D.
Assistant Clinical Professor of Orthopaedics
University of California, Davis
Davis, California

MARTIN A. POSNER, M.D.
Associate Clinical Professor of Orthopaedic Surgery
Mt. Sinai School of Medicine
New York, New York

PATRICIA ANNE POST, B.A.
Coordinator, Orthopaedic Center for
Education and Research
Vanderbilt University School of Medicine
Nashville, Tennessee

DONALD J. PROLO, M.D.
Clinical Associate Professor of Surgery
Stanford University School of Medicine
Stanford, California

MARK PRUZANSKY, M.D.
Assistant Clinical Professor of Orthopaedics
Mt. Sinai School of Medicine
Associate Attending Department of Orthopaedics
Mt. Sinai Medical Center
New York, New York

GEORGE T. RAB, M.D.
Associate Professor of Orthopaedic Surgery
University of California, Davis
Chief, Section of Children's Orthopaedics
University of California, Davis Medical Center
Sacramento, California

RUDOLF RESCHAUER, M.D. PROF.
Prof. Dr. med., University of Graz
Chief, Section of Accident Surgery
Allgemeines Krankenhaus
Linz, Austria

RICHARD S. RIGGINS, M.D.
Professor of Orthopaedics
Emory University School of Medicine
Atlanta, Georgia

LAWRENCE A. RINSKY, M.D.
Associate Professor of Orthopedic Surgery
Stanford University
Chief of Pediatric Orthopedics
Children's Hospital at Stanford
Stanford, California

JOHN M. ROBERTS, M.D.
Professor of Orthopaedics and Pediatrics
Brown University Program in Medicine
Surgeon-in-Charge
Division of Pediatric Orthopaedic Surgery
Rhode Island Hospital
Providence, Rhode Island

JUAN J. RODRIGO, M.D.
Associate Professor of Orthopaedics
University of California, Davis
Chief, Adult Reconstructive Service
University of California, Davis Medical Center
Sacramento, California

WILLIAM L. ROHR, JR., M.D. M.S.M.E.
Chairman, Department of Orthopaedics
Alvarado Hospital Medical Center
Alvarado Orthopaedic Research
San Diego, California

HOWARD ROSEN, M.D.
Clinical Professor of Orthopaedic Surgery
Mt. Sinai School of Medicine
Chief of Fracture-Trauma Service
Hospital for Joint Diseases Orthopaedic Institute
New York, New York

THOMAS D. ROSENBERG, M.D.
Assistant Clinical Professor of Orthopaedic Surgery
University of Utah
Salt Lake City, Utah

THOMAS P. RÜEDI, M.D.
Professor of Surgery
University of Basle
Head, Department of Surgery
Kantonsspital
Chur, Switzerland

MICHAEL F. SCHAFER, M.D.
Ryerson Professor and Chairman
Department of Orthopaedic Surgery
Northwestern University Medical School
Chairman, Department of Orthopaedic Surgery
Northwestern Memorial Hospital
Chicago, Illinois

DOMENIC SCHARPLATZ, M.D.
Head of the Surgical Department
Hospital of Thusis
Thusis, Switzerland

JOSEPH SCHATZKER, M.D., F.R.C.S.(C)
Professor of Surgery
University of Toronto
Chief Division of Orthopaedic Surgery
Sunnybrook Medical Center
Toronto, Ontario
Canada

DAVID J. SCHURMAN, M.D.
Associate Professor of Surgery/Orthopaedics
Stanford University
Chief of Arthritis Surgery
Stanford University Medical Center
Stanford, California

WOLFGANG SEGGL, M.D.
Dr. med., University of Graz
Chief, Department of Accident Surgery
University Clinic for Surgery
Landeskrankenhaus Graz
Graz, Austria

GOTTFRIED SEGMÜLLER, M.D.
Head of Hand Surgery Service
Department of Orthopaedic Surgery
Kantonsspital
St. Gallen, Switzerland

JULES S. SHAPIRO, M.D.
Associate Professor, Orthopedic Surgery
Associate Attending Surgeon
Rush Presbyterian St. Luke's Medical Center
Chicago, Illinois

THOMAS C. SHIVES, M.D.
Assistant Professor of Orthopedic Surgery
Mayo Graduate School of Medicine
Rochester, Minnesota

MARK A. SILVER, M.D.
Hand Fellow
Harvard Medical School
Massachusetts General Hospital
Boston, Massachusetts

FRANKLIN H. SIM, M.D.
Professor of Orthopedic Surgery
Mayo Medical School
Consultant, Department of Orthopedics
Mayo Clinic and Mayo Foundation
Rochester, Minnesota

EDWARD H. SIMMONS, M.D., F.R.C.S. (Tor)
Professor of Orthopaedic Surgery
State University of New York at Buffalo
Head of the Department of Orthopaedic Surgery
Buffalo General Hospital
Buffalo, New York

MICHAEL A. SIMON, M.D.
Professor of Surgery, Section of Orthopaedic Surgery
and Rehabilitation Medicine
Professor of Pathology
University of Chicago Medical Center
Chicago, Illinois

T. DAVID SISK, M.D.
Clinical Associate Professor
Campbell Clinic
University of Tennessee
Department of Orthopedics
Memphis, Tennessee

TAYLOR KING SMITH, M.D.
Clinical Professor
Department of Orthopedic Surgery
University of California, San Francisco
Director of Rehabilitation
Davies Medical Center
San Francisco, California

WAYNE O. SOUTHWICK, M.D.
Professor of Orthopaedics and Rehabilitation
Yale University School of Medicine
New Haven, Connecticut

DAVID L. SPENCER, M.D.
Associate Professor of Orthopaedic Surgery
University of Illinois
Chief of Spine Surgery
Univerity of Illinois and
Lutheran General Hospital
Glenview, Illinois

DAN M. SPENGLER, M.D.
Professor and Chairman
Department of Orthopaedics and Rehabilitation
Vanderbilt University Medical Center
Chief of Orthopaedics
Vanderbilt University Hospital
Nashville, Tennessee

JAMES D. SPIEGEL, M.D.
Chief Resident, Department of Orthopaedic Surgery
University of California, Davis
Davis, California

LYNN T. STAHELI, M.D.
Professor of Orthopaedic Surgery
University of Washington
Director of Orthopedics
Children's Hospital and Medical Center
Seattle, Washington

PETER J. STERN, M.D.
Clinical Professor of Orthopaedic Surgery
University of Cincinnati
College of Medicine
Cincinnati, Ohio

PETER M. STEVENS, M.D.
Clinical Associate Professor
University of Utah Medical Center
Assistant Chief Surgeon
Shriners Hospital for Crippled Children
Salt Lake City, Utah

JAMES W. STRICKLAND, M.D.
Clinical Professor of Orthopaedic Surgery
Indiana University School of Medicine
Chief, Section of Hand Surgery
St. Vincent Hospital and Health Care Center
Indianapolis, Indiana

MARC F. SWIONTKOWSKI, M.D.
Assistant Professor of Orthopaedics and Rehabilitation
Vanderbilt University School of Medicine
Staff Orthopaedist
Vanderbilt University Medical Center
Nashville, Tennessee

ROBERT M. SZABO, M.D.
Assistant Professor of Orthopaedics
University of California, Davis
Chief, Hand & Microvascular Service
University of California, Davis Medical Center
Sacramento, California

RUDOLF SZYSZKOWITZ, M.D.
Professor and Head
Department of Trauma Surgery
School of Medicine
University of Graz
Graz, Austria

JULIO TALEISNIK, M.D.
Clinical Professor
Department of Surgery (Orthopaedics)
University of California, Irvine
Irvine, California

DAVID C. TEMPLEMAN, M.D.
Assistant Professor of Orthopaedics
Department of Orthopaedics
University of Minnesota
Minneapolis, Minnesota

JAMES S. THOMPSON, M.D.
Assistant Professor of Orthopaedic Surgery
Johns Hopkins University School of Medicine
Assistant Professor
Johns Hopkins Hospital
Baltimore, Maryland

JACK W. TUPPER, M.D.
Clinical Professor of Orthopaedic Surgery
University of California, San Francisco
Chief, Hand Division
Orthopaedic Surgery
Samuel Merritt Hospital
Oakland, California

ANTHONY S. UNGER, M.D.
Clinical Instructor of Orthopaedics
George Washington University School of Medicine
Attending Orthopaedic Surgeon
George Washington University Medical Center
Washington, DC
Orthopaedic Consultant
National Institutes of Health
Bethesda, Maryland

JAMES R. URBANIAK, M.D.
Professor, Division of Orthopaedic Surgery
Duke University School of Medicine
Chief, Division of Orthopaedic Surgery
Duke University Medical Center
Durham, North Carolina

MICHAEL I. VENDER, M.D.
Attending Hand and Orthopaedic Surgeon
Department of Orthopaedic Surgery
Edward Hospital
Naperville, Illinois

F. WILLIAM WAGNER, JR., M.D.
Clinical Professor of Orthopaedic Surgery
University of Southern California
School of Medicine
Chief Consultant, Ortho-Diabetes Service
Rancho Los Amigos Medical Center
Downey, California

ROBERT WATERS, M.D.
Clinical Professor of Orthopedic Surgery
University of Southern California
School of Medicine
Chairman, Department of Surgery
Rancho Los Amigos Medical Center
Downey, California

ROBERT G. WATKINS, M.D.
Clinical Associate Professor of Orthopedics
University of Southern California
School of Medicine
Orthopedic Staff
Centinela Hospital Medical Center
Los Angeles, California

H. KIRK WATSON, M.D.
Associate Clinical Professor of Orthopaedics
University of Connecticut Medical School
Farmington, Connecticut
Associate Professor of Orthopaedics and Surgery
University of Massachusetts Medical Center
Worcester, Massachusetts
Assistant Clinical Professor of Plastic Surgery
and Orthopaedics
Yale New Haven Medical School
New Haven, Connecticut
Chief, Connecticut Combined Hand Service
Hartford, Connecticut

BERNHARD GEORG WEBER, M.D.
FMH Orthopaedic and General Surgery
Honorary Professor for Orthopaedic Surgery
University of Berne
Klinik am Rosenberg
Heiden, Switzerland

MICHAEL J. WEBER, M.D.
Orthopaedic Surgeon
McCain Orthopaedic Clinic
North Little Rock, Arkansas

STEPHEN C. WEBER, M.D.
Assistant Clinical Professor of Orthopaedics
University of California, Davis Medical Center
Sacramento, California

ANDREW J. WEILAND, M.D.
Professor, Department of Orthopaedic Surgery
Division of Plastic Surgery and
Department of Emergency Medicine
Chief, Division of Upper Extremity Surgery
Johns Hopkins University School of Medicine
Baltimore, Maryland

TERRY L. WHIPPLE, M.D.
Department of Orthopaedics
Medical College of Virginia
University of Virginia
Chief of Orthopaedics
Humana St. Luke's Hospital
Richmond, Virginia

ROBERT LEE WILSON, M.D.
Chief, Hand Surgery Service
Maricopa Medical Center
Phoenix, Arizona
Associate in Surgery
University of Arizona
Tucson, Arizona

LESTER E. WOLD, M.D.
Assistant Professor of Orthopaedic Surgery
Mayo School of Medicine
Mayo Clinic
Rochester, Minnesota

SAVIO L-Y. WOO, PH.D.
Professor of Surgery and Bioengineering
University of California, San Diego
La Jolla, California

MICHAEL B. WOOD, M.D.
Consultant
Department of Orthopedic Surgery
Section of Hand Surgery
Mayo Clinic
Associate Professor of Orthopedic Surgery
Mayo Medical School
Consultant, Orthopedic Surgery
Saint Mary's Hospital
Rochester, Minnesota

ROBERT E. ZICKEL, M.D.
Clinical Professor, Orthopedic Surgery
Columbia University
Attending Orthopedic Surgeon
St. Lukes-Roosevelt Hospital Center
New York, New York

Contents

Volume 3

PART VII

Infections

CHAPTER 65

Management of Osteomyelitis

MICHAEL J. PATZAKIS

Osteomyelitis, or inflammation of the bone, can result from hematogenous seeding, from direct inoculation (i.e., following open fractures or following open reduction and internal fixation of fractures), or from the contiguous spread of bacteria from infected structures. Early diagnosis and effective surgical and antibiotic management can control the infection; suppression of its activity may last a lifetime. The treatment of osteomyelitis requires the work of a team, consisting of the orthopaedic surgeon, an infectious disease physician, and in complex cases involving soft-tissue defects or inadequate soft-tissue coverage, a plastic surgeon. In many institutions, some orthopaedic nurses are specially trained in the care of orthopaedic infection patients.

INFECTION-CAUSING ORGANISMS

The organisms that cause the infection vary depending on the portal of entry and the type, age, and associated medical conditions of the host. In the past, most infections were caused by *Staphlococcus* and *Streptococcus*. However, the pathophysiology of organisms causing musculoskeletal sepsis has been changing. Gustilo and co-workers and Patzakis and colleagues had reported *Staphylococcus aureus*–coagulase–positive organisms as the most common organisms causing infections in open fractures.[10,23] Subsequent reports by Patzakis, Wilkins, and Moore have shown a significant increase in gram-negative organisms causing infection.[25,26]

Pseudomonas aeruginosa and other gram-negative organisms have been reported by Miskew and colleagues as well as by other researchers to cause osteomyelitis infections in drug addicts.[7,18]

Patients with sickle cell disease are prone to the development of *Salmonella* osteomyelitis. Fungal infections are more likely seen in immune-suppressed hosts. Although viral and parasitic bone infections can occur, they are rare. Antibiotic-resistant organisms, a constant source of concern, are causing infections with increasing frequency.

SYSTEMIC ANTIBIOTIC THERAPY

In the past two decades there has been a surge in the number of effective antibiotics available for the treatment of osteomyelitis. Cephalosporins are effective and relatively safe antimicrobials that can be used to treat both gram-positive and gram-negative microbes. Antimicrobial agents are an adjunct to good surgical management, which includes adequate debridement and wound management.

The questions most often asked about the use of antimicrobials concern choice of agent, dosage, and length of administration. Route of administration is also a question, since antimicrobial agents can be given topically as well as systemically. The Gram stain, culture, and sensitivity tests are important guides in determining the specific antibiotic(s) to be used. In addition, sensitivity tests should be used to select the antimicrobial agent that is most active against the infecting microbe. Finally, some general guidelines on selecting the appropriate antimicrobial can be helpful. Since 90% to 95% of *Staphyloccoc-*

cus aureus gram-positive organisms are resistant to penicillin, a synthetic penicillin is the drug of choice in the treatment of infections caused by these organisms. Other antimicrobial agents that are effective in the treatment of osteomyelitis caused by *Staphylococcus aureus* include the first-generation cephalosporins, vancomycin, and clindamycin. For methicillin-resistant *Staphylococcus aureus* and *Staphylococcus epidermidis*, vancomycin is the drug of choice. In the treatment of an infection caused by a gram-negative organism, an aminoglycoside in combination with a third-generation cephalosporin may be the most effective agent. Infection caused by *Pseudomonas aeruginosa* is best treated with an aminoglycoside in combination with either piperacillin or, if it is more active against *Pseudomonas* than piperacillin, a third-generation cephalosporin. The aminoglycosides most often used are tobramycin and gentamicin, with tobramycin being generally more active against *Pseudomonas* and gentamicin being more active against the other gram-negative organisms. Synergisim is a very important aspect of the treatment of infections caused by microbes, especially those caused by gram-negative organisms. The most commonly administered antimicrobials are shown in Table 65-1.

The cornerstone of tuberculosis therapy used to be the administration of a combination of drugs, including isoniazid (INH), streptomycin, and para-aminosalicylic acid (PAS). Now more active antituberculous antimicrobial agents are available, including rifampin and ethambutol, which may be used either alone or together in combination with INH. Because INH has a tendency to cause peripheral neuritis, pyridoxine is given in daily doses of 50 mg to help prevent this side effect.

The most common and effective antimicrobial agent available for the treatment of fungal infections is amphotericin B. Because renal toxicity is a side effect of this drug, renal function tests should be performed for signs of toxicity.

Antimicrobial agents are complex and may produce harmful side effects; it is therefore imperative that an infectious disease consultant help select specific antibiotic therapy and monitor the patient for undesirable side effects.

TOPICAL ANTIBIOTIC THERAPY

Topical antibiotic therapy is an old concept. Hippocrates and later Galen used medicinal ointments in the treatment of open fractures. Lister introduced carbolic acid. Sulfa powder in wounds was popular among war surgeons. The aspect of topical

TABLE 65-1. COMMONLY ADMINISTERED ANTIMICROBIALS

Antimicrobial	Usual Adult Intravenous Dosage (Lean Body Weight)
Antibiotic	
Penicillin	2 million units every 4 hours
Synthetic Penicillins	
Methicillin, nafcillin, oxacillin	100–200 mg/kg in divided dosages per day, or 1–2 g every 4 hours
Ampicillin	1 g every 4 hours
Piperacillin, ticarcillin	3 g every 4 hours
First-Generation Cephalosporins	
Cephalothin, cephapirin	100–200 mg/kg in divided dosages per day, or 1–2 g every 4 hours
Cefazolin	1 g every 6–8 hours
Second-Generation Cephalosporins	
Cefamandole, cefuroxime, cefoxitin	1–2 g every 4–6 hours
Third-Generation Cephalosporins	
Cefotaxime	2 g every 6 hours
Cefoperazone	2 g every 12 hours
Ceftazidime	2 g every 8 hours
Ceftizoxime	2 g every 8 hours
Vancomycin	500 mg every 6 hours
Clindamycin	600 mg every 6 hours
Aminoglycosides	
Gentamicin, tobramycin	3–5 mg/kg in divided dosages per day, or 80 mg every 8 hours
Amikacin	10–15 mg/kg in divided dosages per day, or 500 mg every 12 hours

therapy that has changed is the agent used and the vehicle of introduction.

Most orthopaedic surgeons use a topical antibiotic solution for irrigation of infected wounds at the time of surgery. Although any antibiotic can be used, the most commonly used agents are polymyxin (1 million units per liter of saline) and bacitracin (50,000 units per liter of saline).

Closed-suction antibiotic ingress and egress irrigation systems using high-volume irrigation have been utilized over a period of 3 to 21 days. The main deterrent to this mode of administration has been secondary contamination and infection with new organisms, generally hydrophilic gram-negative organisms.[14,22] This mode of administration has therefore been abandoned by many surgeons. If this system is used, every means to prevent possible contamination should be adhered to. The risk of secondary contamination increases with the length of usage of the irrigation system. It is advisable to use Silastic drains and to place the tubes on suction or egress for 24 hours before removal of the system; this will remove all of the fluid and hematoma present and will collapse the dead space, thereby precluding the possibility of abscess formation.

The use of antibiotic-impregnated methylmethacrylate at the time of reimplantation of total hip implants into previously infected hips has been advocated by Bucholz and associates and by Murray.[1,19] Antibiotic elution from the methylmethacrylate has been found to be proportional to the surface area of the cement, dosage, and surrounding tissue fluid replacement rate. Murray has reported that 80% of the antibiotic to be eluted is eluted within the first 48 hours.[19]

Klemm and other investigators have reported good results with the use of gentamicin-impregnated methylmethacrylate beads for the treatment of chronic osteomyelitis.[15,16] This method of antibiotic delivery is now under investigation in the United States. These investigators have used antibiotic-impregnated methylmethacrylate beads containing 7.5 mg of gentamicin sulfate with 4.5 mg of free gentamicin per bead string in chains generally containing 30 beads. The pharmokinetics of the elution of antibiotic from these beads have been reported by Wallenkamp and co-workers and by Wahlig and Dingledein.[33,35]

The advantages of this vehicle of antibiotic delivery are very high local antibiotic concentrations; low serum levels, with resultant low systemic toxicity potential; a decreased need for systemic intravenous therapy; and decreased hospitalization time. The disadvantages are that it requires a closed wound; that it may act as a foreign body, especially in the presence of resistant organisms or continued infection; that it may cause organisms to become resistant; and that the organisms present may already be resistant to the gentamicin present in the methylmethacrylate bead. However, the results are encouraging, and the use of this form of treatment in selected cases seems appropriate (Fig. 65-1). A more biologic antibiotic-impregnated vehicle may lessen the disadvantages associated with this treatment.

DIAGNOSIS

The diagnosis of acute osteomyelitis should be considered an emergency. The presenting signs and symptoms may vary with the severity of the infection. Symptoms include fever and chills, general malaise, irritability, pain, and swelling. With lower extremity involvement, there is either a limp or an inability to bear weight. An infant with upper extremity involvement may exhibit pseudoparalysis; older children and adults with upper extremity involvement complain of pain on movement or use of the extremity. It is important to localize the point of maximum tenderness, which is usually also warm and swollen. In children this is generally in the metaphyseal region. It is also important to evaluate the adjoining joint for evidence of an effusion with possible secondary involvement of the septic process from the adjoining osteomyelitis. Osteomyelitis involving the neck of the femur, talus, and humeral head often leads to sepsis of the joint because these foci are located within the capsule of the joint.

Once the point of maximum tenderness has been localized, this area can be aspirated, with the pus or fluid obtained sent for Gram stain, culture, and sensitivity studies. When tuberculosis or a fungal infection is suspected, an acid-fast stain and tuberculosis and fungal cultures should be obtained. When a joint effusion is present or joint involvement is suspected, the joint should be aspirated and an arthrogram obtained. The arthrogram helps document the location of the aspiration and is useful for positive as well as for negative aspirations, since it may also identify joint capsule rupture.

The white blood cell count is generally elevated, depending on the severity of the infection, with an increase in immature or band cells. The erythrocyte sedimentation rate is usually elevated. Blood cultures should be obtained in all cases of acute hematogenous osteomyelitis and in chronic osteomyelitis exacerbated by fever and bacteremia. Roentgenograms taken early in the disease process generally show soft-tissue swelling; bony changes are not present until 7 to 10 days after the onset of the disease process. Radionuclide bone scanning using radioactive-labeled isotopes, such as technetium-99m and, more specifically, gallium citrate-67 and indium-111–labeled white blood cells, is helpful in localizing the area of involvement and in diagnosing the condition. Although aspiration is the basis of the diagnosis, especially when there is no drainage or sinuses, bone biopsy may be necessary.

Sinograms with radiographic documentation should be done whenever there is a sinus tract or open draining area from which the depth and extent of the infection can be determined (Fig. 65-2). Abscessograms should be done whenever an abscess is present and frank pus is aspirated. The abscessogram will help outline the extent of the abscess cavity (Fig. 65-3).

SURGICAL CONSIDERATIONS

Tourniquets

A tourniquet is useful and should be applied whenever possible except in patients with sickle cell disease or with significant peripheral vascular disease. The tourniquet allows for better hemostasis and thus better identification of the infection process. In acute cases with swelling, cellulitis, or abscess formation, the extremity should be elevated for several minutes before the tourniquet is inflated. In chronic osteomyelitis without significant cellulitis or abscess formation, an elastic bandage can be used to extravasate the extremity before the tourniquet is inflated.

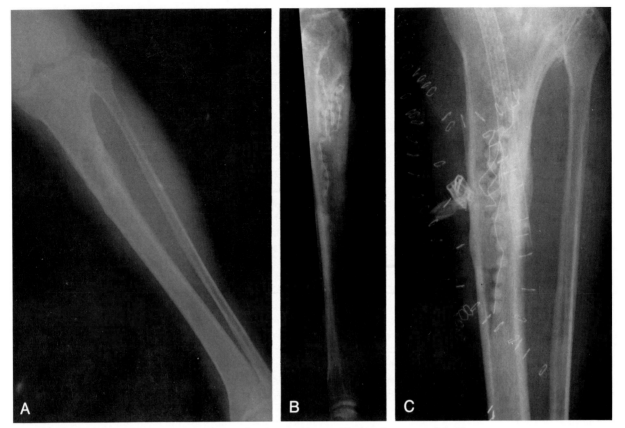

FIGURE 65-1. Anteroposterior roentgenograms of a 46-year-old man with chronic osteomyelitis. The patient was treated with debridement followed by insertion of gentamicin-impregnated methylmethacrylate beads and a local muscle flap.

Debridement

Thorough debridement of all sequestra and necrotic and dessicated bone is essential. Viable infected bone should not be removed lest one create large bony defects. It is not necessary to debride viable infected bone. Some investigators have reported the use of dyes and tetracycline labeling as a means of identifying necrotic bone. However, others have found these techniques unhelpful. Clinically dried out, exposed, dessicated bone is darker than normal in color and should be debrided. Necrotic bone that has not been exposed may appear at surgery more yellowish in color than viable bone, which is whitish. The main finding is that viable bone bleeds, whereas necrotic bone does not. Use of an osteotome to superficially shave the outer cortex of the questionable bone will result in small areas of punctate bleeding. Some bone that may have been exposed to air may be viable; in these cases the exposed outer cortex should be debrided with an osteotome down to good bleeding bone. All pus and abscess should be evacuated, and all necrotic and infected soft tissue should be removed.

Irrigation

Using copious amounts of irrigating fluid is worthwhile. It helps not only to cleanse the area of purulent exudate, small loose soft tissue, and bony fragments, but also to decrease the bacterial count. We use 10 liters of irrigating fluid for most infected wounds. Two liters of antibiotic solution containing 50,000 units of bacitracin per liter of saline and 1 million units of polymyxin per liter are used as the final irrigating solutions.

Wound Management

A decision as to whether a wound should be left open or closed requires clinical judgment, but in the majority of acute infections the wound should be left open. The wound should be left open in all cases in which there is associated abscess formation with cellulitis and swelling. In some cases in which there is an early postoperative infected hematoma or an infection, the wound may be closed over Silastic drainage tubes, provided that the wound has been converted to a clean wound and that the infection is not anaerobic.

In cases of chronic osteomyelitis in which there is no significant cellulitis or abscess formation and in which the wound has been adequately debrided and converted to a clean wound, the wound may be closed over Silastic drainage tubes. In some cases in which bone or metal will be exposed if the wound is left open, a partial closure over the bone or metal may be desirable, provided an adequate pathway has been provided for drainage. When there is any doubt regarding any wound, it is safest to leave the wound open. If the wound is closed, the wound site

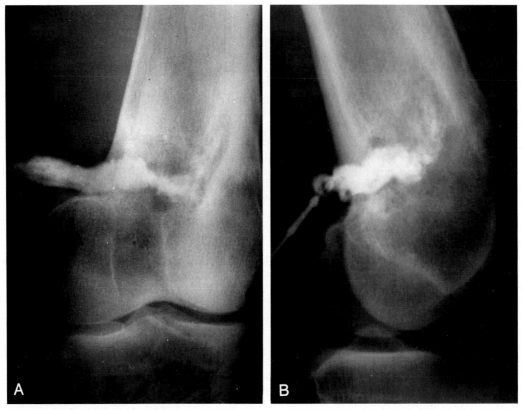

FIGURE 65-2. (*A*) Anterior and (*B*) posterior roentgenograms of a sinogram in a 21-year-old man with chronic osteomyelitis that tracts into an intramedullary cavity.

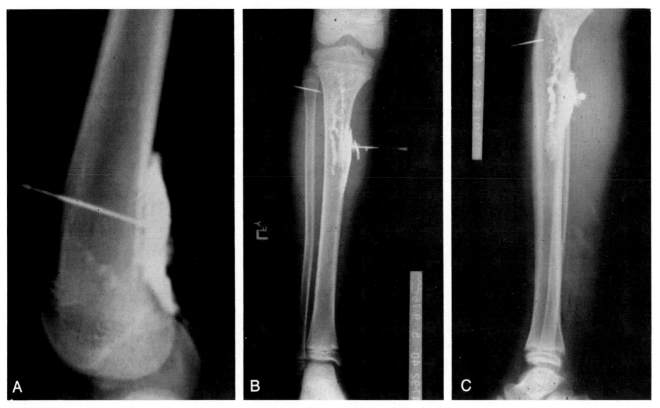

FIGURE 65-3. (*A*) Lateral x-ray film of a 15-year-old male showing a subperiosteal abscess that was aspirated and injected with contrast material. (*B*) Anteroposterior and (*C*) lateral x-ray films of a 9-year-old child showing contrast material in the subperiosteal area and within the medullary cavity after pus had been aspirated. The contrast material demonstrates the extent of the abscess.

must be examined daily for any signs of infection; if such signs appear, the wound must be opened.

Many wounds close by secondary intention. However, in the case of large wounds or in cases in which delayed closure is preferable, closure should not be attempted until two criteria are met. First, the wound should appear clinically healthy, with clean granulating tissue and without any purulent exudate or necrotic tissue. If infected necrotic tissues are present, the wound should be redebrided until the wound appears healthy. Second, once the clinical appearance of the wound is clean, quantitative tissue cultures and Gram stains of the wound should be taken. Wounds with either a positive Gram stain or quantitative tissue cultures with a bacterial count of greater than 10^{-5} organisms should never be closed. (A positive Gram stain implies a bacterial count of greater than 10^{-5} organisms.) These wounds should be considered infected and should be reassessed as to the need for further surgical debridement and the appropriateness of the systemic antibiotic therapy.

In secondary closure of wounds that have satisfied the clinical and laboratory criteria for closure, it is important to redebride the wound at the time of closure. A superficial *en bloc* resection of the granulating tissue should be done for several reasons. First, although the bacterial count is low, these tissues should still be considered contaminated; debridement will further reduce the bacterial count and thereby diminish the chance of infection. Second, debridement allows for cleaner, healthier tissue to be approximated by wound closure.

Drains

When the wounds are closed, Silastic (Jackson-Pratt) drains should be used; they are the least reactive of the drains available today. Polyethelene (Hemovac) drains may be used also, although we prefer Silastic. Penrose drains, which are rubber, are the most reactive, and if left in for long periods can cause foreign body granulomas. Penrose drains should not be used in orthopaedic infection management.

The suction drain should be removed in 48 to 72 hours. The drain allows for removal of all hematoma and tissue fluid and for collapse of the potential dead space. The drains should be removed under sterile conditions and the tip cut off and sent for culture and sensitivity tests. The drain tends to attract whatever bacteria are present because it is a foreign body and because tissue fluids are removed through it. In general, a positive culture of the drain tip is a potentially bad prognostic sign, since it means that bacteria remain behind. The clinical course and wound site should be closely monitored; if any clinical signs of wound infections appear, it may be necessary to consider redebridement or reassessment of antibiotic therapy.

Wound Packing

The purpose of leaving a wound open is to allow for drainage. Therefore, packing of wounds with gauze or other materials must not obstruct drainage. If it does, the purulent exudate will be retained in the wound, possibly causing tissue breakdown and necrosis with secondary cellulitis or even abscess formation. It is best to put wicks perpendicular to the open wound to allow for free drainage. Wicks can be either povidone-iodine (Betadine)–soaked gauze, plain gauze, or fine-mesh gauze. The size will vary with the size of the wound. The ends of the wicks should always protrude through the skin edges to allow for easy access and removal and to prevent retention.

HEMATOGENOUS OSTEOMYELITIS

Hematogenous osteomyelitis is most often seen in infants, children, drug abusers, and immunosuppressed hosts. In 1894 Lexer injected laboratory animals with *Staphylococcus aureus* organisms and then traumatized a bony area, causing infection to appear at that site.[17] Hobo explained that the predilection for the metaphysis in acute osteomyelitis was due to the fact that the arteries in this location are end arteries, that there is slowing of the venous flow in the sinusoids, and that phagocytosis is defective in this area.[13] Trueta later expanded on Hobo's work.[32] Once the metaphyseal region is seeded and exudate or pus forms, the suppurative process may then under pressure travel through the Volkmann canals into the subperiosteal region, extend itself within the medullary cavity, or spread into the epiphysis (Fig. 65-4). It is not uncommon for the joint to be involved secondarily, especially a joint in which the metaphysis is intra-articular, such as the hip or shoulder. Often the abscess extends into the soft tissues as well.[20,34]

In cases in which the disease is not diagnosed promptly or in which either inadequate or no treatment is given, the disease then enters the subacute stage (Fig. 65-5). Because of the introduction of antibiotics and improved diagnostic and operative techniques, the chronic stage and its sequelae are no longer seen as frequently as they used to be.

One question that arises in the treatment of acute hematogenous osteomyelitis is whether to treat all patients surgically. Unless there is clinical evidence of an abscess, we treat patients with systemic antibiotics and without surgery. However, the

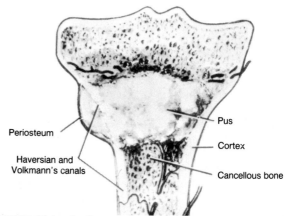

FIGURE 65-4. Outline of the pathophysiology of hematogenous seeding. When under pressure, the exudate or abscess can extend through the Volkmann canals into the subperiosteal region, and from there into the intramedullary cavity or the epiphysis. (Modified from Hobo, T.: Zur Pathogenese der akuten haematogene Osteomyelitis, mit Berücksichtigung der Vitalfarbungslehre. Acta scholae Kioto **4**:1, 1921.)

clinical situation must be repeatedly assessed during treatment. Many osteomyelitic processes are seen early in the disease process or represent a cellulitic process of the bone, and pus or the abscess phase may not occur.

Although some authors have not found it necessary to drill a window in cases of subperiosteal or soft-tissue–extended osteomyelitis, we routinely window the cortical bone for better debridement of the residual intramedullary abscess and necrotic bone and tissue (Fig. 65-6).

Cortical Windowing for an Acute Intramedullary Abscess of the Tibia

Procedure

Using tourniquet control, make a longitudinal incision along the posterior border of the medial tibia and over the affected part of the tibia. If a subperiosteal abscess is present, incise the periosteum longitudinally over the abscess. A subperiosteal abscess is more likely to occur in a child than in an adult.

If no subperiosteal abscess is found, observe the status of the cortex. The infected area is often soft and may be pitted, with or without obvious cortical destruction. Drill several holes through the cortex into the medullary canal. Unless the intramedullary abscess has already decompressed itself into the subperiosteum or soft tissues, pus will exude through these holes. Outline with a drill an elongated cortical window extending along the extent of the intramedullary abscess. The outlined elongated window should be centered in the posterior half of the anterior–posterior diameter of the bone to allow for dependent drainage. The length of the window will depend on the extent of the intramedullary abscess, and the width will depend on the diameter of the bone. For children, a 1- to 2-cm-wide window is generally used. After debridement of any obvious sequestrum and copious irrigation, insert a Betadine gauze into the wound and then leave it open.

A similar type of window of the femur is made for osteomyelitis of the femur.

Helpful Hints

1. Avoid making a cortical window directly under the skin incision. This can lead to the necessity for a muscle transfer, since the soft tissues will not granulate over a cortical defect and skin coverage therefore will not occur.
2. Make the cortical window in the dependent one-half of the anteroposterior diameter of the bone to allow for adequate drainage.
3. Avoid making too large a cortical window, which can lead to pathologic fractures, especially if the width is excessive.
4. In children, in whom the usual location for hematogenous osteomyelitis is in the metaphysis, be careful not to damage the epiphyseal plate. Use roentgenograms intraoperatively to help you locate the epiphyseal plate.

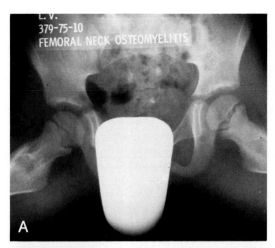

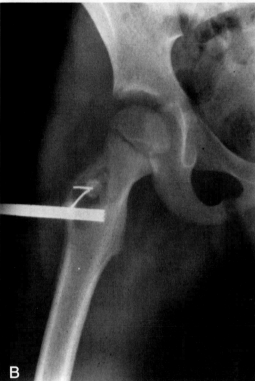

FIGURE 65-5. (*A*) A frogleg lateral view showing a lytic area in the metaphysis of a 7-year-old boy with a 6-month history of pain and a limp. (*B*) Anteroposterior x-ray film taken at the time of biopsy. The lesion was found to be a subacute osteomyelitis caused by a *Staphylococcus aureus* organism.

5. If follow-up cultures are positive or if pus continues to drain, consider performing a second irrigation and debridement.

Aftercare

1. A posterior splint is applied.
2. A wound left open generally closes by secondary intention within 3 weeks.

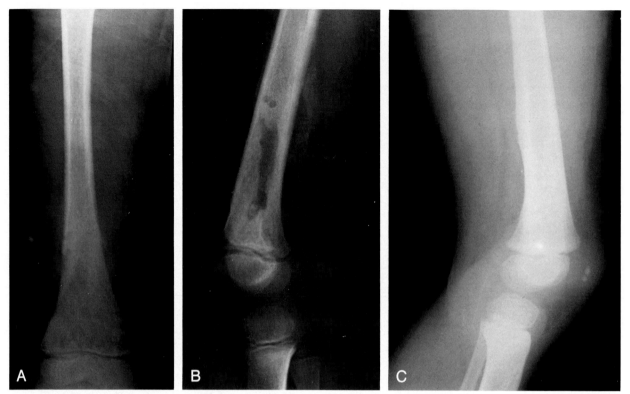

FIGURE 65-6. (*A*) Anteroposterior x-ray film in a child showing destructive lytic changes in the metaphyseal region with periosteal reaction. (*B*) Lateral x-ray film showing the extent of the cortical window made for debridement of the medullary abscess. (*C*) Lateral x-ray film taken 7 months later showing healing of both the cortical window and the osteomyelitic process.

3. Protected weight-bearing in a cast or orthosis is recommended for 6 to 12 weeks whenever a cortical window is used.

OSTEOMYELITIS FOLLOWING OPEN FRACTURES

For acute osteomyelitis following an open fracture, it is important to assess the extent of the infection and to obtain a Gram stain, culture, and sensitivity test. Start appropriate systemic antibiotics, and take the patient to surgery for irrigation, debridement, and stabilization of the fracture if it is not already adequately stabilized (Fig. 65-7). The majority of fractures in the tibia can be stabilized with half-pin external fixation devices with the addition of a delta frame for better immobilization.

Once the open fracture infection has been controlled and the fracture stabilized, cancellous autogenous bone grafting should be done on all remaining unstable fractures and type III open fractures. Fracture healing, which facilitates infection control, is an important principle in the management of infected nonunited fractures and nonunions. Although many fractures heal in the presence of infection, infection interferes with the osteogenic process and may lead to nonunion. Infection does this by a number of mechanisms: the bacteria compete with osteogenic cells for oxygen and nutrients, activate enzymes deleterious to the osteogenic process, lower the pH,

affect oxygen potential, interfere with the differentiation of osteogenic cells, and retard tissue maturation.

For both unstable infected open tibial fractures and type III infected open tibial fractures, early autogenous cancellous bone grafting is recommended. This can be accomplished by a posterior lateral bone graft procedure. Alternatively, if a muscle flap has been made anteriorly for soft-tissue coverage, an autogenous cancellous bone graft can be done anteriorly 6 weeks later, provided there is no evidence of recurrent infection.

Posterolateral Bone Grafting of the Tibia

Posterolateral bone grafting is particularly useful in achieving union of an infected nonunion or an infected fracture of the tibia. Freeland and Mutz have reported a 100% union rate in 26 patients with infected nonunions treated in this manner.[5] We have achieved a union rate of approximately 91% in the treatment of 61 infected tibial nonunions.[24]

The approach is used for the distal two-thirds of the tibia. It was described by Harmon and is also used for tibia–pro–fibula grafting.[11]

Procedure

Place the patient in either a prone or a lateral decubitus position. Identify the posterior border of the fibula and the lateral

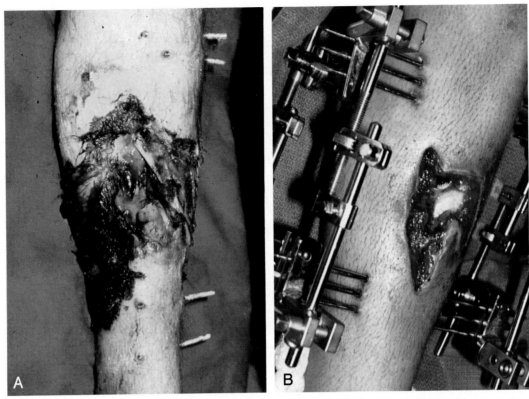

FIGURE 65-7. (*A*) Photograph of a 28-year-old man with an infected open fracture. (*B*) Photograph showing a clean granulating wound. This photograph was taken 12 days after the fracture had been irrigated, debrided, and stabilized with an external fixator and the patient given systemic antibiotic. At this time, biplanar fixation with half-pins rather than full-length pins would be performed.

border of the gastrocnemius muscle. Using tourniquet control, begin an incision of appropriate length along the lateral border of the gastrocnemius and posterior to the fibula.

Once you have cut through the subcutaneous structures, identify the peroneal muscles anteriorly and develop a plane between the peroneals and the posterior muscles consisting of the gastrocnemius, the soleus, and the flexor hallucis longus muscles. Now dissect the soleus and flexor hallucis longus posteriorly and medially to expose the posterior aspect of the fibula. Next dissect the origin of the tibialis posterior muscle from the posterior aspect of the interosseous membrane. Locate the posterior lateral border of the tibia and, using sharp dissection, expose the posterior surface of the tibia by stripping the muscles subperiosteally off the tibia. In the distal one-third of the tibia, approximately 4 to 5 fingerbreadths above the tip of lateral malleolus, an interosseous arteriole branch from the peroneal artery perforates the interosseous membrane and travels anteriorly to anastomose with the anterior tibial artery. Take care to protect this vessel. The posterior tibial neurovascular bundles lie between the tibialis posterior and flexor hallucis longus muscles and are not visible. The muscular branches of the peroneal artery lie within the peroneal muscles. Once the posterior aspect of the tibia is exposed (Fig. 65-8), prepare the tibia and posterior aspect of the fibula for bone grafting by roughening up the cortex with either a burr or an osteotome. Be extremely careful not to disturb the fracture site so as to avoid contamination posteriorly.

Cancellous bone grafts can now be laid posteriorly several inches above and below the fracture site and between the tibia and fibula across the interosseous membrane. The objective is to achieve not only union of the fracture site, but also a tibial–fibular synostosis (Fig. 65-9). A 1½ to 2 oz medicine glass filled with cancellous bone is generally sufficient for a nonunion without bone loss.

At this point release the tourniquet and achieve hemostasis. A Silastic drain should be inserted. Allow the peroneal muscles and posterior muscle mass to return to their anatomic positions. Do not close the deep fascia. Close the subcutaneous tissues and skin with interrupted sutures.

Helpful Hints

1. An arteriogram obtained before this procedure is performed can help determine what vessels are patent and where they are.
2. Be aware of the location of the neurovascular structures.

Aftercare

1. Remove the Silastic drains in approximately 48 hours.
2. Elevate the leg for 72 hours.
3. Full weight-bearing to tolerance should be started 7 days postoperatively if the patient is immobilized in a cast.
4. If an external fixator is used for an unstable fracture, it

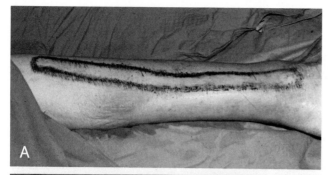

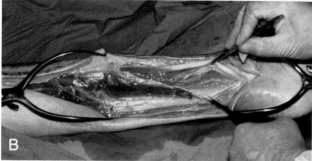

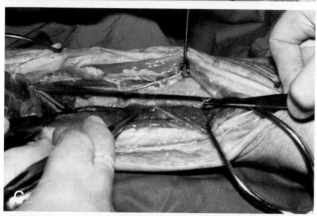

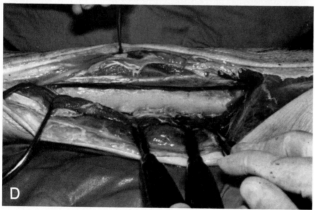

FIGURE 65-8. (*A*) A cadaver specimen outlining the fibula. A skin incision varying with the exposure desired is made just posterior to the fibula along the lateral border of the gastrocnemius and soleus muscles. (*B*) and (*C*) The peroneal muscles are retracted anteriorly, and the border of the fibula is exposed. The tibialis posterior and flexor hallucis muscles are dissected from the interosseus membrane and posterior tibia and retracted posteriorly. The posterior tibialis neurovascular bundle is protected by the tibialis posterior and flexor hallucis longus muscles, which it lies between. (*D*) The posterior aspect of the fibula is now exposed, and the posterior border of the fibula and interosseous membranes are visible.

can generally be removed at 6 to 8 weeks and a walking cast applied.

5. Union generally occurs within 4 to 7 months, median time being 6 months.

DEAD SPACE MANAGEMENT

It is important that soft-tissue and bony defects be filled to reduce the chance of continued infection and loss of function. Advances in microvascular techniques have made possible the transfer of muscle, myocutaneous, osseous, and osteocutaneous flaps to the soft tissue and bony defects. Fitzgerald and his co-workers reported a 93% success rate in the treatment of chronic osteomyelitis with local muscle flaps combined with thorough debridement and specific antimicrobial therapy.[4] Our results using this technique have also been encouraging. In general, for soft-tissue defects involving the proximal third of the tibia, the gastrocnemius muscle is used; for those involving the middle third, the soleus muscle is used; and for those involving the distal third, a free-tissue transfer is used.

In cases of bony defects, autogenous cancellous bone grafting is done 6 or more weeks later. The muscle flap can be elevated and cancellous bone grafting performed underneath, provided there are no signs of infection (Fig. 65-10).

According to Weiland and associates, the highest rate of recurrence of infection in free-tissue transfer in osteomyelitis is found among cases associated with a segmental bone defect.[36]

It has been our experience that the fibula is the key factor in treating osteomyelitis with segmental bone loss of the tibia. If there is a bony defect or segmental loss of both the fibula and tibia with chronic osteomyelitis, an amputation is advisable. If the fibula is intact or without a bony defect, reconstruction of the bony defect is more likely to be successful. For defects up to 6 cm, autogenous cancellous bone grafting can be done (Fig. 65-11). In larger defects, a free vascularized osseous graft is used. A tibia–pro–fibula synostosis using the previously described posterolateral approach can be done when a free vascularized osseous graft or autogenous cancellous bone grafting of the defect is not possible (Fig. 65-12). The fibula will hypertrophy with time, allowing for functional weight-bearing.

Another procedure for dead space management is the open cancellous bone grafting procedure described by Rhinelander and by Papineau and colleagues.[21,28] This procedure is useful when tissue transfer is not possible.

Open Cancellous Bone Grafting

Open cancellous bone grafting has been effective in the treatment of infected bone defects. Papineau, Roy-Camille and colleagues, Rhinelander, Higgs, Knight and Wood, Coleman and associates, Bickel and co-workers, and Green and Dlabal have all reported favorable results.[1a,2a,11a,16a,21,28–30] However, because of the associated long hospitalization time, long healing time, high complication rate, meticulous care required, and resulting unstable scar skin, we have found restricted use for this procedure and use it only if local muscle transfers or free–vascular tissue transfers with secondary cancellous bone grafting cannot be done.

There are three stages to this technique:

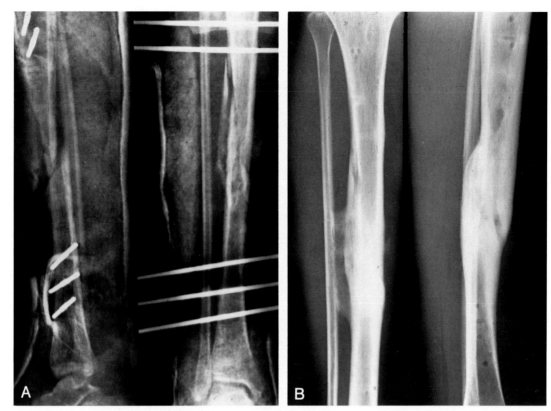

FIGURE 65-9. (*A*) Anteroposterior and lateral x-ray films of the tibia in a 20-year-old woman who had sustained an open fracture and had initially been treated with pins in plaster. The fracture subsequently became infected and was stabilized in an external fixator, and the patient had a posterolateral bone graft. (*B*) Anteroposterior and lateral x-ray films showing healing of the fracture following the posterolateral bone graft. Note the synostosis between the tibia and fibula.

1. Thorough debridement of all infected tissues, repeated as necessary; stabilization of the fracture with an external skeletal fixator
2. Cancellous autogenous bone grafting onto clean uninfected granulation tissue
3. Skin coverage either by secondary epithelialization or, in larger defects, by split-thickness skin grafting

Procedure

Debride all infected soft tissue and sequestra, and debride all necrotic bone to bleeding osseous tissue. Perform stabilization using an external skeletal fixator. When exposed surfaces are covered with clean granulation tissue, pack autogenous cancellous bone chips in the defect created by the bone debridement or previous bone loss. The diameter of the graft should be slightly larger than the diameter of the bone being replaced, since the graft will tend to contract. Rhinelander recommends that the maximum graft thickness be 1.5 cm from the nearest granulation surface.[28] Dress the wound with gauze and keep it moist with a physiologic irrigating solution such as Ringer's lactate, either by intermittent soaking of the dressings or by a slow intravenous drip. The dressing, which should be changed daily, is to be soaked with physiologic solution until the wound is covered by epithelialization or, in some cases, by secondary split-thickness skin grafting (Fig. 65-13).

Helpful Hints

1. Make sure all necrotic soft tissue and bone are debrided.
2. Stabilize the fracture.
3. There must be a clean granulating base before autogenous cancellous bone grafting is performed. Do a quantitative tissue culture and Gram stain. If the quantitative tissue culture yields more than 10^{-5} organisms, or if the Gram stain is positive, which implies the presence of more than 10^{-5} organisms, do not perform the cancellous bone grafting. A count of more than 10^{-5} organisms is consistent with infection, in which case redebridement should be performed.

OSTEOMYELITIS IN THE PRESENCE OF INTERNAL FIXATION FOR FRACTURE STABILIZATION

Osteomyelitis in conjunction with internal fixation for fracture stabilization poses a special problem for the surgeon. Should the metal be removed or left in? The answer to this question is guided by such factors as the stage of fracture healing, the amount of stability provided, the amount of time since surgery, and the location of the fracture. Gristina and Costerton reported that, in 76% of prosthesis-related infections, the micro-

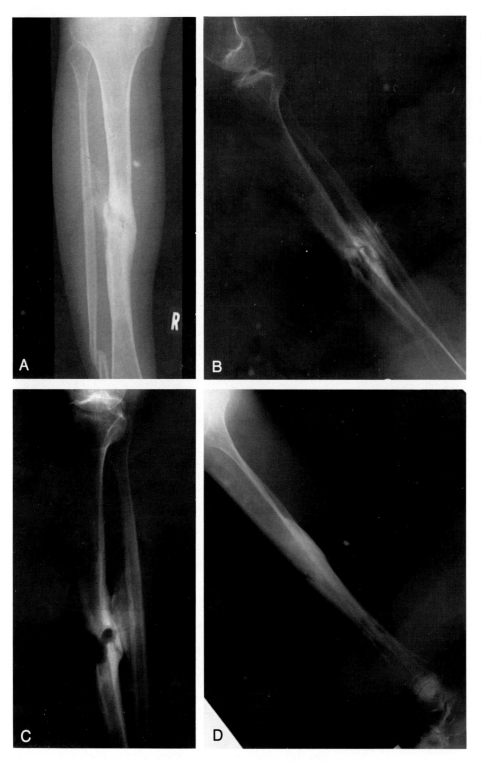

FIGURE 65-10. (*A*) Anteroposterior and (*B*) lateral x-ray films of the tibia and fibula in a 21-year-old man who had a previous posterior bone graft and now shows the presence of a large sequestrum. (*C*) Lateral x-ray film showing debridement of the infection and sequestra. (*D*) Lateral x-ray film taken 10 months after a local flap was followed by an autogenous cancellous bone graft.

organisms grew in a biofilm or glycocalyx that adhered to the surfaces of the biomaterials present.[9] They suggested that infections in the presence of orthopaedic implants may be more resistant than normal to host defense mechanisms and to antimicrobial therapy.

If osteomyelitis develops in the presence of metal with a healed fracture, the metal should be removed. If the fracture is not united and the metal is not providing stability, the metal should be removed and an external fixation device or a plaster cast or splint applied if stabilization is adequate. In the immediate postoperative period (within the first 1 to 6 weeks), the internal fixation device should be retained if it is fulfilling its role and is required. If the internal fixation device is stabilizing a nonunited articular fracture, it should be retained (Fig. 65-14). In general, for late infected nonunion of tibial shaft fractures with internal fixation, we recommend removal of the

FIGURE 65-11. (*A*) Anteroposterior x-ray film of a 34-year-old woman with approximately a 6-cm defect. (*B*) Anteroposterior and lateral x-ray films taken 1 year following performance of an autogenous cancellous bone graft to fill dead space caused by bony defects.

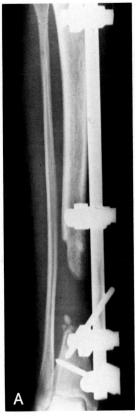

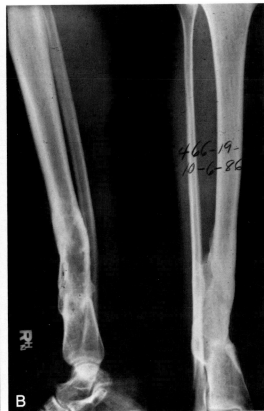

internal fixation device and stabilization with an external fixator. For late nonunion infections of the femur with plate fixation, we recommend removal of the plate and application of a biplane external fixation device. In the case of infected intramedullary nails involving the femoral shaft, except in association with an extensive intramedullary abscess, the metal does not adversely affect eradication of the infection, provided the infection has been appropriately treated with surgical debridement and parenteral antibiotics followed by fracture healing with or without autogenous cancellous bone grafting.[27]

OSTEOMYELITIS OF THE METATARSAL HEADS AND PHALANGES FOLLOWING PUNCTURE WOUNDS OF THE FOOT

Pseudomonas has been reported to be the most common organism causing infection following nail puncture wounds of the foot. The treatment that produces the best results consists of surgical drainage, debridement and curettage of the puncture wound in the bone, and debridement of all necrotic bone, along with specific antibiotic therapy. The antibiotic of choice for *Pseudomonas* infections is generally tobramycin, in combination with either piperacillin or a third-generation cephalosporin, depending on the sensitivity reports. Systemic antimicrobial therapy is continued for approximately 3 weeks. It is important to curette the puncture site, which could be a continued source of seeding and ongoing infection. Because extensive pus is not commonly found in *Pseudomonas* infections,

radiographic evidence of osteomyelitis is an indication for surgical exploration (Figs. 65-15 and 65-16).

The surgical approach is best done plantarward to assure curettage of the puncture site. However, a dorsal incision can be used when there is joint involvement, provided dissection with elevation of the plantar surface of the metatarsal head or proximal phalanx is accomplished for appropriate debridement and curettage.

Procedure

Plantar or Hoffman Approach

Make a plantar transverse incision distal to the weight-bearing area of the metatarsal heads, but proximal to the web space of the toes. Carry the incision down through the subcutaneous tissues and identify the flexor tendons, which should be retracted to expose the involved metatarsal head. Incise the periosteum and elevate it to expose the proximal metatarsal; generally the periosteum has been destroyed and this latter step is not necessary. Identify the area of osteomyelitis, and curette and debride the lytic infected bone. With extensive destruction of the metatarsal head, the head can be excised through this approach.

Dorsal Incision

Make a longitudinal incision over the affected joint. Retract the extensor tendons. Identify the joint capsule and incise the capsule longitudinally. Debride the joint of any necrotic tissue

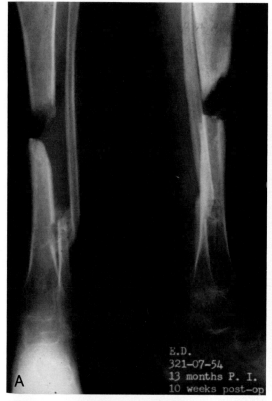

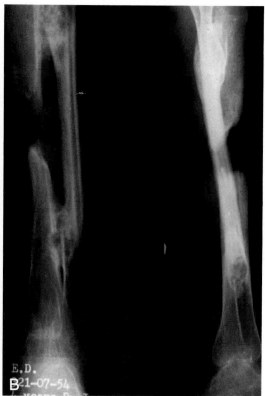

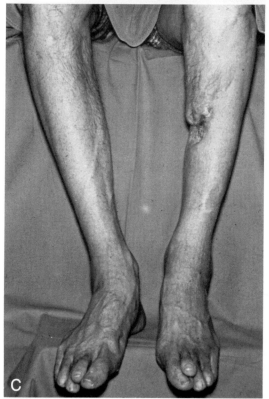

FIGURE 65-12. (*A*) Anteroposterior and lateral x-ray films of a 48-year-old man who developed clostridial myonecrosis following an open fracture of the tibia and treatment with a tibia–pro–fibula synostosis. The distal synostosis site was bone-grafted first and is seen here 10 weeks postoperatively. (*B*) X-ray films taken 4 years following the tibia–pro–fibula synostosis for the segmental defect. Note the synostosis proximally and distally and the hypertrophy of the fibula. (*C*) Photograph of the patient showing healed wounds and no evidence of recurrence of infection. Note the area of defect in the middle calf area.

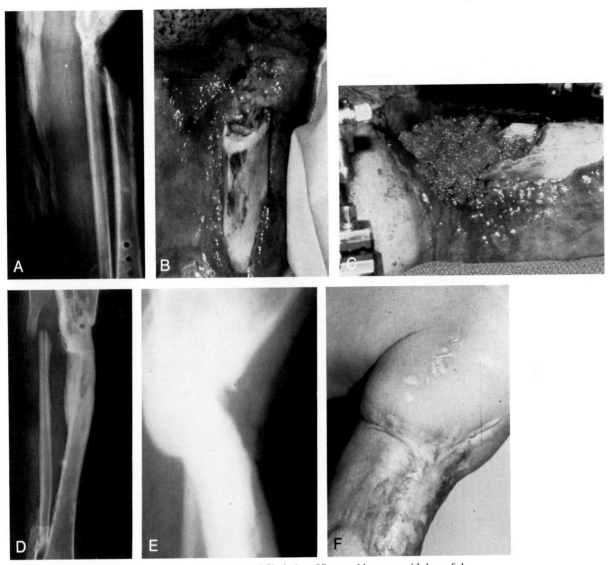

FIGURE 65-13.   (A) Lateral x-ray film of the tibia and fibula in a 37-year-old woman with loss of the tibia following infection. The infection developed after the patient sustained a type III open fracture. (B) Anteroposterior photograph showing the soft-tissue and bone loss and exposed tibial shaft. (C) Photograph taken at the time of autogenous cancellous bone grafting of the dead space. (D) Anteroposterior and (E) lateral x-ray films, taken after the graft had consolidated, showing healing of the fracture. (F) Lateral photograph, taken 3 years after the procedure, showing knee flexion and the appearance of the leg. The patient has been free of infection.

present. Next, free the soft tissue from the plantar surface of the metatarsal, and identify the involved osteomyelitis area to allow for appropriate debridement of necrotic bone and tissue and the curettage of the puncture site. Finally, irrigate the wound with copious amounts of irrigating fluid, and leave a small Betadine gauze or wick in the wound.

Helpful Hints

1. Debride all necrotic tissue.
2. Always curette the bony puncture site when it is identifiable, since this site could be a source of continued seeding of the osteomyelitis.

OSTEOMYELITIS OF THE METATARSAL

The metatarsals are most likely to be infected in diabetics or persons who have open fractures. Depending on the extent of the infection, local debridement of all soft tissue and bone may be satisfactory. In more extensive infections in which the entire metatarsal is necrotic, it may be necessary to remove it.

Procedure

Make a longitudinal incision over the involved bone extending just distal to the distal row of tarsal bones to the middle of the

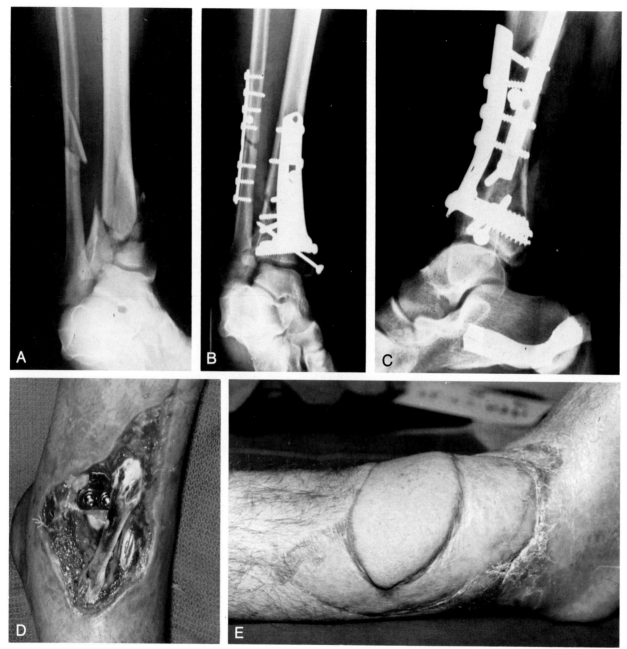

FIGURE 65-14. (A) Anteroposterior x-ray film of the distal tibia and fibula showing a comminuted fracture of the tibia and plafond. (B) Anteroposterior and (C) lateral x-ray films taken following open reduction and internal fixation and showing fractures nonunited at the time of infection. (D) Anterior photograph of the ankle showing exposed metal and ankle joint with a necrotic anterior tibialis tendon after an acute postoperative infection. (E) Photograph taken 9 months following retained metal and a free vascularized latissimus dorsi muscle transfer. There was no evidence of infection at this time.

proximal phalanx of the involved toe. Identify the extensor tendons and retract them. Next identify the involved metatarsal, incise the periosteum longitudinally, and strip it and all soft tissues from the bone. Next, resect the entire shaft or part of the shaft as indicated. In children, avoid injury to the epiphysis. Irrigate the wound with copious amounts of irrigating fluid. Pack the wound loosely with a Betadine gauze or a fine-mesh gauze and leave it protruding from the wound. When the in-

fection is more localized, a smaller longitudinal incision over the involved metatarsal should be used to allow for adequate debridement.

Helpful Hints

Infrequently, especially following open fracture infections, there may be extensive soft-tissue loss with exposed viable

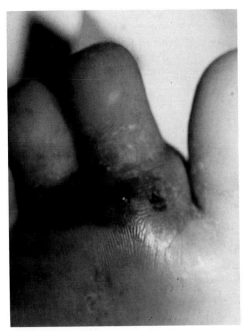

FIGURE 65-15. Photograph of the plantar aspect of the foot of a 5-year-old child, showing swelling, erythrema, and abscess formation following a nail puncture wound to the proximal phalanx of the second toe.

bone. In such a case it may be necessary to perform tissue transfers, including free–vascularized tissue transfers, for coverage.

Aftercare

A below-the-knee splint is applied and the wound is dressed.

OSTEOMYELITIS OF THE CALCANEUS

Osteomyelitis of the calcaneus can be extremely difficult to eradicate and requires adequate, thorough debridement. In early involvement, extensive local debridement and curettage is usually sufficient. With extensive involvement of the calcaneus, resection of the diseased area is necessary to eradicate or control the infection. Osteomyelitis occurring either medially or laterally in the calcaneus usually follows pintrack infections, gunshot wounds, or open fractures.

Medial and lateral approaches to the calcaneus are useful in draining a localized abscess, curetting the infected bone tissue, doing a local resection, and windowing the bone cortex for an osteomyelitic abscess.

In osteomyelitis involving the plantar surface of the calcaneus, a modified approach as described by Gaenslen is used.[6] Gaenslen divided the calcaneus with an osteotome from posterior to anterior, thereby exposing the inside of the bone. He used this technique primarily to treat hematogenous osteomyelitis. However, this technique has a very serious drawback in that it creates a fracture, which could cause an infection to become ongoing and thereby lead to extensive bone loss. Therefore, calcaneus splitting should be avoided.

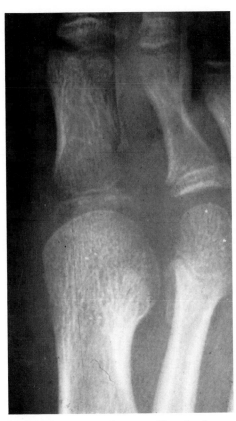

FIGURE 65-16. Anteroposterior x-ray film of a 6-year-old child showing osteomyetic changes of the proximal metaphysis with involvement of the first metatarsal phalangeal joint.

Procedure

With the patient prone, make a longitudinal incision centered in the midline of the heel. Start the incision just inferior to the insertion of the Achilles tendon on the tuberosity, and extend it plantarward approximately to the level of the base of the fifth metatarsal. Next, incise the plantar aponeurosis in a plane between the abductor digiti quinti and flexor digitorum brevis muscles. The lateral plantar artery and nerve can be visualized in the distal aspect of the wound and should be retracted medially. Expose the quadratus plantar muscle and split both it and the long plantar ligament longitudinally. The plantar surface of the calcaneus is now exposed. For localized infection use a curette to remove sequestra, infected tissue, and sinuses. For more extensive involvement use an osteotome to cut the bone parallel to the plantar surface of the foot (Fig. 65-17). Following debridement and copious irrigation, place a Betadine-soaked gauze dressing in the wound and leave the wound open.

Helpful Hints

1. Debridement is the key. Don't be hesitant to resect all infected necrotic bone.
2. Be careful of the lateral plantar neurovascular structures.

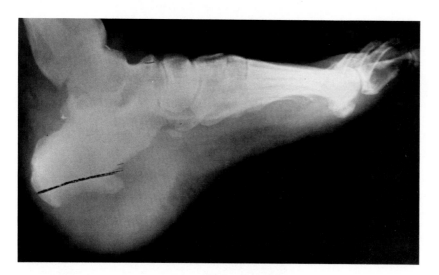

FIGURE 65-17. Lateral x-ray film of a 42-year-old man demonstrating extensive destruction of the calcaneus by osteomyelitis. A marking pen outlines the area of bones to be resected.

Aftercare

1. Dressings should be changed daily.
2. Weight-bearing is allowed after the incision has healed.

OSTEOMYELITIS OF THE FIBULA

Depending on the extent of the infection, it is safe to excise the proximal three-fourths of the fibula, provided the fibular collateral ligament and the biceps femoris tendons are inserted into the tibia when this area of bone is sacrificed. The distal one-fourth should not be excised, since excision would lead to impaired function of the ankle and deformity. If it is necessary to remove this part, a tibial–talar fusion will be necessary later.

Procedure

Make a longitudinal incision, starting on the posterior border of the fibula from the head of the fibula and extending to the length desired. This incision can be carried down the entire length of the fibula. Identify the common peroneal nerve in the proximal part of the wound; it crosses under the peroneus longus just distal to its attachment to the lateral surface of the head of the fibula. Identify the fascial plane between the soleus muscle and peronei anteriorly, and carry the dissection down to the fibula. Retract the peronei muscles anteriorly, and expose the fibula by incising the periosteum. Take care not to injure the deep peroneal nerve branches, which lie on the deep surfaces of the peronei at the neck of the fibula and proximal 2 inches of the fibula. The involved fibula is now exposed, and debridement or resection of the infected area can be accomplished.

The distal one-fourth of the fibula is subcutaneous and can be easily exposed by a longitudinal incision along the posterior border of the fibula.

A Betadine-soaked gauze strip can be loosely placed in the wound.

Aftercare

A long posterior molded splint is applied. The wound is dressed daily.

OSTEOMYELITIS OF THE PATELLA

Expose the patella through a longitudinal skin incision that starts just proximal to the patella and extends distally to the inferior pole. Carry the incision down through the subcutaneous tissue and fascia to the periosteum. Incise the periosteum and elevate it with a periosteal elevator. Curette and debride the involved area of bone.

In cases of extensive involvement of the patella, either part or all of the patella can be removed. In cases in which the knee joint is involved, the knee should be irrigated with 10 liters of irrigating fluid. The joint capsule is then closed over Silastic drainage tubes, which are removed in 48 to 72 hours.

OSTEOMYELITIS OF THE FEMUR

The predisposing factors leading to osteomyelitis of the femur are very important in its management. For hematogenous osteomyelitis, windowing of the cortex as described in this chapter is the preferred method of treatment.

Posterolateral Approach

Either use a lateral decubitus position or turn the patient slightly to elevate the involved extremity. This approach provides access to the entire femoral shaft. Make an incision from the base of the greater trochanter distally to the lateral femoral condyle, depending on the desired length of exposure. Incise the superficial fascia and the fascia lata along the anterior border of the iliotibial band. Expose the vastus lateralis muscle and retract it anteriorly. Continue along the anterior surface of the lateral intermuscular septum, which attaches to the linea aspera. Expose the periosteum and incise it longitudinally. Then use a periosteal elevator to expose the bone. Debride the area of infected necrotic tissue and bone.

In cases of nonunion in which a plate is present and the infection is seen late, the plate should be removed and an external fixation device applied. This should be followed by an autogenous cancellous bone grafting procedure when the infection is controlled.

In the middle third of the thigh, care must be exercised to identify and ligate the second perforating branch of the profunda femoris artery and vein, which travels transversely from the biceps femoris to the vastus lateralis. Avoid damaging the sciatic nerve and profunda femoris artery and vein by not dividing the long and short heads of the biceps femoris muscle.

OSTEOMYELITIS OF THE ILIUM

Infection involving the ilium can occur on either or both the medial, or inner, cortex and the lateral, or outer, cortex. Hematogenous seeding is more common in young persons. In adults, osteomyelitis usually occurs following open fractures, bone-grafting procedures or, in debilitated bed patients, the development of pressure sores.

Procedure

Make an incision along the crest of the ilium extending the length of the infected area. Extend the dissection through the subcutaneous tissues to the crest. Incise the periosteum over the top of the crest and subperiosteally strip the muscles from the lateral cortex of the iliac wing. Identify the abscess, if one is present, and the extent of bone involvement. Drain the abscess and debride all necrotic bone. Window the cortex as necessary. Be careful of the lateral femoral cutaneous nerve, which lies in the vicinity of the anterior superior iliac spine. Perform local resection of the ilium for extensive local involvement, especially in chronic osteomyelitis (Fig. 65-18).

OSTEOMYELITIS OF THE ISCHIUM AND PUBIS

Osteomyelitis involving the ischial tuberosity is usually encountered in paraplegics or patients who are bedridden and develop pressure sores with secondary infection, necrosis, and osteomyelitis. In these infections it is necessary to debride all necrotic tissue, after which the infected ischial tuberosity can be resected with an osteotome and mallet. Copious amounts of irrigation should be used and the wound left open, with Betadine-soaked gauze inserted into it to allow for drainage. In paraplegic patients, soft-tissue transfers are often necessary following infection control.

Abscesses either in the ischiorectal fossa or beneath the obturator externus or internus often develop with osteomyelitis of the pubis and ischium.

OSTEOMYELITIS OF THE RADIUS AND ULNA

The ulna and the radius are most likely to become infected following open reduction and plating of fractures.

Because the posterior surface of the ulna lies subcutaneously essentially throughout its length, the ulna can be exposed by a skin incision carried down through the fascia and periosteum.

The radius is approached in its distal third by the anterior approach as described by Henry.[12] The proximal fourth of the

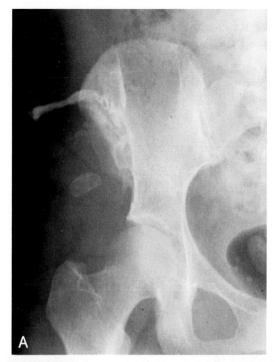

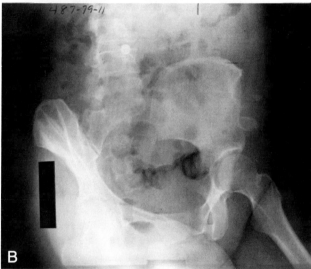

FIGURE 65-18. (*A*) Anteroposterior view of the ilium and hip shortening a sinogram tract down to the ilium of a 44-year-old woman who developed chronic osteomyelitis of the ilium following an open fracture. The patient had undergone multiple previous procedures. (*B*) X-ray film following local resection of the ilium.

radius is exposed by an anterior Henry incision. The middle two-thirds of the radius can then be exposed by the Thompson approach.[31]

OSTEOMYELITIS OF THE HUMERUS

In adults osteomyelitis of the humerus most commonly follows internal fixation of the humerus. Often, draining sinuses are present (Fig. 65-19). After assessing the extent of the infection,

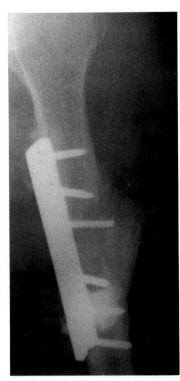

FIGURE 65-19. A sinogram tracts down to metal and bone. The patient had persistent drainage for 7 months following open plating of the humerus. Note that the fracture is healed.

expose the humeral shaft through an anterolateral approach. Make a skin incision from the anterior border of the deltoid muscle, extending it distally along the lateral border of the biceps muscle to within several inches of the elbow joint. Identify the cephalic vein and ligate it. Retract the deltoid laterally and the biceps medially to expose the proximal shaft. Distal to the deltoid insertion, identify the brachialis and split it longitudinally to the bone, retracting the lateral half laterally and the medial half medially. The radial nerve is protected by the lateral half of the brachialis muscle. In the distal third of the exposure, identify the radial nerve, which lies between the brachioradialis and brachialis muscles, and protect it.

REFERENCES

1. Bucholz, H.W., Elson, R.A., and Heinert, K.: Antibiotic-loaded acrylic cement: Current concepts. Clin. Orthop. **190:**96, 1984.

1a. Bickel, W.H., Bateman, J.G., and Johnson, W.E.: Treatment of chronic osteomyelitis by means of saucerization and bone grafting. Surg. Gynecol. Obstet. **96:**265, 1953.

2. Campbell's Operative Orthopaedics, 6th ed. St. Louis, C.V. Mosby, 1980.

2a. Coleman, H.M., Bateman, J. E., Dale, G.M., and Starr, D.E.: Cancellous bone grafts for infected bone defects. Surg. Gynecol. Obstet. **83:**392, 1946.

3. Dombrowski, E.T., and Dunn, A.W.: Treatment of osteomyelitis by debridement and closed wound irrigation—Suction. Clin. Orthop. **43:**215, 1965.

3a. Epps & Copeland

4. Fitzgerald, R.H., Jr., Ruttle, P.E., Arnold, P.G. et al.: Local muscle flaps in the treatment of chronic osteomyelitis. J. Bone Joint Surg. **67-A:**175, 1985.

5. Freeland, A.E., and Mutz, B.: Posterior bone grafting for infected un-united fractures of the tibia. J. Bone Joint Surg. **58-A:**653, 1976.

6. Gaenslen, F.J.: Split-heel approach in osteomyelitis of the os calcis. J. Bone Joint Surg. **13:**759, 1931.

7. Gifford, G.B., Patzakis, M.J., Ivler, D., and Swezey, R.L.: Septic arthritis due to pseudomonas in heroin addicts. J. Bone Joint Surg. **57-A:**631, 1975.

8. Green, S.A., and Dlabal, T.A.: The open bone graft for septic non-union. Clin. Orthop. **180:**117, 1983.

9. Gristina, A.G., and Costerton, J.W.: Bacterial adherence to biomaterials and tissue. J. Bone Joint Surg. **67-A:**264, 1985.

10. Gustilo, R.B., Simpson, L., Nixon, R.A., and Indeck, W.: Analysis of 511 open fractures. Clin. Orthop. **66:**148, 1969.

11. Harmon, P.H.: A simplified surgical approach to the posterior tibia for bone grafting and fibular transference. J. Bone Joint Surg. **27:**496, 1945.

11a. Higgs, S.L.: The use of cancellous chips in bone grafting. J. Bone Joint Surg. **28:**1, 1946.

12. Henry, A.K.: Exposures of long bones and other surgical methods. Bristol, John Wright & Sons, 1927.

13. Hobo, T.: Zur Pathogenese der akuten haematogene Osteomyelitis, mit Berücksichtigung der Vitalfarbungslehre. Acta scholae Kioto **4:**1, 1921.

14. Kelly, P.J., Wilkowske, C.J., and Washington, J.A. II: Musculoskeletal infections due to serratia marcescens. Clin. Orthop. **96:**76, 1973.

15. Klemm, K.: Indikation und Technik zur Einlage von Gentamycin-PMMA-Kugeln bei Knochen- und Wechteilinfekten. In Burri, C., and Rutter, A. (eds.): Lokalbehandlung chirurgischer Infektionen. Aktuelle Probleme in Chirurgie und Orthopädie, Vol. 12. Bern, Huber, 1979.

16. Klemm, K.: Die Behandlung chronischer Knocheninfektionen mit Gentamycin-PMMA-Kugeln. In Contzen H. (ed.): Gentamycin-PMMA-Kettle, Gentamycin-PMMA-Kugeln, Symposium München. Unfallchirurgie **1:**20, 1977.

16a. Knight, M.P., and Wood, G.O.: Surgical obliteration of bone cavities following traumatic osteomyelitis. J. Bone Joint Surg. **27:**547, 1945.

17. Lexer, E.: Zur experimentellen Erzeugung Osteomyelitischer Herdde. Langenbechs Arch. Klin. Chir. **48:**181, 1894.

18. Miskew, D.B.W., Lorenz, M.A., Pearson, R.L., and Pankovich, A.M.: Pseudomonas aeruginosa bone and joint infection in drug abusers. J. Bone Joint Surg. **65-A:**829, 1983.

19. Murray, W.R.: Use of antibiotic-containing bone cement. Clin. Orthop. **190:**89, 1984.

20. Nade, S.: Acute haemotogenous osteomyelitis in infancy and childhood. J. Bone Joint Surg. **65-B:**109, 1983.

21. Papineau, L.J., Alfageme, A., Delcourt, J.P., and Pilon, B.L.: Chronic osteomyelitis of long bones—Resection and bone grafting with delayed skin closure. J. Bone Joint Surg. **52-B:**138, 1976.

22. Patzakis, M.J., Dorr, D.L., Iver, D., Moore, T.M., and Harvey, J.P., Jr.: The early management of open joint injuries. J. Bone Joint Surg. **57-A:**1065, 1975.

23. Patzakis, M.J., Harvey, J.P., Jr., and Ivler, D.: The role of antibiotics in the management of open fractures. J. Bone Joint Surg. **56-A:**532, 1974.

24. Patzakis, M.J., Watkins, R., and Harvey, J.P., Jr.: Posterolateral bone grafting for infected non-unions of the tibia. In Moore T.M. (ed.): American Academy of Orthopaedic Surgeons Symposium on Trauma to the Leg and Its Sequelae, p. 235. St. Louis, C.V. Mosby, 1981.

25. Patzakis, M.J., Wilkins, J., and Moore, T.M.: Considerations in reducing the infection rate in open tibial fractures. Clin. Orthop. **178:**36, 1983.

26. Patzakis, M.J., Wilkins, J., and Moore, T.M.: Use of antibiotics in open tibial fractures. Clin. Orthop. **178:**31, 1983.

27. Patzakis, M.J., Wilkins, J., and Wiss, D.: Infection following intramedullary nailing of long bones. Clin. Orthop. **212:**182, 1986.

28. Rhinelander, F.W.: Minimal internal fixation of tibial fractures. Clin. Orthop. **107:**188, 1975.

29. Roy-Camille, R., Reignier, B., Saillant, G., and Berteaux, D.: Resultants de l'operation de Papineau. Rev. Chir. Orthop. **62:**347, 1976.

30. Roy-Camille, R., Reigner, B., Saillant, G., and Berteaux, D.: Technique et histoire naturelle de l'intervention de Papineau. Rev. Chir. Orthop. **62:**337, 1976.

31. Thompson, J.E.: Anatomical methods of approach in operations on the long bones of the extremities. Ann. Surg. **68:**309, 1918.

32. Trueta, J.: The three types of acute haematogenous osteomyelitis: A clinical and vascular study. J. Bone Joint Surg. **41-B:**671, 1959.

33. Wahlig, H., and Dingledein, E.: Antibiotics and bone cements. Experimental and clinical long-term observations. Acta Orthop. Scand. **51:**49, 1980.

34. Waldvogel, F.A., Medoff, G., and Swartz, M.N.: Osteomyelitis: A review of clinical features, therapeutic considerations and unusual aspects. N. Engl. J. Med. **282:**198, 316, 1970.

35. Wallenkamp, G.H.I.M., Vree, T.B., and Van Rens, T.J.G.: Gentamicin-PMMA beads. Pharmokinetics and nephrotoxicological study. Clin. Orthop. **205:**171, 1986.

36. Weiland, A.J., Moore, J.R., and Daniel, R.K.: The efficacy of free tissue transfer in the treatment of osteomyelitis. J. Bone Joint Surg. **66-A:**181, 1984.

CHAPTER 66

Management of Pyarthrosis

STUART B. GOODMAN and
DAVID J. SCHURMAN

The term *pyarthrosis* is a fusion of two Greek words—*pyon*, meaning pus, and *arthrosis*, meaning joint.[97] Therefore, pyarthrosis by definition denotes a suppurative arthritis. In common medical usage, the term refers to pyogenic infections involving the synovial joints.

PATHOPHYSIOLOGY

Organisms may infect joints by several different mechanisms. These include hematogenous spread from a distant source; spread from an adjacent focus of infection, for example, contiguous osteomyelitis;[4] and direct inoculation through a penetrating injury, an intra-articular injection, or a surgical procedure.

Infection of a synovial joint is an interaction between the host and the infecting organism. Factors that are important to this interaction include (1) general host factors, (2) local host factors, and (3) the quantity and virulence of the infecting organism. General host factors that have been shown to predispose to septic arthritis include defects in the immune system (e.g., hypogammaglobulinemia); quantitative and qualitative white blood cell deficiencies; cancer; immunosuppression caused by chemotherapeutic agents; and severe chronic illness such as liver and kidney disease, rheumatoid arthritis, systemic lupus erythematosus, diabetes mellitus, sickle cell anemia, and alcoholism.[3,16,62,68,75,76,103] Any distant focus of infection that induces recurrent bacteremia may predispose to joint sepsis; this includes chronic sinusitis, bronchiectasis, and intravenous drug abuse.[79]

Local joint factors are also important. Septic arthritis is more common after previous joint trauma,[27,91] and a history of prior arthritis increases the risk of septic arthritis in the same joint.[62,76] In rheumatoid arthritis, the increased risk of superimposed pyogenic arthritis is related to both local factors (e.g., chronic hyperemia, a protein-rich inflammatory exudate within the joint, or local steroid injection) as well as generalized host factors (e.g., humoral and white blood cell deficiencies, the use of systemic immunosuppressive agents, and general debility).[3,32,57,60,62,74,100,103] Other localized arthritides that have been associated with an increased incidence of septic arthritis include degenerative joint disease, Charcot arthropathy, and crystal-induced arthritis (gout and pseudogout).[23,53,55] The incidence of local infection is also increased after the implantation of various biomaterials commonly used in orthopaedic surgery.[72] In particular, methylmethacrylate has been shown to have profound effects on local polymorphonuclear leukocyte chemotaxis and phagocytosis.[70,71]

Synovial infection is dependent not only on host factors, but on the quantity and virulence of the infecting organism. Important factors in this respect include exotoxin, endotoxin, and enzyme production by the bacteria and the synovial membrane. These by-products, as well as bacterial debris, may also play a role by stimulating the host's immune system to produce the "post-infectious" arthritis syndrome.[27,33]

Once the bacteria have reached the synovium, an acute inflammatory response ensues. Proteolytic enzymes are produced that degrade the proteoglycan matrix of the cartilage ground substance and the collagen. These enzymes are released by the polymorphonuclear leukocytes and the lysosomes within

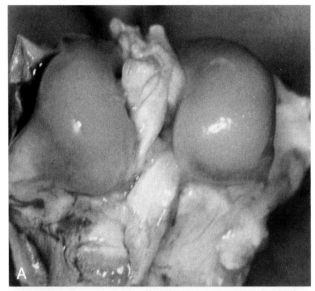

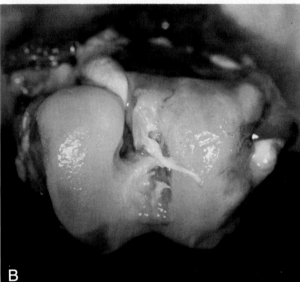

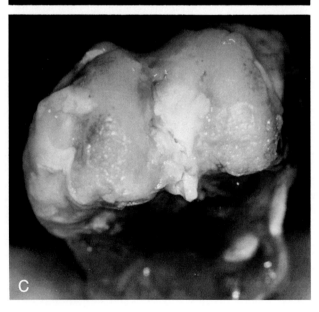

the synovium.[14,15,104] The bacteria themselves may also contribute to this depletion of cell matrix, even in the absence of inflammation.[95] If the septic process can be terminated before collagen loss has begun, the proteoglycan losses may be reversed. Enzymes released by the polymorphonuclear leukocytes and synovium, including collagenase, elastase, cathepsins, and other proteases, remove the proteoglycan matrix from the cartilage, destroy the collagen superstructure, and subject the chondrocytes to increased mechanical stress. As cartilage cells die, matrix formation is decreased, and a vicious cycle ensues. The articular cartilage is eroded away, and the synovium becomes hyperplastic. A pannus of chronic granulation tissue may cover the joint surface. Fibrous or bony ankylosis may be the final result[41] (Fig. 66-1).

CLINICAL PRESENTATION

Septic arthritis may affect any age group, but has a propensity for the neonate and infant, the older adult, and patients who have a chronic, systemic disease or a compromised immune system. Although virtually any joint may be involved, the large weight-bearing joints of the lower extremity are most at risk.[3,4,23,27,41] The joints most commonly involved are the knee, hip, ankle, shoulder, wrist, and elbow.[27] Usually only a single joint is involved; however multiple-joint involvement has been documented.[3,27,45,65]

The classic patient with septic arthritis presents with a single joint that demonstrates the signs of acute inflammation: pain, swelling, heat, erythema, and loss of function. In patients with chronic arthritis, (e.g., rheumatoid arthritis), the diagnosis may be delayed because either the patient or the physician assumes that the clinical picture is a manifestation of an acute exacerbation of the chronic disease. This was the case in four of 13 rheumatoid patients reported by Gristina and associates.[32] In such cases the physician must maintain a high index of suspicion of septic arthritis superimposed on a chronic illness.

Nongonococcal suppurative arthritis is most commonly secondary to hematogenous spread from a distant focus.[3,61] Therefore, signs of systemic sepsis, such as fever and tachycardia, may be present. In one study, during the first 24 hours of hospitalization 78% of patients with septic arthritis were febrile. Chills and rigors are uncommon, and the temperature infrequently goes above 39°.[27,61] The original focus of infection may be discovered after a careful history and physical examination. Special attention should be paid to the ears, nose, throat, chest, integumentary, genitourinary, and gastrointestinal systems.

Gonococcal arthritis is probably the most common cause of bacterial septic arthritis.[66] Whereas nongonococcal septic arthritis affects the very young, the elderly, or the immunocom-

FIGURE 66-1. (*A*) Photograph of the distal femoral articular surface in a normal rabbit. (*B*) Photograph of distal femur of rabbit infected with *Staphylococcus aureus,* and having antibiotic treatment started at 48 hours. Note the irregularity and pitting in the weight-bearing portion of the articular cartilage. (*C*) Distal femoral articular surface of a rabbit that was infected with *Staphyloccocus aureus,* but did not receive antibiotics. Note the severe degenerative arthritis that has developed.

promised, gonococcal arthritis affects healthy males and females, usually younger than 40 years of age. The increasing female preponderance appears to be related to the asymptomatic carrier status. Females often present during pregnancy or just after beginning their menstrual period, implicating local gynecologic/physiologic factors in the production of disseminated disease.[61] Systemic signs and symptoms are variable.[8,13,37,44,96] The clinical picture is classically a migratory polyarthritis, which may eventually become monoarticular. The knees, wrists, ankles, and hands are most often affected, and there may be an associated tenosynovitis. This classic clinical presentation of a migratory polyarthritis, tenosynovitis, and the characteristic vesicopapular skin lesions of gonorrhea is rarely seen in cases of nongonococcal septic arthritis. Other manifestations of gonorrhea, including signs of cardiac (endocarditis or myocarditis), central nervous system (meningitis), hepatic involvement, and conjunctivitis, should always be sought. An examination and cultures of the genitalia, rectum, oral pharynx, and other possible lesions (e.g., of the skin) should be undertaken. Whereas joint aspiration and blood cultures are frequently positive in nongonococcal arthritis, this is not so in the case of gonorrhea.

The pediatric patient poses a special diagnostic problem. Whereas the adult can verbalize his or her pain due to septic arthritis, the neonate and infant cannot. The child with a septic joint is generally systemically ill.[30,31] Pseudoparalysis of the limb and resistance to passive range of motion are frequently present, and often suggest to the unwary that the child has a fracture. It is only after a more in-depth examination that the signs of inflammation are noted and focused to a single joint. The physician must always be suspicious of septic arthritis, especially in the immunocompromised child, the neonate who is small for gestational age, and at any age when invasive monitoring techniques are being used.[30,31,59]

DIAGNOSIS

The history and physical examination pinpointing a monoarticular inflammation should suggest septic arthritis. A white blood cell count from the peripheral blood is >10,000 cells/mm³ in only 50% of patients, and is occasionally helpful. The key diagnostic study is analysis and culture of the synovial fluid.[27,41,61] The fluid should be aspirated under strictly sterile conditions, and the following tests should be performed: gross examination of appearance, viscosity, and color; a white blood cell count; the percentage of polymorphonuclear leukocytes; the glucose concentration of the aspirate; gram stain; and culture. Tables have been published to differentiate the characteristics of normal synovial fluid from those associated with degenerative joint disease, inflammatory arthritis, and septic arthritis.[79a] All specimens should be taken to the laboratory promptly for immediate analysis. The arthrocentesis fluid should be cultured aerobically and anaerobically, and incubated in 5% to 10% CO_2 on chocolate agar plates if gonococcal arthritis is suspected. If tuberculous arthritis is a possibility, a Ziehl–Neelson stain and appropriate culture should be ordered. Fungal infections may be viewed microscopically with potassium hydroxide preparations and cultured on Sabouraud's medium. If the synovial fluid is centrifuged, the concentrated sediment often improves the yield of a Gram's stain or other stain.

In the typical acute bacterial arthritis, the synovial fluid is purulent, being gray, yellow, or green, and usually opaque[79a,85] (Fig. 66-2). The viscosity of the fluid is variable; however the mucin clot is usually very friable. The synovial fluid white blood count is usually >50,000 cells/mm³, and is often >100,000. Polymorphonuclear leukocytes comprise at least 75% of the cellular population, and frequently >90%. Synovial fluid glucose is usually lower than the blood glucose. Frequently, the fasting blood minus synovial fluid glucose is >50 mg/dl.[85] In tuberculous and fungal arthritis, the findings are similar, except there is usually a higher proportion of mononuclear cells (30%–50%).[17] One should also search for the presence of crystals under polarized light to rule out gout or pseudogout in afebrile adults.

Cultures of the blood and other possible portals of entry should be taken. This may include any suspicious skin lesion or wound, the nasal pharynx, sputum, urine, and stool. Approximately 50% of patients with nongonococcal bacterial arthritis will have a positive blood culture.

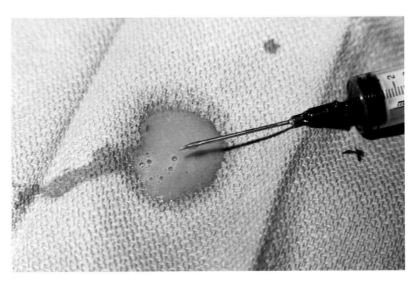

FIGURE 66-2.   Photograph of pus aspirated from a knee joint infected with *Staphyloccocus aureus*.

Various specialized diagnostic studies have been used to detect bacterial antigens,[82] metabolites,[9] and monoclonal antibodies[73] in the synovial fluid in cases of septic arthritis. These procedures are sometimes costly and in practice have had only limited application.

Radiographs of the involved joint should always be taken. The film may show evidence of preexisting disease, and may alert the physician to the possibility of a superimposed septic arthritis. Usually, however, the radiographs show soft tissue swelling and synovial distention and little more. Later radiographs (1–2 weeks) may show osteopenia in the subchondral area or evidence of a coexisting osteomyelitis. Subluxation or dislocation of the joint may be seen early or late. This is more common in the hip of the infant, and may be accompanied by exuberant new periosteal bone formation.[50] Septic arthritis associated with subluxation of the glenohumeral joint has been documented in the adult.[54] If a gas-forming organism (e.g., some gram-negative organisms and anaerobes) is the cause of septic arthritis, the radiograph may disclose gas in the joint and surrounding tissues.[7,56] Late radiographic changes in untreated cases of septic arthritis include progressive joint narrowing and destruction. Fibrous or bony ankylosis may be the final result.

Postoperative hip infections are of particular interest because the appearance of the "classic" radiographic signs may be altered.[47] In a series of proven hip infections after surgical treatment of hip fractures with internal fixation, Lewis and Norman found that pericapsular edema was absent in 50% of patients. Joint space narrowing was the initial and most reliable radiographic sign, and was recognized as early as 4 weeks after surgery. Later acetabular destruction superiorly in the weight-bearing area was often accompanied by subluxation. If septic arthritis is suspected in a prosthetic joint, radiographs should be taken to assess whether there is evidence of new periosteal bone formation, bone lysis, or loosening of the arthroplasty.[77] This subject is discussed in more detail in Chapter 68.

Joint scintigraphy[48,81] using technetium phosphate, gallium citrate, or other radioisotopes is sometimes helpful in the diagnosis of difficult cases of septic arthritis. The scan may localize septic areas that are difficult to examine clinically, and may help differentiate cellulitis from septic arthritis or osteomyelitis. Further localization may also be afforded by plain or computed axial tomography of difficult joints, for example, the sacroiliac or sternoclavicular joints.[58]

Rarely, a synovial biopsy is required for diagnostic purposes to distinguish a case of infectious from noninfectious arthritis, or to provide material for culture and histological analysis in difficult, perplexing cases.[26]

MICROBIOLOGY

Gonococcal arthritis caused by *Neisseria gonorrhoeae* is the most common cause of septic arthritis in the healthy adult population younger than 40 years of age. It has been estimated that two to three cases of gonococcal arthritis are seen for every case of bacterial arthritis.[21]

Staphylococcus aureus continues to be the most common agent responsible for nongonococcal bacterial arthritis. In a recent series from Boston University Medical Center, *S. aureus* comprised 40% of cases of nongonococcal bacterial arthritis

between 1965 and 1982.[27] Various streptococcal species constituted 27% of infections. Recently, gram-negative bacillary septic arthritis has become more prevalent, comprising 23% of cases in the above series; *Diplococcus pneumoniae* (6%) and *Staphylococcus epidermidis* (4%) accounted for the remainder. In two other large series, staphylococcal infections played an even more prominent role, comprising 77% (108 of 141, and 80 of 104 cases) of all bacteria isolated in nongonococcal septic arthritis in adults.[45,65] These bacteria appear to demonstrate increasing penicillin resistance,[91] necessitating the use of newer chemotherapeutic agents.

Streptococcal species, including *Streptococcus pneumoniae* (pneumococcus), almost always cause septic arthritis through hematogenous spread from the upper or lower respiratory tracts or skin; other rare sources have been noted.[10,28,46] Gram-negative bone and joint infections appear to be on the increase in general;[44] this is related to the rise in intravenous drug abuse and to chronic medical problems such as diabetes, cancer, and the use of chemotherapeutic agents.[25,79,92,103] Whereas *Pseudomonas aeruginosa* and *Serratia marcescens* septic arthritis are usually associated with intravenous drug abuse, *Escherichia coli* and *Proteus mirabilis* infections often stem from urinary sepsis.[25,79,92,103] Many other gram-negative organisms have also been implicated in cases of septic arthritis.[25,92]

Septic arthritis in neonates, infants, and children has a slightly different bacteriology. For the first few months of life, the neonate attains passive immunity from maternal antibodies. In this age group, the most common bacteria causing septic arthritis include gram-positive cocci (staphylococcal and beta-streptococcal species) and gram-negative rods.[61,92] These bacteria may emanate from the maternal vaginal flora or from invasive procedures such as intravenous catheters introduced in the hospital nursery. Gonococcal arthritis should always be kept in mind in this age group. Infants older than 6 months of age and children up to several years of age have an increased incidence of *Hemophilus influenzae* infections in addition to the common neonatal organisms. Not infrequently, septic arthritis due to *H. influenzae* is resistant to ampicillin. In children older than 2 years of age, *Staphylococcus aureus* is the usual bacterial organism cultured; however, *H. influenzae*, streptococcal, gonococcal, and other organisms may be the cause.[30,31,59,61] In older children, infection associated with a foreign body in the joint (e.g., the knee) should always be suspected.

Mycobacterial (typical and atypical) and fungal septic arthritis are rare. In general, appropriate cultures should be made to exclude these agents, especially in the case of an immunocompromised host.[29,49] The atypical mycobacteria, including *Mycobacterium kansasii*, *Mycobacterium marinum*, *Mycobacterium intracellulare*, and others, usually cause a mono/pauci-articular arthritis of the hands or knees.[36] Mycotic septic arthritis may include infection with *Sporothrix schenckii*, *Candida* species, the maduromycoses, *Cryptococcus neoformans*, *Coccidiodes immitis*, *Blastomyces dermatitidis*, *Aspergillus fumigatus*, and others.[36]

Viral-associated arthritis may present during infection with any of the more common or uncommon viruses.[84] It frequently appears with infection due to rubella, hepatitis B, and alphavirus, but appears less commonly with infection due to mumps, adenovirus, herpesvirus, and enterovirus. Joint symptoms are transient, often polyarticular, and nondestructive. The etiology of the arthralgia or arthritis may be due to direct synovial invasion of the virus, or to a virus–host interaction involving stimulation of the immune system.[84]

Postoperative infections after orthopaedic procedures are usually due to one predominant organism. Gram-positive bacteria (*Staphylococcus aureus* and *S. epidermidis*) comprise 60% to 80% of the organisms cultured.[1,93] Gram-negative and multiple organisms occur less frequently. After joint replacement, staphylococcal infections take on a new significance.[84,93] *S. epidermidis* infection becomes as common as *S. aureus* and appears to be more difficult to eradicate.[93] In one large series of 137 infected total hip replacements, 68% of cultures grew gram-positive organisms, 18% grew gram-negative organisms, one hip was infected with multiple organisms, and 11% of cultures were sterile (results in two cases were not available).[39] Most authors agree that infection with gram-negative organisms or mixed organisms yield the poorest results.[11,38,39,93] This subject is discussed in greater detail in Chapter 68.

TREATMENT

Any suspicion of the diagnosis of septic arthritis demands an immediate thorough work-up including history, physical examination, appropriate blood work, radiography, joint aspiration with Gram's stain and culture, and an intense search for a primary infective focus.

The principles of treatment of septic arthritis include the following[31]:

1. Sterilize the joint by providing adequate drainage and appropriate antibiotics in sufficient dosages to kill the pathogen.
2. Prevent the occurrence of deformity.
3. Fully rehabilitate the joint and limb.

Aspiration *versus* Surgical Drainage

Perhaps the most controversial aspect in the treatment of septic arthritis is the method of drainage. All agree that adequate drainage is of paramount importance. This would mitigate the ongoing degradation of the cartilage ground sustance by the enzymes of the polymorphonuclear leukocytes and lysosomes within the synovium.[14,15,104] The debate centers around the method of drainage—in other words, whether repeated aspiration or surgical drainage is indicated.

Whereas virtually all physicians believe that septic arthritis of the hip and other less accessible joints requires surgical drainage, the method of treatment in other joints is less clear. In general, internists and pediatricians favor repeated aspiration of an infected joint; most surgeons favor surgical drainage.[3,24,27,31,45,50,65,69,80] Indeed, Paterson has stated, "It is suggested that aspiration has no place in the treatment of suppurative arthritis of the hip, and it is not considered a safe method for any other joint."[69] However, there have been no randomized, prospective studies to document the superiority of one form of treatment over the other. Several retrospective studies, including those by Goldenberg and associates[24] and Rosenthal and co-workers[80] compared the two methods of treatment and concluded that patients undergoing needle aspiration did better than those undergoing surgical drainage and

debridement. However, the controversy has not been settled. Other issues are also involved; for example, consider how difficult it is to convince a pleading, crying child with septic arthritis that he or she must undergo aspiration once (or more) per day.

Aspiration

If aspiration is the chosen mode of treatment, the joint should be aspirated frequently enough to prevent the stagnation and loculation of pus. Initially, this should be once or twice per day.[24,27,80] Careful sterile technique is mandatory. A large bore (at least an 18-gauge needle) should be used for larger joints. The aspirate should be cultured every 1 to 2 days after antibiotic treatment has commenced to assess the efficacy of therapy. Aspirations should continue until little exudate is retrieved and repeat joint fluid cultures are negative. The clinical status also should be closely monitored. It is sometimes useful to inject saline after the aspiration in order to wash the debris and chondrolytic enzymes from the joint.

The specific location of the needle insertion for aspiration is not important,[24,67,80] as long as adequate drainage is attained and the joint and important structures around it (i.e., vessels, nerves, tendons) are not injured. We find it easiest to aspirate the shoulder either anteriorly or posteriorly. In the anterior approach, the needle is directed posteriorly, superiorly, and laterally from a point slightly inferior and lateral to the coracoid process. This maneuver is often facilitated by external rotation of the shoulder. For the posterior approach, enter the shoulder joint 1.5 inches inferior and medial to the acromial angle. The elbow joint can be approached posterolaterally, just below the midpoint connecting the lateral epicondyle and the lateral edge of the olecranon. The elbow should be flexed to 90° during the aspiration.

The dorsal approach to the wrist provides excellent access while avoiding many of the critical structures in the area. The finger joints are entered through a posteromedial or posterolateral stab, just volar to the extensor mechanism. A smaller-bore needle may be necessary. The carpometacarpal joint of the thumb is more difficult because of the large number of tendons, nerves, and vessels passing in the vicinity. It is approached most safely by flexing the thumb across the palm and directing the needle at the base of the first metacarpal volar to the radial artery and snuff box, aiming for the fourth metacarpal base.

The hip joint is one of the most difficult to aspirate. For diagnostic purposes, it behooves the physician to know the proper technique. It is best to perform this procedure in the radiology suite or operating room, with radiographic imaging. The patient lies in the supine position on a radiolucent table. In the anterior approach, the limb is extended and externally rotated. The needle is introduced 1 inch below the anterosuperior iliac spine and 1 inch lateral to the palpable pulsations of the femoral artery. Direct the needle into the joint posteromedially at a 60° angle. For the lateral approach to the hip, the limb is positioned in extension and internal rotation. The greater trochanter is identified. The aspiration needle is directed along the anterior portion of the greater trochanter, parallel to the femoral neck, then medially and cephalad toward the middle of the inguinal ligament.

The knee joint is the easiest joint to aspirate because it

contains the largest synovial cavity in the body. With the patient in the supine position and the knee fully extended, insert the needle from a midlateral or midmedial parapatellar location and direct it posterior and inferior to the patella. Care should be taken not to scratch or scuff the articular surfaces.

The ankle may be approached easily either anteromedially or anterolaterally. In the anteromedial approach, the needle is inserted just distal to the tibial plafond, between the lateral edge of the medial malleolus and the medial edge of the tibialis anterior tendon. For the anterolateral approach, enter the ankle joint just lateral to the extensor digitorum communis tendons. The subtalar joint is readily entered either just below the tip of the lateral malleolus or at the level of the sinus tarsi. The latter is found just below and anterior to the lateral malleolus. If a septic arthritis of this joint is noted, the normal "pitting" landmark of the sinus tarsi may be replaced by bulging synovium. The small joints of the foot and toes are approached in a similar fashion to the small joints in the hand.

Surgical Drainage

Although the indications for surgical drainage of various joints remain controversial, there is general agreement that deeper joints such as the hip and sacroiliac joints, which are less accessible to aspiration, should be treated surgically. Another indication for surgical drainage would include inadequate drainage using aspiration techniques, because of thick purulent material or loculations within the joint. Also, any joint which does not respond to repeated aspirations and appropriate systemic antibiotics in bacteriocidal dosages by 48 hours should be surgically drained. Surgical drainage of a septic hip joint is almost always recommended in the child because of the difficulty in aspiration of this deeply seated joint, the inadvertent damage to the joint surface during the procedure, and the risk of avascular necrosis to the head of the femur. The latter complication may result from compromise of the retinacular vessels caused by increased intracapsular pressures.[31,50,69]

If open surgical drainage of a septic joint is indicated, the operation should be performed promptly. The aims of surgery are to thoroughly debride the joint; excise all dead, infected, nonviable tissue; and assess the articular surface with respect to the possible need for future reconstructive procedures. Some investigators feel that a concomitant synovectomy is indicated, especially if there has been any delay in diagnosis or a poor response to antibiotic treatment and drainage by closed means.[22,98] In one study, synovectomy helped prevent late joint destruction in cases of septic arthritis involving the knee joint, but not the hip.[98] At a minimum, the joint should be thoroughly debrided of all nonviable synovium. During arthrotomy, appropriate specimens for microbiologic and pathologic studies should always be taken.

A surgical approach that will allow wide drainage and complete inspection of the joint should be chosen. Some authors feel that the surgical approach should allow dependent drainage of the joint and that the joint should be left open. This point has never been addressed in a prospective, randomized study. We feel that the joint should *not* be left open to the environment for fear of colonization of the dressings (and joint) with other organisms. We close the debrided joint over suction tubes, which are removed after several days, depending on the patient's clinical response and the amount and type of drainage. Occasionally, suction drainage has been combined with an irrigation system,[12,43] particularly when a great deal of thick, purulent material has been excised. Depending on which joint is involved, a suitably sized inflow catheter is established on one side of the joint, and one or two larger-bore outflow catheters are placed on the opposite side of the joint. (For example, a central venous pressure tubing or small Hemovac drain may be used for inflow irrigation of the knee joint, and a larger-bore Hemovac drain may be used for outflow.) The drains should be placed sufficiently far apart so that distention of the joint and circulation of the fluid will be accomplished. The system should be entirely closed with all tubing joints secured with adhesive tape. A physiological saline solution may be infused at a rate sufficient to provide a constant outflow. Antibiotics need not be added to the irrigant, as sufficient joint levels are attained with systemic antibiotics.[64,86-90] The irrigation tubes are left in place for 2 to 3 days and then withdrawn. The effluent tubes are left in place for approximately 24 hours after the inflow tubes are removed. These time periods have been selected because of experimental evidence which demonstrated changes in the articular cartilage glycosaminoglycan staining after 3 days of constant saline irrigation;[43] these changes reflect deprivation of the nutrients in the synovial fluid which normally bathes the articular cartilage. Furthermore, if drains are left in much longer than several days, they may serve as a portal of entry for bacteria and may contribute to the formation of a synovial fistula.[52,101]

Arthroscopic debridement has been used in conjunction with systemic antibiotics to debride infected joints, most notably the knee. Although most of the reported series are small, this method appears to allow adequate drainage and visualization of the joint with minimal morbidity.[20,40,42]

Specific surgical approaches for open arthrotomy include the standard approaches outlined in Chapters 2 and 4. If the joint is to be left open, then dependent drainage can be facilitated by the surgical approach selected and appropriate postoperative positioning techniques. We routinely close arthrotomy incisions and employ suction (with or without irrigation), so the actual approach may be of less importance because joint dependency is not necessary.

The shoulder joint may be decompressed either anteriorly or posteriorly; we usually select the anterior approach. A deltopectoral approach is made and the shoulder joint is identified beneath the subscapularis muscle, which is reflected medially, allowing a cuff of tendon to remain on the lesser tuberosity for closure.

The elbow joint is most easily debrided posterolaterally through an oblique incision between the extensor carpi ulnaris and anconeus muscles. If a posteromedial approach is selected, the ulnar nerve must be identified and protected.

The wrist joint and carpus are approached dorsally with the forearm pronated. A central incision is made and the wrist joint is entered between the third (extensor pollicis longus) and fourth (extensor digitorum communis) compartments. The extensor retinaculum should be reconstructed before closure. A midlateral or midmedial longitudinal approach to the finger joints is most common. Special care must be exercised to avoid the digital nerves and vessels.

Arthrotomy of the hip joint may be performed through a number of different approaches. We prefer the standard anterior iliofemoral approach in children and the posterolateral, gluteus maximus–splitting approach in adults. If the hip joint is to be left open, the posterolateral approach is recommended, because it allows dependent drainage with the patient supine. A child may be placed in the prone position after an iliofemoral approach.

The anteromedial or anterolateral parapatellar approach allows excellent surgical decompression and visualization of the knee joint. The former approach is most often used. The posteromedial approach just posterior to the medial collateral ligament may be used if dependent drainage is required.

The ankle joint may be exposed by numerous approaches (anteromedial, anterolateral, posteromedial, or posterolateral). We use the anterolateral exposure (lateral to the extensor digitorum longus) or posterolateral exposure (between the fibula and the tendo achilles) most often. In the latter approach, the sural nerve should be identified and protected. This approach allows dependent drainage in the supine position if the wound is left open.

The small joints in the foot and toes are approached dorsally (talus), or midlaterally or midmedially (toes), through exposures similar to those used in the hand.

In each case the joint is thoroughly irrigated, debrided, inspected, and loosely closed over suction tubes. Irrigation tubes may be added if the purulent material is thick. Skin and subcutaneous tissues are loosely closed. If the infection is particularly worrisome (loculated, thick pus, severe joint destruction), the joint should be left open to granulate. Dressing changes 3 to 4 times per day are instituted for open wounds, using hydrogen peroxide or another antiseptic solution.

After surgery, we splint septic joints and begin active assisted and gentle passive range of motion exercises when the inflammatory response subsides, usually after 24 to 48 hours. We have not used postoperative continuous passive motion; however, experimental evidence suggests that this modality may prove useful in maintaining joint range of motion and minimizing cartilage glycosaminoglycan loss.[83] Certainly, prolonged immobilization appears to be contraindicated because it leads to stiffness, atrophy, and poor rehabilitative potential. With respect to lower extremity joints, protected weight-bearing should be maintained until inflammation has ceased, range of motion is pain-free, and rehabilitative endeavors are well under way. In general, extensive bony or soft tissue reconstructive procedures should not be performed during the acute phase of septic arthritis; these procedures should be postponed until the maximal potential of the joint and limb has been realized after extensive rehabilitation.

Antibiotics

The proper selection of antibiotic therapy is an integral part of the treatment of septic arthritis.[23,25,27,36,45,61,65] The immediate Gram's stain of the synovial fluid aspirate may identify specific microorganisms which will determine the choice of antibiotics. If no organisms are seen on the Gram's stain but pus cells are identified in the aspirate, antibiotics should be given according to the "best guess principle," as described below. These are continued until the results of the synovial aspirate and blood cultures become available 24 to 48 hours later. Antibiotics are given intravenously. Bacteriocidal antibiotics are generally preferred over bacteriostatic agents. Intra-articular injection of antibiotic is not necessary because adequate levels are achieved

in synovium and bone with parenteral use; also, a chemical synovitis may result from direct intra-articular inoculation.[27,62,64,86–90] In difficult cases the blood and synovial fluid may be monitored to ensure that antibiotic levels are above the minimal inhibitory concentration for a specific microorganism.

There is no general agreement as to how long to treat a case of septic arthritis with antibiotics. In general, we treat with parenteral antibiotics until systemic toxicity and local swelling are under control. We monitor the white blood cell count and the sedimentation rate in peripheral blood, and perform repeated synovial fluid aspirations in cases treated by needle drainage. The aspirate should be cultured every 1 to 3 days and Gram's stain, glucose concentration, white blood cell, and polymorphonuclear leukocyte counts may be performed. We continue antibiotics orally an additional 2 to 3 weeks after the parenteral course. This may be done on an outpatient basis with close supervision. Longer courses are recommended for gram-negative infections, multiple microorganisms, or in the immunocompromised patient. We frequently confer with our infectious disease colleagues on cases of septic arthritis, especially in the more complex situations.

If gram-positive cocci are noted on the initial Gram's stain, staphylococcal or streptococcal species are the usual microorganism. We employ a semisynthetic, penicillinase-resistant penicillin (e.g., nafcillin, oxacillin, cloxacillin) (8 g–12 g/day, given every 4–6 hours in adults; 150–200 mg/kg/day, given in four to six divided doses in children) until cultures are available. Alternate choices include a cephalosporin (e.g., cefazolin) (1 g–2 g IV every 6 hours in adults; 100–200 mg/kg/day in children), or vancomycin (2 g/day in divided doses in adults; 40 mg/kg/day in two divided doses in children). We continue the above regimen if penicillinase-producing staphylococci are cultured. In penicillin-sensitive cases (e.g., some *Staphylococcus aureus* and streptococcal infections) we switch to penicillin G (10 million units, given in four divided doses in adults; 100–200 mg/kg/day, given in six divided doses in children). Vancomycin may be substituted in patients allergic to penicillin.

Gram-negative cocci in a septic joint in the adult usually signify gonorrheal infection. We recommend the use of parenteral penicillin therapy (penicillin G, 10 million units/day, in four divided doses). The patient can be switched to oral penicillin therapy when signs and symptoms abate, for a 2-week course. Spectinomycin is recommended in patients with penicillinase-producing gonococcal infection.[78] Third-generation cephalosporins can be extremely effective, and long-acting agents such as ceftriaxone are being used with increasing frequency. Gram-negative coccal organisms in an infant's or young child's synovial aspirate may signify *H. influenza* infection. We begin ampicillin (400 mg/kg/day, given every 6 hours) and chloramphenicol (100 mg/kg/day, given every 6 hours). The latter is added because of the ampicillin-resistance of some of these organisms. One could also use cefamandole (700 mg/kg/day, given in four divided doses). The clinical response is monitored closely, and a final choice is made when cultures are available.

Gram-negative bacilli seen on Gram's stain of the joint aspirate require immediate treatment and close observation. A search should be made for infection of the urinary tract, biliary tract, for generalized debilitating disease, and for the possibility of drug abuse.[25,79,91,92,103] We use tobramycin (5 mg/kg/day, given in three divided doses), gentamicin (same dose), or amikacin (15 mg/kg/day) until the cultures are returned. Ticarcillin (300 mg/kg/day given every 4–6 hours) is frequently prescribed by our infectious diseases colleagues in addition to one of the above drugs, especially for pseudomonas infections. If aminoglycosides are used, renal and vestibuloauditory function should be closely monitored, at least on a weekly basis. Antibiotic peak and trough blood levels should also be evaluated in the first few days and repeated later if clinical response is not appropriate, or if aminoglycosides are used.

If the Gram's stain does not show the presence of any bacteria, a "best guess" must be made until the cultures return. The physician must take into account the patient's age, associated disease, and immunocompetence. In the neonate, the most common bacteria causing septic arthritis include gram-positive cocci (staphylococcal and beta-streptococcal species) and gram-negative rods.[61,92] Until the cultures are available, a semisynthetic penicillase-resistant penicillin should be combined with tobramycin, gentamicin, or amikacin. In infants and children from 6 months to 3 years of age, one should consider *Staphylococcus aureus* and *H. influenzae* the most likely pathogens. In such cases we generally combine a semisynthetic penicillinase-resistant penicillin with chloramphenicol; we may substitute cefamandole or ampicillin for one of these, depending on the culture results and sensitivities. In older children and adults, a semisynthetic penicillinase-resistant penicillin active against *Staphylococcus aureus* or a cephalosporin may be used. In the immunocompromised host, we combine an antistaphylococcal agent with tobramycin, gentamicin, or amikacin. We should emphasize once again that an infectious diseases consultation can be very helpful.

In the treatment of tuberculous septic arthritis,[36] combination therapy is most commonly prescribed, including two or more of the following: isoniazid (300 mg/day in adults; 3–5 mg/kg/day in children), ethambutol (1.5–2 g/day in adults; 15–25 mg/kg/day in children), and rifampin (600 mg/day in adults; 10 mg/kg/day in children). Pyridoxine is given to prevent neuritis if isoniazid is used. Liver function should be closely monitored with isoniazid, and one should be aware of the lupus syndromes associated with its use. Thrombocytopenia, hepatitis, and flu-like syndromes may be associated with the use of rifampin, and visual disturbances may be associated with ethambutol. Therapy should continue for at least 18 months. Other drugs that may be useful include streptomycin and aminosalicylic acid.

Antifungal chemotherapy with intravenous amphotericin B (0.6–1.0 mg/kg/day) must be performed with great caution because of the toxicity of this drug. Renal, hematologic, gastrointestinal, and other side-effects should be closely monitored.

REHABILITATION

Spasm of the muscles surrounding an infected joint often accompanies the signs of inflammation. This may lead to pathologic subluxation or dislocation, or the development of contractures.[69] After adequate drainage and the institution of appropriate antibiotic therapy, the limb should be positioned so as to encourage containment of the joint in a position of function while avoiding subluxation or the development of contractures. The hip joint should be positioned in abduction

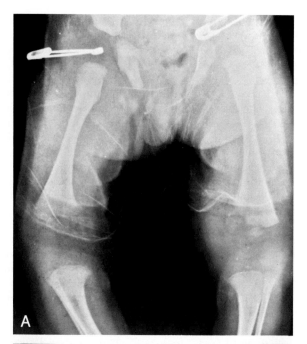

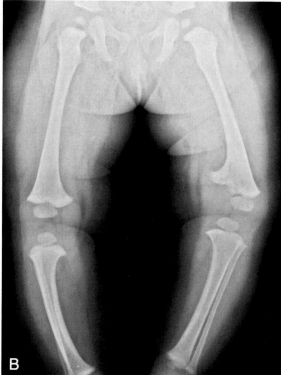

FIGURE 66-3. (*A*) Radiograph of lower extremities in a 2-year-old child with a painful left knee of 2 months' duration. The child was febrile. Notice the soft-tissue swelling over the left distal thigh. Aspiration of the knee joint demonstrated *Staphyloccocus aureus*. (*B*) This septic arthritis of the left knee led to premature closure of the medial half of the left distal femoral epiphysis, resulting in growth abnormality and a varus deformity of the left knee.

and neutral rotation. We have used skin traction in a Thomas splint or a hip spica to maintain this position. After drainage, the knee should be positioned in full extension and the ankle should be placed in neutral dorsiflexion/plantar flexion. A long- or short-leg plaster cast works well for the knee and ankle, respectively. After drainage of the shoulder, a sling, collar and cuff, or Velpeau dressing provides adequate immobilization. We recommend splintage of the elbow in a 90° cast, with the forearm in neutral or mild supination. The wrist should be splinted in slight dorsiflexion and the hand should be placed in the "apple-holding position."

The concept of early joint motion in the treatment of septic arthritis is not a new one. Prior to the use of antibiotics, Willems in 1919 advocated surgical decompression and early active motion for septic joints.[102] This concept was further put to use by Ballard and co-workers, who combined arthrotomy, systemic antibiotics, and early, active range of motion exercises in the treatment of septic arthritis of the knee.[6] They demonstrated an 82% fair/good result rate despite a difficult population composed primarily of prior treatment failures. Perhaps the most elegant experimental study was performed by Salter's group.[83] Using a model of staphylococcal septic arthritis of the rabbit knee, they combined arthrotomy and antibiotic treatment with either plaster immobilization of the knee joint, cage activity, or continuous passive motion (CPM) on a specially designed machine. The CPM group fared the best, showing decreased cartilage ground substance losses compared to the other treatment methods. Our current treatment protocol emphasizes proper splintage during the early stages of treatment, with the institution of active assisted and gentle passive range of motion after 24 to 48 hours, when the inflammation and pain subside. We plan to use CPM in the future for appropriate cases. We delay weight-bearing on septic joints of the lower extremity until range of motion and strength are virtually normal.

PROGNOSIS

Denis Paterson of the Adelaide Children's Hospital has emphasized that "every hour that an acute suppurative process continues within a joint is of urgent significance to prog-

FIGURE 66-4. A 16-year-old patient developed severe pain in the left hip girdle and a temperature of 104°F. (*A*) He developed osteomyelitis of the left iliac wing as well as septic arthritis of the left hip joint. (*B*) A sequestrectomy of the left ilium was performed and the wound was packed open. (*C*) The patient's extremity was placed in a hip spica, which resulted in bony ankylosis of the left hip. (Note: This case is from 1939, the pre-antibiotic era). (Radiographs courtesy of Dr. Henry Jones, Radiology Department, Stanford University Medical Center)

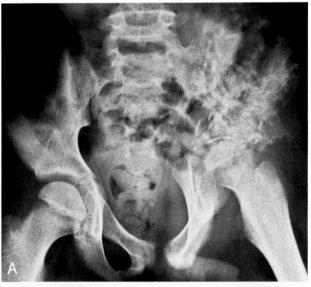

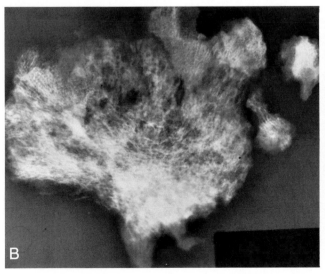

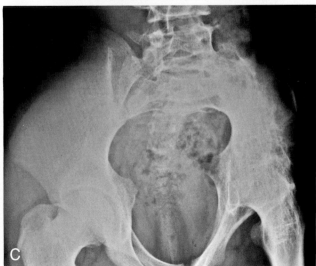

nosis."[69] Lloyd-Roberts agreed that Paterson did "not exaggerate the sense of urgency required of us when confronted by either the certainty, probability or even the possibility of this affection."[50]

Numerous studies have demonstrated a negative correlation between the length of time from onset of symptoms to documentation of a sterile joint and the quality of the outcome.[5,23,27,34,51] Other factors associated with a poor outcome include immunodeficiency in the host (e.g., malignancy, rheumatoid arthritis, or prematurity in neonates), concomitant osteomyelitis, infection involving the hip joint or any prosthetic joint, the presence of positive blood cultures, and infection with *Staphylococcus aureus* or multiple organisms, especially anaerobes or gram-negative rods.[35] In general, gonococcal arthritis has a much better prognosis, if treatment is instituted promptly.[8,13,21,37,44,66,96]

Complications associated with septic arthritis include death, variable destruction of the joint with residual joint stiffness and functional limitation, subluxation and dislocation, avascular necrosis, local growth disturbance (Fig. 66-3), osteomyelitis, and postinfection synovitis.[3,5,18,23,34,50,51,63,69,80,94]

The incidence of death from septic arthritis has ranged from 8% to 15% in three series published since 1975.[23,34,80] Mortality rates are highest in those persons with one or more of the poor outcome factors mentioned above.

The consequences of septic arthritis of a joint, especially the hip, in a growing child can be disastrous.[5,18,50,51,63,69,94] Numerous physicians have documented cases of avascular necrosis, sequestration and absorbtion of the femoral capital epiphysis, chondrolysis of the articular cartilage, destruction of the epiphyseal plate with growth disturbance or arrest, and subluxation or dislocation of the epiphysis or entire hip joint. These complications have a profound effect on a child of any age and may herald a long course of repeated reconstructive surgeries. In the adult, degenerative arthritis with fibrous or bony ankylosis may be the result. These complications may occur in virtually any septic joint, but are most profound in the hip (Fig. 66-4).

Recurrent synovitis may persist despite the eradication of microorganisms from the joint. This complication is most common after intra-articular antibiotic injection.[3] Nonsteroidal anti-inflammatory drugs may aid in the treatment of this puzzling residuum.

Overall, septic arthritis has a favorable outcome in approximately 50% to 80% of cases.[23,34,80] This emphasizes the need for a heightened index of suspicion of this disease, and the immediate institution of appropriate diagnostic and treatment procedures.

REFERENCES

1. Ahlbert, A., Carlsson, A., and Lindberg, L.: Hematogenous Infection in Total Joint Replacements. Clin. Orthop. **137**:69, 1978.
2. Andrews, H.J., Arden, C.P., and Hart, G.M., et al: Deep Infection After Total Hip Replacement. J. Bone Joint Surg. **63-B**:53, 1981.
3. Argen, R.J., Wilson, C.H., and Wood, P.: Suppurative Arthritis. Clinical Features of 42 Cases. Arch. Intern. Med. **117**:661, 1966.
4. Atcheson, S.G., and Ward, J.R.: Acute Hematogenous Osteomyelitis Progressing to Septic Synovitis and Eventual Pyarthrosis: The Vascular Pathway. Arthritis Rheum. **21**:968, 1978.
5. Baitch, A.: Recent Observations of Acute Suppurative Arthritis. Clin Orthop. **22**:157, 1962.
6. Ballard, A., Burkhalter, W.E., Mayfield, G.W., Dehne, E., and Braun, P.W.: The Functional Treatment of Pyogenic Arthritis of the Adult Knee. J. Bone Joint Surg. **57-A**:1119, 1975.
7. Bliznack, J., and Ramsey, J.: Emphysematous Septic Arthritis Due to *Escherichia coli*. J. Bone Joint Surg. **58-A**:138, 1976.
8. Brandt, K.D., Cathcart, E.S., and Cohen, A.S.: Gonococcal Arthritis. Arthritis Rheum. **17**:503, 1974.
9. Brook, I., Reza, M.J., Bricknell, K.S., Bluestone, R., and Finegold, S.M.: Abnormalities in Synovial Fluid of Patients with Septic Arthritis Detected by Gas Liquid Chromatography. Ann. Rheum. Dis. **39**:168, 1980.
10. Brosseau, J.D., and Mazza, J.J.: Group A Streptococcal Sepsis and Arthritis. Origin from an Intra-uterine Device. J.A.M.A. **238**:2178, 1977.
11. Buchholz, H.W., Elson, R.A., Engelbrecht, E., Lodenkamper, H., Rottger, J., and Siegel, A.: Management of Deep Infection of Total Hip Replacement. J. Bone Joint Surg. **63-B**:342, 1981.
12. Compere, E.L., Metyger, W.I., and Mitra, R.N.: The Treatment of Pyogenic Bone and Joint Infections by Closed Irrigation (Circulation) with a Non-toxic Detergent and One or More Antibiotics. J. Bone Joint Surg. **49-A**:614, 1967.
13. Cook, C.L., Owen, D.S., Jr., Irby, R., and Toone, E.: Gonococcal Arthritis. J.A.M.A. **217**:204, 1971.
14. Curtiss, P.H., Jr., and Klein, L.: Destruction of Articular Cartilage in Septic Arthritis. I. *In Vitro* Studies. J. Bone Joint Surg. **45-A**:797, 1963.
15. Curtiss, P.H., Jr., and Klein, L.: Destruction of Articular Cartilage in Septic Arthritis. II. *In Vivo* Studies. J. Bone Joint Surg. **47-A**:1595, 1965.
16. Ebong, W.W.: The Treatment of Severely Ill Patients with Sickle Cell Anemia and Associated Arthritis. Clin. Orthop. **149**:145, 1980.
17. Reference deleted.
18. Eyre–Brook, A.L.: Septic Arthritis of the Hip and Osteomyelitis of the Upper End of the Femur in Infants. J. Bone Joint Surg. **42-B**:11, 1960.
19. Fitzgerald, R.H., Nolan, D.R., Ilstrup, D.M., et al: Deep Wound Sepsis Following Total Hip Arthroplasty. J. Bone Joint Surg. **59-A**:847, 1977.
20. Gainor, B.J.: Instillation of Continuous Tube Irrigation of the Septic Knee at Arthroscopy: A Technique. Clin. Orthop. **183**:96, 1984.
21. Garcia–Kutzbach, A., and Masai, A.T.: Acute Infectious Agent Arthritis (IAA): A Detailed Comparison of Proved Gonococcal and Other Blood-Borne Bacterial Arthritis. J. Rheumatol. **1**:13, 1974.
22. Gerard, Y., Lamarque, B., Segal, P.H., Bedoucha, J.S., and Schernberg, F.: La Place de la Synovectomie dans le Traitement des Arthrites Aigues a Pyogenes. Rev. Rhum. Mal. Osteoartic. **44**:741, 1977.
23. Goldenberg, D.L., and Cohen, A.S.: Acute Infectious Arthritis: A Review of Patients With Non-gonococcal Joint Infections (With Emphasis on Therapy and Prognosis). Am. J. Med. **60**:369, 1976.
24. Goldenberg, D.L., Brandt, K.D., Cohen, A.S., and Cathcart, E.S.: Treatment of Septic Arthritis. Comparison of Needle Aspiration and Surgery as Initial Modes of Joint Drainage. Arthritis Rheum. **18**:83, 1975.
25. Goldenberg, D.L., Brandt, K.D., Cathcart, E.S., and Cohen, A.S.: Acute Arthritis Caused by Gram-negative Bacilli: A Clinical Characterization. Medicine **53**:197, 1974.
26. Goldenberg, D.L., and Cohen, A.S.: Synovial Membrane Histopathology in the Differential Diagnosis of Rheumatoid Arthritis,

Gout, Pseudogout, Systemic Lupus Erythematosus, Infectious Arthritis and Degenerative Joint Disease. Medicine 57:239, 1978.

27. Goldenberg, D.L., and Reed, J.J.: Bacterial Arthritis. N. Engl. J. Med. 312:764, 1985.

28. Good, A.E., Hague, A.M., and Kauffman, C.A.: Streptococcal Endocarditis Initially Seen as Septic Arthritis. Arch. Int. Med. 138:805, 1978.

29. Greene, J.B., Sidhu, G.S., Lewin, S., Levine, J.F., Masur, H., Simberkoff, M.S., et al: Mycobacterium Avium-intracellulare: A Cause of Disseminated Life-threatening Infection in Homosexuals and Drug Abusers. Ann. Intern. Med. 97:539, 1982.

30. Griffin, P.P.: Bone and Joint Infections in Children. Pediatr. Clin. North Am. 14:533, 1967.

31. Griffin, P.P.: Septic Arthritis in Children. Orthopedic Surgery Update Series. Princeton, C.P.E.C., 1982.

32. Gristina, A.G., Rovere, G.D., and Shoji, H.: Spontaneous Septic Arthritis Complicating Rheumatoid Arthritis. J. Bone Joint Surg. 56-A:1180, 1974.

33. Hadler, N.M., and Granovetter, D.A.: Phlogistic Properties of Bacterial Debris. Semin. Arthritis Rheum. 8:1, 1978.

34. Ho, G., Jr., and Su, E.Y.: Therapy for Septic Arthritis. J.A.M.A. 247:797, 1982.

35. Ho, G., Jr., Toder, J.S., and Zimmermann, B.: An Overview of Septic Arthritis and Septic Bursitis. Orthopaedics 7:1571, 1984.

36. Hoffman, G.S.: Mycobacterial and Fungal Infections of Bones and Joints. In Kelley, W.N., Harris, E.D., Ruddy, S., and Sledge, C.B. (eds.): Textbook of Rheumatology. Philadelphia, W.B. Saunders, 1985.

37. Holmes, K.K., Counts, G.W., and Beaty, H.N.: Disseminated Gonococcal Infection. Ann. Intern. Med. 74:979, 1971.

38. Hunter, G.A.: The Results of Reinsertion of a Total Hip Prosthesis After Sepsis. J. Bone Joint Surg. 61-B:422, 1979.

39. Hunter, G.A., and Dandy, D.: The Natural History of the Patient with an Infected Total Hip Replacement. J. Bone Joint Surg. 59-B:293, 1977.

40. Ivey, M., and Clark, R.: Arthroscopic Debridement of the Knee for Septic Arthritis. Clin. Orthop. 199:201, 1985.

41. Infectious arthritis. In Rodman, G.P., and Schumacher, R.H. (eds.): Primer on the Rheumatic Diseases, 8th ed. Atlanta, Arthritis Foundation, 1983.

42. Jackson, R.W., and Parsons, C.J.: Distention Irrigation Treatment of Major Joint Sepsis. Clin. Orthop. 96:160, 1974.

43. Johnson, R.G., Herbert, M.A., Wright, S., Offierski, C., Kellam, J., Goodman, S.B., and Bobechko, W.P.: The Response of Articular Cartilage to the In Vitro Replacement of Synovial Fluid with Saline. Clin. Orthop. 174:285, 1983.

44. Keiser, H., Ruben, F.L., Wolinsky, E., and Kushner, I.: Clinical Forms of Gonococcal Arthritis. N. Engl. J. Med. 279:234, 1968.

45. Kelly, P.J.: Bacterial Arthritis in the Adult. Orthop. Clin. North Am. 6:973, 1975.

46. Kluge, R., Schmidt, M., and Barth, W.F.: Pneumococcal Arthritis. Ann. Rheum. Dis. 32:21, 1973.

47. Lewis, M.S., and Norman, A.: The Earliest Signs of Postoperative Hip Infection. Radiology 104:309, 1972.

48. Lisbona, R., and Rosenthal, L.: Observations on the Sequential Use of 99m Tc-Phosphate Complex and 67Ga Imaging in Osteomyelitis, Cellulitis, and Septic Arthritis. Radiology 123:123, 1977.

49. Lloveras, J., Peterson, P.K., Simmons, R.L., and Najarian, J.S.: Mycobacterial Infections in Renal Transplant Recipients: Seven Cases and a Review of the Literature. Arch. Intern. Med. 142:888, 1982.

50. Lloyd–Roberts, G.C.: Septic Arthritis in Infancy. Int. Orthop. (SICOT) 2:97, 1978.

51. Lunseth, P.A., and Heiple, K.G.: Prognosis in Septic Arthritis of the Hip in Children. Clin. Orthop. 139:81, 1979.

52. Magee, C., Rodeheaver, G.T., Golden, G.T., Fox, J., Edgerton,

M.T., and Edlich, R.F.: Potentiation of Wound Infection by Surgical Drains. Am. J. Surg. 131:547, 1976.

53. Martin, J.R., Root, H.S., Kim, S.O., and Johnson, L.G.: Staphylococcus Suppurative Arthritis Occurring in Neuropathic Knee Joints: A Report of Four Cases with a Discussion of the Mechanisms Involved. Arthritis Rheum. 8:389, 1965.

54. Master, R., Weisman, M.H., Armbuster, T.G., Slivka, J., Resnick, D., and Georgen, T.G.: Septic Arthritis of the Glenohumeral Joint. Arthritis Rheum. 20:1500, 1977.

55. McConville, J.H., Pototsky, R.S., Calia, F.M., and Pachas, W.N.: Septic and Crystalline Joint Disease. J.A.M.A. 231:841, 1975.

56. Meredith, H.C., and Rittenberg, G.M.: Pneumoarthropathy: An Unusual Radiographic Sign of Gram-negative Septic Arthritis. Radiology 128:642, 1978.

57. Mills, L.C., Boylston, B.F., Green, J.A., and Mayer, J.H.: Septic Arthritis as a Complication of Orally Given Steroid Therapy. J.A.M.A. 164:1310, 1957.

58. Morgan, G.J., Jr., Schlegelmilch, J.G., and Spiegel, P.K.: Early Diagnosis of Septic Arthritis of the Sacroiliac Joint by the Use of Computed Tomography. J. Rheumatol. 8:979, 1981.

59. Morrissy, R.T.: Joint Sepsis in the Pediatric Patient: Prevention and Management of Sepsis in Orthopaedic Surgery. Lecture, San Francisco. Aug. 17, 1985. Unpublished Data.

60. Mowat, A.G., and Baum, J.: Chemotaxis of Polymorphonuclear Leukocytes from Patients with Rheumatoid Arthritis. J. Clin. Invest. 50:2541, 1971.

61. Myers, A.R.: Septic Arthritis Caused by Bacteria. In Kelley, W.N., Harris, E.D., Ruddy, S., and Sledge, C.B. (eds.): Textbook of Rheumatology. Philadelphia, W.B. Saunders, 1985.

62. Myers, A.R., Miller, L.M., and Pinals, R.S.: Pyarthrosis Complicating Rheumatoid Arthritis. Lancet 2:714, 1969.

63. Nade, S.: Acute Septic Arthritis in Infancy and Childhood. J. Bone Joint Surg. 65-B:234, 1983.

64. Nelson, J.D.: Antibiotic Concentrations in Septic Joint Effusion. N. Engl. J. Med. 284:349, 1971.

65. Newman, J.H.: Review of Septic Arthritis Throughout the Antibiotic Era. Ann. Rheum. Dis. 35:198, 1976.

66. O'Brien, J.P., Goldenberg, D.L., and Rice, P.A.: Disseminated Gonococcal Infection: A Prospective Analysis of 49 Patients and a Review of Pathophysiology and Immune Mechanisms. Medicine 62:395, 1983.

67. Owen, D.S., Jr.: Aspiration and Injection of Joints and Soft Tissues. In Kelley, W.N., Harris, E.D., Ruddy, S., and Sledge, C.B. (eds.): Textbook of Rheumatology. Philadelphia, W.B. Saunders, 1985.

68. Palmer, D.W.: Septic Arthritis in Sickle-cell Thalassemia: Pathophysiology of Impaired Response to Infection. Arthritis Rheum. 18:339, 1976.

69. Paterson, D.C.: Acute Suppurative Arthritis in Infancy and Childhood. J. Bone Joint Surg. 52-B:474, 1970.

70. Petty, R.W.: The Effect of Methylmethacrylate on Chemotaxis of Polymorphonuclear Leukocytes. J. Bone Joint Surg. 60-A:492, 1978.

71. Petty, W.: The Effect of Methylmethacrylate on Bacterial Phagocytosis and Killing by Human Polymorphonuculear Leukocytes. J. Bone Joint Surg. 60-A:752, 1978.

72. Petty, W., Spanier, S., Shuster, J.J., and Silverthorne, C.: The Influence of Skeletal Implants on Incidence of Infection. J. Bone Joint Surg. 67-A:1236, 1985.

73. Polin, R.A., and Kennett, R.: Use of Monoclonal Antibodies in an Enzyme-linked Inhibition Assay for Rapid Detection of Streptococcal Antigen. J. Pediatr. 97:540, 1980.

74. Pryzanski, W., Leers, W.D., and Wardlow, A.C.: Bacteriolytic and Bactericidal Activity of Sera and Synovial Fluid in Rheumatoid Arthritis and Osteoarthritis. Arthritis Rheum. 17:207, 1974.

75. Quie, P.G., and Mills, E.L.: Microbial-phagocytic Interactions. Clin. Rheum. Dis. **4**:15, 1978.

76. Quismorio, F.P., and Dubois, E.L.: Septic Arthritis in Systemic Lupus Erythematosus. J. Rheumatol. **2**:73, 1975.

77. Rand, J.A., Morrey, B.F., and Bryan, R.S.: Management of the Infected Total Joint Arthroplasty. Orthop. Clin. North Am. **15**:491, 1984.

78. Rinaldi, R.Z., Harrison, W.O., and Fan, P.T.: Penicillin-resistant Gonococcal Arthritis. Ann. Intern. Med. **97**:43, 1982.

79. Roce, R.P., and Yoshikawa, T.T.: Primary Skeletal Infections in Heroin Users: A Clinical Characterization, Diagnosis and Therapy. Clin. Orthop. **144**:238, 1979.

79a.Rodman G.P., Schumacher M.R.: Primer on the Rheumatic Diseases 8th Ed. Atlanta, Arthritis Foundation, 1983, pp 187–188.

80. Rosenthal, J., Bole, G.G., and Robinson, W.D.: Acute Non-gonococcal Infectious Arthritis: Evaluation of Risk Factors, Therapy and Outcome. Arthritis Rheum. **23**:889, 1980.

81. Rosenthal, L., and Hawkins, D.: Radionuclide Joint Imaging in the Diagnosis of Synovial Disease. Semin. Arthritis Rheum. **7**:49, 1977.

82. Rytel, M.W.: Microbial Antigen Detection in Infectious Arthritis. Clin. Rheum. Dis. **4**:83, 1978.

83. Salter, R.B., Bell, R.S., and Keeley, F.W.: The Protective Effect of Continuous Passive Motion on Living Articular Cartilage in Acute Septic Arthritis: An Experimental Investigation in the Rabbit. Clin. Orthop. **159**:223, 1981.

84. Schnitzer, T.J.: Viral Arthritis. *In* Kelley, W.N., Harris, E.D., Ruddy, S., and Sledge, C.B. (eds.): Textbook of Rheumatology. Philadelphia, W.B. Saunders, 1985.

85. Schumacher, R.H.: Synovial Fluid Analysis. *In* Kelley, W.N., Harris, E.D., Ruddy, S., and Sledge, C.B. (eds.): Textbook of Rheumatology. Philadelphia, W.B. Saunders, 1985.

86. Schurman, D.J., Burton, D.S., and Kajiyama, G.: Cefoxitin Antibiotic Concerntration in Bone and Synovial Fluid. Clin. Orthop. **168**:64, 1982.

87. Schurman, D.J., Hirshman, H.P., and Burton, D.S.: Cephalothin and Cefamandole Penetration Into Bone, Synovial Fluid, and Wound Drainage. J. Bone Joint Surg. **62-A**:1981, 1980.

88. Schurman, D.J., Hirshman, H.P., Kajiyama, G., Moser, K., and Burton, D.S.: Cefazolin Concentration in Bone and Synovial Fluid. J. Bone Joint Surg. **60-A**:359, 1978.

89. Schurman, D.J., and Kajiyama, G.: Antibiotic Absorption from Infected and Normal Joints Using a Rabbit Knee Joint Model. J. Orthop. Res. **3**:185, 1985.

90. Schurman, D.J., Kajiyama, G., and Nagel, D.A.: *Escherichia coli* Infections in Rabbit Knee Joints. J. Bone Joint Surg. **62-A**:620, 1980.

91. Schurman, D.J., Mirra, J., Ding, A., and Nagel, D.A.: Experimental *E. Coli* Arthritis in the Rabbit: A Model of Infectious and Post-Infectious Inflammatory Synovitis. J. Rheumatol. **4**:118, 1977.

92. Schurman, D.J., and Wheeler, R.: Gram-negative Bone and Joint Infections. Clin. Orthop. **134**:268, 1978.

93. Schurman, D.J., and Woolson, S.T.: Prophylactic Antibiotics in Orthopaedic Surgery. Orthopaedics **7**:1603, 1984.

94. Sharrard, W.J.W.: Paediatric Orthopaedics and Fractures. Edinburgh, Blackwell Scientific Publications, 1971.

95. Smith, R.L., Merchant, T.C., and Schurman, D.J.: *In Vitro* Cartilage Degradation by *Escherichia coli* and *Staphylococcus aureus.* Arthritis Rheum. **25**:441, 1982.

96. Spink, W.W., and Keefer, C.S.: Diagnosis, Treatment and End Results in Gonococcal Arthritis: Study of Seventy Cases. N. Engl. J. Med. **218**:453, 1938.

97. Stedman's Medical Dictionary, 25th Edition. Baltimore, U.S.A. The Williams and Wilkins Co., 1972, p. 1048.

98. Tarholm, C., Hedstrom, S., Sunden, G., and Lidgren, L.: Synovectomy in Bacterial Arthritis. Acta. Orthop. Scand. **54**:748, 1983.

99. Tesar, J.T., and Dietz, F.: Mechanisms of Inflammation in Infectious Arthritis. Clin. Rheum. Dis. **4**:51, 1978.

100. Turner, R.A., Schumacher, H.R., and Myers, A.R.: Phagocytic Function of Polymorphonuclear Leukocytes in Rheumatic Diseases. J. Clin. Invest. **52**:1632, 1973.

101. Waugh, T.R., and Stinchfield, F.E.: Suction Drainage of Orthopaedic Wounds. J. Bone Joint Surg. **43-A**:939, 1961.

102. Williams, C.: Treatment of Purulent Arthritis by Wide Arthrotomy Followed by Immediate Active Mobilization. Surg. Gynecol. Obstet. **28**:546, 1919.

103. Willkens, R.F., Healey, L.A., and Decker, J.L.: Acute Infectious Arthritis in the Aged and Chronically Ill. Arch. Int. Med. **106**:354, 1960.

104. Ziff, M., Gribetz, H.J., and Lospalluto, J.: Effect of Leukocyte and Synovial Membrane Extracts on Cartilage Mucoprotein. J. Clin. Invest. **39**:405, 1960.

CHAPTER 67

Management of Tuberculosis and Other Granulomatous Infections

TAYLOR KING SMITH

Infectious disease of the skeletal system caused by tuberculosis and other granuloma-forming organisms is considered in this chapter. Granulomatous diseases of the spine are covered in Chapter 162.

TUBERCULOSIS

The causative organism of tuberculosis, *Mycobacterium tuberculosis,* was first identified by Koch in 1882, although the disease has been found in the skeletons of mummies dating from 3400 BC. Indo-Aryan Sanskrit medical records written between 1500 and 700 BC. describe tuberculosis and recommend treatment with diet, rest, and high altitude. Although Aristotle and Galen recognized the contagious nature of tuberculosis, it was not until Koch's discovery that control of the disease began with the use of sanitoria and other public health measures.[26]

Mycobacterium tuberculosis is usually spread by the inhalation of infected, airborne droplets produced by coughing. The primary site of implantation is usually the lung, and 90% of active tuberculosis is pulmonary. From the lung, the disease may spread through lymphatic channels to regional lymph nodes and through the bloodstream to more distant sites. The mobilization of local and systemic immune defense mechanisms may lead to spontaneous healing. However, the disease may subsequently reactivate whenever the host defenses are compromised.

At the beginning of the 20th century, tuberculosis was the leading cause of death in the Western World. Treatment then consisted of rest, diet, sunshine, and limited surgical measures. Even before the discovery of effective chemotherapeutic agents, the mortality rate from tuberculosis was decreasing because of improvements in socioeconomic conditions. At present, 5% to 10% of those who develop tuberculosis die as a result, even though the medical community considers the disease a preventable and curable infection.

Thoracoplasties, drainage of empyemas, lung resections, abscess and joint drainage, and joint arthrodeses were the operative measures used prior to the advent of chemotherapy. Drainage of joints frequently led to secondary infections with pyogenic organisms, resulting in bony ankylosis. It was noted that quiescence of the disease in the skeletal system frequently resulted from these fortuitous ankyloses. Surgical procedures were then devised to arthrodese tuberculous joints, frequently extra-articularly.

In 1944, Schatz and Waksman discovered dihydrostreptomycin, the first truly antituberculous agent.[46] *p*-Aminosalicylic acid and isoniazid were soon discovered, and combinations of these and other drugs became the mainstay of the chemotherapeutic attack on tuberculosis. As more effective and better tolerated drugs were introduced, the ambulatory treatment of tuberculosis became possible, although long-term treatment is still essential.

There were 22,201 cases of tuberculosis reported in the United States in 1985.[15] Worldwide, almost 30 million people have tuberculosis, with 1% to 3% of these having skeletal tuberculosis. Pulmonary tuberculosis has been on the decline in this century, with a corresponding increase in the percentage of extrapulmonary tuberculosis, of which 8.8% is bone and joint tuberculosis, from 7.8% of total cases in 1964 to 16.2% in

1984. The incidence of tuberculosis in the population of the United States fell steadily until recently, when an increase in cases was noted for the first time, mainly in persons with histories of intravenous drug abuse, those having systemic or local immunosuppression as treatment for another disease, and those with acquired immune deficiency syndrome (AIDS).[15,49] Of importance here is the fact that patients with immune deficiency and tuberculosis usually have false-negative results of skin tests.[43] Although the magnitude of the tuberculosis problem in the United States and other well-developed countries has decreased, tuberculosis remains a major cause of morbidity and mortality worldwide. Pockets of tuberculosis persist in this country among the impoverished, recent immigrants, and some groups of Native American Indians. In talking with orthopaedists in major medical centers in the United States, one hears that tuberculosis of the musculoskeletal system is not noted much anymore, but often the orthopaedist just happens to have one or two active cases under treatment at that time. More and more, there are reports of cases of tuberculosis of the musculoskeletal system that went undiagnosed for long periods of time or that were unsuspected but diagnosed by fortuitous biopsy or culture. Suspicion that the disease is present is essential to making an early and definitive diagnosis.

Pathology

Bone and joint tuberculosis results when blood-borne tubercle bacilli lodge in the bone or synovium and form a focus of inflammation.[55] The body reacts to this invasion by forming a granuloma in an attempt to seal off the infection. If the host defense is inadequate, however, the tuberculous infection propagates. Macrophages and monocytes are mobilized and attracted to the inflammation by the lipid that is present in the bacterial cell walls. These white blood cells phagocytize the tubercle bacilli, and the lipid is deposited throughout the cytoplasm of the mononuclear cells, thus turning them into epithelioid cells, which are characteristic of tuberculosis. Langhans' giant cells are formed by the fusing of epithelioid cells. This occurs in the presence of caseous necrosis, and these giant cells serve to phagocytize necrotic tissue and tubercle bacilli. Lymphocytes encircle the mononuclear reactive site, and this forms the typical tubercle, or nodule of inflammation, first described by Laennec, a half-century before Koch identified the tuberculosis organism. Caseation, or central necrosis, occurs, and a large amount of exudate is formed. Bone in the vicinity is rendered necrotic when the granulation tissue interferes with its blood supply, and the sequestrae that are formed become part of the cold abscess that develops. Infections of joints occur by hematogenous spread of the bacteria to the synovium or by direct extension of a focus of osteomyelitis into the joint. The hip, for instance, is frequently infected when tuberculous osteomyelitis in the neck of the femur erodes into the joint.

Synovial reaction causes a pannus to develop, and this may grow over the articular cartilage, depriving it of synovial fluid nutrition and causing it to become necrotic. Where pannus is prevented from developing by articular surfaces being in contact there is preservation of cartilage, but if the subchondral bone is rendered necrotic by the ingrowth of granulation tissue into the subchondral area, "kissing sequestrae" will develop.

These are contiguous sequestrated pieces of preserved cartilage and subchondral bone, which are occasionally seen in tuberculous joints.

Mycobacterium tuberculosis does not form proteolytic enzymes; thus cartilage is not destroyed primarily by the infection, only secondarily by the destruction of its nutritional source by the formation of a pannus. It is not unusual to find large fragments of cartilage and sequestered subchondral bone lying free in a tuberculous joint.

The tuberculous abscess in some instances becomes controlled by the host defenses, in which case, it may fibrose, involute, calcify, and in some cases cause ankylosis of the joint. In some cases, a low-grade chronic state of activity persists, and in some the abscess may spread locally or systemically in the bloodstream. A sinus may spontaneously or iatrogenically develop, evacuating much of the pus and allowing secondary infection by other organisms to develop. Fortunately, this may cause an ankylosis of the joint, often rendering the tuberculous process quiescent.

The introduction of effective antibiotics at any stage of the disease will usually bring the disease under control. Total eradication of the tubercle bacilli, however, is frequently not possible, since the bacteria may be walled off from the antibiotic by fibrosis and necrotic tissue. A decline in host resistance, or an injury, such as a reconstructive surgical procedure, may reactivate the disease at any time, in spite of the patient having received what was considered to be a curative dose of antibiotics. With this in mind, it is suggested that any time a patient with quiescent bone or joint tuberculosis is rendered immunoincompetent or has a surgical procedure on the diseased area, an adequate course of antituberculous medications should be given to prevent reactivation of the disease.

Bone and joint tuberculosis is most frequently located in the spine. Of 980 cases reported by Tuli,[51] 440 cases were spinal, 89 located in the knee, 81 in the hip, 69 in the sacroiliac joint, 51 in the elbow, 44 in the metatarsals and phalanges, 43 in the ankle, and the rest spread throughout the remainder of the skeletal system. Eighty-seven of Tuli's patients had widely disseminated skeletal tuberculosis. Other sites frequently involved are bursae, especially the greater trochanteric bursa of the hip, and the tenosynovium, especially on the dorsum of the wrist.

Clinical Features

Patients will frequently present with long histories of mild bone or joint pain. They may have noted an effusion or a swelling over an extremity, and this usually is not inflamed, warm, or erythematous. Muscle spasms are frequently severe. There may be systemic complaints of weight loss or night sweats. One should inquire as to signs or symptoms of other possible sites of tuberculosis, such as cough, back pain, or blood in the urine.

On physical examination, there may be a cold abscess or a doughy effusion of a joint or a sinus tract may be present. There may be a generalized thickening of a bursa, or tenosynovium, with little inflammatory response. In the later stages of the disease, ankylosis, joint contractures, and joint destruction, with limb shortening and deformity, may all occur. If the disease damages the growth centers in a child, then shortening or angulation of an extremity may result. One should search for old, healed sinus tract scars. They are often found remote from the site of the infection and may indicate the presence of pyogenic organisms complicating the picture.[9]

Laboratory and Radiographic Findings

The only definitive test to document a tuberculous infection is isolation of the tubercle bacillus from the patient. Joint fluid, tissue, sequestrae, and sinus tract drainage from skeletal infections may yield the organism. It may be seen on direct smear with special stains that take into consideration the organism's ability to resist decolorization by an acid–alcohol mixture, thus giving it its acid-fast properties. Culturing of tissues and fluids must be done on special media, and a serious search for the acid-fast bacilli is facilitated by dialogue with the pathologist. Other sources for possibly obtaining positive smears or cultures are sputum, gastric washings, cerebrospinal fluid, urine, and pleural effusions. Attempts to obtain culture material must be made before antituberculous chemotherapy is instituted, if at all possible. It is, however, possible to isolate the organism from abscesses and sequestrae even after the patient has been on antituberculous medication for some period of time. Repeat cultures and sensitivities of persistent sinuses or infected sites may reveal an emergent strain of bacteria that is resistant to the antibiotics that the patient is receiving. All attempts at culturing materials should include studies for pyogenic organisms, atypical mycobacteria, and fungal organisms. Although mycobacterial growth may not be detected on culture media for several weeks, once the material has been obtained for culture, if a high suspicion of tuberculous infection exists, antibiotic therapy should be started.[5]

Tissue biopsy may reveal organisms by culture or by direct examination of tubercles with stains for acid-fast bacteria. If a possible tuberculous infection is encountered at surgery, a frozen section may reveal the typical caseating tubercles and a presumptive diagnosis can be established that might alter the surgical procedure.

Although synovial fluid cultures will be positive in almost 80% of cases of tuberculosis of the joints, open synovial biopsy will be positive in over 90% of the cases.[52] For this reason, synovial biopsy is an excellent method of establishing the diagnosis of tuberculous arthritis. Needle aspiration for synovial biopsy has been believed by some to yield too small a specimen, and it has the fault of perhaps being taken from the wrong location[45] in the joint to be of optimal benefit. To obviate this, open biopsy is advocated by some authors. At the time of open biopsy, a limited synovectomy, or pannus removal, may be done as part of the therapeutic measures.

Joint fluid analysis in tuberculous arthritis will reveal elevated protein levels, a poor mucin clot, and low sugar content of the joint fluid. Ten thousand to 20,000 white blood cells per cubic millimeter may be seen, and these are predominantly polymorphonuclear leukocytes. About 20% of the smears of synovial fluid in active tuberculous arthritis will yield acid-fast bacilli on staining the material with special tuberculous stains.[52]

A complete blood cell count may reveal mild anemia and a slight elevation in the white blood cell count. The sedimentation rate may be elevated or it may be normal. The sedimentation rate, if elevated, is one of the few methods available to plot the course of the disease. Repeat sedimentation rates throughout the treatment should show a return to normal if control of the disease is being obtained.

Blood chemistries should be obtained to document liver function if potentially liver-toxic agents are to be used for treatment of the disease. The total albumin level, taken into consideration with the total lymphocyte count, will give a rough estimate of the patient's nutritional status since it may affect the immune system and perhaps will give some indication as to whether nutritional supplementation or total parenteral nutrition would be indicated.

Urinalysis and urine cultures for acid-fast bacilli may indicate the genitourinary tract as a source of infection. If the patient is going to be placed on streptomycin, then baseline audiograms should be obtained. They should also be obtained on any patient coming under care who has previously had streptomycin, since eighth nerve toxicity is a common complication of streptomycin treatment.

Skin tests, using purified protein derivatives, are becoming even more helpful in the diagnosis of tuberculosis. In the past, when most of the population was exposed to tuberculosis at one time or another, the frequency of positive skin tests lowered the usefulness of this test. Presently, however, in many Western countries, few people under the age of 50 have been exposed to tuberculosis, and if a positive skin test is obtained, this is a valuable piece of information. A patient with a documented negative skin test who converts to a positive skin test will be presumed to have had an exposure to tuberculosis and may require prophylactic treatment even though asymptomatic. One should not start off with an intermediate or full-strength skin test if tuberculosis is highly suspected because of the possibly markedly positive reaction to the skin test. If the weakest strength is negative, then an intermediate skin test can be performed, without fear of a skin slough. In many countries, bacillus Calmette-Guérin (BCG) vaccine has been given routinely as prophylaxis for tuberculosis, and patients receiving this vaccine will exhibit a positive skin test. A negative skin test may be present in the presence of active tuberculous infection if the patient's immune system is depressed from the disease or if they have immune deficiency, such as noted in AIDS.

Radioisotope bone scans, using technetium 99m or gallium citrate 67, may be helpful, but a large number of false-negative studies have been obtained. This is probably related to the low blood flow found in the bone and surrounding tissues of some patients with tuberculous infections. In general, radioisotope studies are not particularly helpful in the workup of a patient with possible tuberculosis of the osteoarticular system.

Plain films of patients with tuberculosis of the skeletal system and joints reveal multiple nonspecific findings. In general, osteopenia is usually seen in areas surrounding tuberculosis in the skeleton. The lesion in bone may reveal a lytic focus, or cavity, surrounded by a mild to moderate amount of reactive sclerosis (Fig. 67-1). The cavity may contain a sequestrum of cancellous bone, the "image en Grelot."[36] Periosteal new bone formation may be quite marked, especially if there has been a superinfection with pyogenic organisms. The typical tuberculous dactylitis finding of spina ventosa, which is a spindle-shaped deformity of the involved phalanx or metacarpal by periosteal new bone formation, is seen frequently in young

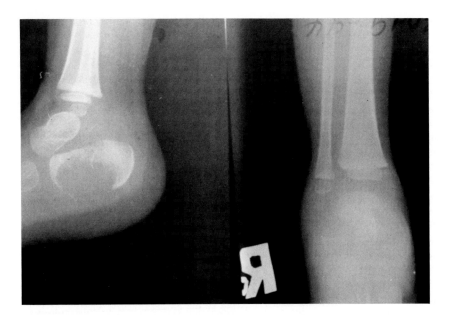

FIGURE 67-1. Tuberculous osteomyelitis of the calcaneus.

patients.[40] Soft tissue swelling, with loss of tissue plane definition, and joint effusions may be evident when there is joint involvement. One should search for a primary focus in the bone adjacent to the joint, since frequently the disease spreads from the metaphysis or epiphysis into the joint by direct extension. There may also be calcification in the bursae, especially over the greater trochanteric area.[13] This represents involution of the abscess, with inspissation and calcification taking place as an attempt to heal the process.

Sinograms and tomograms may be helpful in further defining the extent of disease, and perhaps in discovering sequestrae. Computed tomography (CT scanning) may also further elucidate the extent of disease. The disease almost invariably is more extensive than is seen on the plain radiographs.

Intravenous pyelography, chest films with apical views, and other special studies are ordered as indicated. All patients with osteoarticular tuberculosis should have chest radiographs.

Antituberculous Chemotherapy

The main treatment for tuberculosis is the use of effective antituberculous medication.[50] It has been established that two, and sometimes three, forms of antibiotics are more effective than a single antibiotic to eradicate a tuberculous infection and to prevent the emergence of resistant strains of bacteria. The appropriate antibiotic should be selected by examining the sensitivity to various agents of the obtained organism. The more poorly tolerated triple therapy of streptomycin, isoniazid, and p-aminosalicylic acid has given way now to the use of rifampin, isoniazid, and ethambutol. There are numerous second-line drugs available also, and all these medications have significant advantages and disadvantages that must be taken into consideration before selecting the drugs of treatment for each patient. Failure to respond promptly to what is thought to be adequate antibiotics may indicate the need for a switch in drugs to eradicate resistant strains that have developed. Secondary infection with pyogenic organisms must be considered, especially if si-

nuses have been present, and appropriate antibiotics for these infections must be given. Possibly noncompliant patients, such as alcoholics, may require unusual public health measures to ensure that their medications are taken as prescribed.

As mentioned previously, antibiotics should not be begun until all measures to obtain culture material have been exhausted. Antibiotic coverage prior to surgery has been advocated by some, but if appropriate antibiotics are given following the surgical procedure, they will prevent the spread of the disease and should bring the disease under control rapidly. If diagnosis has not been firmly established, then it is preferred that antibiotics be delayed until after surgery, at which time an empiric choice of antibiotics is used until material obtained in surgery can be analyzed for sensitivities.

Surgery in Osteoarticular Tuberculosis

General Principles

Although effective antibiotics are available for the treatment of tuberculosis, surgery still plays an important role in the diagnosis, in the control of active infection, and in the reconstruction of bones and joints following eradication of the disease.[17] As a general rule, the amount of surgical removal of infected tissue should be kept at a bare minimum. The recuperative and restorative abilities of the skeletal system following eradication of tuberculosis by antibiotics are amazing. It is not unusual for seemingly destroyed bones and joints to recover satisfactory function with antibiotics alone, even when extensive destruction appears on x-ray films. Except for obviously infected synovium or tenosynovium, sequestrae, sinuses, and pockets of pus, debridement should be limited. Reliance on antibiotics, local measures such as immobilization in casts or braces, and general systemic support such as hyperalimentation should generally be the treatment for osteoarticular tuberculosis once the diagnosis is established. If, however, a large abscess is present or a joint is extensively involved with synovial proliferation and pannus formation, then surgery may be used as an adjunct to chemotherapy.

In the past, surgery for osteoarticular tuberculosis consisted of drainage of abscesses and joints and creation of arthrodeses, usually extra-articularly. Fusion of a major joint is rarely indicated as a primary mode of treatment now, and many of the operations described in the literature for the eradication of tuberculosis are no longer necessary. Reconstruction of joints following eradication of the tuberculous infection, however, is a field that is gaining acceptance. Osteotomies and soft-tissue releases to reposition joints destroyed by tuberculosis, late arthrodeses for functional stability, and prosthetic replacement of destroyed joints are all useful measures to reduce the morbidity of tuberculosis of the skeletal system. It should be remembered, however, that any time reconstructive surgery is undertaken in a joint previously treated for tuberculosis, prophylactic antibiotics must be given for an extended period of time, to prevent reactivation of the disease.

If a tuberculous focus is opened surgically, it should be closed without the use of drains. If a sinus is present prior to the operative procedure, then the sinus tract may be excised and the wound closed, followed by the institution of appropriate antibiotics, or the sinus tract may be excised and the wound packed open for a short period of time. Usually when the disease comes under control, the drainage will cease. It is quite gratifying to see how quickly the patient shows dramatic systemic improvement after a tuberculous abscess or joint infection is debrided. Defervescence, return of appetite, and weight gain, as well as a return of motivation and a sense of well-being, are often the rapid result of surgical extirpation of a tuberculous focus.

Tuberculous Osteomyelitis

Tuberculosis of the shafts of long bones is frequently seen in widely disseminated disease. Usually the presenting complaint is a sinus, abscess, local tenderness, or swelling. Delay in diagnosis is frequent. It is extremely important to diagnose and treat juxta-articular tuberculous osteomyelitis to prevent the development of tuberculous arthritis by direct extension of the disease.[36] Almost invariably the disease process responds to adequate antibiotic treatment. Unless tissue is needed for a diagnosis or a large abscess is present in the soft tissue surrounding the bone, treatment is usually limited to antibiotics and protection of the extremity until healing has occurred. Periosteal new bone formation can be quite profuse, especially in the growing child, and remodeling of the bone following the quiescence of the disease is frequent. A superinfection with pyogenic organisms may also elicit a profuse periosteal reaction. If biopsy is undertaken, either by the open method or by a core biopsy, care should be taken to protect the extremity from a pathologic fracture.

Rarely is surgical debridement of the small bones of the foot or hand required, even if a sinus is present.[38] Immobilization of the extremity in a cast and appropriate antibiotic treatment is usually all that is necessary. Even though there appears to be extensive destruction on the x-ray films following control of the disease, the bone will frequently reossify with quite dramatic reconstitution of the anatomy. Large cysts will fill in with bone

as healing takes place, and rarely is excision or bone grafting indicated.

Sternoclavicular Joint

A sinus overlying the anterior chest wall in the child is frequently the only hint that tuberculous involvement of the sternoclavicular joint is present. Once the diagnosis is established, the treatment is with the use of antibiotics. If drainage persists, and resistant bacteria are not present, a very limited curettage of the sinus tract and underlying joint may be necessary to clear up persistant drainage.

Shoulder

Tuberculous infection of the glenohumeral joint or the subdeltoid bursa may come from a focus in adjacent bone spilling into the joint, or from direct hematogenous seeding of the synovium. In most cases, pain is limited and of a dull, aching nature, with limitation of motion being a prominent feature. A doughy swelling in the shoulder region and marked atrophy around the shoulder are the findings most frequently seen in the acute stages.

Treatment, once diagnosis is established, is the use of appropriate antituberculous medication and immobilization. Martini and co-workers[37] advocate the use of a shoulder spica cast with the arm in abduction and external rotation to obviate the frequent sequelae of stiffness in adduction seen in tuberculosis of the shoulder. Immobilization should be limited to 3 or 4 weeks, followed by gentle physical therapy, to maintain the range of motion of the shoulder during resolution of the disease.

Surgery is rarely indicated in tuberculosis of the shoulder. Perhaps massive synovial reaction and joint destruction with sequestrae might call for a limited arthrotomy, synovectomy, and debridement, but usually rest and medication will result in a satisfactory outcome. Arthrodesis of the shoulder, once a mainstay in the control of tuberculosis of the glenohumeral joint, is now indicated only as a salvage procedure for disease that is under control but that has left an unstable or painful shoulder. Extra-articular arthrodesis is not indicated now that antituberculous medications are available. Instead we would prefer an intra-articular arthrodesis with the use of internal fixation and long-term coverage with antituberculous medication. In general, however, tuberculosis of the shoulder is usually best managed with antituberculous medication and immobilization.

Elbow

Tuberculosis of the elbow often is not painful in the early stages. Initially, limitation of motion in extension is seen, but later all motion is restricted by muscle spasm. Swelling of the joint and atrophy of musculature around the joint are seen. When viewed from behind, the elbow appears broad and there is fullness and thickening of the tissues on either side of the triceps tendon. In late untreated stages, the swelling may become extensive and multiple skin sinuses may appear. Tuberculous arthritis of the elbow may masquerade as a chronic olecranon bursitis.[24]

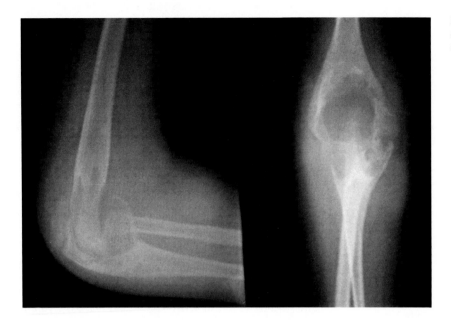

FIGURE 67-2. Tuberculosis of the elbow with extensive destruction and spontaneous fibrous ankylosis at 90° of flexion.

Tuberculosis of the elbow is treated by antituberculous medication and immobilization of the arm in a long-arm cast with the elbow at 90° and the forearm in neutral rotation. Once the pain has resolved, active and gentle passive motions are encouraged and the arm is maintained in a posterior shell at 90° between therapy sessions. If the elbow is allowed to remain in extension the arm may ankylose in extension, a very useless position. Spontaneous ankylosis (Fig. 67-2) frequently occurs in tuberculosis of the elbow, and it is difficult to prevent this occurrence.[37] Synovectomy, debridement, joint excision, and arthrodesis[3] are rarely indicated in the presence of adequate chemotherapy and immobilization.

Wrist and Hand[14]

Tuberculosis of the wrist usually presents as a swollen, slightly warm wrist joint. As destruction of the carpal bones progresses, more stiffness and deformity may occur and the wrist takes on a doughy appearance from synovial proliferation. In neglected cases the hand may be flexed 120° to 130° on the forearm and sinuses may be present. Frequently, as in tuberculosis of other joints, the diagnosis is not suspected until exploratory surgery is performed. In Algeria, where tuberculosis is frequently seen, in 27 cases reported by Benkeddache and Gottesman,[4] the average delay from onset of symptoms to diagnosis was 17½ months. Hodgson and Smith[23] believed that the carpal involvement was an extension of tuberculosis involving the synovium of the wrist primarily. The disease may also extend from or to the tenosynovium adjacent to the wrist joint.

In early cases before extensive synovial or bone involvement occurs, treatment is usually immobilization of the wrist in a position of function and use of antituberculous medication. The immobilization is continued for several weeks until the disease is under control and the pain improves. Then gentle, active range of motion and strengthening exercises are begun, but splinting is continued for several months to avoid deformity and further collapse. If the disease is quite extensive when first seen, synovectomy through a dorsal incision may be indicated. One should be very cautious, however, in the debridement of soft bone or cartilage, since often with adequate chemotherapy the carpal bones will repair themselves dramatically (Fig. 67-3). In most cases this conservative treatment will result in a painless, stable wrist that has an adequate range of motion (Fig. 67-4). If pain persists after the disease is under control, then surgery may be considered. If the pain can be localized to the distal radioulnar joint, then resection of the distal end of the ulna may be all that is required. If there is extensive carpal destruction, instability, and pain, then arthro-

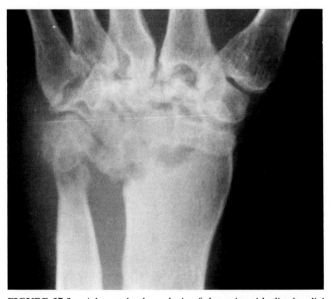

FIGURE 67-3. Advanced tuberculosis of the wrist with distal radial and ulnar and carpal destruction. The disease has been brought under control by antituberculous medication and synovectomy.

FIGURE 67-4. Tuberculosis of the wrist and fifth metacarpal. The wrist infection was an extension of a focus of disease in the radial metaphysis. This patient had multiple sites of osteoarticular tuberculosis and the metacarpal, radial, and wrist lesions healed with antibiotic therapy.

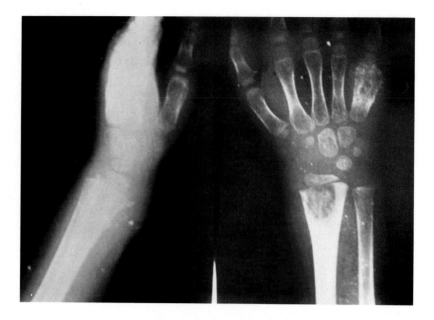

desis of the radius to the carpus and index and long metacarpals with resection of the distal ulna may be necessary.

Tuberculous Tenosynovitis

The most common area for tuberculous tenosynovitis to occur is the forearm, wrist, and hand, but the tendon sheaths about the ankle may also be involved.[20] The radial and ulnar bursae, flexor tendon sheaths of the fingers, and extensor tendon sheaths may all be involved. Both the parietal and visceral tenosynovium is replaced by tuberculous granulation tissue. Ingrowth of granulation tissue into the tendons in the later stages may result in attenuation and rupture of the tendon. Rice bodies or larger melon seed bodies are frequently seen within the swollen tenosynovium, and these represent aggregations of fibrin and cartilage debris.

Swelling is an invariable feature, but pain is rarely severe. Often in areas where tuberculosis is less commonly seen the diagnosis is not suspected prior to surgery.[31] Ganglia and rheumatoid tenosynovitis are frequently confused with tuberculous tenosynovitis.

As in any tuberculous focus, associated tuberculous disease should be sought. In Pimm and Waugh's series,[42] only 6 of 44 patients with tenosynovitis of the wrist had involvement of the wrist joint. Therefore, it seems likely that in most cases tuberculous tenosynovitis is a result of hematogenous spread of the bacillus to the synovium, rather than direct extension from a nearby tuberculous arthritis. Accidental direct inoculation of tubercle bacilli into tendon sheaths by surgeons, pathologists, dairy workers, and others has been the cause of tuberculous tenosynovitis in some cases.

Treatment of tuberculous tenosynovitis should consist of antituberculous medication and excision of the involved tendon sheaths and tenosynovium. Immobilization in a cast for a short period of time with the fingers free to move appears beneficial. If tuberculous tenosynovitis is inadvertently found, then treatment should consist of thorough debridement of the infected material, preservation of the retinaculum and pulleys, and administration of antituberculous medication.[8]

Tuberculous Dactylitis and Metacarpal Involvement

Tuberculosis of the fingers and metacarpals usually manifests itself as a rather painless swelling that is not warm or erythematous. Fistulas may be present in extensive, neglected cases. The radiographic appearance may be that of diffuse, spindle-shaped periostitis, "spina ventosa,"[40] a honeycombed appearance with cysts, sequestrae in cysts, or just bone atrophy. Restoration of bone stock following antituberculous medication is often quite dramatic (Fig. 67-5), but if the small joints of the hand or fingers have been destroyed before drug treatment is started, usually the deformity is permanent. Rarely is arthrodesis indicated, however. The usual treatment for metacarpal and finger involvement is splinting in the position of function and antituberculous medication.

Tuberculosis of the Sacroiliac Joint

Tuberculosis involving the sacroiliac joint is rare and is frequently seen with other foci of tuberculous disease. It rarely is a result of direct extension of a psoas abscess or lumbar spine involvement. The patient presents with pain and an antalgic gait leaning away from the involved side. On palpation over the sacroiliac joint there is pain and usually a mass is present. There may be limitation of motion of the hip with a hip flexion contracture, but this is not as severe as with tuberculosis involving the hip. Stressing the sacroiliac joint with forced *f*lexion, *ab*duction, and *e*xternal *r*otation of the hip (the FABER test) may elicit sacroiliac pain. Computed tomography is particularly helpful in delineating the extent of disease in the sacroiliac joint.

In the past, before antituberculous medication was available, drainage and fusion of the sacroiliac joint was considered

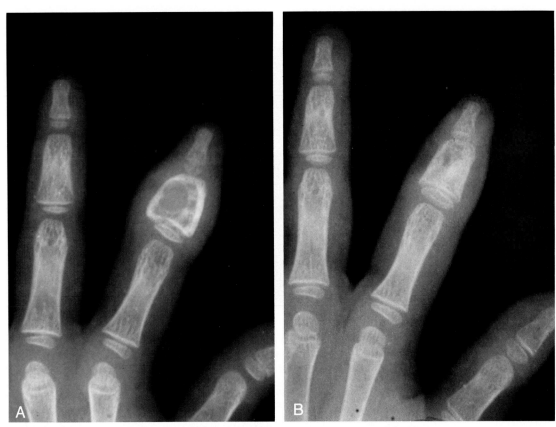

FIGURE 67-5.   Tuberculous dactylitis. (*A*) Appearance prior to antituberculous treatment. (*B*) Appearance following 6 months of antituberculous treatment.

necessary to bring the disease under control. In the growing child, bilateral sacroiliac fusion was considered necessary in unilateral disease to prevent severe pelvic distortion. Rarely now is surgery necessary, however, except to obtain a biopsy for confirmation of the diagnosis or for draining a large abscess extending from the sacroiliac joint. Before antituberculous medication became available there was a 33% mortality rate with sacroiliac joint tuberculosis. The mortality rate fell to 5% after introduction of antituberculous medication, according to Strange.[48]

The treatment of tuberculosis of the sacroiliac joint is antituberculous medication as previously described. Bed rest or crutches until the diseased area becomes less painful may be necessary, and a sacroiliac belt may give relief from pain in the more acute stages. Residual joint disruption after the disease is brought under control may require arthrodesis of the sacroiliac joint if conservative measures fail. This is best performed through a modification of the Smith-Peterson technique.

Technique of Sacroiliac Fusion.   Make a straight, slightly obliqued incision, 10 cm in length directly over the posterosuperior iliac spine. The cluneal nerves are avoided with this incision. Carry the incision down to the outer table of the ilium at the posterosuperior iliac spine, and subperiosteally reflect the gluteus maximus muscle off the outer table of the ilium. Directly over the sacroiliac joint remove a rectangular bicortical piece of ilium approximately 6 cm in length and 2 cm in width. This

exposes the sacroiliac joint. Curette the cartilage, pus, and granulation tissue within the sacroiliac joint as thoroughly as possible. If an abscess is seen on CT scan anterior to the sacroiliac joint, this can frequently be drained through this same incision. After debridement has been conducted, denude the previously removed window of bone of cartilage and cortical bone on one side and place it as a graft into the sacroiliac joint. Close the wound without a drain and give antituberculous medication for 18 to 24 months. Protection from weight bearing should continue for 6 to 8 weeks until there is no pain on weight bearing.

Tuberculosis of the Hip

Except for the spine, the hip is the most common area to be infected with osteoarticular tuberculosis. The reason for this is unclear, but it may be related to the size of the joint or the fact that it bears weight and is subject to repeated trauma. The proximity of the urinary tract and the spine may account for lymphatic, hematogenous, or direct spread to the hip. As seems to be the case most frequently, the disease begins from a focus of osteomyelitis in the femoral head or neck or in the acetabulum. This focus spreads directly into the hip, and a tuberculous synovitis develops. It is not unusual to note a well-established osteitis in the acetabulum or proximal femur at the time that the first symptoms of hip joint irritation are appearing (Figs. 67-6 and 67-7). The earliest symptoms are those of intermittent

FIGURE 67-6.   Dumbbell-shaped lesion seen in the proximal femur of a child presenting with symptoms of hip joint synovitis.

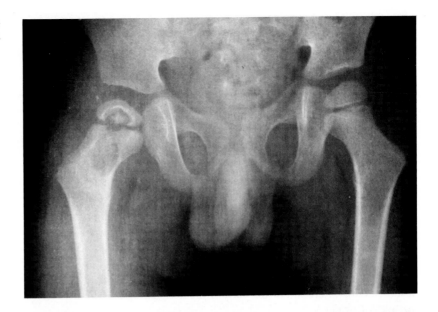

FIGURE 67-7.   (*A*) Tuberculosis of the hip in a 12-year-old child. (*B*) Note extensive acetabular and femoral head destruction with cyst formation.

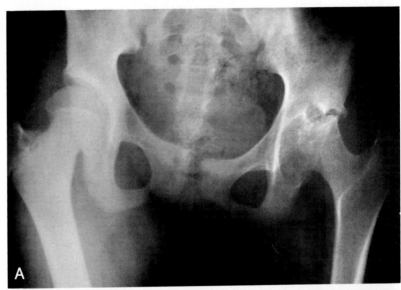

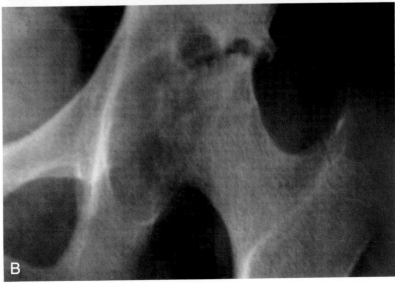

pain and an intermittent limp. Severe pain is rarely seen at initial presentation. The hip develops a flexion and adduction contracture early, and the patient frequently has an antalgic gait, walking on the ball of his foot with the knee and hip flexed. The Thomas test for hip flexion contracture is positive early in the disease. At this early stage, pain may be denied, but a limp may be present, and children will frequently have night cries early in the disease. Night cries occur when the asleep patient, usually a child, cries out in pain as involuntary muscle spasms cause movement in the inflamed joint. As the disease progresses pain becomes more obvious and is often referred to the groin, anterior thigh, or knee. Subconscious attempts to relieve this pain may be seen as the patient lifts the involved leg with the well limb when transferring, or the patient may place traction on the painful hip by pushing down on the dorsum of the foot on the involved side with the opposite foot while recumbant.[9] Muscle spasms around the hip are good indications of the degree of irritability of the hip, and early on lead to flexion contractures and proximal migration of the femoral head, resulting in erosion of the back of the acetabulum and the femoral head.

Atrophy of the muscles of the involved extremity is characteristic and can become quite pronounced. Malposition of the limb may occur, with a position of either flexion, adduction, abduction, or external rotation usually being seen in the later stages of the disease. Shortening and ankylosis in malposition is frequently seen in neglected cases going to spontaneous resolution of the disease.

Palpation around the hip may reveal a doughy thickening anteriorly or posteriorly over the joint. The inguinal nodes may be enlarged or suppurated, and in severe cases may obstruct the venous return from the leg, causing swelling and venous distention. Abscesses may track out through muscular planes and can present anywhere from the popliteal region to above Poupart's ligament. The site of the primary disease cannot be inferred from the site of the abscess or fistula.

In later stages shortening of the extremity may be due to contractures, to resorption of the femoral head or acetabulum, or, in the growing child, to retardation of growth.

Diagnosis is established by isolating the tuberculous organism from the joint fluid, pus, granulation tissue, synovium, sinus tract, or other sites of active disease associated with the hip disease. It is not unusual to make the diagnosis at surgery being performed for what was erroneously presumed to be another disorder. If unusual tissue is encountered at the time of hip arthrotomy, a frozen section of the granulation tissue may give credence to the diagnosis of tuberculosis if a typical granuloma and Langhans' giant cells are seen. The originally planned procedure, synovectomy, debridement, arthroplasty, or fusion, may still be undertaken after thorough debridement if it appears that it would be in the patient's best interest, but postoperative antibiotic treatment must be undertaken as described previously. There are instances in which total hip arthroplasty has been performed with excellent results in the presence of active tuberculous infection.

If diagnosis is established before extensive destruction of the bony architecture of the hip has occurred, treatment with antituberculous medication and limited synovectomy and curettage of bony foci of infection is indicated. Antibiotic therapy alone in the treatment of tuberculosis of the hip in most cases results in a disappointing outcome due to stiffness, contractures, and frequent progression of destruction of the hip. If surgery is contemplated and the patient exhibits contractures and pain of synovitis of the hip, he should be hospitalized and placed in traction (skeletal, if needed) to overcome the muscle spasm and contractures that are quick to develop. When the disease comes under antibiotic control, the pain will frequently resolve and the improved position of the hip can be maintained with bracing or casting as the disease becomes quiescent.

In most cases, however, it is recommended that limited synovectomy, curettage of any foci of tuberculous osteomyelitis, bone grafting of any areas that are significantly weakened by the disease, or debridement be performed.[47,53]

Technique of Synovectomy and Curettage. Approach the hip joint capsule through either an anterior bikini incision or a Smith-Petersen incision, or approach it posteriorly through a posterolateral incision. The decision whether to go anteriorly or posteriorly is based on whether lesions that are to be curetted are more accessible from the anterior or posterior route. Take care not to disrupt the retinacular vessels at the insertion of the capsule onto the base of the neck, nor to dislocate the hip during the debridement procedure. After the capsule is opened and a partial synovectomy has been performed, thoroughly curette cystic lesions. If the cystic lesions are large or are in the weight-bearing portion of the acetabulum or proximal femur, perform a bone graft at this time. Close the wound over a suction drain for several days and protect the hip with a spica cast for 6 to 8 weeks. Possible complications include avascular necrosis of the femoral head, fracture of the femoral neck or acetabulum, and slippage of the proximal femoral epiphysis.

Arthrodesis in Tuberculosis of the Hip. If extensive destruction has occurred, arthrodesis will frequently result in a satisfactory outcome. Marmor and colleagues[35] however, found that there was a high incidence of failure of extra-articular arthrodesis when it was undertaken in the acute stages. They recommend that primary treatment consist of synovectomy and curettage and antibiotic treatment. Once the disease is under control, if the destruction of the hip joint has been considerable, then arthrodesis should be considered. They recommend the method of Brittain.[11,12]

Technique of Brittain Fusion. Preoperative correction of the deformity is obtained with traction. At surgery place the patient supine on the fracture table since intraoperative radiographs or fluoroscopy is helpful. Obtain a corticocancellous graft from the ipsilateral tibia. Expose the proximal femur laterally, taking care to stay out of the involved hip joint capsule. Perform a subtrochanteric osteotomy angling upward toward the ischium beneath the involved acetabulum with a saw or an osteotome. Palpation with a blunt instrument through the osteotomy site will reveal the ischium, and the position of the location on the ischium is confirmed with radiographs. With a curette, fashion a hole in the ischium below the involved hip joint capsule and drive the tibial graft across the osteotomy site into the ischium, angling upward slightly. No internal fixation is used, and the wound is closed with suction drainage.

A hip spica cast is applied, and, if necessary, wedging of the cast can be carried out up to several weeks after surgery. At the eighth week after surgery a single leg hip spica is applied and walking is undertaken in the cast for up to 6 months. When the arthrodesis appears solid, unprotected weight bearing can be resumed. The most common cause of failure of the Brittain arthrodesis is insertion of the graft into a diseased area in the acetabulum. In those joints that are totally destroyed, the osteotomy and grafting must be performed at a lower level to effect an arthrodesis from the femur to the undiseased ischium.

Technique of Abbott-Lucas Fusion.   If there has been extensive destruction of the femoral head and neck or if an arthroplasty attempt has resulted in deficient bone stock, a two-stage arthrodesis in the manner of Abbott and Lucas[1] is an excellent way to accomplish arthrodesis in the tuberculous joint. This procedure is based on the principle that after placement of the denuded greater trochanter into the denuded acetabulum, abduction will cause a compression arthrodesis. As the femur is abducted to 45°, the resting length of the adductor muscles is exceeded and compression of the trochanter into the acetabulum occurs. A second-stage procedure is performed to align the arthrodesed limb in satisfactory position. This can be done in the presence of active sinus drainage and usually results in rapid arrest of the disease and cessation of drainage if antibiotic coverage is adequate.

Preoperative traction is not necessary since tightness of the musculature about the hip is desirable. Expose the hip joint through an anterior Smith-Petersen incision, remove the capsule, and debride the joint. Remove the femoral neck stump and denude the greater trochanter of soft tissue by subperiosteally dissecting the abductor musculature from the greater trochanter. Debride the greater trochanter as well as the acetabulum back to bleeding cancellous bone, and then place the trochanter into the acetabulum with the leg in wide abduction. Thirty to 90° of abduction may be necessary, with the average being about 45°. A 1½ hip spica is applied. Four to 8 weeks later an osteotomy is carried out about 5 cm below the lesser trochanter through the lower end of the previous incision. Create a limited exposure at that time to preserve vascularity to the proximal femur and to preserve stability to the osteotomy site. The distal fragment is usually displaced slightly medially to allow the proximal fragment to fit into the medullary canal of the distal fragment. Apply a bilateral hip spica with the leg in 5° to 10° of external rotation with the hip flexed about 35° and abducted 5° to 10°. The cast is maintained until the osteotomy has healed, and weight bearing is resumed gradually. Any residual limb shortening is compensated for by a heel lift. Antituberculous medication is continued for at least 18 months following the operative procedure (Fig. 67-8).

Arthroplasty in Tuberculosis of the Hip.   Arthroplasty of the tuberculous hip is gaining in popularity as the procedure of total hip arthroplasty is becoming more available in developing countries. If adequate bone stock is available, previous infection did not include pyogenic organisms, and postoperative control of the patient's activities can be ensured, then arthroplasty can be considered.[22,32] Previous successful arthrodesis for tuberculosis can be taken down and converted to total joint arthroplasties in some cases.

In the past, interpositional arthroplasties using metal, amniotic membrane, fascia lata, and other substances have been tried with varying success. Presently, total hip arthroplasty with

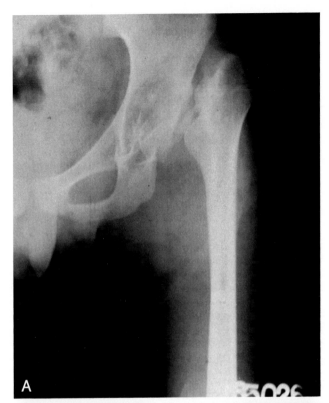

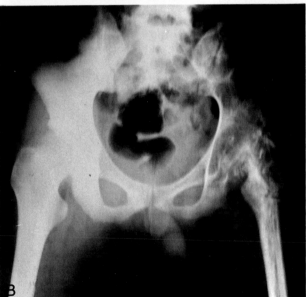

FIGURE 67-8.   (A) Unstable hip joint, destroyed by tuberculosis and draining actively. (B) Arthrodesis of the hip by the Abbott-Lucas method resulting in a stable hip and cessation of drainage.

cemented or uncemented components would be preferable.[29] As in any arthroplasty in the presence of old quiescent tuberculous infection, antituberculous medication must be administered for a prolonged period of time postoperatively to lessen the chance of reactivation of the disease.[25] Other difficulties encountered include difficulty in establishing the correct site for the acetabular component, difficulty with wound healing, extensive scar tissue formation, and lack of adequate postoperative mobility of the joint. Frequently ipsilateral knee problems also require surgery.

Tuberculous Trochanteric Bursitis

The trochanteric bursa is involved in 1% to 2% of patients with musculoskeletal tuberculosis. The disease is thought to spread to the trochanteric bursa by one of three methods: (1) direct hematogenous spread to the trochanteric bursa, (2) spread to the bursa from an adjacent tuberculous osteomyelitis in the proximal femur,[30] or (3) gravitational spread from a paraspinous abscess to the trochanteric region. Unless extensive systemic disease is present the patient is usually not aware of anything more than a mass present in the soft tissue overlying the greater trochanter. Calcification within the trochanteric bursal area and osteoporosis of the adjacent proximal femur with destruction or erosion of the proximal femur can be seen on the radiograph.[13] It is important to look for a remote site of infection such as the hip, pelvis, or lumbar spine because of the frequency of active foci infections elsewhere (Fig. 67-9). The treatment is usually excision of the trochanteric bursal region, debridement of adjacent involved bone, and use of antituberculous medication. The results of treatment are generally quite satisfactory.[2,33,44]

Tuberculosis of the Knee

In the past, tuberculosis of the knee was known as "tumor albus" or "white swelling." In the advanced stages of the disease the knee area became swollen with boggy synovium, and this distention caused the skin to blanch, hence the name.[9]

This affliction begins with a limp and limitation of motion. If the infection is untreated, the synovial proliferation and periarticular abscess combined with marked muscular atrophy gives a fusiform appearance to the knee. Joint destruction, subluxation of the tibia on the femur, and ankylosis may ensue. Sinus tracts may form, and these are frequently secondarily infected with pyogenic organisms. In the growing child with chronic disease, limb overgrowth due to epiphyseal hyperemia may result.

Pain is usually not severe, but night cries occur as they do in tuberculosis of the hip. Contractures of the knee can be quite extreme (Fig. 67-10). Attempts to correct the contractures frequently result in subluxation of the tibia posteriorly on the femur.

The disease usually begins from a focus of infection in the tibial or femoral epiphysis (Fig. 67-11). Rupture of the tuberculous abscess into the synovial reflections of the joint with resultant tuberculous synovitis results in a pannus formation over the articular cartilage. Invasion of the subchondral bone as well as pannus spreading over the articular cartilage results in joint destruction. Where two articular surfaces abut, pannus formation cannot extend over the cartilage so the subchondral destruction results in "kissing sequestrae."

Intra-articular steroids have been implicated as a causative factor in tuberculosis of the knee as well as other joints.[6,41] Either the steroids are given inadvertently to someone with an acute tuberculous knee infection or immunosuppression allows a hematogenous tuberculous infection to become established in that location.

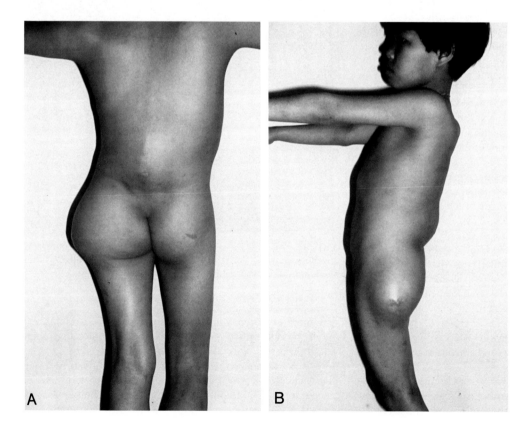

FIGURE 67-9. (*A* and *B*) Tuberculous abscess pointing over the greater trochanter. The origin of the abscess was a focus of tuberculous spondylitis, causing destruction and kyphotic deformity in the lumbar spine.

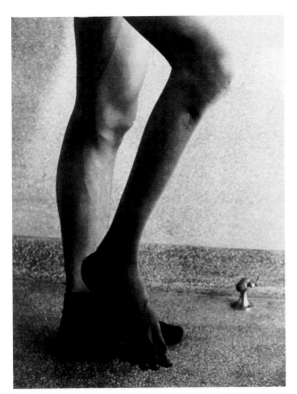

FIGURE 67-10.   Knee contracture resulting from tuberculosis. Note the multiple healed sinus scars where spontaneous drainage occurred.

In the past the treatment of tuberculosis of the knee was aimed mainly at maintaining the knee in a useful position until the disease could be brought under control. One of the earliest uses of the Thomas splint was to overcome the knee contractures of tuberculosis and maintain the limb in a satisfactory position. Often, in the past, extension of the knee under anesthesia was advocated, sometimes resulting in tearing of the popliteal artery or epiphyseal separations.

The current treatment of active tuberculosis of the knee is appropriate chemotherapy combined usually with partial synovectomy.[39,45,54] Extensive debridement is avoided because of the great recuperative ability of the joint once the disease is arrested. As in the hip, however, all cystic areas should be evacuated if possible and bone grafts used if necessary. If secondary infection with pyogenic organisms has occurred, it must be dealt with appropriately.

Although arthrodesis was frequently used in the past to control tuberculosis of the knee, it is rarely indicated now as an initial step. If destruction of the joint has been extensive, however, then an arthrodesis should be considered.

Osteotomy of the femur to correct knee flexion and angulatory deformities frequently results in excellent compromise. The osteotomy is performed to put the residual range of motion of the knee in a position that is functional to the patient.

Total knee replacement has been performed in both acute and arrested tuberculosis of the knee.[6] If scarring is not too serious, if the bone stock is adequate, and if the disease does not reactivate, a satisfactory result can be expected.

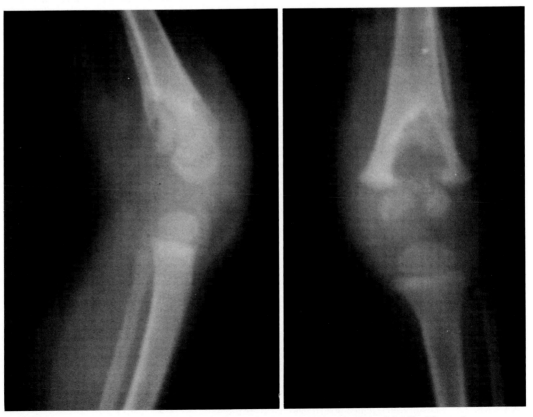

FIGURE 67-11.   Tuberculosis of the knee arising from a tuberculous osteomyelitis of the distal femoral metaphysis.

Tuberculosis of the Ankle

Tuberculosis of the ankle results in a generalized doughy swelling about the ankle, which is not painful; frequently the foot and ankle are contracted into a plantar flexed position (Fig. 67-12). The distal tibia and talus, as well as the other tarsal bones, are usually involved. The treatment is antibiotic medication, limited debridement and synovectomy, and immobilization in a plantigrade position for 4 to 6 weeks until the disease is brought under control. A molded ankle support may be necessary to protect the joint until restoration occurs. Fusion of the ankle may be indicated in extensive disease, if the joint has been destroyed.

NONTUBERCULOUS MYCOBACTERIAL OSTEOARTICULAR INFECTIONS

Occasionally, nontuberculous mycobacteria are isolated from material obtained from bone, joints, or tenosynovium.[27,28] Usually a debridement is performed for a tenosynovitis, synovitis, or osteomyelitis, and granulomatous material is obtained that grows an atypical form of *Mycobacterium* on culture. These atypical infections often respond to debridement or drainage, but when treated with antituberculous medication frequently they do not respond to standard treatment for *M. tuberculosis.*[21,34]

Organisms frequently seen in atypical mycobacterial infections include *M. avium-intracellulae, M. chelonei, M. fortuitum, M. gordonae, M. kansasii, M. marinum,* and *M. terrae.* Often a history of trauma is elicited, such as a puncture wound, steroid injection, or surgery, and in the case of *M. marinum* a history of exposure to contaminated water or fish is frequently found. The *M. marinum* organism grows best at a temperature of 30°C to 33°C and when searched for is often found as a cause of atypical tenosynovitis or bursitis in areas of the body with lower temperatures, such as the hand and wrist and the prepatellar area. The remainder of the nontuberculous mycobacteria grow best at 37°C, as does *M. tuberculosis.*

The role of immunosuppression must be considered in atypical mycobacterial disease. Since the infection frequently follows intra-articular and bursal injections with long-acting steroids, it has been seen as an opportunistic infection in patients with immunosuppression for organ transplantation, in diabetics, and is now showing up in patients infected with human immunodeficiency virus (HIV) virus.[43] Treatment for nontuberculous mycobacterial osteoarticular infections is thorough debridement of the infected tissue. The role of antibiotics has not been well established, since many of these infections clear without antibiotic treatment. If appropriate antibiotics are discerned by culture and sensitivity testing, then I would favor antibiotic coverage for 4 to 6 months in conjunction with thorough surgical debridement.

GRANULOMATOUS OSTEOARTICULAR INFECTIONS CAUSED BY FUNGI

Of the almost 100 types of fungi noted to be pathogenic in humans, only a few cause osteoarticular disease. These fungi are all dimorphic and may have a unicellular yeast form or a mycelial form. Fungal infections of the bones and joints usually gain their entrance into the body through the respiratory tract and are spread to the bones and joints like tuberculosis through the bloodstream. The body develops hypersensitivity to the fungus, and an inflammatory reaction, usually in the form of granulomatous material with abscess formation, occurs.

The diagnosis of fungal infection is made by visualization of the organism with special stains or growth of the organism on special media. Presumptive diagnosis can be established with the determination of specific serum complement-fixation antibody titers, and these titers can be used to plot the effect of treatment.

Once diagnosis is established, most of the fungal infections of bones and joints can be brought under control with aggressive debridement of contaminated tissue and appropriate antifungal agents. New, less toxic, and more easily administered antifungal agents are becoming available, and these show great promise for controlling diseases that once in the past were frequently fatal.

Coccidioidomycosis

Coccidioidomycosis is a fungal disease caused by *Coccidioides immitis.* This fungus is found principally in the San Joaquin Valley of California, the southwestern United States, and Central and South America. Inhalation of the spores of *C. imitis* usually causes an acute respiratory tract infection that is easily conquered by the body's defenses. There appears to be a predilection to blacks and Filipinos, the elderly, pregnant women, those with immunoincompetence such as from diabetes, and immunosuppressed patients.

Skin testing for reactivity to coccidioidin may give a false-negative result in a patient with serious widely disseminated disease since the patient may be anergic. Likewise, the cocci-

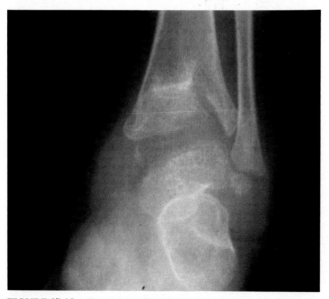

FIGURE 67-12. Extensive ankle joint destruction with massive proliferation of the synovium. Epiphyseal injury resulted in a leg length inequality.

dioidal complement-fixation antibody titer, while usually highly indicative of the activity of the disease, may fall when the patient's humoral immune system is overwhelmed by a large number of organisms.

The disease as seen in the osteoarticular system usually is a benign low-grade inflammation of joints, tenosynovium, bursa, or bone. Cystic destructive areas are seen in the bone, and soft tissue granulomatous masses often accompany the osseous lesions. Sequestrae are seen late in the disease. There seems to be a predilection for the ends of the long bones and bony prominences. In the spine, disc space sparing is common.

The treatment of coccidioidomycosis of the bones and joints consists of surgical debridement of as much contaminated tissue as possible combined with appropriate antibiotic treatment.[10,19,56] In the past amphotericin B given systemically and locally was the mainstay of treatment. The toxicity of this drug, however, limited its use. Recently, excellent results have been achieved with the use of ketoconazole or itraconazole. In most cases surgically removing as much of the infected tissue as possible decreases the antigen load, thereby facilitating the control of the disease by the patient's immune system. Attention should be focused on the patient's nutritional status to provide the optimal environment for immunologic recovery.

In the past, mutilative surgery including amputations and joint fusions were commonly necessary to bring the disease under control. In most cases now, however, joint function can be preserved with aggressive synovectomy and appropriate antibiotic treatment. For the time being, surgery remains a mainstay in the treatment of coccidioidomycosis of the osteoarticular system.

North American Blastomycosis

North American blastomycosis is caused by *Blastomyces dermatitidis*. The systemic form of the disease usually begins as a respiratory tract infection. The fungus spreads to the bones and synovial tissue by the bloodstream, and frequently patients dying of blastomycosis will show bone and joint involvement. The clinical appearance is that of other granulomatous diseases of the osteoarticular system, and the diagnosis is made by identification of the organism by direct visualization or growth on Sabouraud's agar. Debridement and treatment with ketoconazole is the treatment of choice.

Cryptococcosis

Cryptococcosis is caused by *Cryptococcus neoformans*.[16,18] This dimorphic fungus usually attacks the central nervous system but can involve the skeletal system in a patient with disseminated systemic infection. The fungus spreads from the lungs to other tissues in the body through the bloodstream, and local immune reaction causes the formation of granulomas. Almost all osseous infections with cryptococcosis are part of a systemic infection that may not be clinically apparent. The axial skeleton, vertebrae, pelvis, and ribs are most frequently involved. The cryptococcal antigen determination is usually positive, and definitive diagnosis is made by biopsy. The refractile bodies of *C. neoformans* can be seen on routine hematoxylin and eosin stains, but mucicarmine stains are more specific for cryptococcosis. The fungus may be grown on Sabouraud's media. Treat-

ment by surgical debridement of infected tissue and antifungal systemic therapy with flucytosine are recommended.

Histoplasmosis

Histoplasmosis is a very common pulmonary infection that is by and large asymptomatic. It is caused by *Histoplasma capsulatum*, which will on occasion spread from the lungs to the bones and joints. This occurs usually in patients who are immunosuppressed. The organism may be seen on direct microscopic examination or by culturing the organism on Sabouraud's agar. Skin tests and immune titers are helpful also in establishing the diagnosis.

The *Histoplasma* organism causes a synovitis or osteomyelitis similar to other fungal infections, and the treatment is thorough debridement and chemotherapy with ketoconazole or amphotericin B.

Sporotrichosis

Systemic sporotrichosis, although rare, is being seen with increasing frequency in patients who have immunosuppression.[7] This is an opportunistic fungal infection that is typically lymphocutaneous in location. Inoculation from contaminated soil or plants may occur, but the most likely means of entry is through the lungs. Sporotrichosis is caused by the organism *Sporotrix schenckii*. This is an indolent infection that frequently involves the upper extremity (mainly the wrist and elbow) when bones and joints are involved. If unrecognized, extensive destruction of the involved joints occurs.

The organism should be sought for by culturing appropriate biopsy material on Sabouraud's ager or by recognizing the cigar-shaped organism of *S. schenckii* on periodic acid–Schiff stain.

Treatment consists of systemic treatment with amphotericin B and debridement of skin, lymphatic, synovial, and osseous lesions.

REFERENCES

1. Abbott, L.C., and Lucas, D.B.: Arthrodesis of the Hip in Wide Abduction. J. Bone Joint Surg. **36-A:**1129, 1954.
2. Alvik, I.: Tuberculosis of the Greater Trochanter. Acta Orthop. Scand. **19:**247, 1949.
3. Arafiles, R. P.: A New Technique of Fusion for Tuberculous Arthritis of the Elbow. J. Bone Joint Surg. **63-A:**1396, 1981.
4. Benkeddache, Y., and Gottesman, H.: Skeletal Tuberculosis of the Wrist and Hand: A Study of 27 Cases. J. Hand Surg. **7:**594, 1982.
5. Berney, S., Goldstein, M., and Bisko, F.: Clinical and Diagnostic Features of Tuberculous Arthritis. Am. J. Med. **53:**36, 1972.
6. Besser, M.I.: Total Knee Replacement in Unsuspected Tuberculosis of the Joint. Br. Med. J. **280:**1434, 1980.
7. Bibler, M.R., Luber, H.J., Glueck, H.I., and Estes, S.A.: Disseminated Sporotrichosis in a Patient with HIV Infection after Treatment for Acquired Factor VIII Inhibitor. J.A.M.A. **256:**3125, 1986.
8. Bickle, W.H., Kimbrough, R.F., and Dahlin, D.C.: Tuberculous Tenosynovitis. J.A.M.A. **151:**31, 1953.
9. Bradford, E.H., and Lovett, R.W.: Orthopaedic Surgery, 5th ed. New York, William Wood & Co., 1915.

10. Bried, J.M., and Galgiani, J.N.: *Coccidioides Immitis* Infections in Bone and Joints. Clin. Orthop. **211**:235, 1986.

11. Brittain, H.A.: Ischiofemoral Arthrodesis. Br. J. Surg. **29**:93, 1941.

12. Brittain, H.A.: Architectural Principles in Arthrodesis, 2nd ed. Edinburgh, E. & S. Livingstone, 1952.

13. Brown, N.L.: Tuberculosis of the Greater Trochanter and Its Bursa. Orthopedics **9**:1276, 1986.

14. Bush, D.C. et al.: Tuberculosis of the Hand and Wrist. J. Hand Surg. **9**:391, 1984.

15. Centers for Disease Control: Leads from the MMWR: Tuberculosis—United States, 1985. J.A.M.A. **256**:3335, 1986.

16. Chleboun, J., and Nade, S.: Skeletal Cryptococcosis. J. Bone Joint Surg. **59-A**:509, 1977.

17. DeRoy, M.S., and Fisher, H.: The Treatment of Tuberculous Bone Disease by Surgical Drainage Combined with Streptomycin. J. Bone Joint Surg. **34-A**:299, 1952.

18. Fialk, M.A., Maracove, R.C., and Armstrong, D.: Cryptococcal Bone Disease: A Manifestation of Disseminated Cryptococcosis. Clin. Orthop. **158**: 219, 1981.

19. Gillespie, R.: Treatment of Cranial Osteomyelitis from Disseminated Coccidioidomycosis. West. J. Med. **145**:694, 1986.

20. Goldberg, I., and Avidar, I.: Isolated Tuberculous Tenosynovitis of the Achilles Tendon, a Case Report. Clin. Orthop. **194**:185, 1985.

21. Gunther, S.F., Elliott, R.C., Brand, R.L., and Adams, J.P.: Experience with Atypical Mycobacterial Infection in the Deep Structures of the Hand. J. Hand Surg. **2**:90, 1977.

22. Hardinge, K., Cleary, J., and Charnley, J.: Low-Friction Arthroplasty for Healed Septic and Tuberculous Arthritis. J. Bone Joint Surg. **61-B**:144, 1979.

23. Hodgson, A.R., and Smith, T.K.: Tuberculosis of the Wrist. Clin. Orthop. **83**:73, 1972.

24. Holder, S.F., Hopson, C.N., and VonKuster, L.C.: Tuberculous Arthritis of the Elbow Presenting as Chronic Bursitis of the Olecranon: A Case Report. J. Bone Joint Surg. **67-A**:1127, 1985.

25. Johnson, R., Barnes, K.L., and Owen, R.: Reactivation of Tuberculosis After Total Hip Replacement. J. Bone Joint Surg. **61-B**:148, 1979.

26. Keers, R.Y.: Pulmonary Tuberculosis: A Journey Down the Centuries. London, Balliere Tindall, 1978.

27. Kelly, P.J., and Karlson, A.G.: Granulomatous Bacterial Arthritis. Clin. Orthop. **96**:165, 1973.

28. Kelly, P.J., Karlson, A.G., Weed, L.A., and Lipscomb, P.R.: Infection of Synovial Tissues by Mycobacteria Other Than *Mycobacterium Tuberculosis*. J. Bone and Joint Surg. **49-A**:1521, 1967.

29. Kim, Y.Y., Ohn, B.H., Bae, D.K., Ko, C.U., Lee, J.D., Kwak, B.M., and Yoon, Y.S.: Arthroplasty Using Charnley Prosthesis in Old Tuberculosis of the Hip. Clin. Orthop. **211**:116, 1986.

30. Lampe, C.E.: Tuberculous Osteomyelitis of the Greater Trochanter: A Report of Eight Cases. J. Bone Joint Surg. **64-B**:185, 1982.

31. Lee, K.E.: Tuberculosis Presenting as Carpal Tunnel Syndrome. J. Hand Surg. **10**:242, 1985.

32. Lin, E., Oliver, S., Caspi, I., Ezra, E., Bubis, J.J., and Nerubay, J.: Hip Arthroplasty in Quiescent Mycobacterial Infection of the Hip. Orthop. Rev. **15**:73, 1986.

33. Lynch, A.F.: Tuberculosis of the Greater Trochanter: A Report of Eight Cases. J. Bone Joint Surg. **64-B**:185, 1982.

34. Marchevsky, A.M., Damsker, L.B., Green, S., and Tepper, S.: The Clinicopathological Spectrum of Non-Tuberculous Mycobacterial Osteoarticular Infections. J. Bone Joint Surg. **67-A**:925, 1985.

35. Marmor, L., Chan, K.B., Ho, K.C., and Justin, M.: Surgical Treatment of Tuberculosis of the Hip in Children. Clin. Orthop. **67**:135, 1969.

36. Martini, M., Adjrad, A., and Boudjemaa, A.: Tuberculous Osteomyelitis. Int. Orthop. **10**:201, 1986.

37. Martini, M., Benkeddache, Y., Medjani, Y., and Gottesman, H.: Tuberculosis of the Upper Limb Joints, Int. Orthopaedics, **10**:17, 1986.

38. Meltzer, R.M. et al.: Tuberculous Arthritis: A Case Study and Review of the Literature. J. Foot Surg. **24**:30, 1985.

39. Misgar, M.S., Mir, N.A., and Narbu, T.: Partial Synovectomy in the Treatment of Tuberculosis of the Knee. Int. Surg. **67**:53, 1982.

40. Pepersack, F., and Yourassowsky, E.: Spina Ventosa, A Forgotten Form of Tuberculosis. Acta Clin. Belg. **34**:360, 1979.

41. Peterson, C.A.: Tuberculous Arthritis Following Intra-articular Steroid. J. Bone Joint Surg. **58-A**:278, 1976.

42. Pimm, L.H., and Waugh, W.: Tuberculous Synovitis. J. Bone Joint Surg. **39-B**:91, 1957.

43. Pitchenik, A.E., Cole, C., Russell, B.W., Fischl, M.A., Spira, T.J., and Snider, D.E.: Tuberculosis, Atypical Mycobacteriosis, and the Acquired Immunodeficiency Syndrome Among Haitian and non-Haitian Patients in South Florida. Ann. Intern. Med. **101**:641, 1984.

44. Rehm-Graves, S., Weinstein, A.J., Calabrese, L.H., Cook, S.A., and Boumphrey, F.R.S.: Tuberculosis of the Greater Trochanteric Bursa. Arthritis Rheum. **26**:77, 1983.

45. Rose, G.K.: Tuberculosis of the Knee Joint. Br. J. Clin. Pract. **13**:241, 1959.

46. Schatz, A., and Waksman, S.A.: Effect of Streptomycin and Other Antibiotic Substances Upon *Mycobacterium Tuberculosis* and Related Organisms. Proc. Soc. Exp. Biol. Med. **57**:244, 1944.

47. Stevenson, F.H., Cholmeley, J.A., and Jory, H.I.: Tuberculosis of the Hip in Children: Seven Years of Chemotherapy. Tubercle **38**:164, 1967.

48. Strange, F.G.: The Prognosis in Sacro-Iliac Tuberculosis. Br. J. Surg. **50**:561, 1963.

49. Sunderam, G., McDonald, R.J., Maniatis, J.O., Kapila, R., and Reichman, L.B.: Tuberculosis as a Manifestation of the Acquired Immunodeficiency Syndrome (AIDS). J.A.M.A. **256**:362, 1986.

50. Tager, I.B.: Current Concepts in the Treatment of Tuberculosis. West. J. Med. **146**:461, 1987.

51. Tuli, S.M.: Tuberculosis of the Spine. Lucknow, India, Prem Printing Press, 1975.

52. Wallace, R., and Cohen, A.S.: Tuberculous Arthritis. Am. J. Med. **61**:277, 1976.

53. Wilkinson, M.C.: Partial Synovectomy and Curettage in the Treatment of Tuberculosis in the Hip. J. Bone Joint Surg. **39-B**:66, 1957.

54. Wilkinson, M.C.: Partial Synovectomy in the Treatment of Tuberculosis of the Knee. J. Bone Joint Surg. **44-B**:34, 1962.

55. Wilson, G.S., and Miles, A.: Topley and Wilson's Principles of Bacteriology, Virology and Immunity, 6th ed. London, Edward Arnold, 1975.

56. Winter, W.G. Jr., Larson, R.K., Honeggar, M.M., Jacobsen, D.T., Pappagianis, D., and Huntington, R.W. Jr.: Coccidioidal Arthritis and its Treatment—1975. J. Bone Joint Surg. **57-A**:1152, 1975.

CHAPTER 68

Management of Infected Implants

LEWIS D. ANDERSON and
FREDERICK N. MEYER

The two most common examples of infected implants in orthopaedic surgery are (1) metallic devices used in fracture and nonunion treatment, and (2) the various components, including metal, plastic, and cement, used in joint replacement. Noncorrosive metal devices have been used for fixation of fractures for about 50 years.[35] Modern unipolar joint replacement was reported by Thompson in 1955[34] and Moore in 1959;[23] Charnley reported his first 450 total joint replacements in 1963.[8]

These two relatively new procedures—internal fixation of fractures with noncorrosive metals and joint replacement—have now been used long enough that we can understand the management of infection, which is one of the most serious complications common to both operations.

There are many factors that determine whether or not a bone infection will develop in a given situation. These include general host factors such as the state of nutrition, concomitant disease, and immunosuppression. Local wound factors include the size of the wound, the length of time the wound is open, the vascularity and nutrition, the presence or absence of dead bone and necrotic soft tissue, and the presence or absence of foreign material. Also important are the type and virulence of bacteria present and the number of bacteria.

Rhinelander and associates have shown that reaming of the proximal femur in dogs followed by implantation of methylmethacrylate cement directly against cortical bone leads to devascularization and bone death that may persist for at least a year.[32]

Bowers, Wilson, and Green[4] studied infection in surgical windows in dog femurs. In the dogs given preoperative antibiotics, no infections developed even though approximately 500,000 *Staphylococcus aureus* organisms were inserted into the bone defect at the time of surgery. On the other hand, if the same number of bacteria were placed in the defect and antibiotics were not begun until 6 hours after surgery, all dogs developed infection.

Elek and Conen[10] showed experimentally that both the number of organisms and the presence of foreign material affect the incidence of infection. A single subcutaneous injection of up to one million staphylococci will not produce an infection; however, two million to eight million organisms similarly injected will overwhelm the host and produce infection. In the presence of a foreign body (e.g., sutures) only 100 staphylococci produced an infection.

It is most interesting that these three experimental studies demonstrated facts well known to most orthopaedists:

1. Dead bone is produced by reaming and cement.
2. Antibiotics, to be effective, must be in adequate concentration when the hematoma forms.
3. The likelihood of infection is affected by the size of the wound and the amount of time it is open (i.e., the number of bacteria) as well as the presence of foreign material.

When one considers these factors, it is amazing that infection is not more frequent after internal fixation of fractures, and especially after total joint replacement.

Early Infection After Internal Fixation

If an infection develops in the first month or so after internal fixation of the fracture, obtain a culture as soon as possible.

Aspiration should be done if necessary. Start the patient immediately on the appropriate intravenous antibiotics, and take him to the operating room for a thorough debridement and irrigation of the infected wound.[13,21]

Fracture stability is very important to the treatment of infection; rarely does infection resolve in an unstable fracture or nonunion. Loose implants promote infection, and must be removed or replaced. If they are removed, fracture stability is maintained with external fixation.

In acute infections the internal fixation device is almost always stable. (Fig. 68-1), in which case it is usually better to leave it in place.[2,21] This is particularly true in intra-articular fractures where limited internal fixation with screws and wires is present. Plates on most long bones, if stable, can also be left *in situ*.

Acutely infected plates on the tibia present a special problem in that skin loss is common, and leaving the wound open exposes the plate and bones. There is no question that bone union is achievable with an exposed plate and bone, but the risk of chronic osteomyelitis is high. If the plate is stable but exposed, conversion to external fixation should be considered.

Acute infection of fractures fixed by intramedullary nails often involves the medullary cavity, which requires debridement. In most cases this can be achieved by opening and debriding the fracture site directly, removing the nail, and reaming the medullary canal to debride it. If the infection is low-grade and due to a gram-positive organism, immediate renailing with a reamed nail is often possible. If the infection is severe, particularly with gram-negative bacteria, conversion to external fixation is advisable.

The prognosis is worse with gram-negative or mixed gram-negative–gram-positive infections. These often require conversion to external fixation. Although it is difficult to totally eradicate infection with implants in place, it is most important to achieve fracture union and maintain function. After achieving union, infection often resolves when the implant is removed.

After debridement use irrigation suction or pack the wound open for possible later closure. This decision will depend on many factors including the type of bacteria and the location of the wound. In general irrigation suction works best with infections caused by gram-positive bacteria.[3] Intravenous antibiotics should usually be continued for 6 weeks.

In our experience, the success rate of early debridement and antibiotics for fractures with retained metal is not high in terms of total clearing of the infection.[3] However, it is worthwhile in helping to control the spread of infection and preventing systemic manifestations of infection.[1,13]

Late Infection After Internal Fixation

Most often, late infection after internal fixation is a residual of an earlier infection. Occasionally a smoldering, low-grade infection may become clinically apparent only long after internal fixation. When late infection is present, the metal internal fixation devices should be left in place as long as they provide fixation.[13,21] The hope is that fracture union will eventually take place, even though some drainage continues (Fig. 68-2). At times the sinus tract may seal over, causing an abscess to form. If this occurs, drain the abscess and pack the wound open to recreate the sinus tract.[1]

Once union has taken place and the callus has matured, perform a thorough debridement, removing any sequestrae, along with infected soft tissues and the metal implants.[21] Do this with appropriate intravenous antibiotic coverage, using irrigation suction for the local wound if necessary. This will result in healing of the wound and clearing of the infection in a high percentage of cases.[1,21] If a skin slough develops over a metal plate, clinical infection can be circumvented by covering the wound with a muscle pedicle or free vascularized muscle flap. (Fig. 68-3)

When the fixation device loosens before the fracture has healed, there is no point in delaying removal of the metal. Remove the internal fixation and thoroughly debride the bone and soft tissues. An external fixator is helpful in stabilizing the fracture and controlling infection. At times an intramedullary nail that has become loose should be replaced with a larger one to provide better fixation. According to MacAusland, this can be done without undue danger.[21] Plates should be avoided in the presence of established infection. In our experience, they tend to lose fixation earlier and more frequently than either external fixators or tight intramedullary nails. Generally, bone grafting is delayed until the wound is well healed and has been free of drainage for 3 to 6 months. However, cancellous bone grafting of open wounds using the Papineau technique can be carried out whenever there is a clean granulating bed that is free of drainage.[26] Skin grafting over the cancellous bone is done later.

Antibiotics alone appear to have little effect on chronically infected fractures, especially when metal is present.[3] Therefore, their use should be reserved for episodes of cellulitis or septicemia or for use in conjunction with surgical procedures.

Infected Total Joint Implants

In 1969 Charnley and Eftekhar reported that the infection rate in the first 190 patients undergoing low-friction arthroplasty was 9.8%.[8] Their concern over this high rate of deep infection led directly to Charnley's "green house" or vertical laminar flow operating room. This, along with the use of cleaner operating rooms with more rapid turnover of air, better drapes, intravenous prophylactic antibiotics and antibiotic-impregnated cement, has significantly lowered the infection rate in most medical centers for total hip and knee replacement procedures to about 1% to 2%.[16,24,27,30]

Infection Following Total Hip Arthroplasty

According to Murray, pain is the most frequent symptom of infection following total hip arthroplasty, and occurs in 75% of patients with infection.[24] Drainage is present in 21%, and the sedimentation rate is elevated in only 57%. Murray obtained a positive preoperative culture in 57%.

It is very important to aspirate a hip suspected of being infected under strict aseptic technique. Knowing the organism and its sensitivity pattern is extremely helpful in choosing the best antibiotics and deciding on the most appropriate operative procedure (Fig. 68-4).

The choices of treatment for infection following total hip arthroplasty include (1) antibiotics alone, (2) debridement with irrigation suction, (3) debridement with direct reimplantation,

(Text continues on p. 880)

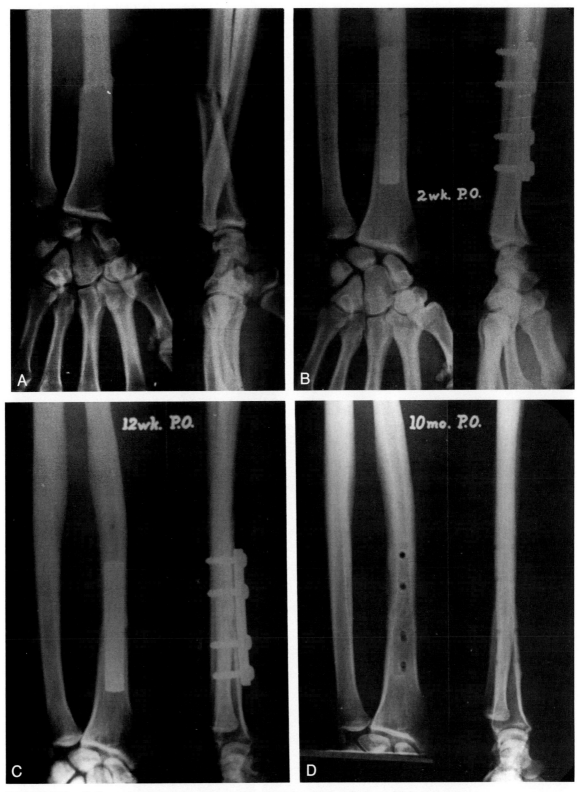

FIGURE 68-1. Radiographs of wrist in a 20-year-old male with a Galeazzi fracture. (*A*) Anteroposterior and lateral films obtained before surgery. (*B*) Two weeks after reduction and fixation with a compression plate. Drainage developed at 10 days and cultures were positive for *Staphylococcus aureus*. Debridement and irrigation suction were performed. (*C*) By 12 weeks after surgery the infection had been controlled but slight drainage persisted. The fracture showed early signs of healing. (*D*) Ten months after surgery the fracture was healed. The plate was removed and irrigation suction was repeated. There was excellent function and no further drainage.

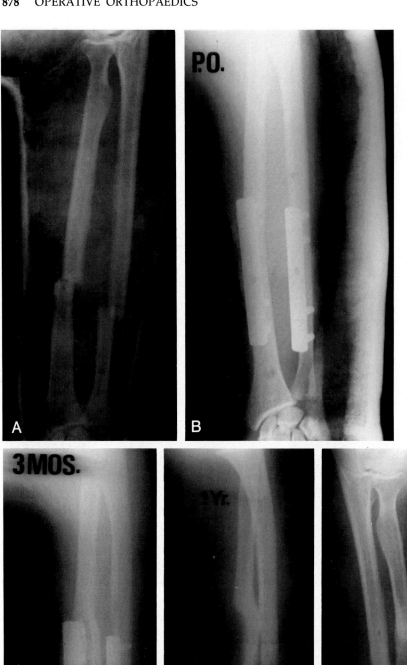

FIGURE 68-2. (*A*) Preoperative and (*B*) postoperative radiographs in a 35-year-old female with closed fracture of the radius and ulna. The fractures were internally fixed with compression plates. (*C*) A severe postoperative infection developed. At 3 months involucrum was noted about the radius. The fractures healed slowly in spite of the infection. (*D* and *E*) At 1 year the plates were removed and irrigation suction was performed. The infection cleared entirely but pronation and supination were limited.

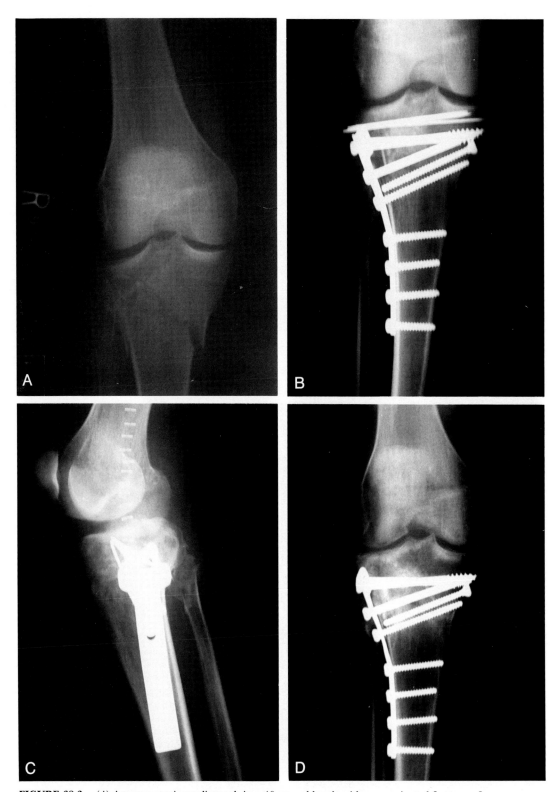

FIGURE 68-3. (*A*) Anteroposterior radiograph in a 40-year-old male with a comminuted fracture of the tibial plateau. (*B*) Anteroposterior and (*C*) lateral films obtained 10 days after open reduction and internal fixation. A full-thickness skin slough developed, exposing 2 inches of the plate. Before clinical infection could develop, a gastrocnemius muscle flap was rotated to cover the plate. Split-thickness skin graft was applied over the muscle. (*D*) Anteroposterior radiograph obtained 1 year later. Infection was prevented by the gastrocnemius flap. The fracture healed and there was excellent function.

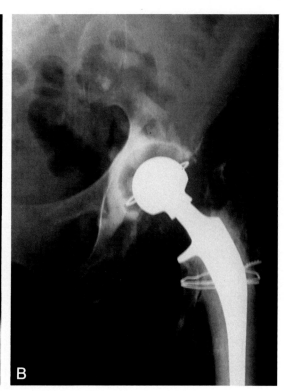

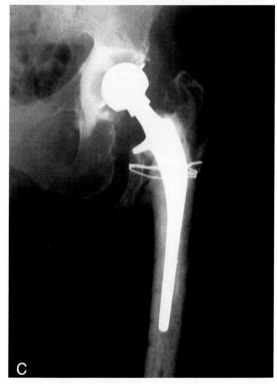

FIGURE 68-4. (*A*) Radiograph of the hip obtained in a 78-year-old female who had incurred a trochanteric fracture 14 months earlier. The fracture had been fixed with a Jewett nail but had failed to unite. Aspiration of the hip grew *Staphylococcus epidermidis*. (*B*) Debridement of the hip was carried out with copious irrigation. Under intravenous antibiotic coverage a total hip replacement was done at the same operation. This radiograph was obtained 2 weeks after surgery. (*C*) Eighteen months after arthroplasty, the patient was free of pain and had no sign of infection.

(4) debridement with removal and delayed reimplantation, (5) removal (Girdlestone) as definitive procedure, and (6) hip disarticulation.

Antibiotics Alone. Antibiotics alone have very little place in the treatment of an infected total hip arthroplasty. They almost never cure the infection and may lead to resistance of the organisms. Occasionally the use of antibiotics without surgery may be justified in a patient who is septic and is too medically ill to undergo an operation.

Debridement with Irrigation Suction. Debridement with irrigation suction is used primarily in early infections within the first 3 months after hip replacement. Murray does not recommend this method when the infecting organism is *Staphylococcus aureus* or any of the gram-negative bacteria, and finds it successful only when the infecting bacteria is of relatively low virulence.[24] Most surgeons report a relatively low percentage of complete success (approximately 20%) in eradicating the infection with this method.[7] However, the morbidity is relatively low and it is probably worth trying under the circumstances outlined above. When this method is used, appropriate intravenous antibiotics should be started during surgery as soon as gram stains and cultures have been obtained. Intravenous antibiotics should be continued for 6 weeks.[14,24] When intravenous antibiotics are discontinued, oral antibiotics are started and given for an additional 6-week period.[14,24] This same antibiotic regimen is followed for all surgical procedures described in the following text for treatment of infected total hip and knee replacements.

Salvati and associates at the Hospital for Special Surgery recommend using tube dilution studies to determine the amount of antibiotics to be administered.[33] They attempt to give doses sufficient to attain peak bacterial serum titers of at least 1:8. When drugs that are nephrotoxic are used, renal function must be carefully monitored. Patients receiving ototoxic drugs should have audiograms done twice weekly.[24]

Some orthopaedists do not use irrigation suction for fear of retrograde infection. On the other hand, Murray advocates copious irrigation of the wound at the time of surgery with a solution of 1 gram of kanamycin per 500 ml of saline.[24] After surgery he uses the low volume–high concentration method of irrigation suction as described by Jergesen and Jawetz, and instills a solution of 1% kanamycin and 0.1% polymyxin.[20] Twelve ml to 20 ml of the solution is instilled in the tubes twice daily. The suction is then turned off for 3 hours, after which it is turned on again for 9 hours before the next cycle is begun. This is continued for 7 days. Using this method, Murray has had no case of retrograde infection.[24]

Others prefer the high volume–low concentration method advocated by Compere[9] and modified by Anderson and Horn.[3] In 75 patients with bone and joint infections treated by this method, Anderson found no retrograde infection.[3]

With either type of irrigation suction, a careful debridement must be performed. All infected and necrotic soft tissues must be removed, along with as much granulation tissue as possible, and any loose cement. Sinus tracts must be carefully excised. For up to 3 months after implantation, the femoral and acetabular components are usually not loose and are normally not removed.

Debridement with Direct Reimplantation. Harris states that when debridement with direct reimplantation is to be performed, careful patient selection is imperative.[14] Except for the infected joint, the patient should be in good health, should not have a debilitating disease, and should not be on immunosuppressive therapy (usually steroids). Direct reimplantation has not generally been successful in gram-negative infections and is not recommended. Harris reported two successful direct reimplantations when the infection was caused by *Staphylococcus aureus*.[14] On the other hand, Murray advises against this method with *Staphylococcus aureus* infection.[24]

When the above criteria are met and direct reimplantation is decided on, a trochanteric osteotomy should be performed.[14] This greatly aids the radical debridement and the complete removal of cement that is necessary. Both components are removed, along with all cement from the acetabulum and femur, even though only one component may be loose.[24] All scar tissue and necrotic and infected tissue must be excised. The wound should be copiously irrigated with kanamycin solution as outlined previously. The new components should be cemented with antibiotic-impregnated cement. Harris and Murray both recommend the addition of 1 g of erythromycin and 300 mg of colistin to 40 g to 60 g of polymethylmethacrylate powder.[14,24] Irrigation suction is carried out for 5 to 7 days.[24]

The success rate for patients selected as outlined is reasonably good. Several reported series in the recent literature give success rates ranging from 50% to 90%.[4,6,14,24]

Debridement with Removal and Delayed Reimplantation. When debridement with removal of the implant is performed, followed by later reimplantation, everything is done exactly as outlined for direct reimplantation except that no new components are initially inserted. The wound is closed over irrigation suction tubes. A Kirschner wire is placed in the tibial tubercle and the extremity is placed in balanced skeletal traction. Intravenous antibiotics are continued for 6 weeks. Oral antibiotics are then begun, traction is discontinued, and the patient is allowed up on crutches or a walker touching down with the foot. Oral antibiotics are usually stopped after 6 weeks and crutch-walking is continued. After a period of 3 to 6 months without antibiotics, the patient is evaluated to determine if he or she is free from infection. Examination of the wound, laboratory work, cultures from an arthrogram and often a gallium scan should be evaluated. If there is no evidence of infection, reimplantation of a total hip prosthesis is performed using antibiotic-impregnated cement. Intravenous antibiotics are avoided until the wound is open and tissue samples can be taken for cultures. Antibiotics are then started based on previous cultures. If the cultures taken at the time of reimplantation are negative, the antibiotics can be stopped after 7 to 10 days. If the intraoperative cultures are positive, then the most appropriate antibiotics should be continued for 6 weeks intravenously followed by 6 more weeks orally.[24]

The expense, morbidity, and especially the time of hospitalization required for the delayed reimplantation method is obviously much greater than when direct reimplantation can be done. On the other hand, delayed reimplantation is safer and gives a much higher rate of success for gram-negative infection, mixed infection, and probably for infections with *Staphylococcus aureus*.[11,14,33] Using antibiotic-impregnated cement along with the other measures, two-stage reimplantation has averaged over 90% success in Fitzgerald's report from the Mayo Clinic and Murray's report from the University of California at San Francisco.[11,14]

Removal (Girdlestone) as Definitive Procedure. Removal of implants without subsequent reimplantation is most often indicated in lieu of one of the previous methods, when the overall health of the patient is poor or the resistance of the infecting organisms is high. Removal is performed exactly as described above. Considerable relief of pain is usually afforded by the procedure, but function is usually poor. Most patients require at least two walking canes and often two crutches are necessary.[15,22,25] The average limb shortening is 3.7 cm, and may be as much as 5.5 cm or more with significant loss of bone stock.[22]

The resection arthroplasty combined with the use of antibiotics as outlined above appears to be successful in eliminating clinical infection in about 90% of cases.[22,25] It is especially important to remove all cement and infected tissues.

Hip Disarticulation.   Disarticulation of the hip after hip replacement fortunately is seldom required. It is used only in the face of severe sepsis that cannot be controlled by other means. As with any amputation done for infection, it should be performed as a two-stage procedure. The wound is packed open initially and usually can be closed after 5 to 7 days.

Infected Total Knee Arthroplasties

The deep infection rate in most large series of total knee replacements is in the range of 1.0% to 2.5%.[12,16,29,30] In one series the average time from surgery to discovery of the infection was 8.3 months.[12] However, some infections are discovered in the early postoperative period and some may not appear for years after surgery. The organisms causing knee infection are similar to those causing infection after total hip replacement, and *Staphylococcus aureus* is probably the most common. Mixed infections and those caused by gram-negative bacteria are the most difficult to treat.

Treatment choices include (1) antibiotics alone, (2) debridement with irrigation suction, (3) resection arthroplasty, (4) debridement with removal and delayed reimplantation, (5) arthrodesis, and (6) amputation.

Antibiotics Alone.   Antibiotics alone are almost never successful in treating an infected total knee. This form of treatment should be reserved for patients who are septic and too ill to undergo surgery.

Debridement with Irrigation Suction.   Debridement combined with irrigation suction and carefully managed intravenous antibiotic coverage does not enjoy a high rate of success. With this technique the components are left in place, and the procedures are similar to those detailed previously for the total hip. Petty and co-workers reported eight knees salvaged by this procedure.[27] Woods and associates were able to successfully treat only three of 27 infected total knee replacements.[36] This method has no place in the treatment of a chronically infected knee. It should be used almost entirely in acute infection soon after surgery, and even then with the realization that the chances of success are not great.

Resection Arthroplasty.   Kaufer and Matthews have reported on 30 infected total knee arthroplasties in 28 patients treated by replacement arthroplasty.[18] These were done most often in patients with multiarticular arthritis who spent most of their time sitting or recumbent, and in whom a knee fused in extension was thought to be a disadvantage. A few patients who refused arthrodesis were also treated by this method.[18]

This technique requires careful debridement with removal of the components, all cement, and any infected tissues.[18] The tibia and femur are allowed to collapse together to close the dead space. Transarticular Steinmann pins may be used for initial stability, or suture loops may be passed through drill holes in the distal femur and proximal tibia. If Steinmann pins are used, they are removed in 2 to 4 weeks. A long-leg cast is worn for 4 to 10 months. Care should be taken to place the tibia securely on the end of the femur. The extremity is aligned with 7° of valgus and 15° of flexion. Antibiotic management is similar to that outlined previously for infected total hips.[18]

Kaufer and Matthews advocate weight-bearing to tolerance in the cast as soon as possible.[19] Their average cast time was 7 months. Braces are used if needed after casts are discontinued. In their series, systemic sepsis was controlled in all cases. Twelve of the 30 (40%) knees healed primarily with no further drainage. Ten knees drained for 3 to 6 months and then had no further drainage. Overall, 17% had small, intermittent drainage and 83% had no drainage. The authors point out that if the patient is unhappy with the result, fusion can be performed secondarily. There were six such fusions done with trochanter-to-malleolus medullary nails and all were successful. Some patients with resection arthroplasty had surprisingly stable and functional knees.

Debridement with Implant Removal and Delayed Reimplantation.   Another option is debridement with removal of the implant and later reimplantation. Under suitable antibiotic coverage, meticulous debridement of the infected knee component, cement, and infected tissues is carried out as previously described. Insall points out that if the infection is relatively recent, the components will still be tightly cemented and will be difficult to remove without sacrificing bone stock.[16] However, it is essential to preserve as much healthy bone as possible. Allow the tibia and femur to come together. Place one or two absorbable sutures through drill holes in the tibia and femur to maintain general alignment. Then apply a bulky dressing with plaster splints.[16] We prefer to use irrigation suction on these cases, although some orthopaedists, including Insall, do not favor irrigation suction because of the fear of retrograde infection.

Insall believes that if there has been a good response to the above procedure and antibiotics, and if the patient is healthy and robust, reimplantation of another prosthesis may be indicated.[16] The exact timing is based on the appearance of the wound, the white blood cell count, and the sedimentation rate. If there is doubt about the wound, antibiotics should be discontinued, the knee aspirated, and the wound observed for a further period of time. Reimplantations cannot be successfully done much beyond 3 months. After this the soft tissues become contracted to the point that the operation becomes very difficult and knee motion is not regained.

If the wound appears benign and other signs of infection are absent, reimplantation can then be performed. At the time of reimplantation, do not start antibiotics until specimens have been obtained for culture and gram stain. Postoperatively, antibiotic therapy should be the same as outlined previously for a reimplanted total hip.

In a series of 30 patients with infected total knees who were treated by removal of the components and delayed reimplantation, Insall had only one patient (3%) with recurrent infection who was considered a failure.[16] Seventy-eight percent had good or excellent results. The 19% that were fair were so rated because of quadriceps weakness. They were, however, free of infection.[16]

Rand and co-workers from the Mayo Clinic reported 14 patients with infected total knee replacements who were treated by antibiotics, debridement, and removal of the components.[30] Reimplantation was done within 2 weeks. Of the seven patients with low-virulence organisms, six achieved a good functional result without infection. In the other seven patients, high-virulence organisms were identified (i.e., *Staphylococcus aureus* or gram-negative bacteria). Only two of these operations were successful. These authors concluded that a period of time greater than 2 weeks should elapse between removal of an infected total knee and reimplantation of a new one. They also pointed out that the success rate is much higher if the infection is caused by a low-virulence bacteria.[30,31]

Arthrodesis. Arthrodesis is the method most often recommended for the treatment of an infected total knee. If successful, it gives the patient a stable, painless extremity, although there are obvious disadvantages. Arthrodesis after infected total knee replacement is not always easy to achieve. Success depends, in large part, on how much bone stock can be preserved. The success rate for arthrodesis at the Mayo Clinic was 56% after hinged arthroplasty and 81% after nonhinged arthroplasty.[5] Johnson reported successful bony ankylosis in six of 12 infected total knee replacements using Charnley compression clamps.[17] Both Rand at the Mayo Clinic and Knutson and his group in Lund, Sweden now prefer the Ace–Fischer Fixator if external fixation is to be used.[19,28]

Probably the most successful series of arthrodeses following infected total knee replacement is that reported by Knutson and associates.[19] They described 20 consecutive patients (15 with infections) in whom successful bony ankylosis was eventually achieved. However, several patients required more than one attempt.

These authors advise a two-stage procedure. Systemic antibiotics are begun before surgery. Initially thoroughly debride the knee and remove the components as well as all cement. Excise and close all fistulas. If there is good bone stock, apply an external fixator. If there is poor bone stock, an intramedullary nail is preferred. If an intramedullary nail is decided on, ream the femur from the trochanter to the knee. Then ream the tibia from the knee to below the isthmus. Knutson states that it is usually possible to use a nail with at least a 14-mm diameter. Insert a nail of appropriate length from the greater trochanter past the isthmus of the tibia. Whether the nail or a fixator is used, place gentamicin-impregnated polymethylmethacrylate beads about the knee and close the wound.[19]

The second stage is carried out after the wound is well healed, usually after an interval of 4 to 6 weeks. At this time remove the gentamicin beads. Shape the condyles of the tibia and femur for their best possible contact, and freshen the cortices. If an external fixator had been applied, compress it. With either an external fixator or an intramedullary nail, place a large amount of cancellous iliac bone about the knee after freshening the cortices of the femurs and tibia.

Crutch-walking is allowed after a few days, and weight-bearing after 6 weeks. Antibiotics are continued until fusion is documented. In Knutson's series, shortening ranged from 2 cm to 8 cm and averaged 4 cm.[19]

Kaufer and Matthews also report good success using intramedullary nail fixation for infected total knee replacements.[18] Six of their patients who underwent resection arthroplasty as described earlier subsequently required arthrodesis for instability. All six achieved bony arthrodesis and had good results.[18]

Amputation. Fortunately, amputation after an infected total knee replacement is not often necessary. The principal indication is sepsis that cannot be controlled by other methods. Most commonly it is required when a long-stemmed, hinged prosthesis becomes infected. These are rarely used at the present time.

REFERENCES

1. Anderson, L.D.: Fractures. *In* Crenshaw, A.H. (ed.): Campbell's Operative Orthopaedics, 5th ed., Vol. 1, p. 477. St. Louis, C.V. Mosby, 1971.
2. Anderson, L.D.: Infections. In Edmonson, A.S., and Crenshaw, A.H. (ed.): Campbell's Operative Orthopaedics, 6th ed., Vol. 1, p. 1031. St. Louis, C.V. Mosby, 1980.
3. Anderson, L.D., and Horn, L.G.: Irrigation-Suction Technic in the Treatment of Acute Hematogenous Ostomyelitis, Chronic Osteomyelitis, and Acute and Chronic Joint Infections. South. Med. J. **63**:745, 1970.
4. Bowers, W.H., Wilson, F.C., and Greene, W.B.: Antibiotic Prophylaxis in Experimental Bone Infections. J. Bone Joint Surg. **55-A**:795, 1973.
5. Brodersen, M.P., Fitzgerald, R.H., Peterson, L.F.A., Coventry, M.B., and Bryan, R.S.: Arthrodesis of the Knee following Failed Total Knee Arthroplasty. J. Bone Joint Surg. **61-A**:181, 1979.
6. Buchholz, H.W., Elson, R.A., Engelbrecht, E., Lodenkamper, H., Rottger, J., and Siegel, A.: Management of Deep Infection of Total Hip Replacement. J. Bone Joint Surg. **63**:342, 1981.
7. Canner, G.C., Steinberg, M.E., Heppenstall, R.B., and Balderston, R.: The Infected Hip after Total Hip Arthroplasty. J. Bone Joint Surg. **66-A**:1393, 1984.
8. Charnley, J., and Eftekhar, N.S.: Postoperative Infection and Total Hip Prosthetic Replacement Arthroplasty of the Hip Joint with Reference to the Bacterial Content of the Area of the Operating Room. Br. Med. J. **56**:641, 1969.
9. Compere, E.L.: Treatment of Osteomyelitis and Infected Wounds by Closed Irrigation with a Detergent-Antibiotic Solution. Acta Orthop. Scand. **32**:324, 1962.
10. Elek, S.D., and Conen, P.E.: The Virulence of Staph. Pyogenes for Man. A Study of Problems of Wound Infection. Br. J. Exp. Pathol. **38**:573, 1957.
11. Fitzgerald, R.H., and Jones, D.R.: Hip Implant Infection. Treatment with Resection Arthroplasty and Late Total Hip Arthroplasty. Am. J. Med. **78**(Suppl. 6B):225, 1985.
12. Grogran, T.J., Dorey, F., Rollins, J., and Amstutz, H.C.: Deep Sepsis following Total Knee Arthroplasty. Ten-Year Experience at the University of California at Los Angeles Medical Center. J. Bone Joint Surg. **68-A**:226, 1986.
13. Gustilo, R.B.: Management of Infected Fractures. AAOS Instr. Course Lect. **XXXI**:18, 1982.
14. Harris, W.H.: One-staged Exchange Arthroplasty for Septic Total Hip Replacement. AAOS Instr. Course Lect. **XXXV**:226, 1986.
15. Hunter, G.A.: Natural History of the Patient with an Infected Total Hip Replacement. AAOS Instr. Course Lect. **XXXI**:38, 1982.
16. Insall, J.N.: Infection of Total Knee Arthroplasty. AAOS Instr. Course Lect. **XXXV**:319, 1986.
17. Johnson, D.P., and Bannister, G.C.: The Outcome of Infected Arthroplasty of the Knee. J. Bone Joint Surg. **68-B**:289, 1986.
18. Kaufer, H., and Matthews, L.S.: Resection Arthroplasty: An Alternative to Arthrodesis for Salvage of the Infected Total Knee Arthroplasty. AAOS Instr. Course Lect. **XXXV**:283, 1986.
19. Knutson, K., Lindstrand, A., and Lidgren, L.: Arthrodesis for Failed Knee Arthroplasty. A Report of 20 Cases. J. Bone Joint Surg. **67-B**:47, 1985.

20. Leach, R.E., Hoaglund, E.T., and Rerzborough, E.J.: Controversies in Orthopaedic Surgery. Philadelphia, W.B. Saunders, 1982.

21. MacAusland, W.R.: Treatment of Sepsis after Intramedullary Nailing of Fractures of Femur. Clin. Orthop. **60**:87, 1968.

22. McElwaine, J.P., and Colville, J.: Excision Arthroplasty for Infected Total Hip Replacements. J. Bone Joint Surg. **66-B:**168, 1984.

23. Moore, A.T.: The Moore Self-locking Vitallium Prosthesis in Fresh Femoral Neck Fractures. A New Low Posterior Approach (The Southern Exposure). AAOS Instr. Course Lect. **XVI:**688, 1959.

24. Murray, W.R.: Treatment of the Infected Total Hip Arthroplasty. AAOS Instr. Course Lect. **XXXV:**229, 1986.

25. Nelson, C.L., Evarts, C.M., Andrish, J., and Marks, K.: Results of Infected Total Hip Replacement Arthroplasty. Clin. Orthop. **147:**258, 1980.

26. Papineau, L.J., Alfageme, A., Dalcourt, J.P., and Pilon, L.: Osteomyelite Chronique: Excision et Greffe de Spongieux a l'Air Libre Apres Mises a Plat Extensives. Int. Orthop. **3:**165, 1979.

27. Petty, W., Brian, R.S., Coventry, M.B., and Peterson, L.F.A.: Infection After Total Knee Arthroplasty. Orthop. Clin. North Am. **6:**1005–1014, 1975.

28. Rand, J.A.: Knee Arthrodesis. AAOS Instr. Course Lect. **XXXV:**325, 1986.

29. Rand, J.A., and Bryan, R.S.: Reimplantation for the Salvage of an Infected Total Knee Arthroplasty. J. Bone Joint Surg. **65-A:**1081, 1983.

30. Rand, J.A., Bryan, R.S., Morrey, B.F., and Westholm, F.: Management of Infected Total Knee Arthroplasty. Clin. Orthop. **205:**75, 1986.

31. Rand, J.A., Peterson, L.F.A., Bryan, R.S., and Ilstrup, D.M.: Revision Total Knee Arthroplasty. AAOS Instr. Course Lect. **XXXV:**305, 1986.

32. Rhinelander, F.W., Nelson, C.L., Stewart, R.D., and Stewart, C.L.: Experimental Reaming of the Proximal Femur and Acrylic Cement Implantation: Vascular and Histologic Effects. *In* The Hip: Proceedings of the Seventh Open Scientific Meeting of the Hip Society. St. Louis, C.V. Mosby, 1979.

33. Salvati, E.S., Callaghan, J.J., and Brause, B.D.: Prosthetic Reimplantation for Salvage of the Infected Hip. AAOS Instr. Course Lect. **XXXV:**234, 1986.

34. Thompson, F.R.: Indications and Contraindication for the Early Use of an Intramedullary Hip Prosthesis. Clin. Orthop. **6:**690, 1955.

35. Venable, C.S., Stuck, W.G., and Beach, A.: The Effects on Bone of the Presence of Metals: Based upon Electrolysis. An Experimental Study. Ann. Surg. **105:**917, 1937.

36. Woods, C.W., Lionberger, D.R., and Tullos, H.S.: Failed Total Knee Arthroplasty. Clin. Orthop. **173:**184, 1983.

PART VIII

Tumors

CHAPTER 69

Clinical Evaluation, Biopsy, and Staging of Bone Tumors

THOMAS C. SHIVES

Although the literature is replete with information regarding tumors of bone, evaluation and management of these lesions remain somewhat troublesome. Diagnostic difficulties arise for several reasons. First, tumors of the skeleton are rare, accounting for only a small fraction of the benign and malignant lesions of the body. Benign primary bone tumors significantly outnumber malignant lesions, and primary malignant bone tumors are only approximately 1% as common as metastatic lesions of bone.[4] Therefore, few physicians encounter tumors of the skeletal system in sufficient numbers to feel comfortable in their evaluation and management. Second, the clinical presentation of these lesions is often insidious, making prompt recognition difficult. Third, the wide variety of radiographic and histologic presentations of bone tumors and nonneoplastic lesions that simulate bone tumors creates difficult diagnostic and therapeutic challenges.

Because no one individual can be well versed in all areas of the preoperative evaluation of these lesions, orthopaedic oncology demands a high degree of teamwork to arrive at a valid diagnosis and provide effective treatment. Many pitfalls can be avoided by combining the talents and expertise of a team of physicians which includes an orthopaedist, radiologist, pathologist, medical oncologist, and radiotherapist.

CLASSIFICATION

Neoplasms of bone may arise from essentially all of the cellular elements that normally constitute osseous and epiphyseal tissues (Table 69-1). A large number of lesions have been identified based on the cytology or the recognizable products of the proliferating cells.

In addition, lesions are further subdivided as to whether they are primary or secondary. A primary bone tumor is one that arises from one of the connective tissue elements found in osseous tissue. These lesions may be either benign or malignant. However, it should be remembered that a bone tumor may be heterogeneous, containing not only frankly malignant areas but also areas similar to those seen in benign lesions.

A secondary bone tumor is one that arises within a previously benign condition (e.g., enchondroma) or from a distant metastatic source. Inherent in this definition is the fact that secondary bone tumors are malignant.

Benign tumors are localized lesions that grow by expansion and direct extension but do not metastasize. However, they may be quite aggressive, causing extensive skeletal destruction and local invasion.

CLINICAL EVALUATION

In recent years, newer techniques in clinical assessment, diagnosis, surgery, reconstruction, and adjunctive medical and radiotherapeutic management have altered, to some extent, the traditional approach of prompt pathologic diagnosis followed by ablative surgery.

More emphasis is now placed on alternative combinations of surgery, radiation therapy, chemotherapy, and even immunotherapy. In order to select the best therapeutic approach, the lesion must be accurately assessed for not only its histologic

TABLE 69-1. CLASSIFICATION OF BONE TUMORS

Histologic Type	Type of Lesion	
	Benign	*Malignant*
Hematopoietic	——	Myeloma
		Lymphoma
Chondrogenic	Osteochondroma	Chondrosarcoma and variants
	Chondroma	
	Chondroblastoma	
	Chondromyxoid fibroma	
Osteogenic	Osteoid osteoma	Osteosarcoma and variants
	Osteoblastoma	
Unknown origin	Giant cell tumor	Malignant giant cell tumor
	(?) Fibrous histiocytoma	Ewing's tumor
		Adamantinoma
		(?) Malignant fibrous histiocytoma
Fibrogenic	Desmoplastic fibroma	Fibrosarcoma
Notochordal	——	Chordoma
Vascular	Hemangioma	Hemangioendotheliosarcoma
		Hemangiopericytoma

(Wold, L. E., Unni, K. K., and Dahlin, D. C.: Pathology and Classification. *In* Sim, F. H. (ed.): Diagnosis and Treatment of Bone Tumors: A Team Approach (A Mayo Clinic Monograph). Thorofare, NJ, Charles B. Slack, 1983.)

type but also its degree of aggressiveness, its precise anatomic setting, and the presence or absence of metastasis. Because open biopsy may significantly distort interpretation of CT scans, isotope scans, and other diagnostic images, these parameters should be evaluated before biopsy.

The clinical evaluation of patients with known or suspected bone tumors may be divided into four phases. First is the discovery phase, when the bone tumor is found; second is the diagnostic phase, in which all of the relative diagnoses are considered and a differential diagnosis is formulated; third is the planning phase, in which preoperative evaluations are performed; and fourth is the actual biopsy, the final step in obtaining a definitive diagnosis.

Discovery Phase

As noted, one of the difficulties in diagnosing bone tumors is their rarity. However, most physicians should be able to assess the patient and find the lesion. Generally, the patient's medical history is of limited diagnostic value. However, a past history of treatment for a carcinoma should increase the index of suspicion in a patient with suspected skeletal abnormalities. Most patients with primary bone tumors present with pain which is characteristically described as deep, boring or, aching, and of a constant nature, sometimes accentuated at night. The hallmark of tumor-related pain is that it is usually progressive. It is not uncommon for a patient to experience an injury at the site of a previously unsuspected tumor and then seek medical attention because of the injury. If a patient is sufficiently symptomatic to seek medical attention, then the site in question should certainly be examined. Occasionally, a bone tumor may remain essentially asymptomatic until fracture occurs through the lesion. Fractures resulting from insignificant trauma should be considered pathologic until proven otherwise.

In addition, one must keep in mind the patterns of referred pain, because discomfort is sometimes referred to a site remote from the actual tumor. This is especially true with lesions in the region of the hip joint, which may cause pain referred to the knee. It is always necessary to maintain a high index of suspicion and to proceed with prompt and complete medical investigation of the patient with persistent pain in an extremity.

Systemic inquiry should be made during the discovery phase to detect symptoms indicative of infection, lymphoma, or leukemia, or symptoms of another organ system that might suggest metastases.

Physical findings are rarely diagnostic. The presence of a soft tissue mass suggests an aggressive lesion. Large bone lesions may be accompanied by increased skin temperature, dilated superficial veins, or a sympathetic effusion in a neighboring joint.

Diagnostic Phase

Once a bone lesion has been found, the next task is to focus on the diagnostic possibilities. Usually, a reasonable differential diagnosis can be established based on the radiographic appearance of the lesion and the patient's history. However, it is important to recognize that certain conditions of bone may simulate true neoplastic disease, benign or malignant. While the mistaken identity of the underlying pathologic process may, on one hand, result in a delay of appropriate treatment, it may also result in tragic amputation of a limb for benign disease. The attending physicians must therefore be aware of the reactive, traumatic, infectious, and other conditions of bone that may simulate neoplasia. Typical examples include osteomyelitis mistaken for Ewing's sarcoma, hyperparathyroidism misdiagnosed as giant cell tumor, and myositis ossificans misinterpreted as osteosarcoma.

A number of factors may be of help in arriving at a reasonable differential diagnosis of a suspected bone tumor. The age of the patient is probably the most important clinical piece of information in formulating a differential diagnosis (Fig. 69-1).

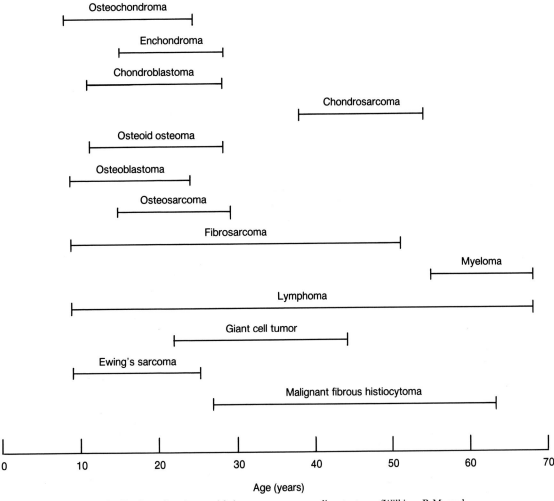

FIGURE 69-1.   Age distribution of patients with bone tumors according to type. (Wilkins, R.M, and Sim, F.H.: Evaluation of Bone and Soft Tissue Tumors. *In* D'Ambrosia R.D. (ed.): Musculoskeletal Disorders. Philadelphia, J. B. Lippincott, 1986.)

Elderly patients are prone to develop metastatic cancer or myeloma. Lesions in young children are most likely to represent primary tumors. Chondrosarcomas and fibrosarcomas tend to occur in older individuals, whereas osteosarcoma and Ewing's sarcoma generally occur in childhood. Certain conditions are likely to be seen in certain age groups. For example, 80% of aneurysmal bone cysts and chondroblastomas, which may be confused with giant cell tumors, occur in patients who are younger than 20 years of age.[1]

The sex of the patient is usually not helpful. However, bone tumors are more common in males than in females, with the exception of giant cell tumor, which has a slight predilection for the female.[1]

The site of the lesion is another helpful parameter in the differential diagnosis in that certain lesions occur more commonly in a particular bone or a particular site within a bone. For example, giant cell tumors and chondroblastomas almost always occur in the epiphyseal region of the bone. Osteosarcoma is almost always metaphyseal in location with a peculiar tendency to extend to the physis without violating the epiphysis. Chondrosarcomas, aneurysmal bone cysts, osteochon-

dromas, osteoblastomas, and nonossifying fibromas are usually metaphyseal. Ewing's sarcoma and adamantinoma generally involve the diaphysis.

Enchondromas tend to occur in the small bones of the hands and feet, and most lesions of the hands and feet are benign. Conversely, tumors which involve the sternum have almost always been malignant in our experience. Multiple myeloma tends to spare the pedicles of the spine and involve the mandible, unlike metastatic carcinoma, in which the opposite is true.

Fundamental to the clinical evaluation of a suspected neoplasm are the screening radiographs. Despite the ever-increasing availability of new radiologic techniques, plain roentgenograms provide the basis for differential diagnosis, particularly when combined with the clinical factors already mentioned. Following initial radiologic screening, more information may be necessary. Tomograms may demonstrate more clearly the characteristics of the tumor and help to delineate its exact location and extent. Computed tomography (CT) may also be valuable in providing further information with regard to the intramedullary or extramedullary extent of the lesion. The role of angiography in evaluating neoplastic disease remains controversial; in the vast majority of cases, we have found it to be unnecessary and have been able to obtain the same information by ordering a CT scan with contrast material.

Information regarding the potential usefulness of magnetic resonance imaging (MRI) is relatively scarce but this modality is rapidly proving itself to be useful, particularly for lesions distal to the elbow or knee (Fig. 69-2). Technetium-99m bone scans are only occasionally of help in formulating a differential diagnosis; for example, an older patient with a destructive, malignant-appearing lesion of bone with a negative scan is likely to have myeloma. However, for most osseous neoplasms, the bone scan is helpful only in determining the extent of the disease.

Conventional serologic, biochemical, and immunologic laboratory studies have limited value in the diagnosis and staging of bone tumors. However, they may occasionally provide clues to an appropriate diagnosis. For example, if there is a destructive lesion in the end of a long bone, the serum calcium level may be elevated, suggesting the possibility of hyperparathyroidism. The sedimentation rate is nonspecific but may be elevated in the patient with marrow cell tumors such as Ewing's sarcoma, lymphoma, and myeloma as well as metastatic bone tumors. In a male older than 60 years of age, a normocytic, normochromic anemia and elevated sedimentation rate are suggestive of myeloma.

Preoperative Phase

Once the lesion has been found and the differential diagnosis has been formulated, a therapeutic plan should be devised. If it is clear that a biopsy is necessary and that subsequent surgery may be indicated based on the results of the biopsy, then detailed preoperative planning should be done. The major considerations are the location, extent, and nature of the tumor. It is important that the preoperative work-up be individualized.

Ordering every available test for each patient with a suspected neoplasm is not only uneconomical, but also wastes valuable time and effort. However, certain circumstances do warrant extensive tests before biopsy. If, for example, the lesion has radiographic features suggestive of a primary malignant bone tumor, it is wise to try to rule out systemic metastatic disease. In such an instance, a technetium bone scan may be useful and a CT scan of the chest may reveal occult metastatic disease that is not visible on a plain film of the chest. For neoplasms involving the pelvis, a CT scan of the pelvis is usually very useful. In addition, excretory urography, barium enema study, or proctoscopic examination may be necessary before biopsy and definitive therapy.

Biopsy

After having taken a careful history, performed a physical examination, and accomplished the initial staging on the basis of clinical and radiographic information, biopsy of the lesion is performed. Unfortunately, the importance of the biopsy is sometimes overlooked. It is not a simple surgical procedure that can be relegated to a junior member of the team. In 1982 Simon stated that "the biopsy is crucial to the treatment outcome of aggressive, benign, and malignant tumors."[5] Paramount to providing good surgical oncologic care is a thorough understanding of the principles of biopsy outlined below:

1. The placement of t e incision and the technique of execution must be done with a clear view of the subsequent incisions that may be required to accomplish definitive treatment. The correctly placed biopsy incision must allow for *en bloc* excision of a malignant tumor when a local surgical procedure or amputation is performed. *Always* avoid transverse incisions on an extremity.

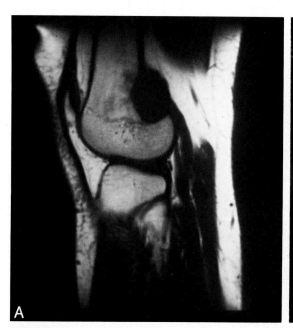
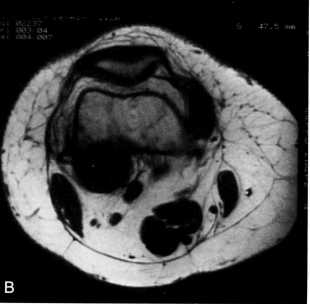

FIGURE 69-2.   MRI scan of an osteosarcoma of the distal femur taken in sagittal (*A*) and coronal (*B*) planes. Note the clear delineation of both the osseous and soft-tissue extent of the lesion.

2. If intraosseous biopsy is necessary, the cortical window should be round or oval. Stress-concentrating biopsy defects in load-bearing bones may initiate pathologic fractures and preclude possible limb salvage. Avoid the tension side of a bone wherever possible.

3. If possible, always biopsy the soft tissue rather than the osseous component of the lesion. At least 90% of bone tumors have soft portions that can be sectioned and examined for immediate diagnosis. In most cases, the soft portions afford the best material for diagnosis. The soft tissues usually contain the most rapidly growing area of the tumor and provide the pathologist with the most useful tissue for making a diagnosis.

4. Always use a separate set of instruments, gowns, gloves, and drapes when performing a biopsy procedure. This will help provide insurance against contamination of previously uninvolved tissues.

5. There are certain indications for needle and trochar biopsy, but in our experience these situations are uncommon. An inadequate or small sample of tissue may turn a difficult job into one of guesswork for the pathologist. In addition, it is well known that some tumors are not homogeneous and a small sample may easily lead to underinterpretation of the true character of the tumor.

6. The frozen-section technique of evaluation of the biopsy specimen has several advantages over conventional permanent-section techniques. First and foremost, it allows immediate appraisal of adequacy of the specimen for biopsy. Edematous tissue around the tumor, necrotic neoplastic tissue, or benign portions of the lesion with frankly malignant foci may otherwise be considered representative of the pathologic process. Second, if the lesion proves to be inflammatory, the surgeon is guided to proper bacteriologic studies. Third, frozen section allows immediate evaluation of the adequacy of resection or the level of amputation.

The importance of the biopsy technique and the complications associated with it have been documented by Mankin and colleagues[3] in an extensive analysis of cases provided by members of the Musculoskeletal Tumor Society. They commented on the results of misapplication of the principles of biopsy discussed above. The highlights of their article were as follows:

1. The incidence of significant problems in patient management caused by inappropriate biopsy technique is currently 20%.

2. The incidence of wound healing complications after biopsy is also 20%.

3. Eight percent of biopsies produced a significant adverse effect on prognosis.

4. Five percent of biopsies can cause or significantly contribute to an otherwise unnecessary amputation.

5. Errors in diagnosis leading to inadequate treatment occur twice as often when the biopsy is done in a community hospital prior to referral as opposed to when the biopsy is done after referral to an oncology center.

These authors concluded that if a surgeon or institution is not prepared to do accurate diagnostic studies and proceed with definitive surgical management, the outcome will be significantly enhanced by transfer to a referral center before biopsy rather than afterwards. This conclusion certainly agrees with our experience.

STAGING

One of the recent major advances in the management of tumors of the skeletal system has been the development of a useful staging system by Enneking and other members of the Musculoskeletal Tumor Society.[2] This staging system, shown in Table 69-2, is based on surgical site, either intracompartmental (A) or extracompartmental (B); and surgical grade, either low (I) or high (II). If there is evidence of metastasis, including regional lymph nodes, the disease is graded as Stage III. Thus, there are five stages: low-grade intracompartmental (IA); low-grade extracompartmental (IB); high-grade intracompartmental (IIA); high-grade extracompartmental (IIB); and metastatic

TABLE 69-2. SURGICAL STAGING SYSTEM OF THE MUSCULOSKELETAL TUMOR SOCIETY FOR BONE AND SOFT TISSUE TUMORS

Stage	Histologic Grade	Site	Metastasis
I			
A	Low (G_1)	Intracompartmental (T_1)	None (M_0)
B		Extracompartmental (T_2)	
II			
A	High (G_2)	Intracompartmental (T_1)	None (M_0)
B		Extracompartmental (T_2)	
III			
A	Low (G_1)	Either (T_1 or T_2)	Regional or distant (M_1)
B	High (G_2)		

(Enneking, W. F.: Musculoskeletal Tumor Surgery. New York, Churchill Livingstone, 1983.)

(III). For example, a low-grade chondrosarcoma confined to the medullary canal of the proximal humerus is a G_0, T_1, M_0 and hence, is a Stage IA lesion. A patient with an osteosarcoma of the distal femur that has broken out of the bone is a G_2, T_2, M_0 lesion that is therefore designated Stage IIB. If, in the same patient, there is evidence of pulmonary metastasis, the condition is designated G_2, T_2, M_1 and is a Stage III lesion.

The staging system is simple in application and useful in assessing prognosis, choosing treatment protocols, and enhancing communication among clinicians and investigators from different institutions. Its use is becoming widespread and should be encouraged.

REFERENCES

1. Dahlin, D.C.: Bone Tumors: General Aspects and Data on 6,221 Cases. Springfield, IL, Charles C. Thomas, 1978.
2. Enneking, W.F., Spannier, S.S., and Goodman, M.A.: A System for the Surgical Staging of Musculoskeletal Sarcoma. Clin. Orthop. **153:**106, 1980.
3. Mankin, H.J., Lange, T.A., and Spannier, S.S.: The Hazards of Biopsy in Patients with Malignant Primary Bone and Soft Tissue Tumors. J. Bone Joint Surg. **64-A:**1121, 1982.
4. Silverberg, E.: Cancer Statistics. Cancer **34:**7, 1984.
5. Simon, M.A.: Biopsy of Musculoskeletal Tumors. J. Bone Joint Surg. **64-A:**1253, 1982.

CHAPTER 70

Principles of Limb Salvage Surgery

JAMES O. JOHNSTON

The concept of limb-sparing procedures in managing primary bone tumors of the extremities is not new. The first orthopaedists to explore these techniques—in the 1930s—included Lexer,[4] Meyerding,[5] and Phemister.[6] Most of the tumors treated by these pioneers were low-grade lesions such as giant cell tumors, fibromas, and chondrosarcomas. Limb-sparing procedures consisted primarily of massive bone grafts to replace the defect created by wide local resection. Smaller grafts were harvested from the patient if possible or from cadaver skeletons if large grafts were needed. Some of these large allografts replaced major joint surfaces, especially those about the knee. Prosthetic implants were not available at that time; as a result, many tumors about a major joint were managed by a technique of excisional arthrodesis still used today.

Two events in the last 20 years dramatically changed our approach to managing extremity tumors. First came the technology of total joint implantation using bone cement. Shortly thereafter came adjuvant chemotherapy for systemic management of high-grade sarcomas such as round cell tumors and osteosarcoma. With these major breakthroughs, the stage was set for limb salvage procedures for a wider range of tumors, even high-grade (Stage II) tumors such as osteosarcoma. Before 1970, it was standard to amputate limbs afflicted with osteosarcoma, and patients nevertheless faced a grim 25% chance of survival. Today, with the use of adjuvant chemotherapy, most large treatment centers recommend limb salvage procedures which give patients a 75% chance of surviving their disease.

Indications for Various Types of Limb Salvage Procedures

Allografts

Allografts are large, whole-bone grafts (including joints and ligaments) that are stored in large tissue banks which are expensive to maintain. In general, these large grafts are used for management of younger patients with low-grade tumors that do not require adjuvant irradiation or chemotherapy. The procedure allows a favorable prognosis: patients can be expected to live many years at a fairly high activity level. The complication rate during the first 2 years after an allograft is quite high; infection, delayed union, and repeated stress fractures commonly occur. However, patients who survive longer than 2 years tend to improve over time as the host bone gradually incorporates and strengthens the dead bone. This procedure is discussed more completely in Chapter 71.

Prostheses

By far the most commonly used techniques for limb salvage involve prosthetic joint replacement. At first, orthopaedic oncologists had to adapt the early joint-replacement prostheses designed primarily for older patients with arthritis. Problems arose when larger amounts of juxta-articular bone were resected with the tumor or when these devices were placed in younger patients who had higher activity levels. For this reason, many tumor surgeons advanced to larger and stronger customized implants with stronger intramedullary stems. Recently, porous surfaces have been incorporated to help decrease the chance of later loosening. The problem with custom implants is the time required to design and fabricate the implant (frequently as long as 4 weeks). Another problem is the considerable expense involved, especially now that increasing financial constraints are being placed on the medical community.

A recent trend—and outlook for the future—lies in modular-design prostheses such as the system shown in Figure 70-1.[2] This is a commercial system designed for tumors about the knee and hip, which comprise about 80% of extremity tumors. The standard knee joint used is a modified rotating hinge; a bipolar device for the hip has the option of being converted to a total hip if indicated. A series of titanium pipe spacers 25 mm wide and 75 mm to 150 mm long connect the joint implant to a variety of intramedullary stems ranging from 10 mm to 16 mm in diameter (see Fig. 70-1A, right). In the operating room, after choosing the proper resection level for a given tumor, the surgeon can simply ask the nurse for the appropriate pipe length and stem diameters from off-the-shelf sterile packaged components. The surgeon can then assemble the components by means of secure Morse taper fittings and place the implant into the limb, thus avoiding the complexity, time loss, and expense of a custom implant. Surgeons can also opt to make semicustomized implants by modifying the stem design or applying porous or hydroxyapatite surfaces to the components.

Figure 70-1B shows the most commonly assembled modular system, which uses a 5-inch-long pipe for a tumor resection that requires removing 8 inches of the distal end of the femur. With this system, the surgeon can even link the knee unit with the hip system so as to construct a total femur. A recent advance in prosthetic design has been the adaptation of an expandable implant for use in children younger than 13 years of age.

In contrast to the allografts discussed above, a prosthesis is easy to implant and gives excellent function immediately and for the first 2 years. However, late complications in the form of mechanical breakdown and stem loosening do occur, especially in younger patients with high activity levels and long survival potential.

Excisional Arthrodesis

Compared with the newer prosthetic implants used for tumors about a major joint, excisional arthrodesis has stood the test of time for nearly half a century. The technique is difficult, however, because of the large amount of bone sacrificed in removing a tumor with safe margins. Large amounts of allograft are required along with heavy metallic fixation devices to hold the joint until union occurs, over a period of nearly a year or more. As with large allografts, early complications of excisional arthrodesis—infection, skin breakdown, and failure of fusion—are common. However, once a solid union is established, the patient has a strong leg that can tolerate higher levels of stress and over longer periods of time than a prosthetic joint.

For these reasons, excisional arthrodesis should be reserved for younger patients with low-grade tumors that do not require adjuvant irradiation or chemotherapy. Excisional arthrodesis is well suited in patients with heavily physical occupations or in uncooperative patients who might not restrict their activities with a prosthetic joint. In any case, the surgeon must be aware of the functional demands expected of the salvaged limb before making a final decision with the patient.

Vascularized Bone Grafts

Some institutions have been adapting new microvascular technologies for use in limb salvage. The fibula, used most commonly in these procedures, provides suitable graft material in cases of diaphyseal tumors where the joint above and below can be preserved. Use of the fibula is also appropriate in cases where postoperative irradiation or chemotherapy is not required. One problem, however, is the small size of the fibula as compared with the shaft size of the femur, humerus, or tibia which the fibula frequently replaces. For this reason, fibular bone is frequently augmented with adjacent struts of dead allograft and metal side-plates. The major advantages are that the viable graft can heal itself in the event of fracture and can tolerate infection better than can dead bone. Vascularized bone grafts are discussed further in Chapter 79.

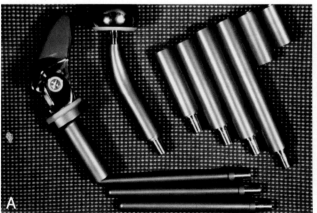 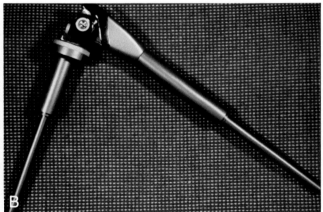

FIGURE 70-1. (A) Modular system designed for resection of tumors about the hip and knee uses various lengths of 1-inch-diameter titanium pipe and a variety of intramedullary stems. (B) Assembled unit which I designed and built for resection of tumor in distal femur.

Combined Techniques

The tumor surgeon must have wide knowledge and expertise in the field of limb salvage to adapt or combine the techniques discussed above. Perhaps the best application of combined systems is the use of diaphyseal allografts placed over long-stemmed prostheses in the hip and shoulder area. This combination eliminates the severe joint surface degeneration related to breakdown of cartilage in large joint allografts. At the same time, it gives excellent intramedullary strength to the diaphyseal allograft during the first 2 years, when delayed union and stress fractures are major concerns.

Contraindications to Salvage

In order to justify a limb-sparing procedure, the surgeon must be reasonably sure that the local recurrence rate is no greater than that with ablative surgery (i.e., <10%). At the same time, the surgeon must feel secure that patient survival will not be influenced by attempts to save the limb. Large comparative studies have already suggested that limb-sparing procedures are safe.[1,3] Furthermore, the function of the spared limb should be superior to that of an artificial limb. With these thoughts in mind, there are several situations in which it is probably best to amputate the limb and not attempt a salvage procedure.

Neurovascular Involvement

Most surgeons are reluctant to attempt limb salvage if there is a major involvement of the significant neurovascular structures of the affected limb. In the case of the leg, the major concern is with the femoral artery and the sciatic nerve. If the sciatic nerve must be sacrificed to obtain safe margins, amputation is probably advisable. In the case of femoral artery involvement, a vein graft could be considered; however, this further complicates a difficult procedure and introduces a high risk of failure, especially if postoperative irradiation or chemotherapy is needed.

Pathologic Fracture

In the case of low-grade lesions such as giant cell tumors, pathologic fracture is not a serious concern. However, with high-grade tumors such as osteosarcoma, widespread contamination of the entire fracture hematoma area is a major problem. In the case of the femur, the tumor-contaminated hematoma affects all of the surrounding thigh muscle compartments.

Infection

Infection is not usually a problem before a patient is considered for limb salvage. However, infection may occur occasionally after initial biopsy or perhaps after an early attempt at marginal resection. This unfortunate complication virtually precludes attempts to place large allografts or prosthetic implants. The surgeon may consider waiting for the infection to clear and then attempt a major procedure at a later date.

Improper Biopsy Technique

Inexperienced surgeons sometimes make biopsy incisions in compromising areas that severely decrease the chances of a successful limb salvage procedure. For example, biopsy of a high-grade lesion in the femur through a posterior or medial approach could result in contamination of the sciatic nerve or femoral artery by the biopsy hematoma.

Another problem with biopsy technique occurs when the initial surgeon performs a marginal excisional biopsy of an apparently benign lesion through a large incision: several adjacent compartments may become contaminated and thus negate the chances for limb salvage.

Even the placement of a transverse biopsy incision can make removal of the entire biopsy scar difficult during longitudinal exposure for massive wide local resection and limb salvage reconstruction.

Extensive Skin Involvement

With most bone tumors, skin integrity is not a problem unless surgery was previously done or the tumor involves subcutaneous bone, as in the proximal end of the tibia. In the case of soft tissue tumors, however, skin involvement can be a more frequent problem.

If the surgeon attempts to resect a large amount of contaminated skin requiring a skin grafting procedure, serious wound healing problems result—especially if the skin graft is to cover a large allograft or prosthesis. Skin grafting is particularly risky in high-grade lesions requiring adjuvant irradiation or chemotherapy.

Principles of Surgical Technique by Region

Distal Femur

The most common area for primary tumors of bone is the distal end of the femur. For low-grade tumors such as a Stage IA or IB chondrosarcoma in young, active adults who have a favorable prognosis for living another 20 to 40 years, an ideal procedure would be excisional arthrodesis (Fig. 70-2). The radiographic appearance of primary chondrosarcoma in the lateral femoral condyle is shown in Figure 70-2A. This Stage IB lesion has minimal breakthrough into soft tissue, which makes it suitable for a limb salvage procedure. Figure 70-2B shows the resected specimen, including the entire knee joint and a 1-inch safety margin at transfemoral resection. Figure 70-2C shows the sharp interface of a typical chondrosarcoma and its surrounding metaphyseal bone. After resection, the surgeon must take care not to leave any satellite lesions in the surrounding soft tissue which could result in local recurrence. A strong and solid intramedullary nail is placed across the knee area (see Fig. 70-2D). The patella and portions of the proximal tibia can be used to help fill the void left by the tumor resection. Additional bone can be obtained from the pelvis—being careful not to cross-contaminate—or freeze-dried allograft can supplement the autograft.

For the past decade, the more common approach to limb salvage in cases of high-grade sarcoma has been the use of

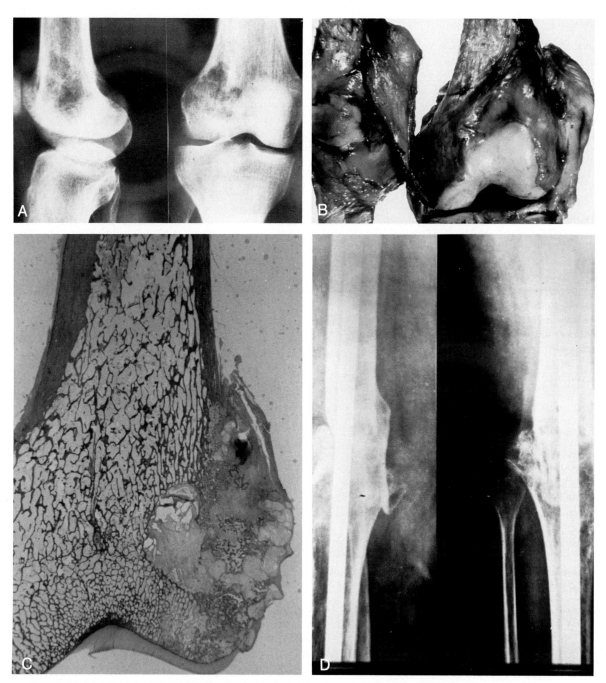

FIGURE 70-2. (*A*) Radiographic appearance of Stage IB primary chondrosarcoma in a 35-year-old man. (*B*) Photograph of resected specimen, including entire knee joint and cuff of normal soft tissue surrounding extraosseous portion of tumor. (*C*) Gross sagittal section of resected distal femur demonstrates safe bony margins around eccentrically located cartilage tumor. (*D*) Postoperative radiograph taken after successful excisional arthrodesis using large intramedullary nail.

custom-design or semicustom modular systems to replace the defect left after massive *en bloc* resection of the distal femur. Figure 70-3 illustrates a typical high-grade (Stage IIB) osteosarcoma in the distal femur of a 19-year-old woman. Figures 70-3*A* and 70-3*B* show the radiographic appearance of this lesion, which has a moderate amount of breakthrough into the popliteal space. The resection margin is therefore very close to the popliteal artery, which must be carefully dissected away

from the posterior margin of the tumor. Figure 70-3*C* shows the technetium-99 isotope study of the tumor that helps determine the upper pole of the tumor's bony extent. In high-grade lesions, at least 2 inches of clear margin should be obtained at this upper pole. If a skip metastasis in the upper femur were noted on the isotope study, a better choice of treatment would be hip disarticulation or total femoral replacement. Figure 70-3*D* shows a well-placed 1-inch vertical biopsy site in an anterolateral position that allows easy resection with 7 inches of the distal end of the femur, including the proximal tibial plateau. Figure 70-3D shows the resected specimen, with forceps marking the biopsy site. Figure 70-3E shows the sagittal section of the same specimen. In most cases such as this one, the tumor does not directly invade the knee joint; the patellar tendon, quadriceps tendon, and retinaculum over the front of the knee can therefore be preserved for better function. The remaining joint ligaments and posterior capsule should be transected as far distally as possible at the level of the tibial plateau. In this case, the off-the-shelf modular system used was similar to that shown in Figure 70-1B. This implant was designed and constructed in the operating room at the time of resection. Figure 70-3G shows the implanted device prior to wound closure; the radiographic appearance is shown in Figure 70-3H. Nearly all patients with high-grade sarcomas are placed on adjuvant chemotherapy such as the T-10 high-dosage methotrexate protocol advocated by Rosen and colleagues.[7]

Proximal Tibia

As mentioned above, the indications for limb-sparing procedures involving tumors of the proximal tibia are limited because of anatomic difficulties. The proximal end of the tibia has minimal muscle cover, which creates problems with wound closure and healing over a large allograft or prosthesis. A second anatomic problem is discovered when attempting to reconstruct the quadriceps insertion mechanism below the knee. Surgeons periodically find that patients with proximal tibial limb salvage have greater functional limitations than do patients treated by simple supracondylar amputation and a suction-socket prosthetic limb.

Patients commonly refuse amputation for reasons that are not scientific or logical. As with the distal end of the femur, excisional arthrodesis might be the preferred procedure, especially in young patients with good chances for long survival. For older patients with high-grade lesions, however, the surgeon might elect a prosthetic implant. Figure 70-4 shows a 60-year-old patient with a Stage IIB malignant fibrous histiocytoma located in the proximal tibial metaphysis. Figure 70-4A shows the radiographic appearance with complete, diffuse infiltration of the proximal 4 inches of the tibia.

Figure 70-4B shows the technique of combining a large allograft with the 12-inch tibial component of a spherocentric knee, which allows the surgeon to suture the patellar tendon down onto the allograft. The illustration shows the heavy wires positioned in the graft prior to cementing back intothe leg; Figure 70-4C shows the final position with the tendon secured. Figure 70-4D shows the retinacular structures sutured over the exposed allograft. The postoperative radiographic appearance is shown in Figure 70-4E. Because of the high-grade nature of this tumor, the patient received 5500 rads of irradiation starting 2 weeks after surgery to reduce chances of local recurrence to about 10%.

Distal Tibia

Primary tumors of the distal end of the tibia are rare and are usually low-grade lesions. In high-grade sarcomas of the lower end of the tibia, most authorities advocate ablative surgery—ei-ther at or just below the knee—which leaves the patient with a very functional limb with greater function than provided by most procedures for limb salvage. However, in the case of a low-grade sarcoma such as adamantinoma, attempted limb salvage might be worth considering. No standard prosthesis about the ankle area has stood the test of time, and the surgeon must for this reason rely on massive bone grafts with or without ankle fusion, depending on the exact location of the distal tibial tumor.

Figure 70-5 shows a typical low-grade sarcoma in the distal end of the tibia, treated with limb salvage technique. Figure 70-5A is a radiograph of an adamantinoma in the distal tibial diaphysis of a 25-year-old man. The lesion was resected widely by segmental removal with the lower cut coming very close to the ankle joint but sparing it. Figure 70-5B shows the tumor opened to check margins. A diaphyseal allograft was then placed into the surgical defect and fixed into position with an intramedullary rod. The adjacent fibula was synostosed to the allograft in a stepladder fashion, with large amounts of autograft taken from the iliac crest. The final result 5 years later (see Fig. 70-5C) was excellent incorporation of the grafts and nearly normal ankle function. The tumor did not recur and the patient had nearly normal function of the leg.

Proximal Femur

Second only to the distal end of the femur, the proximal end of the femur is a common site for limb salvage. A fair number of primary tumors are seen in this area, as well as metastatic tumors (see Chap. 74) which frequently lead to pathologic fractures. The functional advantage of limb salvage in the proximal femoral area is apparent when problems related to hip disarticulation are considered along with the poor functional control of artificial limbs after ablative surgery. Another major advantage of proximal femoral limb salvage is the availability of advanced total hip replacement technology, which lends itself well to massive bone resection from the hip area. Furthermore, the operating surgeon can usually find good muscle flaps to close over the prosthetic device, thus reducing the chances of wound breakdown and infection common in the proximal tibia.

As with the knee, excisional arthrodesis is a time-proven technique for limb salvage in cases of low-grade tumors that are close to the acetabulum and do not require postoperative irradiation therapy. Figure 70-6 illustrates this technique as applied to a 40-year-old patient who had a low-grade central fibrosarcoma in the femoral head and neck. Figure 70-6A shows the preoperative radiographic appearance of the tumor. A macroscopic photomicrograph (Fig. 70-6B) shows the upper end of the femur fused to the lower acetabular lip; extra support comes from a fibular strut placed laterally with loose cancellous autograft from the ipsilateral ilium. The leg is held in moderate abduction in a spica cast until fusion is solid. Internal stabilization can be increased by cobra plates or even curved intramedullary Schneider nails placed down through the ilium into the femoral canal.

A second example of proximal femur limb salvage involves a 30-year-old female patient with a high-grade malignant fibrous histiocytoma at the lesser trochanteric level (Fig. 70-7). This condition can complicate excisional arthrodesis: in younger

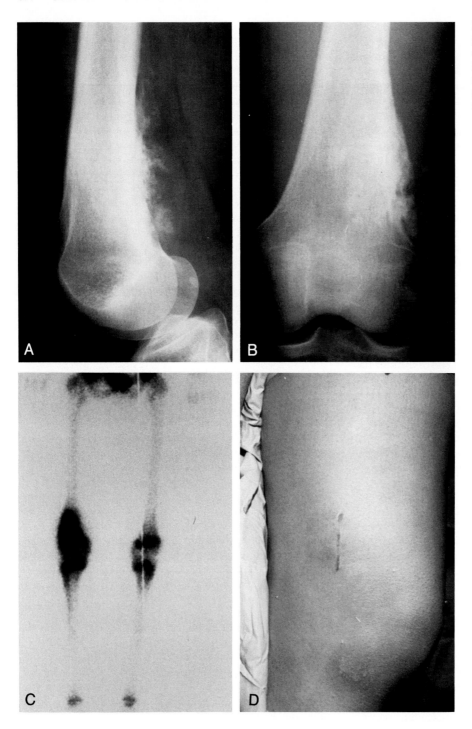

FIGURE 70-3. (*A*) Lateral and (*B*) antero-posterior radiographs show typical osteosar-coma of distal femur in a 19-year-old female. (*C*) Isotope study was done to help delineate the proximal extent of the tumor. (*D*) Photo-graph of well-planned preoperative biopsy site.

patients, massive bone resection as well as postoperative irra-diation and chemotherapy are required for treating high-grade lesions. Figure 70-7*A* shows the preoperative radiographic ap-pearance of the tumor. Figure 70-7*B* shows the resected proxi-mal 7 inches of femur with a wide cuff of normal muscle and the entire biopsy-skin ellipse marked with a hemostat. This resection was performed 4 weeks after biopsy using an exten-sive posterolateral approach to reduce the chances of invading the biopsy hematoma. Figure 70-7*C* shows the tumor in the resected femoral fragment with a 4-cm safety margin at the

lower edge of the tumor. A long, titanium bipolar prosthesis for calcar replacement was selected to replace the defect (see Fig. 70-7*D*). In this case, the entire joint capsule was retained for postoperative stability. Further stability is given by closing the iliotibial band and abductor–vastus complex over and into the fenestrated portion of the prosthesis so as to maintain active control of hip abduction and rotation. Figure 70-7*E* is a photograph taken during closure of the deep muscle and fascia just before placement of strong number 2 sutures; Figure 70-7*F* shows the postoperative radiographic appearance. Addi-

(*E*) Photograph of resected specimen, including entire biopsy site. (*F*) Sagittal section of distal 7 inches of resected femur with 2-inch safety margin at upper pole of the tumor. (*G*) Photograph of modular-design titanium implant prior to closure. (*H*) Postoperative radiographic appearance of the prosthesis in position.

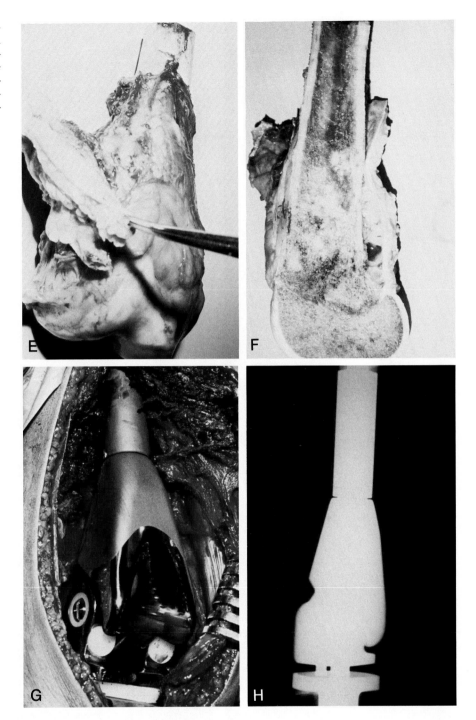

tional stability can be obtained by using porous surfaces near the point of femoral shaft attachment augmented by autogenous bone graft.

Pitfalls and Complications.   Two cases will be used to demonstrate some of the potential problems encountered with proximal femoral resection. The first case involves the problem of pathologic fractures occurring through a primary sarcoma prior to attempted limb salvage. In this unfortunate situation, the fracture creates a large fracture hematoma similar to a biopsy hematoma and spreads tumor cells into all adjacent compartments, making a safe wide local resection more difficult. For this reason, I usually advise hip disarticulation. In the patient shown in Figure 70-8, however, the patient refused ablative surgery and insisted on limb salvage despite the risk of local recurrence. The usual approach in this situation is to place the leg in tibial pin traction for about 6 weeks to allow healing of soft tissue around the fracture hematoma and thereby facilitate wide local resection. Figure 70-8*B* shows the resected fracture complex, including biopsy site. The im-

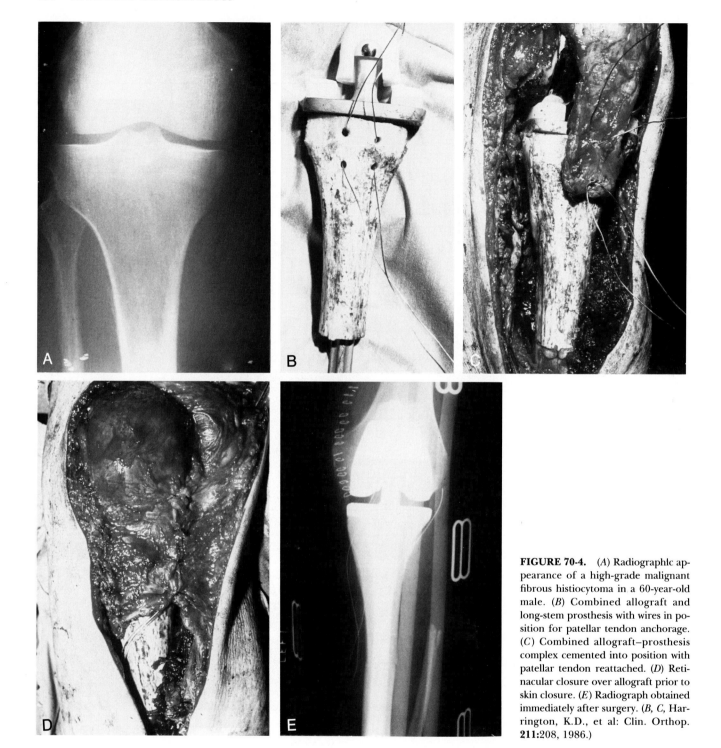

FIGURE 70-4. (*A*) Radiographic appearance of a high-grade malignant fibrous histiocytoma in a 60-year-old male. (*B*) Combined allograft and long-stem prosthesis with wires in position for patellar tendon anchorage. (*C*) Combined allograft–prosthesis complex cemented into position with patellar tendon reattached. (*D*) Retinacular closure over allograft prior to skin closure. (*E*) Radiograph obtained immediately after surgery. (*B, C,* Harrington, K.D., et al: Clin. Orthop. **211**:208, 1986.)

planted bipolar prosthesis with a porous-coated 8-inch-long calcar replacement is shown in Figure 70-8C. Because of the high risk of local recurrence in high-grade malignant fibrous histiocytoma, postoperative irradiation and chemotherapy were used. Local recurrence did not develop; however, liver and pulmonary metastases resulted in death 1 year later for this 35-year-old man.

The major concern about late complications with large prosthetic implants is related to stem loosening and stem-related fracture. Figure 70-9 illustrates a patient for whom wide local resection was performed and a large, bipolar prosthesis was used for calcar replacement. During the intramedullary broaching technique, the area from distal femur down to the supracondylar area exploded into ten large bone fragments.

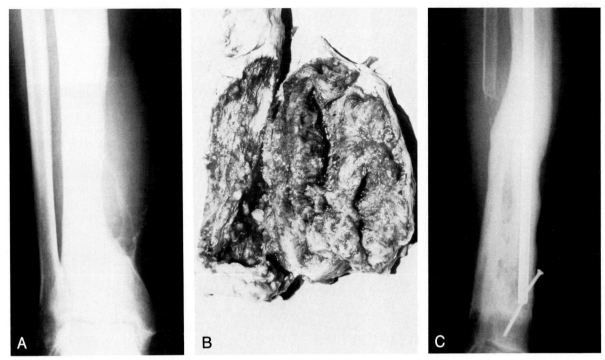

FIGURE 70-5. (*A*) Radiograph shows adamantinoma of the distal tibia in a young man. (*B*) Gross appearance of tumor after successful segmental limb salvage resection. (*C*) Radiograph taken five years after surgery shows well-incorporated allograft supplemented with autograft.

Immediate amputation was considered; instead, however, the fracture was reconstructed around the prosthetic stem and cement, and a combination of circumferential bands and a long blade plate with the fixation screws were placed tangentially around the titanium stem.

Midshaft of Femur

Primary bone tumors are not commonly found at the midshaft of a long bone. However, if this does occur—especially with low-grade sarcoma such as chondrosarcoma or parosteal osteogenic sarcoma—an ideal opportunity is provided for limb salvage using segmental resection. This type of limb salvage is perhaps the most ideal because it preserves the major joints at either end of the involved long bone and therefore allows excellent function over a long span of time. In order for the patient to qualify for this technique, the surgeon must develop safe margins of 1 inch to 2 inches on either side of the resected specimen and still have 3 inches of remaining normal medullary space on either side to gain secure fixation with either a cemented intramedullary nail or a strong side-plate. I prefer the large, solid, intramedullary Schneider nail (instead of side-plates) because of the reduced chances for fatigue fracture in the hardware. The diaphyseal defect can be filled by placing an allograft over the intramedullary nail as a length-maintaining spacer. Alternatively, if the original bone has not been damaged too badly by the tumor, the surgeon can simply autoclave the resected specimen for 5 minutes, place it back into the defect over the nail, and augment the fixation with bone cement. The upper and lower juncture points should be rein-

forced with autogenous cancellous bone. Over a period of 2 years, new bone will grow as a reactive involucrum over and into the allograft and give long-lasting stability and excellent function.

One illustration of this technique is seen in Figure 70-10. This 13-year-old boy had a parosteal osteogenic sarcoma at the midshaft of the femur (Fig. 70-10*A*). The middle third of the femur was segmentally resected; a wide margin of normal muscle tissue was included. The tumor was debulked on a separate table, and the bone was autoclaved for 5 minutes. A 15-mm solid Schneider nail was placed through the autoclaved segment and secured into the neighboring segments of remaining viable femur as might be done in a segmental femoral fracture. Figure 70-10*B* shows the autoclaved segment returned to the thigh and ready for additional cancellous bone to be placed about the ends of the autograft; Fig. 70-10*C* shows the postoperative radiographic appearance. The nail will remain in place indefinitely.

Acetabulum

Technically, perhaps the most challenging area for limb salvage is the supra-acetabular area of the pelvis. Metastatic tumors commonly seen in this area are relatively easy to deal with by intralesional debridement (see Chap. 72). In the case of primary sarcoma, however, the entire hip joint and surrounding muscle must be resected widely, leaving a large defect which may or may not be reconstructed. This general technique has been referred to as *internal hemipelvectomy* because of its similarity to the ablative hemipelvectomy considered an option for

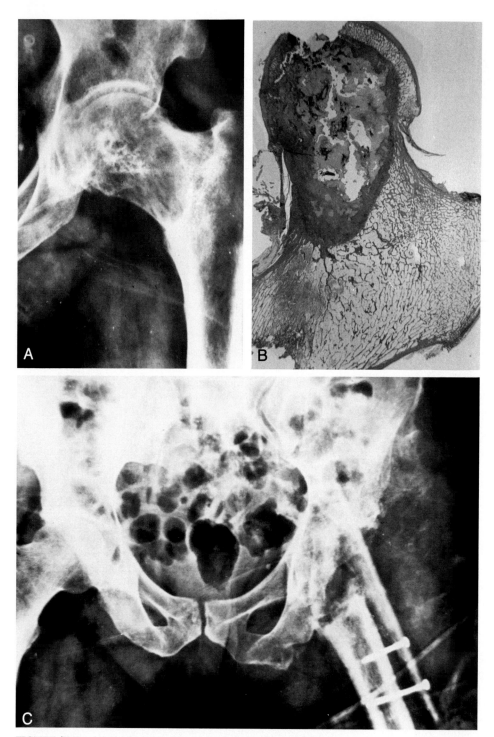

FIGURE 70-6.   (*A*) Radiograph shows low-grade fibrosarcoma of the femoral head and neck in a 40-year-old patient. (*B*) Macrosection of resected specimen. (*C*) Postoperative radiographic appearance after time-proven excisional arthrodesis.

treating sarcomas in the supra-acetabular pelvic area. In order for a patient to fit the oncologic criteria for internal hemipelvectomy, the surgeon must be able to achieve the same safety margins as provided by the time-proven ablative hemipelvectomy. Once the tumor is resected, the surgeon can elect any of three alternatives: (1) fuse the remaining upper femur to a portion of the remaining pelvis; (2) perform a complicated reconstruction of the resected pelvic area, combining prosthetic material and allografts; or (3) simply allow the hip to become flail and stabilized with scar tissue.

By way of illustration, consider the fairly simple situation of a chondrosarcoma arising from the medial and inferior por-

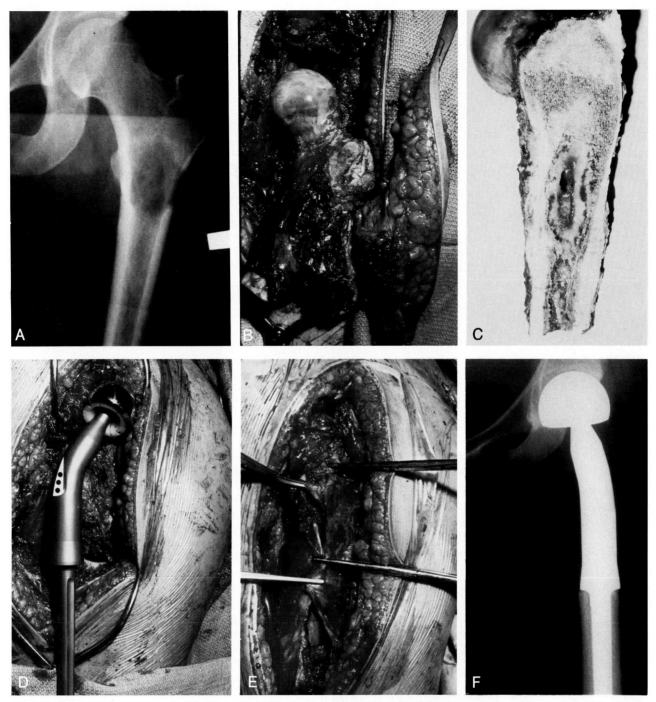

FIGURE 70-7. (*A*) Radiographic appearance of high-grade malignant fibrous histiocytoma of the lesser trochanter in a 30-year-old patient. (*B*) Intraoperative photograph shows widely resected specimen, including biopsy site marked with hemostat. (*C*) Photograph of sagittal section of bone specimen demonstrates 4-cm safety margin at lower edge of centrally located tumor. (*D*) Intraoperative photograph shows bipolar prosthesis for calcar replacement with holes for attachment of intertrochanteric abductor complex at time of closure. (*E*) Intraoperative photograph shows final closure of intertrochanteric band and vastus–abductor complex over the prosthesis for increased stability of soft tissues. (*F*) Postoperative radiograph shows the prosthesis ready for full weight-bearing.

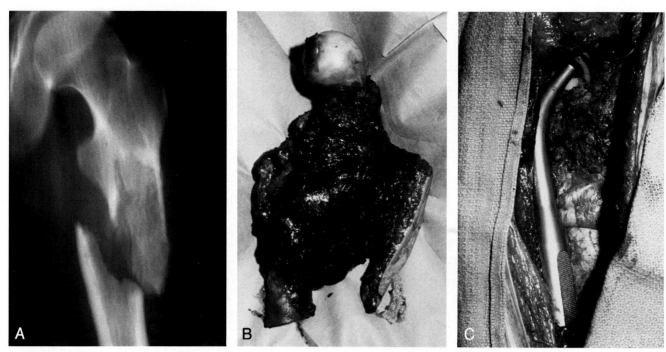

FIGURE 70-8. (*A*) Radiographic appearance of a pathologic fracture through a high-grade malignant fibrous histiocytoma in 35-year-old man. (*B*) Gross appearance of attempted wide local resection of entire fracture hematoma six weeks after fracture. (*C*) Surgical appearance of custom calcar-replacement titanium implant with bipolar head and porous shoulder.

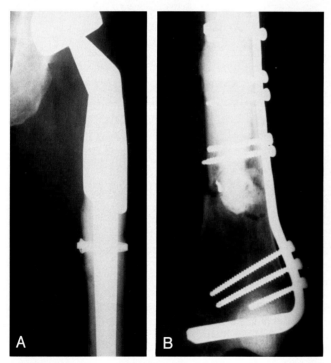

FIGURE 70-9. (*A*) Radiographic appearance of a calcar-replacement prosthesis for sarcoma complicated by iatrogenic fracture of the distal femur during broaching of the femoral canal. (*B*) Radiograph of the lower half of the same femur shows blade plate fixation for the comminuted supracondylar fracture.

tions of the acetabulum and extending out toward the pubic symphysis. Figure 70-11*A* shows the preoperative radiographic appearance of this tumor in a 40-year-old female patient. The entire tumor was removed with wide margins, leaving behind a large portion of weight-bearing ilium and femoral head and neck. The femoral head could therefore be easily fused up into the body of the ilium, with a blade-plate used for internal fixation. Figure 70-11*B* is a postoperative radiograph taken after the successful procedure. This reconstruction is excellent for low-grade lesions in young patients who have excellent chances for survival.

Several surgeons have attempted aggressive reconstruction with large custom implants in a few selected patients but have had a high failure rate because of loosening of the synthetic component over time. Perhaps the best-known reconstruction at present is a combination of conventional total hip implants and large allografts that have less chance of loosening with time. This is illustrated by the case of a 45-year-old female with a central IA chondrosarcoma in the supra-acetabular area (Fig. 70-12). This lesion was exposed through a generous Gibson posterior approach. The entire belly of the middle gluteal muscle was reflected posteriorly with its neurovascular bundle intact and the sciatic nerve lifted from the sciatic notch. The ilium was cut transversely at the level of the mid-sacroiliac joint, which cleared the upper pole of the tumor by 1 inch. The lower margins of the anterior and posterior acetabular columns were transected at the obturator foramen level, and the femoral neck was transected to complete the entire wide margin. The tumor was then debulked on a separate table and the resected

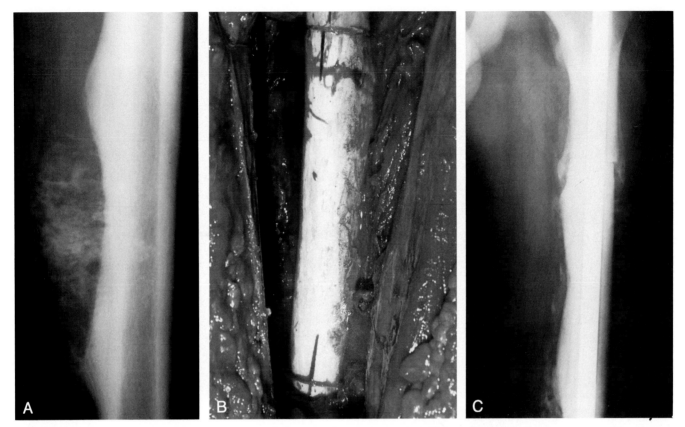

FIGURE 70-10. (A) Radiographic appearance of midshaft parosteal osteosarcoma in a 13-year-old boy. (B) Intraoperative photograph of segmentally resected middle third of the femur, placed back into the thigh over the intramedullary nail after a five-minute tumor-killing autoclave procedure. (C) Postoperative radiograph shows nail and graft in stable position for early weight-bearing.

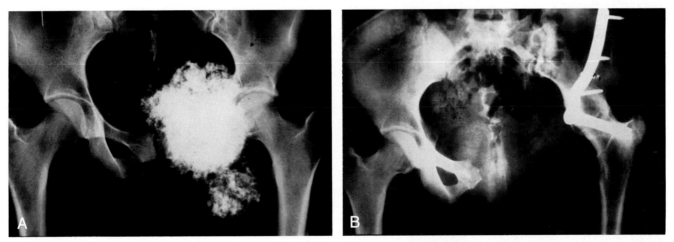

FIGURE 70-11. (A) Preoperative radiograph shows low-grade chondrosarcoma arising from inferomedial aspect of the acetabulum in a 40-year-old woman. (B) Postoperative radiograph taken after successful excisional arthrodesis.

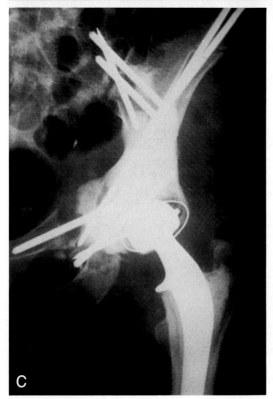

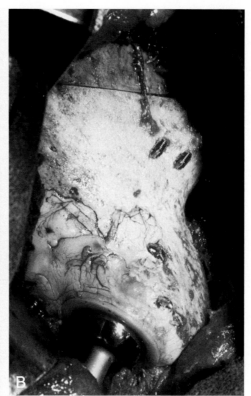

FIGURE 70-12.   (*A*) Radiographic appearance of low-grade chondrosarcoma in the supra-acetabular area in a 45-year-old female. (*B*) Intraoperative appearance following reinsertion of autoclaved bone specimen combined with coventional total hip replacement system. (*C*) Radiograph obtained five years after surgery.

FIGURE 70-13. (*A*) Radiographic appearance of dedifferentiated chondrosarcoma in the upper part of the humerus in a 40-year-old female. (*B*) Gross appearance of resected specimen with biopsy site at time of wide local resection. (*C*) Photograph shows composite device fashioned from a large-bone allograft cemented over an 11-inch, long-stem Neer prosthesis. (*D*) Postoperative radiograph shows the composite device cemented into distal part of humerus.

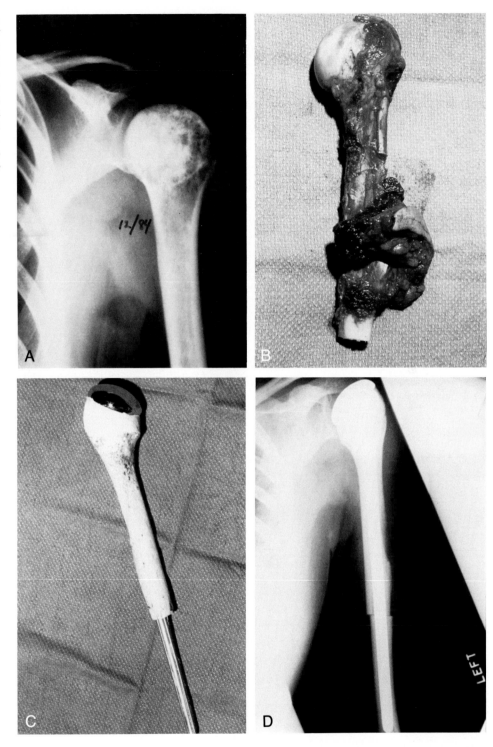

bone autoclaved for 5 minutes. The bone was placed back into the pelvic area and secured with multiple ³⁄₁₆-inch threaded Steinmann pins, cement, and a conventional total hip system. Figure 70-12*A* shows the preoperative radiographic features of the tumor; the intraoperative appearance of the completed internal reconstruction is shown in Figure 70-12*B;* final radiographic appearance 5 years after surgery is shown in Figure 70-12*C.* The tumor did not recur and the patient was walking

well but with a moderate limp because of weak abduction. In such cases, bone bank allografts that fit well are difficult to find and require complicated custom fitting at surgery.

Proximal Humerus

Tumors in the upper extremity are much less common than those in the leg. Most upper extremity tumors occur in the

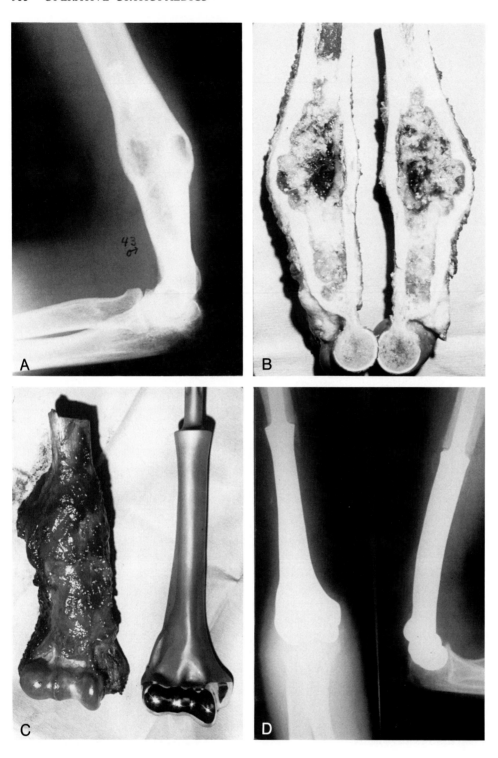

FIGURE 70-14. (*A*) Preoperative radiographic appearance of a distal humeral chondrosarcoma in a 43-year-old male. (*B*) Photograph shows sagittal section through resected surgical specimen. (*C*) Photograph of custom titanium prosthesis shows excellent anatomic matching of resected specimen. (*D*) Postoperative radiograph shows composite device cemented into distal humerus.

proximal humerus, which is one of the most ideal anatomic areas for limb salvage for three reasons: (1) reduced stress is placed on this area because the arm is a non–weight-bearing structure; (2) sarcomas arising from this area, including osteosarcoma, have a lower rate of local recurrence and a better overall survival rate (about 90%) than when the same tumor is found in the lower extremity; and (3) in contrast to the more complicated total hip and knee systems, the long-stem Neer

prosthesis can be easily adapted to the proximal humerus area for stable reconstruction with minimal late complications.

One of the earliest limb salvage procedures for proximal humeral tumors was the Tikhor–Linberg procedure. This technique used wide local resection of the upper part of the humerus, the glenoid cavity, and the distal part of the clavicle, allowing the arm to hang free with an unstable pseudarthrosis. With the advent of modern technology, the procedure became rare and has been replaced by more popular allografts and prosthetic devices.

A common tumor seen in the upper part of the humerus is the low-grade chondrosarcoma. This tumor usually requires resection of the upper third of the humerus along with the rotator cuff mechanism and possibly the undersurface of the deltoid muscle. The glenoid cavity is most often spared in low-grade tumors, which helps to stabilize either a Neer prosthesis or a large allograft that might be selected to replace the surgical defect. For more aggressive tumors such as osteosarcoma, many surgeons prefer to resect the entire glenoid cavity and deltoid muscle to reduce the chances of local recurrence. In this situation, it becomes necessary to create a stabilizing sling about the upper end of the allograft or prosthesis using the tendinous remains of the latissimus dorsi, teres major, and pectoralis major muscles.

The following is a typical example of how surgeons can combine the technologies of a long-stem Neer prosthesis and a large bone allograft to gain desired functional stability. Figure 70-13*A* shows the radiographic appearance of a dedifferentiated chondrosarcoma in the humeral head of a 40-year-old female with extensive infiltration of the tumor in the medullary canal. The upper half of the humerus was resected widely, as demonstrated by the surgical specimen (see Fig. 70-13*B*), which includes the biopsy site. An allograft of appropriate length was prepared and cemented onto the 11-inch stem of a Neer prosthesis. Figure 70-13*C* shows the composite device ready for cementing into the distal humeral canal. After this procedure, the tendons that normally attach to the upper humerus were reconstructed as a stabilizing sling around and into the allograft. The postoperative radiograph is shown in Fig. 70-13*D*. In my experience, this combined technology is far superior to the old-fashioned fibular grafts, which had a high failure rate because of fracture through dead bone. Newer, vascularized fibular grafts show promise in a few centers but are demanding, time-consuming procedures.

Distal Humerus

The distal end of the humerus is the least common location for primary sarcoma. This area is also one of the more difficult to manage by limb salvage techniques because of the lack of adequate, standard prosthetic devices for the elbow. Whether a distal humeral allograft or a prosthesis is used, a common problem is created by having to stabilize the complex surface anatomy of the distal end of the humerus against the proximal ends of the radius and ulna. In my experience, synthetic articulation should not be attempted with the opposite side of the elbow joint because of the high incidence of stem loosening.

Figure 70-14 illustrates a low-grade chondrosarcoma in the distal humerus of a 43-year-old male. The preoperative radiograph (Fig. 70-14*A*) shows chronic dilatation and sclerotic changes in the distal humerus. Figure 70-14*B* shows a sagittal section through the surgical specimen after wide local resection. Figure 70-14*C* shows the appearance of the custom distal humeral prosthesis and excellent replication of the surface anatomy of the adjacent resected specimen. The postoperative radiographic appearance is seen in Figure 70-14*D*. Five years postoperatively, the patient had no recurrence of tumor and had excellent elbow function.

REFERENCES

1. Eilber, F.R., Mirra, J.J., Grant, T.T., Weisenburger, T., and Morton, D.L.: Is Amputation Necessary for Sarcomas? A Seven-Year Study with Limb Salvage. Ann. Surg. **192:**431, 1980.
2. Johnston, J.: A Custom-Like Modular Design Prosthesis for Tumor Resection Surgery About the Knee. *In* Kotz, R. (ed.): Proceedings of the Second International Workshop on the Design and Application of Tumor Prostheses for Bone and Joint Reconstruction, Vienna, September 5–8, 1983. p. 214. Vienna, Egermann Druckereigesellschaft, 1983.
3. Lane, J.M., Hurson, B., Boland, P.J., and Glasser, D.B.: Osteogenic Sarcoma. Clin. Orthop. **204:**93, 1986.
4. Lexer, E.: Die Gesamte Wiederherstellungs-Chirurgie. Leipzig, Barth, 1931.
5. Meyerding, H.W.: Treatment of Benign Giant-Cell Tumors. J. Bone Joint Surg. **18-A:**823, 1936.
6. Phemister, D.B.: Bone Transplantation in the Treatment of Tumors and Dystrophies of Bones. *In* Onzième Congrès de la Société Internationale de Chirurgie, Vol. 1, p. 357. Brussels, Imprimerie Medicale et Scientifique, 1939.
7. Rosen, G., Caparros, B., Huvos, A.G., Kosloff, C., Nirenberg, A., Cacavio, A., Marcove, R.C., Lane, J.M., Mehta, B., and Urban, C.: Preoperative Chemotherapy for Osteogenic Sarcoma: Selection of Postoperative Adjuvant Chemotherapy Based on the Response of the Primary Tumor to Preoperative Chemotherapy. Cancer **49:**1221, 1982.

CHAPTER 71

Allografts

JUAN J. RODRIGO and
DONALD J. PROLO

GENERAL CONSIDERATIONS

The clinical application of bone allografting became prevalent in the first two decades of the 20th century, after the experimental work of Ollier and Axhausen.[23] Lexer was the first to perform allogeneic whole joint transplantation, in 1907, and had performed 25 by 1925.[79,80] Inclan, in 1942, reported the storage of autogeneic and allogeneic bone, and this stimulated many similar clinical efforts at preservation, sterilization, and delayed reimplantation.[8,24,73] Although the superiority of fresh autogeneic grafts has repeatedly been confirmed in experimental studies and clinical experiments,[15,16,74,104,120] allogeneic implants preserved by freezing, by freeze-drying after sterilization with ethylene oxide, by chemical sterilization, or by gamma irradiation are widely being used.[119] Recent polls indicate that 69% of practicing orthopaedic surgeons in the United States would use allografts if they were available, and 55% of the program directors in orthopaedic surgery are using preserved allografts.[29,97] Bone is more commonly transplanted in the body than any other tissue or organ except blood. Only recently has attention been paid to other musculoskeletal tissues for allografting, such as cartilage, tendons, ligaments, and menisci.

The terminology of bone grafting and other musculoskeletal grafting has been confusing. In current terminology, an "autograft" is transplanted from one part of the body to another; "autogeneic" is the corresponding adjective, now replacing "autogenous" or "autologous." An "allograft" (replacing the previous term, "homograft") is transplanted between genetically nonidentical members of the same species; the corresponding adjective is "allogeneic." A "syngraft" (replacing "isograft") is transplanted between genetically identical members of a species (adjective, "syngeneic"). A "xenograft" (previously, "heterograft") is transplanted between members of different species (adjective, "xenogeneic"). Urist[155] recommends the term "implant" for nonviable bone; an example is frozen, freeze-dried, sterilized bone, a derivative of whole bone that lacks viable cellular components but potentially contains inductive protein that can stimulate osteogenesis.

A graft may be 'orthotopic' (transplanted to the same site in the recipient that it occupied in the donor, e.g. distal femur to distal femur); 'heterotopic' (transplanted to a different site but one occupied by the same tissue as in the donor, e.g. fibula to spine); or ectopic (transplanted to a site in the recipient normally occupied by a different type of tissue, e.g. bone into a muscle pouch). Ectopic sites for bone grafting have been used mainly in investigating osteogenesis, and, rarely, for temporary clinical storage of bone.

In general, bone grafting operations are performed to stabilize painful joints, to promote healing of nonunited fractures, and to restore structure and cosmetic appearance. Cancellous bone or morcellized cortical bone is most often used for filling cysts or cavities (Fig. 71-1); cortical bone is optimal for reconstructing defects that require a certain form and strength (Fig. 71-2). Although a cortical bone graft is strong when first implanted, the incorporation process frequently weakens it, so that a fatigue fracture occasionally occurs 6 to 8 months after implantation.[14] Therefore, plates or intramedullary devices are frequently used to augment the strength of the graft during incorporation.[72]

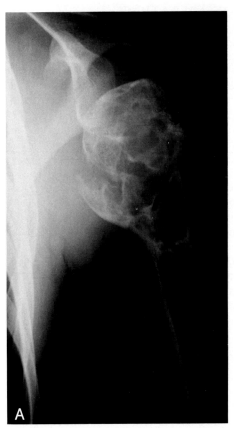
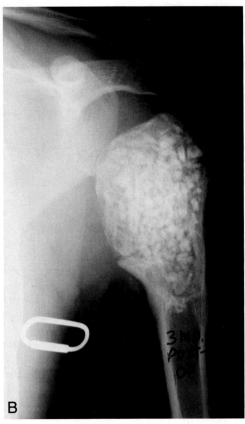
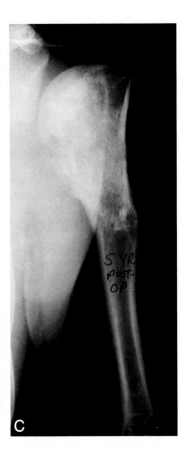

FIGURE 71-1. (*A*) Unicameral bone cyst in a young adult with a pathologic fracture. (*B*) Four months after freeze-dried and partially decalcified allograft (AAA bone) packing. (*C*) Five years after allograft packing. The graft rapidly became incorporated and remodeled.

Bone Tissue Banking

Guidelines for the procurement, processing, and clinical use of bone have recently been established by the American Association of Tissue Banks.[48] The goals of bone banking are to preserve the physical integrity of the implant and the inductive protein, to reduce immunogenicity, and to ensure sterility. In general, a minimal interval (less than 24 hours) between the death of the donor and the time of procurement is desirable. Proper consents are essential.

Harvested bone is fashioned quickly in various sizes and shapes, and then all possible soft tissues and cells are removed to reduce immunogenicity. Freezing to −70°C in a sterile state effectively decreases immunogenicity and maintains sterility, and is generally recommended for osteoarticular allografts.[87] This method of storage decreases the strength of the allograft to only a small extent (about 10%).[9] Ethylene oxide sterilization is also effective and does not destroy the bone morphogenetic protein (BMP).[119,154] The bone is then preserved by freeze-drying, after removal of ethylene oxide.[73,119] Freezing to −70°C and freeze-drying both reduce the immunogenicity of the implant, but with some compromise in its mechanical strength. Freezing bone decreases its tensile and compressive strength by about 10% each, while freeze-drying decreases torsional strength by about 50% and compressive strength by about 10%.[116] These decreases in strength are probably not signifi-cant, however, since both compressive and tensile strength fall by about 50% in vivo during the process of replacement.

Sterilization of bone by heating to over 60°C, by autoclaving, or by gamma irradiation all disrupt the physical and chemical nature of bone and impair its mechanical properties.[18,35] Experience argues against the effectiveness of bone implants subjected to these physically damaging processing methods. Bone subjected to freeze-drying, to freeze-drying and partial demineralization, or to freezing will show some decrease in incorporation as compared to fresh autografts or syngeneic grafts;[7,104] nonetheless, these techniques are superior to the more damaging techniques mentioned above, and are the current standard techniques.

Quality control measures must be enforced to avoid the transfer of bacterial, fungal, or viral pathogens to the recipient. Such measures should include patients' histories and screening tests for hepatitis, AIDS, and syphilis.

Figure 71-3 represents storage techniques commonly used and recommended for various types of musculoskeletal allografts.

Biology of Incorporation

A successful bone graft will eventually be incorporated into the skeletal system of the host. In the process of incorporation, new bone deposited by the recipient envelops and replaces the donor bone tissue. How rapidly the graft is incorporated depends on its size, structure, position, fixation, and genetic composition. The role of the graft in stimulating incorporation may encompass osteoconduction, osteoinduction, and osteogenesis.

Osteoconduction (Trellis Formation)

Grafts share with biologic and nonbiologic materials a three-dimensional structure into which sprouting capillaries, perivascular tissue, and osteoprogenitor cells can grow. Glass tubes, ceramics, plastics, and autoclaved deproteinized bone all provide a scaffold into and around which bone formation can occur.[155] This function of the graft as a scaffold for ingrowth is referred to as "osteoconduction."

Osteoinduction

Induction occurs when "two or more tissues of different natures or properties become intimately associated, [and] alterations of the developmental course of the interactivants results."[55] Urist defines osteoinduction as "the process of recruitment of mesenchymal-type cells into cartilage and bone under the influence of a diffusible bone morphogenetic protein (BMP)."[155] Urist has characterized BMP as a glycoprotein with a predominant component having a molecular weight of 17,500 and with variable quantities of 14,000, 24,000, and 34,000 proteins. It is an acidic polypeptide, degraded by acid alcohol, trypsin, and chymotrypsin, but not by nuclease (RNAse, DNAse) or collagenase. Its concentration is greater in cortical than in cancellous bone in quantities of 1 mg/kg of wet weight of fresh bone.[159] It is lost if collection time is delayed, and is destroyed by irradiation sterilization over 2.0 Mrad, by heating to over 60°C, by exposure to chemicals (including hydrogen peroxide, β-propiolactone, and benzalkonium chloride), and by cryolysis (thrice freezing and thawing).[161] Disso-

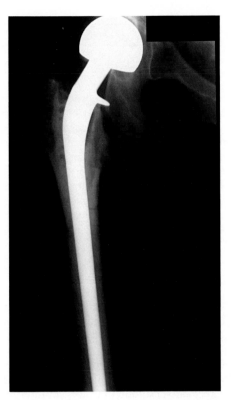

FIGURE 71-2. Proximal femoral allograft to replace the proximal femur in a patient with a giant-cell tumor. A custom metallic prosthesis was threaded through the allograft.

ciated BMP diffuses across as many as five membranes, across distances of 450 to 1000 μm, and through pores as small as 25 nm in diameter, and will induce bone formation on a millipore chamber implanted in muscle.[82,109]

Bone grafts in which preparation of the graft has not destroyed the BMP are capable of osteoinduction in addition to

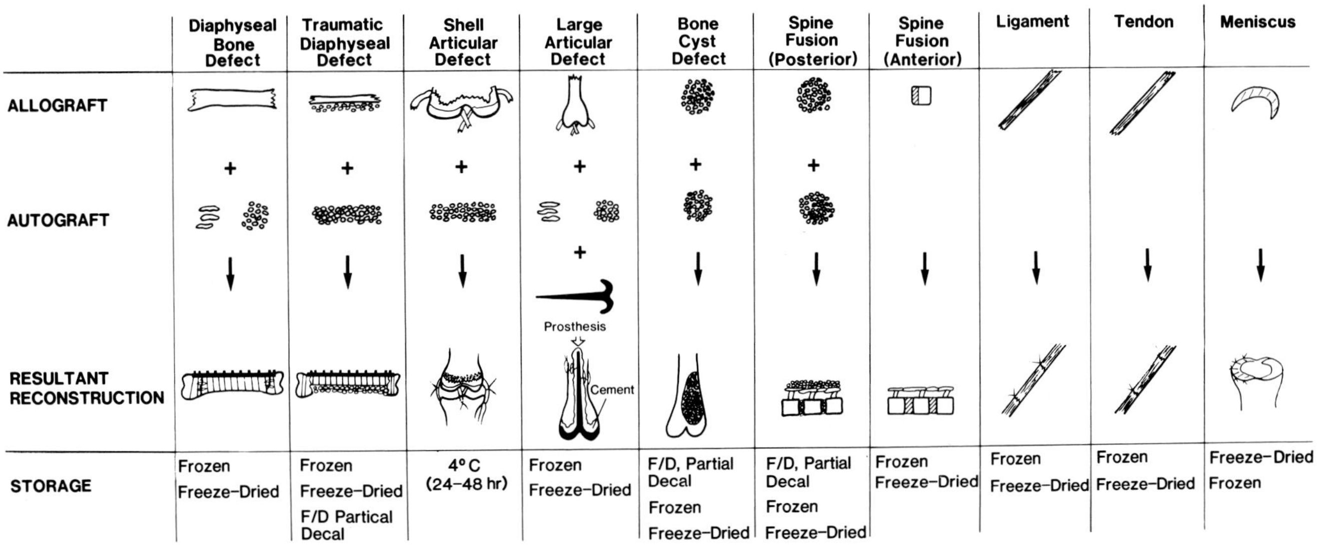

	Diaphyseal Bone Defect	Traumatic Diaphyseal Defect	Shell Articular Defect	Large Articular Defect	Bone Cyst Defect	Spine Fusion (Posterior)	Spine Fusion (Anterior)	Ligament	Tendon	Meniscus
ALLOGRAFT										
AUTOGRAFT										
RESULTANT RECONSTRUCTION										
STORAGE	Frozen Freeze–Dried	Frozen Freeze–Dried F/D Partical Decal	4°C (24–48 hr)	Frozen Freeze–Dried	F/D, Partial Decal Frozen Freeze–Dried	F/D, Partial Decal Frozen Freeze–Dried	Frozen Freeze–Dried	Frozen Freeze–Dried	Frozen Freeze–Dried	Freeze–Dried Frozen

FIGURE 71-3. Methods of storing and using musculoskeletal allografts for different orthopaedic needs.

osteoconduction. An osteoinductive graft is incorporated more rapidly than one that is merely osteoconductive.[18,154,157,158]

Osteogenesis

Osteogenesis, together with the absence of an immune response, is the basis for the superior clinical performance of autografts. Osteogenesis from surviving donor cells is characteristic only of fresh autogeneic bone. Whereas autogeneically transplanted osteocytes die and leave empty lacunae, preosteoclasts, preosteoblasts, and osteoclasts can survive.[155] By contrast, cells from a fresh allograft quickly elicit antibody production and cell-mediated immunity, and are destroyed by the recipient. Osteoclast precursor cells may migrate into the graft by transport through the blood stream from the host's bone marrow.[155]

Revascularization

Revascularization of a fresh autograft seldom occurs by microanastomosis with existing microvessels. This process is more common in cancellous bone, and is aided in cortical bone by removal of the periosteum.[18] Most autografts and alloimplants revascularize only by invasion of capillary sprouts from the host bed during the resorption of the old matrix ("creeping substitution"). Creeping substitution involves invasion of the allograft by osteoclasts, and these are in turn followed by a blood vessel bud. New osteons are laid down around the many blood vessels which invade the graft.

Selection and Preparation of the Graft

The criteria that characterize an ideal graft follow from the goal of restoring structural stability to bones or joints, with mechanical properties equal to adjacent bone and an acceptable cosmetic result. The graft should therefore be strong, potentially viable, nonreactive (nontoxic, nonimmunogenic, noncarcinogenic), sterile, and cosmetically pleasing; it should also be controlled in growth, storeable, capable of being shaped during surgery, and affordable.

The eventual choice of a graft will depend on the type of structural osteogenic functions one desires, the size and shape of various donor bones, and whether viable articular cartilage needs to be transplanted. The morbidity attendant upon procuring an autogeneic graft is often a difficult limiting factor in bone graft surgery. The removal of large masses of bone from a patient's iliac crest is potentially mutilating and is associated with at least eight possible complications: massive hematoma or blood loss, fatigue fractures, pelvic instability, donor site pain, heterotopic bone formation, iliac hernia, sepsis, and deformity. However, the use of some autogeneic corticocancellous bone is almost essential in certain applications (such as posterolateral lumbar and cervical fusions, and to supplement allografts at the osteosynthesis site). Alloimplants seldom result in fusion across transverse processes or posterior arch structures; autolyzed, antigen-extracted allogeneic (AAA) bone may be an exception. Some autograft bone must be used along with allografts because it helps to avoid nonunion and stimulates incorporation.

Types of Grafts and Their Indications

Autografts

Fresh autogeneic bone still remains the "gold standard" to which all other grafts are compared. If a patient has an adequate supply of donor bone of appropriate configuration, the fresh autograft would be the graft of choice, since the fresh autograft is the most likely to achieve all the optimal characteristics in bone transplantation. The fresh autograft is likely to contain BMP and cells that will survive transplantation, and it is, of course, immunologically identical with the host.

Frozen autografts are often used in neurosurgery where portions of the cranium are exteriorized because of cerebral swelling and are later replaced.[118] Occasionally, in the presence of tumor, autogeneic bone is removed, autoclaved, and then replaced.[61]

Allografts and Alloimplants

Fresh allogeneic bone is no longer used in clinical transplantation because of the major immune response to the transplanted tissues. Most alloimplants contain some cortical and cancellous areas. As discussed under Bone Tissue Banking, freezing and freeze-drying are both useful storage measures, and reduce the immunogenicity of the implant; the compromise in mechanical strength that also results is probably not clinically significant, since both grafts lose about 50% of strength during incorporation in the recipient from the process of creeping substitution.

Alloimplants may be successfully used in many applications, from craniofacial restoration to spinal operations and whole joint transplantation. Donor bone is either removed aseptically or secondarily sterilized with gaseous ethylene oxide or gamma irradiation.[119] The bone is then frozen or freeze-dried for preservation and reduction of immunogenicity.

Urist emphasizes that frozen or freeze-dried bone contains numerous transplantation alloantigens.[155] Further, while in the frozen or freeze-dried state, bone loses its BMP due to enzymic autodigestion by intra- and extracellular enzymes, and the concomitant preservation of BMPases in tissue degrades the bone. Accordingly, Urist developed a protocol for the preparation of chemosterilized, autolyzed, antigen-extracted allogeneic (AAA) bone that would preserve the BMP.[155]

In this method, chloroform-methanol is used to extract lipids and cell membrane lipoproteins (4 hours), 0.6 N hydrochloric acid extracts acid-soluble proteins and demineralizes the surface (24 hours), and neutral phosphate buffer autodigestion in the presence of sulfhydryl-group enzyme inhibitors removes endogenous intra- and extracellular transplantation antigens (72 hours). The bone is then frozen and freeze-dried.

For this treatment, bone must be excised from the donor within 8 to 12 hours of death (minimal biodegradation time) if the donor has not been stored in a morgue environment (4°C). If morgue storage has been used, 12 to 24 hours is acceptable. Prolonged storage at −18° to 0°C and immediate freeze-drying must both be avoided, since both reduce the BMP through autodigestion. Sterilization by irradiation with more than 2.0 Mrad further denatures the BMP. The principal disadvantage of AAA bone is a decreased strength; therefore, it is rarely used where strength is an important consideration. Urist has used AAA bone in 40 patients undergoing posterolateral lumbar fusion with a clinical success rate of 80% and a pseudarthrosis rate of 12%.[156] He also reported its successful application in eight of ten patients who underwent arthrodesis of the knee, ankle, and wrist.[157] The addition of fresh autogeneic cancellous bone (including marrow) to AAA bone created a composite graft with enhanced osteogenic capacity.

Urist and co-workers were also the first to discover, in the early 1960s, the osteoinductive capacity of demineralized bone.[153] Urist reported his clinical results in 1968.[154] More recently, others have used demineralized alloimplants in craniofacial restoration.[52] AAA bone and demineralized bone are not generally available for clinical use at this time.

Other Allograft Tissues

Cartilage as Allograft

Allogeneic cartilage, in theory, should not trigger an immune response after transplantation, because the potentially immunogenic chondrocytes are buried in the cartilage matrix and therefore are inaccessible to the host's immune system. However, late immune responses, such as lymph node hyperplasia, have been noted, and the role of cartilage in eliciting an immune response remains controversial.[33,34,39–41,44,63,74–76,113,167] If this immune response is strong, it can lead to destruction of cartilage by a pannus-like reaction and a joint fluid inflammatory response.[130,131,133]

The late deterioration in allograft cartilage[20,60,62,115,121] is not clearly understood, but again this could be an immune response, cellular or humoral, to histocompatibility antigens. Deterioration of the joint surfaces may also be the result of misfit and eventual mechanical degeneration. Correction of this problem requires exacting surgical technique[108] and excellent matching of donor and recipient sites.

Tendon as Allograft

Fresh autogeneic tendon grafts have been employed for many years, but tendon allografts have been attempted only recently.[64,112] In animal studies, it appears that allografts are as successful as autografts, but the healing time is longer.[85] Various methods of tendon preservation did not seem to alter the results.[117] Some studies, using skin grafts and complement fixation assays, demonstrated no antigenicity after allogeneic transplantation.[113] The donor cells in the tendon then apparently disappear and are replaced by recipient cells. The exact immune mechanisms are not well worked out.[98] Clinically, the healing of freeze-dried allograft tendon appears to be very satisfactory.[10]

Shino and co-workers[144] compared allograft and autograft patellar tendon for reconstructing the anterior cruciate ligament in dogs. Both the allograft and the autograft tendons underwent a similar revascularization and remodeling. Both grafts attained approximately 30% of the tensile strength of the control side. The tendons were reorganized over time, and resembled normal ligament histology after 30 and 52 weeks, including no evidence of immune rejection.

Ligament and Fascia Lata as Allograft

Allografts have been used for ligament replacement in a number of sites, including the ankle, knee, shoulder, and hip. Substitution with freeze-dried fascia lata gave good results in 73% of patients.[10] Studies in monkeys[4] and in dogs[117] confirm the healing potential of frozen ligament allografts. Freeze-dried ligament or fascia lata does not appear to generate an immune response in the host,[144] although studies have not been done on antigens altered by the freeze-drying process. Freezing to −80°C does not appear to change the tensile strength of allograft ligament.[4] However, Vasseur and others,[163] using frozen allogeneic cruciate ligament in a bone–ligament–bone preparation in the dog, obtained a strength of only 14% of control ligaments at 9 months. An immune response to the histocompatibility antigens was noted in the synovial fluid of all six dogs at 9 months. Hydroxyproline uptake was significantly decreased in the allograft ligaments as compared to the autograft ligaments; this was considered a delay in the reconstitution of the ligament due to the early immune response and secondary inflammatory response. Replacement of the allograft ligament was expected to catch up with the autografts, because long-term studies by Shino and others[2,36,144] showed that long-term reconstitution was as good as with autografts.

Large Composite Allografts

Allograft replacement of diseased segments of the limbs and long bones has long been a goal of physicians. The goal was in part realized in 1908, when Lexer reported the use of whole-joint or hemijoint bone and soft tissue transplants to replace damaged knees.[79] Despite the crudity of the technique, the results, carefully reviewed some 20 years later, suggested a success rate of approximately 50%.[80] In the years following Lexer's original work, only occasional case reports indicated the interest of orthopaedists in allograft transplantation until the early 1960s, when large series of allograft transplantation of bony segments were reported separately by Parrish in this country,[109–111] Ottolenghi in Argentina,[107] and Volkov in the USSR.[164] Most of the patients in these series had a malignant tumor of the midsection or end of a long bone and, after its excision, the allograft was inserted as a scaffolding for subsequent replacement by host bone. The results of the procedures depended in part on technique and on location of the tumor, but all grafts showed complications resulting from an unpredictable rate of incorporation of the bone and degradation of the cartilage, leading to a failure of normal joint function. Despite the complications and occasional late failures, it was apparent that the technique of allograft transplantation had potential usefulness in the surgery of malignant tumors and that it was possible to utilize cadaver segments for replacement of long bones which are excised for malignant disease. Recently, Mankin and colleagues[90] reported preliminary results of 19 massive resections and allograft transplantations performed for malignant or aggressive bone tumors. Their improved allograft procurement technique involved freezing of the segments to decrease the immunogenicity of the bony portion, and glycerinization of the cartilage to maintain chondrocyte viability during freezing and thawing. Fifteen of the patients were followed for an average of almost 2 years and, despite numerous complications (related to both tumor and surgery), none showed local recurrence or major functional impairment, except for two whose grafts became infected. Koskinen[72] proposed the addition of autograft material at the osteosynthesis site and noted an improvement in the nonunion and delayed union rates. He also advocated strong internal fixation throughout the entire length of the allograft to protect it from delayed fatigue fracture.

Since some whole-joint or half-joint allografts have tended to deteriorate, one speculates as to the mechanism. Is there loss of cartilage viability during storage before transplantation? Is there avascular necrosis of subchondral bone, with subsequent collapse of the joint surface? Is there failure of creeping substitution and non-development of good subchondral bone? Is there mechanical failure of the joint due to ligamentous laxity or due to a poor fit of the allograft surface on the recipient surface? Is there destruction of articular cartilage secondary to an immune mechanism? Is there loss of joint stability due to ligament and tendon absorption? It seems important to examine these questions in order to better the definition of possible failure mechanisms.

Immunologic Considerations

The antigen–antibody response to allografts varies considerably in reported series. Studies of small osteoarticular fresh human allografts performed by Urovitz and co-workers[162] have demonstrated little evidence for anti-histocompatibility (anti-HLA) antibodies in the serum of the hosts, whereas patients receiving massive frozen allografts in the series reported by Rodrigo and co-workers[129] showed high titers of anti-HLA antibodies that remained positive as long as 5 years after transplantation.

In osteochondral grafting, one transplants fresh cartilage of low immunogenicity and fresh subchondral bone that is highly immunogenic. With the use of a free avascular osteochondral allograft for replacement of the end of a long bone, one hopes that creeping substitution will remodel the devitalized bone at an appropriate rate[54,131] and that the cartilaginous surface will remain viable. Cartilage is transplanted for destroyed joints primarily in the form of shell allografts (joint cartilage plus 2 to 3 mm of subchondral bone). A strong immune response to the bone can also destroy the adjacent cartilage, even though cartilage resists destruction by antibody and cellular resorptive mechanisms.[33,34] If the recipient launches an immune response against donor histocompatibility antigens, this protection of cartilage from destruction is only relative, and a low-grade, slow, immunologically mediated inflammatory response ensues, characterized by increased synovial fluid, increased synovial fluid white cell counts, an antibody response, and pannus reactions that can destroy the cartilage.[134,135]

Transplantation of allogeneic cortical and cancellous bone elicits an immune response that delays, but does not prevent, healing at the osteosynthesis site, and that blocks revascularization, resorption, and appositional new bone formation. However, long-term studies show no difference in the morphology of eventual repair of autografts and allografts.[70,123,166] Decalcified allografts repair at a faster rate than those merely frozen, although they are mechanically weaker.[102]

Recently, allogeneic tendons and ligaments have been grafted, occasionally with bone attachments. As with allogeneic bone, healing is delayed, but eventually the graft is replaced by cells of the recipient.[113] Freezing storage methods do not speed up this slow repair, as there also appears to be an immune response to foreign histocompatibility antigens if a frozen bone–ligament–bone allograft is used, and this is the probable cause for the delayed healing.[163] But healing of freeze-dried allogeneic tendons appears satisfactory.[10]

Over the past 10 years, attempts have been made, using animals, to inhibit the immune response to musculoskeletal allografts. Inasmuch as antigens in the bone persist for only 2 to 3 months after transplantation, temporary systemic immunosuppression may be used. Burchardt and his colleagues[15,16] used azathioprine to induce a temporary nonspecific inhibition of the immune response in the dog; this resulted in improved healing, incorporation, and replacement of avascular canine fibular allografts. Allografts were replaced at the same rate as autografts.[15,74] Other drugs and techniques (cyclosporin A,[135] cyclophosphamide,[130,142] steroids,[168] and total lymphoid irradiation[128]) have been tried in the rat. While most of these experimental methods have been successful in inhibiting the immune response, toxic side effects negate their routine use in human musculoskeletal transplantation, although they are occasionally indicated.

Recent research has focused on a more specific inhibition of only the immune reaction against donor antigens. This would have the advantage of being less toxic, because it would not suppress the entire immune system. One promising technique uses a temporary biodegradable cement to coat the donor bone, thus hiding the histocompatibility antigens until the donor cells have died and their antigens have deteriorated.[75,124,132]

Alternatives to Bone for Grafting

Various synthetic bone substitutes are now being evaluated as alternatives to allografts. The biodegradable ceramics (tricalcium and tetracalcium phosphates, hydroxyapatite) have the highest success rate and are superior to biodegradable polymers, such as polylactic acid and polyglycolic acid.[18,65,100] Calcium hydroxyapatite and tricalcium phosphate are more successful implants in bone repair than calcium aluminate. The structural formation and porosity of a ceramic is important in facilitating interface activity with the host and potentiating bony ingrowth[105]; the specific clinical application may dictate the use of a ceramic over bone for a graft. Tricalcium and tetracalcium phosphate differ structurally from hydroxyapatite as well as chemically; only hydroxyapatite is identical with bone mineral. Different preparative methods lead to either compact hydroxyapatite or to a porous material with interconnective macropores that is structurally and spatially similar to cancellous bone. In a biologic system, greater crystal formation and greater density result in resistance to dissolution and promote long-lasting stability; by contrast, an amorphous ultrastructure and greater porosity enhance interface activity and bone ingrowth, but also speed the biodegradation of the implant.

APPLICATIONS AND SPECIFIC TECHNIQUES

Allografts for Spine Surgery

The choice of grafting material depends on the anatomic and spatial constraints of the area to be stabilized and the osteogenic capacity of the host bed. In general, vertebral bodies, rich in cancellous bone and marrow, provide far greater numbers of osteoprogenitor cells for remodeling a graft than do spinous processes, facets, and transverse processes, which are composed mostly of cortical bone. Hence, demands placed upon a graft destined for posterolateral areas of the spine are greater than those imposed on bone grafted to an intervertebral body location. For posterolateral grafting of the spine, therefore, fresh autogeneic bone is considered essential because such a graft provides surviving osteogenic precursor cells and BMP. An exception to this rule is the use of AAA bone augmented with fresh autogeneic corticocancellous bone fragments.[158] Frozen or freeze-dried devitalized allogeneic cortical and cancellous bone may be used for cervical and lumbar interbody fusions, where less is demanded of the graft. At these locations the incidence of fusion is the same with allogeneic bone and fresh autografts, although the allograft fuses more slowly.[3,27,92,149] The failure to achieve a solid fusion by roentgenographic criteria can still be associated with a satisfactory clinical result.[30,150]

Interbody fusions of the cervical spine have long been used since the pioneering efforts of Cloward[27] and Smith and Robinson.[148] In the lumbar spine, Cloward first performed a posterior lumbar interbody fusion in 1943.[26] Recently there has been a resurgence of interest in this technique.[28,81] The instantaneous axis of rotation of the lumbar motion segment is within the intervertebral disc space,[165] and immediate rigidity of the spine is most easily achieved by positioning a graft under tension at this axis of rotation.[46,165] Fully 80% of the biomechanical load of the motion segment is sustained at the intervertebral disc.[11] In the upright position, compressive forces act upon blocks tightly fitted into the disc space and promote fusion through the ingrowth of vascular buds and proliferative mesenchymal cells from the cancellous bone of the host into the cancellous donor bone. In this application, sterilized frozen or freeze-dried allogeneic bone from a cadaver donor can be used instead of fresh autogeneic bone, since it results in a comparable fusion rate.[28]

At times vertebral bodies of the cervical, thoracic, and lumbar spine are lost because of degenerative processes, infection, or neoplasia. Fibular struts of allogeneic bone can be used effectively to restore stability. Allogeneic fibula is incorporated and remodeled in time. Even in the presence of recent osteomyelitis, devitalized allogeneic bone can fuse and provide homostructural support for the weakened spine.[11] For large, multilevel defects of several vertebral bodies, a femoral allo-graft will frequently fill the defect and provide the correct curvature.

Allogeneic bone is frequently used in the long fusions required in operations for scoliosis. These procedures are often done in young children whose iliac crests can not provide enough bone for an autograft fusion. In these cases, allograft bone (frozen, freeze-dried, or AAA bone) may be morcellized and mixed with the child's own bone to provide adequate amounts of graft material.

Allografts for Spine Surgery—Specific Techniques

During an operation, protect the sterility of the graft at all stages. Prolonged exposure to air and saline and prolonged heating can destroy cells and BMP within fresh autogeneic corticocancellous bone and must therefore be avoided.[5,120,155] Create an optimal host bed, preferably with marrow-rich cancellous bone margins. Heating the recipient bed with power burrs or coating a bleeding interface with bone wax can destroy viable host cells and impair subsequent incorporation.

Fashion the graft during the operative procedure to mortise implants tightly into host bone. "Butter" the allograft contact sites with autograft, and apply supplemental "barrel-stave" strips of bone graft to the osteosynthesis site. Orient the graft *in situ* so as to provide axial alignment of donor cortical bone in the erect patient and maximum exposure of the cancellous areas of donor bone to the host's marrow-rich cancellous bone. Forces across the host–graft interface should maximize contact compression when the patient becomes ambulatory.

Use of continuous suction for the first 48 hours after surgery reduces hematoma formation within periosseous soft tissues, thereby reducing pain and preventing donor bone from floating in a large blood clot. Early postoperative ambulation and mild exercise stimulate blood flow and osteogenesis within the graft, provided the graft is secure within the recipient bed. External splinting appliances, as well as the patient's muscle spasm and pain, tend to stabilize the graft. Educating the patient with respect to proper posture, weight bearing, turning, and exercises, especially when the graft is most vulnerable, is critical in avoiding fatigue fractures and pseudarthrosis.

Allografts for Tumor Surgery

Large Diaphyseal Defects

When large diaphyseal bone losses are present, the alternatives for replacement include the following: sliding cortical autografts from the remaining bone above or below the defect, large corticocancellous bone grafts from the iliac crest, vascularized fibular autografts, morcellized autograft placed around an intramedullary rod,[22] and allograft bone with or without an autograft.[72,88] Autogeneic bone alone is always preferable to an unsupplemented allograft. When autograft sources are insufficient, allogeneic bone should be used in combination with the autograft. When allograft bone is used alone, it should be protected by a plate or rod throughout its entire length, in order to prevent a fatigue fracture when the allograft bone weakens because of remodeling. Many years later, when the plate or rod begins to weaken, the allograft bone will have been replaced sufficiently to provide the needed strength (Fig. 71-4). In many cases, gradual step-wise removal of the plates and screws is advisable to dynamize the allograft. In cases where devitalized or inadequate skin would overlie the graft, a preliminary or simultaneous skin-grafting operation must be performed.

Large Composite Defects

When bone and joint losses together are present, the alternatives for replacement include the following: a large osteoarticular allograft, a large diaphyseal allograft with a customized metallic joint replacement threaded through the allograft, and a joint fusion using sliding autografts with or without allograft bone. Preliminary evidence suggests that using diaphyseal allografts in combination with joint replacements is superior to using large osteoarticular allografts for replacement of large osteoarticular defects.[6]

Transplantation of large whole-joint or half-joint allografts has been reported over the past several decades.[37,88,90,99,107,109,110] Results were varied, and in all cases, complications led to a failure of normal joint function, but the operations worked well as salvage procedures. The more recent technique of threading a long-stem customized joint replacement through a large diaphyseal allograft[6] (see Fig. 71-2) appears to give better results, at least in the short term.

Acetabular allografts can be fashioned from morcellized iliac crests, from femoral heads, or from an allogeneic acetabulum itself (Fig. 71-5). All of these are best protected by screws, a porous fixed acetabular component, a plate, or some combination of these.

Large Cystic Defects

When large cysts are present in diaphyseal bone, they can be filled with autografts in most cases. However, when the cysts are so large that there is inadequate autogeneic bone available from the iliac crests, morcellized allogeneic bone (preferably AAA bone) may be used to supplement the autograft, in order to fill the cyst cavity (see Fig. 71-1).

Allografts in Sports Medicine

Perhaps the most commonly used allograft for sports medicine is the anterior cruciate ligament. Now and again it has been found to be successful in a large number of cases, but its general acceptance and place in anterior cruciate ligament reconstructions is not yet well defined because there has not been a controlled study comparing its use to the standard autogenous reconstruction techniques. If a patient is deemed an acceptable candidate for an allograft reconstruction, the following is my recommendation for the technique to be used.

Anterior Cruciate Ligament Reconstruction

The graft of choice is an iliotibial allograft that is freeze-dried after it is harvested from a cadaver that has been dead no longer than 24 hours and has been in a 4°C morgue environment after death. Move the cadaver from the morgue to the operating room and perform a sterile preparation and draping of the iliotibial band region. Harvest the graft through a longitudinal incision over the iliotibial band. The graft is approximately 2.5 cm wide, and it is approximately 25 to 30 cm long, beginning at Gerdy's tubercle and extending along the lateral aspect of the leg; this ensures that the strongest part of the ligament has been obtained. After obtaining the graft, roll it into a tubelike structure, fold it, and place it in a sterile tube for freeze-drying. Freeze-dry the graft by standard techniques in a lyophilizer as a sterile specimen, and store it for later use. Carry out a thorough donor evaluation to ensure that there is no significant risk of disease transmission.

Prepare and drape the recipient in the usual fashion, and perform an arthroscopic reconstruction of the anterior cruciate ligament, as follows. After making a standard arthroscopic evaluation of the knee joint, isolate the semitendinosus muscle tendon, using a one-inch medial incision alongside the tibial tubercle and ending at the insertion of the semitendinosus tendon. Expose the proximal medial tibia and drill a hole into the insertion area of the old anterior cruciate ligament inside the joint under arthroscopic control. Enlarge the hole to a size that will accept both the reconstituted iliotibial band allograft and the semitendinosus graft. The semitendinosus graft is used to augment the allograft with the idea that this will help to stimulate early acceptance and healing of the allograft. Cut the

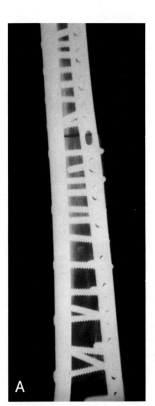
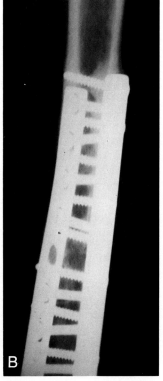

FIGURE 71-4. (*A*) Midshaft femoral freeze-dried allograft for a central chondrosarcoma. (*B*) The allograft showed good revascularization at 8 years postoperatively when one plate was removed for bursitis.

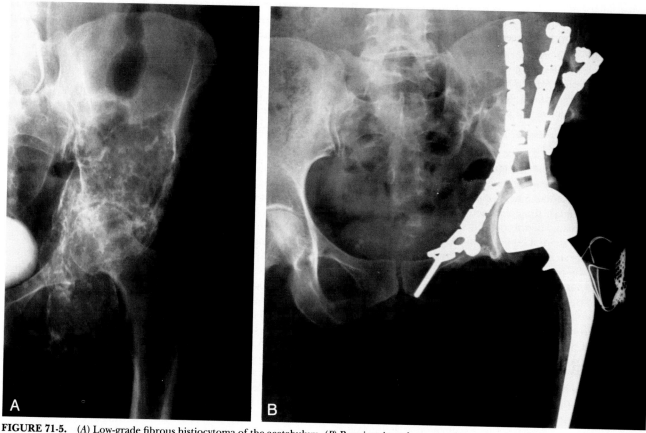

FIGURE 71-5. (*A*) Low-grade fibrous histiocytoma of the acetabulum. (*B*) Repair using a large acetabular allograft.

semitendinosus tendon graft longitudinally, open it to form a sheath, and wrap it around the tubular allograft specimen, leaving the ends of the allograft extending out of the semitendinosus sheath so that the allograft can be sewn to the insertion of the semitendinosus and other pes anserinus tendons.

Next, make a lateral incision in the lateral femur approximately 5 to 6 inches above the joint line and carry it down through the iliotibial band, anterior to the thick substance of the band. Continue the incision down through the anterior margin of the vastus lateralis onto the side of the femur. Under arthroscopic control, and using a guide to place the drill bit accurately, drill a hole into the femoral origin of the old anterior cruciate stump on the inside of the knee. Enlarge the hole to accept the iliotibial band allograft surrounded by the semitendinosus tube.

Pass the iliotibial band allograft through the tibial hole, through the knee joint, and out through the femoral hole. It is useful to use no. 2 or no. 3 Tevdek sutures at either end of the allograft in a Bunnell-type suture for passing the allograft through the knee joint and eventually sewing it to its respective sites of insertion. Denude an area of bone at the proximal medial tibia, just underneath the pes anserinus tendons and at the insertion of the semitendinosus. Sew the distal end of the allograft to the insertion of the semitendinosus tendon, and add a few additional sutures through the pes anserinus tendon.

Pass the proximal end of the allograft underneath the iliotibial band and sew it to the iliotibial band insertion at Gerdy's

tubercle, after denuding the bone in this area to promote healing of the allograft to the bone. If there is anterolateral rotatory instability due to deficiencies and laxity of the posterolateral capsule, then route the allograft first to the posterolateral capsule and sew it into this region; then route it to Gerdy's tubercle for distal attachment. Augment the sutures at the posterolateral capsule with sutures into the lateral collateral ligament.

The incision may need to be extended from 5 inches above the joint line down to Gerdy's tubercle if a reconstruction of the posterolateral corner of the knee is necessary. However, if the posterolateral capsule does not need to be reinforced, then a proximal lateral incision and a small distal lateral incision over Gerdy's tubercle are all that is needed.

Close the wounds and apply a posterolateral Robert Jones dressing. This is kept on until bleeding has been controlled postoperatively; then place the patient in a moveable knee splint which restricts the range of motion to the middle ranges, in order to prevent stress on the allograft repair at its origin or insertion. This restricted range of motion is maintained for 6 weeks, after which time the patient may progress to a full range of motion by 3 months. Additional protection of the allograft is then provided by a brace, which is worn for another 6 months to a year. Full weight bearing is allowed at 6 months.

Other ligaments about the knee and other joints can be reconstructed, as well as the anterior cruciate ligament. In general, the principle of augmenting the allograft with a nearby smaller autograft is advisable, if possible. Extra-articular allograft ligament reconstructions can be expected to do much better than those that need to be passed through the center of the joint. The extra-articular environment appears much more conducive to rapid and complete allograft replacement.[10] Nonetheless, brace protection of extra-articular grafts for 3 to 6 months is advised, as the allograft ligaments heal more slowly than autograft reconstructions.

Meniscal Allografts

Meniscal allografts are intriguing, but their applicability to sports medicine replacements is ill-defined. Our experience, using a canine medial compartment knee joint allograft as a model,[131,133] suggests that fresh meniscal allografts suffer some damage as a result of the immune response that develops against the subchondral bone and cartilage of the medial compartment allograft. The characteristic findings in our studies were loss of the central proteoglycan staining of the meniscus and some pannus reaction around the edge of the meniscus. These findings were not apparent in the autograft group; however, the autograft menisci did not appear to be as healthy as fresh unoperated menisci.[126] The allograft menisci showed some reconstitution, apparently by new cell invasion from the recipient bed. Preliminary studies in our laboratory have shown that frozen menisci do reconstitute well and appear to become viable and healthy. In summary, at the present time, the meniscal allograft must be considered experimental: it has not been tried in humans and it is in various stages of animal experimentation. However, it deserves future evaluation as an innovative procedure in certain human experimental situations. It is recommended that human menisci be transplanted as frozen or freeze-dried material, as it appears from our experiments that frozen menisci show good reconstitution, and freezing or freeze-drying the menisci should decrease the HLA antigenicity. Again, since they do contain some foreign material, after surgery the grafts would probably need longer protection from mediolateral, anterior, and rotatory stresses, as well as from weight bearing, than would a regular meniscal repair.

Allografts for Joint Surface Defects (Shell Allografts)

Since abrasion chondroplasty and arthroplastic reconstruction for joint surface defects can yield poor results,[23,25,31,51,57,78,89] biologic resurfacing of joint defects is being tried. The concept of an autogenous free periosteal graft coupled with continuous passive motion[101] is a promising one, but development of this technique is still in the preliminary stages. The use of autogenous osteoarticular autografts is an acceptable means of reconstruction;[134,145,146] however, this technique has the disadvantage that the available graft materials seldom have a suitable shape for reconstructing a given defect.

Somewhat better known is the use of shell allografts, involving the transplantation of a devascularized, osteoarticular allograft with a small bony component. Studies of osteoarticular shell allografts in humans have not been followed long enough or often enough to determine their eventual outcome, but several authors have reported promising early results.[56–58,96] Of those shell allografts that have failed, some appear to have had a significant pannus reaction,[69] suggesting that an immune response was induced by the cells of the subchondral bone.[38]

Shell Allografts—Specific Techniques

The specific techniques in performing shell allografts vary to a certain extent, as there is always considerable variation in the defect that exists. If a small joint surface defect exists, then an attempt is made to resect only that part of the joint surface. Press fit a clear plastic or wax material over the joint surface defect, to use as a template, and make a cut in the cartilage approximately 3 to 4 mm around the defect. In this way, a circumferential cut is made in good viable cartilage just to the edge of the defected cartilage. Then cut approximately 3 mm into subchondral bone with an osteotome, and remove the entire joint surface defect. Inspect the subchondral bone, and curette any remaining defective subchondral bone. If there is a large crater, as in avascular necrosis of the hip, pack it with a fresh autogenous iliac crest bone graft.

Prepare the small allograft piece from a donor joint that has recently been procured. (Procurement requires taking the specimen in a sterile fashion and keeping it stored at 4°C, soaking in a plastic bag of Ringer's lactate and sitting on ice.) The end of a long bone is sufficient for small defects. Place the plastic template that was used to mark the size of the defect over the donor cartilage surface, mark the donor surface cartilage with a knife, and cut a corresponding piece from the donor surface, being sure to make the piece slightly larger than that which was removed from the recipient. Remove approximately 1 cm of subchondral bone with the donor cartilage. Press fit the perfectly sized donor piece into the defect.

If there is good fixation at this point, no further fixation is needed. However, it is better to err on the side of obtaining good fixation if possible. Small threaded Steinmann pins may be drilled from the side into the subchondral bone, and small screws may also be used for this purpose. Either would be a better procedure than to pass screws across the cartilaginous surface through the tidemark. If the anatomy of the joint does not allow this technique, then drill four small (2.7-mm) holes in the four quadrants of the graft, bringing the drill holes out through cortical bone at some place distant from the graft along the metaphyseal region of the bone. Pass one absorbable suture (such as polyglycolic acid) through two of the holes and tie it over the cortical bone. Pass another suture in a crisscross fashion through the other two holes and tie it over bone. This provides fixation of the graft until the subchondral bone heals, and by that time the suture will dissolve. The latter method is not as good as using screws or small pins, as it involves drilling through the tidemark as well as the pressure of suture across the donor cartilaginous surface.

Place the patient's joint in a temporary splint after adequate closure has been obtained, and allow the joint to rest for 2 to 3 days. Once the bleeding has stopped and the wound has begun good healing, start continuous passive motion if adequate fixation of the graft has been obtained at surgery. The continuous passive motion is continued for 3 months if the patient's insurance allows for the additional expense of this machine, or if the patient can rent such a machine through his own resources. Otherwise, a second-best option would be to recommend intermittent passive movement of the joint ten times every 10 minutes. The patient is not allowed full weight bearing for 6 to 9 months, when radiographs should show adequate healing of the subchondral bone interfaces. This process will take longer than normal, because there most likely will be a mild immune and inflammatory response at these interfaces that will delay healing of the bone. It is important to evaluate the graft approximately one year after surgery, using diagnostic arthroscopy in order to look for an immune rejection phenomenon, which will be characterized by pannus covering the graft. If this occurs, the prognosis for the graft is poor.

Pre- and postoperative serum studies can help to predict an immune response. Serum samples should be obtained before surgery and at 6 weeks, 12 weeks, and one year after the surgery. These serum samples can be tested against donor lym-

phocytes or a panel of typed lymphocytes in a standard lymphocyte toxicity assay, if the donor lymphocytes were obtained at the time of the graft procurement. A strong immune response does not necessarily mean that the graft will be destroyed, and although it is helpful to know in advance whether this may occur, diagnostic arthroscopy is the only sure way to determine the health of the graft.

If a large shell allograft is needed, such as in replacement of the entire hemijoint surface of a given joint, or in replacing a medial or lateral side of both the proximal and distal joint surfaces, then different techniques are needed. In these cases, there is usually a large defect due to a severe traumatic episode, such as a gunshot wound.

Procure the allograft specimen as an entire joint specimen, and transport it to the operating room in sterile saline at 4°C

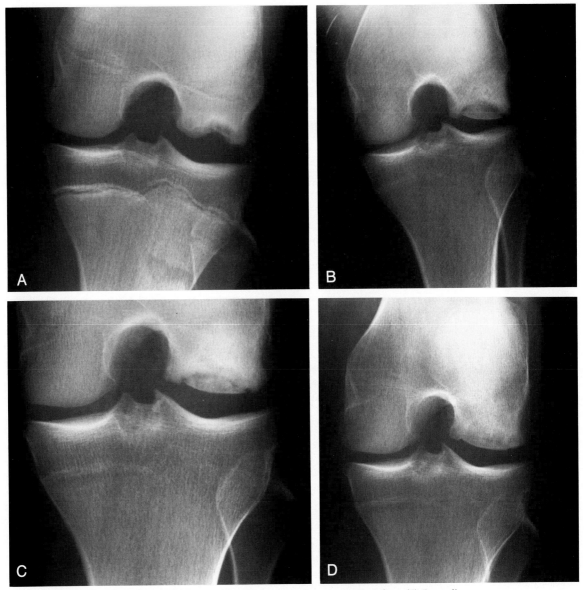

FIGURE 71-6.   Femoral condyle shell allograft. (*A*) Preoperative traumatic defect. (*B*) Immediate postoperative radiograph. (*C*) Replacement of subchondral bone in progress. (*D*) Full replacement of subchondral bone at 2 years after surgery. (Courtesy of Dr. Frank Palumbo.)

with the capsule intact. Transplantation of the joint surfaces should be done at approximately 24 hours from the time of procurement. There is evidence to suggest that, with this type of storage, the subchondral bone cells will die before the cartilage cells, and this may be advantageous in trying to prevent an immune response against the subchondral bone that could eventually damage the donor cartilage.[132] For this reason, the specimens are not transplanted fresh and "warm."

Debride the defect in the joint of all scar tissue down to good bleeding bone. Fashion the shell allograft pieces to fit the defect, leaving intact on the graft any ligaments needed to replace ligaments missing in the recipient. Fix the graft through subchondral bone with threaded Steinmann pins, screws, or staples placed from the side and not passing the donor cartilage surface. If good fixation is obtained at the time of surgery, then begin continuous passive motion within a short time after surgery. However, if only marginal fixation is obtained, then immobilize the entire joint for 6 weeks or, at most, allow a few degrees of motion in a protective brace. Partial weight bearing is allowed for 3 to 6 months until adequate healing of the subchondral bone interfaces is evident on radiography; this may require tomographic evaluation. A second look with an arthroscope at one year after surgery is desirable to determine whether or not a severe immune reaction is occurring. Serial pre- and postoperative serum histocompatibility testing should also be done to monitor the immune response.

Shell Allografts—Results and Prognosis

As shown by the results of McDermott and co-workers[93] (Table 71-1), shell allografts have been most successful in those patients who have suffered traumatic damage to their joint surfaces. These patients have had a success rate of 69% to 92%.[93] Patients with osteoarthritis have also fared satisfactorily, with a success rate of 42%. Patients with osteochondritis dissecans and avascular necrosis have had the poorest results, with a success rate of only about 25%. The reason for this poor show-

TABLE 71-1. EFFECTS OF ETIOLOGY ON THE RESULTS OF SHELL ALLOGRAFTS

	No. of Patients	No. (Percent) Successful
Trauma		
Tibial plateau	36	25 (69)
Femoral condyle	12	11 (92)
Osteoarthritis	24	10 (42)
Osteochondritis dissecans	4	1 (25)
Osteonecrosis		
SONK	11	3 (27)
Steroids	3	0 (0)
TOTALS	90*	50 (56)

* Five patients had a second graft and results listed are for the final graft, and five patients had grafts of the patella (two) or talus (three) and are not included, thus accounting for 90 patients of an initial 100 grafts. (From McDermott, A. G., Langer, F., Pritzker, K. P., and Gross, A. E.: Fresh Small-Fragment Osteochondral Allografts. Long-Term Follow-Up Study on First 100 Cases. Clin. Orthop. **197:**96, 1985.)

ing may be that there is inadequate healing of the osteosynthesis site because of a poor blood supply to the subchondral bone.

Allografts for Revision Arthroplasties

Allografts for revision arthroplasties have been used primarily in the hip. Major segmental defects in acetabulum as well as in the proximal femur may occur after multiple revision arthroplasties, and these defects may be reconstructed with allografts.

Acetabular defects may be divided into rim defects, medial wall defects, and global defects. The rim defects can be subcategorized into superior rim, posterior rim, or combinations of the superior and posterior rim defect. Most of the superior or posterior rim defects can be reconstructed using a bicortical piece of autogenous iliac crest. If the defect is large, as in the case of the combined superior and posterior rim defect, it is usually better to reconstruct the defect with a proximal femoral head allograft. In these cases, cut and shape the proximal femoral head to provide the bone stock that is necessary, and fix it to the pelvis with two to three screws. It is advantageous to use a porous ingrowth type of acetabular component that has screw holes, particularly near the rim, so that the screws securing the component can be used as additional fixation of the allograft. Butter the allograft with autogenous marrow and morcellized iliac crest bone to stimulate healing at the osteosynthesis site. These grafts may take up to 2 years to be completely resorbed and replaced by recipient bone, and, therefore, they should be protected with partial weight bearing during this time.

In acetabular medial wall defects, if there is simply thinning of the medial wall, then using morcellized autograft under a fixed porous acetabular component is recommended. If there is ballooning of the medial wall, morcellized autograft with a fixed porous component is usually satisfactory. If the medial wall defect is segmental and large, then it may be adequate to use a large outer table of autogenous iliac crest, plus morcellized graft in a fixed porous component, or it may be necessary also to use a femoral head allograft fashioned to fill the defect. Again, a porous acetabular component is desirable as it will fix the allograft to the recipient autogenous surfaces.

The combination of a medial wall defect and a rim defect may constitute a very large defect to be replaced. In these cases, use a large femoral head allograft. Debride the femoral head allograft of all cartilage and soft tissue, and fix it with a few screws to the recipient pelvic wall. Butter the surfaces of the femoral head allograft with autogenous bone and marrow before fixation. Once it is in position, ream the allograft, using standard reaming techniques, and then place a porous ingrowth type of acetabular component. Fastening additional screws through the porous component into the allograft as well as into the remaining recipient pelvic wall will improve graft fixation. Prolonged protection with partial weight bearing for up to 2 years is recommended to allow complete incorporation of the allograft material.

For very large global defects, a complete acetabular allograft is necessary. In harvesting the allograft for these cases, preserve the ischial ramus, pubic ramus, and superior acetabular bone. Fix the graft with screws and plates to the recipient pelvic bone. If a bipolar proximal femoral component is to be used, then use an anterior as well as a posterior column plate to fix the allograft. Again, butter the surfaces of the allograft with autograft to stimulate healing and union. If a total hip replacement is to be used, then install a posterior column plate plus a fixed porous acetabular component, after reaming the allograft acetabulum and coating it with autogenous bone. Place the screws fixing the acetabular component so that they pass through the allograft and into recipient autogenous bone. Take care to place the posterior column plate slightly anterior on the recipient's ischial tuberosity to protect the sciatic nerve from irritation as it passes near the plate.

Proximal femur defects may be categorized into three types. The first is an intramedullary defect due to diffuse focal resorption of intramedullarly bone around the bone cement interface; the second is a medial calcar defect; and the third is a global proximal femoral defect. The intramedullary defect is best treated with autogenous morcellized bone plus a porous ingrowth type of prosthesis. If, however, the amount of bone lost is too great to be replaced with autogenous bone, then mix autogenous iliac crest bone with morcellized allograft bone as a slurry and pack the defect with this combination autograft and allograft before seating the proximal femoral component. Use a proximal femoral component that has porous coating throughout most of its length to allow maximum ingrowth. For medial calcar defects, cut and fashion a medial calcar allograft to fit the defect. Fix this graft with wires, screws, or a combination of both, prior to seating the proximal femoral component. In these cases, the porous coating need only be in the proximal third of the femoral component, where ingrowth is to be enhanced.

A global defect of the proximal femur may encompass bone loss of several centimeters in length. In these cases, cut an entire proximal femur allograft and fashion it to fit the defect, making a step cut at the osteosynthesis site. If the allograft is worked on the back table until it has been reamed, cement the proximal femoral component into place in the allograft as a separate procedure on the back table. Remove all excess cement from the osteosynthesis step cut site on the allograft, and then cement the distal stem into place. Additional fixation is usually necessary at the osteosynthesis site in the form of a plate, screws, or cerclage wires. In addition, place strips of autogenous iliac crest around the circumference of the osteosynthesis site and hold them in place with cerclage wires. This stimulates healing at the osteosynthesis site.

Postoperative management of these patients includes suction drainage of any postoperative hematomas and bed rest for 3 to 4 days until bleeding has stopped. At this time the patient is allowed mobilization and partial weight bearing, using a walker or crutches for several months until adequate healing of the osteosynthesis site has occurred. Follow graft healing on serial radiographs. Healing of the osteosynthesis site can be expected to take twice as long as normal bone healing; that is, 3 to 6 months rather than 6 weeks to 3 months. Replacement of large grafts may take several years, and for this reason patients should use a cane for several years to protect the prosthesis and the graft until it has been solidly incorporated and replaced by recipient bone. Serial bone scans are helpful in interpreting this replacement process. The allograft will become "hot" on bone scan within a few weeks to a few months after the operative procedure, and will remain hot for several years. If quanti-

tative bone scans can be done, when the scan turns "colder" it is probably an indication that sufficient strength has been regained to allow full weight bearing.

Allografts for Trauma

The use of bone and joint allografts after severe traumatic destruction of skeletal parts presents many more difficult problems than replacement of tumor or arthritic defects. Severe soft tissue injuries usually accompany the bony trauma, and, in addition, the wounds have often been previously infected. Therefore, the surgeon is frequently operating in an area with a decreased blood supply, poor skin coverage, and a few persisting organisms from previous infections. Most of the use of allografts for traumatic defects has come from wartime experience, and the following important prerequisites should be adhered to:[12]

1. The distal anatomic parts must be functionally intact.
2. Good skin coverage must be present or obtainable at the time of surgery (remembering that a collapsed soft tissue space is going to be filled with bone, creating a stress on the previous skin coverage).
3. Infection must be controlled.
4. Circulation must be adequate.
5. Abundant cancellous autograft must be used to supplement the bony surfaces of the allograft.
6. The graft must be immobilized until healing is complete.

Failure to adhere to these principles places the graft at significant risk of failure.

Diaphyseal Bone Defects

A number of technical principles have been developed in the treatment of diaphyseal defects. First, morcellized bone appears to incorporate faster than large segmental allografts. Jeshrani and Bencivenga[66] found that 5 of 5 cortical grafts without morcellized grafts failed, 3 of 3 cortical grafts with morcelized graft succeeded, and 17 of 17 grafts with only morcellized bone healed well. Osteogenesis and revascularization of the morcellized bone begins to occur within 10 days, and bacteria are much less likely to survive in these small, rapidly revascularized pieces than in a large, nonviable piece of allograft bone.[17]

Second, when a large cortical graft is needed to bridge a gap in the femur, humerus, or other isolated long bone, it is recommended that half of an allograft shaft be used with morcellized autologous bone packed around it.[12] This has two advantages: it maximizes the morcellized graft material, and it decreases the volume of cortical bone that might overdistend the already shrunken surrounding soft tissue. Extreme care must be taken to protect the large cortical allograft until it has been incorporated; this may take as long as two to three years. The protection can be provided by a cast, brace, internal fixation with rods or plates, or a combination of these techniques.

Third, it is usually not advisable to use a large cortical allograft for tibial bone loss. In this case, a proximal and distal

TABLE 71-2. RESULTS OF ALLOGRAFT–AUTOGRAFTS FOR TRAUMATIC BONE LOSS

Involved Bone	No. of Grafts	Results			
		Good	Satisfactory	Poor	Failure
Upper extremity					
Humerus	7	2	3	2	0
Ulna	4	2	1	1	0
Radius	3	1	1	1	0
TOTALS	14	5	5	4	0
		70%			
Lower extremity					
Femur	7	2	2	2	1
Tibia	9	2	2	2	3
TOTALS	16	4	4	4	4
		50%			

(Adapted from Brown, R. H., and Townsend, G. B.: Segmental Defects in Open Fractures of Long Bones. Med. Ann. D. C. **39:**555, 1970.)

tibiofibular synostosis is obtained first; then progressive grafts made of morcellized, mixed autograft and allograft bone are used to bridge the defect.[94] This may require a number of successive grafts. It is possible that synthetic bone materials mixed with autogenous graft may prove to be at least as good as allograft material for filling such defects.

If one follows the principles of attention to soft tissues and protection from infection, and if one emphasizes the maximal use of morcellized autografts with allografts, the results[12] shown in Table 71-2 can be expected. A good result is defined as restored bone continuity and no need for a brace. Satisfactory results are those with restored bone continuity but with the need for bracing. A failure is defined as an amputation for persistent infection.

Articular Surface Defects

When articular surface defects are due to trauma, replacement requires the use of a fresh allograft, because the cartilage must be viable to provide a good joint surface. With a fresh shell allograft (a fresh allograft taken within 24 hours after death and stored at 4°C for several hours until it is transplanted), the results can be expected to be good in 80% of the cases.[93] An immune response routinely occurs after these grafts, most likely induced by the exposed subchondral bone,[77] but the extent of damage to the graft from this response is not known. The success rate is considerably better when shell allografts are used for traumatic defects than when used for primary arthritic conditions such as osteoarthritis and avascular necrosis (see Table 71-1).

The success rates of large fresh osteochondral allografts has not yet been determined for post-traumatic conditions. The success rates would probably be considerably lower, owing to problems with avascular necrosis, collapse of subchondral bone, and a more severe immune response. Using artificial joints threaded through the allograft may prove to be a better method to treat post-traumatic defects of the ends of long bone, as has been the case with large tumors or failed total joint replacements.

REFERENCES

1. Andersson, G.B.J., Lereim, P., Galante, J.O., and Rostoker, W.: Segmental Replacement of the Femur in Baboons with Fiber Metal Implants and Autologous Bone Grafts of Different Particle Size. Acta Orthop. Scand. **53:**349, 1982.
2. Arnoczky, S., Warren, R.F., Ashlock, M.A.: Replacement of the Anterior Cruciate Ligament Using a Patellar Tendon Allograft. J. Bone Joint Surg. **68-A:**376, 1986.
3. Aurori, B.F., Weierman, R.J., Lowell, H.A., Nadel, C.I., and Parsons, J.R.: Pseudarthrosis After Spinal Fusion for Scoliosis. Clin. Orthop. **199:**153, 1985.
4. Barad, S., Cabaud, H.E., and Rodrigo, J.J.: Effects of Storage at −80°C as Compared to 4°C on the Strength of Rhesus Monkey Anterior Cruciate Ligaments. Trans. Orthop. Res. Soc. **7:**378, 1982.
5. Bassett, C.A.L.: Clinical Implications of Cell Function in Bone Grafting. Clin. Orthop. **87:**49, 1972.
6. Borja, F.J., and Mnaymneh, W.: Bone Allografts in Salvage of Difficult Hip Arthroplasties. Clin. Orthop. **197:**123, 1985.
7. Bos, G.D., Goldberg, V.M., Gordon, N.H., Dollinger, B.M., Zika, J.M., Powell, A.E., and Heiple, K.G.: The Long-Term Fate of Fresh and Frozen Orthotopic Bone Allografts in Genetically Defined Rats. Clin. Orthop. **197:**245, 1985.
8. Boyne, P.T.: Review of the Literature on Cryopreservation of Bone. Cryobiology **4:**341, 1968.
9. Bright, R.W., and Burchardt, H.: The Biomechanical Properties of Preserved Bone Grafts. *In* Friedlaender, G.E., Mankin, H.J., and Sell, K.W. (eds.): *Osteochondral Allografts.* Boston, Little, Brown, 1983, p. 241.
10. Bright, R.W., and Green, W.T.: Freeze-dried Fascia Lata Allografts: A Review of 47 Cases. J. Pediatr. Orthop. **1:**13, 1981.
11. Brown, M.D.: Lumbar spine fusion. *In* Finneson, B.E. (ed.): *Low Back Pain,* 2nd ed. Philadelphia, J.B. Lippincott, 1980, p. 379.
12. Brown, R.H., and Townsend, G.B.: Segmental Defects in Open Fractures of Long Bones. Med. Ann. D.C. **39:**555, 1970.

13. Burchardt, H.: Biology of Cortical Bone Graft Incorporation. *In* Friedlaender, G.E., Mankin, H.J. and Sell, K.W. (eds.): *Osteochondral Allografts.* Boston, Little, Brown, 1983, p. 51.

14. Burchardt, H., and Enneking, W.F.: Transplantation of Bone. Surg. Clin. North Am. **58:**403, 1978.

15. Burchardt, H., Glowczewskie, F.P., and Enneking, W.F.: Allogeneic Segmental Fibular Transplants in Azathioprine-Immunosuppressed Dogs. J. Bone Joint Surg. **59-A:**881, 1977.

16. Burchardt, H., Glowczewskie, F.P., and Enneking, W.F.: Short-Term Immunosuppression with Fresh Segmental Fibular Allografts in Dogs. J. Bone Joint Surg. **63-A:**411, 1981.

17. Reference deleted.

18. Burwell, R.G.: The Fate of Bone Grafts. *In* Apley, A.G. (ed.): *Recent Advances in Orthopaedics.* London, Churchill, 1969, p. 115.

19. Cameron, H.U.: Evaluation of a Biodegradable Ceramic. J. Biomed. Mater. Res. **11:**179, 1977.

20. Campbell, C.J.: Homotransplantation of Half and Whole Joints. Clin. Orthop. **87:**146, 1972.

21. Cautilli, R.A.: Theoretical Superiority of Posterior Lumbar Interbody Fusion. *In* Lin, P.M. (ed.): *Posterior Lumbar Interbody Fusion.* Springfield, Ill., Charles C Thomas, 1982, p. 82.

22. Chapman, M.W.: Closed Intramedullary Bone-Grafting and Nailing of Segmental Defects of the Femur. J. Bone Joint Surg. **62-A:**1004, 1980.

23. Chappell, G.E.: Current Trends in the Treatment of the Young Adult with Disabling Hip Disease. Clin. Orthop. **106:**35, 1975.

24. Chase, S.W., and Herndon, C.H.: The Fate of Autogenous and Homogenous Bone Grafts. J. Bone Joint Surg. **37-A:**809, 1955.

25. Childers, J.C., and Ellwood, S.C.: Partial Chondrectomy and Subchondral Bone Drilling for Chondromalacia. Clin. Orthop. **144:**114, 1979.

26. Cloward, R.B.: The Treatment of Ruptured Lumbar Intervertebral Discs by Vertebral Body Fusion. J. Neurosurg. **10:**154, 1953.

27. Cloward, R.B.: The Anterior Approach for Removal of Ruptured Cervical Discs. J. Neurosurg. **15:**602, 1958.

28. Cloward, R.B.: Posterior Lumbar Interbody Fusion Updated. Clin. Orthop. **193:**16, 1985.

29. Cobey, M.C.: A National Bone Bank Survey. Clin. Orthop. **110:**333, 1975.

30. Collis, J.S.: Total Disc Replacement: A Modified Posterior Lumbar Interbody Fusion. Clin. Orthop. **193:**64, 1985.

31. Collis, D.K., and Johnston, R.C.: Comparative Evaluation of the Results of Cup Arthroplasty and Total Hip Replacement. Clin. Orthop. **86:**102, 1972.

32. Cook, S.D., Anderson, R.L., Kester, M.A., Thomas, K.A., Reynolds, M.C., and Haddad, R.J., Jr.: Articular Cartilage Degeneration as a Function of Material and Fixation. Trans. Orthop. Res. Soc. **10:**92, 1985.

33. Craigmyle, M.B.: Antigenicity and Survival of Cartilage Homografts. Nature **182:**1248, 1958.

34. Craigmyle, M.B.: Regional Lymph Node Changes Induced by Cartilage Homo- and Heterografts in the Rabbit. J. Anat. **92:**74, 1958.

35. Craven, P.L., and Urist, M.R.: Osteogenesis by Radio-Isotope Labelled Cell Populations in Implants of Bone Matrix under the Influence of Ionizing Radiation. Clin. Orthop. **76:**231, 1971.

36. Curtis, R.J., Delee, J.C., and Drez, D.J., Jr.: Reconstruction of the Anterior Cruciate Ligament with Freeze Dried Fascia Lata Allografts in Dogs. A preliminary report. Am. J. Sports Med. **13:**408, 1985.

37. Czitrom, A.A., Langer, F., McKee, N., and Gross, A.E.: Bone and Cartilage Allotransplantation. Clin. Orthop. **208:**141, 1986.

38. Czitrom, A.A., Axelrod, T., and Fernandes, B.: Antigen Presenting Cells and Bone Allotransplantation. Clin. Orthop. **197:**27, 1985.

39. Elves, M.W.: Immunological Studies of Osteoarticular Allografts. Proc. R. Soc. Med. **64:**644, 1971.

40. Elves, M.W.: A Study of the Transplantation Antigens on Chondrocytes from Articular Cartilage. J. Bone Joint Surg. **56-B:**178, 1974.

41. Elves, M.W.: Humoral Immune Responses to Allografts of Bone. Int. Arch. Allergy Appl. Immunol. **47:**708, 1974.

42. Elves, M.W.: Transplantation of Osteoarticular Tissues. *In* Ali, S.Y., Elves, M.W., and Leaback, D.H. (eds.): *Normal and Osteoarthritic Articular Cartilage.* Stanmore Institute of Orthopaedics, University of London, 1974, p. 233.

43. Elves, M.W., and Ford, C.H.: The Development of Humoral Cytotoxic Antibodies after the Allografting of Articular Surfaces at the Knee Joint in Sheep. J. Bone Joint Surg. **53-B:**554, 1971.

44. Elves, M.W., and Ford, C.H.: A Study of the Humoral Immune Response to Osteoarticular Allografts in Sheep. Clin. Exp. Immunol. **17:**497, 1974.

45. Emerson, R.H., Jr., and Potter, T.: The Use of the McKeever Hemiarthroplasty for Unicompartmental Arthritis. J. Bone Joint Surg. **67-A:**208, 1985.

46. Evans, J.H.: Biomechanics of Lumbar Fusion. Clin. Orthop. **193:**38, 1985.

47. Friedlaender, G.E.: Immune Responses to Preserved Bone Allografts in Humans. *In* Friedlaender, G.E., Mankin, H.J., and Sell, K.W. (eds.): *Osteochondral Allografts.* Boston, Little, Brown, 1983, p. 159.

48. Friedlaender, G.E., and Mankin, H.J.: Bone Banking: Current Methods and Suggested Guidelines. AAOS Instructional Course Lectures **30:**36, 1981.

49. Friedlaender, G.E., Mankin, H.J., and Langer, F.: Immunology of Osteochondral Allografts: Background and General Considerations. *In* Friedlaender, G.E., Mankin, H.G., and Sell, K.W. (eds.): *Osteochondral Allografts.* Boston, Little, Brown, 1983, p. 133.

50. Friedlaender, G.E., Strong, D.M., and Sell, S.W.: Studies in the Antigenicity of Bone. J. Bone Joint Surg. **58-A:**854, 1976.

51. Friedman, M.J., Berasi, C.C., Fox, J.M., Del Pizzo, W., Synder, S.J., and Farkel, R.D.: Preliminary Results with Abrasion Arthroplasty in the Osteoarthritic Knee. Clin. Orthop. **182:**200, 1984.

52. Glowacki, J., Kaban, C.B., Murray, J.E., Folkman, J., and Mulliken, J.B.: Application of the Biological Principle of Induced Osteogenesis for Craniofacial Defects. Lancet **1:**959, 1981.

53. Goldberg, V.M., Herndon, C.H., Lance, E.M., Heiple, K.G., and Powell, A.E.: Fate of Transplanted Whole Joints. *In* Friedlaender, G.E., Mankin, H.J., and Sell, K.W. (eds.): *Osteochondral Allografts.* Boston, Little, Brown, 1983, p. 103.

54. Goldberg, V.M., and Lance, E.M.: Revascularization and Accretion in Transplantation. Quantitative Studies of the Allograft Barrier. J. Bone Joint Surg. **54-A:**807, 1972.

55. Grobstein, C.: Inductive Tissue Interactions in Development. Adv. Cancer Res. **4:**187, 1956.

56. Gross, A.E., McKee, N.H., Pritzker, K.P.H., and Langer, F.: Reconstruction of Skeletal Deficits at the Knee. Clin. Orthop. **174:**96, 1983.

57. Gross, A.E., McKee, N.H., Langer, F., and Pritzker, K.: Surgical Techniques and Clinical Experience with Articular Allografts at the Knee, *In* Friedlaender, G.E., Mankin, H.J., and Sell, K.W. (eds.): *Osteochondral Allografts.* Boston, Little, Brown, 1983, p. 289.

58. Gross, A.E., Silverstein, E.A., Fal, J., Falk, R., and Langer, F.: The Allotransplantation of Partial Joints in the Treatment of Osteoarthritis of the Knee. Clin. Orthop. **108:**7, 1975.

59. Grotz, R.T., Rodrigo, J.J., Thompson, E.C., and Travis, C.: Inhibition of the Immune Response to Fresh Osteocartilaginous Distal Femur Allografts by Preadministration of Sensitized Serum in the Rat. Trans. Orthop. Res. Soc. **5:**281, 1980.

60. Hagerty, R.F., Braid, H.L., Bonner, W.M., Jr., Henningar, G.R., and Lee, W.H., Jr.: Viable and Non-Viable Human Cartilage Homografts. Surg. Gynecol. Obstet. **125:**485, 1967.

61. Harrington, K.D., Johnston, J.O., Kaufer, H.N., and Luck, J.V., Jr.: Limb Salvage and Prosthetic Joint Reconstruction for Low-Grade and Selected High-Grade Sarcomas of Bone after Wide Resection and Replacement by Autoclaved Autogeneic Grafts. Clin. Orthop. **211:**180, 1986.

62. Herndon, C.H., and Chase, S.W.: Experimental Studies in the Transplantation of Whole Joints. J. Bone Joint Surg. **34-A:**564, 1952.

63. Heyner, S.: The Antigenicity of Cartilage Grafts. Surg. Gynecol. Obstet. **136:**298, 1973.

64. Hueston, J.T., Hubble, B., and Rigg, B.R.: Homografts of the Digital Flexor Tendon System. Aust. N.Z. J. Surg. **36:**269, 1967.

65. Jarcho, M.: Calcium Phosphate Ceramics as Hard Tissue Prosthetics. Clin. Orthop. **157:**259, 1981.

66. Jeshrani, M.K., and Bencivenga, A.: Comparative Value of Cortical and Cancellous Bone as Grafting Material in Bone Defect of Different Origins. East Afr. Med. J. **55:**228, 1978.

67. Johnson, C.A., Brown, B.A., and Lasky, L.C.: Rh Immunization Caused by Osseous Allograft. N. Engl. J. Med. **312:**121, 1985.

68. Judet, H., and Padovani, J.P.: Transplantation d'articulation complète avec rétablissement circulatoire immediat par anastomoses arterielles et veineuses. Mem. Acad. Chir. (Paris) **94:**520, 1968.

69. Kandel, R.A., Gross, A.E., Ganel, A., McDermott, A.G.P., Langer, F., and Pritzker, K.P.H.: Histopathology of Failed Osteoarticular Shell Allografts. Clin. Orthop. **197:**103, 1985.

70. Kingma, M.J., and Hampe, J.F.: The Behavior of Blood Vessels after Experimental Transplantation of Bone. J. Bone Joint Surg. **46-B:**141, 1964.

71. Kirkaldy-Willis, W.H., and Farfan, H.F.: Instability of the Lumbar Spine. Clin. Orthop. **165:**110, 1982.

72. Koskinen, E.V.S.: Wide Resection of Primary Tumors of Bone and Replacement with Massive Bone Grafts. An Improved Technique for Transplanting Allogeneic Bone Grafts. Clin. Orthop. **134:**302, 1978.

73. Kreuz, F.P., Hyatt, G.W., Turner, T.C., and Bassett, A.L.: The Preservation and Clinical Use of Freeze-Dried Bone. J. Bone Joint Surg. **33-A:**863, 1951.

74. Lance, E.M., and Fisher, R.L.: Transplantation of the Rabbit Patella. J. Bone Joint Surg. **52-A:**145, 1970.

75. Langer, F., and Gross, A.E.: Immunogenicity of Allograft Articular Cartilage. J. Bone Joint Surg. **56-A:**297, 1974.

76. Langer, F., Gross, A.E., and Greaves, M.F.: The Auto-Immunogenicity of Articular Cartilage. Clin. Exp. Immunol. **12:**31, 1972.

77. Langer, F., Gross, A.E., West, M., and Urovitz, E.P.: The Immunogenicity of Allograft Knee Joint Transplants. Clin. Orthop. **132:**155, 1978.

78. Laskin, R.S.: Unicompartment Tibiofemoral Resurfacing Arthroplasty. J. Bone Joint Surg. **60-A:**182, 1978.

79. Lexer, E.: Die Verwendung der freien Knockenplastik nebst Versuchen über Gelenkverstiefung und Gelenktransplantation. Arch. Klin. Chir. **86:**939, 1908.

80. Lexer, E.: Joint Transplantation and Arthroplasty. Surg. Gynecol. Obstet. **40:**782, 1925.

81. Lin, P.M.: Posterior Lumbar Interbody Fusion Technique: complications and Pitfalls. Clin. Orthop. **193:**90, 1985.

82. Lindholm, T.S., and Urist, M.R.: A Quantitative Analysis of New Bone Formation by Induction in Composite Grafts of Bone Marrow and Bone Matrix. Clin. Orthop. **150:**288, 1980.

83. Lipson, R.A., Kawano, H., Halloran, P.F., McKee, N.H., Pritzker, K.P.H., and Langer, F.: Vascularized Limb Transplantation in the Rat. I. Results with syngeneic grafts. Transplantation **35:**293, 1983.

84. Lipson, R.A., Kawano, H., Halloran, P.F., Pritzker, K.P.H., Kandal, R., and Langer, F.: Vascularized Limb Transplantation in the Rat. II. Results with allogeneic grafts. Transplantation **35:**300, 1983.

85. Liu, T.K.: Transplantation of Preserved Composite Tendon Allografts. J. Bone Joint Surg. **57-A:**65, 1975.

86. Makley, J.T.: The Use of Allografts to Reconstruct Intercalary Defects of Long Bones. Clin. Orthop. **197:**58, 1985.

87. Malinin, T.I., Martinez, O.V., and Brown, M.D.: Banking of Massive Osteoarticular and Intercalary Bone Allografts—12-Year Experience. Clin. Orthop. **197:**44, 1985.

88. Mankin, H.J.: Complications of Allograft Surgery. *In* Friedlander, G.E., Mankin, H.J., Sell, K.W., (eds.): *Osteochondral Allografts.* Boston, Little, Brown, 1983, p. 259.

89. Mankin, H.J.: The Response of Articular Cartilage to Mechanical Injury. J. Bone Joint Surg. **64-A:**460, 1982.

90. Mankin, H.J., Fogelson, F.S., Thrasher, A.Z., and Jaffer, F.: Massive Resection and Allograft Transplantation in the Treatment of Malignant Bone Tumors. New Engl. J. Med. **294:**1247, 1976.

91. Marmor, L.: Unicompartmental and Total Knee Arthroplasty. Clin. Orthop. **192:**75, 1985.

92. McCarthy, R.E., Peek, R.D., Morrissy, R.T., and Hough, A.J.: Allograft Bone in Spinal Fusion for Paralytic Scoliosis. J. Bone Joint Surg. **68-A:**370, 1986.

93. McDermott, A.G., Langer, F., Pritzker, K.P., and Gross, A.E.: Fresh Small-Fragment Osteochondral Allografts. Long-Term Follow-Up Study on First 100 Cases. Clin. Orthop. **197:**96, 1985.

94. McMaster, P.E., and Hohl, M.: Tibiofibular Cross-Peg Grafting. J. Bone Joint Surg. **47-A:**1146, 1965.

95. Mellonig, J.T., Bowers, G.M., and Cotton, W.R.: Comparison of Bone Graft Materials. II. New Bone Formation with Autografts and Allografts: a Histological Evaluation. J. Periodontol. **52:**297, 1981.

96. Meyers, M.H., Bucholtz, R.W., and Jones, R.E.: Surgical Techniques and Clinical Experience with Fresh Osteochondral Allografts of the Hip. *In* Friedlander, G.E., Mankin, J.H., and Sell, K.W. (eds.): *Osteochondral Allografts.* Boston, Little, Brown, 1983, p. 287.

97. Miller, F., Sussman, M., and Stamp, W.: The Use of Bone Allograft: a Survey of Current Practice. In Jacobs R.R. (ed.): Pathogenesis of Idiopathic Scoliosis: Proceedings of an International Conference: Chicago, Scoliosis Research Society, 1984.

98. Minami, A., Ishii, S., Ogino, T., Oikawa, T., and Kobayashi, H.: Effect of the Immunological Antigenicity of the Allogeneic Tendons on Tendon Grafting. Hand, **14:**111, 1982.

99. Mnaymneh, W., Malinin, T.I., Makley, J.T., and Dick, H.M.: Massive Osteoarticular Allografts in the Reconstruction of Extremities Following Resection of Tumors not Requiring Chemotherapy and Radiation. Clin. Orthop. **197:**76, 1985.

100. Nelson, J.F., Stanford, H.G., and Cutright, D.E.: Evaluation and Comparisons of Biodegradable Substances as Osteogenic Agents. Oral Med. Oral Pathol. **43:**836, 1977.

101. O'Driscoll, S.W., and Salter, R.B.: The Induction of Neochondrogenesis in Free Intra-Articular Periosteal Autografts Under the Influence of Continuous Passive Motion. J. Bone Joint Surg. **66-A:**1248, 1984.

102. Oikarinen, J.: Experimental Spinal Fusion with Decalcified Bone Matrix and Deep Frozen Allogeneic Bone in Rabbits. Clin. Orthop. **162:**210, 1982.

103. Oikarinen, J., and Korhonen, L.K.: The Bone Inductive Capacity of Various Bone Transplanting Materials Used for Treatment of Experimental Bone Defects. Clin. Orthop. **140:**208, 1979.

104. Oklund, S.A., Prolo, D.J., Gutierrez, R.V., and King, S.E.: Quantitative Comparisons of Healing in Cranial Fresh Autografts, Frozen Autografts, and Processed Autografts and Allografts in Canine Skull Defects. Clin. Orthop. **205:**269, 1986.

105. Osborn, J.F., and Newesley, H.: Dynamic Aspects of the Implant-Bone Interface. *In Symposium of the European Society of Biomaterials*, Heidelberg, March 1974.

106. Osterman, K., and Lindholm, T.S.: Reconstruction of Articular Surface Using a Homogenous Osteochondral Fragment. An Experimental Study. Scand. J. Rheumatol. [Suppl.] **44:**21, 1982.

107. Ottolenghi, C.E.: Massive Osteoarticular Bone Grafts. Technic and Results of 62 Cases. Clin. Orthop. **87:**156, 1972.

108. Pap, K., and Krompecher, S.: Arthroplasty of the Knee: Experimental and Clinical Experiences. J. Bone Joint Surg. **43-A:**523, 1961.

109. Parrish, F.F.: Treatment of Bone Tumors by Total Excision and Replacement with Massive Autologous and Homologous Grafts. J. Bone Joint Surg. **48-A:**968, 1966.

110. Parrish, F.F.: Homografts of Bone. Clin. Orthop. **87:**36, 1972.

111. Parrish, F.F.: Allograft Replacement of All or Part of the End of a Long Bone Following Excision of a Tumor: report of 21 cases. J. Bone Joint Surg. **55-A:**1, 1973.

112. Peacock, E.E., Jr., and Madden, J.W.: Human Composite Flexor Tendon Allografts. Ann. Surg. **166:**624, 1967.

113. Peacock, E.E., Jr., and Petty, B.S.: Antigenicity of Tendon. Surg. Gynecol. & Obstet. **110:**187, 1960.

114. Peacock, E.E., Weekes, P.M., and Petty, J.M.L.: Some Studies on the Antigenicity of Tendon. Ann. N.Y. Acad. Sci. **87:**175, 1960.

115. Peer, L.A.: Cartilage Grafting. Br. J. Plast. Surg. **7:**250, 1954.

116. Pelker, R.R., Friedlaender, G.E., Markham, T.C., Panjabi, M.M., and Moen, C.J.: Effects of Freezing and Freeze-Drying on the Biomechanical Properties of Rat Bone. J. Orthop. Res. **1:**405, 1984.

117. Potenza, A.D., and Malone, C.: Evaluation of Freeze-Dried Flexor Tendon Grafts in the Dog. J. Hand Surg. **3-A:**157, 1978.

118. Prolo, D.J., and Oklund, S.A.: Composite Autogeneic Human Cranioplasty: Frozen Skull Supplemented with Fresh Iliac Corticocancellous Bone. Neurosurgery **15:**846, 1984.

119. Prolo, D.J., Pedrotti, P.W., and White, D.H.: Ethylene Oxide Sterilization of Bone, Dura Mater and Fascia Lata for Human Transplantation. Neurosurgery **6:**529, 1980.

120. Puranen, J.: Reorganization of Fresh and Preserved Bone Transplants: an Experimental Study in Rabbits Using Tetracycline Labelling. Acta Orthop. Scand. [Suppl.] **92:**9, 1966.

121. Rasi, H.B.: The Fate of Preserved Human Cartilage. Plast. Reconstr. Surg. **24:**24, 1959.

122. Reeves, B.: Orthotopic Transplantation of Vascularized Whole Knee Joints in Dogs. Lancet **1:**500, 1969.

123. Reynolds, F.C., and Oliver, D.R.: Experimental Evaluation of Homogenous Bone Grafts. J. Bone Joint Surg. **32-A:**283, 1950.

124. Reynolds, H.M., Rodrigo, J.J., Gray, J.M., and Thompson, E.C.: Cement Coating of Distal Rat Femur Allografts to Inhibit the Immune Response. Trans. Orthop. Res. Soc. **9:**377, 1974.

125. Richmond, J.J., Gambardella, P.G., Schelling, S., McGinty, J.B., and Schwartz, E.C.: A Canine Model of Osteoarthritis with Histologic Study of Repair Tissue Following Abrasion Chondroplasty. Trans. Orthop. Res. Soc. **10:**61, 1985.

126. Rodrigo, J.J.: The Problem of Fit in Osteocartilaginous Allografts. *In* Friedlaender, G.E., Mankin, H.J., and Sell, K.W.: *Osteochondral Allografts*. Boston, Little, Brown, 1983, p. 249.

127. Rodrigo, J.J.: Modulation of Immune Responses Associated with Bone Allografts. *In* Friedlaender, G.E., Mankin, H.J., and Sell, K.W.: *Osteochondral Allografts*. Boston, Little, Brown, 1983, p. 363.

128. Rodrigo, J.J., Chism, S., and Thompson, E.: Total Lymphoid Irradiation to Inhibit the Immune Response after Femur Allografts in the Rat. Trans. Orthop. Res. Soc. **5:**282, 1980.

129. Rodrigo, J.J., Fuller, T.C., and Mankin, H.J.: Cytotoxic HL-A Antibodies in Patients with Bone and Cartilage Allografts. Trans. Orthop. Res. Soc. **1:**131, 1976.

130. Rodrigo, J.J., Gray, J.M., and Thompson, E.C.: Temporary Suppression of Humoral Cytotoxic Antibodies with Double Dose Cyclophosphamide Treatment in Rats Receiving Distal Femur Allografts. Trans. Orthop. Res. Soc. **9:**265, 1984.

131. Rodrigo, J.J., Leathers, M.W., Thompson, E.C., Biggart, J.F., Fu, J.C.C., and Gray, J.M.: Osteocartilaginous Shell Allografts in Dogs. Trans. Orthop. Res. Soc. **8:**319, 1983.

132. Rodrigo, J.J., Reynolds, H., Thorson, E., Gray, J., Thompson, E., and Heitter, D.: Cement Coating of Osteoarticular Allografts in Rats to Prevent the Immune Response. Trans. Orthop. Res. Soc. **12:**274, 1987.

133. Rodrigo, J.J., and Sakovich, L.: Osteocartilaginous Allografts as Compared with Autografts in the Treatment of Knee Joint Osteocartilaginous Defects in Dogs. Trans. Orthop. Res. Soc. **2:**92, 1977.

134. Rodrigo, J.J., Sakovich, L., Travis, C., and Smith, G.: Osteocartilaginous Allografts as Compared with Autografts in the Treatment of Knee Joint Osteocartilaginous Defects in Dogs. Clin. Orthop. **134:**342, 1978.

135. Rodrigo, J.J., Thompson, E.C., and Gray, J.M.: Inhibition of the Antibody Response with Cyclosporin A after Distal Femur Allografts in Rats. Trans. Orthop. Res. Soc. **8:**165, 1983.

136. Rodrigo, J.J., Thompson, E.C., and Travis, C.: 4° Preservation of Avascular Osteocartilaginous Shell Allografts in Rats. Trans. Orthop. Res. Soc. **5:**72, 1980.

137. Rodrigo, J.J., Thompson, E.C., and Travis, C.R.: Correlation of the Immune Response in a Rat Distal Femur Allograft Model with Previous Blood Transfusions. Trans. Orthop. Res. Soc. **4:**306, 1979.

138. Rodrigo, J.J., Thompson, E.C., and Travis, C.R.: Deep-Freezing Versus 4° Preservation of Avascular Osteocartilaginous Shell Allografts in Rats. Clin. Orthop. **218:**268–275, 1987.

139. Ronningen, H., Solheim, L.F., and Langeland, N.: Bone Formation Enhanced by Induction. Bone Growth in Titanium Implants in Rats. Acta Orthop. Scand. **56:**67, 1985.

140. Salter, R.B., Simmonds, D.F., Malcolm, B.W., Rumble, E.J., MacMichael, D., and Clements, N.D.: The Biological Effect of Continuous Passive Motion on the Healing Full-Thickness Defects in Articular Cartilage. J. Bone Joint Surg. **62-A:**1232, 1980.

141. Sato, K., and Urist, M.R.: Bone Morphogenetic Protein-Induced Cartilage Development in Tissue Culture. Clin. Orthop. **183:**180, 1984.

142. Schnaser, A.M., Rodrigo, J.J., and Travis, C.R.: Suppression of Humoral Cytotoxic Antibodies with Single Dose Cyclophosphamide Treatment of Rats Receiving Distal Femur Allografts. Trans. Orthop. Res. Soc. **2:**152, 1978.

143. Scott, R.D., Joyce, M.J., Ewald, F.C., and Thomas, W.H.: McKeever Metallic Hemiarthroplasty in Unicompartmental Degenerative Arthritis. J. Bone Joint Surg. **67-A:**203, 1985.

144. Shino, K., Kawasaki, T., Hirose, H., Gotoh, I., Inoue, M., and Ono, K.: Replacement of the Anterior Cruciate Ligament by an Allogeneic Tendon Graft. An Experimental Study in the Dog. J. Bone Joint Surg. **66-B:**672, 1984.

145. Shively, R.A., Maylack, F.H., and Simmons, D.J.: Autogenous Articular Cartilage and Osteochondral Grafts. Trans. Orthop. Res. Soc. **11:**281, 1986.

146. Skoog, T., and Johansson, S.H.: The Formation of Articular Cartilage From Free Periochondral Grafts. Plast. Reconstr. Surg. **57:**1, 1976.

147. Sloame, D., and Reeves, B.: Experimental Homotransplantation of the Knee Joint. Lancet **2:**205, 1966.

148. Smith, G.W., and Robinson, R.A.: The Treatment of Certain Cervical-Spine Disorders by Anterior Removal of the Intervertebral Disc and Interbody Fusion. J. Bone Joint Surg. **40-A:**607, 1958.

149. Stabler, C.L., Eismont, F.J., Brown, M.D., Green, B.A., and Ma-

linen, T.I.: Failure of Posterior Cervical Fusions Using Cadaveric Bone Graft in Children. J. Bone Joint Surg. **67-A:**370, 1985.

150. Stauffer, R.N., and Coventry, M.B.: Anterior Interbody Lumbar Spine Fusions. J. Bone Joint Surg. **54-A:**756, 1972.

151. Stevenson, S., Danucci, G., and Sharkey, N.: Fresh and Cryopreserved DLA-Matched and Mismatched Massive Osteochondral Allografts: The Fate of Articular Cartilage. Trans. Orthop. Res. Soc. **2:**274, 1986.

152. Strub, J.R., Gaberthuel, T.W., and Firestone, A.R.: Comparison of Tricalcium Phosphate and Frozen Allogeneic Bone Implants in Man. J. Periodontol. **50:**624, 1979.

153. Urist, M.R.: Bone: Formation by Autoinduction. Science **150:**893, 1965.

154. Urist, M.R.: Surface-Decalcified Allogeneic Bone (SDAB) Implants. Clin. Orthop. **56:**37, 1968.

155. Urist, M.R.: Bone Transplants and Implants. *In* Urist, M.R. (ed.): *Fundamental and Clinical Bone Physiology.* Philadelphia, J.B. Lippincott, 1980, p. 331.

156. Urist, M.R.: New Bone Formation Induced in Post-Fetal Life by Bone Morphogenetic Protein. *In* Becker, R.O. (ed.): *Mechanisms of Growth Control.* Springfield, Ill., Charles C Thomas, 1981, p. 406.

157. Urist, M.R.: Chemosterilized Antigen-Extracted Surface-Demineralized Autolysed Allogeneic (AAA) Bone for Arthrodesis. *In* Friedlaender, G.E., Mankin, H.J., and Sell, K.W. (eds.): *Osteochondral Allografts.* Boston, Little, Brown, 1983, p. 193.

158. Urist, M.R., and Dawson, E.: Intertransverse Process Fusion with the Aid of Chemosterilized Autolyzed Antigen-Extracted Allogeneic (AAA) Bone. Clin. Orthop. **154:**97, 1981.

159. Urist, M.R., Delange, R.J., and Finerman, G.A.M.: Bone Cell Differentiation and Growth Factors. Science **220:**680, 1983.

160. Urist, M.R., and Hudak, R.T.: Radioimmunoassay of Bone Morphogenetic Protein in Serum: A Tissue-Specific Parameter of Bone Metabolism. Proc. Soc. Exp. Biol. Med. **176:**472, 1984.

161. Urist, M.R., Silverman, B.F., Buring, K., Dubuc, F.L., and Roseberg, J.M.: The Bone Induction Principle. Clin. Orthop. **53:**243, 1967.

162. Urovitz, E.P., Langer, F., Gross, A.E., and West, M.: Cell Mediated Immunity in Patients Following Joint Allografting. Trans. Orthop. Res. Soc. **1:**132, 1976.

163. Vasseur, P.B., Rodrigo, J.J., Stevenson, S., Clark, G., and Sharkey, N.: Replacement of Canine Anterior Cruciate Ligament With a Bone-Ligament-Bone Anterior Cruciate Ligament Allograft. Clin. Orthop. **219:**268, 1987.

164. Volkov, M.: Allotransplantation of Joints. J. Bone Joint Surg. **52-B:**49, 1970.

165. White, A.A., and Panjabi, M.M.: *Clinical Biomechanics of the Spine.* Philadelphia, J.B. Lippincott, 1978, pp. 192, 396, 398, 408.

166. Wilson, P.D.: Follow-Up Study of the Use of Refrigerated Homogenous Bone Transplants in Orthopaedic Surgery. J. Bone Joint Surg. **33-A:**307, 1951.

167. Yablon, I.G.: Immune Responses to Matrix Components. *In* Friedlaender, G.E., Mankin, H.J., and Sell, K.W. (eds.): *Osteochondral Allografts,* Boston, Little, Brown, 1983, p. 165.

168. Yang, Q-M, Rodrigo, J.J., Gray, M., and Thompson, E.C.: Temporary Suppression of Humoral Cytotoxic Antibodies with an Azathioprine/Steroid Regime after Distal Femur Allografts in the Rat. Trans. Orthop. Res. Soc. **9:**347, 1984.

CHAPTER 72

Benign Bone Tumors

JOSEPH M. LANE,
KAREN DUANE, and
DALE B. GLASSER

Osteoid Osteoma
Osteoblastoma
Giant Cell Tumor
Osteochondroma
Enchondroma
Chondroblastoma
Nonossifying Fibroma
Fibrous Dysplasia
Solitary Bone Cyst
Aneurysmal Bone Cyst
Eosinophilic Granuloma

The staging system for benign bone tumors allows the establishment of principles for the treatment of these tumors. These principles are only general guidelines, which must be individualized for each tumor, anatomic site, and specific patient; however, they allow comparison of results between different histologic types and planning of either surgical or nonsurgical treatment based on the anticipated natural history of the lesion. The following discussion is based on the surgical staging system adopted by the Musculoskeletal Tumor Society.

Stage 1 benign lesions (Fig. 72-1) are latent, have little growth potential, and are often discovered incidentally. They may be treated by observation alone in many instances or by intralesional procedures, which result in a negligible recurrence rate.

Stage 2 benign lesions (Fig. 72-2) are actively growing lesions treated by intralesional procedures that excise the reactive margin. This can be achieved by curettage into normal osseous tissue or by physical adjuvants to extend the surgical margins such as phenol, polymethylmethacrylate, or cryosurgery utilizing liquid nitrogen.

Stage 3 benign lesions are aggressive tumors (Fig. 72-3); they must be treated by procedures that obtain wide surgical margins. The most reliable means of achieving this margin is by *en bloc* excision. However this may not be the most reasonable method of treatment where *en bloc* excision would create significant disability. In such instances, wide margins are obtained by an intralesional approach with adjuvant procedures as for stage 2 lesions, recognizing that the potential for recurrence is increased over that which would be obtained by a primary wide *en bloc* excision.

OSTEOID OSTEOMA

Osteoid osteoma is a benign bone-forming tumor which constitutes 11% of all benign bone tumors.[8] These lesions are characteristically found in the second decade, with most occurring in patients under 30 years of age. A majority are found in the lower extremities, especially in the region of the hip; however, up to 18% may occur in the spine. In the spine the posterior elements are preferentially involved, and the mode of presentation may be that of a painful scoliosis.[26]

The clinical history usually involves pain, which may be worse at night and may respond dramatically to salicylates or other nonsteroidals.[16] The typical radiographic picture is that of a central, lucent nidus surrounded by dense sclerosis (Fig. 72-4). Radiographic localization, however, may prove quite difficult. Radionuclide scanning (^{99m}Tc), triaxial tomography, and computed tomography (CT) may be useful in localizing the nidus, not only in difficult locations such as the spine, but also when the surrounding sclerosis is dense. Conservative management with salicylates or, preferably, long-acting nonsteroidals may obviate the need for surgical resection. To date there exist no studies clearly demonstrating a medical cure for osteoid osteoma. The goal for surgical treatment is complete removal of the nidus, since this is the most reliable method of preventing recurrence. Removal of the surrounding sclerotic bone is not necessary, although a greater portion of this sclerosis is removed when dealing with recurrent lesions. The difficulty at

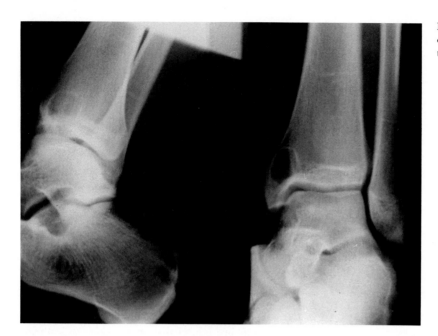

FIGURE 72-1. Anteroposterior lateral radiograph of a stage 1 benign tumor (intraosseous ganglion) of the medial maleolus.

surgery is in localizing the nidus, since the overlying cortical bone and periosteum are usually normal in appearance.

Preoperatively, the lesion is evaluated by plane radiographs and either trispiral tomograms or CT scan to localize the nidus. In difficult cases, 1 g oxytetracycline (previous day) or ^{99m}TC diphosphenate (for 2 to 3 hr before surgery) may be given.

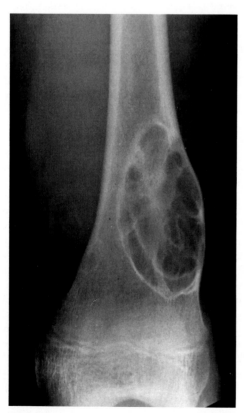

FIGURE 72-2. Anteroposterior radiograph of stage 2 benign tumor of the distal femur. The nonfibroma demonstrates expansion and margination.

Intraoperative localization is then performed by using a hand-held ultraviolet lamp or a geiger counter, respectively.

If technically possible, a block excision that includes the nidus is done. Where minimal bone can be sacrificed, such as in the spine, intralesional curettage is preferred. No fusion is performed for spine lesions unless instability has been created by the resection. Intraoperative confirmation of removal of the osteoid osteoma can be provided by radiograph of the specimen, loss of radioactivity when Technetium has been administered, or removal of fluorescent bone. In most instances, removal of the inner nest of osteoid osteoma with thorough curettage of the perilesional bone will result in a cure.[17]

OSTEOBLASTOMA

Osteoblastoma, although histologically similar to osteoid osteoma, is a progressively growing lesion of larger size (>2 cm), is sometimes painful, and is characterized by missing or only slight perifocal osseous reaction[16] (Fig. 72-5). The average patient age at presentation is 17, but its range extends through all decades. Some 75% of lesions occur in the second and third decades.[17]

Osteoblastoma most commonly involves the vertebral column (34%), long bones of the appendicular skeleton (30%), or the small bones of the hands and feet (13.5%). The preferential sites in the spine are the spinous and transverse processes. Involvement of the vertebral body is usually secondary to extension from the posterior elements.

When the lesion is of small to moderate size, surgical treatment is similar to that for osteoid osteomas, and consists of thorough curettage, with or without autogenous bone grafting. Since there is rarely a perilesional zone of sclerosis, no wide margin of intact bone resection is indicated. Even if removal of the tumor by curettage is incomplete, the residual tumor may remain dormant and asymptomatic for many years.[23] Camepa reported a recurrence rate of less than 20%.[2] Radiation from

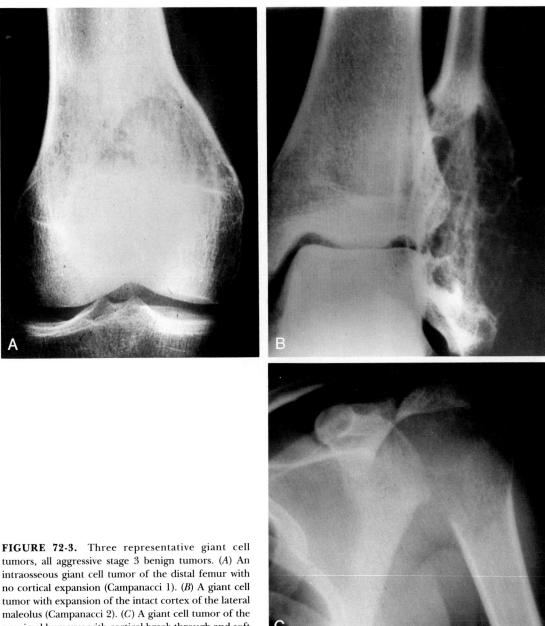

FIGURE 72-3. Three representative giant cell tumors, all aggressive stage 3 benign tumors. (*A*) An intraosseous giant cell tumor of the distal femur with no cortical expansion (Campanacci 1). (*B*) A giant cell tumor with expansion of the intact cortex of the lateral maleolus (Campanacci 2). (*C*) A giant cell tumor of the proximal humerus with cortical break through and soft tissue extension (Campanacci 3).

3000 up to 6000 cGy has been utilized for the unresectable recurrent tumor. Rarely, malignant osteoblastomas may develop in the recurring lesions, even in the absence of intervening radiation treatment.[24]

GIANT CELL TUMOR

Conventional giant cell tumor represents approximately 5% of primary bone tumors. The lesions are generally eccentrically located in the ends of long bones, originating in the metaphysis, with extension into the epiphysis down to the subchondral bone (see Fig. 72-3). Fifty percent of lesions are located at the knee; the distal radius and proximal humerus are also com-

mon locations. The sacrum is involved in approximately 10%, and the spine may be involved, with the vertebral body as the preferential site. Patient age at the time of involvement is from 20 to 40 years in about 80% of patients; the diagnosis prior to skeletal maturity is suspect.[30]

On radiograph, giant cell tumor is usually translucent and lacks stippling or calcifications. The metaphyseal extension may be marginated but is not sclerotic. Campanacci has defined three stages: (1) The lesion is confined totally within the bone, (2) the lesion is contained within a bony envelope but with cortical thinning and bulging, and (3) the lesion has broken through the cortex.[4] These lesions represent perhaps the most difficult management problems of the benign bone tumors, in part because of the location next to the articular surface, and in

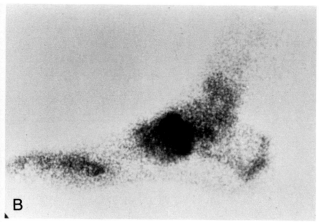

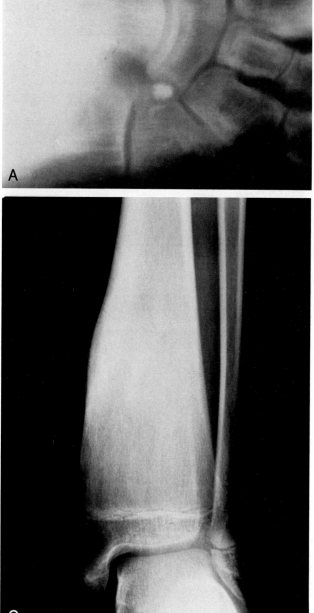

FIGURE 72-4.   Osteoid osteomas. (*A*) Oblique radiograph of an osteoid osteoma of the cuboid, demonstrating a nidus. (*B*) Radionuclide scan of the same patient highlighting the tarsal lesion. (*C*) Anteroposterior radiograph of a distal tibial osteoid osteoma with significant expansion of the metaphysis and cortical thickening.

part because of the difficulty in accurately predicting the natural history, as histologic grading has little relevance to prognosis except for the malignant giant cell tumors.[11]

Treatment depends on the stage of the lesion at presentation; more aggressive lesions should not be treated in the same way as latent lesions. The high recurrence rates following curettage alone or curettage and bone graft undoubtedly are the result of analyzing pooled results for all stages of disease.[15] In planning the surgical approach, weigh the risk of local recurrence against the anticipated functional result; many times a marginally adequate procedure is chosen in order to attempt to preserve the patient's own joint and bone stock.

Nonoperative treatment is rarely employed, except in surgically inaccessible lesions. The incidence of sarcomatous change following therapeutic radiation therapy is reported as approaching 20%, although this figure may change with newer methods of radiation delivery.[9]

The most common approach to Stage 1 lesions (see Fig. 72-3*A*) (intraosseous lesions without expansion) is thorough curettage to normal bone that requires wide unroofing of the lesion to allow complete visualization. The use of high speed burrs aids in achieving a complete curettage. Bone grafting of the defect can be carried out at the same time. A recurrence rate of less than 10% should be expected for these latent le-

FIGURE 72-5. An osteoblastoma of the long metacarpal, with expansion and mineral sclerosis.

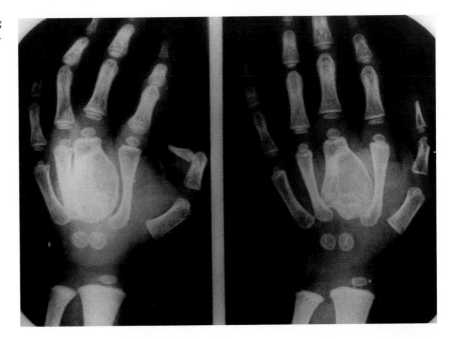

sions. Enhanced cure rates have been reported with the use of polymethylmethacrylate,[29] phenol,[10] or cryosurgery,[22] but these are not necessary if curettage reaches normal bone in all direction.

Stage 2 lesions are more aggressive, exhibiting expansion and extreme thinning of the cortex (Fig. 72-3B). Most favor thorough curettage, filling of the cavity with polymethylmethacrylate, and a "second look" procedure 3 to 6 months later.[29] At this time the polymethylmethacrylate is removed and bone grafting is carried out if there is no evidence of recurrent disease. The recurrence rate can be lowered substantially with the addition of cryosurgery,[29] although it does add a significant complication rate, most notably from delayed fractures. Cryosurgery is indicated for Stage 2 lesions that have not been adequately curetted, particularly at the subchondral area (Fig. 72-6). The technique involves three freeze-thaw cycles with liquid nitrogen and is illustrated in Figure 72-4. Not only can the pour method be used, but adjacent soft tissues can be frozen using a controlled (Brymyl) spray of fine liquid nitrogen. The same principle of extending the surgical margins by chemical or physical means has been proposed utilizing phenol or polymethylmethacrylate.[10,29] These methods can only extend the "kill" 1 to 2 mm, as compared with 1 to 2 cm with liquid nitrogen. The apparent advantage to the use of liquid nitrogen is the predictability of the depth of the freeze. The late fracture complication rate can be decreased by using internal fixation.

Stage 3 lesions that have reached the cortex and extended into adjacent soft tissue are best treated by *en bloc* resection; using this technique a 7% to 13% recurrence rate has been reported (see Fig. 72-3C). A 30% recurrence rate occurs in Stage 3 lesions using curettage and cryosurgery; however, these are the lesions which have extended beyond the cortex and are impossible to curette thoroughly. It may be an acceptable risk, however, if it allows one to avoid the problems of reconstruction following resection. Resection, of course, requires subsequent reconstruction such as arthrodesis, allograft, or endoprosthetic reconstruction.

The short-term use of polymethylmethacrylate is especially beneficial in those instances where the subchondral bone is so involved as to give poor support to the articular cartilage, or when an intra-articular fracture occurs. Healing will occur around the cement. Delaying bone grafting should allow revascularization of the bone previously frozen and cemented. Additionally, the use of cement allows early identification of recurrence, since interpretation of radiographs is not confused by resorption of bone graft material.

OSTEOCHONDROMA

The solitary and multiple forms of osteochondroma are the most common primary benign bone tumors, representing 40% of benign tumors[8,17] (Fig. 72-7).

These lesions are typically discovered in the second decade and may enlarge until closure of the epiphyseal plates. They are primarily located in long bones, with the femur, tibia, and humerus the most common sites. The majority of lesions are asymptomatic and require only observation. Symptoms may occur due to nerve compression or mechanical irritation of adjacent structures, and simple excision is the treatment of choice in these instances. The lesion is removed at its base or stalk at the level of the normal cortical bone, taking care to excise periosteum along with the lesion to prevent recurrence (Fig. 72-8). Since the stalk provides minimal mechanical strength to the bone, protective weight-bearing need be for only a limited period.

ENCHONDROMA

Solitary enchondroma is a common hyaline cartilage growth with lesions appearing within the medullary cavity of bones. Enchondromas represented 11% of benign tumors in Dahlin's series.[8] They occur most commonly in the hand (35%) (Fig.

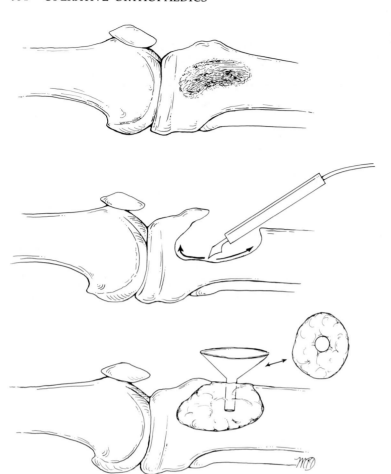

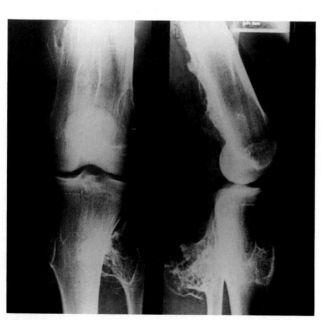

FIGURE 72-6. The stages of cryosurgery include the isolation of the tumor (*top*), thorough curettage through a large cortical window (*middle*), and cryosurgery with liquid nitrogen through a funnel surrounded by Gelfoam insulation (*bottom*).

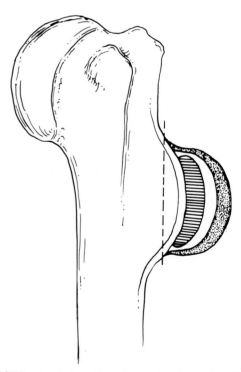

FIGURE 72-7. Multiple osteochondromatosis, demonstrating sessile and pedunculated lesions.

FIGURE 72-8. Surgical excision of osteochondroma should be proximal to the perichondral extension onto the bony stalk. The *dashed line* demonstrates the cleavage plan through cortical bone.

72-9A), followed by the femur (Fig. 72-9B), humerus, and ribs. The average patient age at presentation is in the third or fourth decade, often with pain caused by trauma or fracture; incidental radiographic discovery is not uncommon.[17]

The indications for biopsy of these lesions are often difficult to determine, particularly since the pathologist has difficulty in defining the fine line between the enchondroma and low grade chondrosarcoma.[17] The radiographic appearance of these lesions may be variable and is not a reliable means of determining benignity. The typical lesion is centrally located with sclerotic margins; spotty calcifications occur within the center of the lesion. However, the cortex may be expanded and thinned, with the margins of the lesions indistinct, and the matrix may lack calcifications in a histologically benign lesion. The bone scan is of limited diagnostic value except when no increased uptake is present, or when used serially to confirm a suspected malignant transformation.[10]

Generally, a bone scan is favored as part of the evaluation of a lesion which presents for treatment. In the absence of symptoms, if the radiographic picture is characteristic and the bone scan shows no increased uptake, observation alone is sufficient treatment. Observation is also sufficient if the bone scan is positive for the lesion if all of the above criteria are met. No definitive guidelines for following these lesions have been established, but one radiograph at 3 to 6 months and then yearly is adequate in the absence of symptoms.

In the presence of a positive lesion in which the patient has symptoms or the radiographic picture is unusual, intralesional curettage with adjuvant phenol cauterization followed by bone grafting is the preferred treatment. The technique of phenol cauterization follows: Develop a wide window into the lesion, and thoroughly curette to "normal" bone. Carefully isolate the opening from the adjacent tissues with vaseline gauze and fill the defect with full strength phenol; leave it in place for 2 min. Remove the phenol with suction, and neutralize it by washing the site with 4 volumes of 95% ethylalcohol, followed by bone grafting.

Pathologic fracture as the mode of presentation is most common in the hand. Some authors advocate immediate curettage and bone grafting so as to lessen the total period of disability.[33] The major problem with this method is a lack of stability, which may require internal fixation. We immobilize the fracture by external means for approximately 3 weeks until stability is achieved before proceeding with thorough curettage and bone grafting. This obviates the necessity for internal fixation.

One must recognize that after delayed curettage the histologic appearance of the curetted material may appear more aggressive, owing to the presence of callus. A separate cortical window is used to curette the lesion so that the fracture callus is not disturbed; in most instances a midlateral approach to the phalanx can be used. Most hand surgeons do not follow a policy of nonoperative treatment of these pathologic fractures, for they consider the lesions active.[19] Observation alone may lead to further growth of the lesion and destruction of the phalanx, making for a difficult reconstruction instead of a simple curettage and grafting procedure.

CHONDROBLASTOMA

Chondroblastoma is an unusual benign bone tumor of immature cartilage tissue with preferential anatomic localization in the epiphysis. The tumor is most common in adolescents and young adults (<25 yr). Symptoms are nonspecific. Pain and swelling may be noticed.[32]

Some 75% of the tumors occur in the femur, humerus, tibia, and tarsal or innominate bones. The lesions, which occur in the epiphysis or apophysis (Fig. 72-10), are lytic and round. Occasionally fuzzy stippling may occur. Chondroblastoma may be associated with an aneurysmal component (see below).[17]

Treatment of these lesions involves thorough curettage and bone grafting. In the hip, internal fixation (Fig. 72-10C and D) may be warranted to prevent pathologic fracture.

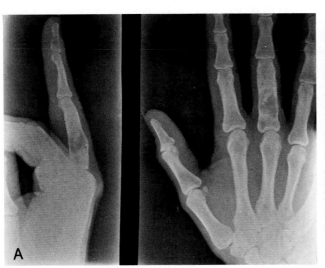
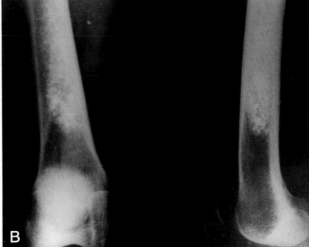

FIGURE 72-9. Enchondromas of bone. (A) Anteroposterior and lateral radiographs of an enchondroma of the proximal phalynx of the long digit. (B) Anteroposterior and lateral radiographs of an enchondroma of the distal diaphysis of the femur.

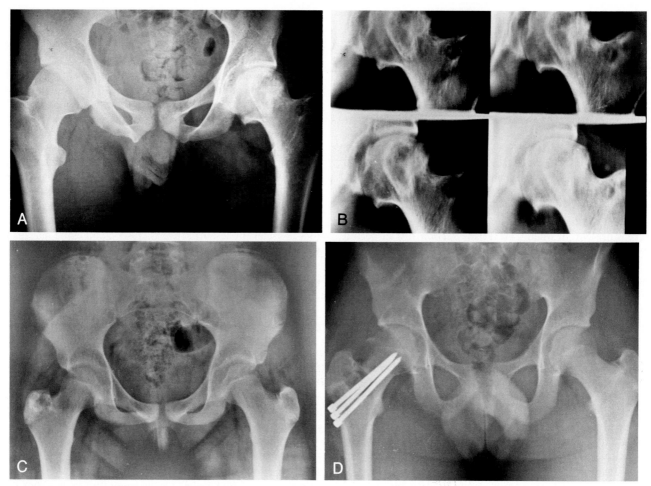

FIGURE 72-10. Chondroblastoma. (*A*) Anteroposterior view of a chondroblastoma of the left femoral hip epiphysis. (*B*) Tomogram of the same femoral chondroblastoma. (*C*) Chondroblastoma of the right femoral greater trochanteric epiphysis. (*D*) Chondroblastoma has been curetted and the femoral neck reinforced with several pins.

Chondroblastomas without an aneurysmal bone cyst (ABC) component treated by curettage have a 20% recurrence rate, but coexistence of an ABC lead to 100% recurrence rate in one series. Consequently, in those cases associated with an aneurysmal bone cyst, we use cryosurgery in an effort to prevent recurrence.[18]

NONOSSIFYING FIBROMA

Nonossifying fibromas are felt to represent a part of the spectrum of benign fibrous lesions ranging from the fibrous cortical defect to the benign fibrous histiocytoma. According to Dahlin's series,[8] nonossifying fibromas represent 5% of benign bone tumors. These lesions are rarely symptomatic and are usually discovered when radiographs are taken for unrelated reasons. The lesions are generally found in the juxtaepiphyseal metaphysis of the long bones in the second decade. The radiographic appearance is usually characteristic, showing a 1 to 5 cm lesion eccentrically located with a thin sclerotic border. The cortex may be thinned or expanded, but intact (see Fig. 72-2).

Observation alone may suffice if the lesion is found incidentally. If the lesions is painful, has an unusual radiographic appearance, or an unusual location, we advocate curettage followed by bone grafting. Curettage and bone grafting are also recommended if the lesion is in a weight-bearing bone and 50% of the diameter is involved, even in the absence of symptoms. Internal fixation is generally not needed. If the presentation is that of a pathologic fracture, our preference is to allow enough healing to provide stability before proceeding with surgical treatment.

FIBROUS DYSPLASIA

Fibrous dysplasia is a benign developmental condition, which may be monostotic or polyostotic.[8,17] The disease begins in childhood but usually becomes clinically apparent in young adulthood during an incidental radiographic examination. The appearance is that of a radiolucent cystic lesion with deformity and diffuse enlargement of the bone contour. The patient may present with pain or progressive deformity. The hip, an area under great loads, may give rise to a special form of deformity known as the shepherd's crook.

The treatment is indicated for pathologic fracture or progressive deformity. Curettage, bone grafting, and stabilization either with bracing or internal fixation are required until the osseous remodeling has been completed. The spongy bone has high vascularity and large amounts of blood may be needed during surgical correction. The triad of café au lait skin lesions, polyostotic fibrous dysplagia, and endocrinopathy constitute Albright's syndrome.

SOLITARY BONE CYST

Solitary or unicameral bone cysts are benign, non-neoplastic lesions that occur in children.[3] Eighty to 90% of all lesions are found in proximal metaphysis of the femur or humerus (Fig. 72-11). The cysts may be adjacent to the epiphyseal plate, and such cysts have been called "active." These lesions should be observed while growth increases the distance between the lesion and the epiphyseal plate. However, this does not reliably occur, and the recurrence rate appears to be related as much to the patient's age as to proximity to the epiphyseal plate.[27] Fracture through a cyst seldom results in spontaneous healing of the lesion.[1]

Various methods of treatment have been advocated, from curettage and bone graft, subtotal resection with[13] and without graft,[25] to methylprednisolone injection.[31] The main complication of all of these treatment methods has been recurrence or incomplete healing.

The current approach to treating these lesions is multiple steroid injections. Under radiographic control, two large bore needles are introduced into the cyst. Diluted Renographin is then injected to assure free flow into the cavity and to identify any localization which will need separate injections. At this point, 80 to 200 mg of Depo medrol is injected, depending on the size of the cyst. This procedure is repeated every 4 to 6

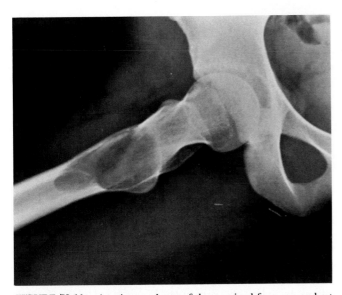

FIGURE 72-11. A unicameral cyst of the proximal femur, seen best on this lateral radiograph.

weeks for a total of five injections or until healing occurs. Follow-up must be continued after healing begins, as incomplete healing and recurrence may occur. One can expect approximately 50% to heal completely and 30% to heal partially.[3,5] The results of curettage and bone graft are similar. A trial is underway using a similar technique with the injection of autologous bone marrow instead of the methylprednisolone. The early results of this method appear to be superior to steroids.

Cysts that present with pathologic fractures are immobilized and treated in a similar manner. One exception to this is a pathologic fracture of the proximal femur, which we treat by curettage to normal bone and autologous bone graft, without internal fixation but with external support (1½ spica).

ANEURYSMAL BONE CYST

Aneurysmal bone cyst is a hemorrhagic and cystic lesion of bone. It can occur primarily, or secondary to chondroblastoma, osteoblastoma, osteosarcoma, giant cell tumor, fibrous dysplasia, hemangioendothelioma, or brown tumors of hyperparathyroidism.[3] The tumors have a slight predilection for females, and occur most frequently in children (specifically adolescents); rarely do they occur past age 30 (9.95%). Long bones are the most frequent site: tibia (42%), femur (18%), humerus (7.5%), fibula (7%), ulna (3%), and radius (1.5%). The most common localization is in the metaphysis of long bone. Twelve percent occur in the posterior elements of the spinal column.

The tumor course is usually rapid. There is frequently painful swelling and an increase in local temperature. In spinal lesions, spinal cord and root compression frequently occur.

There are five radiographic presentations. Type I cysts occupy the center of the bone with little or no expansion. Type II lesions substitute for the entire bone segment (Fig. 72-12 A and B). Type III lesions appear as eccentric intraosseous lesions showing no or minimal cortical expansion (Fig. 72-12C). Type IV cysts are subperiosteal with a superficial erosion of the underlying cortex (Fig. 72-12D). In Type V lesions, the periosteum is elevated with expansion of the cyst into soft tissues. The lesion also penetrates into the cancellous bone[3] (Fig. 72-12E).

Treatment of aneurysmal bone cyst has traditionally utilized thorough curettage with or without bone graft. A recurrence rate of 20% follows such procedures. In unresectable lesions, radiotherapy with or without partial curettage can similarly cure 80%. The addition of light cryosurgery can further decrease the local recurrence rate, particularly in aneurysmal bone cyst with soft-tissue extension. Expendable bones such as the fibula should be resected; in highly vascular situations, presurgical embolization may enhance the surgery.[6]

EOSINOPHILIC GRANULOMA

This rare condition has previously been grouped under the spectrum of diseases termed Histiocytosis X. Although the histogenesis remains unproved, it appears that both solitary and multifocal forms of the disease are reactive processes and not neoplastic. The term Langerhans cell granulomatosis is a more accurate description, since histologically the lesions contain

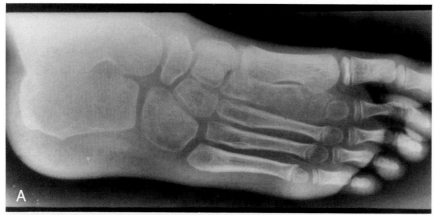

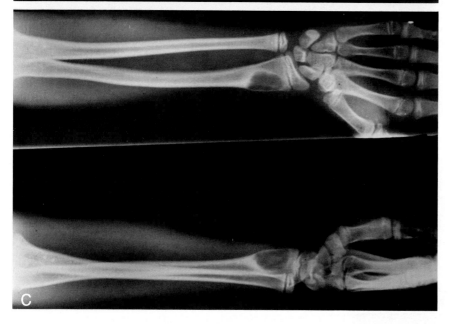

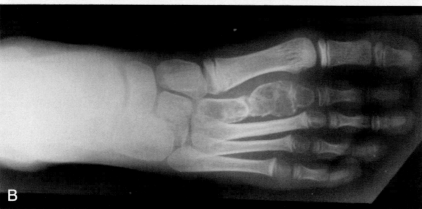

FIGURE 72-12. Aneurysmal bone cysts. (A) A type II aneurysmal bone cyst of the second metatarsal. (B) The same patient following curettage and cryosurgery spray of the cyst. (C) Anteroposterior and lateral radiographs of a type III aneurysmal bone cyst of the distal radius.

eosinophils, multinucleated giant cells, and the mononuclear Langerhans cell.[20]

The lesions are characteristically found in the skull, ribs, and long bones.[21] Usually the patient presents in the first decade with pain, tenderness, and swelling as the most common symptoms; occurrence after 30 years of age is rare. The usual radiographic picture is a lytic lesion that may be expansile. The margins of the lesion may be well defined; however, periosteal reaction and indistinct margins are not unusual and may give the appearance of a more aggressive lesion such as Ewing's sarcoma.

Various treatment options are available for the long-bone lesions, including observation alone, curettage, curettage and cryosurgery, and low-dose radiation therapy. As the lesions

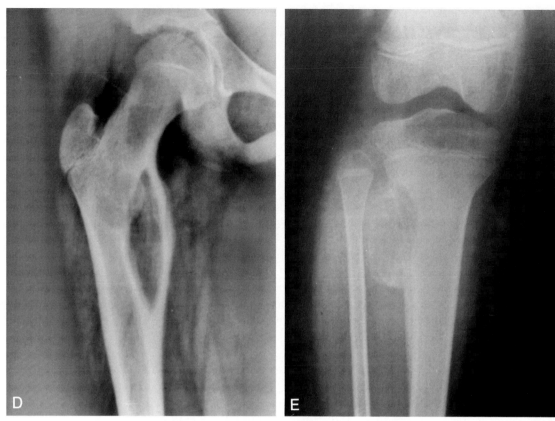

FIGURE 72-12. (*continued*) (*D*) Anteroposterior radiograph of a type IV aneurysmal bone cyst of the proximal femur. (*E*) Anteroposterior radiograph of type V aneurysmal bone cyst of the proximal tibia.

appear to resolve spontaneously, relief of pain with minimal morbidity is the ideal treatment goal. A limited number of cases has been reported which were successfully treated with steroid injection.[7] Lesions in the vertebral column usually present with collapse or vertebra plana, and partial reconstitution of height is the rule, regardless of the treatment given.[28]

These lesions are approached by open biopsy following a bone scan to identify additional lesions. Unless the lesion is in a dangerous location and at high risk for fracture, bone graft is not carried out. Following biopsy, 300 to 600 cGy are given to the lesion. If no additional lesions have developed within 12 months of the appearance of the first lesion, the probability of developing the multifocal form of the disease is quite low.[20]

The multifocal form may develop other manifestations such as diabetes insipidis, hepatosplenomegaly, and adenopathy. This form is best treated with low dose chemotherapy; methotrexate, prednisone, and vinblastine have been found effective.

REFERENCES

1. Baker, D.M.: Benign Unicameral Bone Cyst. A Study of Forty-Five Cases with Long-term Follow Up. Clin. Orthop. **71:**140–151, 1970.
2. Camepa, G., and Defabiani, F.: Osteoblastoma del Radio. Minerva Orthop. **16:**645–648, 1965.
3. Campanacci, M., Capanna, R., and Picci, P.: Unicameral and Aneurysmal Bone Cysts. Clin. Orthop. **204:**25–36, 1986.
4. Campanacci, M., Giunti, A., and Olmi, R.: Giant Cell Tumors of Bone. A Study of 209 Cases with Long Term Follow Up in 130. Ital. J. Orthop. Traumatol. **1:**249–277, 1975.
5. Campanna, R., DalMonte, A., Gitelis, S., and Campanacci, M.: The Natural History of Unicameral Bone Cyst after Steroid Injection. Clin. Orthop. **166:**204–211, 1982.
6. Chuang, V.P., Soo, C.S., Wallace, S., and Benjamin, R.S.: Arterial Occlusion. Management of Giant Cell Tumor and Aneurysmal Bone Cyst. Am. J. Roentgenol. **136:**1127–1130, 1981.
7. Cohen, M., Zornoza, J., Cangir, A., Murray, J., and Wallace, S.: Direct Injection of Methylprednisolone Sodium Succinate in the treatment of Solitary Eosinophilic Granuloma of Bone. Radiology **136:**289–293, 1980.
8. Dahlin, D.C.: Bone Tumors, 3rd ed. Springfield, Ill., Charles C Thomas, 1967.
9. Dahlin, D.C., Crupps, R.E., and Johnson, E.W.: Giant-Cell Tumor. A Study of 195 Cases. Cancer **25:**1061–1070, 1970.
10. Eckardt, J.J., Cooper, K.L., Unni, K.K., and Sim, F.H.: Mayo Clinic Rounds: Benign Giant Cell Tumor of Bone. Orthopedics **3:**1142–1152, 1980.
11. Eckardt, J.J., and Grogan, T.J.: Giant Cell Tumor of Bone. Clin. Orthop. **204:**45–58, 1986.
12. Enneking, W.F.: A system of Staging Musculoskeletal Neoplasms. Clin. Orthop. **204:**9–24, 1986.
13. Fahey, J.J., and O'Brien, E.T.: Subtotal Resection and Grafting in Selected Cases of Solitary Unicameral Bone Cyst. J. Bone Joint Surg. **55-A:**59–68, 1973.

14. Ghelman, B., Thompson, F.M., and Arnold, W.D.: Intraoperative Radioactive Localization of an Osteoid Osteoma. J. Bone Joint Surg. **63-A:**826–827, 1981.

15. Goldenberg, R.R., Campbell, C.J., and Bonfiglio, M.: Giant Cell Tumor of Bone: An Analysis of Two Hundred and Eighteen Cases. J. Bone Joint Surg. **52-A:**619–664, 1970.

16. Healey, J.H., and Ghelman, B.: Osteoid Osteoma and Osteoblastoma. Current Concepts and Recent Advances. Clin. Orthop. **204:**76–86, 1986.

17. Huvos, A.: Bone Tumors: Diagnosis, Treatment and Prognosis. Philadelphia, W.B. Saunders, 1979.

18. Huvos, A., and Marcove, R.: Chondroblastome of Bone. A Critical Review. Clin. Orthop. **95:**300–312, 1973.

19. Lane, J.M., McCormack, R.R., Jr., Hurson, B., and Glasser, D.: Tumors of the Upper Extremity. *In* Bora, F.W., Jr. (ed): The Upper Extremity. Philadelphia, W.B. Saunders, 1986.

20. Lieberman, P.H., Jones, C.R., Dargeon, H.W.K., and Begg, L.F.: A Reappraisal of Eosinophilic Granuloma of Bone, Hand-Schuller-Christian Syndrome and Letterer-Siwe Syndrome. Medicine **48:**375–400, 1969.

21. Makley, J.J., and Carter, J.R.: Eosinophilic Granuloma of Bone. Clin. Orthop. **204:**37–44, 1986.

22. Marcove, R.C., Lyden, J.P., Huvos, A.G., and Bullough, P.G.: Giant Cell Tumors Treated by Cryosurgery. J. Bone Joint Surg. **55-A:**1633–1644, 1973.

23. Marsh, B.W., Bonfiglio, M., Brady, L.P., and Enneking, W.F.: Benign Osteoblastoma, Range of Manifestations. J. Bone Joint Surg. **57-A:**1–9, 1975.

24. Mayer, L.: Malignant Degeneration of So-Called Benign Osteoblastoma. Bull. Hosp. Joint Dis. **28:**4–13, 1967.

25. McKay, D., and Nason, S.S.: Treatment of Unicameral Bone Cysts by Subtotal Resection without Grafts. J. Bone Joint Surg. **59-A:**515–519, 1977.

26. McLellan, D.I., and Wilson, F.C., Jr.: Osteoid Osteoma of the Spine. J. Bone Joint Surg. **49-A:**111–121, 1967.

27. Neer, C.S., Francis, K.D., Johnston, A.D., and Kiernan, H.A.: Current Concepts on the Treatment of Solitary Unicameral Bone Cyst. Clin. Orthop. **97:**40–51, 1973.

28. Nesbit, M.E., Kieffer, S., and D'Angio, G.J.: Reconstitution of Vertebral Height in Histiocytosis X: A Long Term Follow-up. J. Bone Joint Surg. **51-A:**1360–1368, 1969.

29. Persson, B.M., and Wouters, J.W.: Curettage and Acrylic Cementation in Surgery of Giant Cell Tumors of Bone. Clin. Orthop. **120:**125–133, 1979.

30. Picci, P., Manfrini, M., Zucchi, V., Gherlinzoni, F., Rock, M., Bertoni, F., and Neff, J.R.: Giant-Cell Tumor of Bone in Skeletally Immature Patients. J. Bone Joint Surg. **65-A:**486–490, 1983.

31. Scaglietti, O., Marchette, P.G., and Bartolozzi, P.: The Effects of Methylprenisolone Acetate in the Treatment of Bone Cysts. J. Bone Joint Surg. **61-B:**200–204, 1979.

32. Schajowicz, F., and Gallardo, N.: Epiphyseal Chondroblastoma of bone. A Clinical-Pathological Study of 69 cases. J. Bone Joint Surg. **52-B:**205–226, 1970.

33. Smith, R.J., Koniuch, M.P.: Tumors of the Hand. *In* Evarts, C.M. (ed.): Surgery of the Musculoskeletal System, Vol. 2. New York, Churchill Livingstone, 1983, pp. 71–122.

CHAPTER 73

Malignant Bone Tumors

FRANKLIN H. SIM,
DOUGLAS J. McDONALD,
and LESTER E. WOLD

Osteogenic Sarcoma
Chondrosarcoma
Fibrosarcoma
Ewing's Sarcoma
Myeloma
Malignant Lymphoma of Bone
Malignant Fibrous Histiocytoma
Chordoma
Adamantinoma

OSTEOGENIC SARCOMA

Clinical Features

Osteogenic sarcoma is a primary neoplasm of bone characterized by the formation of tumor osteoid by a frankly sarcomatous connective tissue stroma. It is the second most common primary malignant bone tumor (myeloma is first) and accounts for 20% of all bone sarcomas. Although the tumor can occur in any bone, the appendicular skeleton is most frequently involved; approximately 50% of the lesions occur about the knee.[9,18,22] Most lesions appear to arise *de novo;* however, secondary lesions may occur following irradiation or at the site of preexisting benign lesions, such as fibrous dysplasia, bone infarcts, and Paget's disease.[121,123] Bone involvement at many sites in the same patient is rare.

Most patients present with a short history of pain and swelling in the involved limb. The pain may be intermittent at first, later becoming constant and often accentuated at night. Occasionally, the patient may present with a pathologic fracture.

Hematogenous metastasis is normally to the lungs and develops in approximately half the patients.[116]

Pathologic Features

Osteosarcoma is not a homogeneous disease.[19,20,25] Various clinical and pathologic subtypes exist, and the prognoses differ. Conventional osteosarcoma is a high-grade intramedullary lesion and accounts for approximately 85% of tumors. The tumor usually is located in the metaphyseal area of a long bone and may have extracortical extension or intra-articular invasion. Variable amounts of soft friable tissue, firm fibrous tissue, cartilaginous tissue, and foci of ossification or sclerosis may be present in any given tumor. Microscopically, three usual subtypes have been identified, depending on the predominant histologic pattern: osteoblastic, chondroblastic, and fibroblastic.

An intramedullary lesion that has a better prognosis than the conventional osteosarcoma is the low-grade central or intraosseous osteosarcoma.[118] Telangiectatic osteosarcoma, a subtype of the intramedullary lesions, has a poor prognosis, possibly worse than that of a conventional lesion; it accounts for approximately 3% of lesions. Grossly it looks like a blood-filled cyst and can be mistaken for an aneurysmal bone cyst.[73]

Periosteal or juxtacortical osteosarcoma is a rare subtype that arises on the surface of a bone. There is no intramedullary involvement, and a chondroblastic histologic pattern predominates. It has a slightly better prognosis than conventional osteosarcoma. Parosteal osteosarcoma is another surface subtype. Accounting for 3% of osteosarcomas, it commonly occurs on the posterior aspect of the distal femur. It tends to be heavily ossified with a well-differentiated histologic appearance, and the prognosis is distinctly better than with the conventional lesion.

Radiographic Features

On plain radiographs, osteogenic sarcoma appears as a mixed lytic and sclerotic lesion. The tumor appears aggressive with indistinct margins, evidence of cortical destruction, and periosteal reaction (Fig. 73-1A). Variable amounts of new bone formation may be present, often giving the typical "sunburst" appearance. Some lesions may be purely lytic, particularly the telangiectatic subtype. Other lesions may be heavily ossified, as the parosteal type. Computed tomography (CT) and magnetic resonance imaging (MRI) are useful modalities, especially in determining local soft-tissue boundaries and proximity to adjacent structures. Radionuclide scans can aid in determining intraosseous extent or identifying skip lesions.

Treatment

A multidisciplinary approach is necessary for the patient with osteosarcoma. Careful preoperative staging, including a well-planned, adequate biopsy forms the basis of the overall treatment plan.

For high-grade extraosseous osteosarcoma, amputation remains the standard recommended treatment (Fig. 73-2). However, recent advances may be changing this standard. Some controversy once existed over the proper level of amputation; some authors suggested that it was safer to leave a joint between the tumor site and the amputation level. Most now agree that amputation 8 to 10 cm above the most proximal margin of the tumor, as determined by radiographs and bone scans, is adequate (see Fig. 73-2). Historically, this approach gave an overall 5-year survival of 20% in most patients. Pulmonary metastasis developed in some patients despite adequate local tumor control.[22,40,41,70,77] Clearly, for survival to be improved, an effective means of treating the systemic disease is needed.

Enthusiasm for adjuvant chemotherapy was generated in the early 1970s with reports of 5-year survival increasing to the 45% to 60% range.[17,39,51,52,98] Other reports comparing chemotherapy with concurrent surgical controls showed no apparent survival benefit for patients treated with chemotherapy, whereas survival after surgical treatment alone had improved.[32,69,114,115] Thus, considerable controversy developed over the effectiveness of chemotherapy for osteosarcoma. A number of clinical trials with various chemotherapeutic agents, usually including high-dose methotrexate, doxorubicin, or cisplatin, are in progress. Some protocols utilize preoperative (neoadjuvant) chemotherapy; the extent of tumor necrosis at the time of definitive operation is used as a measure of the effectiveness.[31,94] Currently, these advances in chemotherapy are thought to make an important contribution to the improved survival being reported in patients with osteosarcoma.[106]

Limb Salvage

Increased enthusiasm for chemotherapy combined with improved techniques of oncologic reconstruction has stimulated an interest in limb salvage, as outlined in Chapter 70. Often, a surgical margin can be achieved with a limb-sparing resection that is comparable to the margin with an amputation. Thus, proper patient selection is important. A number of factors need to be considered. Age is important because many of the techniques generally apply to patients with closed physes. However, the development of expandable prostheses holds promise for extending the possibilities of limb salvage to younger age

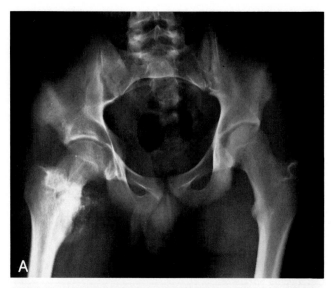
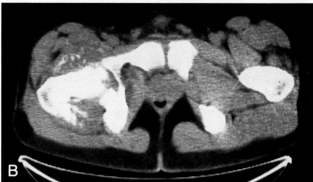
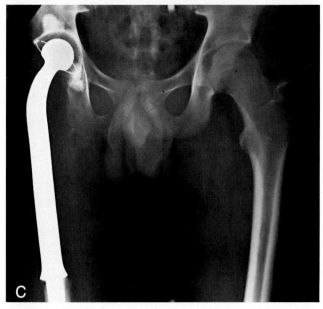

FIGURE 73-1. Osteogenic sarcoma. (*A*) Anteroposterior radiograph. (*B*) CT scan showing stage IIB osteosarcoma involving the proximal femur. (*C*) After resection and proximal femoral replacement arthroplasty. (Sim, F.H., Bowman, W.E., Jr., Wilkins, R.M., and Chao, E.Y.S.: Limb Salvage in Primary Malignant Bone Tumors. Orthopedics **8:**574–581, 1985.)

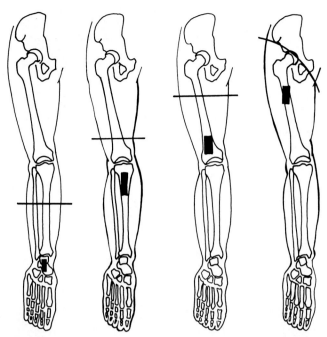

FIGURE 73-2. Levels of amputation for osteogenic sarcoma at various sites in the lower extremity. (Sim, F.H., Ivins, J.C., and Pritchard, D.J.: Surgical Treatment of Osteogenic Sarcoma at the Mayo Clinic. Cancer Treat. Rep. **62:**205–211, 1978.)

groups. A rotation-plasty may be useful in preserving function in younger patients (Fig. 73-3).[59] The location and extent of the tumor must be favorable to allow an adequate margin of resection that does not preclude restoration of useful limb function. Preferably, the tumor should be entirely intraosseous (stage IIA). However, because many osteosarcomas have extraosseous extension, the patient can be a candidate if this extension is small and away from vital neurovascular structures. Ultimately, a viable limb-salvage technique must provide local tumor control comparable to that from an amputation yet maintain a functional status of the extremity superior to that after amputation and prosthesis fitting.

The techniques used for reconstruction after resection depend on the location of the tumor and the function expected by the patient. The alternatives include custom prosthesis replacement, allograft replacement as an osteochondral graft, or resection arthrodesis.[105] For lesions about the hip, prosthesis replacement has been particularly effective in restoring the function of the joint (see Fig. 73-1).[102] For lesions of the pelvis, limb salvage is important not only because of the mutilating functional effect of a hemipelvectomy but also because the surgical margin achieved often may be the same as that achieved by an amputation. Current techniques vary depending on the location and extent of pelvic resection. With complete iliosacral joint resection, fusion of the remaining ilium to the sacrum can be achieved by hinging the pelvis on the sym-

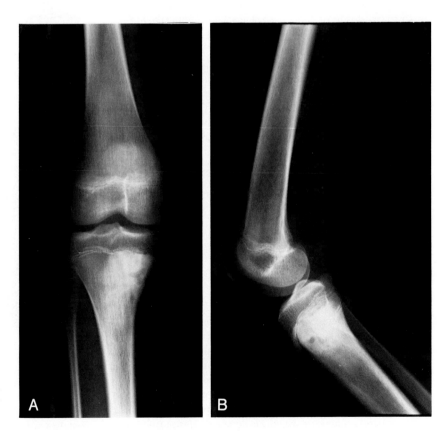

FIGURE 73-3. Osteosarcoma of right tibia in a 13-year-old girl. Anteroposterior and lateral radiographs of the right knee.

physis pubis. After periacetabular resection, fusion of the proximal femur to the ilium is the preferred technique (Fig. 73-4). This can be enhanced by the use of vascularized fibular grafts or intercalary allograft segments.

When a lesion involves the knee, our preferred technique is a segmental arthrodesis. This can be accomplished by various methods. Use of hemicylindrical femoral turn-down or tibial turn-up grafts combined with ipsilateral fibular grafts and a long Küntscher rod for stabilization is the optimal technique. A fiber-metal ingrowth fusion prosthesis or intercalary allograft segments also can be used, particularly to span large defects (Fig. 73-5). However, when the lesion is a life-threatening tumor with a high incidence of metastasis, custom total knee arthroplasty is often utilized because of the immediate restoration of function.

Reconstruction for osteosarcoma of an upper extremity primarily involves the shoulder. Resection of the proximal humerus and often portions of the scapula usually requires sacrifice of the rotator cuff muscles, overlying deltoid, and axillary nerve. Reconstructive alternatives include prosthetic replacement, allograft, and arthrodesis. Current custom prosthesis replacements use a modular design with a porous coating for potential biologic fixation (Fig. 73-6). Arthrodesis using dual fibular grafts, vascularized fibular grafts, or allografts has also been successful.[63,71,81,100,103]

Results of Treatment

With advances in chemotherapy and surgical techniques, the outlook for patients with osteosarcoma has improved. Current 5-year survival rates after a multidisciplinary approach are 40% to 60%. The results of limb salvage have been equally encouraging. Local recurrence rates are reported as 3.8% to 6%, comparable to those obtained with amputation.[31] Moreover, overall survival is not compromised by limb-salvage surgery: 5-year survival was 49% compared with 54% in 160 patients with osteogenic sarcoma who underwent amputation from 1970 to 1981.[105] The challenge remains for treating those patients who have pulmonary metastasis, but advances in treatment have been made for them as well. In a recent report, approximately one-third of the patients with pulmonary metastasis were salvaged with an aggressive surgical approach, often including multiple thoracotomies in attempts to eradicate the pulmonary lesions.[116]

CHONDROSARCOMA

Clinical Features

Chondrosarcoma of bone is a malignant tumor of proliferating cartilage tissue devoid of osteoid. It accounts for approximately 10% of malignant bone tumors and tends to occur in older adults (peak incidence is in the fifth to sixth decades of life). More than three-fourths of these lesions are located in the trunk or proximal portions of the femur or humerus. The inner wall of the acetabulum is a particularly common site.[18] The lesions tend to grow slowly and pain may be present for months or years before a mass or swelling is detected. Metastasis is rare

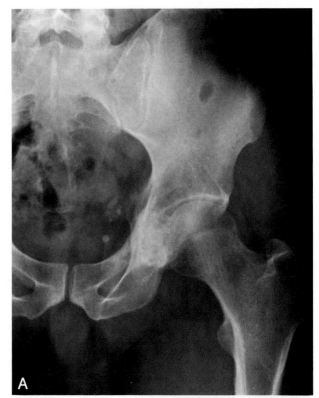

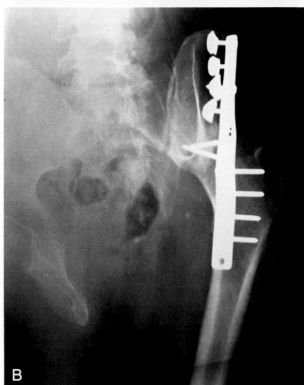

FIGURE 73-4.   (*A*) Anteroposterior view of left hemipelvis, showing chondrosarcoma involving innominate bone and acetabulum. (*B*) After *en bloc* resection and reconstruction with femoral iliac arthrodesis. (Sim, F.H., Bowman, W.E., Jr., and Chao, E.Y.S.: Limb Salvage and Reconstructive Techniques. In Sim, F.H. (ed.): Diagnosis and Treatment of Bone Tumors: A Team Approach. Rochester, Minn., Mayo Foundation, 1983, pp. 75–104.)

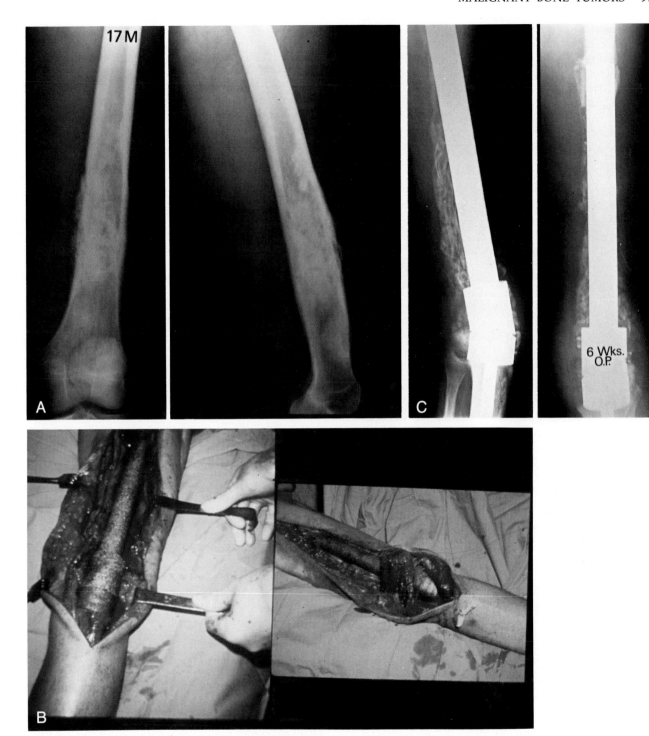

FIGURE 73-5. (*A*) Anteroposterior and lateral views of distal femur, showing extensive osteosarcoma extending into diaphysis. (*B*) Operative photographs after resection, showing intercalary fiber-metal prosthesis (*left*) and transfer of both gastrocnemius muscles over the implant to supply soft tissue coverage (*right*). (*C*) Anteroposterior and lateral views 6 weeks after reconstruction, showing early incorporation of bone grafts and fixation of prosthesis.

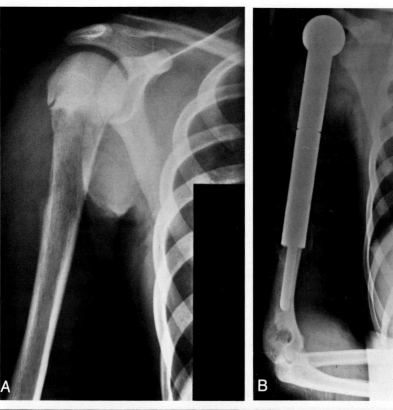

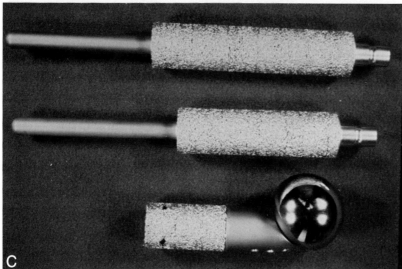

FIGURE 73-6. (*A*) Anteroposterior view of right humerus, showing osteosarcoma involving the metaphysis and extending into the diaphysis. (*B*) After resection of upper two-thirds of the humerus and replacement with fiber-metal prosthesis. (*C*) Interchangeable components of proximal humerus prosthesis. (Sim, F.H., Ivins, J.C., Taylor, W.F., and Chao, E.Y.S.: Limb-Sparing Surgery for Osteosarcoma: Mayo Clinic Experience. Cancer Treat. Symp. **3:**139–154, 1985.)

and often occurs late in the course of the disease; however, the tumor has a distinct tendency to recur locally.

Pathologic Features

Chondrosarcomas may arise *de novo* as primary lesions or occur secondarily at the site of a previous benign lesion, usually an osteochondroma but also enchondromas. Approximately 75% are primary tumors.

Grossly, primary chondrosarcomas occur centrally within the intramedullary portion of the bone. They tend to be lobular with a matrix of varying consistency. The center of the lobules often undergoes myxoid degeneration. Cortical destruction with soft tissue extension and calcific densities within the chondroid matrix are common.

Microscopically, the tumors have been divided into three histologic grades. Approximately 90% are well-differentiated (grade 1 or 2) tumors. An important subtype of chondrosarcomas is the dedifferentiated lesion. This subtype accounts for approximately 10% of chondrosarcomas and is characterized by regions of highly anaplastic (grade 3 or 4) tissue within the tumor immediately adjacent to areas of ordinary low-grade chondrosarcoma. This subtype carries a poor prognosis.[21,38,74]

Other subtypes include a clear cell variant and a mesenchymal chondrosarcoma. The clear cell chondrosarcoma is rare and sometimes is referred to as "atypical" chondrosarcoma or malignant chondroblastoma. Its malignant potential is low and it is characterized by the presence of cells with clear cytoplasm. Occasionally, benign giant cells or reactive bone formation may be evident. Mesenchymal chondrosarcoma is another uncommon variant; approximately one-third of these tumors arise in the soft tissues. Considered to be highly malignant, it is characterized by a combination of rather benign chondroid islands with highly cellular areas of small round to ovoid cells arranged in a hemangiopericytomatous pattern.[35,45,46,62]

Radiographic Features

On plain film radiographic examination, chondrosarcomas appear as predominantly lytic lesions with cortical destruction combined with areas of calcification that give a mottled appearance (Fig. 73-7A). Endosteal scalloping and cortical expansion are helpful in differentiating chondrosarcomas from benign enchondromas. Tumors arising in the pelvis are less distinctive unless associated with a characteristic large mass and mottled mineralization. The use of CT and, more recently, MRI is of particular aid in defining soft-tissue margins and cortical de-

struction in pelvic tumors. Both are useful in detection of recurrent lesions.

Treatment

Surgical resection remains the mainstay of therapy for chondrosarcoma because these tumors are considered to be resistant to routine chemotherapy and radiotherapy.[10,34] Two important principles apply in surgical management. First, a well-planned and adequate biopsy that is representative of the entire tumor is necessary. Second, a wide margin must be achieved at initial resection to ensure the best chance of cure for this tumor, which is notorious for local recurrence.

Accurate preoperative staging with determination of the histopathologic grade as well as regional tumor extent will dictate the aggressiveness needed at operation. For higher grade lesions with extensive soft-tissue involvement, amputation may be required to gain control. If a limb-sparing procedure is feasible, the reconstructive techniques described for osteosarcoma apply equally well for chondrosarcoma (Fig. 73-7B). Because many lesions involve the proximal femur or pelvis, custom prosthesis replacement for proximal femoral resection or internal hemipelvectomy and fusion for pelvic lesions has yielded satisfactory results.

Results of Treatment

The overall 5-year survival rate after chondrosarcoma is approximately 50%.[87] For lower grade lesions, a rate approaching 85% is possible; for the higher grade lesions, a survival rate of 15% can be expected. Because local recurrence affects survival adversely and recurrences after 5 years are not uncommon, 5-year survival rates are unreliable indicators of long-term results. Nevertheless, with adequate surgical therapy, long-term survival can be expected in more than half of the patients.

Results of treatment of the highly malignant dedifferentiated chondrosarcoma are poor despite radical surgery; the 5-year survival is less than 10%.[38]

FIBROSARCOMA

Clinical Features

Fibrosarcoma of bone is a malignancy characterized by the proliferation of fibroblastic cells without any discernable matrix production. This tumor accounts for less than 4% of primary osseous malignancies and occurs over a wide age range, from the second through sixth decades. Thus, as a group, patients with fibrosarcomas have an age distribution different from those with fibroblastic osteosarcoma although the tumors are similar histologically. Males and females are affected equally. The skeletal distribution is similar to that of osteosarcoma, with more than 50% occurring in long bones (usually the femur or tibia).[18,23,36] Most of these lesions arise *de novo*, yet more than 25% can be considered secondary, arising at sites of preexisting disease or after irradiation.[29,47,78]

Symptoms of fibrosarcoma include pain and swelling, similar to symptoms of other malignancies, which on occasion may be present for a long time before diagnosis.

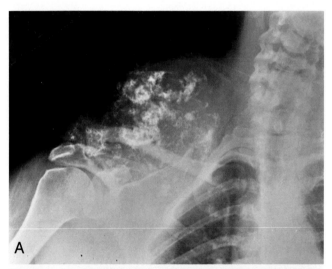

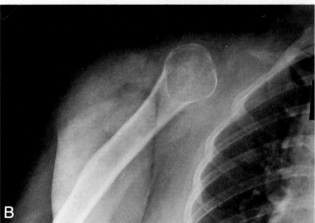

FIGURE 73-7. (*A*) Anteroposterior view of right shoulder, showing extensive chondrosarcoma arising from the upper scapula. (*B*) After scapulectomy.

Pathologic Features

Grossly, fibrosarcomas vary in appearance. Some well-differentiated lesions may be firm, dense, and seemingly well circumscribed. Poorly differentiated lesions tend to be soft and friable with regions of myxoid degeneration. Areas of hemorrhage and necrosis are frequently evident. Cortical destruction is common and soft-tissue involvement may be extensive.

Microscopically, fibrosarcomas are characterized by spindle cells that show varying degrees of cytologic atypia and are arranged in a herringbone pattern. The degrees of cellular anaplasia and stroma production can vary significantly. Some lesions appear to be so well differentiated that confusion with benign fibrous lesions can occur. Other tumors are highly anaplastic with little or no recognizable collagenous stroma being produced. Approximately 68% of the lesions are grade 3 or 4, and 32% are grade 1 or 2.[18]

Radiographic Features

There are no pathognomonic radiographic features of fibrosarcoma. Generally, the presence of osteolytic bone destruction with cortical and soft-tissue extension suggests a malignant process, yet distinction from other malignancies, particularly an osteolytic osteosarcoma, is difficult. Periosteal new bone formation may be seen and permeative destruction may be evident well beyond the principal area of lysis. Occasionally, a fibrosarcoma may originate on the periosteal surface; however, most lesions appear to arise from the intramedullary portion of the bone. Radionuclide scans, CT, and MRI aid in determining osseous extent as well as in defining regional margins.

Treatment

Adequate treatment requires surgical removal with a wide or radical margin through uninvolved tissue. As with other high-grade extraosseous lesions (stage IIB), amputation may be required. With lower grade lesions or stage IIA lesions, consideration can be given to limb-sparing surgery to preserve function and still achieve local tumor control (Fig. 73-8). The principles of limb-sparing surgery and reconstructive techniques are discussed above.

Radiation therapy generally is ineffective, although it may have a palliative role in lesions deemed unresectable. Adjuvant multidrug chemotherapy programs similar to those used for osteosarcoma are being evaluated in a number of centers for dealing with systemic disease. The overall 5-year survival for fibrosarcoma is approximately 30%.[23,36] As with other spindle cell sarcomas, prognosis relates to histologic grade, with well-differentiated lesions carrying a distinctly better prognosis than osteogenic sarcoma.[18]

EWING'S SARCOMA

Clinical Features

Ewing's sarcoma of bone is a highly anaplastic, small, round cell tumor of unknown histiogenesis but presumably arising from a primitive mesenchymal cell. Although originally thought to possibly be of endothelial origin,[28,99] recent studies have suggested a neuroectodermal origin.[53] Ewing's sarcoma accounts for approximately 5% of primary bone sarcomas and a slight

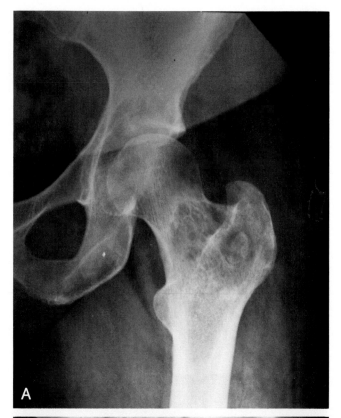

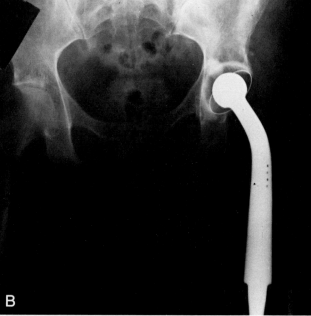

FIGURE 73-8. (*A*) Anteroposterior view of left proximal femur, showing large destructive lesion involving the intertrochanteric area. Biopsy revealed grade 3 fibrosarcoma; surgical stage was IIb. (*B*) After wide resection and proximal femoral replacement.

male predominance is found. The tumor occurs typically in the first and second decades of life, and more than 90% of patients are less than 30 years of age. It can arise in any bone of the body, but more than 60% of the lesions occur in the pelvic girdle and lower extremity. Other common sites include the proximal humerus and scapula.[18,86]

FIGURE 73-9. (*A*) Anteroposterior view, showing extensive destruction of proximal femur secondary to Ewing's sarcoma in 7-year-old boy; a pathologic fracture is evident. He was treated with hip disarticulation. (*B*) Pathologic specimen after amputation.

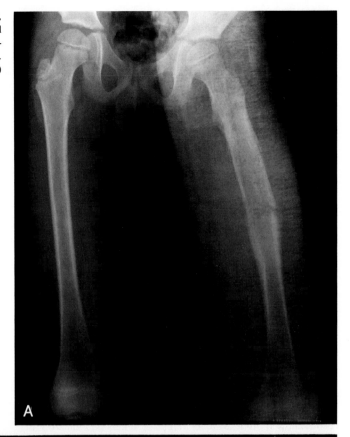

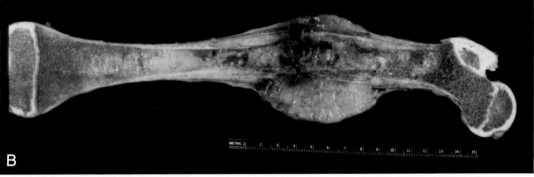

Pain and swelling are the most common symptoms; they may be present for several months before diagnosis. Occasionally, systemic signs and symptoms are present, such as low-grade fever, increased erythrocyte sedimentation rate, leukocytosis, and anemia.

Approximately 50% of the metastatic lesions occur in the lungs, but other skeletal sites, including the skull and vertebral column, are affected.

Pathologic Features

Ewing's sarcoma appears to originate in the intramedullary cavity. It usually involves the metaphysis and commonly a significant portion of the shaft of a long bone. The tumor is characteristically gray or white and is very soft, almost liquid, suggesting purulence. Microscopically it is a cellular sheetlike proliferation without matrix production. However, fibrous strands may be identified traversing the lesion. The cells have indistinct cytoplasmic borders with round to oval nuclei. It may be difficult to differentiate Ewing's sarcoma from other round cell tumors histologically, particularly lymphoma. However, the cytologic monotony of the cells in Ewing's sarcoma and the absence of reticulum fibers are helpful factors in making the diagnosis. The presence of glycogen within tumor cells is not a constant finding in Ewing's sarcoma of bone.

Radiographic Features

Combined lytic destruction and blastic areas in a mottled or motheaten pattern is the most common radiographic appearance. The margins are indistinct and the tumor may extend through the entire bone (Fig. 73-9). Cortical destruction with periosteal elevation and multiple layers of subperiosteal new bone gives the classic "onionskin" appearance; however, this is not pathognomonic for Ewing's sarcoma. Radiating spicules of new bone in a "sunburst" pattern also can occur, making radiographic distinction from osteosarcoma difficult. In rare lesions with little or no intramedullary involvement (subperiosteal Ewing's sarcoma), saucer-shaped destruction of the exterior cortex is a fairly characteristic feature, if present. As in other malignant tumors, CT and MRI are helpful in defining the soft-tissue extension that is common in Ewing's sarcoma.

Treatment

As a small round cell tumor, Ewing's sarcoma is considered relatively radiosensitive. Thus, until recently the standard recommended treatment consisted of irradiation of the primary lesion, with chemotherapy directed at occult systemic metastasis. Most radiotherapy protocols consisted of 4000 to 6000 cGy delivered to the whole affected bone with effort to avoid irradiating an actively growing physis.

Radiation alone, however, is inconsistent in controlling the primary tumor. Local recurrence rates of 15% to 20% after radiation therapy alone have been reported, with microscopic viability present in 65% of cases in an autopsy study.[88,117] In addition, the late morbidity associated with irradiation, such as limb-length inequality, pathologic fracture, fibrosis, and ankylosis, as well as an increased awareness of radiation-induced sarcoma, has led to a renewed interest in the role of surgical treatment for Ewing's sarcoma.

Currently, surgical resection is recommended as the primary treatment for isolated rib lesions or lesions located in an expendable bone such as the proximal fibula. Although not recommended often, primary amputation may be indicated for distal extremity lesions in a growing child or large, destructive tumors about the knee with extensive soft tissue involvement (see Fig. 73-9). For pelvic lesions or when limb salvage is considered, careful preoperative planning will aid in determining the feasibility of surgical treatment. Although still somewhat controversial, preoperative chemotherapy followed by resection with or without postoperative irradiation, depending on the surgical margin achieved, may be an effective therapeutic regimen.

Results of Treatment

Prior to effective chemotherapy, Ewing's sarcoma was considered one of the most lethal sarcomas, with a 5-year survival rate of less than 20%. With a modern approach to treatment utilizing all known effective modalities, 5-year survival rates have improved to approximately 40%.[13,55,68,125] The addition of surgery to the therapeutic regimen has been shown to have a favorable result.[4,64,86,96,97] Poor prognostic variables include pelvic lesions, young age in males, and development of local recurrence. Overall, the role of surgical treatment is expanding. Hopefully, with combined surgery, irradiation, and effective chemotherapy, the once dismal outlook associated with Ewing's sarcoma can further be improved.

MYELOMA

Clinical Features

Myeloma is a neoplastic disease of plasma cells which characteristically involves the bone marrow. It has a wide clinical spectrum of disease, accounting for the variety in clinical presentations. The most common type is multiple myeloma, manifested by widespread skeletal involvement with marked overproduction of monoclonal immunoglobulins. Presentation with a solitary osseous lesion occurs in approximately 25% of patients with myeloma; subsequent dissemination of the disease occurs in most of these patients. Solitary extramedullary infiltrates (plasmacytomas), often located in the upper airway passages, also can occur alone or in patients in whom multiple myeloma later develops.[5]

Myeloma is the most common primary malignancy of bone, accounting for approximately half of all bone tumors. It is considered to be a disease of middle age and older; most patients are between 50 and 70 years old. The most common tumor locations are in bones containing active hematopoietic elements; more than 85% of the lesions involve the axial skeleton and proximal portions of the femur and humerus. More than half of the solitary osseous lesions are located in the vertebral column.[6,18,60,72]

Pain is a prominent feature of myeloma, particularly if a pathologic fracture occurs. Systemic symptoms (weakness, fatigue) along with various abnormal laboratory findings are helpful in establishing a diagnosis. Patients have characteristic immunoglobulins that can be demonstrated with immunoelectrophoretic techniques.

Pathologic Features

Myeloma is typically soft, gray to red, and friable. The gross boundaries are indistinct, and often the medullary and extraosseous involvement is greater than anticipated. Microscopically, the tumor consists of sheets of closely packed plasma cells. Abundant granular cytoplasm is present, and multinucleated cells are occasionally seen. Variable amounts of pink, amorphous amyloid is present in approximately 10% of myelomas.[18]

Radiographic Features

The classic plain film appearance is that of purely lytic "punched-out" areas of bone destruction. Typically, there is no reactive zone of sclerosis. Occasionally, a balloon-like expansion of bone may occur, particularly in rib lesions. Pathologic fractures are a common feature in vertebral lesions. In 15% to 25% of patients, no discrete lysis occurs, and diffuse osteopenia and osteoporosis are the only skeletal manifestations. Technetium-99m bone scans are less reliable in identifying myeloma lesions because of a lack of osseous response to the tumor. A skeletal survey together with plain or computed tomography is more helpful in identifying additional lesions or defining extent of osseous destruction.

Treatment

The primary treatment modality for patients with multiple myeloma is chemotherapy. Most protocols include the use of melphalan (L-phenylalanine mustard) and cyclophosphamide; prednisone occasionally is used to enhance the response to these agents.[30,42,75] A positive response to treatment can be monitored objectively by noting a decrease in M-type proteins, hematologic recovery, and, occasionally, resolution of the skeletal disease.

For localized lesions that are causing disabling pain or limitation of activity, radiation in doses of 2000 cGy is very effective. Radiation tends to slow the growth of the tumor, allowing microfractures to heal and thus relieving pain. Occasionally, the lesion reossifies with a return of structural integrity. For patients with solitary myeloma—as defined by positive biopsy of an isolated lesion with negative bone marrow aspirate and no laboratory evidence of myeloma for 2 years—a more aggressive approach to therapy is warranted. Radiation doses up to 5000 cGy to the solitary lesion are indicated along with a more aggressive surgical approach to resection.

Surgical intervention in multiple myeloma is most commonly indicated in patients with vertebral involvement who have neurologic symptoms and in patients with impending or actual pathologic fractures. Myeloma is the second most common malignancy, after metastatic carcinoma, producing compressive paraplegia.[43,91] Decompressive laminectomy is indicated in this circumstance, and moderate to excellent return of function can be expected in many patients. Spinal stabilization is occasionally warranted, and recent advances in the techniques of anterior and posterior instrumentation have improved the effectiveness in restoring stability.

Pathologic fractures require aggressive surgical management in order to relieve pain and maintain ambulatory status (Fig. 73-10). The principles of open reduction and internal fixation, often utilizing supplemental methylmethacrylate, will achieve skeletal stability in a majority of these fractures. For pathologic fractures involving the femoral neck, resection and prosthetic replacement are effective. For subtrochanteric lesions, our preferred technique for treatment is use of a Zickel nail with methylmethacrylate augmentation (Fig. 73-11).

The indications for prophylactic internal fixation of an impending pathologic fracture are the same as in metastatic disease. Generally, if a lesion is larger than 3 cm, destroys more than 50% of the cortex of a weight-bearing bone, or fails to respond to irradiation, prophylactic fixation may be indicated.[2,16,27,44,54,57,61,66,104]

Results

The overall prognosis for patients with multiple myeloma continues to be poor. However, significant advances in chemotherapy have increased the median survival over the last 20 years from 12 months to up to 32 months in more recent reports.[30,56,60] Poor prognostic variables include the presence of M proteins, pancytopenia, hypercalcemia, diffuse skeletal lesions, and renal failure.

Patients with solitary myeloma may often have a protracted course, with survival for more than 10 years being reported.[43,76,120]

MALIGNANT LYMPHOMA OF BONE

Clinical Features

Malignant lymphoma of bone is a neoplasm of the reticuloendothelial system. Most often, it is composed of a proliferation of lymphoid cells, at various stages of differentiation, as well as histiocytes. It accounts for approximately 3% of primary os-

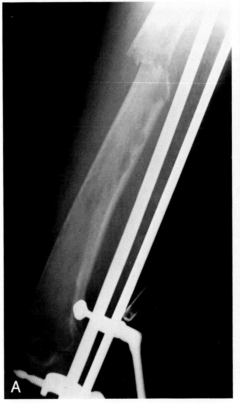
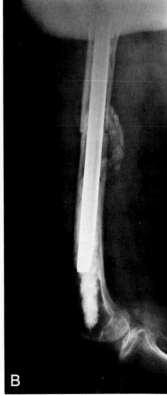

FIGURE 73-10. Lateral radiographs of left femur in patient with myeloma. (*A*) Pathologic fracture. (*B*) After reduction and internal fixation with intermedullary rod and adjuvant use of methyl methacrylate. (From Sim, F.H.: Myeloma of Bone. Orthop. Surg. Update Series **4:**1–12, 1986.)

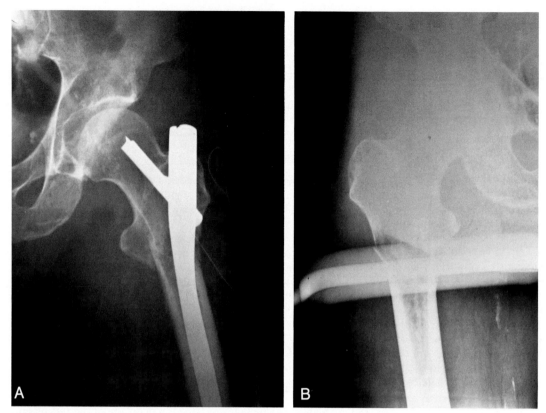

FIGURE 73-11. Anteroposterior radiographs of right hip in patient with myeloma. (*A*) Lytic destruction involving subtrochanteric area. (*B*) After internal fixation with Zickel nail. (Sim, F.H.: Myeloma of Bone. Orthop. Surg. Update Series **4**:1–12, 1986).

seous malignancies; an equal number of cases represent secondary osseous involvement. Any age group can be affected, but it is rare in the very young and peaks in the fifth to seventh decades of life. When located in long bones, the lesions tend to be metaphyseal, occurring primarily in the proximal femur, proximal humerus, and distal femur. The pelvis and spinal column are also common sites.[7,18,82,83]

Pain, often present for many months or years, is a constant feature. Neurologic symptoms are common with spinal lesions, as are pathologic fractures.

Pathologic Features

Grossly, the primary lymphoma of bone tends to be located in the metaphyseal region although diffuse osseous involvement may be present. Soft-tissue extension of the tumor is frequently found. The tumors are generally soft when they have destroyed the bone but are firm where residual osseous trabeculae are present. Areas of necrosis may be apparent. Extraosseous masses are usually soft and friable.

The tumor most commonly consists of an admixture of large and small cells amid a fine reticulin meshwork. Various degrees of fibrosis also may be present. Occasionally, the multinucleated Reed-Sternberg cells are seen, suggesting primary Hodgkin's disease of bone. Histologically, primary malignant lymphoma of bone is indistinguishable from lymphoma lesions originating elsewhere.

Radiographic Features

Extensive bony involvement, often 25% to 50% of the involved bone, in a mottled or patchy fashion is evident on plain film radiographs. The margins are indistinct, with marked cortical destruction and soft-tissue extension being apparent. Occasionally, irregular sclerosis is seen, confusing the radiographic picture. Distinction from Ewing's sarcoma, metastatic carcinoma, osteomyelitis, and occasionally Paget's disease may be difficult in some cases.

Treatment

The primary treatment of lymphoma is radiation therapy because these lesions, as other round cell tumors, are considered to be radiosensitive. Doses of 5000 to 5500 cGy are directed at the primary lesion, and usually this is the only local treatment indicated.[85,112,113] The role of chemotherapy for systemic or metastatic disease is less clear, although some authors advocate it.[89,111] Operation is reserved for pathologic fractures that cannot reasonably be managed by other means. Some authors believe that operation also is indicated for isolated, uncontrolled lesions of a distal extremity that have failed to respond to radiation treatment.[18]

The overall 5-year survival with lymphoma approaches 50%.[7,82,89] This is in contrast to Ewing's sarcoma, although they are closely related tumors. Metastasis or recurrence may occur many years later, making 5-year survival values less reliable. The clinical staging of lymphoma has important prognostic significance.[101,113] Proper treatment design requires thorough evaluation, not only of the primary lesion but also of potential systemic and metastatic disease.

MALIGNANT FIBROUS HISTIOCYTOMA

Clinical Features

Malignant fibrous histiocytoma of bone is a highly malignant neoplasm derived from primitive mesenchymal cells and demonstrating both fibrous and histiocytic cytologic features. It is similar to its soft-tissue counterpart but is less common, accounting for approximately 5% of malignant bone tumors. Arising at any age, its peak incidence lies in the fourth and fifth decades with males outnumbering females 1.5 to 1.[11,18,26,37,49]

Secondary tumors arising from preexisting benign conditions (e.g., bone infarcts) after radiation therapy or as the prominent histologic component of dedifferentiated chondrosarcomas have also been reported.[38]

The lesions are seen with greatest frequency in the appendicular skeleton, particularly in the proximal and distal metaphyses of the femur and the proximal metaphysis of the tibia. Metastasis occurs hematogenously, usually to the lungs but also to other osseous sites.

Pathologic Features

Grossly, the tumors vary in consistency from firm to soft, depending on the amount of fibrous tissue present. Typically gray to yellow in color, areas of necrosis and hemorrhage may also be present. Cortical destruction and soft-tissue extension are prominent features.

Malignant fibrous histiocytoma in general shows a pleomorphic pattern at low magnification. The spindle cell regions show the matted or "storiform" pattern typical of soft-tissue primary lesions. Considerable cytologic variation is identifiable at high magnification. The indentation of nuclei and large, well-defined cytoplasm gives them their histiocytic appearance. Other cells show a spindle cell arrangement with ovoid to ellipsoid nuclei. Differentiation from fibrosarcoma may be difficult.

Radiographic Features

Radiographically, malignant fibrous histiocytoma shows geographic lysis but occasionally will have a permeative picture. Cortical destruction and indistinct margins suggest an aggressive malignancy. Little reactive periosteal or sclerotic bone is seen. Radionuclide scans are helpful in determining osseous extent of the primary lesion as well as in detecting other lesions. CT and MRI confirm the cortical destruction and aid in determining soft-tissue margins and the relationship of the tumor to adjacent neurovascular structures.

Treatment

The preoperative staging and surgical treatment plan for a malignant fibrous histiocytoma are similar to those for fibro-

sarcomas and all other high-grade radioresistant tumors. The goals of adequate surgical control with maximal preservation of limb function determine the feasibility of limb-sparing surgery. Adjuvant chemotherapy has been introduced recently in an effort to control systemic disease and has given encouraging results.[95,119,122] Prognosis is similar to that with fibrosarcoma, with 5-year survival approaching 30%.

CHORDOMA

Clinical Features

Chordoma is a malignancy that originates from primitive notochord remnants and accounts for approximately 1% to 4% of primary osseous malignancies. These tumors arise in the midline of the axial skeleton; half are located in the sacrococcygeal region, approximately 35% are at the base of the skull, and the remainder are within the true vertebrae, usually cervical. They occur in males twice as often as in females and the peak incidence is in the fifth to sixth decades; they are rare in patients less than 30 years old.[18,24,48] Characteristically thought to be slow-growing locally invasive tumors, they do metastasize in approximately 10% of patients.[12,110] The symptoms vary depending on the location; however, pain and neurologic dysfunction are common. Sacral lesions often create a palpable presacral mass on rectal examination.

Pathologic Features

Grossly, chordomas are lobulated, usually soft tumors but may be variable in consistency. Soft tissue extensions often will form a pseudocapsule; intraosseous margins usually are indistinct. Microscopically, the cells are arranged in lobules. Characteristic cytoplasmic vacuoles of mucus are identified within the cells. Other cells have indistinct boundaries with considerable variation in nuclear size and chromatin content. Cells are arranged in clusters and cords amid the extracellular mucoid matrix, which often forms the predominant component of the tumor.

Radiographic Features

Sacral lesions are characterized on plain radiographs by irregular lytic destruction, often of several sacral segments. Residual osseous trabeculae and calcification may be present within the lesion. A presacral mass is usually visible, although overlying shadows of bowel gas can obscure the radiographic picture. Cranial lesions usually produce osseous destruction in the spheno-occipital or hypophyseal region. CT scans offer excellent advantages in the visualization and determination of soft tissue extension of this tumor, often identifying the amorphous peripheral calcification common to these tumors.

Treatment

The principal management of chordomas includes both surgical resection and radiation therapy.

For tumors of the sacrum, *en bloc* resection provides the best chance for cure. Thorough preoperative evaluation often in-

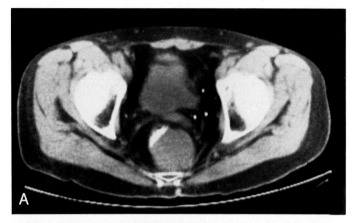

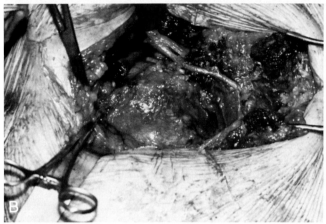

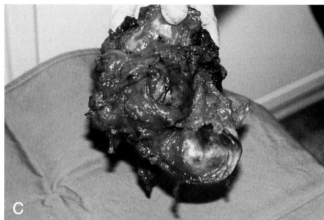

FIGURE 73-12. Chordoma. (*A*) CT scan of pelvis, showing soft tissue extension of chordoma in the presacral region. (*B*) Surgical photograph after resection. Dural sac has been ligated and S-2 nerve roots are salvaged bilaterally. (*C*) Surgical photograph of pathologic specimen. A combined anterior/posterior approach was utilized, removing the rectum *en bloc* with the specimen.

cludes myelography, CT scanning, and intravenous pyelography to assess the soft-tissue extent and involvement of nearby structures. Transrectal biopsy should be avoided because this contaminates the presacral tissue as well as the rectum, necessitating their inclusion in the resected specimen.

For smaller tumors, resection can be accomplished strictly through a posterior approach as described by MacCarty et al.[67] Attempts should be made to save at least the S2 nerve roots bilaterally in order to preserve useful bladder and rectal function. For more extensive lesions or when the rectum is to be included in the resection, a combined anterior and posterior approach has been advocated (Fig. 73-12).[15,65] Through an anterior laparotomy, the bladder and ureters can be mobilized from the tumor and a colostomy can be performed prior to tumor resection. In addition, hemorrhage can be controlled with ligation of one or both of the internal iliac vessels, depending on the extension of the tumor.

Reconstruction is not thought to be needed if pelvic continuity can be maintained through preservation of S1.[107] The response of chordomas to irradiation is variable, and therefore irradiation generally is advocated for unresectable lesions or for palliation of recurrent tumors. Doses of 5000 to 6000 cGy are generally required if cure is sought; smaller doses are given for palliation. Tumors located in the high cervical or cranial region may require irradiation if inaccessible to operation. However, recent advances in technique have permitted a number of successful resections.[3,108,109,124]

Results

Survival is most closely related to the ability to achieve a wide surgical margin. After a definite wide excision, the recurrence rate is probably less than 10%, and approximately 85% of the patients are alive at 10 years.[33] The difficulty arises when curative resection is precluded owing to initial tumor extent at diagnosis or when the surgical resection results in a lesional or marginal margin. In this circumstance, recurrence rates and subsequent mortality increase sharply. Thus, the actual 10-year survival with sacral chordoma is approximately 40%.[110]

ADAMANTINOMA

Clinical Features

Adamantinoma of the appendicular skeleton is rare. It is considered by most authors to be of epithelial origin.[58,80,84,92,93] Others support an angioblastic origin, as suggested by Changus and colleagues in 1957.[14] It has a distinct tendency to occur in the tibial diaphysis, which accounts for more than 90% of the lesions. The tumors most often occur in the second to fifth decades of life and have a slight male predominance.[18]

Pain is the usual presenting feature, often for long duration (months to years), coinciding with the tumor's prolonged indolent course.

Metastasis occurs late, most often to the lungs, and accounts for 70% of the reported deaths.[79]

Pathologic Features

Grossly, the tumor varies in consistency, tends to be lobulated, and may contain spicules of bone as well as cystic areas. Various patterns are seen microscopically; however, an epithelial quality predominates. Commonly, epithelial cells at the periphery of neoplastic islands, are arranged in a palisaded fashion. At the center of the islands, the cells are arranged in a loose spindled manner, termed "stellate reticulum." Areas of fibroblastic tissue predominate, causing these tumors to be confused with fibrous dysplasia or osteofibrous dysplasia, which they simulate radiographically as well.

Radiographic Features

Multiple osteolytic defects of different sizes are seen radiographically, usually in the mid-diaphysis of the tibia. The cortex is locally expanded and thinned. Deformity of the bone and cortical sclerosis are also common.

Treatment

Because of the rarity of the tumor, there are few specific recommendations on treatment. In the past, the malignant potential of this tumor was underestimated, with numerous cases reported as being treated with local excision or curettage.[1] Most authors now think that initial *en bloc* resection to a wide margin is required, with amputation used for unresectable or recurrent lesions. Other authors have advocated amputation as the primary form of treatment.[8,50,90] Irradiation alone or in combination with surgical resection does not seem to influence results. Reconstruction after resection of a tibial lesion can be achieved by using local, iliac, or fibular bone grafts. Mankin and colleagues[71] described excellent early results after treatment by large segmental tibial resection followed by intercalary allograft replacement.

Results

In an excellent review of all documented cases of adamantinoma by Moon and Mori,[79] mortality was 18% and known metastasis was present in 70% of the patients who died. It is important not to underestimate the malignant potential of these tumors. Strict adherence to the principles of oncologic surgery will ensure an optimal result.

REFERENCES

1. Allegreni, R., and Dell'Orto, R.: Adamantinoma Delle Ossa Lunghe: Presentazione di un Caso. Arch. Ortop. **80:**465–471, 1967.
2. Altman, H.: Intramedullary Nailing for Pathological Impending and Actual Fractures of Long Bones. Bull. Hosp. Joint Dis. **13:**239–251, 1952.
3. Arbit, E., and Patterson, R.H., Jr.: Combined Transoral and Median Labiomandibular Glossotomy Approach to the Upper Cervical Spine. Neurosurgery **8:**672–674, 1981.
4. Bacci, G., Picci, P., Gitelis, S., Borghi, A., and Campanacci, M.: The Treatment of Localized Ewing's Sarcoma: The Experience at the Istituto Ortopedico Rizzoli in 163 Cases Treated With and Without Adjuvant Chemotherapy. Cancer **49:**1561–1570, 1982.
5. Bataille, R.: Localized Plasmacytomas. Clin. Haematol. **11:**113–122, 1982.
6. Blattner, W.A., Blair, A., and Mason, T.J.: Multiple Myeloma in the United States, 1950–1975. Cancer **48:**2547–2554, 1981.
7. Boston, H.C., Jr., Dahlin, D.C., Ivins, J.C., and Cupps, R.E.: Malignant Lymphoma (So-Called Reticulum Cell Sarcoma) of Bone. Cancer **34:**1131–1137, 1974.
8. Braidwood, A.S., and McDougall, A.: Adamantinoma of the Tibia: Report of Two Cases. J. Bone Joint Surg. **56-B:**735–738, 1974.
9. Campanacci, M., and Cervellati, G.: Osteosarcoma: A Review of 345 Cases. Ital. J. Orthop. Traumatol. **1:**5–22, 1975.
10. Campanacci, M., Guernelli, N., Leonessa, C., and Boni, A.: Chondrosarcoma: A Study of 133 Cases, 80 With Long Term Follow Up. Ital. J. Orthop. Traumatol. **1:**387–414, 1975.
11. Capanna, R., Bertoni, F., Bacchini, P., Bacci, G., Guerra, A., and Campanacci, M.: Malignant Fibrous Histiocytoma of Bone: The Experience at the Rizzoli Institute; Report of 90 Cases. Cancer **54:**177–187, 1984.
12. Chambers, P.W., and Schwinn, C.P.: Chordoma: A Clinicopathologic Study of Metastasis. Am. J. Clin. Pathol. **72:**765–776, 1979.
13. Chan, R.C., Sutow, W.W., Lindberg, R.D., Samuels, M.L., Murray, J.A., and Johnston, D.A.: Management and Results of Localized Ewing's Sarcoma. Cancer **43:**1001–1006, 1979.
14. Changus, G.W., Speed, J.S., and Stewart, F.W.: Malignant Angioblastoma of Bone: a Reappraisal of Adamantinoma of Long Bone. Cancer **10:**540–559, 1957.
15. Cody, H.S., III, Marcove, R.C., and Quan, S.H.: Malignant Retrorectal Tumors: 28 Years' Experience at Memorial Sloan-Kettering Cancer Center. Dis. Colon Rectum **24:**501–506, 1981.
16. Coley, B.L., and Higinbotham, N.L.: Diagnosis and Treatment of Metastatic Lesions in Bone. Instr. Course Lect. **7:**18–25, 1950.
17. Cortes, E.P., Holland, J.F., Wang, J.J., Sinks, L.F., Blom, J., Senn, H., Bank, A., and Glidewell, O.: Amputation and Adriamycin in Primary Osteosarcoma. N. Engl. J. Med. **291:**998–1000, 1974.
18. Dahlin, D.C.: Bone Tumors: General Aspects and Data on 6,221 Cases, 3rd ed. Springfield, Ill., Charles C Thomas, 1978.
19. Dahlin, D.C.: Osteosarcoma of Bone and a Consideration of Prognostic Variables. Cancer Treat. Rep. **62:**189–192, 1978.
20. Dahlin, D.C.: The Problems in Assessment of New Treatment Regimens of Osteosarcoma. Clin. Orthop. **153:**81–85, 1980.
21. Dahlin, D.C., and Beabout, J.W.: Dedifferentiation of Low-Grade Chondrosarcomas. Cancer **28:**461–466, 1971.
22. Dahlin, D.C., and Coventry, M.B.: Osteogenic Sarcoma: A Study of Six Hundred Cases. J. Bone Joint Surg. **49-A:**101–110, 1967.
23. Dahlin, D.C., and Ivins, J.C.: Fibrosarcoma of Bone: A Study of 114 Cases. Cancer **23:**35–41, 1969.
24. Dahlin, D.C., and MacCarty, C.S.: Chordoma: A Study of Fifty-Nine Cases. Cancer **5:**1170–1178, 1952.
25. Dahlin, D.C., and Unni, K.K.: Osteosarcoma of Bone and Its Important Recognizable Varieties. Am. J. Surg. Pathol. **1:**61–72, 1977.
26. Dahlin, D.C., Unni, K.K., and Matsuno, T.: Malignant (Fibrous) Histiocytoma of Bone: Fact or Fancy? Cancer **39:**1508–1516, 1977.
27. Devas, M.B., Dickson, J.W., and Jelliffe, A.M.: Pathological Fractures: Treatment by Internal Fixation and Irradiation. Lancet **2:**484–487, 1956.
28. Dickman, P.S., Liotta, L.A., and Triche, T.J.: Ewing's Sarcoma:

Characterization in Established Cultures and Evidence of Its Histogenesis. Lab. Invest. **47**:375–382, 1982.

29. Dorfman, H.D., Norman, A., and Wolff, H.: Fibrosarcoma Complicating Bone Infarction in a Caisson Worker: A Case Report. J. Bone Joint Surg. **48-A**:528–532, 1966.

30. Durie, B.G.M., and Salmon, S.E.: The Current Status and Future Prospects of Treatment of Multiple Myeloma. Clin. Haematol. **11**:181–210, 1982.

31. Eckardt, J.J., Eilber, F.R., Grant, T.T., Mirra, J.M., Weisenberger, T.H., and Dorey, F.J.: The UCLA Experience in the Management of Stage IIB Osteogenic Sarcoma. *In* Proceedings of the National Institutes of Health Consensus Development Conference on "Limb-Sparing Treatment: Adult Soft Tissue and Osteogenic Sarcomas," December 3–5, 1984, pp. 61–63.

32. Edmonson, J.H., Green, S.J., Ivins, J.C., Gilchrist, G.S., Creagan, E.T., Pritchard, D.J., Smithson, W.A., Dahlin, D.C., and Taylor, W.F.: A Controlled Pilot Study of High-Dose Methotrexate as Postsurgical Adjuvant Treatment for Primary Osteosarcoma. J. Clin. Oncol. **2**:152–156, 1984.

33. Enneking, W.F.: Musculoskeletal Tumor Surgery, Vol. 2. New York, Churchill Livingstone, 1983, pp. 1435–1540.

34. Eriksson, A.I., Schiller, A., and Mankin, H.J.: The Management of Chondrosarcoma of Bone. Clin. Orthop. **153**:44–66, 1980.

35. Evans, H.L., Ayala, A.G., and Romsdahl, M.M.: Prognostic Factors in Chondrosarcoma of Bone: A Clinicopathologic Analysis With Emphasis on Histologic Grading. Cancer **40**:818–831, 1977.

36. Eyre-Brook, A.L., and Price, C.H.G.: Fibrosarcoma of Bone: Report of Fifty Consecutive Cases From the Bristol Bone Tumour Registry. J. Bone Joint Surg. **51-B**:20–37, 1969.

37. Feldman, F., and Lattes, R.: Primary Malignant Fibrous Histiocytoma (Fibrous Xanthoma) of Bone. Skeletal Radiol. **1**:145–160, 1977.

38. Frassica, F.J., Unni, K.K., Beabout, J., and Sim, F.H.: Dedifferentiated Chondrosarcoma: A Report of the Clinicopathologic Features and Treatment in Seventy-Eight Cases. J. Bone Joint Surg. **68-A**:1197–1205, 1986.

39. Frei, E., Jaffe, N., Link, M., and Abelson, H.: Adjuvant Chemotherapy of Osteogenic Sarcoma: Progress, Problems and Prospects. In Jones, S.E., and Salmon, S.E. (eds.): Adjuvant Therapy of Cancer II. New York, Grune & Stratton, 1979, pp. 355–363.

40. Friedman, M.A., and Carter, S.K.: The Therapy of Osteogenic Sarcoma: Current Status and Thoughts for the Future. J. Surg. Oncol. **4**:482–510, 1972.

41. Gehan, E.A., Sutow, W.W., Uribe-Botero, G., Romsdahl, M., and Smith, T.L.: Osteosarcoma: The M.D. Anderson Experience, 1950–1974. Prog. Cancer Res. Ther. **6**:271–282, 1978.

42. Goodman, M.A.: Plasma Cell Tumors. Clin. Orthop. **204**:86–92, 1986.

43. Griffiths, D.L.: Orthopaedic Aspects of Myelomatosis. J. Bone Joint Surg. **48-B**:703–728, 1966.

44. Harrington, K.D., Sim, F.H., Enis, J.E., Johnston, J.O., Dick, H.M., and Gristina, A.G.: Methylmethacrylate as an Adjunct in Internal Fixation of Pathologic Fractures: Experience With Three Hundred and Seventy-Five Cases. J. Bone Joint Surg. **58-A**:1047–1055, 1976.

45. Harwood, A.R., Krajbich, J.I., and Fornasier, V.L.: Mesenchymal Chondrosarcoma: A Report of 17 Cases. Clin. Orthop. **158**:144–148, 1980.

46. Henderson, E.D., and Dahlin, D.C.: Chondrosarcoma of Bone: A Study of Two Hundred and Eighty-Eight Cases. J. Bone Joint Surg. **45-A**:1450–1458, 1963.

47. Hernandez, F.J., and Fernandez, B.B.: Multiple Diffuse Fibrosarcoma of Bone. Cancer **37**:939–945, 1976.

48. Huvos, A.G.: Bone Tumors: Diagnosis, Treatment and Prognosis. Philadelphia, W.B. Saunders, 1979, p. 373.

49. Huvos, A.G., Heilweil, M., and Bretsky, S.S.: The Pathology of Malignant Fibrous Histiocytoma of Bone: A Study of 130 Patients. Am. J. Surg. Pathol. **9**:853–871, 1985.

50. Huvos, A.G., and Marcove, R.C.: Adamantinoma of Long Bones: A Clinicopathological Study of Fourteen Cases With Vascular Origin Suggested. J. Bone Joint Surg. **57-A**:148–154, 1975.

51. Jaffe, N., Frei, E., III, Traggis, D., and Bishop, Y.: Adjuvant Methotrexate and Citrovorum-Factor Treatment of Osteogenic Sarcoma. N. Engl. J. Med. **291**:994–997, 1974.

52. Jaffe, N., Frei, E., III, Watts, H., and Traggis, D.: High-Dose Methotrexate in Osteogenic Sarcoma: A 5-Year Experience. Cancer Treat. Rep. **62**:259–264, 1978.

53. Jaffe, R., Santamaria, M., Yunis, E.J., Tannery, N.H., Agostini, R.M., Jr., Medina, J., and Goodman, M.: The Neuroectodermal Tumor of Bone. Am. J. Surg. Pathol. **8**:885–898, 1984.

54. Johnson, E.W., Jr.: Intramedullary Fixation of Pathological Fractures. J.A.M.A. **163**:417–419, 1957.

55. Johnson, R.E., and Pomeroy, T.C.: Evaluation of Therapeutic Results in Ewing's Sarcoma. Am. J. Roentgenol. **123**:583–587, 1975.

56. Kapadia, S.B.: Multiple Myeloma: A Clinicopathologic Study of 62 Consecutively Autopsied Cases. Medicine **59**:380–392, 1980.

57. Kavanaugh, J.H.: Multiple Myeloma, Amyloid Arthropathy, and Pathological Fracture of the Femur: A Case Report. J. Bone Joint Surg. **60-A**:135–137, 1978.

58. Knapp, R.H., Wick, M.R., Scheithauer, B.W., and Unni, K.K.: Adamantinoma of Bone: An Electron Microscopic and Immunohistochemical Study. Virchows Arch. **398-A**:75–86, 1982.

59. Kotz, R., and Salzer, M.: Rotation-Plasty for Childhood Osteosarcoma of the Distal Part of the Femur. J. Bone Joint Surg. **64-A**:959–969, 1982.

60. Kyle, R.A.: Multiple Myeloma: Review of 869 Cases. Mayo Clin. Proc. **50**:29–40, 1975.

61. Laha, R.K., and Rao, S.: Replacement of Vertebral Body With Acrylic in Plasma Cell Myeloma. Int. Surg. **64**:59–61, 1979.

62. Le Charpentier, Y., Forest, M., Postel, M., Tomeno, B., and Abelanet, R.: Clear-Cell Chondrosarcoma: A Report of Five Cases Including Ultrastructural Study. Cancer **44**:622–629, 1979.

63. Lettin, A.W.F.: Fibular Replacement of the Upper Humerus After Segmental Resection for Chondrosarcoma. Proc. R. Soc. Med. **57**:90–92, 1964.

64. Li, W.K., Lane, J.M., Rosen, G., Marcove, R.C., Caparros, B., Huvos, A., and Groshen, S.: Pelvic Ewing's Sarcoma: Advances in Treatment. J. Bone Joint Surg. **65-A**:738–747, 1983.

65. Localio, S.A., Eng, K., and Ranson, J.H.C.: Abdominosacral Approach for Retrorectal Tumors. Ann. Surg. **191**:555–559, 1980.

66. MacAusland, W.R., Jr., and Wyman, E.T., Jr.: Management of Metastatic Pathological Fractures. Clin. Orthop. **73**:39–51, 1970.

67. MacCarty, C.S., Waugh, J.M., Mayo, C.W., and Coventry, M.B.: The Surgical Treatment of Presacral Tumors: A Combined Problem. Proc. Staff Meet. Mayo Clin. **27**:73–84, 1952.

68. Macintosh, D.J., Price, C.H.G., and Jeffree, G.M.: Ewing's Tumour: A Study of Behaviour and Treatment in Forty-Seven Cases. J. Bone Joint Surg. **57-B**:331–340, 1975.

69. Makley, J.T., Ertel, I., Baum, E., Weetman, R., Yunis, E., Bleyer, A., Fryer, C., Krailo, M., Leikih, S., and Hammond, D.: CCSG 741, Osteogenic Sarcoma Study (Submitted for Publication).

70. Malawer, M.N.: Surgical Technique and Results of Limb Sparing Surgery for High Grade Bone Sarcomas of the Knee and Shoulder. Orthopedics **8**:597–607, 1985.

71. Mankin, H.J., Doppelt, S.H., Sullivan, T.R., and Tomford, W.W.: Osteoarticular and Intercalary Allograft Transplantation in the Management of Malignant Tumors of Bone. Cancer **50**:613–630, 1982.

72. Martin, N.H.: The Incidence of Myelomatosis. Lancet **1**:237–239, 1961.

73. Matsuno, T., Unni, K.K., McLeod, R.A., and Dahlin, D.C.: Telangiectatic Osteogenic Sarcoma. Cancer **38**:2538–2547, 1976.

74. McCarthy, E.F., and Dorfman, H.D.: Chondrosarcoma of Bone With Dedifferentiation: A Study of Eighteen Cases. Hum. Pathol. **13**:36–40, 1982.

75. McIntyre, O.R.: Current Concepts in Cancer: Multiple Myeloma. N. Engl. J. Med. **301**:193–196, 1979.

76. Meyer, J.E., and Schulz, M.D.: "Solitary" Myeloma of Bone: A Review of 12 Cases. Cancer **34**:438–440, 1974.

77. Miké, V., and Marcove, R.C.: Osteogenic Sarcoma Under the Age of 21: Experience at Memorial Sloan-Kettering Cancer Center. Prog. Cancer Res. Ther. **6**:283–292, 1978.

78. Mirra, J.M., and Marcove, R.C.: Fibrosarcomatous Dedifferentiation of Primary and Secondary Chondrosarcoma: Review of Five Cases. J. Bone Joint Surg. **56-A**:285–296, 1974.

79. Moon, N.F., and Mori, H.: Adamantinoma of the Appendicular Skeleton—Updated. Clin. Orthop. **204**:215–237, 1986.

80. Mori, H., Yamamoto, S., Hiramatsu, K., Miura, T., and Moon, N.F.: Adamantinoma of the Tibia: Ultrastructural and Immunohistochemic Study With Reference to Histogenesis. Clin. Orthop. **190**:299–310, 1984.

81. Packard, A.G., Jr.: Prosthetic Replacement of the Proximal Half of the Humerus. Clin. Orthop. **93**:250–252, 1973.

82. Parker, F., Jr., and Jackson, H., Jr.: Primary Reticulum Cell Sarcoma of Bone. Surg. Gynecol. Obstet. **68**:45–53, 1939.

83. Pear, B.L.: Skeletal Manifestations of the Lymphomas and Leukemias. Semin. Roentgenol. **9**:229–240, 1974.

84. Pieterse, A.S., Smith, P.S., and McClure, J.: Adamantinoma of Long Bones: Clinical, Pathological and Ultrastructural Features. J. Clin. Pathol. **35**:780–786, 1982.

85. Pritchard, D.J.: Small Cell Tumors of Bone. Instr. Course Lect. **33**:26–39, 1984.

86. Pritchard, D.J., Dahlin, D.C., Dauphine, R.T., Taylor, W.F., and Beabout, J.W.: Ewing's Sarcoma: A Clinicopathological and Statistical Analysis of Patients Surviving Five Years or Longer. J. Bone Joint Surg. **57-A**:10–16, 1975.

87. Pritchard, D.J., Lunke, R.J., Taylor, W.F., Dahlin, D.C., and Medley, B.E.: Chondrosarcoma: A Clinicopathologic and Statistical Analysis. Cancer **45**:149–157, 1980.

88. Razek, A., Perez, C.A., Tefft, M., Nesbit, M., Vietti, T., Burgert, E.O., Jr., Kissane, J., Pritchard, D.J., and Gehan, E.A.: Intergroup Ewing's Sarcoma Study: Local Control Related to Radiation Dose, Volume, and Site of Primary Lesion in Ewing's Sarcoma. Cancer **46**:516–521, 1980.

89. Reimer, R.R., Chabner, B.A., Young, R.C., Reddick, R., and Johnson, R.E.: Lymphoma Presenting in Bone: Results of Histopathology, Staging, and Therapy. Ann. Intern. Med. **87**:50–55, 1977.

90. Rock, M.G., Beabout, J.W., Unni, K.K., and Sim, F.H.: Adamantinoma. Orthopedics **6**:472–477, 1983.

91. Rogers, L.: Plasmocytomas Producing Paraplegia. Br. J. Surg. **41**:54–56, 1953.

92. Rosai, J.: Adamantinoma of the Tibia: Electron Microscopic Evidence of Its Epithelial Origin. Am. J. Clin. Pathol. **51**:786–792, 1969.

93. Rosai, J., and Pinkus, G.S.: Immunohistochemical Demonstration of Epithelial Differentiation in Adamantinoma of the Tibia. Am. J. Surg. Pathol. **6**:427–434, 1982.

94. Rosen, G.: Preoperative (Neoadjuvant) Chemotherapy for Osteogenic Sarcoma: A Ten Year Experience. Orthopedics **8**:659–664, 1985.

95. Rosen, G., Caparros, B., Huvos, A.G., Kosloff, C., Nirenberg, A., Cacavio, A., Marcove, R.C., Lane, J.M., Mehta, B., and Urban, C.: Preoperative Chemotherapy for Osteogenic Sarcoma: Selection of Postoperative Adjuvant Chemotherapy Based on the Response of the Primary Tumor to Preoperative Chemotherapy. Cancer **49**:1221–1230, 1982.

96. Rosen, G., Caparros, B., Mosende, C., McCormick, B., Huvos, A.G., and Marcove, R.C.: Curability of Ewing's Sarcoma and Considerations for Future Therapeutic Trials. Cancer **41**:888–899, 1978.

97. Rosen, G., Caparros, B., Nirenberg, A., Marcove, R.C., Huvos, A.G., Kosloff, C., Lane, J., and Murphy, M.L.: Ewing's Sarcoma: Ten-Year Experience With Adjuvant Chemotherapy. Cancer **47**:2204–2213, 1981.

98. Rosenberg, S.A., Chabner, B.A., Young, R.C., Seipp, C.A., Levine, A.S., Costa, J., Hanson, T.A., Head, G.C., and Simon, R.M.: Treatment of Osteogenic Sarcoma. I. Effect of Adjuvant High-Dose Methotrexate After Amputation. Cancer Treat. Rep. **63**:739–751, 1979.

99. Sage, H., Balian, G., Vogel, A.M., and Bornstein, P.: Type VIII Collagen: Synthesis by Normal and Malignant Cells in Culture. Lab. Invest. **50**:219–231, 1984.

100. Salzer, M., Knahr, K., Locke, H., Stärk, N., Matejovsky, Z., Plenk, H., Jr., Punzet, G., and Zweymüller, K.: A Bioceramic Endoprosthesis for the Replacement of the Proximal Humerus. Arch. Orthop. Trauma Surg. **93**:169–184, 1979.

101. Shoji, H., and Miller, T.R.: Primary Reticulum Cell Sarcoma of Bone: Significance of Clinical Features Upon the Prognosis. Cancer **28**:1234–1244, 1971.

102. Sim, F.H., and Chao, E.Y.S.: Hip Salvage by Proximal Femoral Replacement. J. Bone Joint Surg. **63-A**:1228–1239, 1981.

103. Sim, F.H., Chao, E.Y.S., Pritchard, D.J., and Salzer, M.: Replacement of the Proximal Humerus With a Ceramic Prosthesis: A Preliminary Report. Clin. Orthop. **146**:161–174, 1980.

104. Sim, F.H., Daugherty, T.W., and Ivins, J.C.: The Adjunctive Use of Methylmethacrylate in Fixation of Pathological Fractures. J. Bone Joint Surg. **56-A**:40–48, 1974.

105. Sim, F.H., Ivins, J.C., Taylor, W.F., and Chao, E.Y.S.: Limb-Sparing Surgery for Osteosarcoma: Mayo Clinic Experience. Cancer Treat. Symp. **3**:139–154, 1985.

106. Sim, F.H., Wold, L.E., Beabout, J.W., Amadio, P.C., and McDonald, D.J.: Osteosarcoma: State of the Art. Minn. Med. **69**:442–448, 1986.

107. Stener, B., and Gunterberg, B.: High Amputation of the Sacrum for Extirpation of Tumors: Principles and Technique. Spine **3**:351–366, 1978.

108. Suit, H.D., Goitein, M., Munzenrider, J., Verhey, L., Davis, K.R., Koehler, A., Linggood, R., and Ojemann, R.G.: Definitive Radiation Therapy for Chordoma and Chondrosarcoma of Base of Skull and Cervical Spine. J. Neurosurg. **56**:377–385, 1982.

109. Sundaresan, N., Galicich, J.H., Bains, M.S., Martini, N., and Beattie, E.J.: Vertebral Body Resection in the Treatment of Cancer Involving the Spine. Cancer **53**:1393–1396, 1984.

110. Sundaresan, N., Galicich, J.H., Chu, F.C.H., and Huvos, A.G.: Spinal Chordomas. J. Neurosurg. **50**:312–319, 1979.

111. Sweet, D.L., and Golomb, H.M.: The Treatment of Histiocytic Lymphoma. Semin. Oncol. **7**:302–309, 1980.

112. Sweet, D.L., Golomb, H.M., Kinzie, J., Ferguson, D., Gaeke, M.E., and Ultmann, J.E.: Survival in Localized Diffuse Histiocytic Lymphoma (DHL) (Abstract). Proc. Am. Assoc. Cancer Res. Am. Soc. Clin Oncol. **21**:465, 1980.

113. Sweet, D.L., Mass, D.P., Simon, M.A., and Shapiro, C.M.: Histiocytic Lymphoma (Reticulum-Cell Sarcoma) of Bone: Current Strategy for Orthopaedic Surgeons. J. Bone Joint Surg. **63-A**:79–84, 1981.

114. Taylor, W.F., Ivins, J.C., Dahlin, D.C., Edmonson, J.H., and Pritchard, D.J.: Trends and Variability in Survival From Osteosarcoma. Mayo Clin. Proc. **53**:695–700, 1978.

115. Taylor, W.F., Ivins, J.C., Dahlin, D.C., and Pritchard, D.J.: Os-

teogenic Sarcoma Experience at the Mayo Clinic, 1963–1974. Prog. Cancer Res. Ther. **6:**257–268, 1978.

116. Telander, R.L., Pairolero, P.C., Pritchard, D.J., Sim, F.H., and Gilchrist, G.S.: Resection of Pulmonary Metastatic Osteogenic Sarcoma in Children. Surgery **84:**335–340, 1978.

117. Telles, N.C., Rabson, A.S., and Pomeroy, T.C.: Ewing's Sarcoma: An Autopsy Study. Cancer **41:**2321–2329, 1978.

118. Unni, K.K., Dahlin, D.C., McLeod, R.A., and Pritchard, D.J.: Intraosseous Well-Differentiated Osteosarcoma. Cancer **40:**1337–1347, 1977.

119. Urban, C., Rosen, G., Huvos, A.G., Caparros, B., Cacavio, A., and Nirenberg, A.: Chemotherapy of Malignant Fibrous Histiocytoma of Bone: A Report of Five Cases. Cancer **51:**795–802, 1983.

120. Valderrama, J.A.F., and Bullough, P.G.: Solitary Myeloma of the Spine. J. Bone Joint Surg. **50-B:**82–90, 1968.

121. Weatherby, R.P., Dahlin, D.C., and Ivins, J.C.: Postradiation Sarcoma of Bone: Review of 78 Mayo Clinic Cases. Mayo Clin. Proc. **56:**294–306, 1981.

122. Weiner, M., Sedlis, M., Johnston, A.D., Dick, H.M., and Wolff, J.A.: Adjuvant Chemotherapy of Malignant Fibrous Histiocytoma of Bone. Cancer **51:**25–29, 1983.

123. Wick, M.R., Siegal, G.P., Unni, K.K., McLeod, R.A., and Greditzer, H.G.: Sarcomas of Bone Complicating Osteitis Deformans (Paget's Disease): Fifty Years' Experience. Am. J. Surg. Pathol. **5:**47–59, 1981.

124. Wold, L.E., and Laws, E.R., Jr.: Cranial Chordomas in Children and Young Adults. J. Neurosurg. **59:**1043–1047, 1983.

125. Zucker, J.M., and Henry-Amar, M.: Therapeutic Controlled Trial in Ewing's Sarcoma: Report on the Results of a Trial by the Clinical Cooperative Group on Radio- and Chemotherapy of the E.O.R.T.C. Eur. J. Cancer **13:**1019–1023, 1977.

CHAPTER 74

Metastatic Diseases of Bone

KEVIN D. HARRINGTON

Cancer is the second leading cause of death in the United States, accounting for 21% of deaths in 1981 and 24% in 1984. In 1985, there were 482,000 deaths and 910,000 new cancer cases reported.[31] A statistical analysis of these trends reveals that a child born in the United States in 1985 has a more than 1 in 3 chance of eventually developing invasive cancer (excluding epidermal skin cancer and carcinoma *in situ*). Breast cancer alone strikes between 1 in 10 and 1 in 14 women worldwide. Incidence and mortality parallel each other and have changed little in the past half century. Although these statistics seem discouraging at first glance, they must be balanced against the fact that more aggressive palliative treatment of patients with established metastases, using sophisticated combinations of hormonal manipulation, chemotherapy, and radiotherapy have been successful in markedly prolonging these patients' lives and improving their general wellbeing. Almost half of newly diagnosed cancer patients are alive 5 years later. Of women with breast carcinoma diagnosed between 1977 and 1979, 81% were alive 5 years later and 34% of these were alive with metastases. These percentages had increased from 63% and 18% respectively in 1960.[31] Well over half a million women in the U.S. will be living with metastatic breast carcinoma during the next 5 years. The number of patients alive with metastases from other cancers will be in excess of 2 million.

Unfortunately, coincident with such improved overall cancer palliation comes an increasing incidence of clinically apparent bony metastases, with an attendant increase in pathologic long-bone fractures. Simply stated, as patients survive for progressively longer periods after developing cancer metastases, the incidence of metastatic involvement of bone increases accordingly. Metastatic carcinoma is the most common malignancy of bone, affecting more than 40 times as many patients as are affected by all other types of bone cancer combined.[4,25] It has been estimated that more than 60% of women with disseminated breast cancer have radiographic evidence of bone metastases and that the incidence is much higher when measured by bone scanning techniques.[15,21] Statistics on the prevalence of pathologic fractures among these patients are difficult to find. Higinbotham reported that of 1800 patients treated for skeletal metastases between 1931 and 1964, 9.5% developed pathologic fractures.[25]

Between 1960 and 1970, the published mean survival for patients following their first long-bone pathologic fracture was 7.8 months.[6,7] This figure has since risen to 18.8 months. When analyzed by primary origin, those patients suffering pathologic fractures from metastatic carcinoma of the breast had a mean survival of 22.6 months, and those with primaries in the prostate and kidney had mean survivals of 29.3 and 11.8 months respectively. In contrast, patients with lung primaries still have a mean survival of only 3.6 months.[21]

Approximately 75% of pathologic fractures requiring operative fixation or reconstruction occur in the proximal femur or acetabulum. From a technical viewpoint, these may be subdivided into fractures of the acetabulum, fractures of the femoral neck, intertrochanteric fractures, and subtrochanteric fractures. The remaining fractures requiring stabilization are equally divided between the spine and the upper extremities. In addition, consideration must be given to prophylactic fixation of destructive lesions in the pelvis or long bones where the risk of fracture is high.

FRACTURES OF THE ACETABULUM

Displaced pathologic acetabular fractures reflect the culmination of two simultaneous destructive processes leading to joint instability. The first of these is the phenomenon of gradual softening of the periacetabular bone, both from the tumor process and also often from superimposed irradiation osteolysis, both conditions resulting in progressive deformity of the acetabular walls. The second process is the ablation of the subchondral blood supply by the gradually expanding tumor focus, which eventually results in a frank disruption of the joint surfaces (Fig. 74-1). The loss of periacetabular bone resulting from both processes seriously interferes with attempts at joint stabilization or reconstruction. When the femoral head has become displaced significantly, conventional total hip replacement is likely to fail because there is insufficient structurally adequate bone around the acetabular component to prevent its loosening and migration. Simply removing gross tumor tissue and filling the resultant cavity with excess cement will not prevent medial and superior migration of the acetabular compo-

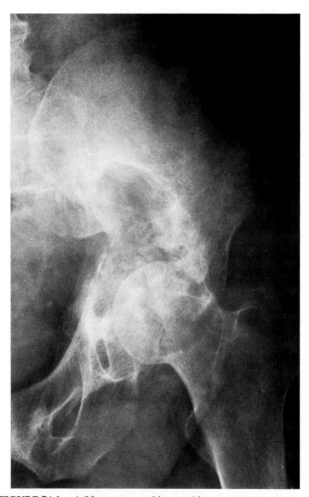

FIGURE 74-1. A fifty-one-year-old man with metastatic carcinoma of the adrenal cortex and Class III involvement. Extensive lytic destruction of the supra-acetabular bone is apparent, with migration of the femoral head proximally. The patient, although evidencing no other metastatic foci, had been confined to a wheelchair a year earlier after being advised that the hip joint was not reconstructable.

nent (Fig. 74-2). The cement is much harder than the surrounding tumor-infiltrated bone, and the prosthetic component with its attached acrylic will become loosened as soon as weight-bearing is attempted. Meshes of various materials do not enhance acetabular component stability or limit this tendency towards migration. Attempts to attach the acetabular component to the lateral pelvic wall in the absence of an intact roof are equally ineffective and will result in rapid component loosening and migration.

Bearing in mind these considerations, acetabular pathologic fractures or impending fractures are subdivided into four groups,[18,20] based on the location of the fracture within the periacetabular bone, the extent of tumor or radiation osteolysis, and the specialized technical requirements needed to accomplish a secure arthroplasty:

Class I: Lateral cortices, superior and medial walls structurally intact
Class II: Medial wall deficient
Class III: Lateral cortices, superior wall and medial wall all deficient
Class IV: Resection for cure

Class I The patients in this group, although often showing extensive invasion of bone by metastases (Fig. 74-3A) have sufficient unaffected periacetabular bone to predict that conventional fixation of the prosthetic acetabular component will result in an incidence of loosening or migration not exceeding that seen in routine total hip arthroplasty. For these patients conventional total hip arthroplasty is performed by a posterolateral approach. Avoid osteotomy of the greater trochanter because of the high risk of trochanteric nonunion after postoperative irradiation. Chromium-cobalt mesh is placed along the medial part of the acetabular wall, primarily to minimize the escape of cement into the pelvis through bony defects created by tumor lysis (Fig. 74-3B). No other specialized techniques are considered necessary to secure the acetabular component in these hips.[18,20,21]

Class II The patients in this group have in common a loss of structural continuity of the medial wall of the acetabulum (Fig. 74-4A). However, the superior part of the wall (roof) of the acetabulum and the lateral cortices of the ilium, ischium, and pubis adjacent to the acetabulum (acetabular rim) remain intact. The aim of reconstruction is to transmit the stresses of weight-bearing away from the deficient medial wall and out onto the intact acetabular rim. The Oh-Harris protrusio shell is the most effective and versatile example of the many similar devices now available (Fig. 74-4B and C). In small women, it is often necessary to use the smallest available protrusio shell and then the small 42 mm acetabular component that will fit within it. We have encountered no evidence of loosening, instability, polyethylene wear, or any other problems attributable to the use of such a small component.

The rim of the protrusio shell must rest firmly on the superior and the anteroinferior margins of the bony acetabulum in order to be stable. If bone along the rim is deficient in these areas, it may still be possible to obtain secure seating of the protrusio shell by rotating it slightly. If there is extensive bone loss, however, particularly along the inferior rim, use of the

FIGURE 74-2. A conventional hip replacement arthroplasty was attempted on this 62-year-old-man with metastatic carcinoma of the prostate. The acetabular rim was intact, but the medial wall had been destroyed by tumor (Class II). The acetabular component loosened rapidly and migrated medially. This case demonstrates that simply using an abundance of methylmethacrylate to secure the acetabular component does little to enhance its stability under such circumstances.

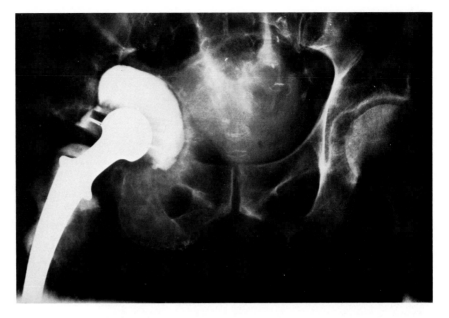

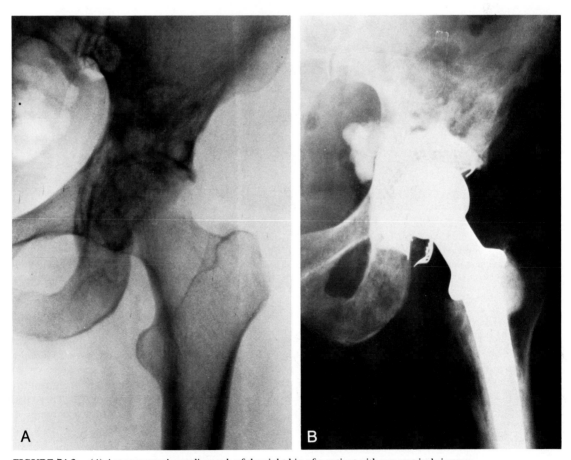

FIGURE 74-3. (*A*) Anteroposterior radiograph of the right hip of a patient with progressively increasing pain with weight-bearing but minimal changes apparent on convention plain radiographs. The medial wall and the acetabular rim are intact, but an area of the acetabular roof has been destroyed. This is a Class I fracture. (*B*) The hip has been reconstructed as a conventional hip replacement arthroplasty, acetabular mesh having been used to minimize escape of methylmethacrylate into the pelvis.

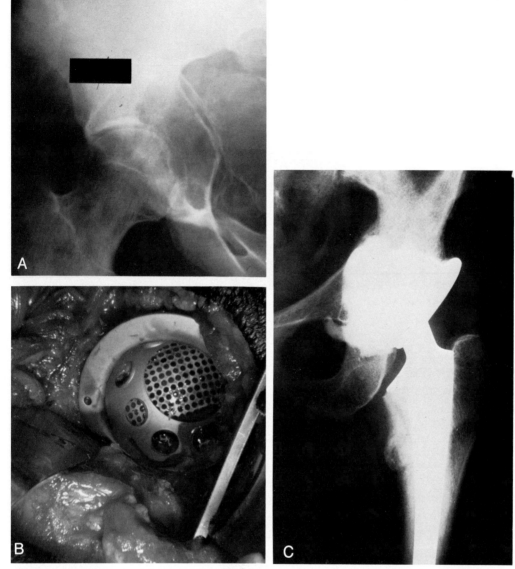

FIGURE 74-4. (*A*) Class II fracture of the medial wall, with a large aneurysmal metastasis having destroyed the medial wall of the acetabulum. (*B*) Intraoperative photograph of a Class II reconstruction, showing proper lining of the acetabular cavity by mesh and subsequent positioning of the protrusio shell. (*C*) Thirteen months after reconstruction of the hip and postoperative irradiation. The protrusio: acetabuli ring effectively transfers weight-bearing stresses onto the intact acetabular rim.

protrusio shell alone is not sufficient and more extensive measures must be used in order to transmit weight-bearing loads into an area of intact bone (Fig. 74-5). It is important to remember that if the rim extensions of the protrusio shell are properly in contact with the acetabular rim, the shell will be aligned quite obliquely in approximately 65° of valgus. The prosthetic acetabular component must be aligned independently within the shell at approximately 45° of abduction and 25° of anteversion.

The femoral intramedullary canal should be prepared for a conventional hip replacement prosthesis, unless there is evidence either radiographically or scintigraphically of significant tumor lysis within the femoral cortices. In such an instance, a long-stemmed femoral prosthesis should be used.

Class III This is the largest and most challenging group of candidates for reconstruction. These patients have in common a loss of structural continuity not only of the medial acetabular wall but also of the acetabular roof and rim (Figs. 74-6 and 74-7). Attempts at acetabular reconstruction by bridging the large tumor defect with rods or pins placed horizontally have failed because of the deficiency of strong bone laterally, inferiorly, or medially to the acetabulum. If however, the weight-bearing loads can be transmitted along a line 15° medial to the

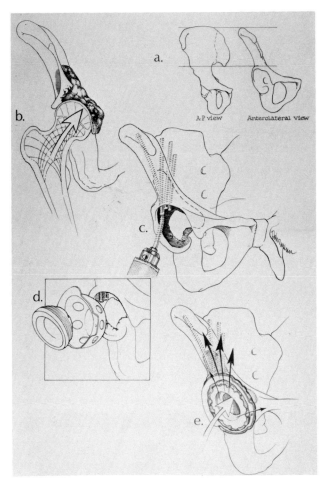

FIGURE 74-5. A schematic concept for reconstruction of Class III acetabular deficiency. (*A*) Anterolateral view of the pelvis demonstrates the thinness of the ilium superior to the acetabulum. Attempting to anchor the acetabular prosthetic component superior to its normal position would provide very poor fixation because of the thinness of the ilium there. (*B*) The tumor has destroyed the superior and medial areas of acetabular bone, leaving minimal intact cortex for fixation of the acetabular component. (*C*) After resection of tumor tissue, a large cavity is apparent, as is the destruction of the acetabular roof, medial part of the wall, and most of the rim. Steinmann pins can be drilled into structurally sound bone of the superior part of the ilium and across the sacroiliac joint. (*D*) The acetabular component as it is positioned in the protrusio acetabuli shell. (*E*) The combination of the acetabular cup, protrusio shell, and Steinmann pins all incorporated into methylmethacrylate effectively transmits weight-bearing stresses into strong bone of the iliac wing and sacrum.

true vertical, the line of normal weight-bearing stress across the pelvis, the likelihood of fixation failure will be reduced markedly.

The most effective means of such weight transmission is to drill several large threaded Steinmann pins from the bone above the acetabular roof through the medial-superior ilium and across the sacroiliac joint. In addition, drill two or three large pins down into the acetabulum from the anterior superior iliac crest through a separate small incision (Fig. 74-6*C*). Ideally, these latter pins are drilled across the open acetabular

defect and into the ischial bone below (Fig. 74-6*B* and *C*). This allows rigid pin fixation in bone both above and below the tumor defect and minimizes the risks of pin loosening. During the drilling of all these pins, move the index finger in and out of the pelvis through the greater sciatic notch to guard against inadvertent penetration of the cortex and potential injury to soft-tissue structures including the sciatic nerve (Fig. 74-6*D*). Once the pins are positioned properly, use a heavy bolt cutter to cut them off within the acetabular defect just deep enough to allow secure seating of the protrusio ring. Ideally, the rim flanges on the ring will seat firmly against the remaining intact bone of the acetabular rim, and the deepest portion of the ring will rest against the pins crossing the acetabular defect from the anterosuperior iliac spine (Figs. 74-5*D* and 74-6*F*).

After cleansing the acetabular bed, inject methylmethacrylate from a gun into the exposed bony interstices and about the Steinmann pins while pressing a finger from within the pelvis against the medial wall defect to minimize cement extrusion intrapelvically. Two or three packages of methylmethacrylate are usually required. Press the protrusio ring and the acetabular component firmly into position, taking care again to position the acetabular component at a less oblique angle than the protrusio ring.[18,20]

Some bony metastatic lesions in the pelvis, particularly those from myeloma and metastatic carcinomas of the colon, pancreas, and kidney, tend to be highly vascular. Blood loss at the time of attempted hip replacement may be prohibitive. When a sharp sclerotic rim is apparent on radiograph (see Figs. 74-1*C* and 74-6*A*), the likelihood of excessive intraoperative blood loss is minimal. However, when extensive reticulated osteolysis exists and extends irregularly and vaguely into the iliac ring, one should consider arteriographic evaluation and possible embolization of the tumor bed to minimize operative blood loss. When the arteriogram demonstrates excessive vascularity of the tumor bed (Fig. 74-7*A*), one should selectively catheterize the major arterial trunk from which the tumor vessels arise and occlude that vessel by embolization (Fig. 74-7*B*). Small strips of Gelfoam (2 × 2 mm) are morselized in sterile saline into a syrup of a consistency that can just be forced through the catheter by injection. Although much of the devascularized tumor tissue presumably becomes necrotic, we have seen no evidence of late ill effects, even when the subsequent tumor resection and joint reconstruction were delayed for more than 1 week after embolization.

Class IV On rare occasions, solitary metastases may be resected locally *en bloc* with a reasonable anticipation of cure (Fig. 74-8*A*). For example, patients with solitary metastases from a hypernephroma or from a thyroid carcinoma, who are more than 4 years postresection of the primary lesion, have a good prognosis for cure if the metastasis can be resected completely with good tumor margins. The most common locations for such resectable metastases are the proximal humerus and the supraacetabular portion of the pelvis. At the time of the resection, the adequacy of tumor margins should not be compromised in an effort to allow pelvic reconstruction. After such a resection the patient may be left with an internal partial hemipelvectomy, and limb stability may be surprisingly good, particularly after postoperative irradiation. When the solitary metastasis within

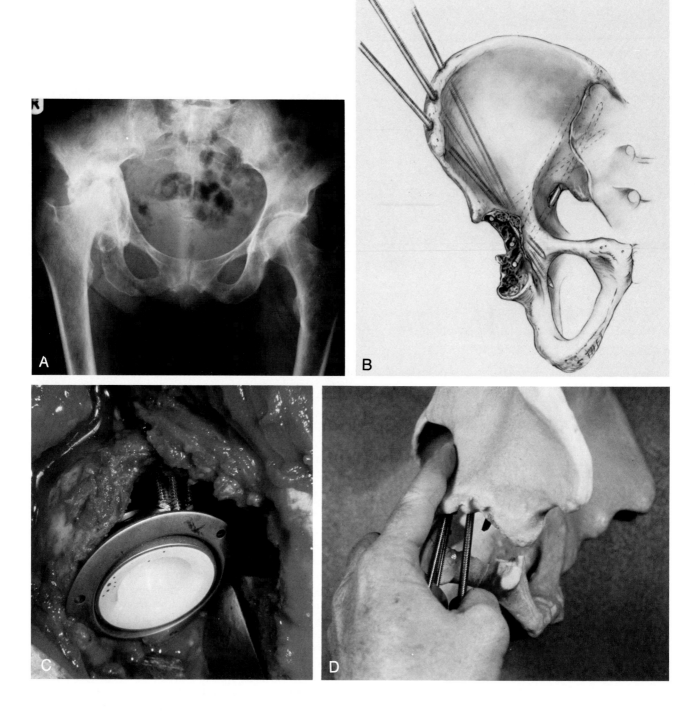

the resected pelvic segment has not weakened the bone so much that that bone can no longer support weight-bearing, it is possible to autoclave the segment and then use it to reconstruct the pelvic ring as a prelude to hip joint arthroplasty (Fig. 74-8B).

After a wide resection of the affected periacetabular bone is accomplished, and the margins of the specimen have been determined to be free of tumor tissue, autoclave the specimen at 135°C for 10 min. Once sterilized, remove extraneous soft tissues and remaining intraosseous tumor, leaving the bony

model to be fit back exactly into the pelvic defect. Affix the implant to the adjacent viable ischium, ilium, and pubis by a combination of threaded pins, cancellous bone screws, and bone plates (Fig. 74-8B). Complete reaming and drilling of the acetabulum and cement fixation of an acetabular component as with conventional total hip arthroplasty. Healing across the bone interspaces occurs rapidly and can be assessed radiographically (Fig. 74-8B). Because the nonviable segment of bone appears radiographically to be no different from the adjacent viable bone, however, creeping replacement of the au-

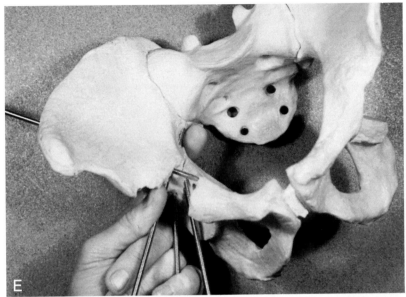
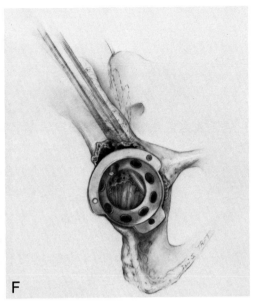

FIGURE 74-6. (A) A Class III acetabular fracture from lung cancer metastases. The medial wall, superior dome, and much of the acetabular rim have been destroyed, but the femoral bone appears unaffected After irradiation of the hip, the medial wall fracture appeared to heal and the patient enjoyed several months of improved mobility and diminished pain. Eventually, however, the patient again began to experience progressively increasing joint pain and gradually lost the ability to walk because of that pain. (B) Three large threaded Steinmann pins are drilled retrograde from the acetabular roof into the intact bone of the superior ilium and sacroiliac joint. These retrograde pins are cut off within the resected tumor bed. A 3-cm incision is then made over the anterosuperior iliac spine and three additional large Steinmann pins are drilled antegrade through the ilium and into the acetabular cavity. An attempt should be made to bury their tips into the bone of the ischium and pubis as shown. So positioned, these six Steinmann pins create an excellent latticework for support of the Oh-Harris protrusio shell. (C) With the pins properly positioned, the rim of the protrusio shell rests against and is partially supported by them. (D) By rotating the hand, the index finger can be inserted into the notch and the sciatic nerve palpated. (E) By further supination, it is possible to palpate the anterior surface of the sacrum and the sacroiliac joint to ensure that the Steinmann pin does not penetrate the cortex. (F) The protrusio shell is seated. Its rim flanges should rest on whatever bone remains of the acetabular rim. The depths of the cup should rest against the latticework of crossed Steinmann pins.

toclaved segment by bony ingrowth must be evaluated by serial bone scans.

LOWER EXTREMITY FRACTURES

Femoral Neck Fractures

Pathologic fractures of the femoral neck will almost never heal, even if undisplaced, and should be managed by prosthetic replacement (Fig. 74-9A and B). Whether a total hip arthroplasty, a femoral endoprosthesis, or a bipolar femoral prosthesis is used, a long-stemmed femoral component (140 to 200 mm) should be installed in most cases in order to prophylactically reinforce the remaining proximal femur, almost invariably also weakened by lytic metastases. It should be remembered that the extent of metastatic tumor lysis is almost always considerably in excess of that appreciable from conventional radiographs. Moreover, reactive hyperemia, typically occurring at the periphery of a progressive lytic lesion, contributes to weakening of the bone even outside the area of immediate destruction.

Some authors have advocated replacement of both sides of the hip joint if periacetabular metastases are detected by bone scan or by direct biopsy at the time of operation, even with minimal radiographic evidence of periacetabular metastatic disease.[14,32] We have not found such an aggressive approach necessary. The presence of metastases in the acetabular region does not ensure that they will become symptomatic, particularly if the area is irradiated postoperatively. Routine replacement of the acetabular side of the joint subjects the patient to additional operative time and risks, including acetabular loosening and hip dislocation.

Proximal femoral prosthetic replacement is performed with the patient in a lateral decubitus position, using a posterolateral Gibson operative approach. Avoid transection of the greater trochanter whenever possible to obviate the risk of subsequent trochanteric nonunion after irradiation. After the femoral canal has been rasped and curretted, fit the prosthesis into place and reduce the hip. Check the correct seating of the prosthesis within the shaft by direct vision for both limb length and joint stability. Bony defects between the prosthesis collar and remaining femoral bone can be reconstructed either by

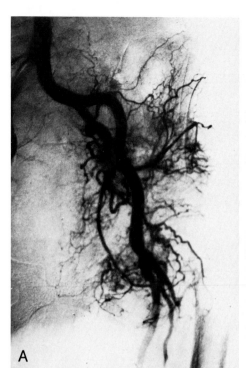
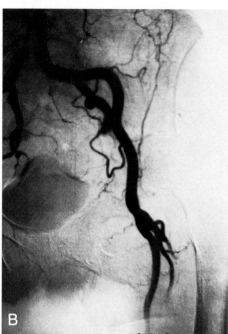

FIGURE 74-7. (*A*) Arteriogram demonstrates hypervascularization of the metastatic focus from multiple tumor vessels all originating from the hypogastric artery (*arrow*). (*B*) Arteriographic appearance after selective embolization of the hypogastric artery using Gelfoam. Joint reconstruction using pins and methylmethacrylate was accomplished thereafter with minimal blood loss.

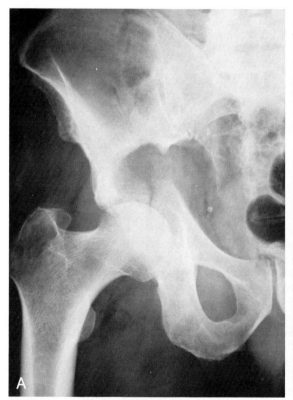
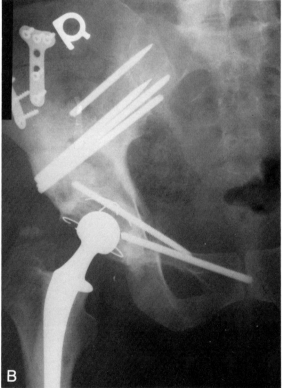

FIGURE 74-8. (*A*) Radiograph of the pelvis of a 58-year-old man with a solitary metastasis from a renal carcinoma. A nephrectomy had been performed 6 years earlier and careful screening failed to reveal any other evidence of metastatic disease. The patient, therefore, was a candidate for a Class IV resection and reconstruction. (*B*) A Class IV supra-acetabular lesion without a fracture through the involved segment. Five years after resection of the involved ilium, with wide margins, autoclaving of the segment, and reconstruction of the pelvis with a total hip arthroplasty.

using a custom femoral prosthesis (Fig. 74-9*C* and *D*) or by reconstitution of the bony deficit using methylmethacrylate molded *in situ*.

After establishing the proper length-tension relationships of the joint, remove the prosthesis. Mix methylmethacrylate for only 80 sec, and inject it by a cement gun as far as possible down the medullary canal in an effort to surround the prosthesis stem with cement as far distally as possible (Fig. 74-9*E*). One may drill a ¼-inch hole percutaneously through the distal femoral cortex and create a vacuum in the medullary canal by suction in order to encourage the cement to fill the canal completely. If this technique is used, however, the drill holes should be made well above the level where the prosthesis stem tip ultimately will rest in order to avoid creating a stress riser below the level of diaphyseal reinforcement. Finally, mold the cement about the flanged upper stem of the prosthesis by wrapping a malleable hard rubber dam around and above the proximal part of the femoral shaft in order to hold the acrylic in a form approximating the upper end of the femur. This dam also protects adjacent soft tissues during the exothermic phase of polymerization.

Peritrochanteric Fractures

Pathologic peritrochanteric fractures of the femur are difficult to manage operatively because there are usually extensive lytic changes extending proximally into the femoral neck, at the same time destruction of the cortical bone distal to the intertrochanteric line prevents proximal femoral replacement except by using a custom prosthesis. Many surgeons have advocated using just such a custom prosthesis, feeling that this allows the patient to regain the ability to walk more rapidly and that it also enhances nursing care in the more debilitated cancer patients who will never regain ambulatory status.[15,28] Although the use of a custom prosthesis does diminish the risk of fixation device failure, it also introduces new variables and risks not encountered if the femoral head and neck are salvaged. These include the necessity for stocking a wide variety of different sized prostheses, attempting to relocate the greater trochanter or its attached abductors to the neck of the prosthesis, and the risks of hip dislocation or instability inherent in any proximal femoral prosthesis. For these reasons, whenever possible we prefer to stabilize the fracture internally by the combination of a compression hip screw and intramedullary methylmethacrylate (Fig. 74-10).

The technique for such fixation is similar to that used for conventional hip fracture fixation. Obtain a closed manipulative reduction, anatomic if possible, using traction under image intensifier control on a fracture table. Using a conventional lateral approach, create a 1.5 cm window in the lateral femoral cortex just distal to the greater trochanter. Resect tumor tissue and structurally inadequate bone with a rongeur and currette, and remove any cancellous bone remaining within the distal femoral neck or trochanters (Fig. 74-11*A*). Insert a calibrated guide pin into the center of the femoral neck and confirm its position radiographically. Ream the femoral head and neck and the lateral cortex to accept the corkscrew portion of a compression hip screw as well as its sideplate. Twist the compression screw into place, positioning its tip as proximal as possible into the subchondral bone of the femoral head (Fig. 74-11*B*).

With a long, medium-angled currette complete hollowing out the femoral neck as far proximally as the first threads of the hip screw and as far distally in the femoral shaft as possible.

Fit a four-holed 130° sideplate over the hip screw, position it along the femoral shaft, and fix it there with a Lowman clamp to ensure that the fracture reduction is acceptable and that the fixation components can be articulated easily, even after the medullary canal has been filled with methylmethacrylate. Remove the sideplate and inject the liquid cement using a cement gun. Hand pressure exerted against the medial thigh by an assistant allows the adductor muscles to be pressed against the medial cortical defect to prevent any extrusion of cement. Then reposition the sideplate over the hip screw and affix it loosely to the shaft with a Lowman clamp. Release traction and impact the femoral shaft proximally sufficiently to ensure maximal bony contact between the major fragments. Remove excess cement, taking care to minimize interposition of methylmethacrylate between the bony cortices. When bone union of such a fracture occurs, it is through the apposition of periosteal new bone, and this process can be adversely affected by the presence of cement extracortically. After the intramedullary cement is solidly polymerized make drill holes for fixation of the sideplate, tap the holes, and insert the sideplate screws.

Postoperatively, patients are encouraged to begin full and unrestricted weight-bearing as soon as pain allows. There is no need to restrict stress across the fracture site, and the few failures that have occurred with this technique did not become apparent for many months or even years after operative fixation. They resulted then only because of metal fatigue finally developing across a fracture defect where ultimate bony union had been prevented by postoperative irradiation. On several occasions when bony union was delayed markedly by irradiation, the intramedullary cement alone has prevented deformity at the fracture site until healing finally occurred even though the metal fixation device itself had failed.

The use of condylocephalic nails for fixation of pathologic fractures in the intertrochanteric region has been advocated by some because fixation can be achieved without the necessity of opening the fracture site.[16] However, the technique has been effective only rarely for such basically unstable fractures. There has been a high incidence of loss of reduction, particularly with malrotation and also numerous complications related to distal migration of the Ender nail tips toward the knee. Even when the fracture site is exposed laterally and methylmethacrylate is injected, the stability achieved by the combination of flexible pins with cement is rarely adequate.

Subtrochanteric Fractures

Pathologic fractures in the subtrochanteric area of the femur are the most difficult to manage because both the surface area of cortical contact and the vascularity of the bone are poorer than in the proximal intertrochanteric area. At the same time, however, the proximal fragment remains relatively small and difficult to control by conventional fixation techniques. These fractures are not ideally suited for nail-plate fixation, even if the device is reinforced at the nail-plate junction and its use is augmented by intramedullary cement. Rather than being concentrated at the reinforced nail-plate junction, as in an intertrochanteric fracture, maximal stress here is focused on the

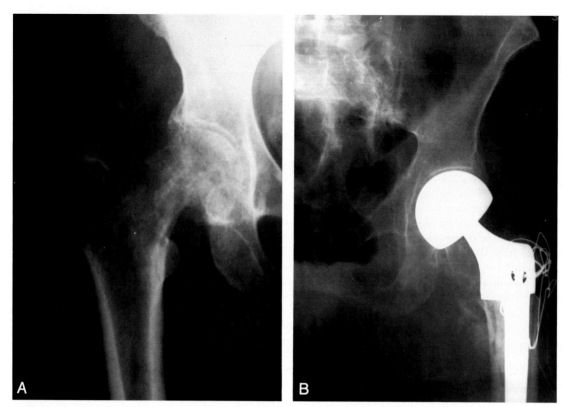

FIGURE 74-9. (A) Pathologic, minimally displaced fracture of the femoral neck in a patient with metastatic breast carcinoma. The chances of such a fracture healing after internal fixation are slight. Prosthetic replacement of the proximal femur is appropriate. (B) Subcapital pathologic fracture with tumor lysis extending into the intertrochanteric area has been managed by proximal femoral replacement using a bipolar prosthesis. The decision was made to use a prosthesis that replaced not only the femoral head and neck but the intertrochanteric bone as well. (C) Some surgeons have advocated prosthetic replacement of the proximal femur for all intertrochanteric or subcapital pathologic fractures, using the type of custom prosthesis shown here. (D) Operative view taken during prosthetic replacement of the left proximal femur. Tumor and structurally weak bone have been resected and a Moore prosthesis has been inserted. Note the lack of a cortical margin upon which the prosthesis might seat. (E) The prosthesis was removed, the medullary canal was plugged, and methylmethacrylate was injected. The prosthesis was replaced and cement was then molded about the upper stem to give axial and rotatory stability.

sideplate at its weakest point, the position of the first screw hole. If such a fracture does not progress ultimately to bony union, and many do not in the face of perioperative irradiation, metal fatigue and plate failure will inevitably occur despite the presence of acylic cement. From a biomechanical viewpoint, the most practical position for a subtrochanteric fixation device is within the medullary canal of the femur. There is eccentric loading of the femur at the subtrochanteric level with the magnitude of forces higher than at any other level. The medial cortex has been shown to have compressive forces in excess of 1200 lb/in^2 while the lateral cortex must resist tension stresses exceeding 900 lb/in^2. An intramedullary device affords some degree of balanced resistance midway between the cortices.

Conventional intramedullary Küntscher nail fixation has been used for pathologic subtrochanteric fractures but suffers from the major disadvantage of offering no reinforcement to the femoral neck. The ideal device for such fixation is the Zickel nail. We have never seen a failure of either the main

intramedullary Zickel nail or its triflanged cross nail extending into the femoral head and neck. In situations where there is extensive lysis of bone about the fracture site and extending into the proximal fragment (Fig. 74-12), however, we advocate reinforcement of fixation by intramedullary methylmethacrylate. This augmentation prevents rotation of the distal femoral fragment about the tapered and relatively short distal rod segment, reinforces fixation of the femoral head and neck fragment, and prevents shortening of the femur caused by collapse of weakened bone to either side of the fracture and subsequent progressive telescoping of the distal fragment proximally. Zickel et al.[36] and Michelson et al.[29] reported a significant incidence of femoral shortening and loss of rotational alignment when pathologic subtrochanteric fractures were initially fixed with a Zickel nail but without augmentation by acrylic cement. The technique of Zickel nailing is described in Chapter 29.

The Zickel nail can be a difficult device to use if care is not taken to avoid certain pitfalls during insertion. We prefer the

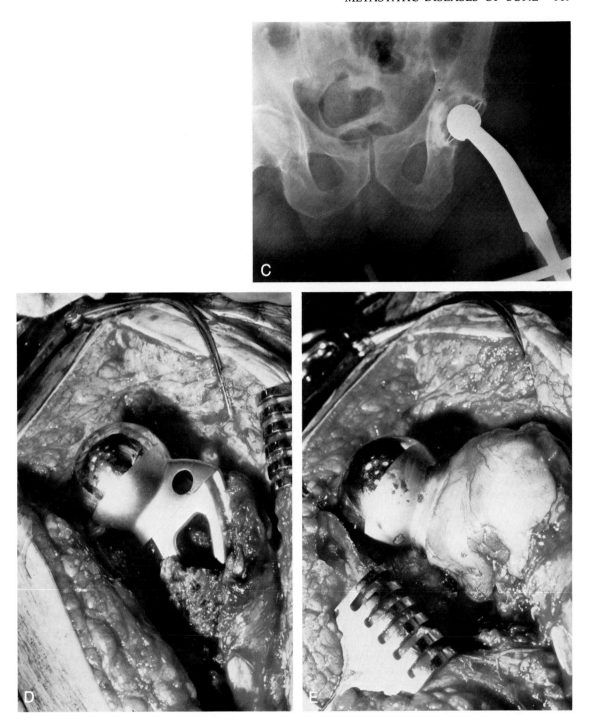

use of a standard operating table, placing the patient in a lateral decubitus position. This allows easy access to the greater trochanteric area, yet allows adequate radiographs of the proximal fragment by rotating the femur internally and externally.

Incise the skin along the posterior border of the greater trochanter, extending the incision approximately 6 cm proximal to its tip. It is important that the incision curve slightly behind the trochanter so that the trochanteric tip is accessible with the femur flexed. Expose the fracture site directly and create a 2 cm hole in the lateral femoral cortex through which tumor tissue and bony debris are removed with an angled curette. Split the gluteus muscle fibers sufficiently to expose the tip of the greater trochanter, and use a pointed awl to penetrate the bone there (Fig. 74-13A). Reduce the fracture and insert a blunt-tipped guide down the medullary canal. Ream the canal beginning with a 9 mm cannulated reamer. The proximal fragment must be reamed serially up to 17 mm, and the distal fragment to between 11 and 15 mm, depending on the size of the bone.

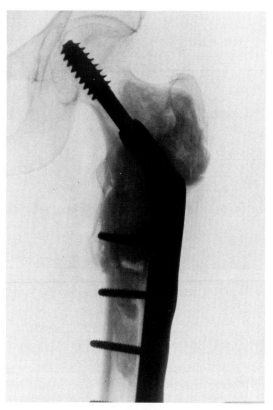

FIGURE 74-10. A pathologic intertrochanteric fracture has been internally stabilized by a compression hip screw reinforced by methylmethacrylate. The acrylic cement effectively reinforces the thinned cortices by extending from the level of the first screw thread proximally to the third side plate screw distally. This degree of filling of the intramedullary and tumor space is ideal.

It is important to recognize that the upper end of the rod is angulated slightly laterally in order to allow the cannulated nail to enter the femoral neck at an angle of 130°. Although the tip of the Zickel nail must be inserted into the sulcus just medial to the greater trochanter in order to be directed down the medullary canal, the upper end of the nail must eventually end within the tip of the greater trochanter in order to ensure that the tunnel locator guide will pass freely around the trochanter during impaction. Sangeorzen has developed a technique for accomplishing both aims during insertion of the nail.[30] Create a slotted groove from posterior medial to anterior lateral in the proximal femur (Fig. 74-13*B*). Such a groove allows the nail tip to be inserted initially through the trochanteric sulcus, yet allows the laterally angled and anteverted upper nail to pass through the trochanter laterally without comminuting the weakened bone. Once the nail has been inserted, assemble the tunnel locator guide, and pass a guide pin through its arm, through the intramedullary nail, and into the femoral neck to insure correct assembly (Fig. 74-13*C*). Mix methylmethacrylate and inject it in a liquid consistency through the lateral cortical window, well proximal and distal into the femoral canal. Take care to remove any cement that has escaped extracortically in an effort to minimize interference with periosteal bony union.

Fractures of the Femoral Shaft

Pathologic fractures of the femoral shaft are most appropriately treated by intramedullary nail fixation. Closed femoral nailing rarely is indicated because of the high likelihood of femoral fragments telescoping together as tumor-destroyed bone on either side of the fracture site collapses under the axial stress imposed by weight-bearing. Even when preoperative radiographs suggest that cortical bone is well maintained to either side of the fracture, it is likely that there will be some collapse or resorption of that bone after closed rod fixation if the fracture is irradiated perioperatively. Consequently, all pathologic fractures of the femoral shaft should be managed by open intramedullary rod fixation. At the time of open fracture reduction, gross tumor tissue and cortical bone obviously rendered structurally inadequate can be removed under direct vision. The cavity thus created can then be filled with methylmethacrylate before the rod is advanced into the distal fragment in a manner similar to that used with the Zickel nail. When this technique is used, progressive shortening of the femur does not occur, the fracture fragments do not telescope, and the nail does not migrate proximally, even in the face of marked cortical bone loss (Fig. 74-14). An alternative method of managing the pathologic femoral shaft fracture where there is extensive loss of bone stock is to employ an interlocking nail for fixation.[1,27] The procedure is technically difficult because insertion of the distal cross bolts must be performed under x-ray control. In addition, the cross bolts are of limited strength and they are likely to migrate or break eventually in the face of weight-bearing and a prolonged failure of fracture union after irradiation. For this reason, we advocate open resection of tumor and destroyed bone at the time of such fixation followed by filling the cavity with methylmethacrylate to discourage telescoping of the major fragments.

Supracondylar Femur Fractures

Metastatic foci of the distal femoral metaphysis frequently will break through the relatively thin cortical bone and form a palpable mass in the soft tissues (Fig. 74-15*A*). There is almost always extensive destruction of cortical bone apparent before the actual fracture occurs. The two alternatives for fixation include the use of an angled blade-plate and the use of an intramedullary device. An angled blade-plate affords excellent resistance to torque and shear stresses, and when augmented by methylmethacrylate filling the defect created by tumor lysis, it resists varus and valgus deforming loads, as well. However, a laterally applied plate in the supracondylar area is subject to tension loads, as is a compression hip screw and plate in the proximal femur, and is just as apt to suffer fatigue failure in patients who survive fracture fixation for years if progression to a true bony union is frustrated by irradiation. Moreover, a major stress riser is created just proximal to the tip of the side plate, increasing the likelihood of a secondary fracture there.

For these reasons use of an intramedullary device that encourages continuing impaction of the major fragments with weight-bearing is preferred. Small multiple rods such as Ender nails or Rush rods rarely are adequate to stabilize a distal fragment. Similarly, the use of an intramedullary rod offers tenu-

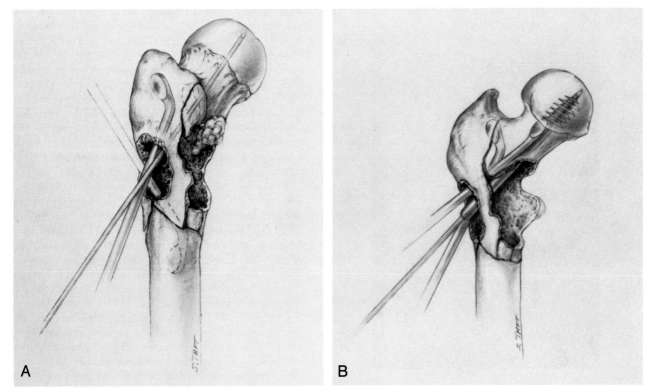

FIGURE 74-11. (A) Pathologic intertrochanteric femur fractures are reduced as anatomically as possible by closed manipulation on a conventional fracture table under image intensifier control. A standard straight lateral incision is made, centered over the greater trochanter. The lateral femoral shaft is exposed as for any hip fracture, by incising the vastus lateralis and reflecting its bulk anteriorly as shown. Tumor tissue may be exposed as it escapes through the typical medial cortical defect. A 2 × 1.5 cm window is made in the lateral cortex through which tumor may be removed and the fixation device may be inserted. Through the lateral cortical window, a large angled curette is used to remove tumor tissue as well as remnants of intramedullary fat and bone extending from the midfemoral neck and the greater trochanter proximally to well below the fracture level distally. A calibrated guide pin is inserted under x-ray control into the center of the femoral head. (B) A stepcut reamer is inserted over the guide pin to create channels for the compression hip screw proximally and its side plate sleeve distally. The corkscrew portion of a compression hip screw is inserted over the guide pin until its threads come within approximately 1 mm of the femoral head cortical margin. Remaining intramedullary tumor and bone then are removed up to the level of the distalmost threads on the screw.

ous fixation of the distal fragment if bony union does not occur promptly.

Zickel supracondylar nails afford excellent intramedullary fixation, yet because they transfix both femoral condyles by a combination of rods and screws, they ensure secure resistance to rotational forces as well[8,37] (Fig. 74-15B). Although these can be inserted by a semiclosed technique using small medial and lateral epicondylar incisions, usually an anterior medial parapatellar incision is required to resect tumor tissue that has broken through the cortex intra- or extrasynovially. Obviously, such an approach allows tumor cells to contaminate the joint, even if the knee had not been invaded already, but we have never seen a situation where this resulted in metastases within the joint or any other functional disability.

Expose the entire extent of the extracortical tumor mass; by flexing the knee, both epicondyles also are easily approachable. Remove as much tumor tissue as possible, together with bone obviously destroyed by the lytic process. Drill a ¼-inch hole through the anterior portion of the epicondylar prominence medially or laterally in line with the long axis of the femoral canal. Use the largest diameter Zickel supracondylar nail that will fit within the medullary canal, long enough so that at least two-thirds of the length will be above the proximal extent of obvious tumor lysis. Advance the rods together and impact them within the medullary canal, forcing their ends against the femoral cortex as they spring against each other. Then insert the horizontal intercondylar screws after drilling of the bone. Often the tip of one screw, the end of one nail, or both will not engage cortical bone because of the extent of tumor lysis, but all components of the fixation system should be of a length and in a position that would be appropriate if the cortex were intact.

Fill the bony defect with methylmethacrylate injected from a cement gun while in a liquid consistency, and digitally pack it to fill the confines of the tumor cavity and to extend as proximally as possible. It may be necessary to reattach a portion of the

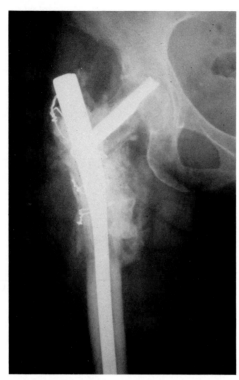

FIGURE 74-12. Extensive destructive changes are apparent involving most of the proximal half of the right femur. Prophylactic fixation has been accomplished using a Zickel nail. The femur was irradiated.

medial or lateral capsular complex to the cement mass with a barbed staple before polymerization is complete. The capsule then will scar down to adjacent soft tissues and restore amazingly good collateral stability, even in the absence of actual attachment to bone. Immediate weight-bearing and early range of motion exercises for the knee are encouraged, as are exercises for strengthening adjacent muscles.

Fractures of the Tibia

Metastatic pathologic fractures of the tibia are uncommon, accounting for only 36 of 399 long bone fractures in our series.[7] The great majority involve the proximal tibial metaphysis. They occur either as minimally displaced "rotten wood" fractures through sclerotic and often irradiated bone or as fractures through thin plateau cortices weakened by a vascularized lytic lesion. In the former instance, the Zickel supracondylar nails can be inserted effectively for fixation and often can be inserted by a "closed" technique not requiring exposure of the fracture or augmentation by methylmethacrylate. When a fracture of one or both plateaus has occurred, internal fixation is usually impossible because the remaining bone is too thin. Under such circumstances, and in a patient with an acceptable prognosis for prolonged survival, the fracture is best managed by prosthetic knee replacement using a semiconstrained device with a long-stemmed tibial component.

UPPER EXTREMITY FRACTURES

In decades past, upper extremity fractures were managed only by external splintage because their stability was considered un-

important in a patient's ability to move in bed or walk, and because few patients survived long enough to warrant internal fixation. As survival statistics improved and as techniques for irradiation of metastases changed, a complete reversal in attitude towards these fractures occurred. It was recognized that once a displaced fracture occurred, healing rarely followed in the absence of internal fixation, and in the absence of healing pain relief was difficult to obtain. Moreover, as patients survive for longer periods after developing bony metastases, they are likely to become increasingly dependent on their upper extremities for transfer in and out of bed, ambulation, or participation in even minimal activities of daily living.

Upper extremity pathologic fractures requiring internal fixation involve the humerus in the great majority of instances. Biomechanical considerations pertaining to humeral fractures differ significantly from those pertaining to lower extremity fractures. To begin with, the humerus is a bone subjected to distractive forces at least as often as compressive forces. Thus, external functional braces of various sorts are less effective in the upper extremity than in the lower extremity, and appear to afford little stability or relief of pain for activities such as lifting, reaching, or even walking with the arms extended. It is also important to recognize that the medullary canal of the humerus varies widely in diameter from patient to patient. In most women, the mid-diaphyseal medullary canal is too small to allow intramedullary fracture fixation except by a relatively small device such as a Rush rod. Such fixation is rarely secure, even when augmented by methylmethacrylate. Consequently, in such patients extracortical fixation by a compression plate is advisable whenever possible. At the other extreme, in large men the intramedullary canal often is large and will allow fixation by an intramedullary rod with good stability in most instances.

Fractures of the Humerus

Metastatic lesions of the humerus have a good prognosis for bony healing after irradiation so long as an actual fracture has not supervened. Once a fracture occurs, however, the likelihood of eventual bony union is significantly poorer than for lower extremity long bone fractures, probably because of the distractive forces that tend to pull the major fracture fragments apart even after internal fixation. Consequently, if there is any doubt about the likelihood of a fracture occurring through a humeral lytic lesion, it is advisable to splint the bone internally before irradiation is commenced. This is best accomplished by extending the extremity overhead using olecranon pin traction, and accomplishing closed pin stabilization of the humerus under image intensifier control.

For lesions involving the middle and distal thirds of the humerus, make a small triceps-splitting approach to the posterior humerus just proximal to the olecranon process but well distal to the spiral groove and radial nerve. Drill a hole through the posterior cortex. Using a high speed burr, enlarge this hole until it is approximately 1 cm wide and 1.5 cm long. With a hole of this size, attempts at subsequent Rush rod insertion will not require unnecessary force, and the risk of creating an iatrogenic fracture can be minimized. Usually two Ender or Rush rods of between 23 and 30 mm are required. Take care not to use rods that are too long for fear of penetrating the humeral

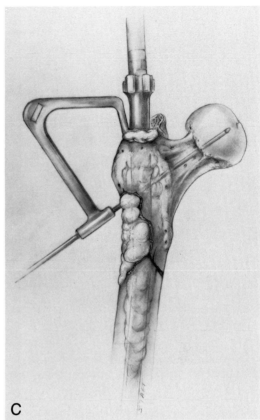

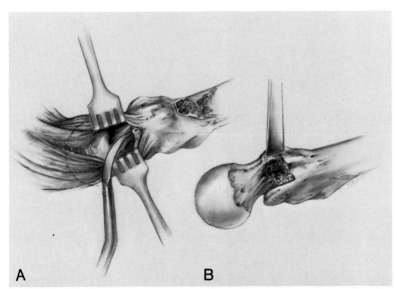

FIGURE 74-13. (*A*) For insertion of the Zickel nail, the patient is placed in a lateral decubitus position. Using an image intensifier, acceptable anteroposterior and lateral views of the femoral neck may be obtained simply by rotating the femur after the intramedullary portion of the nail has been inserted under direct vision. Some surgeons prefer to reduce the fracture on a conventional fracture table and to insert the nail under continuous fluoroscopic control. The only disadvantage of this technique is that the affected leg is difficult to adduct fully, and thus exposure of the greater trochanteric tip is limited. A curved incision is made extending just posterior to the greater trochanter. The fracture is exposed by an incision through and a forward displacement of the vastus lateralis. Using a curved curette, the medullary canal is cleaned of gross tumor tissue, fat, and bone fragments. (*B*) The abductor tendon is split longitudinally. Using a curved awl, the sulcus just medial to the tip of the greater trochanter is located and broached. A notch is then cut in the superior and lateral aspect of the greater trochanter extending from anterolateral to posteromedial. (*C*) A blunt-tipped guide pin is inserted down the medullary canal of the proximal fragment. The fracture is reduced under direct vision and the guide pin then is inserted down the distal fragment canal. Using serial reamers, the medullary canal is enlarged to accept the appropriate sized Zickel nail. The proximal fragment must be reamed to 17 mm. The intramedullary portion of the Zickel nail then is inserted to insure that it can be positioned as far distally as necessary and with approximately 12° of anteversion. The nail then is withdrawn until its tip is just visible through the lateral cortical defect. The proximal and distal canals are filled with methylmethacrylate in a liquid consistency, and the nail is driven back into its final position. The Zickel cross nail guide is fitted over the proximal tip of the nail and held firmly in place while a guide pin is inserted down the center of the femoral neck. If the cement still is soft, the guide pin can be inserted directly. If not, a $^5/_{64}$-inch drill can be used to create a tract for the pin. A cannulated drill is inserted over the pin, its tip extending proximally to the center of the femoral head. The cross nail then is inserted as shown and held firmly within the intramedullary nail by a friction-stabilized longitudinal pin.

head. Prebend the rods in an effort to allow their tips to bounce off the opposite humeral cortex without penetrating the often soft cortical bone at the tumor focus. More proximal lesions can be fixed prophylactically by Ender or Rush rods inserted antegrade through a cortical hole placed well distal to the prominence of the greater tuberosity. This prevents impingement of the proximal rod tip against the acromion during

shoulder abduction. Stern reported a 56% incidence of adhesive capsulitis of the shoulder when such impingement was allowed to occur with antegrade fixation using a Rush rod inserted in the more conventional manner through the proximal tip of the greater tuberosity.[33]

Once prophylactic fixation has been accomplished, irradiation of the metastatic focus can be commenced. Generally, a

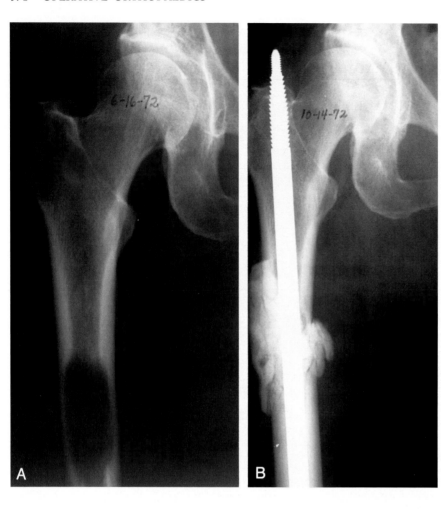

FIGURE 74-14. (*A*) A large myelomatous lesion of the femoral shaft. (*B*) Fixation has been accomplished using a Schneider nail augmented by packing the tumor cavity with acrylic cement. Greater care should have been exercised to keep the acrylic cement within the confines of the cortical defect. Nevertheless, the patient continues with a stable, pain-free extremity despite the absence of a bony union 14 years after surgery.

course of between 2000 and 2500 rads is sufficient to prevent local recurrence and yet will not prevent bone healing of the focus so long as a fracture has not occurred. External splintage of the humerus is favored using a functional sleeve-type brace during the period of irradiation and for approximately 3 weeks thereafter. The limb should also be protected for an additional 6 weeks after removal of the splint.

Fractures of the proximal humerus ordinarily require prosthetic replacement, although occasionally there may be sufficient bone stock remaining in the humeral head to consider internal fixation of the fracture (Fig. 74-16*A*). In such circumstances a short, right-angled blade-plate, of the type used for proximal femoral osteotomy in pediatric patients, is the most secure means of stabilizing the proximal segment. The ideal technique for replacement of the proximal humerus is to use a custom proximal humerus prosthesis, fashioned directly from preoperative radiographs (Fig. 74-16*B*). Manufacture of such a prosthesis ordinarily requires between 6 and 8 weeks, however, and many patients with severe postfracture pain and a limited life expectancy are not best served by such a delay. With few exceptions, the results in terms of restoration of function and relief of pain are as good if one simply uses a conventional Neer proximal humeral prosthesis and recreates continuity with the humeral metaphysis using methylmethacrylate (Fig. 74-16*C*).

A fracture of the humeral diaphysis must be analyzed carefully before any decision is made regarding the technique to be used for fixation. The alternatives include the use of an intra-

medullary nail or the use of a compression sideplate. When a fracture occurs through a well-circumscribed metastasis, particularly in the midhumeral diaphysis, a heavy compression plate is ideal for fixation. A longitudinal incision paralleling the palpable interval between the biceps and brachialis muscles is used and the humeral shaft is approached by blunt dissection through the midportion of the brachialis muscle. The underlying radial nerve frequently is displaced from its normal anatomic position either by the tumor mass or by the fracture fragments themselves. Consequently, the nerve should be identified and gently retracted before an attempt is made to reduce and stabilize the fracture.

When there is extensive destruction of cortical bone to either side of the fracture, the conventional technique of using screw fixation of six cortices above and six below the fracture is inadequate. Effective alternatives include the use of a large heavy compression plate, allowing at least six cortices of fixation into good bone to either side of the fracture or, in patients with a sufficiently large medullary canal the use of an intramedullary nail of the Küntscher type (Fig. 74-17). When a Küntscher nail is used, it must be inserted proximally through the point of attachment of the rotator cuff tendons. It is essential that the nail tip be buried beneath the cortical surface and that the rotator cuff insertion be reestablished directly to bone. With either alternative, methylmethacrylate should be injected and packed within the intramedullary canal to enhance fixation by minimizing varus angulation strains (in the case of a plate)

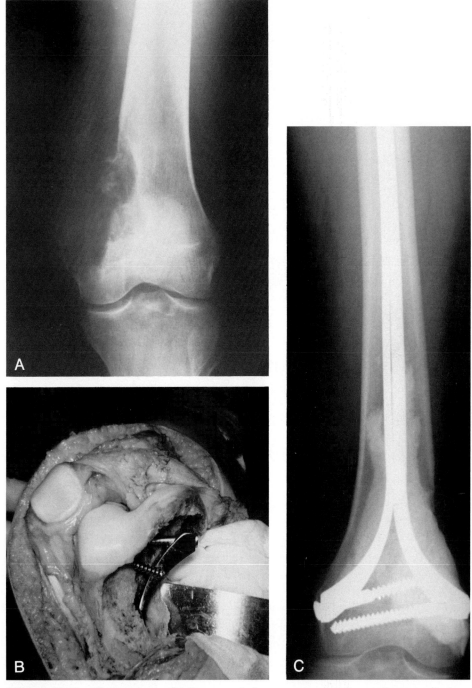

FIGURE 74-15. (*A*) An aneurysmal lytic metastasis from a cutaneous melanoma has created a large extracortical mass. (*B*) Fixation is accomplished using two Zickel supracondylar nails inserted retrograde after having been bent to allow full seating of the squared tips flush with the epicondylar cortex. The cross screws then are inserted as shown. The two nails have differing angles for these screws so that they do not interfere with each other. As shown here, the screws rarely are seated entirely in intact bone. However, because they have large cancellous threads throughout most of their length, fixation still can be achieved. (*C*) Methylmethacrylate then is injected while quite liquid to fill the curetted cavity and to reinforce the stability afforded by the Zickel nails.

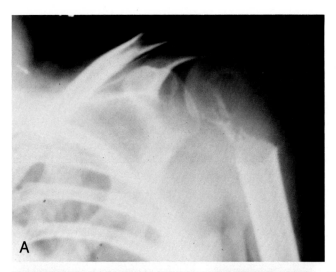

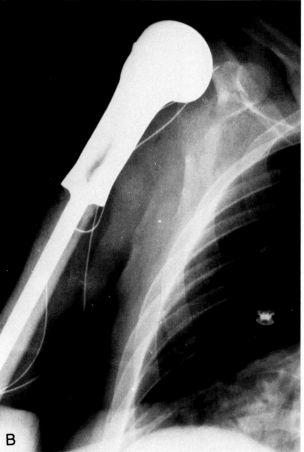

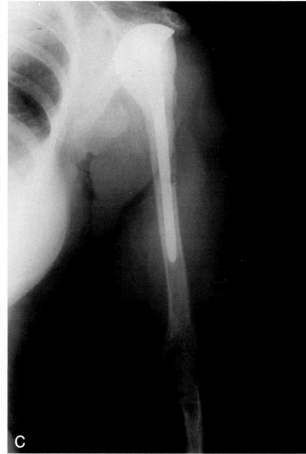

FIGURE 74-16. (*A*) Aneurysmal metastatic hypernephroma destroying the proximal humerus in a 52-year-old male with no other demonstrable metastases. A nephrectomy had been performed 3 years before this radiograph was obtained. The proximal humerus was resected with wide margins and was replaced by a custom prosthesis. The patient enjoyed excellent relief of pain and regained 60° of glenohumeral abduction and 70° of flexion despite the resection of the rotator cuff. (*B*) An aggressive lytic metastasis in the proximal humerus, again from a primary hypernephroma, has been resected and replaced by a custom-fitted prosthesis. Such a prosthesis can be fashioned from properly measured preoperative radiographs (Courtesy of Franklin H. Sim, M.D.). (*C*) A similar lesion of the proximal humerus has been resected and replaced by a conventional Neer prosthesis. The junction between the articular margin of the prosthesis and the remaining shell of humeral metaphysis has been recreated by molded methylmethacrylate.

and to increase resistance to torque stresses (in the case of the rod). On occasion, it may be necessary to resect some structurally inadequate bone and then to bring the intact cortices of the major fragments together by shortening the humerus slightly.

Supracondylar humeral fractures are particularly difficult to stabilize because the marked flattening of bone at the olecranon fossa precludes both direct intramedullary fixation and the use of an angled blade-plate of any sort. The most effective means for stabilization such a fracture is to insert two Rush rods retrograde through the medial and lateral epicondyles,

respectively. Some degree of three-point fixation is achieved by each rod, and the combination of both rods effectively prevents varus or valgus malalignment of the fracture fragments. The construct is minimally resistant to torque stresses, however, because the rods usually cross each other at the level of the fracture-tumor defect. Consequently, it is essential that the medullary canal be thoroughly debrided of residual tumor tissue and then filled well both proximal and distal to the fracture site with methylmethacrylate. By hollowing out the distal fragment well beyond the metaphyseal flare, and if possible down

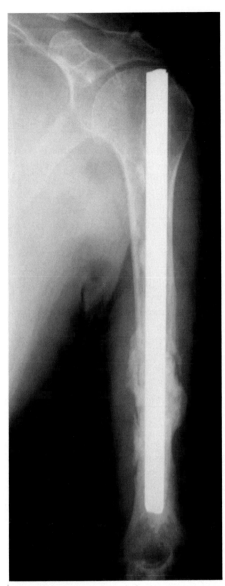

FIGURE 74-17. When the involved humerus has a large intramedullary canal, fixation is best accomplished by a slight shortening of the bone and the use of a Kuntscher nail augmented by cement. The nail was inserted through a small incision in the supraspinatus tendon, and its tip was buried beneath the cortical surface.

along either side of the olecranon fossa, the cement filling that defect will also diminish the risk of distraction of the fracture fragments by gravity or lifting-traction stresses. Despite the rather tenuous radiographic appearance of these constructs, they function in a remarkably stable manner and almost invariably afford excellent relief of pain.

Another alternative is dual reconstruction plates.

IMPENDING PATHOLOGIC FRACTURES: EVALUATION AND MANAGEMENT

It is impossible in this space to cover the topic of pathologic fracture management with any completeness, and the reader is

referred elsewhere if more detail is required.[24] However, the basic indications for prophylactic long bone stabilization are summarized here:

1. Cortical bone destruction of 50% or more
2. Lesion of 2.5 cm or more of proximal femur
3. Pathologic avulsion fracture of the lesser trochanter
4. Persisting stress pain despite irradiation

Fidler has demonstrated a technique for estimating the percentage of cortical bone destruction at any level of a long bone using the conventional anteroposterior and lateral radiographs (Fig. 74-18). This technique usually is as accurate a prognosticator of an impending pathologic fracture as is a cross sectional CT scan. When cortical destruction progresses in a patchy or spiral distribution, however, it may be difficult to assess the circumferential bone loss accurately by this technique, and a cross sectional CT scan of the extremity may be more accurate.

Once tumor lysis has progressed to the point that 50% or more of the cortex has been destroyed at any given level, the incidence of a spontaneous pathologic fracture increases dramatically. In the proximal femur a lytic lesion in excess of 2.5 cm on either the anteroposterior or the lateral view almost always can be seen to have an associated cortical disruption in excess of 50%.

The finding of a pathologic avulsion fracture of the lesser trochanter also suggests that at least 50% of the femoral cortex has been destroyed locally and that the patient has a significant

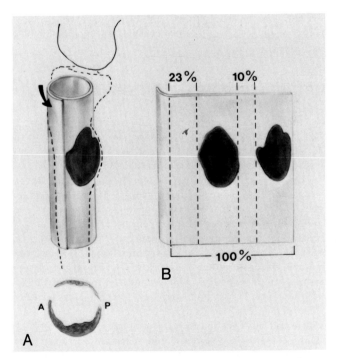

FIGURE 74-18. With well-circumscribed lesions, the extent of cortical destruction can be estimated with surprising accuracy from conventional anteroposterior and lateral radiographs. The tube is then turned 90° and the outline from the lateral radiograph is copied (A). When the sheet is unfurled (B), an accurate assessment can be made of the extent of circumferential cortical destruction. In this instance, only 33% of the circumferential cortex remains intact. This patient is at high risk for a spontaneous pathologic fracture and should have prophylactic fixation.

chance of developing a pathologic fracture across the femur at the intertrochanteric or subtrochanteric level. Unfortunately, all of these criteria are based on the assessment of lytic lesions where the size of the tumor focus or the extent of its destruction can be determined radiographically. In fact, however, the majority of bony metastases ultimately resulting in pathologic fractures combine both blastic and lytic changes or show radiographic evidence of diffuse or difficult to quantify lytic changes. For patients who experience focal limb pain that is aggravated by weight-bearing, where conventional radiographs, CT scans, or tomograms do not demonstrate a clear cut risk of an impending fracture, a combination of these studies with radioisotope scanning may afford a better concept of balance between tumor aggressiveness and host response. Such patients typically are treated by local irradiation, and in most instances effective pain control can be achieved. However, the physician must realize that the initial response of bone to irradiation is focal hyperemia leading to a localized osteopenia, which actually weakens the host bone temporarily. For the first 10 to 18 days after the beginning of a course of radiotherapy, the patient is actually at a higher risk of fracturing through the tumor focus than before radiation was commenced.

The vagaries of assessing fracture risk in patients with mixed blastic and lytic lesions and the increase in risk of fracture created by the initial response to irradiation prompt the establishment of another relative indication for prophylactic fixation. This is the presence of persistent or increasing local pain, particularly when aggravated by weight-bearing, despite completion of at least 2 weeks of radiotherapy. Most such patients probably have microfractures that will progress to displacement even in the face of restricted weight-bearing if the bone is not internally splinted.

METASTATIC DISEASE OF THE SPINE

The spine is a very complex and controversial area of pathologic fracture management and can be covered only briefly in this chapter. For a more detailed analysis of the principles and practicalities involved, the reader is referred elsewhere.[23]

The spine is the most common site for skeletal metastases, irrespective of the primary tumor involved. The vertebral body typically is affected first, although the initial roentgenographic finding often is destruction of a pedicle. This discrepancy is explained by the fact that in the absence of a blastic or sclerotic reaction within the vertebral cancellous bone, between 30% and 50% of the vertebral body must be destroyed before any changes can be recognized radiographically. In contrast, minimal lysis of pedicular bone can be appreciated because the cortex of the pedicle tends to be involved early and because the pedicle can be seen well in cross section on anteroposterior roentgenograms. The vertebral bodies contain active red marrow throughout life, unlike the peripheral skeleton which in adulthood contains a relatively avascular yellow marrow. The vascular sinusoidal system within red marrow is particularly vulnerable to cancer cells, allowing them to escape from the circulation and become established within the network of cancellous bone. The ability of these cells to form a protective fibrin sheath and to secrete osteoclast-activating factors and perhaps lytic prostaglandins also appear to be enhanced within the red marrow of vertebrae.[11,12] This explains, perhaps, why more than 70% of patients who die from cancer have evidence of vertebral metastases.

Vertebral metastases in themselves are often asymptomatic and may be discovered only by routine bone scans. When symptoms do develop they are a consequence of one or more of the following: (1) an enlarging mass within the vertebral body, which may break through the cortex and invade paravertebral soft tissues; (2) compression or invasion of adjacent nerve roots; (3) the development of a pathologic fracture secondary to vertebral destruction; (4) the development of spinal instability from such a fracture, particularly associated with lytic destructive changes in the posterior elements; and (5) compression of the spinal cord. Such compression has been reported to occur in approximately 5% of patients with widespread cancer.[5,9,10,18,19]

The most common cause of compression of the spinal cord or the nerve root is the extrusion of tumor tissue and detritus of bone into the spinal canal following the partial collapse of a vertebral body that was infiltrated and weakened by a metastatic deposit. On occasion, tumor tissue may break into the canal and compress the cord without causing significant destruction or collapse of the vertebral body. Rarely, compression of the cord or root results from a soft tissue mass growing into the spinal canal through a neural foramen, from intradural metastases, or from carcinomatous meningitis. It is uncommon for the dura to be penetrated by metastatic tumor tissue, although a reactive dural thickening is commonly encountered.

Because the metastatic tumor mass typically invades the canal from the vertebral body, the motor functions of the anterior part of the spinal cord are usually compromised first, with sensory disturbances following as the cord is displaced posteriorly and impinges on the lamina. Although the lumbar vertebrae are most commonly affected by tumor metastases, it is in the thoracic spine that compromise of the spinal cord occurs most often. This is because the cord is largest at that point relative to the diameter of the canal and thus is compressed earliest by a given tumor mass. Histologic examination of spinal cords removed from patients who died with clinical evidence of metastatic compression of the spinal cord have revealed no consistent pattern. The pathologic alterations often are slight, despite severe, longstanding clinical disease. Edema and cellular degeneration have been noted in the myelinated tissue at the level of the compression, but the gray matter is generally well preserved. The distribution of pathologic changes usually does not conform to the arterial supply or venous drainage of the cord, although it has been suggested that venous occlusion is the most important factor leading to neuronal degeneration.[2,3]

About half of all patients in whom impingement of the spinal cord ultimately develops complain of radicular pain for weeks or months before long tract signs become apparent. Loss of sphincter control is a late phenomenon, and usually occurs in patients with the most profound neurologic deficits. The sensory level is not a reliable indicator of the level of compression of the spinal cord, as this usually is recorded several segments below in myelographically demonstrable subarachnoid block.

The rapidity of onset of muscular weakness has considerable bearing on the ultimate prognosis. When there is a delay of less

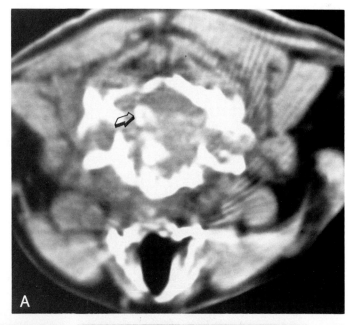

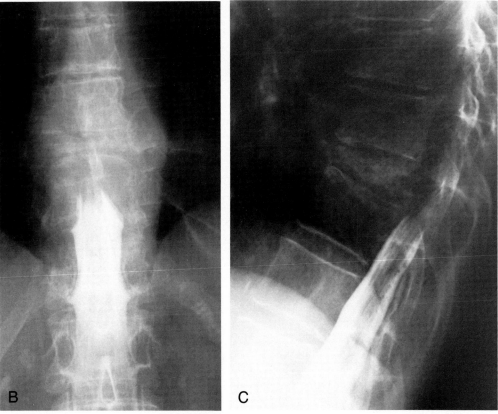

FIGURE 74-19. (*A*) CT scan of the cervical spine in a patient with metastatic breast carcinoma. The patient had minimal left-sided C5 root symptoms but showed no evidence clinically of spinal cord compromise. Because the density (attenuation number) of the tumor is almost identical to that of the spinal cord, this scan is not particularly helpful in quantitating how much if any spinal cord compromise exists. However, one large bony fragment (*arrow*) is seen to be extruded into the area of the C5 nerve root. A myelogram showed minimal canal compromise but displacement of the root by the bony fragment. Anteroposterior (*B*) and lateral (*C*) metrizamide myelographic views of the thoracolumbar spine in a patient with metastatic breast carcinoma. The patient had a severe (Frankel Grade B) paraparesis and a complete myelographic block. The anteroposterior view shows that the spinal cord is compressed eccentrically from the left. The lateral view confirms that the compression comes from in front at the level of the collapsed vertebral body.

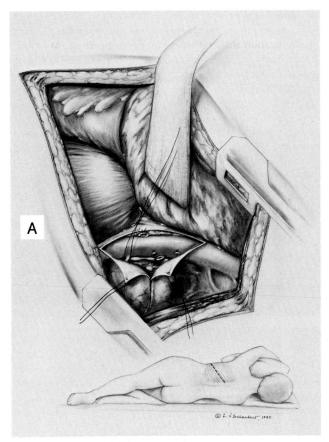

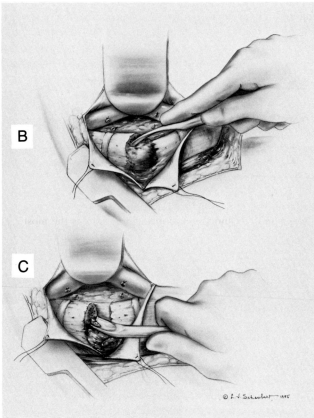

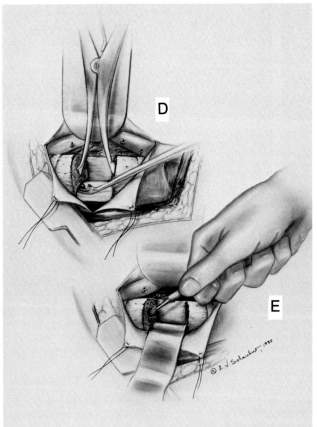

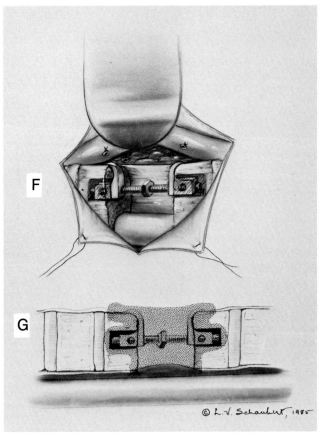

than 24 hr between the onset of symptoms and the appearance of a full blown neurologic syndrome, the prognosis for recovery is poor no matter what treatment is offered. Conversely, most patients whose neurologic deficit has developed over a period of 7 to 10 days will respond favorably to decompression of the cord or radiotherapy.

Once an individual is suspected of harboring a significant spinal metastasis, studies must be initiated to determine the level or levels of involvement, the likelihood of vertebral collapse and progressive neurologic impairment, and the most reasonable approach to treatment. Laboratory studies rarely are of much value in defining these parameters but may be critical in preparing a patient for surgical intervention. Such studies include white cell and platelet determinations, particularly in patients on chemotherapy, clotting studies, and calcium and phosphate determinations. Bone scintigraphy is the most sensitive diagnostic tool available for detecting spinal metastases. However, it will often reflect multiple areas of vertebral involvement without clarifying which level, if any, is associated with progressive pain, neurologic compromise, or vertebral collapse. In contrast, computed tomography allows visualization of even small areas of vertebral destruction, assessment of the extent of paravertebral soft tissue masses, and, most importantly, a clear visualization of the extent and direction of the impingement of the spinal cord by bone debris or tumor. On occasion, computed tomography may fail to demonstrate the extent or configuration of displacement of the spinal cord when the attenuation value (CT number) of the soft tissue mass in the spinal canal closely approximates that of the spinal cord itself (Fig. 74-19A). This problem can be overcome by injecting a small amount of water-soluble metrizamide into the subarachnoid space before scanning.

The principle limitation of computed tomography is its potential failure to disclose a second site of compression of the spinal cord, an event that occurs in approximately 10% of affected patients. Consequently, myelography is still an important means of clarifying the extent of intraspinal pathology (Fig. 74-19B and C), particularly in patients with a potential for more than one level of involvement. Bernat[3] reported that the symptoms of patients who had a myelographically demonstrable complete block often were indistinguishable from the symptoms of patients who had free flow intrathecally.[3] In fact, the myelographic demonstration of an intraspinal block has

little clinical significance; rather, evidence of progressive neurologic compromise, irrespective of the myelographic picture, is the indication for irradiation or decompression. Magnetic resonance imaging (MRI) is still in its infancy, and the extent of its value in assessing these patients has not been determined fully. To date, it appears that MRI rarely offers significant diagnostic advantages over CT, particularly when the latter is enhanced with intrathecal metrizamide.

Patients who have spinal metastases can be divided into five categories, depending on the extent of neurologic compromise or bone destruction:

Class I: No significant neurologic involvement
Class II: Involvement of bone without collapse or instability
Class III: Major neurologic impairment (sensory or motor) without significant involvement of bone
Class IV: Vertebral collapse with pain due to mechanical causes or instability but without significant neurologic compromise
Class V: Vertebral collapse or instability combined with major neurologic impairment.

Patients who are in Class I or Class II, with little or no neurologic impairment and without evidence of vertebral collapse or instability, generally obtain relief from pain by chemotherapy or hormonal manipulation, or, in the absence of success with these modalities, from local irradiation. Those in Class III, with neurologic compromise and the absence of major destruction of bone or spinal instability, usually respond to treatment with radiotherapy alone. If the neurologic compromise is of acute onset and relatively rapid in progression, the radiotherapy should be augmented by systemic administration of steroids.[5]

When metastatic tumor has destroyed enough bone to result in vertebral collapse and progressive pain in the spine due to mechanical causes (Class IV), or when that collapse has caused fragments of bone, ligament, or disc to compress the cord directly (Class V), it is illogical to assume that any improvement can result from irradiation alone, no matter how radiosensitive the malignant disease itself may be.

The indications for surgical intervention can be summarized as follows:

FIGURE 74-20. (A) Anterior decompression of the thoracic spine is accomplished by a thoracotomy with the patient in the lateral decubitus position. The aorta can be retracted gently, segmental vessels ligated and transected and the affected vertebral body easily approached. Often a prominent paravertebral extrapleural tumor mass exists and assists in localizing the focus of destruction. (B) Most of the tumor and bone disc debris can be removed using a small periosteal elevator. (C) As the level of the posterior cortical margin is approached, further decompression should be accomplished using an angled gouge or curette. All this material adherent to the adjacent vertebral body is removed. (D) The vertebral space is recreated using a lamina spreader, and a small angled curette is used to complete decompression of the spinal canal and to round off the edges of the posterior cortex of the adjacent vertebrae. (E) The end-plates of adjacent vertebrae are undercut using a high-speed burr in order to allow the ends of the Knodt rod and the bodies of its hooks to be buried within the vertebral bone. (F) The Knodt rod has been positioned within the resected space. As the rod is twisted, the hooks are distracted, and their bodies are firmly impacted within the adjacent vertebral bone. Only the tips of the hooks extend anterior to the vertebral cortex. (G) The defect is filled with methylmethacrylate polymerizing *in situ* and incorporating the rods and hooks. A malleable retractor has been placed between the expanding mass and the spinal canal in order to avoid compression of the cord.

1. Progressive impingement on the spinal canal and compression of the spinal cord by radioresistant tumor, by recurrent tumor in an area that has already been subjected to maximum irradiation, or by bone or soft tissue detritus that has been extruded into the canal as a result of progressive spinal deformity. These patients require decompression anteriorly, anterolaterally, or posteriorly, with or without spinal stabilization.
2. Progressive kyphotic spinal deformity with intact posterior structures but with intractable pain due to mechanical causes. These patients require anterior decompression and anterior stabilization.
3. Progressive kypohotic deformity associated with disruption of the posterior elements and progressive shear deformity. These patients require anterior and posterior decompression and stabilization.

In general, when spinal canal compromise originates from the vertebral body, the diseased anterior structures can be resected, the spinal canal can be decompressed, and the stability of the spine can be restored by bone grafting or artificial constructs. However, if there is advanced destruction of the posterior elements by tumor, the greatly increased tensile loads posteriorly cannot be resisted and a forward shearing deformity will develop, further compromising the spinal canal. This situation necessitates both anterior and posterior decompression and stabilization.

The technique of anterior decompression involves a complete vertebrectomy. The anterior two-thirds of the vertebrae are removed with relative ease using a rongeur or large currette (Fig. 74-20A to C). In approaching the posterior third of the vertebral body, and therefore the spinal canal, however, take great care to remove debris of tumor and bone without in any way increasing the already existing impingement on the spinal canal. An angled currette usually is the most effective instrument and allows material to be pulled forward out of the canal and away from the dura (Fig. 74-20D and E).

For lesions of the cervical spine, employ an anterior approach through the avascular interval between the sternocleidomastoid muscle and the carotid sheath laterally and the strap muscles, trachea, and esophagus medially. The middle thyroid vein is the only structure requiring ligation and transection, although care must be taken to avoid injury to the recurrent laryngeal nerve running obliquely through the lower field. Anterior decompression and stabilization of the thoracic spine requires a thoracotomy, but once the heart, lung, and great vessels have been retracted, the vertebral bodies are readily approachable from the third thoracic to the second lumbar level. The upper part of the thoracic spine from the first to the third thoracic vertebra are exposed using a thoracoplasty approach by mobilizing the scapula anteriorly and resecting the second rib. The major advantage of this anterior approach is the ability to resect the tumor directly, decompress the neurologic structures from the side of their compromise, and jack open the collapsed vertebral body, thereby correcting the kyphotic deformity at its source.

Once the cord and roots have been decompressed completely, stabilization is performed. Some surgeons advocate the use of an anterior interbody graft of corticocancellous bone, keyed into the adjacent vertebral end-plates and stabilized by external immobilization until incorporation.[26] The rationale for this technique is that once incorporation of the graft is complete there need be no further concern about spinal instability. In patients who are chronically debilitated and face a limited life expectancy, however, the requirement for external immobilization for more than 10 weeks postoperatively is a major drawback of this technique. In addition, in patients who have received or will receive local irradiation within 3 or 4 months after operation, the likelihood of a bone graft becoming incorporated at any point is markedly reduced.[19,22]

In an effort to achieve instantaneous internal stability that is not dependent on incorporation of a graft and does not require external immobilization, many surgeons have begun using methylmethacrylate to create an artificial vertebral construct. The most adjustable and effective technique of stabilization is the use of a Knodt distraction rod and hooks to jack open the collapsed vertebral space to its appropriate height, the device then being incorporated into the acrylic vertebral replacement (Fig. 74-20F and G). Penetrate the end-plates of the intact vertebral bodies above and below the area of decompression using a high-speed power burr, and enlarge the cavity thus created to accept both the rod and the body of the hook (see Fig. 74-20E). The tip of the hook protrudes slightly anterior to the vertebral body; incorporate the remainder of the distraction device into the acrylic cement, which is injected to fill the vertebrectomy space. A malleable retractor is held between the spinal canal and the back of the polymerzing cement to prevent expansion of the cement into the canal and thus recreation of cord impingement.

For patients with a projected survival of more than 2 years, reinforce the vertebral replacement by anterior grafting with cancellous bone. Pack the graft over the remaining lateral elements of the resected vertebrae as well as proximally and distally over the exposed cortices of the intact vertebrae beyond the level of decompression. If a patient is irradiated within 2 months of this operation, it is unlikely that the cancellous graft will be incorporated. In patients who do not require further irradiation, however, the incidence of incorporation of the grafts and the development of a mature arthrodesis is better than 50%.

Decompressive laminectomy of the spine is no more effective than radiation alone.[9,13] Moreover, destruction of the vertebral body by tumor leads to a progressive kyphotic deformity that can only be accentuated by surgical destruction of the remaining stability of the posterior elements. It is all but impossible to decompress the anterior part of the cord, where invasion by tumor usually originates, from the posterior approach. The best that one can hope to accomplish is to remove enough bone—ordinarily a minimum of four laminae—to allow the cord to bulge posteriorly and escape the effects, if not the presence, of the anterior mass of tumor. Thus, the idea that a posterior decompression often is preferable to an anterior decompression in the cancer patient because the procedure is less extensive has little validity. On occasion, however, posterior spinal decompression is indicated for a patient who has compression of the spinal cord or a root originating from a focus of tumor in the lamina or in a pedicle, or in whom a circumferential napkin ring constriction by tumor or inflammatory tissue can not be relieved entirely from the front (Fig. 74-21A and B).

After wide decompressive laminectomy, posterior stabilization is essential. In the cervical spine this is best accomplished by posterior wire stabilization, and in the thoracic and lumbar spine by Luque rod stabilization with sublaminar wiring. The rod should extend three levels above and three levels below the extent of the decompression (Fig. 74-21*C*). Some authors have advocated reinforcing this fixation with methylmethacrylate, incorporating the rods and laminae and perhaps augmented by bone grafting. The major difficulty with using posteriorly placed acrylic cement to enhance stabilization, particularly in the mobile cervical spine, is that the stresses imposed on this construct attack its greatest weakness. Methylmethacrylate is minimally able to withstand torque and shear loads, and these are the exact stresses to which it is subjected when used for posterior stabilization. Whitehill and others[34,35] have demonstrated that a fibrous tissue interface invariably forms between the posterior surface of the lamina and the mass of cement, and that the apparently solid construct that was created at operation degenerates quickly into separately moving segments shortly after motion of the spine is resumed.

In summary, operative decompression, usually anteriorly, and stabilization are appropriate for certain patients who have spinal metastases and intractable pain due to mechanical

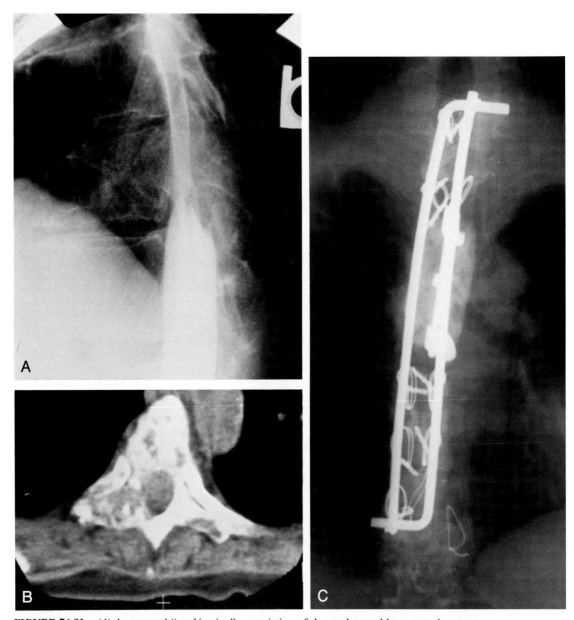

FIGURE 74-21. (*A*) An unusual "napkin ring" constriction of the cord caused by metastatic tumor within the spinal canal growing around the dura to compress the cord circumferentially. (*B*) A CT scan of the spine demonstrating both anterior and posterior bony destruction and canal compromise. Under such circumstances, both anterior and posterior decompression and stabilization probably will be necessary. (*C*) Anteroposterior radiograph of the spine taken 1 year after decompression and stabilization both anteriorly and posteriorly.

causes, spinal instability, or neurologic compromise. This is a small percentage of all patients who have spinal metastases, however. Most patients do not have persistent pain after an initial period of rest and a course of local radiotherapy. Most do not have neurologic compromise of any degree. Most Class III patients, even with major neurologic compromise, will respond as favorably to local irradiation as they will to operative decompression. Many patients who have vertebral collapse or instability, even if it is associated with severe local or neurologic compromise, do not have a sufficient projected life expectancy to warrant such major operative intervention. Finally, the operative technique is not easy, and the anterior approach, particularly in the thoracolumbar area, subjects the patient to a variety of potentially serious complications.

REFERENCES

1. Acker, J.H., Murphy, C., D'Ambrosia, R.: Treatment of Fractures of the Femur with the Grosse-Kempf Rod. Orthopedics **8**:1393, 1985.
2. Barron, K.D., Hirano, A., Araki, S., and Ferry, F.D.: Experience with Metastatic Neoplasms Involving Spinal Cord. Neurology **9**:91, 1959.
3. Bernat, J.L., Greenberg, E.R., and Barrett, J.: Suspected Epidural Compression of the Spinal Cord and Cauda Equina by Metastatic Carcinoma. Clinical Diagnosis and Survival. Cancer **51**:1953, 1983.
4. Bickel, W.H., and Barber, J.R.: Pathologic or Spontaneous Fractures. G.P. **3**:41, 1951.
5. Boland, P.J., Lane, J.M., and Sundaresan, N.: Metastatic Disease of the Spine. Clin. Orthop. **169**:95, 1982.
6. Bremner, R.A., and Jelliffe, A.M.: The Management of Pathological Fracture of the Major Long Bones from Metastatic Cancer. J. Bone Joint Surg. **40-B**:652–659, 1958.
7. Campbell, C.J.: Palliation of Metastatic Bone Disease. In Hickey, R.C. (ed.): Palliative Care of the Cancer Patient. Boston, Little, Brown, 1967, pp. 313–340.
8. Clancey, G.J., Smith, R.F., and Madenwald, M.B.: Fractures of the Distal End of the Femur Below Hip Implants in Elderly Patients. Treatment with the Zickel Supracondylar Device. J. Bone Joint Surg. **65-A**:491, 1983.
9. Constans, J.P., deDivitiis, E., Donzelli, R., Spaziante, R., Meder, J.P., and Hayge, C.: Spinal Metastases with Neurological Manifestations. J. Neurosurg. **59**:111, 1983.
10. Edelson, R.N., Deck, M.D., and Posner, J.B.: Intramedullary Spinal Cord Metastases: Clinical and Radiographic Findings in Nine Cases. Neurology **22**:1222, 1972.
11. Galasko, C.S.B., and Bennett, A.: Relationship of Bone Destruction in Skeletal Metastases to Osteoclast Activation and Prostaglandins. Nature **263**:508, 1976.
12. Galasko, C.S.B.: Mechanisms of Bone Destruction in the Development of Skeletal Metastases. Nature **263**:507, 1976.
13. Gilbert, R.N., Kim, J.M., and Posner, J.B.: Epidural Spinal Cord Compression from Metastatic Tumors: Diagnosis and Treatment. Ann. Neurol. **3**:40, 1978.
14. Gustilo, R.B.: Management of Open Fractures and Their Complications. Philadelphia, W.B. Saunders, 1982.
15. Habermann, E.T., Sachs, R., Stern, R.E., Hirsh, D.M., and Anderson, W.J., Jr.: The Pathology and Treatment of Metastatic Disease of the Femur. Clin. Orthop. **169**:70, 1982.
16. Harper, M.C., and Walsh, T.: Ender Nailing for Peritrochanteric Fractures of the Femur. J. Bone Joint Surg. **67-A**:79, 1985.
17. Harrington, K.D., Johnston, J.O., Turner, R.H., and Green, D.L.: The Use of Methylmethacrylate as an Adjunct in the Internal Fix-ation of Malignant Neoplastic Fractures. J. Bone Joint Surg. **54-A**:1665, 1972.
18. Harrington, K.D.: Management of Unstable Pathologic Fracture-Dislocations of the Spine and Acetabulum Secondary to Metastic Malignancy. Instructional Course Lectures of the American Academy of Orthopaedic Surgeons. St. Louis, C.V. Mosby, 1980, Vol. 29.
19. Harrington, K.D.: The Use of Methylmethacrylate for Vertebral Body Replacement Anterior Stabilization of Pathological Fracture Disclocations of the Spine due to Metastatic Disease. J. Bone Joint Surg. **63-A**:36, 1981.
20. Harrington, K.D.: The Management of Acetabular Insufficiency Secondary to Metastatic Malignant Disease. J. Bone Joint Surg. **63-A**:653, 1981.
21. Harrington, K.D.: New Trends in the Management of Lower Extremity Metastases. Clin. Orthop. **169**:53, 1982.
22. Harrington, K.D.: Anterior Cord Decompression and Spine Stabilization for Patients with Metastatic Lesions of the Spine. J. Neurosurg. **61**:107, 1984.
23. Harrington, K.D.: Current Concepts Review. Metastatic Disease of the Spine. J. Bone Joint Surg. **68-A**:1110, 1986.
24. Harrington, K.D.: Impending Pathologic Fractures from Metastatic Malignancy: Evaluation and Management. Instructional Course Lectures of The American Academy of Orthopaedic Surgeons, St. Louis, C.V. Mosby, 1987, Chapter 37.
25. Higinbotham, N.L., and Marcove, R.C.: The Management of Pathological Fractures. J. Trauma **5**:792–798, 1965.
26. Johnson, J.R., Leatherman, K.D., and Holdt, R.T.: Anterior Decompression of the Spinal Cord for Neurological Deficit. Spine **8**:396, 1983.
27. Johnson, K.D., Johnston, D.W.C., and Parker, B.: Comminuted Femoral Shaft Fractures: Treatment by Roller Traction, Cerclage Wires with an Intramedullary Nail, or an Interlocking Nail. J. Bone Joint Surg. **66-A**:1222, 1984.
28. Lane, J., Senko, T., and Zolan, S.: Treatment of Pathological Fractures of the Hip by Endoprosthetic Replacement. J. Bone Joint Surg. **62-A**:954, 1980.
29. Mickelson, M.R., and Bonfiglio, M.: Pathological Fractures in the Proximal Part of the Femur Treated by Zickel-Nail Fixation. J. Bone Joint Surg. **58-A**:1067, 1976.
30. Sangeorzan, B.J., Ryan, J.R., and Salciccioli, G.G.: Prophylactic Internal Fixation of the Femur with the Zickel Nail: A Retrospective Analysis and Recommendation for Modification of the Described Technique. J. Bone Joint Surg. **68-A**:991, 1986.
31. Silverberg, E.: Cancer Statistics, 1985. CA **35**:19, 1985.
32. Sim, F.H., Hartz, C.R., and Chao, E.Y.S.: Total Hip Arthroplasty for Tumors of the Hip. In The Hip: Proceedings of the Fourth Open Scientific Meeting of the Hip Society. St. Louis, C.V. Mosby, 1976, pp. 246–259.
33. Stern, P.J., Mattingly, D.A., Pomeroy, D.L., Zenni, E.J. Jr., and Kreig, J.K.: Intramedullary Fixation of Humeral Shaft Fractures. J. Bone Joint Surg. **66-A**:639, 1984.
34. Whitehill, R., Reger, S.I., Fox, E., Payne, R., Barry, J., Cole, C., Richman, J., and Bruce, J.: The Use of Methylmethacrylate Cement as an Instantaneous Fusion Mass in Posterior Cervical Fusions: A Canine In Vivo Experimental Model. Spine **9**:246, 1984.
35. Whitehill, R., and Barry, J.C.: The Evolution of Stability in Cervical Spinal Constructs using either Autogenous Bone Graft or Methylmethacrylate Cement. A Follow Up Report on a Canine In Vivo Model. Spine **10**:32, 1985.
36. Zickel, R.F., and Mouradian, W.H.: Intramedullary Fixation of Pathological Fractures and Lesions of the Subtrochanteric Region of the Femur. J. Bone Joint Surg. **58-A**:1061, 1976.
37. Zickel, R.E., Fietti, V.G., Jr., Lawsing, J.F., III, and Cochran, G.V.B.: A New Intramedullary Fixation Device for the Distal Third of the Femur. Clin. Orthop. **125**:185–191, 1977.

CHAPTER 75

Soft–Tissue Sarcomas of the Extremities: Surgical Techniques for Limb–Salvage Resection

HENRY A. FINN and
MICHAEL A. SIMON

Soft-tissue sarcomas of the extremities are derived from the mesodermal tissues. An understanding of their local pattern of growth is integral to the successful surgical management of these tumors. Pseudoencapsulation by surrounding fibrous connective tissues as the sarcoma grows and enlarges in a centripetal fashion is a consistent finding.[5,9,18,24,26,27] This encapsulation is a result of compression and layering of normal tissue cells at the expanding border of the growing sarcoma and constitutes the host's reaction to the neoplasm. Microscopic extensions of tumor are usually found in the reactive-tissue zone, or the periphery of the pseudocapsule. In addition, satellite colonies of malignant cells may be found at some distance from the main tumor.

Soft-tissue sarcomas are known to be contained by major fascial planes as they grow and spread. The spread is usually centripetal in a subcutaneous site or longitudinal in a deep muscular compartment bounded by fascia or bone. The sarcoma generally remains limited to a well-defined anatomic compartment, except late in the course or upon disruption by a surgical procedure. Sarcomas may also arise outside well-defined anatomic compartments and can spread over considerable distances when there are no natural anatomic boundaries; this is the case in the popliteal fossa, groin, and antecubital fossa. Extracompartmental sarcomas may also spread over great distances along neurovascular planes. In this process, major neurovascular structures are usually displaced rather than invaded. Metastatic spread to the lungs by a hematogenous route may be seen in approximately 10% of cases at the time of diagnosis.[18] Rarely, distant nonpulmonary metastases are found in bone and other soft tissues. Adult soft-tissue sarcomas only infrequently spread to regional lymph nodes.

DEFINITIONS OF SURGICAL MARGINS

Armed with a knowledge of the biologic growth behavior of soft-tissue sarcomas in the extremities, one must understand the following surgical procedures and apply them in an appropriate fashion.

1. *Incisional Biopsy.* A portion of the tumor is removed by incision through the pseudocapsule. This procedure is appropriate for diagnosis only and leaves residual gross tumor *in situ.* There is seeding in any anatomic plane contaminated by the postoperative hematoma.
2. *Marginal (Capsular) Excision.* The tumor is removed by dissection through a plane in its surrounding pseudocapsule. This procedure frequently leaves microscopic tumor not only locally, but also in all planes contaminated by the hematoma.
3. *Wide Excision.* In this procedure, the tumor and, in addition, a variable amount of "normal" tissue are removed. Afterwards, microscopic regions containing tumor cells may be present in the remaining "normal" tissue. It implies no specific distance. It is difficult to measure the distance away from the tumor accurately, since the surgical specimen contracts when it is removed. Thus, measurements of the surgical specimen *ex vivo* by pathologists or surgeons are inaccurate.
4. *Radical Resection.* This procedure includes the tumor

and surrounding tissue extending at least one major anatomic plane beyond the dimensions of the tumor. The resected specimen includes appropriate musculoaponeurotic structures from their origins to their insertions as well as all neurovascular structures within the compartment.

GENERAL PRINCIPLES OF SURGICAL MANAGEMENT

In the absence of metastases, the prognosis for patients with soft-tissue sarcomas of the extremities depends on the histologic grade and the success of local control of the tumor.[2,24,27] These tumors are a histologically heterogeneous group, but the surgical management is similar for all types. At the time of diagnosis, sarcomas may be subcutaneous, deep and intracompartmental, or deep and extracompartmental. They may be small or large relative to their specific location in the extremity, and they may be of high grade (Broder's grade 3 and 4) or low grade (Broder's grade 1 and 2) histologically[3,6,8,25] (see Figs. 75-1 to 75-3). Although the size of the tumor and its anatomic location are important practical considerations, the histologic grade and the adequacy of the surgical margin obtained are the primary determinants for successful local control.[1,3,8,21,27]

High-grade, deep sarcomas require radical margins and are associated with local recurrence rates of approximately 10% to 15%.[9,20,27] Tumors that are deep and of low grade may be treated adequately with a wide margin.[9,27] In general, all subcutaneous tumors of high or low grade may be treated with a wide margin, and the prognosis is favorable.[9,12]

An appropriate surgical margin can be achieved either by a limb salvage resection or by amputation. In general, subcutaneous and small, deep intracompartmental tumors are potential candidates for limb salvage by surgery alone and do not require adjuvant radiation therapy. Extracompartmental tumors, large intracompartmental tumors adjacent to vital neurovascular structures or bone, or intracompartmental tumors in unexpendable compartments require adjuvant treatment if amputation is to be avoided. The technical aspects of amputation are discussed in chapters 47 and 48. In the attempt to avoid amputation, good results have been reported with large tumors, and with tumors adjacent to neurovascular structures or unexpendable bones, when they were treated with more limited surgical margins in combination with radiation therapy, chemotherapy, or both.[4,7,13,17,19,29,31]

STAGING AND INDICATIONS FOR LIMB SALVAGE

Great emphasis has been placed on limb preservation in the treatment of sarcomas of the extremities.[4] The resulting function after radical compartment excision in certain locations is better than that after amputation.[9,11,15,16,27] Patient selection is critical because of the prolonged recovery and increased postoperative surgical morbidity associated with limb salvage procedures. Preoperative staging and surgical planning are necessary for definition of the anatomic extent of the tumor and determination of the feasibility of limb salvage.[6,8,23,25,30] Rou-

tine staging of soft-tissue sarcomas of the extremity requires physical examination, radiography of the lungs and the involved limb, technetium-99m phosphonate and gallium-67 citrate scintigraphy, and computed tomography (CT) of the lungs and the limb. Because of superior image contrast and the ability to provide sagittal and coronal images, magnetic resonance imaging (MRI) is superior to CT in demonstrating the size and local extent of soft-tissue sarcomas.[32] An open biopsy is generally indicated so that the histogenesis and histologic grade of the tumor can be evaluated.[22,26] Biopsy technique and possible pitfalls have been reported in the past and are discussed in chapter 19.[14,22]

If there is no evidence of distant metastases, potential candidates for limb salvage by surgery alone include most patients with subcutaneous lesions and most of those with small, deep intracompartmental lesions. In most cases, tumors that are very large, bicompartmental, extracompartmental, or recurrent, and those that involve unexpendable bones or adjacent vital neurovascular structures, or that arise in an unexpendable compartment should not be treated with local surgery alone because it is technically impossible to attain adequate margins. Either adjuvant therapy or amputation is necessary in these situations. The addition of an adjuvant to surgery (pre- or postoperative radiation therapy) allows limb salvage resection with more limited surgical margins.[7,13,19,29,31]

In one study at a primary referral center, the authors found that one-third of sarcomas in the extremity were subcutaneous, one-third were deep to the fascia and intracompartmental, and one-third were extracompartmental[25] (Figs. 75-1 and 75-2). A small percentage of the extracompartmental tumors involved two deep muscular compartments (i.e., they were bicompartmental) (Figs. 75-3). Most of the subcutaneous tumors were treated with a wide excision. However, only one-half of the patients with deep tumors were candidates for radical compartmental excision as the sole form of local treatment, either because the tumors were very large or because the compartment was not expendable (e.g., the volar forearm).[25] Thus, of all patients with soft-tissue sarcomas of the extremity, somewhat more than half are candidates for limb salvage without

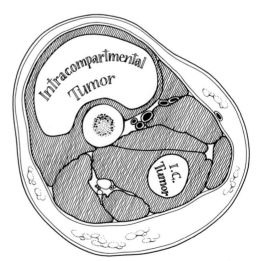

FIGURE 75-1. Cross section through the upper thigh, showing two deep intracompartmental tumors of different sizes.

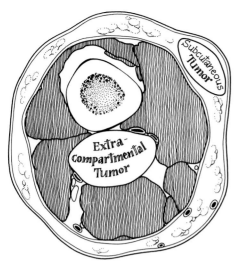

FIGURE 75-2. Cross section through the distal thigh, showing a subcutaneous intracompartmental tumor and an extracompartmental tumor arising in the popliteal space.

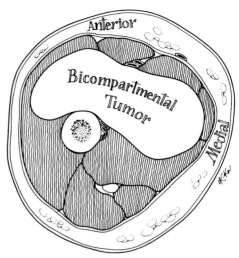

FIGURE 75-3. Cross section through the upper thigh, demonstrating a large tumor involving two muscular compartments (bicompartmental).

adjuvant therapy. If amputation is to be avoided in the other 50% of patients, adjuvant treatment will be necessary for extension of the surgical margins.

In all techniques of limb salvage, the biopsy tract and surrounding contaminated tissue will require *en bloc* excision, in which an appropriate margin of skin and fat (usually 3 cm) is left intact with the surgical specimen. This is necessary for prevention of a local recurrence in tissue that may have been contaminated with sarcoma cells during the biopsy. In addition, if the definitive procedure is to follow the incisional biopsy immediately, the patient must be reprepped and draped, and separate instruments are necessary so that contamination with tumor is avoided.

The thigh is an anatomic location that serves as an excellent model for limb salvage. Not only is there an adequate amount of soft tissue, but the thigh contains two expendable compartments. In addition, approximately one-third of soft tissue sarcomas of the extremity arise in the thigh.[25] Therefore, we will use the thigh to demonstrate the techniques employed in three types of resection.

WIDE EXCISION OF SUBCUTANEOUS TUMOR

Wide excision is indicated for most subcutaneous sarcomas of an extremity. Irrespective of their histologic grade, subcutaneous sarcomas may confer a more favorable prognosis than do their deep counterparts, probably because they are small when they are first diagnosed. Usually a wide margin that includes a cuff of "normal" skin, subcutaneous fat, and superficial muscle fascia is adequate for local surgical control. Depending on the size and location of the tumor, a cuff of 3 to 5 cm surrounding the tumor is used as a wide margin. Unfortunately, there are no anatomic planes or landmarks that prevent centripetal spread of the sarcoma, and the surgeon must use palpation and inspection of the mass in determining the necessary extent of

dissection. One should also remove about 1 to 2 cm of deep muscle under the deep fascia. Frozen sections obtained intraoperatively may serve to show whether tumor-free margins have been obtained.

If a lesion is very small and is located where there is redundant soft tissue, a primary closure might be attempted. In almost all cases, however, if an adequate wide margin is to be achieved, a split-thickness skin graft will be necessary to cover the remaining muscular bed. A special situation exists when a subcutaneous sarcoma arises over a subcutaneous bony prominence. A candidate for wide excision should have a normal bone scintigram, which indicates that the underlying bone is not involved. Also, a CT scan or MRI should demonstrate a plane of tissue between the tumor and the periosteum. If it does not, wide excision should include a portion of the underlying bone. Muscle transfers with a split-thickness skin graft may be used in most cases for covering of the defect over bone.

The surgical technique involves an elliptical incision 3 to 5 cm beyond and encompassing the palpable tumor mass and the entire biopsy tract (Fig. 75-4). At no time should the pseudocapsule of the tumor be visualized or inadvertently violated surgically. While the skin incision is deepened, take care to avoid beveling toward the tumor; use palpation as a guide (Fig. 75-5). When the superficial muscle fascia becomes visible, incise it in line with the original incision, and not with the retracted skin and fat (Fig. 75-6). To complete the resection, retract the mass with your hand and excise the superficial fascia and a few centimeters of underlying muscle with the electrocautery (Fig. 75-7). Be careful not to pull the tumor away from the underlying fascia inadvertently. Penetrating rake retractors should never be used on the tumor mass, as they may accidentally enter the pseudocapsule with resulting spillage of tumor cells.

Frozen sections of the muscular bed and subcutaneous tissue should not contain any tumor cells. After hemostasis is obtained in the muscle bed, apply a split-thickness skin graft. In harvesting the skin graft, avoid cross contamination with tumor cells.

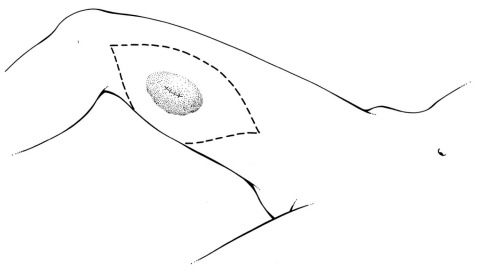

FIGURE 75-4. Elliptical excision for biopsy of a subcutaneous sarcoma of the medial thigh.

RADICAL COMPARTMENTAL EXCISION OF THE QUADRICEPS MUSCLE GROUP

Radical excision of the quadriceps muscles is indicated for intracompartmental soft-tissue sarcomas that arise within this group of muscles. The tensor fasciae latae, sartorius, rectus femoris, vastus lateralis, vastus intermedius, and vastus medialis, along with the tumor and the elliptically excised biopsy tract, are included in the resected specimen. Generally, unless the tumor is low grade and small, the entire muscle group is excised. As a prerequisite for this procedure, all bone margins including the anterior-superior iliac spine, patella, and femur should be free of tumor. This is best demonstrated by a combination of computed tomography and bone scintigraphy. In addition, the superficial femoral vessels must be separated from the tumor by the fascia of the anterior compartment. Computed tomography and, occasionally, arteriography may be used for evaluation of the vascular structures.

With the patient in the supine position, incise the skin from the anterior superior iliac spine to the midportion of the patella. Include the previous biopsy tract in an elliptical incision, to be excised in continuity with the specimen (Fig. 75-8). Develop full-thickness skin flaps, extending laterally from the tensor fasciae latae and the iliotibial tract to the lateral intermuscular septum, and medially to the anterior border of the gracilis

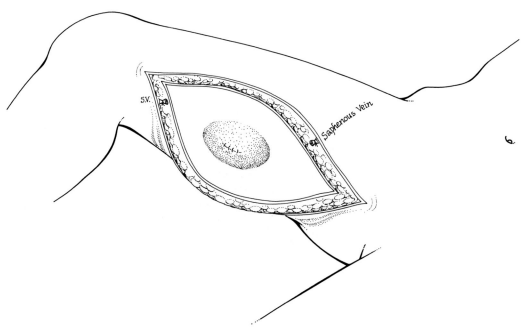

FIGURE 75-5. Incision is carried through the subcutaneous tissue by beveling of the knife away from the tumor.

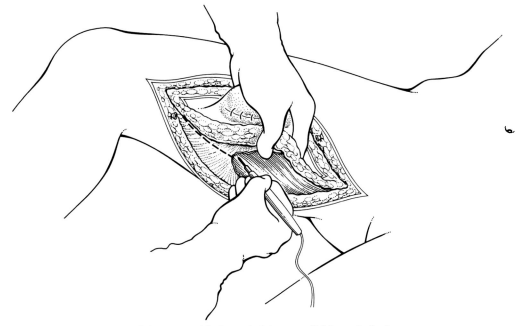

FIGURE 75-6. Excision of the tumor with the underlying superficial muscle fascia.

(Fig. 75-9). In developing the medial flap, preserve the saphenous vein in the flap and dissect it to the fossa ovalis, where the femoral vein is identified.

Just beneath the inguinal ligament, expose the contents of the femoral triangle. From the lateral to the medial aspect, identify the femoral nerve, common femoral artery, and femoral vein. Dissect the femoral vessels over the entire length of the incision, so that they are mobilized from the tissue to be excised (see Fig. 75-9). With gentle medial traction, and proceeding from proximal to distal, preserve the deep femoral artery and vein. However, carefully identify and ligate small muscle branches of the deep femoral artery (see Fig. 75-9). Proceeding distally, retract the sartorius laterally and expose the roof of

Hunter's canal. For completion of the vascular dissection, it is necessary to unroof Hunter's canal by incising the fibers that arise from the adductor magnus muscle, which are coursing over the vessels. Sacrifice branches of the femoral nerve to the quadriceps muscle just distal to the inguinal ligament (Fig. 75-10). Try to preserve the saphenous vein.

Attention is then turned to the origins of the muscles to be excised (see Fig. 75-10). Develop an interval between the tensor fasciae latae and gluteus medius muscle as a lateral margin. Excise the avascular origins of the tensor fasciae latae, sartorius, and rectus femoris from the wing of the ilium, anterior superior iliac spine, and anterior inferior iliac spine, respectively. Continue dissection of the muscular compartment dis-

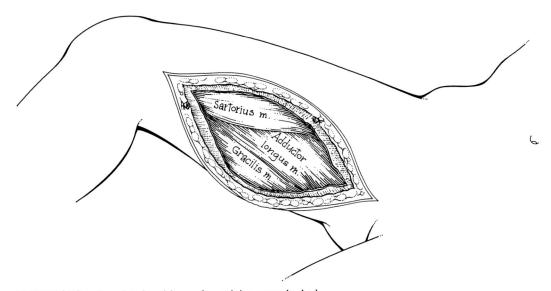

FIGURE 75-7. Completed excision and remaining muscular bed.

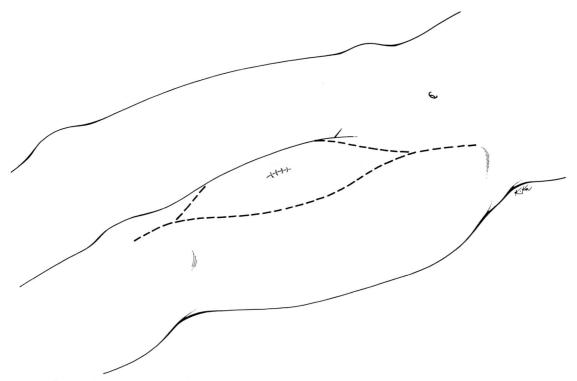

FIGURE 75-8.   Skin incision from the anterior superior iliac spine to the superior pole of the patella, including site of elliptically excised biopsy specimen, for a deep intracompartmental tumor of the anterior thigh.

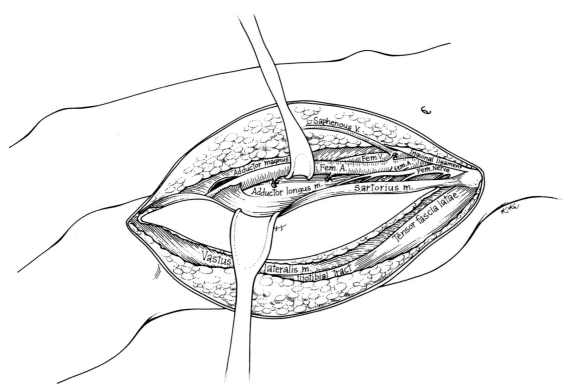

FIGURE 75-9.   Creation of skin flaps and dissection of superficial femoral vessels.

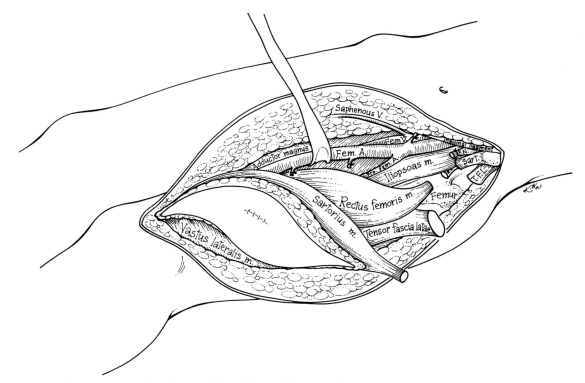

FIGURE 75-10. Release of tendinous origins of the quadriceps muscle group.

tally, with the electrocautery releasing the origins of the vastus lateralis, vastus intermedius, and vastus medialis from the anterior surface of the femur (Fig. 75-11). With upward traction, carry the dissection to the insertions of the vastus laterallis, vastus medialis, vastus intermedius, and rectus femoris, and into the superior portion of the patella, where it is divided. Then deliver the specimen by division of the insertion of the vastus medialis and sartorius into and over the medial collateral ligament, while taking care to avoid damage to the medial supporting structures of the knee (Fig. 75-12). At no time during the dissection is the pseudocapsule of the sarcoma visualized or surgically violated.

After copious irrigation and meticulous hemostasis, attempt reconstruction by releasing the insertions of the gracilis and the short head of the biceps and suturing them into the patella. In addition to covering the anterior aspect of the femur and decreasing the dead space, the transferred muscles may aid knee extension. Place two large drains with their exit sites distal to and in line with the incision, and carefully approximate the skin flaps. Apply a sterile bulky dressing and a knee immobilizer.

Rehabilitation is begun after the drains are removed and initial soft-tissue healing has occurred. It is necessary to be careful to keep even compression on the wound and to leave the drains in place until the drainage has ceased. The knee should be protected from flexion for 6 weeks. Most patients can ambulate without assistance by changing their gait pattern, after they learn to stabilize their knee. However, some older patients may require a cane that assists with balance or is used for ambulation outside the household. Younger adults will have difficulty riding a bike or swimming the crawl stroke.

RADICAL COMPARTMENTAL EXCISION OF THE ADDUCTOR MUSCLE GROUP OF THE THIGH

Radical excision of the adductor muscles is indicated for an intracompartmental soft-tissue sarcoma that arises within this group of muscles. The pectineus, adductor minimus, adductor brevis, adductor longus, adductor magnus, and gracilis, along with the tumor and the elliptically excised biopsy tract, are included in the resected specimen. Again, it is a prerequisite that all bone margins are uninvolved by tumor, as demonstrated by bone scintigraphy, MRI, or computed tomography. In addition, a cuff of "normal" tissue should exist between the tumor and the superficial femoral vessels and it should be demonstrated by computed tomography or MRI. In the absence of direct involvement of the inguinal lymphatic system, its removal is not recommended.[28] Spread of sarcoma to the lymphatics is uncommon, and their dissection and excision are associated with increased postoperative wound complications and distal edema.

With the patient in the supine position, and with the knee and hip flexed and externally rotated, make a skin incision from the pubic tubercle to the medial joint line of the knee (Fig. 75-13). The previous biopsy tract is resected *en bloc* with the tumor by being encompassed in an elliptical incision. Fashion the proximal portion of the incision into a "T," which extends along the superior and inferior pubic rami. Then develop full-thickness skin flaps superior to the sartorius and inferior to the hamstring muscles (Fig. 75-14).

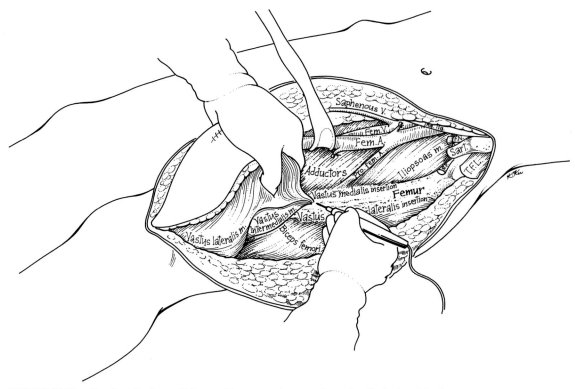

FIGURE 75-11. Continued release of the quadriceps muscle group from the diaphysis of the femur.

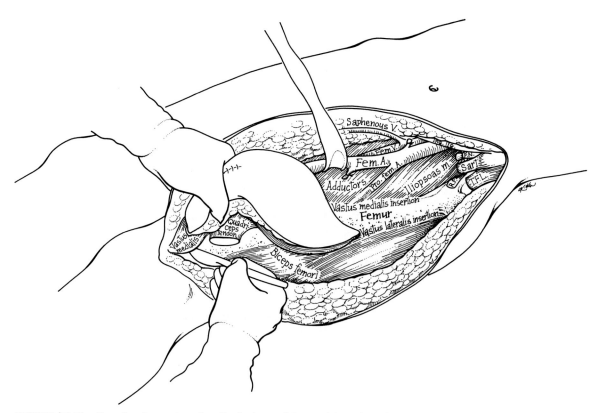

FIGURE 75-12. Completed resection after distal release of the quadriceps insertions.

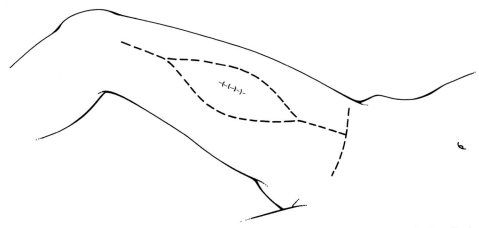

FIGURE 75-13. Skin incision from the pubic tubercle to the medial femoral condyle, including elliptically excised biopsy site, for a deep intracompartmental tumor of the medial thigh.

Expose the femoral artery and vein in the proximal extent of the wound by developing the superior skin flap along the superior pubic ramus. The lymphatic structures and usually the saphenous vein can be carefully preserved. The superficial femoral vessels must be mobilized from the adductor muscles between the femoral triangle and a point just distal to Hunter's canal (see Fig. 75-14). Proceeding from proximal to distal, ligate the medial circumflex femoral vessels, but the deep femoral vessels may be preserved. Carry the dissection distally to the roof of Hunter's canal.

After the superficial femoral vessels are dissected and retracted superiorly, attention is turned to the origins of the adductor muscles. Starting superiorly, release the pectineus, adductor group, and gracilis from their origins on the pubic rami (Fig. 75-15). Leave the obturator externus, quadratus femoris, and hamstring muscles undisturbed, as they, along

with the pelvic bones, form the proximal and inferior margins. Take care to identify and ligate the obturator vein and artery as they exit from the pelvis and enter the medial compartment of the thigh. The obturator nerve should also be isolated and divided.

Continue the dissection distally, with traction applied to the muscle mass and release of the insertions of the adductor muscles from the linea aspera of the femur (Fig. 75-16). The sciatic nerve can be seen; bluntly mobilize it in the inferior portion of the dissection. Bleeding can be minimized by use of the electrocautery. To deliver the specimen, divide the insertions of the adductor magnus from the femur and gracilis at Hunter's canal, where they form a roof over the superficial femoral vessels (Figs. 75-16 and 75-17).

Irrigate the wound copiously, and obtain meticulous hemostasis. Place two large drains with their exit distal to and in line

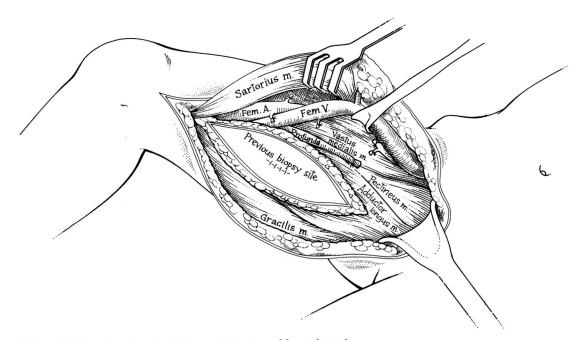

FIGURE 75-14. Creation of skin flaps and dissection of femoral vessels.

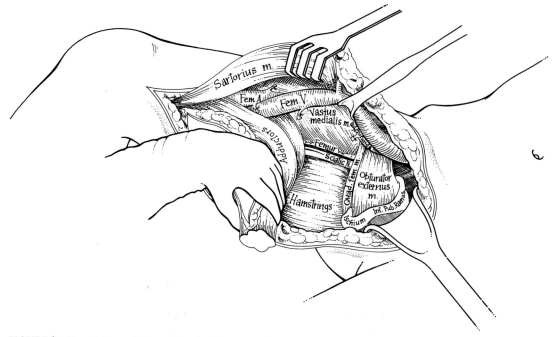

FIGURE 75-15. Release of the origins of adductor muscles.

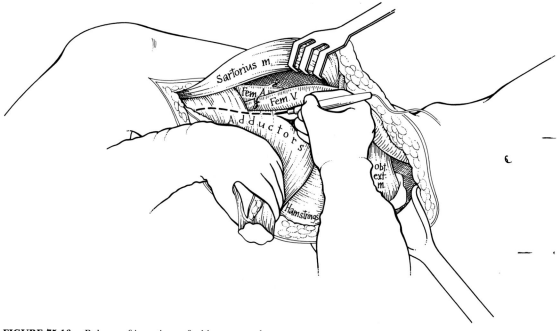

FIGURE 75-16. Release of insertions of adductor muscles.

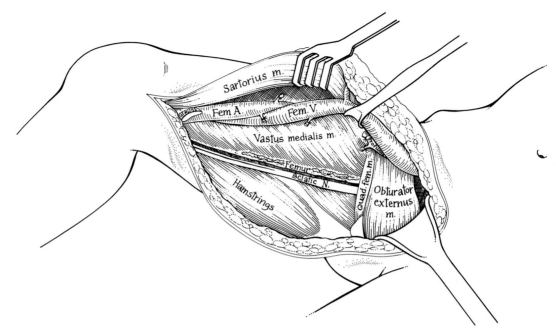

FIGURE 75-17. Completed excision, with remaining femoral vessels, femur, sciatic nerve, and anterior and posterior muscle compartments.

with the skin incision. Approximate the skin flaps, and apply a sterile bulky dressing. Drains should remain in place for at least 3 to 5 days, and a compression dressing should remain in place for 1 to 2 weeks. In general, no specific rehabilitation or bracing is needed, and the patient can expect fairly normal function.

REFERENCES

1. Bowden, L., and Booher, R.J.: The Principles and Techniques of Resection of Soft Parts for Sarcoma. Surgery **44**:963–977, 1958.
2. Cantin, J., McNeer, G.P., Chu, F.C., and Booher, R.J.: The Problem of Local Recurrence after Treatment of Soft Tissue Sarcomas. Am. Surg. **168**:47–53, 1968.
3. Costa, J., Wesley, R.A., Glatstein, E., and Rosenberg, S.A.: The Grading of Soft Tissue Sarcomas. Results of a Clinicohistopathologic Correlation in a Series of 163 Cases. Cancer **53**:530–541, 1984.
4. Eilber, F.R., Eckhardt, J., and Morton, D.L.: Advances in Treatment of Sarcomas of the Extremity. Current Status of Limb Salvage. Cancer **54**:2695–2701, 1984.
5. Enneking, W.F.: Musculoskeletal Tumor Surgery, Vol. 1. New York, Churchill Livingstone, 1983.
6. Enneking, W.F.: Preoperative Staging of Sarcomas. Cancer Treatment Symp. **3**:67–71, 1985.
7. Enneking, W.F., and McAuliffe, J.A.: Adjunctive Preoperative Radiation Therapy in Treatment of Soft Tissue Sarcomas: A Preliminary Report. Cancer Treatment Symp. **3**:37–43, 1985.
8. Enneking, W.F., Spanier, S.S., and Goodman, M.A.: A System for the Surgical Staging of the Musculoskeletal Sarcoma. Clin. Orthop. Rel. Res. **153**:106–120, 1980.
9. Enneking, W.F., Spanier, S.S., and Malawer, M.M.: The Effect of the Anatomic Setting on the Results of Surgical Procedures for Soft Parts Sarcoma of the Thigh. Cancer **47**:1005–1022, 1981.
10. Finn, H.A., Simon, M.A., Darakjian, H., and Martin, W.: The

11. Clinical Utility of Gallium-67 Citrate Scintigraphy in the Staging of Soft Tissue Sarcomas of the Extremities. J. Bone Joint Surg. **69-A**:886–891, 1987.
11. Gunterberg, B, Markhede, G., and Stener, B.: Function after Anterolateral Resection of the Lower Leg for Extirpation of Tumors. Extension and Pronation of the Foot Restored by Transfer of the Tibialis Posterior Muscle. Acta Orthop. Scand. **54**:95–98, 1981.
12. Kearney, M.M., Soule, E.H., and Ivins, J.C.: Malignant Fibrous Histiocytoma. A Retrospective Study of 167 Cases. Cancer **45**:167–178, 1980.
13. Lindberg, R.D., Martin, R.G., Romsdahl, M.M., and Barkley, H.T.: Conservative Surgery and Postoperative Radiotherapy in 300 Adults with Soft Tissue Sarcomas. Cancer **47**:2391–2397, 1981.
14. Mankin, H.J., Lange, T.A., and Spanier, S.S.: The Hazards of Biopsy in Patients with Malignant Primary Bone and Soft Tissue Tumors. J. Bone Joint Surg. **64-A**:1121–1127, 1982.
15. Markhede, G., and Nistor, L.: Strength of Plantar Flexion and Function after Resection of Various Parts of the Triceps Surae Muscle. Acta Orthop. Scand. **50**:693–697, 1979.
16. Markhede, G., and Stener, B.: Function after Removal of Various Hip and Thigh Muscles for Extirpation of Tumors. Acta Orthop. Scand. **52**:373–395, 1981.
17. Morton, D.L., Eilber, F.R., Townsend, C.M., Grant, T.T., Mirra, J., and Weisenburgery, T.H.: Limb Salvage from a Multidisciplinary Treatment Approach for Skeletal and Soft Tissue Sarcoma of the Extremity. Ann. Surg. **184**:268–278, 1976.
18. Rosenberg, S.A.: Soft Tissue Sarcoma of the Extremities. In Sugarbaker, P.H., and Nicholson, T. H. (eds.): Atlas of Extremity Sarcoma Surgery. Philadelphia, J.B. Lippincott, 1984, Chapter 1.
19. Rosenberg, S.A., Kent, H., and Costa, J.: Prospective Randomized Evaluation of the Role of Limb-Sparing Surgery, Radiation Therapy, and Adjuvant Chemotherapy in the Treatment of Adult Soft Tissue Sarcomas. Surgery **84**:62–69, 1978.
20. Rosenberg, S.A., Suit, H.D., Baker, L.H., and Rosen, G.: Sarcomas of Soft Tissue and Bone. In DeVita, V.C., Hellman, S., and Rosenberg, S.A. (eds.): Principles and Practice of Oncology, 2nd ed. Philadelphia, J.B. Lippincott, 1982, pp. 1037–1093.
21. Rydholm, A.: Management of Patients with Soft Tissue Tumors.

Strategies Developed at a Regional Oncology Center. Acta Orthop. Scand. **54** (Suppl.):203, 1983.

22. Simon, M.A.: Current Concepts Review. Biopsy of Musculoskeletal Tumors. J. Bone Joint surg. **64-A:**1253–1257, 1982.

23. Simon, M.A.: Diagnostic and Staging Strategy for Musculoskeletal Tumors. In Evarts, C.M. (ed.): Surgery of the Musculoskeletal System, Vol. 4. New York, Churchill Livingstone, 1983.

24. Simon, M.A., and Enneking, W.F.: The Management of Soft Tissue Sarcomas of the Extremities. J. Bone Joint Surg. **58-A:**317–327, 1976.

25. Simon, M.A., and Finn, H.A.: Anatomic Location of Soft Tissue Sarcomas of the Extremity: Implications for Staging and Treatment. Unpublished data, 1986.

26. Simon, M.A., and Kerns, L.L.: Diagnostic Strategy for Adult Soft Tissue Sarcomas. In Baker, L.H. (ed.): Soft Tissue Sarcomas. Boston, Martinus Nijhoff, 1983, pp. 29–47.

27. Simon, M.A., Spanier, S.S., and Enneking, W.F.: Management of Soft Tissue Sarcomas of the Extremities. In Nyhus, L.M. (ed.): Surgery Annual. Norwalk, Conn., Appleton-Century-Crofts, 1979, pp. 363–402.

28. Sugarbaker, P.H.: Adductor Muscle Group Excision. In Sugarbaker, P.H., and Nicholson, T.L. (eds): Atlas of Extremity Sarcoma Surgery. Philadelphia, J.B. Lippincott, 1984, Chapter 9.

29. Sugarbaker, P.H.: The Treatment of Extremity Soft Tissue Sarcoma by Wide Local Excision plus High Dose Radiation Therapy. In Sugarbaker, P.H., and Nicholson, T.L. (eds.): Atlas of Extremity Sarcoma Surgery. Philadelphia, J.B. Lippincott, 1984, Chapter 15.

30. Suit, H.D., Mankin, H.J., Schiller, A.L., Wood, W.C., and Tepper, J.E.: Staging Systems for Sarcoma of Soft Tissue and Sarcoma of Bone. Cancer Treatment Symp. **3:**29–37, 1985.

31. Suit, H.D., Mankin, H.J., Wood, H.J., and Proppe, K.L.: Preoperative, Intraoperative and Postoperative Radiation in the Treatment of Primary Soft Tissue Sarcoma. Cancer **55:**2659–2667, 1985.

32. Totty, W.G., Murphy, W.A., and Lee, J.K.T.: Soft Tissue Tumors: MR Imaging. Radiology **160:**135–141, 1986.

PART IX

Microvascular Surgery

CHAPTER 76

Management of Arterial Injuries

L. ANDREW KOMAN

Success in the management of arterial injuries has changed dramatically over the last 45 years. During World War II only 3 of 2,471 acute arterial repairs by end-to-end anastomosis were successful.[4] Today, vascular patency following replantation of complete upper extremity amputations is the rule rather than the exception. Thrombosis following the delayed repair of "noncritical" arterial injuries is common, however, even with sophisticated microvascular techniques performed by experienced vascular surgeons.[1,3,10,12,20,22] This chapter presents the techniques necessary to optimize patency following arterial repair, delineates the indications for arterial reconstruction, outlines regimens of postoperative care, and points out potential pitfalls and complications associated with arterial reconstruction.

INDICATIONS FOR ARTERIAL RECONSTRUCTION

Although pulseless extremities may survive on small-collateral and subdermal-plexus flow, there is uniform agreement that revascularization of one or both forearm vessels should be performed if the vessels in the distal extremity are suitable and the patient's overall condition permits. In the reports of World War II arterial injuries reviewed by DeBakey, the rate of amputation of the forearm after ligation of both the radial and ulnar arteries was 39%.[4] Fortunately, isolated injuries to the radial or ulnar artery cause partial or complete distal necrosis ("critical injuries") in less than 5% of extremities.[6,10,13,15,17]

"Critical" arterial injuries always require vascular reconstruction if the portion distal to the injury is to survive. The majority of isolated radial or ulnar artery injuries are not associated with signs of acute vascular compromise, however, and absolute indications for reconstruction of acute noncritical injuries are not so well defined.[7,8,11,13,15,18]

Relative indications for arterial repair, assuming the absence of additional injuries or problems, include objective evidence of inadequate collateral flow; associated transection distal to major collateral inflow; previous injury to major collateral flow; associated major nerve injury (i.e., median or ulnar nerve); and the ability of the surgeon to perform the repair without compromising the extremity should that repair fail.[17] This last relative indication may, in fact, be the most important—we have observed two patients in whom the significant morbidity that occurred was related primarily to the surgical repair of the vessel, not to the injury itself (Table 76-1).

Following unrepaired noncritical forearm arterial injury, there is a slight to moderate decrease in digital blood pressure in spite of a consistent compensatory increase in the flow of the parallel artery. Symptoms depend on associated injuries and the ability of the remaining vasculature to respond appropriately to stress.[9,14,15,20] Associated major nerve injury makes stress-related adverse symptoms more likely.[9]

At the present time, acute arterial reconstruction of "noncritical" injuries should *not* be considered the standard of care. While thrombosis following repair of noncritical injuries remains high (50% to 100%) even after repair by experienced vascular surgeons,[10,12,20] functional disability without repair is generally minimal, often being more dependent upon concomitant injuries than upon the arterial flow.[10,16] Extremities with

TABLE 76-1. "NONCRITICAL" ARTERIAL INJURY: RELATIVE INDICATIONS FOR RECONSTRUCTION

1. Objective evidence of inadequate collateral flow
   a. Poor back bleeding
   b. Low back pressure
2. Transection distal to major collateral inflow
3. Previous injury to collateral vessel
4. Associated major nerve injury
5. Repair performance without compromise of extremity

good capillary refill, good turgor of the digits, and objective evidence of adequate collateral circulation are candidates for revascularization, depending, of course, upon the type of injury, the damage to surrounding associated tissue and vital structures, the timing of repair, the experience and capabilities of the surgeon, and the hospital facilities available. Symptomatic noncritical injuries can be revascularized electively.

PRINCIPLES OF ANASTOMOSIS

In order to obtain reliably patent anastomoses, proper instruments, appropriately sized needles, suture materials of appropriate diameter, adequate magnification, and meticulous microsurgical technique must be employed.

Instrumentation

Numerous microsurgical instruments are available commercially, and which to choose is, in part, at the discretion of the operating surgeon. In general, however, instruments should be simple, corrosion-resistant, and composed of nonglare material, and they should approximate accurately (Fig. 76-1). Scissors and needle holders should have nonlocking spring mechanisms and should be long enough to rest comfortably in the thumb–index finger web space. Sufficient length, by minimizing intrinsic muscle fatigue, will decrease hand tremors and help to minimize technical errors (Fig. 76-2).

Forceps

Smoothly functioning forceps capable of holding without tearing are essential. Their tips should vary in size from 0.2 mm to 0.6 mm. Jewelers' forceps (straight No. 5 and No. 3) traditionally have been used as microsurgical forceps, but unfortunately their tips are easily distorted, which makes them ineffective, and they are not available in lengths greater than 8 to 10 cm. Forceps made specifically for microsurgery are longer and their tips are of forged metal to ensure greater durability (see Fig. 76-1B). A variety of specialized forceps is available for vessel dilatation, stretching, and tissue manipulation (see Figs. 76-1A and B and Fig. 76-3).

Scissors

Microscissors are extremely important. Ideally, they should be 15 to 18 cm long, and their tips should be of forged or case-hardened metal. Adventitial scissors are straight; dissecting

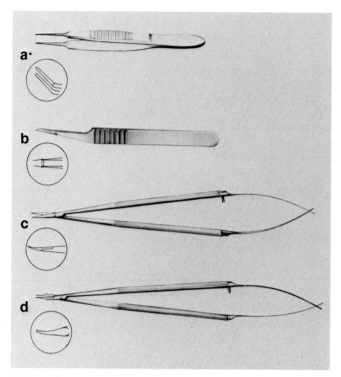

FIGURE 76-1. Basic microsurgical instruments. (*A*) Tying forceps may be used for tissue manipulation and suture handling and tying. (*B*) Specialized forceps may be used to dilate vessels as well as to manipulate tissue and to handle sutures. (*C*) Straight or adventitial scissors and curved or dissecting scissors (*inset*) are used for dissection, tissue preparation, and suture transection. Needles may be manipulated with curved or straight forceps or specialized needle holders (*D*).

scissors have a gentle curve. Tips may be pointed or slightly blunted; the latter will decrease inadvertent vessel damage and may be preferable for the less experienced surgeon. Handles may be straight, rounded, or flared. Many of the newer microscissors are counterbalanced for better "feel" and maneuverability (see Fig. 76-1C and D).

Needle holders

In the past, microsurgical needles were maneuvered with straight or curved jewelers' forceps (see Fig. 76-3A and C).

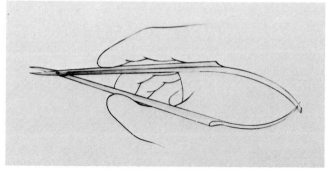

FIGURE 76-2. Technique of manipulating microinstruments of sufficient length to rest in the thumb-index space.

FIGURE 76-3. Microforceps. Tip size, shape and configuration, and length vary. Smooth tips (0.2–0.8 mm) may be used for fine tissue handling, needle manipulation, vessel control, or dilatation (A to D). Specialized tips facilitate tissue manipulation but are inappropriate for suture or needle handling (E to G). Specialized forceps with longer handles and forged tips are easier to manipulate and more durable (G).

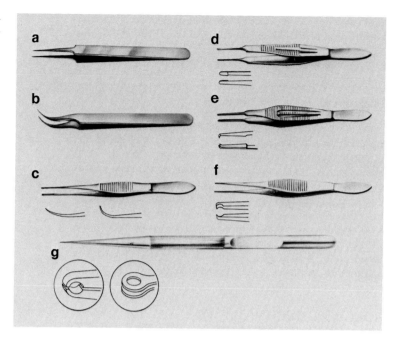

Most microsurgeons prefer specialized needle holders with finely forged tips and smooth action. Longer lengths (15 to 18 cm) improve handling and help to minimize false needle passes, inadvertent vessel wall penetration, and trauma. Needle holders come with straight or curved jaws (see Fig. 76-1D). A gently curved jaw facilitates handling, allowing rotation of the needle through the vessel wall by rolling the handle between the thumb and forefinger. Locking needle holders should be avoided when needles smaller than 150 to 200 μm are used.

Clamps

Microvascular clamps have become more specialized over the years and are available at reliable pressures. Single and double clamps in several sizes are available for vessel approximation or hemostasis (Fig. 76-4). Vessel clamps are designed to hold the vessel, to prevent bleeding, and to allow rotatory approximation. Clamps are available to hold even 0.4-mm (Fig. 76-4A) to 2.0-mm (Fig. 76-4D, center) vessels without damage. Specialized clamps may include stay suture–holding frames, adjustable tension devices, or clamps with variably angled blades. The perfect clamp has enough tension to hold the vessel without damage and jaws 1.5 to 2.0 times the diameter of the vessel. A clamp with excessive pressure will result in damage to the intima and media, and will thus increase the incidence of thrombosis. The use of bar clamps to overcome tension during vessel approximation should be avoided. Clamps are designed as anastomotic aids to facilitate vessel positioning, hemostasis, and suture management.

Special Instruments

Custom-made vessel dilators or smooth probes (lacrimal duct probes, etc.) are often helpful, but they may damage the intima if their surfaces are rough or if they are mishandled. Counterpressors to facilitate needle passes in difficult situations or to avoid the back wall may be useful, and are available from most instrument manufacturers.

Suture Material and Needles

As a basic rule, the smallest needle capable of passing through the vessel wall without bending and the smallest suture strong

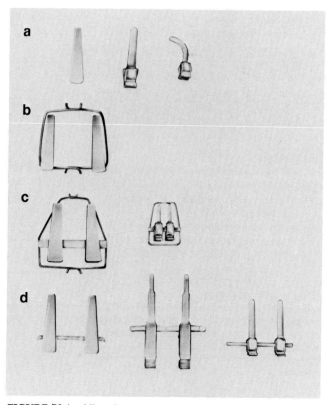

FIGURE 76-4. Microclamps. A large variety of microclamps capable of holding 0.3- to 2.0-mm vessels is available.

enough to approximate the vessel should be chosen. Standard needle sizes range in diameter from 50 to 135 μm and in cord length from 2 to 5 mm. Suture material in sizes 8-0 to 11-0 (35 to 14 μm) is available on most needles (Table 76-2).

Magnification

The choice of magnification relates to vessel size, and large vessels in the proximal forearm or arm may be repaired reliably by many surgeons using loop magnification (2.5× to 6.0×). Since magnification requires concomitant increases in light in order to be effective, it is often simpler to use an operating microscope than the "easier" loops and headlamp when higher power is necessary. It is preferable to do gross dissection using loop magnification of 3.5× to 4.5× and the actual repair using the operating microscope at 6.0× to 30.0×. Inspection of the vessel under high power is essential to prevent inadvertent anastomosis of a too severely damaged vessel.

SURGICAL TECHNIQUE OF ANASTOMOTIC REPAIR

The importance of resecting all damaged tissue cannot be overstated, and failure to identify vessels with severe intimal or medial disruption may be the most significant factor in preventing long-term patency.[16] To minimize inadvertent trauma, the vessel should be identified in relatively normal tissue planes proximal and distal to the transection or thrombosis and then dissected toward the damaged areas. At the same time, associated damaged structures, such as tendons, should be identified and tagged for later retrieval and repair. I place sutures in the lacerated flexor tendons but do not tie them, so that following the anastomoses those tendons can be repaired without additional dissection, thus minimizing the possibility of damaging the vessel repair. Tendon repair carried out before vessel anastomosis may make exposure of the anastomotic site more difficult because of finger, hand, or wrist position, or because of the tendon itself.

Dissection

Identify the periadventitial plane proximal and distal to the transection to allow rapid and safe dissection. Ligate branches from the damaged artery in the proximity of the transection, or cauterized them with bipolar cautery, leaving a 0.5-mm stump. Take care to minimize manipulation of the media or intima.

TABLE 76-2. CHOICE OF MICROSUTURE AND MICRONEEDLE

Anatomic Level	Vessel Size (mm)	Needle Diameter (μm)	Suture Material
Forearm	2.0–3.5	100–135	8-0
Wrist	1.5–2.5	100–135	8-0, 9-0
Hand	1.0–1.8	70–135	8-0, 9-0, 10-0
Digit	0.2–1.5	50–100	9-0, 10-0, 11-0

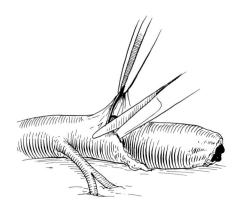

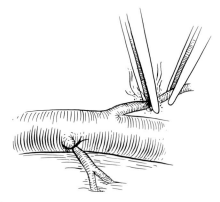

FIGURE 76-5. Periadventitial tissue may be dissected safely after identification of the vessel lumen in the area of dissection. Avoidance of direct manipulation of the lumen minimizes trauma. Branches may be ligated with 8-0 nylon sutures or cauterized using a bipolar cautery.

Periadventitial tissue must be removed so that the vessel wall and lumen can be visualized easily and debris does not interfere with passing or tying the sutures (Fig. 76-5).

Examine the proximal portion of the vessel first. If that end of the vessel can be visualized, probe the lumen gently with a vessel dilator or a lacrimal duct probe. If the lumen cannot be visualized, partially transect the vessel 0.3 to 0.5 mm from the end while applying traction to the vessel stump. The interior of the vessel can then be visualized and dilated safely (Fig. 76-6). Remove the remaining periadventitial debris and transect the end sharply. Prepare the distal segment similarly.

Inspect both portions of the vessel to determine if the intima and media are suitable for anastomosis. Hemorrhage within the media, intimal disruption and multiple stellate tears, or telescoping of the intima, are ominous findings and require additional resection. Intimal damage of itself is an important but not definitive factor in long-term patency. Intimal damage, however, is the most easily recognizable external sign of local trauma; it may indicate significant additional damage, and its presence is associated with a high rate of thrombosis. It is, therefore, good practice to resect the vessel until relatively normal intima is visualized.

Gently reapproximate the vessel ends to assess the degree of tension present. If tension is excessive, additional mobilization of the vessel is necessary by dissection and transection and ligation of collaterals. If there is any question of excessive ten-

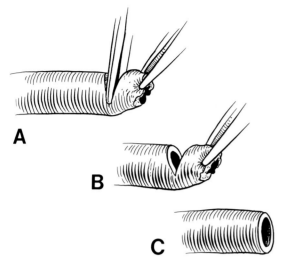

FIGURE 76-6. Blind probing of a transected vessel may cause additional damage. If the lumen of the vessel cannot be visualized easily, grasp the end with a forceps and partially transect the vessel (*A*). The lumen can then be inspected (*B*). If it is suitable for anastomosis at this area, complete the transection (*C*). If the vessel is severely damaged, repeat the process.

sion, then the plan to reanastomose the vessel must be dropped and preparations made to insert a reversed interposition vein graft. Excessive tension at the anastomotic suture line will result in tearing and in intimal and medial damage, and will increase the likelihood of thrombosis.

Vessel ends may be placed in a vessel-approximating clamp or the anastomosis can be done without a clamp. Colored background material makes suture handling easier, by decreasing glare and by improving contrast. Vessel-approximating clamps should be used only to hold the vessel in position, not to overcome excessive tension. I prefer bar clamps oriented initially with the open end away from the primary surgeon. The tension is then adjusted. Irrigate the lumens with heparinized saline and remove any debris from the lumens. Additional loose adventitial tissue should be removed at this time. Make a final inspection of the intima, and if the vessel is suitable, the anastomosis may begin (Fig. 76-7).

Anastomosis

After ensuring that the vessel is not twisted and that tension is not excessive, place stay sutures at 120°. Then place sutures to approximate the "front wall" by halving the distance with each suture, employing a triangulation technique (Fig. 76-8*A*). Rotate the vessel-approximating clamp 180° and similarly approximate the "back wall" (Fig. 76-8*B*). Size or spacing discrepancies should be minimized by applying tension to the adjacent sutures as the first throw of the knot is tied (Fig. 76-9).

When the anastomosis is completed, inspect it and remove the clamp. Additional sutures may be necessary, but early leaks will often stop spontaneously or can be stopped by placing fat over the anastomosis. Spaces of 0.3 mm or less between sutures generally do not require additional sutures. Patency may be confirmed by direct observation or by patency testing (Fig. 76-10).

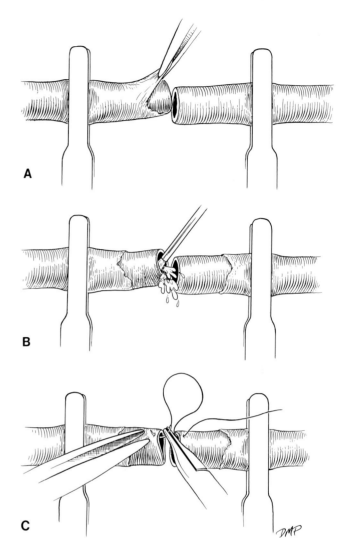

FIGURE 76-7. Vessels may be placed in a bar clamp to facilitate positioning, control bleeding, and maximize ease of repair. (*A*) Periadventitial tissue, which is highly thrombogenic if left within the lumen, is debrided to prevent clot formation and to facilitate visualization of the lumen. The vessel interior should then be irrigated with heparinized saline (*B*) and inspected under high power magnification before the repair (*C*).

Size Discrepancies

Minor discrepancies in size are handled by gentle dilatation of the end of the smaller vessel, oblique cutting of the end of the smaller vessel (not to exceed 30°), end-to-side anastomosis (Fig. 76-11*A*), V-section and closure of the end of the larger vessel (Fig. 76-11*B*), longitudinal slit opening of the end of the smaller vessel (Fig. 76-11*C*), or interposition of appropriate graft material (Fig. 76-11*D*).

Vein Grafting

Vein grafting should be used without hesitation if excessive tension is present or if too much tissue is injured to achieve end-to-end reapproximation after appropriate debridement. Although two anastomoses are necessary with vein grafting,

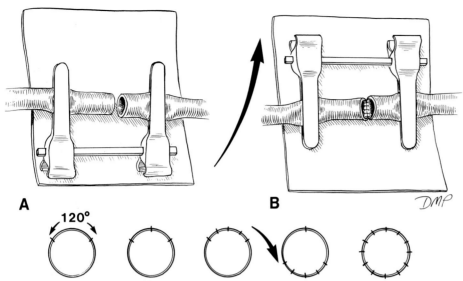

FIGURE 76-8. The vessel ends should be positioned within a bar clamp to facilitate access during vessel repair. Background material is placed beneath the clamp and leveled using saline-soaked sponges. Keeping the entire vessel on a uniform level and in focus will improve visualization during the anastomosis. (*A*) Placement of initial stay sutures at 120° and subsequent "front wall" suture placement. (*B*) The clamp is then flipped 180° and the "back wall" is repaired. Vessel illustrated is 1.5 to 1.8 mm; significantly fewer sutures are needed for smaller vessels.

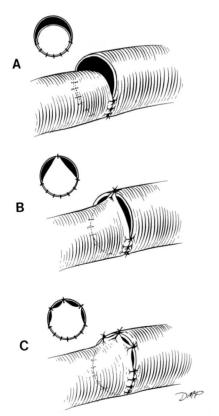

FIGURE 76-9. (*A*) Minimal size discrepancies (10–20%) may be managed by careful triangulation. The first suture is placed, halving the distance between stay sutures. (*B*) As the knot is tied, tension on the stay suture will ensure intimal apposition without buckling. (*C*) Additional sutures are placed similarly.

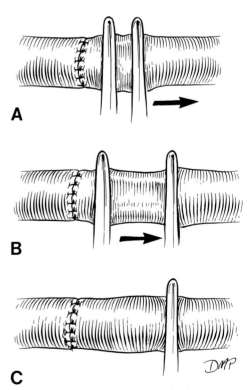

FIGURE 76-10. Technique for patency testing. (*A*) Using minimal pressure, the vessel is occluded distal to the anastomosis. (*B*) Blood is milked from the vessel, which flattens between the forceps. (*C*) The proximal forceps is released and blood will fill the flattened area.

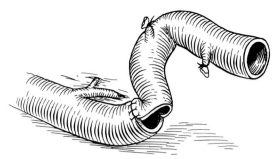

FIGURE 76-12. Vein grafts may be used to overcome deficits in vessel length. The vein must be reversed, but either anastomosis may be performed first and this advantage should be utilized if either anastomosis will be technically more difficult.

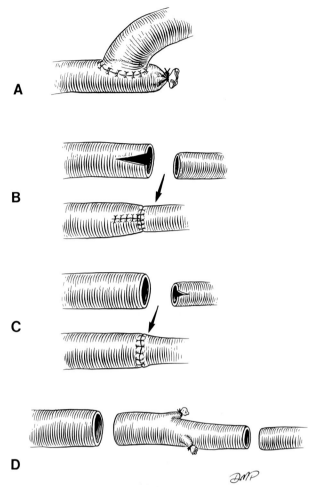

FIGURE 76-11. Compensatory technique for size discrepancy. (*A*) end-to-side, (*B*) V excision and closure, (*C*) V opening, (*D*) vein graft.

patency rates are not significantly less and, in severe injuries, they will be better. For radial artery, ulnar artery, or proximal superficial arch injuries, use the distal saphenous vein or a dorsal vein from the foot. For digital vessels, veins from the volar forearm are excellent donor sources.

Veins must be harvested meticulously, and all branches must be ligated or appropriately cauterized to prevent leakage. A few moments spent in marking the veins before exsanguination of the extremity and inflation of the tourniquet facilitates vein harvest and helps to identify proximally branching veins. If the length of the vein is measured before it is removed, problems related to estimating the resting length should be eliminated.

Reverse the vein graft and place it in position. Performing the more difficult anastomosis first facilitates the repair because of the extra degree of freedom allowed by the mobility of the vein graft. Discrepancies in size are common with vein grafting and may be overcome by the techniques previously discussed (Fig. 76-12).

POSTOPERATIVE CARE

Postoperative care begins with wound closure and application of the dressing. Arterial injuries generally occur in conjunction with open wounds and may be associated with periods of relative tissue anoxia. The former predispose to infection, hemorrhage, and direct tissue damage; the latter may precipitate reperfusion edema. Wound closure must be predicated on sound surgical principles and, if done immediately, should be in conjunction with adequate drainage. Suction drainage is often indicated. Bulky, nonocclusive, compressive dressings reinforced with plaster splints provide the best protection of the injured extremity. The presence of an anastomosis does not require wound closure, and grossly contaminated wounds or wounds that could only be closed under excessive tension should be left open for delayed closure or coverage. If possible, the anastomosis should be covered with skin or muscle. If this is impossible, an artificial membrane or a split-thickness skin graft may be applied directly over the anastomosis. The wrist and fingers should be placed in a functional position, and the elbow flexed to 90° if above-elbow support is indicated.

Fasciotomy

Excessive elevation of interstitial pressure secondary to direct trauma or associated with reperfusion edema results in tissue anoxia and, if untreated, in progression to ischemic necrosis. Any suspicion of a compartment syndrome should be confirmed by tissue pressure measurements. Fasciotomy of the forearm, hand, and digits as necessary should be performed if interstitial pressure is sufficient to compromise nutrient blood flow (i.e., if interstitial pressure is greater than 50% of diastolic pressure).

Antibiotic Prophylaxis and Therapy

In patients with repair of open injuries, broad spectrum antibiotics (cephalosporins) are generally indicated for 5 to 10 days. Whether to use the parenteral or oral route and how long to continue the antibiotics depend on the clinical situation. If the arterial injury occurred through an open injury, the use of antibiotics should be considered therapeutic and not prophylactic. Use of prophylactic antibiotics in repair of closed injuries is not mandatory, and should be left to the discretion of the operating surgeon. Prophylactic antibiotics are usually continued for only 1 to 2 days.

Antithrombotic Prophylaxis and Therapy

The role of and specific indications for anticoagulant or antithrombotic therapy following noncritical or critical arterial injuries have not been defined. Most recommendations are based upon the empiric use of different regimens rather than on scientifically controlled evaluations. In general, sharp lacerations should require minimal antithrombotic agents,[10] while the patency rate following high-energy, crush, or avulsion injuries in which widespread vessel damage might have occurred may be improved by the use of these agents.[10,12,17,20] The antithrombotic agents most frequently employed are heparin, coumadin, low molecular weight dextran (Dextran 40), salicylates, dipyridamole, and ibuprofen.

Our current program, based on clinical experience and scientific considerations but without statistical corroborative data, is as follows: Intraoperatively, we give heparin from the time the initial anastomosis is performed until the dressing has been applied. An initial dose of 2000 to 5000 units of heparin is given immediately before removal of the clamp or deflation of the tourniquet, and 600 to 1000 units are given each hour while the tourniquet is in intermittent use. We do not use heparin postoperatively. If the patient has early evidence of thrombosis following critical artery repair, we reexplore the wound and either reestablish the anastomosis after removing the clot, or interpose a reversed vein graft. In the postoperative period, we give low molecular weight dextran at 20 ml/hr for 1 to 5 days; over the same period, the patient is also given oral salicylates (325 mg twice daily). On discharge, the patient is asked to take one 325 mg aspirin per day for 3 months and ibuprofen 600 mg four times a day for 2 weeks.

Drains

The use of drains following vascular surgery is controversial; many surgeons maintain that proper technique does not require wound drainage. Properly positioned, appropriately chosen drains are rarely a problem, and we have never been sorry that we have placed a drain. Drains may prevent the wound problems and pressure problems that can compromise the repair. In closed wounds, we prefer suction drains made of silicone; in open wounds, stent type drains. Drains should be brought out through separate stab wounds rather than through suture lines.

Monitoring

Postoperative monitoring of capillary refill, turgor, digital temperature, and changes in neurologic function is important and is mandatory for repaired critical injuries. In more proximal limb injuries, periodic palpation of the distal pulses is useful. Repaired noncritical injuries should be observed for signs of ischemia, embolization, or impending compartment syndromes; retrograde pulsations may exist even when thrombosis blocks the repaired artery or the integrity of the anastomotic site has been compromised.[9]

Trained nursing personnel are prerequisite for proper monitoring, and frequent periodic clinical evaluations are crucial. In addition, use of small surface temperature probes,[21] fluorescein monitoring,[19] and periodic Doppler evaluations[2] may be of value.

Salvage Technique

Thrombosis of arterial repairs may be manifested by a sudden and dramatic pallor with loss of capillary refill, decreased tissue turgor, and a rapid fall in limb temperature. Acute arterial thrombosis in repaired critical injuries or with any evidence of inadequate tissue perfusion indicates the need for immediate reexploration. Arterial vasospasm, however, may mimic acute arterial thrombosis and may be precipitated by changes in the local environment (cold drafts or exposure to nicotine) by mechanical or systemic factors, or by centrally mediated factors. Local mechanical difficulties, such as edema, hemorrhage, or external compression, may result in arterial insufficiency by either direct compression or reflex vasospasm. Relief of local pressure may be effected by loosening the dressings, removing skin sutures, or reexploring the site and evacuating the hematoma. Adverse environmental factors must be recognized and changed—patients should be moved away from air conditioning vents, and room temperature should be elevated. Anxiety may be relieved by appropriate medications.

Acute thrombosis occurring between 3 and 10 days after surgery may be treated pharmacologically by anticoagulants such as heparin or by thrombolytic agents such as urokinase or streptokinase. Aberrations in sympathetic tone may be decreased by the use of stellate or axillary blocks, chemical sympathectomy, or continuous peripheral autonomic blockade using a catheter placed on the appropriate nerve with periodic instillation of local anesthetics.

COMPLICATIONS AND PITFALLS

Most vascular complications can be avoided by adhering rigidly to basic principles of technique and avoiding shortcuts. Thrombosis following arterial reconstruction may be divided into intraoperative and postoperative causes. Prompt recognition of potential impending problems and rapid institution of corrective measures will decrease the incidence of complications and increase the patency rates.

Intraoperative Complications

Intraoperative complications include those caused by errors in judgment and errors in technique, and those that are systemic. Judging the extent of vessel damage is extremely difficult, but close inspection of vessels under high-power magnification will minimize inadvertent repair of irreversibly damaged vessels.[17] The surgeon performing the repair is the only judge of the quality of repair. False needle passes, malalignment, intimal inversion, and excessive tension must be realistically assessed, and if any are in question, then the repair must be resected and redone or a vein graft must be inserted. The degree of associated injuries and the quality of soft-tissue coverage are important, since anastomoses left exposed or placed beneath necrotic skin or adjacent to necrotic muscle have a high thrombosis rate.

Assessment of the entire limb, proper debridement, and proper planning before attempted repair will decrease the number of complications. Vessels can be rerouted with vein grafts to undamaged areas; appropriately mobilized myocutaneous or cutaneous flaps or split-thickness skin grafts can be

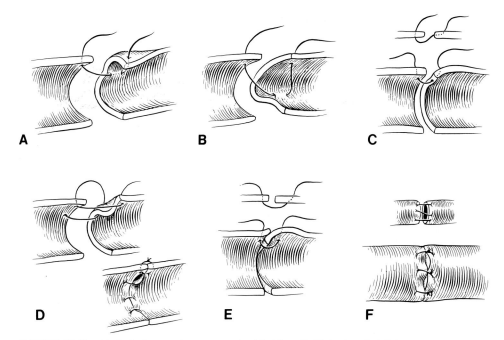

FIGURE 76-13. Technical errors in anastomosis. (*A*) side wall, (*B*) back wall, (*C*) failure to penetrate full vessel, (*D*) uneven lateral placement, (*E* and *F*) uneven approximation of intima.

employed to cover exposed vessels. Dead space must be eliminated and wounds appropriately drained. The development of a compartment syndrome must be kept in mind, and prophylactic or therapeutic fasciotomy performed as necessary.

Technical errors are unforgiving and must be recognized early. Twisted anastomoses or those under excessive tension will not function. Vessels crushed by clamps may function transiently but are predisposed to postoperative thrombosis. The most common errors in anastomotic technique include sutures inadvertently catching the side wall or the back wall of the vessel (Fig. 76-13*A* and *B*); sutures not penetrating the vessel wall (Fig. 76-13*C*); uneven intimal apposition and uneven spacing of sutures (Fig. 76-13*D* to *F*); intimal or adventitial flaps (Fig. 76-13*D*); excessive discrepancy in size without compensation; and intimal and medial damage from needle tears, "false passes," or probes and forceps.

Systemic complications of hypothermia, hypovolemia, or acidosis[5] will result in excessive vasoconstriction and will potentiate thrombosis formation. Low-flow states or "stasis" secondary to these systemic complications may result in thrombosis without pharmacologic protection. If the tourniquet is to be inflated after an anastomosis, protection by heparinization (2000 to 5000 units as an intravenous bolus followed by 600 to 1000 units/hr until the end of the operation) is an effective prophylactic precaution. Vascular spasm is often the result of systemic problems, but may be secondary to local factors. Initial attempts to decrease spasm should be by correction of systemic causes (e.g., giving bicarbonate), or by nonpharmacologic manipulation of the local environment (i.e., raising the room temperature, warm saline bath, adventitial stripping). Pharmacologic intervention with local vasodilators is effective in decreasing spasm but may mask vasoconstriction secondary to abnormal (e.g., twisted) vessels or technical errors. Topical or intravascular agents, including lidocaine, papaverine,

and nitroprusside are rapid and may last 20 min to 2 hr (Table 76-3).[2]

Postoperative Complications

Postoperative causes of thrombosis include environmental factors, systemic problems, pressure phenomena, localized edema, hematoma, external constriction, and infection. Recognition of the problem when it occurs is essential to correction.

Changes in environmental conditions can have a significant effect on peripheral vasoconstriction or vasodilatation. Cold drafts, ambient temperatures below 70°F, and excitement or anxiety decrease peripheral blood flow and should be avoided. Systemic complications, including hypothermia, acidosis, hypovolemia, shock, and vascular disease, may decrease tissue perfusion with resultant thrombosis. Local increases in pressure may result from too tight a wound closure, edema, external compression from "blood casts," or hematoma. Compartment syndromes may occur secondary to concomitant local damage or from more proximal ischemia. Fasciotomy should be per-

TABLE 76-3. LOCAL VASODILATORS

Product	Volume (ml)	Route	Systemic Effects
Lidocaine	1–5	Topical	None
Nitroprusside	5–10	Topical	None
Magnesium sulfate	5–10	Topical	None
Tolazoline	5–10	IA*	None
Papaverine	5–10	IA	None
Nitroglycerin	5–10	IA	Minimal
Prostaglandin (PGE₁)	?	IA	None

* IA = intra-arterial

formed if necessary. Hematoma formation is best prevented by meticulous hemostasis before wound closure and by adequate postoperative drainage.

REFERENCES

1. Ashbell, T.S., Kleinert, H.E., and Kutz, J.E.: Vascular Injuries About the Elbow. Clin. Orthop. **50:**107–127, 1967.
2. Baker, D.W., and Hollaway, G.A., Jr.: Assessment of Viability in Transplanted Tissue. Doppler Techniques Using Acoustic (Ultrasound) and Optic (Laser) Techniques. In Serafin, D., and Buncke, H. (eds.): Microsurgical Composite Tissue Transplantation. St. Louis, C. V. Mosby, 1979.
3. Boswick, J.A.: Injuries of the Radial and Ulnar Arteries. In Proceedings of the American Society for Surgery of the Hand. J. Bone Joint Surg. **49-A:**582, 1967.
4. DeBakey, M.E., and Simeone, F.A.: Battle Injuries of the Arteries in World War II: An Analysis of 2,471 Cases. Ann. Surg. **123:**534–579, 1946.
5. Dell, P.C., Seaber, A.V., and Urbaniak, J.R.: The Effect of Systemic Acidosis on Perfusion of Replanted Extremities. J. Hand Surg. **5:**433–442, 1980.
6. Gelberman, R.H., and Blasingame, J.P.: The Timed Allen Test. J. Trauma **21:**477–479, 1981.
7. Gelberman, R.H., Blasingame, J.P., Fronek, A., and Dimick, M.P.: Forearm Arterial Injuries. J. Hand Surg. **4:**401–408, 1979.
8. Gelberman, R.H., Gould, R.N., Hargens, A.R., and Vande Berg, J.S.: Lacerations of the Ulnar Artery: Hemodynamic, Ultrastructural, and Compliance Changes in the Dog. J. Hand Surg. **8:**306–309, 1983.
9. Gelberman, R.H., Menon, J., and Fronek, A.: The Peripheral Pulse Following Arterial Injury. J. Trauma **20:**948–950, 1980.
10. Gelberman, R.H., Nunley, J.A., Koman, L.A., Gould, J.S., Hergenroeder, P.T., MacClean, C.R., and Urbaniak, J.R.: The Results of Radial and Ulnar Arterial Repair in the Forearm. J. Bone Joint Surg. **64-A:**383–387, 1982.
11. Gross, W.S., Flanigan, D.P., Kraft, R.O., and Stanley, J.C.: Chronic Upper Extremity Arterial Insufficiency. Etiology, Manifestations, and Operative Management. Arch. Surg. **113:**419–423, 1978.
12. Kleinert, H.E., and Kasdan, M.L.: Restoration of Blood Flow in Upper Extremity Injuries. J. Trauma **3:**461–476, 1963.
13. Koman, L.A.: Current Status of Noninvasive Techniques in the Diagnosis of Upper Extremity Disorders. In Evarts, C.M. (ed.): American Academy of Orthopaedic Surgeons: Instructional Course Lectures. St. Louis, C. V. Mosby, 1983, pp. 61–76.
14. Koman, L.A., and Nunley, J.A.: Thermoregulatory Control After Upper Extremity Replantation. J. Hand Surg. **11-A:**548–552, 1986.
15. Koman, L.A., Nunley, J.A., Goldner, J.L., Seaber, A.V., and Urbaniak, J.R.: Isolated Cold Stress Testing in the Assessment of Symptoms in the Upper Extremity: Preliminary Communication. J. Hand Surg. **9-A:**305–313, 1984.
16. Koman, L.A., Nunley, J.A., Wilkinson, R.H., Jr., Urbaniak, J.R., and Coleman, R.E.: Dynamic Radionuclide Imaging as a Means of Evaluating Vascular Perfusion of the Upper Extremity. A Preliminary Report. J. Hand Surg. **8:**424–434, 1983.
17. Koman, L.A., and Urbaniak, J.R.: Ulnar Artery Thrombosis. Hand Clin. **1:**311–325, 1985.
18. Lawrence, H.W.: The Collateral Circulation in the Hand—After Cutting the Radial and Ulnar Arteries at the Wrist. Indust. Med. **6:**410–411, 1937.
19. Lund, F.: Fluorescein Angiography Especially of the Upper Extremities. Acta Chir. Scand. **465**(Suppl.):60–70, 1976.
20. Nunley, J.A., Goldner, R.D., Koman, L.A., et al.: Arterial Stump Pressure as a Determinant of Arterial Patency. J. Hand Surg. **12A:**245–249, 1987.
21. Stirrat, C.R., Seaber, A.V., Urbaniak, J.R., and Bright, D.S.: Temperature Monitoring in Digital Replantation. J. Hand Surg. **3:**342–347, 1978.
22. Trumble, T., Seaber, A., and Urbaniak, J.R.: Patency After Repair of Forearm Arterial Injuries in Animal Models. J. Hand Surg. **12A:**47–53, 1987.

CHAPTER 77

Replantation

JAMES R. URBANIAK

Successful clinical replantation of completely severed limbs has been possible for a quarter of a century. The first successful reattachment of a completely severed human limb was reported by Malt and associates in Boston in 1962.[30] Komatsu and Tamai have been accredited with successful replantation of a completely severed digit in 1965.[25] Zhong-Wei reported the successful replantation of a severed digit in the same year.[66] Over the past 20 years several microsurgery centers throughout the world have achieved greater than 80% success rate in replantation of severed digits, hands, and major limbs.[4,7,9,15,23,24,26,27,29,32,33,40,42,44,45,46,49,50,62,64,65] Additional experience, upgrading in proficiency of microvascular anastomosis, and improvement in microscopes, ultrafine needles, microsuture materials, and instruments, have made replantation the procedure of choice for the management of many amputations.[1,5,6,11,35,57,58]

The most important factor determining the patency of the anastomosis and survival of the replanted or revascularized part is the technical adequacy of the microvascular repair.[48] Successful microsurgery requires familiarity with the operating microscope and microsurgical instruments, and the careful handling of small vessels and surrounding tissues. These skills must be learned in the animal laboratory—not in the clinical operating room. After the surgeon has demonstrated proficiency in the animal laboratory in the repair of microvessels and nerves, then these skills may be transposed to the operating room. In addition, replantation of amputated parts should be done by surgeons who are thoroughly trained in surgery of the upper extremity and hand, and who have had sufficient experience to be able to predict the outcome following replantation of a severed part.

INDICATIONS FOR REPLANTATION

Among the factors that must be considered in deciding to replant an amputated extremity are the predicted morbidity to the patient, survival of the replanted part, functional outcome of the reconstructed limb, and the overall financial outlay of the patient, insurance carrier, or society.[51] The predicted function after replantation should be better than that of a prosthesis or amputation revision. Because the ultimate functional result may be unpredictable, the decision of whether or not to replant an amputated part is often difficult, even for the experienced reconstructive surgeon. Replantation experience does help in the selection process. Based on experience of more than 1200 attempted replantations over a 15-year period, we have developed criteria for proper patient selection. The surgeon must understand that viability alone does not determine success in replantation, but whether the patient achieves useful function.

Factors that influence the selection process include:

1. Level of amputation.
2. Severity of injury (guillotine *versus* crush or avulsion).
3. Warm and cold ischemic times.
4. Age of patient.
5. Segmental injuries.
6. General health of patient.
7. Vocation.
8. Predicted rehabilitation.

Although the final decision regarding replantation rests with the patient and the surgeon, it is generally not wise to allow the patient or the family to make the decision, for they will usually request replantation in cases where there is little chance of survival or function of the replanted part. However, social, ethnic, and religious beliefs about the significance of loss of the amputated part do influence the decision regarding replantation. No listing of indications or contraindications for replantation is rigid or absolute, and the criteria, although generally similar for most replantation surgeons, do vary with individual experience.[51] Future experience with replantation and technologic advances in externally powered prostheses will likely further alter these criteria.

Based on this information, good candidates for replantation are those with amputations of the following types:

1. Wrist (Fig. 77-1).
2. Partial hand (through metacarpal level of palm) (Fig. 77-2).
3. Thumb (Fig. 77-3).

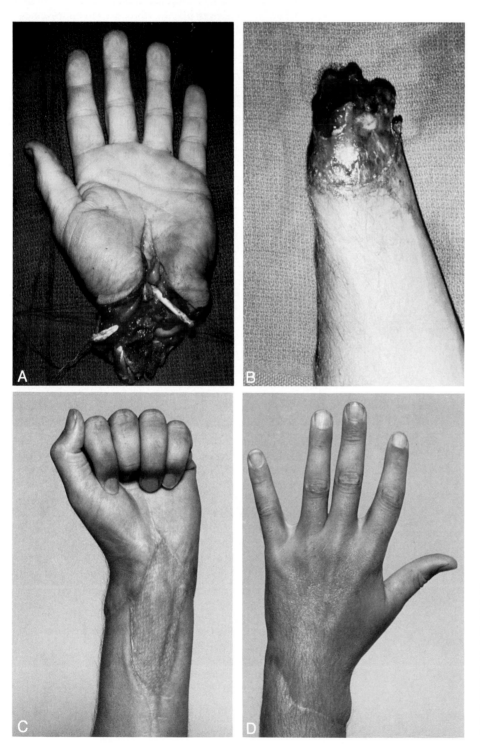

FIGURE 77-1. Good candidates for replantation include amputations at the level of the wrist. (*A* and *B*) A complete amputation at the wrist level in a 21-year-old man. (*C*) The amount of digital flexion and (*D*) extension is seen in this patient 3 years following successful replantation. (Porubsky, G.L., and Urbaniak, J.R.: Limb and Digital Replantation. In Flye, M.W. (ed.): Principles of Organ Transplantation. Philadelphia, W. B. Saunders, In press.)

FIGURE 77-2. (*A* and *B*) Complete amputation of the left index and long finger through the metacarpals in a 20-year-old male. The amputated part was reattached as a composite. (*C*) Flexion and (*D*) extension is shown 1 year later. The patient lacks 5 mm of touching the distal palmar crease with the index finger and 4 mm with the long finger. He returned to work as a meatcutter 3.25 months after the injury.

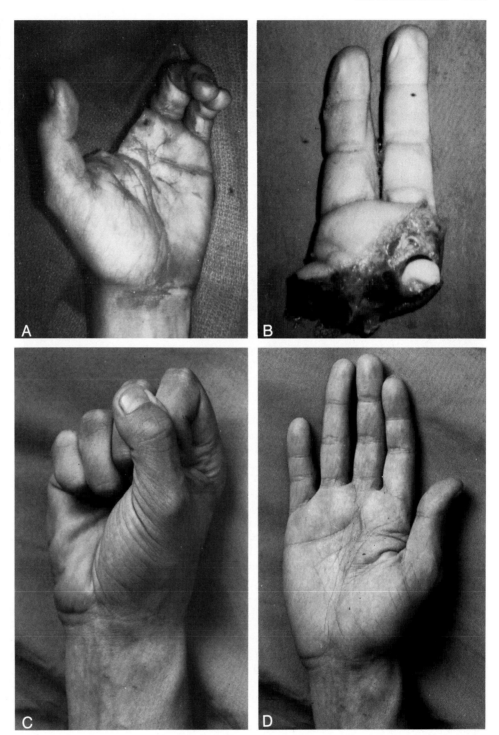

4. Multiple digits.
5. Forearm.
6. Almost any body part of a child.
7. Elbow and above elbow (only sharply severed or moderately avulsed).
8. Individual digit distal to the flexor superficialis insertion.

Although these are not necessarily rigid indicators for replantation, if all other factors are favorable, an attempted replantation of the amputated part should be undertaken. Suc-cessful replantations at the level of the palm, wrist, and distal forearm result in good hand function[26,40,46,61] (see Fig. 77-1). Usually, amputations proximal to the midforearm level are of a crushing or avulsing nature, which produces considerable muscle trauma. Myonecrosis and subsequent infection are frequent problems with this type of replantation, particularly at the elbow or brachial level, and therefore, the surgeon must be extremely selective if choosing replantation at these levels.

Every effort should be made to salvage the amputated thumb in patients of all ages. A replanted thumb is far better

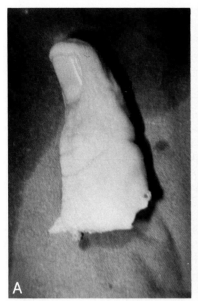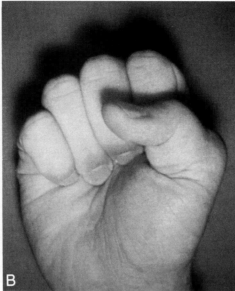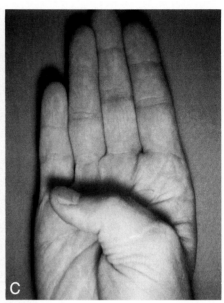

FIGURE 77-3. (*A*) Dominant thumb of a 16-year-old boy was avulsed by a nylon rope. (*B* and *C*) Replantation resulted in less than 5 mm of two-point sensory discrimination and individual interphalangeal and metacarpophalangeal flexion and extension. (Urbaniak, J.R.: Replantation of Amputated Hands and Digits. American Academy of Orthopaedic Surgeons Instructional Course Lectures, Vol. 27., St. Louis, C. V. Mosby, 1978.)

than any type of reconstructed thumb to replace one that has been amputated[10,14,20,34,41,56,60] (see Fig. 77-3). Replantation even as far distal as the nail base should be attempted if vessels for revascularization can be located. If the patient is healthy, there is no upper age limit.[28]

When multiple digits are amputated, a decision must be made about whether to replant all of the digits or just some of them.[39,50] The digits that are least damaged may be transposed to the most useful or least injured amputation stumps. As an example, if the thumb and index finger have been completely amputated in a crushing injury and the distal thumb has irreparable distal vessels, the amputated index finger should be transposed to the thumb stump. This alteration should result in excellent thumb function and cosmetic acceptability.

The level of the amputated digit influences the decision for replantation. Amputations at or distal to the distal interphalangeal joint of the fingers or the interphalangeal joint of the thumb can be successfully replanted if dorsal veins can be located on the amputated part. As a general rule, at least 4 mm of dorsal skin proximal to the base of the nail plate must be present for locating veins suitable for repair.

We replant amputations distal to the superficialis insertion, for an excellent functional result can be achieved and the operating time is not long (usually less than 4 hours).[56] Replantations at this level are usually successful (over 90% viability rate), provide a good appearance, are not painful, allow good function, eliminate the potential for painful neuromas, and permit early return to work (usually less than 3 months).[56,63]

In children, an attempt should be made to replant almost any amputated body part, for if the reattached part survives, useful function can be predicted.[52]

Just as indications for replantation are not absolute, neither are contraindications. Injuries that are generally not considered ideal for replantation include:

1. Amputations in patients with other serious injuries or diseases
2. Amputations at multiple or segmental levels
3. Severely crushed or avulsed parts
4. Amputations in which the vessels demonstrate arteriosclerosis
5. Amputations in mentally unstable patients
6. Amputations with prolonged warm ischemic time
7. Individual finger amputations in the adult at a level proximal to the superficialis insertion (proximal interphalangeal joint or proximal)

Severe crushing or avulsing amputations can frequently be salvaged with the use of vein grafts to replace the injured vessels; however, there are no methods of replacing the most distal vessels in the amputated part. Since arteriosclerotic plaques on the intima frequently preclude functional patency following the reanastomosis of small vessels, the arteries of older patients must be thoroughly evaluated beneath the microscope prior to the reattachment. In addition, patients with diabetes mellitus may have diseased blood vessels, which would lessen the likelihood of repaired vessels remaining patent. Again, the experienced microsurgeon can determine the potential success of an anastomosis by studying the vessel structure beneath the high-powered microscope.

Although it is possible to reconstruct amputations that have been severed at multiple levels,[2] for example, in the phalanges and midpalm or at the elbow and above the elbow, in the same patient, replantation is usually not recommended because the time commitment is large, but the predicted outcome is uncertain.

The patient's mental stability is important when making the decision regarding replantation. Mental instability is not uncommon in patients who sustain completely amputated upper extremities. However, it is frequently difficult to determine the patient's stability during the limited preoperative assessment stage.

Based on assessment of isolated digital replantation, we recommend *not* replanting the isolated finger amputation proximal to the flexor superficialis tendon insertion. Although the cosmetic result is excellent, the overall function of the hand is usually not improved. In fact this digit sometimes "gets in the way." Special considerations, such as in musicians, young females, and children, do influence selection.[56] The patient with a replanted index finger that is amputated at the base of the finger will usually bypass the replanted digit to oppose the thumb to the long finger.

The surgeon must explain to the patient and family the chances of viability, length of surgery and hospitalization, anticipated functional outcome, predicted loss time from work, and cost compared with an amputation revision. Equipped with all of this information most patients and their families will insist on replantation; therefore, the ultimate decision rests with the surgeon. On many occasions the final decision cannot be made until the vessels of the amputated part are carefully evaluated beneath the operating microscope.

PREPARATION OF THE AMPUTATED PART AND PREOPERATIVE CARE

Preservation of the Amputated Part

Preoperative physiologic storage of amputation parts is essential to achieve success in replantation. Generally, if the warm ischemic time of the amputated part exceeds 6 hours, replantation should not be attempted. If the amputated part contains muscle, the ischemic time is much more critical. Muscle is extremely sensitive to ischemia, compared with tissues such as skin, bone, and tendon.[12,13]

Cooling reduces metabolic acidosis, muscle autolysis, and bacterial growth. All amputated parts should be cooled during the transportation to a replantation center. If the part is cooled, successful replantation is possible with cold ischemic times up to 12 hours or even longer if it is a digit, since we have performed successful replantation of amputated digits with cold ischemic times up to 30 hours.[9] However, transportation of the amputated part and the patient should be as rapid as possible.

There are two basic methods of preserving the amputated part:

1. Wrapping the part with gauze moistened with Ringer's lactate or saline solution and placing the package in a plastic bag, which is then placed on ice.
2. Immersion of the amputated part in one of these solutions in a plastic bag and placing this bag on ice.

Either method results in equal viability rates at 24 hours.[59] We prefer the immersion method for the following reasons:

1. The part is less likely to become frozen (frostbitten).
2. The part is less likely to be strangled by the wrappings.

3. Instructions are easier to explain to the primary care physician.
4. Maceration secondary to immersion is not a problem.

Instruments

Since the microsurgery instruments are described in detail in the previous chapter, only the equipment essential for replantation surgery is mentioned here. It is not necessary for the replantation surgeon to have a great variety of expensive microsurgery instruments, but the appropriate instruments must be available, with the working ends well maintained for precision handling of the small microstructures, fine needles, and suture material[35] (Fig. 77-4).

Surgical loupes of 3.5 to 4.5 power are necessary for the initial debridement, exploration, and dissection of the amputated part and injured extremity. It is essential to have an operating microscope with magnification to at least 20 power. Preferably, the operating microscope should have a beam splitter and a double head that allows the surgeon and the first assistant to visualize the same microfield. A foot control for focusing, zoom magnification, and horizontal XY movement are ideal. We use the microscope for the repair of any vessels distal to the axilla.

All of the microinstruments should be at least 10 cm long to allow the handles to rest comfortably in the thumb-index web space. Instrument handles at least 15 cm in length are recommended for all microsurgery instruments to increase the versatility of the instruments when operating in deep fields. Essential instruments include a spring-loaded needle holder and scissors, two sets of jeweler's forceps, a microtipped dilator (lacrimal duct dilator), a microirrigator (30 gauge smooth tipped needle), and various-sized microclips mounted on some type of bar. The less complex the microclip the better. I prefer the type with two tips mounted on a sliding bar.

Other helpful equipment includes small hemoclips to tag the vessels and nerves and to use when isolating or harvesting vessels. A small tipped bipolar cautery is essential in isolating and mobilizing the vascular structures to be repaired. Some type of colored rubber background material is useful in highlighting the vessels and suture material. I prefer a yellow background material, particularly if the lighting is diminished.

The level of the replantation determines the selection of needle and suture size for the vascular repairs. Table 77-1 suggests the appropriate needle and suture size for amputations at the wrist level or distal. The 8-0 or even 7-0 suture may be used proximal to the elbow.

SURGICAL TECHNIQUE

Initial Management of the Amputated Part and Patient

It is advantageous for the replantation team to divide into two subteams when the patient and the amputated part arrive in the emergency room. Particularly with major limb replantations, one subteam immediately transports the amputated part to the operating room for the initial cleansing with Hibiclens and sterile Ringer's lactate solution. The other subteam conducts

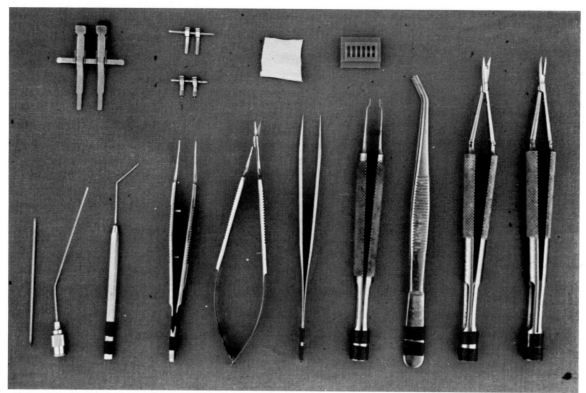

FIGURE 77-4. Basic microsurgery instruments for replantation. *Left* to *right, bottom row:* Kirschner wire, 30-gauge needle, lacrimal duct dilator, tying forceps, spring-loaded straight-blade scissors, jeweler's forceps, Seaber forceps, microclip applier, spring-loaded curved scissors, and needle holder. *Top row:* Large microclip, small microclip (*above*), Van Beek nerve approximator (*below*), blue rubber background material, and hemoclips. (Urbaniak, J.R.: Replantation in Children. In Serafin, D., and Georgiade, N.G. (eds.): Pediatric Plastic Surgery. St. Louis, C. V. Mosby, 1984.)

the patient assessment, with routine physical examination and other studies. The prepped amputated part is the placed on a bed of ice covered with a sterile plastic drape. If multiple digits are involved, these may be cooled by keeping them in a refrigerator or under ice packets until the appropriate time for replantation. Care must be taken not to freeze them.

Using the operating microscope or operating loupes (depending on the size of the amputated part), carefully debride the part or parts and identify and tag the nerves and vessels with small hemoclips. This identification and tagging of the neurovascular structures will save time when working in a bloody field at a later time. The ease in locating the tagged structures, particularly in multiple amputations, is definitely beneficial in the later stages of replantation, particularly if the procedure is lengthy and fatiguing.

TABLE 77-1. NEEDLE AND SUTURE SIZES FOR WRIST AMPUTATION

Location	Needle Size	Suture Size
Wrist and forearm	130	9-0
Palm	100	10-0
Proximal digit	50-75	10-0
Distal digit	50	11-0

Bilateral longitudinal midlateral incisions provide the most rapid and best exposure of the neurovascular structures on the digits (Fig. 77-5). Place the incisions slightly toward the dorsum so that both the dorsal and palmar skin flaps can be reflected to locate the veins, nerves, and arteries with ease. Using magnification, isolate the digital nerves and vessels for 1.5 to 2 cm and tag them. Identify the dorsal veins on the amputated part by reflecting the entire dorsal flap of skin and dissecting the subdermal tissue. In the amputated digit, locating and labeling the veins may be delayed until after arterial anastomosis, which makes identification of veins easier because of the backbleeding, particularly if the patient and amputation stump are ready to receive the amputated part. If the patient is not yet prepared to receive the amputated part, however, then search for the veins at this time in order to diminish the overall operating time. Continue additional debridement after isolation and labeling of the neurovascular bundles.

Shorten and trim the bone appropriately on the amputated digit. Insert an intramedullary Kirschner wire retrograde in the amputated part so the part is prepared for immediate reattachment. If the bone is closely surrounded by soft-tissue structures, a 16-gauge hypodermic needle serves as an excellent protector guide for the 0.45 Kirschner wire. Concurrently, the other subteam thoroughly evaluates the patient in the emergency room with a physical examination, radiographs of the chest and injured extremity, electrocardiogram, complete blood count, blood chemistries, urinalysis, blood type and cross-match, and activated partial thromboplastin time. Intravenous fluids are begun and the patient is given intravenous antibiotics and tetanus prophylaxis if it is indicated. If a long procedure is anticipated, then an in-dwelling urethral catheter is inserted.

Most replantations can be performed under axillary block with bupivacaine (Marcaine), a long-acting local anesthetic. Regional anesthesia is favored because of the peripheral autonomic block, which increases vasodilatation and peripheral blood flow.[19] Some inhalation anesthetics may result in vasospasm and diminished peripheral blood flow. General anesthesia is necessary in the uncooperative patient or for children 12 years or under. The operating room should be kept warm at all times to diminish peripheral vasospasm caused by cooling the body temperature.

Using magnification and tourniquet ischemia, the second subteam debrides the stump and locates and labels the neurovascular structures in a manner similar to the preparation used on the amputated part. The subcutaneous veins on the stump may be difficult to locate, particularly for the inexperienced. Since successful replantation depends on the patency of an adequate number of veins, this is a critical point of the operation. Vein harvesting in the digit may be tedious, and requires meticulous dissection and careful handling of these small structures. After one good vein is located in the subcutaneous layer, this vein may serve as a guide to direct the surgeon to similar veins in the same subdermal plane.

Surgeons without microsurgical experience may be employed in the preparation of the amputated part and patient; however, they must be experienced in dissecting the small vessels lest irreparable damage occur. They may, however, be quite helpful in the bone trimming, bone fixation, and tendon repair and subsequent wound coverage.

Operative Sequence

The sequence of repair of the severed structures in replantation will vary slightly, depending on the level of amputation (digit *versus* levels proximal to the wrist) and type of injury (sharp *versus* avulsion). The technique of replantation of amputated digits is described first, since these amputations are much more common than the more proximal amputations. The variations in technique used for major limb replantations are described subsequently.

The order of repair for digit and hand replantation follows.

1. Vessels and nerve identification and labeling.
2. Tissue debridement.
3. Bone shortening and stabilization.
4. Extensor tendon repair.
5. Flexor tendon repair.
6. Arterial anastomoses.
7. Nerve repair.
8. Venous anastomoses.
9. Skin coverage (fasciotomies when indicated).

Once the vessels and nerves are located and tagged, protect these neurovascular structures during the debridement, which must be thorough. Do not, in haste to reestablish blood flow,

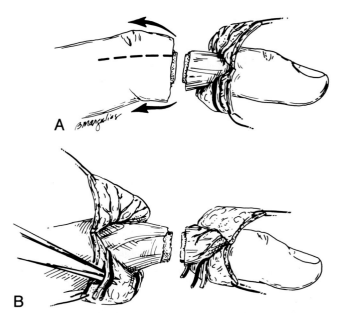

FIGURE 77-5. (*A*) Bilateral longitudinal midlateral incisions provide the most rapid and best exposure of the neurovascular structures of the digit. (*B*) The neurovascular bundles are exposed palmarly and the veins dorsally. (Urbaniak, J.R.: Replantation in Children. In Serafin, D., and Georgiade, N.G. (eds.): Pediatric Plastic Surgery. St. Louis, C. V. Mosby, 1984.)

interfere with the procedures of thorough wound debridement. A pulsating jet lavage is useful in severely contaminated major limb replantations. Excise all necrotic and potentially necrotic tissue, particularly muscle.

All of these structures are repaired primarily, even if primary nerve grafting is necessary for approximation of the severed nerves. It is much easier to make repairs at the time of the initial reconstruction rather than to reoperate secondarily through the repaired structures of the replanted part.

Bone Shortening and Stabilization

The connection of arteries, veins, and nerves should never be performed under tension.[48] Therefore, sufficient bone must be resected to ensure the ease of approximation of normal intima in the vascular anastomosis. Additionally, bone shortening allows easier skin coverage of the repaired veins, particularly on the dorsum of the digits. The amount of resected bone depends on the type of injury. In an avulsion or crushing type of injury, a greater amount of bone must be resected until normal intimal coaptation is possible without tension. For the digit, it is usually necessary to resect 5 to 10 mm of bone, and in amputations proximal to the hand, 2 to 3 cm of bone resection may be indicated. In the avulsion type of injury, even more bone resection is chosen.

If it appears that a great amount of bone must be resected in the digit or in partial hand amputations, the surgeon should use vein grafts to make up the deficit rather than excessive bone shortening.

Many replantation surgeons emphasize that bone shortening is seldom necessary, and recommend vein grafting when there is considerable intimal damage.[47] Bone shortening should usually be chosen over vein grafting, however, because there is frequently concomitant damage to the nerves and other soft tissues. These injured structures can be more easily managed after bone shortening. However, do not hesitate to perform vein grafts when they are indicated, for example when the loss of a potentially functional joint may result from bone shortening. This is particularly true in a child, when excessive bone resection should be avoided as it results in the excision or potential damage to the epiphysis and joint. Every effort must be made to protect the potential epiphyseal growth when trimming bone near the epiphyseal plate. Do not hesitate to perform interposition vein grafts when they are necessary; certainly it is quicker, easier, and less frustrating to perform an interposition graft rather than to redo a difficult anastomosis several times, or even one time.

In replantation of the thumb, the major portion of bone shortening is conducted on the amputated part to preserve maximal length on the stump in the event that replantation fails. This is not always possible, as for example, when attempting to preserve joint function. Several methods of bone fixation are available[20,55] (Fig. 77-6).

1. Longitudinal intramedullary Kirschner wire or wires.
2. Longitudinal intramedullary Kirschner wire plus oblique Kirschner wire to prevent rotation.
3. Crossed Kirschner wires.
4. Interosseous wiring.
5. Intramedullary screw or bone peg.
6. Mini-plates and screws.
7. Tension band technique.

All these methods may be used to stabilize amputations; however, certain methods may be preferred in specific areas, such as near the joint or epiphyseal plates. When possible it is preferable to perform bone stabilization in a digit with double axial Kirschner wires. This is the easiest and quickest method when a motorized drill is used for the careful pin placement. A large bore hypodermic needle (16 gauge) is frequently used as a guide retractor to prevent the surrounding soft tissue from wrapping up near the bone ends. In more than 1200 replantations, we have experimented with all methods of bone stabilization but prefer single or double axial Kirschner wire fixation for the following reasons:

1. Speed and simplicity of the technique.
2. Minimal bone exposure required.
3. Minimal skeletal mass needed for fixation.
4. Ease of reshortening or readjusting the bone approximation if this is deemed necessary.
5. In children, the likelihood of epiphyseal damage is minimal with a single well centered intramedullary longitudinal pin. A second axial intramedullary pin is frequently used for better stability.[21]

Crossed Kirschner wires can cause potential damage in the repaired neurovascular bundles, either by contact or by tethering of the vessels or the protective retaining ligaments. Crossed Kirschner wires are favored for arthrodesis at the joint level. A chevron type of bone cutting for stabilization is recommended in the bone stabilized with crossed Kirschner wire fixation or the tension band principle (that is, two longitudinal Kirschner wires with figure-of-eight wire). Intramedullary screw fixation is ideal for thumb metacarpal stabilization in the complete amputation at this level. This method is easy and rapid, and it provides immediate stability. Its use is limited in arthrodesis of other joints, since some flexion is usually desired. Intramedullary screw fixation provides immediate fixation and allows early motion of the digits; however, it is difficult to remove if the replanted digit becomes infected. Bone pegs or other intramedullary devices can be substituted for the screw. Intramedullary devices are not favored in contaminated wounds. Every effort should be made to preserve the joints in children.

Intraosseous wiring through four drill holes at 12, 3, 6, and 9 o'clock in each end of the bone allows two strains of 24-gauge wire to be placed perpendicular to each other. This type of wiring provides good stability.[31] It is particularly useful for

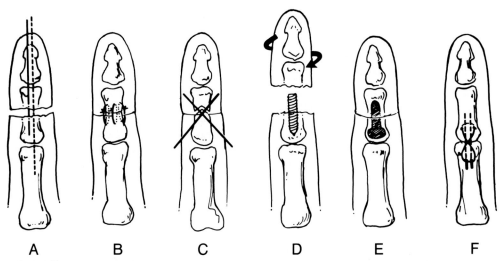

FIGURE 77-6. Methods of bone fixation in replantation. (*A*) Longitudinal intramedullary Kirschner wire or wires (an oblique Kirschner wire may be added to prevent rotation). (*B*) Interosseous wiring. (*C*) Crossed Kirschner wires. (*D*) Intramedullary screw or bone peg. (*E*) Mini plates and screws. (*F*) Tension band technique.

fractures in the metaphyseal areas or even for primary joint fusions. This method also allows immediate or early motion. It does require slightly more time than intramedullary pins, but the amputated part can be prepared by having the wires inserted in one end by one of the teams.

Plate and screw fixation is seldom indicated, since nonunion is rarely a significant problem in replantation of digits. This method requires extensive bone exposure, with the possibility of further soft-tissue damage, and it also requires more time. In major limb replantation, however, it is the preferred method because of the precision and rigid fixation obtained.[36,50]

One of the most difficult problems, even for the experienced hand surgeon, is obtaining proper digital alignment when replanting multiple digits. This may even present a problem when replanting a single digit. The relationships of the digits must be checked frequently in extension and flexion. The cascade and rotation of fingertips must be observed, and in general, when flexed the fingertip should point to the scaphoid bone. Since most replantations do survive, great care must be taken to achieve anatomic alignment and rotation of the replanted parts. In adults there are occasional indications for primary silicone implant arthroplasty with replantations at the joint level, such as an effort to save proximal interphalangeal joint function in a musician. This is particularly true if one of the central digits (long or ring finger) are amputated at the proximal interphalangeal joint level. It is actually quicker and easier to perform a silicone implant arthroplasty than a primary fusion; however, the indications are not common. In addition to bone stabilization, whenever possible an effort should be made to repair the periosteum, capsule, and ligamentous structures to provide better gliding of joints and tendons and to promote joint stability.

Extensor Tendon Repair

Extensor tendons are always repaired primarily, just after bone stabilization, to provide additional stability. Using surgical loupes, two horizontal mattress sutures of 4-0 polyester or absorbable suture are sufficient. It is important to repair the entire extensor mechanism, which may include repair of the extensor hood or lateral band.

In some instances of severe avulsion injuries, no extensor tendons are available for repair. Under these circumstances, extensor tendon grafting is usually recommended as a secondary procedure. In the digits it is usually advisable to perform interphalangeal joint arthrodesis because of the difficulty in reconstructing the extensor mechanism as well as dealing with other injuries. In children, however, primary extensor tendon grafting is favored over interphalangeal joint fusion.[52]

Flexor Tendon Repair

Primary flexor tendon repair is attempted in essentially all replantations. Secondary repair is rather difficult, because of the excessive scarring around the repaired nerves, vessels, and joints. Secondary flexor tendon repair in replanted digits usually requires a two-stage silicone rod procedure in digits other than the thumb. Since this amounts to two additional surgical procedures, it is wise to attempt primary repair.

The Tajima suture method is excellent for primary flexor tendon repair in replantation surgery (Fig. 77-7).[43] With this

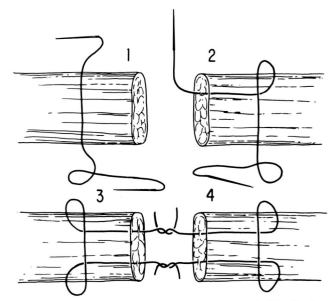

FIGURE 77-7. The Tajima suture method. (Urbaniak, J.R.: Replantation in Children. In Serafin, D., and Georgiade, N.G. (eds.): Pediatric Plastic Surgery. St. Louis, C. V. Mosby, 1984.)

method, sutures can be placed in each end of the tendon initially, and the approximation secured at any time during the procedure. This delayed coaptation has the advantage of allowing the digit to be held in full extension for better vascular and nerve repair, particularly in the area of the proximal phalanx. The type of suture material best suited for this repair is 4-0 polyester on a double-armed curved needle.

Some primary repairs of flexor tendons in replanted digits may require subsequent tenolysis. This should not be performed for at least 3 to 6 months after the primary repair. If a delayed flexor tendon repair is necessary, this may be safely performed as long as 3 months after the initial replantation or revascularization. Usually the two-stage silicone rod method is indicated.

Take care, in retrieving the proximal stumps of the flexor tendons, not to provoke spasm or damage to the proximal arteries. Try to retrieve the proximal stumps by flexing the wrist, massaging the palm, or extending the other digit. If one of these methods does not produce the proximal stump, then insert wall suction tubing in the proximal portion of the flexor sheath, turn on the suction and withdraw the proximal stump. If none of these methods proves profitable, make proximal incisions to locate the tendons.[34] Line grasping with some type of tendon retriever must *not* be performed, because this may produce irreversible damage to the vital proximal vessels.

Another reason for performing primary flexor tendon repair is to relieve any undue compression or tethering of the proximal vascular tree that could be caused by proximal retraction of the severed flexor tendons.

Vascular Repair

Arterial Repair

The details of microvascular technique are not discussed in this section, since there are many excellent descriptions of this subject in other sources[37,58] (see Chapter 76).

The arteries are anastomosed after bone fixation and extensor and flexor tendon repair. With the digit, it is advisable to repair both arteries when possible. If an amputation occurs through the palm or at the wrist level, all available arteries should be anastomosed to increase the chances of survival. Some microsurgeons recommend the repair of only one digital artery to diminish the operating time; however, we have clinically demonstrated that both vessels, even in multiple digital amputations, should be anastomosed to increase the survival rate.[56]

Free the arteries from their surrounding connective tissue for a distance of 1.5 to 2 cm. This dissection should be carried out under the microscope with microsurgical instruments. Small branches from the arteries may be safely coagulated with bipolar cautery. Dissect a severed artery until normal intima is visualized under high-power magnification. Only normal intima must be reconnected (Fig. 77-8). If vessels with normal intima cannot be approximated, further bone shortening is necessary, but preferably interpositional vein grafting is used. The two most critical factors in achieving successful microvascular anastomosis are (1) the skill and expertise of the microsurgeon, and (2) the ease of coaptation of normal intima to normal intima with minimal tension.

Assess the most distal and proximal portions of the exposed vessels to be certain there is no damage to the media or surrounding adventitia. If such injury is detected, further arterial resection and vein grafting are indicated. After sharply trimming the opened end of the proximal stump and enlarging it with jeweler's forceps or a dilator, an excellent pulsating blood flow must occur. Active spurting blood in a digital vessel should produce a persistent stream of at least 10 cm for about 20 to 30 seconds. If such flow cannot be obtained, do not use this vessel for repair. Next, take steps to relieve the proximal vasospasm that is present. Be certain that the patient is not hypotensive, hypovolemic, cold, acidotic, or in pain. All of these factors introduce unwanted vasospasm. Thorough irrigation of the proximal lumen with *warm* heparinized Ringer's lactate solution will frequently relieve vasospasm. If it is certain that no proximal mechanical block exists, papaverine in a 1:20 solution

with normal saline may be placed directly on the proximal vessel or gently inserted into the lumen. This maneuver usually provides an excellent pulsatile flow that lasts for at least 30 minutes. The use of papaverine or similar dilating agents must be attempted with caution, because temporary flow occurs after their use, even from vessels with some damaged intima.

After excellent flow is established in the proximal stump, insert the two vessel stumps into the approximating microclip. Their ends should be coapted without tension. If undue tension is present, use an interpositional vein graft (obtained from the palmar forearm). Trim the vessel ends with sharp straight scissors so that no adventitia is covering the ends of the lumen. Carefully dilate the lumen of each end with jeweler's forceps or a lacrimal duct dilator. After irrigation with heparinized Ringer's lactate solution, reinspect the intima for complete normalcy. Just before beginning the anastomosis, an intravenous bolus of 3,000 to 5,000 units of heparin is given by the anesthesiologist. This dose may be decreased in young children.

Apply two stay sutures of 10-0 monofilament nylon 180° apart. Do not tie the sutures too tightly, because this will produce necrosis of the vessel wall. The distance from the needle insertion to the cut end of the vessel should be about once or twice the thickness of the arterial wall. Do not pinch or touch the intima with the jeweler's forceps. After the application of each knot, carefully irrigate the anastomosis site with heparinized Ringer's lactate and examine it to ensure the suture does not pierce the back wall. After the anterior wall is repaired, turn over the clip approximator and again examine the lumen under high-powered magnification to ensure that all sutures are properly placed. Then place additional sutures in the back wall in a similar manner. Usually six to nine sutures are required to repair an artery 1 mm in diameter. In the small distal vessels, particularly in children, sometime only four or five sutures are necessary for the anastomosis.

A pneumatic tourniquet around the upper arm may be used safely for each vascular anastomosis. If the microsurgery is skillfully and rapidly performed, the patency rate will not be affected by the ischemia. The tourniquet is helpful in diminishing blood loss as well as operating time. The tourniquet should be released at the conclusion of each anastomosis to be certain that the anastomosis is patent and blood flow is strong. The tourniquet may be inflated or deflated many times during the procedure for nerve, artery, and vein repair. If all is going well and the operating field is not obscured by blood, then a tourniquet is not necessary.

Because all available microclips do produce some amount of vessel wall damage, they should not be applied for more than 30 minutes.[57] In a crushing or avulsion injury, and if the procedure is lengthy, serial doses of heparin, 500 to 1000 units every hour, may be given intravenously. Adjust this dosage for children. After completion of the anastomosis and release of the microclips, the blood flow across the anastomosis site should be immediate.

In some avulsion or crush injuries undamaged arteries may be shifted. For example, in a ring finger avulsion the proximal ulnar digital artery may be shifted to the distal radial digital artery if these ends are less traumatized. However, in most instances a vein graft is used if the distal artery is salvageable.[53]

For replantation of thumbs that have been avulsed or amputated, I prefer to use an interpositional vein graft from the

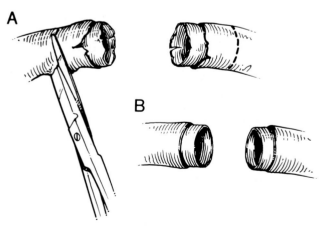

FIGURE 77-8. Preparation of the vessel. (*A*) The damaged portion must be resected until normal intima is visualized under high power magnification. (*B*) Minimal adventitia is stripped to make the lumen clearly visible.

ulnar digital artery of the amputated thumb to the first dorsal metacarpal artery, or to the dorsum of the hand, for an end-to-side anastomosis into the radial artery at the wrist. For expediency, the reversed vein graft is often anastomosed to the ulnar digital artery of the detached thumb prior to bone fixation.[8] The final stage is the proximal end of the vein graft into the artery.

Interposition vein grafts are used in approximately 20% of our replantations to obtain reapproximation of healthy arteries and veins. The palmar aspect of the wrist contains veins of 1 to 2 mm in diameter, which are appropriate for replantation of digits. If the use of vein grafts is anticipated, then the vein grafts are harvested from the forearm in the initial steps of replantation, using loupe magnification before the operating microscope, in an effort to save time.

Within a few minutes after completion of the arterial anastomosis the fingertip will begin to turn pink if there is adequate perfusion. Capillary refill should be excellent and pulp turgor good. If the amputated part has been without blood flow for several hours and has been cooled for a prolonged period, a return of adequate perfusion to the distal part will be delayed. Under these circumstances, the surgeon should proceed with repair of the digital nerve, and repair of the opposite digital artery. In addition to warming the replanted part, this waiting period is often all that is necessary to allow adequate distal perfusion.

Some surgeons prefer to repair the veins prior to the arteries to decrease blood loss and maintain a bloodless field for better vision.[11,37,39] By judicious use of the tourniquet, however, the artery may be repaired first and a dry field maintained. This sequence provides the advantage of earlier revascularization and allows easier location of the most functional veins, detected by their spurting backflow. Additionally, if the veins are repaired first, and a subsequent arterial anastomosis fails to show adequate arterial inflow, the surgeon has wasted valuable time on a nonsalvageable part.

In some difficult replantations, such as distal to the interphalangeal joint, or deep in the thumb index web space, the back wall "inside-out" technique is favored over the conventional two-stage microanastomosis.[58] This method is used in cases where limited exposure of the vessel ends may preclude the possibility of inverting the vessel for back wall repair. The needle is introduced into one vessel end from the outside in, withdrawn, and passed from inside out on the other vessel. Repair begins with the back wall, and by alternating sutures, the knots are worked towards the front wall.

Various "coupling devices," laser methods, and even tissue cements have been developed for small vessel repair, but none have proven as favorable as interrupted suture methods.

Venous Repair

In general, an attempt is made to repair two veins for each artery. It may be necessary to mobilize or harvest veins to achieve the ratio (Fig. 77-9). Perhaps the greatest error in venous anastomosis is attempting to repair veins under tension. If vein harvesting does not allow coaptation without undue tension, then vein grafts must be used. Following this principle will elevate the patency rate and diminish the surgeon's frustration, as well.

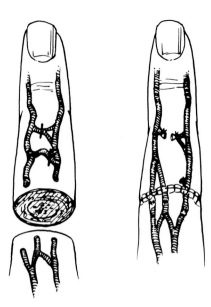

FIGURE 77-9. The mobilization or "harvesting" of veins is a useful method of achieving ease of approximation for vein reconstruction in a completely amputated digit. An attempt is made to repair two veins for each artery.

The technique of vein repair is similar to arterial repair with only a few exceptions. Since the blood flow through the venous system is not as strong as the arterial system, generally fewer sutures are necessary at the anastomosis site. Since the walls of the veins are more fragile than those of the arteries, the application time of microclips must be minimized. The distance from the needle insertion to the cut in the vessel should be two to three times the thickness of the wall. The anastomosis is made easier by constant irrigation of the suture line with warm heparinized lactate solution to float the thin walls apart. Do not waste time repairing the very small veins: instead connect only the largest veins. One large repaired vein is more reliable than two smaller repaired veins.

Nerve Repair

Nerve repair in replantation is usually not difficult, since the bone has been shortened and no tension should be present at the suture line. When feasible, attempt primary repair in all replantations. If direct end-to-end repair is not possible, then use primary nerve grafts. The median antebrachial cutaneous nerve of the ipsilateral extremity is ideal for primary nerve grafting in the digital nerve. Nerve grafts may also be achieved when a portion of the amputated part, such as a severely damaged digit, is to be discarded. The nerves from this discarded segment may be used to bridge the gap. The Van Beek nerve approximator is extremely helpful in repair of nerves in difficult areas.

Cut the nerve ends sharply until pouting fascicles are visualized on each stump. Using the operating microscope align the fascicles on the freshly cut nerve ends and approximate the ends without undue tension.

Repair the nerves with 8-0 to 10-0 monofilament nylon or polypropylene (prolene) by epineurial repair after geographic fascicular alignment has been obtained. In the digital nerves, only two or three epineurial sutures are necessary; more sutures are used in proximal injuries.

Skin Coverage and Dressing

After all of these structures have been repaired and successful revascularization of the replanted part has been ensured, meticulous hemostasis is essential. Failure to obtain complete hemostasis can lead to multiple postoperative problems and failure of the replant. Loosely approximate the skin with a few interrupted nylon sutures. Usually the midlateral incisions are *not* closed to allow for decompression of the digital vessels. Excise all potentially necrotic skin, and place no tension on the skin during the closure. It is important to cover the vessels without constriction from the overlying skin or sutures. A local flap or split thickness graft may be necessary, even for digital vessel coverage. Fasciotomies are indicated if the slightest pressure or constriction occurs. Cover the wounds with small strips of gauze impregnated with petrolatum or antibacterial grease. These strips should *never* be placed in a continuous or circumferential manner around the replanted part.

Although the replanted part should not be covered with any dressing or splint to allow free drainage and early active motion, this is usually not feasible because some type of protective dressing is necessary. The ideal dressing is bulky in nature and uniformly compressive, but not constrictive. The plaster splints

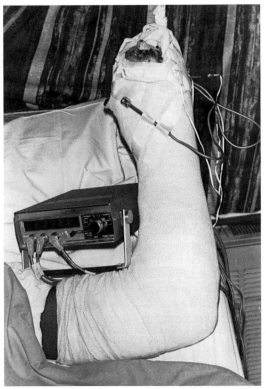

FIGURE 77-10. The postoperative dressing should be bulky in nature and uniformly compressive, but not constrictive. Plaster splints should extend above the elbow to prevent proximal slippage while the hand is being elevated. (Urbaniak, J.R.: Replantation in Children. In Serafin, D., and Georgiade, N.G. (eds.): Pediatric Plastic Surgery. St. Louis, C. V. Mosby, 1984.)

extend above the elbow to prevent proximal slippage while the hand is being elevated (Fig. 77-10). Plaster splints are applied on one side of the hand, usually on the palmar aspect, so that the dorsum of the hand can be inspected if there is a problem after surgery. If flexor tendons have been repaired, however, then the splints must be placed dorsally to prevent unwanted pull of the flexors against the rigid plaster. The extremity in the bulky compressive dressing is then elevated by a rope attached to the dressing. The fingertips remain exposed for application of temperature probes and frequent clinical observation. The environment of the bulky compressive dressing seems to be well suited to the replanted part, as frequently evidenced by increase of blood flow to the fingertips at the conclusion of the dressing application.

The dressing is not changed for about 2 weeks (particularly in children) since anxiety and discomfort produced by the dressing change will frequently incite potentially irreversible vasospasm in the replanted part.[17] If there is excessive bleeding into the dressing, the dressing is changed immediately to prevent constriction from the "blood casts."

Major Limb Replantation

The amputation of major limbs (proximal to the wrist or lower extremity) is less common than amputation of digits or parts of the hand. Replantation of limbs amputated proximal to the wrist level or amputations of a lower extremity below or above the knee employ similar principles with minor modifications. The major difference is related to the increased amount of muscle tissue involved. Because more muscle mass is present in a major limb amputation, the duration of ischemia of the detached part is more critical. While amputated digits that have been detached for 30 to 36 hours may be replanted with a high degree of success, an amputated arm at the elbow area is in jeopardy if it has been avascular for 10 to 12 hours, even with appropriate cooling. Rarely are major limbs cleanly severed, and therefore, the muscle damage is usually quite severe. Extensive muscle debridement of both the detached part and the proximal stump is essential to prevent myonecrosis and subsequent infection. This is a problem in major limb replantation, but it seldom occurs in digital reattachment.[36]

If the amputated part and the patient arrive in the operating room more than 4 hours after injury, it is desirable to initiate immediate blood flow into the detached part. This is best accomplished by using some form of shunt, such as a Sundt or ventriculoperitoneal shunt, to obtain rapid arterial inflow from the proximal vessel to the detached part (Fig. 77-11).[43] Shunting should be performed before bone fixation unless the bone can be rapidly stabilized and early blood flow obtained. After establishment of temporary blood flow, further debridement can be continued, the bone stabilized, and the shunts removed, and a direct arterial repair or interposition vein graftings of the vessels performed.

For major limb replantation, the best bone fixation is obtained by plates and screws. Cross pin fixation is usually the best method of managing the amputations at the joint level. Adequate bone shortening must be carefully planned relative to the type of injury, tissue damage, proximity of the epiphysis, and the particular limb involved. Usually, the plate may be secured to the amputated part after the initial debriding and

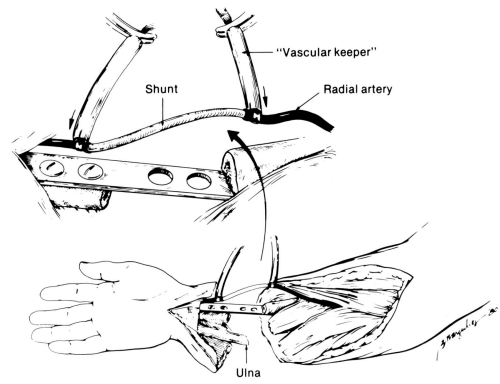

FIGURE 77-11. A Sundt or ventriculoperitoneal shunt is used to obtain rapid arterial inflow from the proximal vessel to the amputated part. This is particularly useful for major limb amputations that arrive in the operating room more than 4 hours after injury. (Urbaniak, J.R.: Replantation in Children. In Serafin, D., and Georgiade, N.G. (eds.): Pediatric Plastic Surgery. St. Louis, C. V. Mosby, 1984.)

then fixed to the stump after blood flow has been established through the shunts (if the ischemic time has been longer than 10 to 12 hours).

Since major limb amputations are usually severe injuries with extensive muscle and other soft tissue damage, a great amount of soft tissue, including skin, muscle, tendon, and nerve must be excised if the replanted part is to survive without infection. It is, therefore, prudent to shorten the bone considerably when possible.

In major limb replantation it is critical to perform the arterial anastomosis before the venous anastomosis. This sequence permits a physiologic washout of noxious agents, such as lactic acid, in the distal part. If this order is reversed, with venous repair first, the return of toxic metabolites to the systemic circulation can cause serious consequences, even death. Administration of intravenous sodium bicarbonate before venous anastomosis is beneficial.[13]

Fasciotomies are almost always necessary in major limb replantation. The most common error of failure of this type of replantation is failure to adequately decompress the replanted limb, leading to myonecrosis with subsequent infection. Meshed split-thickness skin grafts provide some coverage of exposed vessels. Other areas may be closed primarily or grafted several days later.

In replantations of major limbs the patient should be returned to the operating room within 48 to 72 hours to evaluate the state of the muscle tissue. The dressing should be changed with the patient under general or regional block, and any ne-

crotic tissue must be further debrided to prevent infection. In general, no anticoagulation is used for major limb replantations. Most digital replantations are hospitalized for 7 or 8 days, and major limb replantations, of course, require longer periods, depending on the severity of the injury.

POSTOPERATIVE MANAGEMENT AND REHABILITATION

Intelligent and careful postoperative management is essential in achieving a high success rate in replantation surgery.[17] The replanted part in the elevated bulky dressing must be kept warm at all times. It is important to keep the entire patient in a warm comfortable environment during the first week. If the recovery room is cooler than normal room temperature, a patient heater or a warmer is placed over the patient. The patient's room temperature is kept at a minimum of 72°F, and no cool air drafts are allowed in the area.

Anticoagulation therapy remains controversial during the postoperative period. A few surgeons use none, or perhaps only aspirin and dipyridamole (Persantin), and some use all or various combinations of anticoagulations.[11,23,32,45,49] We prefer some type of anticoagulation for all patients. Heparin is generally not indicated in clean cut amputations that are replanted or in cases in which the anastomosis was technically easy and the blood flow was immediately brisk. In these types of patients aspirin, 300 mg bid, dipyridamole, 50 mg bid, and 500 mg of low molecular weight dextran are given for 1 week. In addition, chlorpromazine, 25 mg tid or qid, is added for a tranquilizing effect as well as a peripheral dilator. This drug is valuable in relieving vasospasms secondary to anxiety, which particularly occurs in children.

If the injury is of the avulsing or crushing type, intravenous heparin, 1000 units every hour, is given in adults for 7 days. This dosage is adjusted for children in the range of 100 units per kilogram for 4 hours and is regulated according to the activated partial thromboplastin time, which is maintained 1.5 times normal. If bleeding occurs into the dressing, the dosage is adjusted and the dressing is changed immediately to prevent constriction by a blood cast. Heparin prophylaxis should not be used in amputations proximal to the wrist level.

Capillary refill, pulp turgor, color, and warmth are all useful aids in monitoring the replant, but quantitative skin temperature measurements have proved the most reliable indicators.[16] Digital temperature is monitored with a telethermometer and small surface probes (Fig. 77-12). The normal skin temperature of the digits is 31° to 35°C. The ambient temperature may influence the interpretation of the recordings. Probes are usually placed on the replanted digits, on a normal digit for control, and on the dressing for measurement of the ambient temperature. An abrupt or even gradual change in temperature indicates that the replant may be failing, and steps must be taken to improve the blood flow. If the temperature drops below 30°C or shows more than a 2° drop when compared with the normal digit, appropriate methods of management must be undertaken immediately.

Antibiotics are administered for 7 days. Bed rest or ambulation is determined by the activity level or desire of the patient. If the patient is anxious and choses to remain in bed or appears to be having difficulty with blood flow to the replanted part, then bed rest is advised for 3 to 5 days. However, if the patient is vigorous or energetic, activity is allowed a day or two after the replantation. No smoking is allowed for the patient nor in the patient's room, and all efforts should be made to keep the patient tranquil.

Relatively early active motion is encouraged in most replantations. Since the dressing is not changed for at least 2 weeks, however, immediate early motion is limited. In the patient who has had a replantation distal to the superficialis insertion, movement of the digit is encouraged the following day, since there is really no stress on the flexor or extensor tendons. Otherwise, protective active motion against rubber bands and flexor and extensor outriggers, supervised by a hand therapist, is begun 2 to 3 weeks after the replantation. Since many replantation patients may live at great distances from the treatment center, if more than one digit has been replanted or a major limb has been replanted, the patient is kept in the hospital or maintained in a nearby motel so that daily therapy can be supervised by hand therapists.

COMPLICATIONS

Acute Complications

Acute failures are secondary to inadequate perfusion. Frequently, the surgeon can predict which replantation will have a postoperative problem with perfusion. Some examples are replantation in children under 10 years of age, crush and avulsion injuries, ring avulsion injuries, poor proximal flow observed prior to the arterial anastomosis, and intermittent or inconsistent distal flow despite a technically good anastomosis. When these signs of jeopardy are present, extra postoperative efforts are recommended to enhance the chances of survival.

Intravenous heparin is particularly beneficial in these difficult replantations. The use of an indwelling silicone catheter to administer a regional sympathetic block is particularly helpful.[38] Insert a number 5 silicone urethral stent beside the median or ulnar nerve (depending on the digits revascularized or replanted) to permit regional block to be administered in the postoperative course. The catheter exits from the dressing and has a stop-cock attached so that a nurse can give 5 ml of bupi-

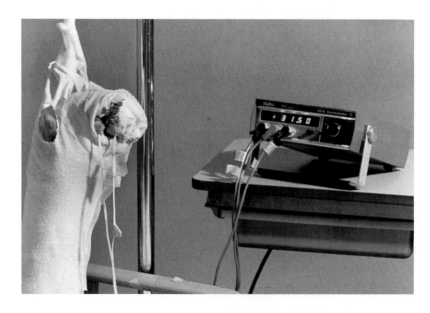

FIGURE 77-12. Digital temperature is monitored with a telethermometer and small surface probes. These quantitative skin temperature measurements have proven to be the most reliable indicators of replantation's status.

vacaine hydrochloride (Marcaine), .025% every 6 to 8 hours. This drug provides regional block anesthesia to diminish vasospasm as well as alleviate pain. This procedure is particularly rewarding in children, because it obviates the use of axillary or brachial block if postoperative spasm develops. We have not administered an axillary nor brachial block in more than 10 years on our service.

If the reattached part appears in jeopardy in the immediate postoperative period as indicated by decreased skin temperature, loss of capillary refill, diminished pulp turgor, or abnormal color, immediate rectifying steps must be taken. Inspect the dressing to rule out any type of constriction. Depression or elevation of the hand may improve the vascular status, depending on whether the problem is arterial or venous. If the patient complains of pain, intramuscular narcotics are helpful, and in fact, should be given prior to any dressing inspection. An intravenous bolus of heparin (3000 to 5000 units) often incites recovery. Chlorpromazine may be given to diminish anxiety and decrease vasospasm. Be sure that the patient is adequately hydrated and that his hematocrit is normal or near normal.

The environment of the patient's room may need to be altered, for example, increasing the temperature, or removing smokers or other agitating factors. All efforts are made to calm the patient, especially children, as pain, fear, and anxiety may initiate peripheral vasospasm.

If normal perfusion does not return after these measures, the decision is made to return the patient to the operating room. Once this decision is made, it should be done within the first 4 to 6 hours after the loss of adequate perfusion. Seldom have we found reexploration to benefit the patient if it occurs more than 1 to 2 days after replantation. If the patient is returned to the operating room within the first 12 to 48 hours, however, many potential failures can be salvaged by redoing the vein graft, removing the thrombus, and usually grafting a previously unrecognized damaged vessel segment.

Subacute Complications

Although infections occur frequently in digital replantations, loss of a replanted digit is rare secondary to infection. The most common infections are pin tract infections, which usually occur more than 4 weeks after the replantation and are easily managed by the removal of pins and the placement of the patient on antibiotics. We have seldom found it necessary to admit a patient to the hospital for pin tract infections.

Infection is both more common and more serious in major limb replantations. The presence of large amounts of muscle that have been rendered ischemic increases the likelihood of infection. To ensure muscle debridement, all major limb replantations should be returned to the operating room in 48 hours for a "second look" procedure. At this time, the wounds are thoroughly inspected and any muscle necrosis that was overlooked during the first procedure is debrided. Infections in major limb replantations may not become apparent until the second week (most commonly 8 to 10 days), and if the infection involves the vascular anastomosis, failure is almost inevitable.

Chronic Complications

The most common chronic complications are:

1. Cold intolerance.
2. Tendon adhesions.
3. Malunion.

Cold intolerance is an almost universal complaint in patients who have undergone digital replantations. However, cold intolerance is not unique to digital replantation and occurs with almost equal incidence in other severe hand injuries, including the amputations that are not replanted.[22] Cold intolerance is related to the adequacy of digital reperfusion, and for this reason an effort should be made to maximize the number of arterial repairs. Cold intolerance improves with time and usually resolves by 2 years. Pain is rare in successful replanted limbs.

Since both the flexor and extensor tendons are usually repaired in replantations, tendon adhesions are frequent, with diminished motion occurring. If this is severe, then tenolysis may be performed as early as 3 months after replantation.

Malunion is most frequently seen after transmetacarpal replantation. These are complex injuries that require multiple tendon, vessel, and nerve repairs, and if care is not taken during bone fixation, rotational malunion may occur. Every effort should be made to properly align digits prior to replantation. Another form of malunion can occur in multiple digit replantations when it is difficult to identify the various digits at the time of surgery. It may become apparent that one digit has been "exchanged" for another. This is primarily a cosmetic problem and does not result in any diminished function.

Nonunion is not a common problem following replantation and it has been reported to occur in 2% to 9% of digital replantations,[32,55,62] but usually nonunions are asymptomatic and I have yet to operate on a patient for a nonunion of a digital replantation.

RESULTS

Most replantation centers are now able to achieve better than 80% viability in replantation of completely severed parts. Our team has achieved 84% viability in replantations of completely amputated parts in 1224 replantations.

By applying the principles presented in this chapter, the experienced and proficient microsurgeon should be able to achieve at least an 80% overall viability rate in replantations. The results, based on our long-term follow-up as well as the reports from major replantation centers, should be as follows:

1. The active range of joint motion should be approximately 50% of normal, depending on the level of injury.
2. Cold intolerance is a definite problem that usually subsides within 2 years.
3. Nerve recovery is comparable to the repair of an isolated, severed peripheral nerve.
4. Cosmetic acceptability is usually better than any amputation revision or prosthesis.
5. Near normal growth may be anticipated in amputations through the diaphyseal region of children. If the injury involves the epiphyseal plate, growth will most always be retarded, although excessive growth has been reported.

6. The best results are obtained in replantations of the thumb, a finger distal to the insertion of the superficialis tendon, and the hand at the wrist level.

REFERENCES

1. Acland, R.D.: Microsurgery Practice Manual. St. Louis, C.V. Mosby, 1980.

2. Belsky, M.R., and Ruby, L.K.: Double Level Amputation: Should it be Replanted? J. Reconstr. Microsurg. **2:**159–162, 1986.

3. Berger, A., Millesi, H., Mandl, H., and Freilingr, G.: Replantation and Revascularization of Amputated Parts of Extremities: A Three-Year Report from the Viennese Replantation Team. Clin. Orthop. **133:**212, 1978.

4. Biemer, E.: Replantation von Fingern und Extremitatenteilen: Technik und Ergebnisse. Chirurgie **48:**353, 1977.

5. Bright, D.S.: Microsurgical Techniques in Vessel and Nerve Repair. American Academy of Orthopaedic Surgeons Instructional Course Lectures, Vol. 27. St. Louis, C.V. Mosby, 1978, pp. 1–15.

6. Bright, D.S.: Techniques of Microsurgery. American Academy of Orthopaedic Surgeons Symposium on Microsurgery Practical Use in Orthopaedics. St. Louis, C.V. Mosby, 1979, p. 40.

7. Buncke, H.J., Alpert, B.S., and Johnson-Giebink, R.: Digital Replantation. Surg. Clin. N. Am. **61:**383–394, 1981.

8. Caffee, H.H.: Improved Exposure for Arterial Repair in Thumb Replantation. J. Hand Surg. **10-A:**416, 1985.

9. Chiu, M.-Y., and Chen, M.-T.: Revascularization of Digits after Thirty-Three Hours of Warm Ischemic Time: A Case Report. J. Hand Surg. **9-A:**63, 1984.

10. Chow, J.A., Bilos, Z.J., and Chunprapaph, B.: Thirty Thumb Replantations. Plast. Reconstr. Surg. **64:**626–630, 1979.

11. Daniel, R., and Terzis, J.: Reconstructive Microsurgery. Boston, Little, Brown, 1977.

12. Dell, P.C., Seaber, A.V., and Urbaniak, J.R.: Effect of Hypovolemia on Perfusion after Digit Replantation. Surg. Forum **31:**503, 1980.

13. Dell, P.C., Seaber, A.V., and Urbaniak, J.R.: The Effect of Systemic Acidosis on Perfusion of Replanted Extremities. J. Hand Surg. **5-A:**433–442, 1980.

14. Early, M.J., and Watson, J.S.: Twenty-Four Thumb Replantations. J. Hand Surg. **9-B:**98–102, 1984.

15. Ferreira, M.C., Marques, E.F., and Azze, R.J.: Limb Replantation. Clin. Plast. Surg. **5:**211, 1978.

16. Gelberman, R.H., Urbaniak, J.R., Bright, D.S., and Levin, L.S.: Digital Sensibility Following Replantation. J. Hand Surg. **3:**313–319, 1978.

17. Goldner, R.D.: Postoperative Management. Hand Clin. **1:**205–215, 1985.

18. Hamilton, R.B., O'Brien, B.McC., Morrison, A., and MacLeod, A.M.: Survival Factors in Replantation and Revascularization of the Amputated Thumb—10 Years Experience. Scand. J. Plast. Reconstr. Surg. **18:**163–173, 1984.

19. Harmel, M.H., Urbaniak, J.R., and Bright, D.S.: Anesthesia for Replantation of Severed Extremities. Anaesthesiologie und Intensivmedizin, Band 138, Neue Aspekte in der Regionalanaesthesia 2, Herausgegeben von H.J. Wust und M. Zindler. Springer-Verlag, Berlin, pp. 161–166, 1981.

20. Hayes, M.C., and Urbaniak, J.R.: Management of Bone in Microvascular Surgery. American Academy of Orthopaedic Surgeons Symposium on Microsurgical Practical Use in Orthopaedics. St. Louis, C.V. Mosby, 1979, p. 96.

21. Ikuta, Y.: Method of Bone Fixation in Reattachment of Amputations in the Upper Extremities. Clin. Orthop. **133:**169, 1978.

22. Jones, J. M., Schenck, R.R., and Chesney, R.B.: Digital Replanta-

tion and Amputation—Comparison of Function. J. Hand Surg. **7:**183–189, 1982.

23. Kleinert, H.E., Juhala, C.A., Tsai, T.-M., and Van Beek, A.: Digital Replantation—Selection, Technique, and Results. Orthop. Clin. N. Am. **8:**309–318, 1977.

24. Kleinert, H.E., and Tsai, T.-M.: Microvascular Repair in Replantation. Clin. Orthop. **133:**205, 1978.

25. Komatsu, S., and Tamai, S.: Successful Replantation of a Completely Cut-off Thumb: Case Report. Plast. Reconstr. Surg. **42:**374, 1968.

26. Kutz, J.E., Hanel, D., and Scheker, L., et al.: Upper Extremity Replantation. Orthop. Clin. N. Am. **14:**873, 1983.

27. Lendvay, P.G.: Replacement of the Amputated Digit. Br. J. Plast. Surg. **26:**398, 1973.

28. Leung, P.-C.: Hand Replantation in an 83-year-old Woman: The Oldest Replantation? Plast. Reconstr. Surg. **64:**416, 1979.

29. MacLeod, A.M., O'Brien, B.M., and Morrison, W.A.: Digital Replantation: Clinical Experiences. Clin. Orthop. **133:**26–34, 1978.

30. Malt, R.A., and McKhann, C.: Replantation of Severed Arms. J.A.M.A. **189:**716, 1964.

31. Massengill, J.B., Alexander, H., Langrama, N., and Mylod, A.: A Phalangeal Fracture Model—Quantitative Analysis of Rigidity and Failure. J. Hand Surg. **7-A:**264–270, 1982.

32. Morrison, W.A., O'Brien, B.M., and McLeod, A.M.: Evaluation of Digital Replantation—A Review of 100 Cases. Orthop. Clin. N. Am. **8:**295–308, 1977.

33. Morrison, W.A., O'Brien, B.M., and McLeod, A.M.: Digital Replantation and Revascularisation: A Long Term Review of One Hundred Cases. Hand **10:**125–134, 1978.

34. Morrison, W.A., O'Brien, B.McC., and McLeod, A.M.: The Surgical Repair of Amputations of the Thumb. Aust. N.Z. J. Surg. **50:**237–243, 1980.

35. Nunley, J.A.: Microscopes and Microinstruments. Hand Clin. **1:**197–204, 1985.

36. Nunley, J.A., Koman, L.A., and Urbaniak, J.R.: Arterial Shunting as an Adjunct to Major Limb Revascularization. Ann. Surg. **193:**271–273, 1981.

37. O'Brien, B.M.: Microvascular Reconstructive Surgery. London, Churchill Livingstone, 1977.

38. Phelps, D.B., Rutherford, R.B., and Boswick, J.A., Jr.: Control of Vasospasm Following Trauma and Microvascular Surgery. J. Hand Surg. **4:**109–117, 1979.

39. Rose, E.H., and Buncke, H.J.: Selective Finger Transposition and Primary Metacarpal Ray Resection in Multidigit Amputations of the Hand. J. Hand Surg. **8-A:**178, 1983.

40. Russell, R.C., O'Brien, B.M., Morrision, W.A., Pamamull, G., and MacLeod, A.: The Late Functional Results of Upper Limb Revascularization and Replantation. J. Hand Surg. **9-A:**623, 1984.

41. Schlenker, J.D., Kleinert, H.E., and Tsai, T.-M.: Methods and Results of Replantation Following Traumatic Amputation of the Thumb in Sixty-Four Patients. J. Hand Surg. **5:**63–69, 1980.

42. Sixth People's Hospital, Shanghai: Replantation of Severed Fingers: Clinical Experience in 162 Cases Involving 270 Severed Fingers. July, 1963.

43. Tajima, T.: History, Current Status, and Aspects of Hand Surgery in Japan. Clin. Orthop. Rel. Res. **184:**41–49, 1984.

44. Tamai, S.: Digit Replantation: Analysis of 163 Replantations in an 11-Year Period. Clin. Plast. Surg. **5:**195, 1978.

45. Tamai, S., Hori, Y., Tatsumi, Y., Okuda, H., Nakamura, Y., Sakmato, H., Takita, T., and Fukui, A.: Microvascular Anastomosis and its Application on the Replantation of Amputated Digits and Hands. Clin. Orthop. **133:**106–121, 1978.

46. Tamai, S.: Twenty Years Experience of Limb Replantation—Review of 293 Upper Extremity Replants. J. Hand Surg. **7:**549–556, 1982.

47. Tupper, J.W.: Vascular Defects and Salvage of Failed Vascular

Repairs. American Academy of Orthopaedic Surgeons Symposium on Microsurgery Practical Use in Orthopaedics. St. Louis, C.V. Mosby, 1979, p. 111.

48. Urbaniak, J.R.: Replantation of Amputated Hands and Digits. American Academy of Orthopaedic Surgeons Instructional Course Lectures. St. Louis, C.V. Mosby, 1978, pp. 15–26.

49. Urbaniak, J.R.: Digit and Hand Replantation: Current Status. Neurosurgery **4:**551, 1979.

50. Urbaniak, J.R.: Replantation of Amputated Parts—Technique, Results and Indications. American Academy of Orthopaedic Surgeons Symposium on Microsurgery Practical Use in Orthopaedics. St. Louis, C.V. Mosby, 1979, p. 64.

51. Urbaniak, J.R.: To Replant or Not to Replant? That Is Not the Question. J. Hand Surg. **8-A:**507–508, 1983.

52. Urbaniak, J.R.: Replantation in Children. In: Serafin, D., and Georgiade, N.G. (eds.): Pediatric Plastic Surgery. St. Louis, C.V. Mosby, 1984, p. 1168.

53. Urbaniak, J.R., Evans, J.P., and Bright, D.S.: Microvascular Management of Ring Avulsion Injuries. J. Hand Surg. **6:**25–30, 1981.

54. Urbaniak, J.R., and Goldner, J.L.: Laceration of the Flexor Pollicis Longus Tendon: Delayed Repair by Advancement, Free Graft or Direct Suture. A Clinical and Experimental Study. J. Bone Joint Surg. **55-A:**1123–1148, 1973.

55. Urbaniak, J.R., Hayes, M.G., and Bright, D.S.: Management of Bone in Digital Replantation: Free Vascularized and Composite Bone Grafts. Clin. Orthop. **133:**184–194, 1978.

56. Urbaniak, J.R., Roth, J.H., Nunley, J.A., Goldner, R.D., and Koman, L.A.: The Results of Replantation after Amputation of a Single Finger. J. Bone Joint Surg. **67-A:**611–619, 1985.

57. Urbaniak, J.R., Soucacos, P.N., Adelaar, R.S., Bright, D.S., and Whitehurst, L.A.: Experimental Evaluation of Microsurgical Techniques in Small Artery Anastomoses. Orthop. Clin. N. Am. **8:**249–263, 1977.

58. Urbaniak, J.R., Steichen, J.B., Weiland, A.J., Wood, M.B., and Seaber, A.V.: Microsurgical Skills Development. Laboratory Manual. American Academy of Orthopaedic Surgeons, 1985.

59. Van Giesen, P.J., Seaber, A.V., and Urbaniak, J.R.: Storage of Amputated Parts Prior to Replantation. J. Hand Surg. **8-A:**60–65, 1985.

60. Vlastou, C., and Earle, A.S.: Avulsion Injuries of the Thumb. J. Hand Surg. **11-A:**51–56, 1986.

61. Wang, S.-H., Young, K.-F., and Wei, J.-N.: Replantation of Severed Limbs—Clinical Analysis of 91 Cases. J. Hand Surg. **6:**311, 1981.

62. Weiland, A.J., Villarreal-Rios, A., Kleinert, H.E., Kutz, J., Atasoy, E., and Lister, G.: Replantation of Digits and Hands: Analysis of Surgical Techniques and Functional Results in 71 Patients with 86 Replantations. J. Hand Surg. **2-A:**1–12, 1977.

63. Yamano, Y.: Replantation of the Amputated Distal Part of the Fingers. J. Hand Surg. **10-A:**211–218, 1985.

64. Yoshizu, T., Katsumi, M., and Tajima, T.: Replantation of Untidy Amputated Finger, Hand and Arm: Experience of 99 Replantations in 66 Cases. J. Trauma **18:**194–200, 1978.

65. Zhong-Wei, C., Meyer, V.E., Kleinert, H.E., and Beasley, R.W.: Present Indications and Contraindications for Replantations as Reflected by Long-term Functional Results. Orthop. Clin. N. Am. **12:**849, 1981.

66. Zhong-Wei, C., Ch'ien, Y.-C., P.Y.S., and Lin, C.T.: Further Experiences in the Restoration of Amputated Limbs. Chin. Med. J. **84:**225, 1965.

CHAPTER 78

Free Tissue Transfers

MICHAEL B. WOOD

Microvascular techniques allow the revascularization, at a distant site, of virtually any tissue mass that can be isolated on a defined nutrient arteriovenous system. Free tissue transfer procedures have proved to be an important addition to the management options for orthopaedic reconstruction.[27,28,30] Although these procedures may involve digits, bone segments, joints, or composite grafts, this chapter is concerned with soft-tissue flaps. Emphasis is placed on the role and technical aspects of microvascular free flap transfer for specific orthopedic reconstructive problems.

INDICATIONS

The indications for free soft-tissue flap transfer in orthopaedic reconstruction are becoming better defined as clinical experience increases. The selection of a free flap for a specific situation should follow a review of available management options, beginning with the most simple and reliable procedures and proceeding to the more complex methods. In general, the most predictable and straightforward procedure expected to satisfy the reconstructive goal should be selected. Therefore, a free-tissue transfer procedure should be chosen only when other methods will likely be inadequate, less reliable, or associated with a higher incidence of complications.

Recipient Site Considerations

Distal Leg and Foot

The most common areas for the consideration of free soft-tissue flaps probably are the foot, ankle, and distal third to middle of the tibial region (Fig. 78-1). These locations usually lack reliable regional or muscle pedicle flaps. The option of skin grafting may exist, but for stable coverage over the distal pretibial surface or over the plantar aspect of the foot, a luxuriant bed of granulation tissue is requisite. Available distant pedicle flaps for the distal tibia, ankle, and foot include ipsilateral thigh flaps, cross-leg flaps, or staged, carrier-mediated tube flaps. The first is almost exclusively indicated in children. Cross-leg flaps may be indicated in children or young adults; however, a cross-leg flap probably should be considered a second choice to free flaps in most adults because of the required immobilization period and the risk of thromboembolic complications. This choice is particularly important when risk factors for venous thrombosis coexist. Multistaged carrier flaps are associated with various complications, including partial skin necrosis, at each stage and thromboembolic risks. Furthermore, prolonged hospitalization is often necessary, so that the multistaged carrier flap is seldom preferred over a free tissue transfer.

Upper Leg, Knee, and Distal Thigh

The indications for free flaps in the upper half of the tibia, knee region, or distal part of the thigh occur substantially less often. In these locations, the more generous girth of soft tissue often provides an excellent bed for skin grafting. When there is not enough soft tissue, an assortment of versatile muscle pedicle flaps is usually available. The typical circumstances for a free

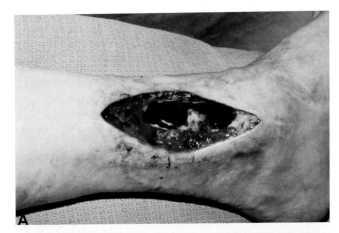

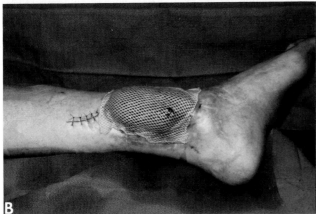

FIGURE 78-1. (*A*) Soft tissue defect with saucerized area of distal tibia, resulting from osteomyelitis. This is an ideal indication for free tissue transfer because of lack of available local muscle pedicle flap in this distal location. (*B*) After obliteration of bony dead space and closure by free muscle flap transfer and skin graft.

tissue transfer in these locations are extensive regional scarring, a prior failed gastrocnemius (or other muscle) pedicle flap, exposure of a knee arthroplasty endoprosthesis, or a massive dead space associated with chronic osteomyelitis.

Pelvis and Upper Thigh

The upper thigh, hip, pelvis, and lower spine regions are infrequent recipient sites for free flaps. Most defects in these regions can be effectively managed by pedicled muscle flaps, rotational groin flaps, or omentum brought out through the abdominal wall. Generally, management by free tissue transfers has been associated with radionecrosis for neoplastic conditions or chronic sepsis of the sacrococcygeal region.

Upper Limb

The indications for free soft-tissue transfer in the upper limb are not well defined. Many surgeons advocate the use of free flaps in preference to distant pedicle flaps, citing the advantages of more rapid limb mobilization and shorter periods of hospital confinement.[8] Although these points may be true in select patients, in general, most soft-tissue defects in the upper

limb can be effectively managed by regional pedicle flaps or a standard groin pedicle flap, with high reliability, a relatively brief period of joint immobilization, and few associated donor site problems.[29] Most patients with defects involving the upper brachium and elbow region are candidates for coverage by an ipsilateral pedicled latissimus dorsi or pectoralis muscle or myocutaneous flap (Fig. 78-2). These flaps can be raised and transferred with little shoulder immobilization and with disfigurement similar to that after most free flap alternatives. Forearm coverage may be managed by a regional radial or ulnar forearm fasciocutaneous flap or occasionally by a local muscle shift. However, if a regional flap is not available for forearm coverage, a free tissue transfer may be indicated in preference to a distant pedicle thoracoepigastric flap (Fig. 78-3). Most defects about the wrist and hand may be managed by a retrograde-based radial forearm flap (Fig. 78-4) or a standard pedicle groin flap (Fig. 78-5). The groin flap is particularly well suited to wrist or hand coverage, while still permitting a reasonable range of motion of all joints in the upper limb.

Reconstructive Goal Considerations

In addition to the location of the soft-tissue defect, the intended reconstructive goal or requirement is an indication for a free tissue transfer in orthopaedic reconstruction.

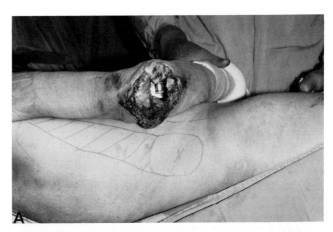

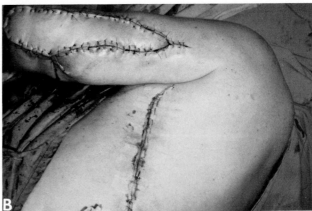

FIGURE 78-2. (*A*) Soft tissue defect over posterior aspect of the elbow, with exposure of total elbow arthroplasty endoprosthesis. (*B*) Closure of defect with ipsilateral vascular island latissimus dorsi flap. Free tissue transfer is not usually required for defects in this location.

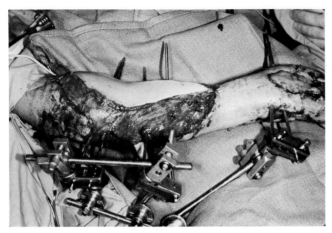

FIGURE 78-3. Free myocutaneous flap transfer for coverage of large soft tissue defect of the forearm.

Primary Soft-Tissue Coverage

In general, a free flap is indicated for primary soft tissue coverage in patients in whom a direct closure, split-thickness skin graft, or local muscle flap is not a reasonable option. Such a situation frequently exists when the defect is massive and particularly when the patient has a joint, nerve, tendon, denuded bone, or endoprosthesis (Fig. 78-6) exposed. Primary coverage by free tissue transfer should also be considered in patients in whom secondary reconstructive operative intervention is anticipated in the field of injury.

Unstable Wound Resurfacing

A closed wound covered by skin graft or one that reepithelialized spontaneously—that is, one likely to have repeated episodes of breakdown—may warrant excision and skin or muscle flap replacement (Fig. 78-7). Such replacement is particularly necessary over the weight-bearing areas of the foot or over the pretibial surface. The ideal patient for flap resurfacing is one who lacks adequate soft-tissue padding over a bony prominence or tendon. At times, instability may be related to venous hypertension. Resurfacing by free tissue transfer in such patients is a less favorable indication and may be followed by continued episodes of epidermolysis.

Obliteration of Dead Space

Perhaps one of the greatest advantages of a free tissue transfer procedure is that it permits the design of a tissue flap of virtually any size and shape. Therefore, this procedure is ideal for patients who require a vascularized flap to obliterate dead space in a cavity with an irregular contour and difficult access. Such a situation arises when there is a saucerized bony defect after debridement for chronic osteomyelitis (see Fig. 78-1). Although a muscle flap appropriately contoured and inset will suffice in most instances, a free flap of omentum in an extremely irregular and narrow cavity occasionally can be used for maximal dead space obliteration.

Sensibility Requirements

An ideal feature of several available free skin flap donor sites is an identifiable sensory nerve with the pedicle that may be neurotized to provide cutaneous sensibility. This feature may be the major consideration that prompts the selection of a free tissue transfer in certain patients. Skin flaps with sensibility seem to be particularly indicated about the heel, sacrum, or digit tips (Fig. 78-8). Most reports indicate that sensory-innervated flaps are reliable for providing protective sensibility and may provide two-point discriminatory ability and stereognosis.

Esthetics

Occasionally, the use of a free flap may be warranted for esthetic reasons only. This possibility occurs when the patient has a significant contour defect despite having stable overlying skin coverage. In such patients, muscle contoured to restore shape and bulk may be indicated.

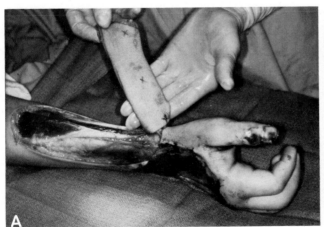
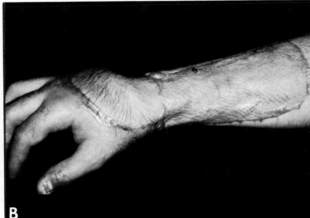

FIGURE 78-4. (*A*) Retrograde vascular island radial forearm flap for coverage of dorsal defect of hand and wrist. The flap is fully isolated on the distal vascular pedicle of the radial artery and venae comitantes. (*B*) Late healed radial forearm flap over dorsum of hand and healed skin graft over donor defect.

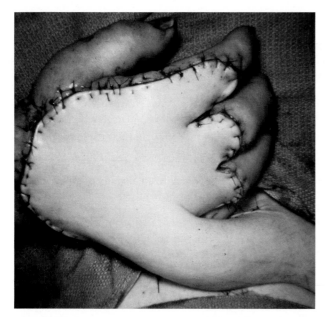

FIGURE 78-5. Pedicle groin flap to cover large soft tissue defect over the dorsum of the hand. In this case, the dorsal defect was too large for closure by a retrograde-based radial forearm flap.

CONTRAINDICATIONS

The chief contraindication to free tissue transfer procedures in orthopaedic reconstruction is the availability of simpler, more reliable treatment options. An additional and also common contraindication is when reconstruction involves an extremity of poor or absent salvage potential. In some patients, a well-conceived amputation and prosthesis may be a better choice of surgical management than to use a free tissue transfer in an attempt to provide coverage of a stiff, short, insensate, painful limb. A final but infrequent contraindication for free tissue transfer is the unavailability of recipient site vessels. The availability of multiple major arteries and veins was once considered a prerequisite for free tissue transfer, although this is no longer true. The liberal use of end-to-side arterial anastomoses has made even the single-vessel limb a reasonable candidate for free tissue transfer. Furthermore, even in patients who do not have an identifiable major vessel near the recipient site, the use of long vein grafts from more proximal vessels, well above the site of vascular occlusion, may allow for a successful free tissue transfer.

PRINCIPLES OF TREATMENT

Free tissue transfer procedures in general have their most important applications for difficult reconstructive problems. For this reason, consistent success regarding flap survival or limb salvage (or both) is most unlikely. However, despite the complexity of the reconstructive challenge, a reasonably high rate of success can be achieved by close adherence to a few well-substantiated principles of preoperative, perioperative, and postoperative treatment.

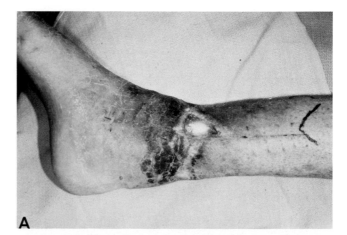

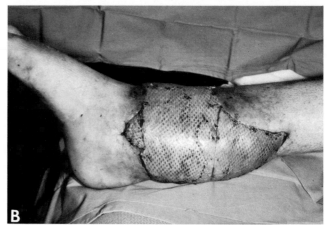

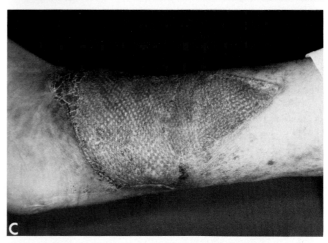

FIGURE 78-6. (*A*) Skin necrosis and slough over distal tibia region 2 weeks after open reduction and fixation of tibia plafond fracture. Note exposure of internal fixation hardware. (*B*) Excision of marginal tissue and coverage by latissimus dorsi free muscle flap and skin graft. (*C*) One year after operation. Fracture healed without sepsis. Note atrophy of muscle and improved soft tissue contour about the distal tibia region.

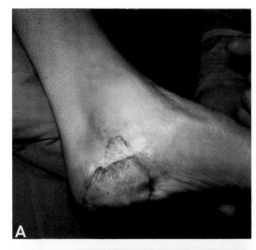

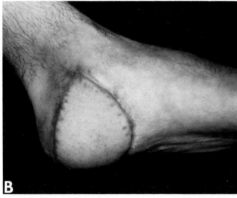

FIGURE 78-7. (*A*) Unstable skin graft over calcaneus. Recurrent episodes of skin breakdown with weight-bearing. (*B*) Three months after excision of skin graft and free cutaneous flap transfer.

Preoperative Care

Before operation, the selection of a free tissue transfer for a specific patient must be guided by proper indications. Once these indications are established, the patient should be well informed as to the procedural risks. In general, the most significant risk is flap failure and necrosis. The reported success rate of various free tissue transfer series is not consistent. However, the lowest success rates involve lower extremity reconstruction, particularly when there is extensive scarring, as is typical for chronic osteomyelitis. I generally advise the patient that the procedure involves a 20% rate of failure or significant complication. The patient should be further advised of alternative treatment options available in the event of failure, including amputation. If a significant complication does occur, preoperative discussion is often invaluable for maintaining patient rapport, confidence, and morale.

Before the actual flap transfer, the patient's vascular anatomy should be defined and his general medical condition and local wound condition stabilized. In most patients, satisfactory vascularity of the recipient site can be confirmed by the presence of the usual major peripheral pulses accompanied by a normal Doppler audible signal. If adequacy of the vascular status of the recipient site is in doubt or if clarification of the patient's vascular anatomy will influence the planning and execution of the procedure, arteriography should be performed. Approximately one-third of patients undergoing free tissue transfer will require preoperative arteriography.

In addition to the usual general medical considerations of a patient undergoing major surgery, patients who are to undergo a free tissue transfer should be advised to abstain completely from nicotine before and for 2 weeks after operation. Moreover, antiplatelet drugs (aspirin and dipyridamole) and drugs to inhibit the formation of superoxide reperfusion products (allopurinol) should be given, beginning 3 to 4 days before operation.

Apart from the patient's general state of health and preparation, fastidious wound care is mandatory before flap transfer. This is particularly important in patients with chronic osteomyelitis. Complete debridement of all necrotic and marginally viable tissue is required. There should be no active suppuration, and, ideally, topical wound cultures should be sterile or yield a scant growth of surface contaminant organisms. If active wound sepsis is present at some time in the patient's clinical course, antibiotics, guided by wound culture results, should be administered systemically. In general, the presence of a progressive growth of healthy granulation tissue over the wound surface is an encouraging indication that wound preparation and debridement is adequate. Skeletal stabilization, if required by fracture union, internal fixation, or exoskeletal fixation, should be obtained either before or concurrent with free tissue transfer.

Perioperative Management

In general, free tissue transfers are lengthy procedures that may require extraordinary periods of anesthesia. Patient positioning and padding of bony prominences, therefore, are very important. Moreover, an indwelling urinary catheter should be placed in most patients undergoing a free tissue transfer.

Although the surgeon usually defers specific decisions regarding anesthesia technique to the anesthesiologist, free tissue transfer procedures have unique anesthesia requirements that merit attention. Whenever possible, regional anesthesia supplemented by intermittent or light general anesthesia or sedation are used. For operations on the lower extremity, epidural anesthesia is induced. This technique is effective for surgical anesthesia as far cephalad as the nipple line. Thus, with this technique, harvest of a rectus abdominis or lower extremity muscle flap and transfer to a lower extremity recipient site can be accomplished without a supplemental general anesthetic. For operations on the upper extremity, an axillary or supraclavicular brachial block is preferred. Both epidural and brachial blocks produce a sympathectomy effect that decreases problems related to vasospasm during the procedure.

Whether regional or general anesthesia or a combination of both is used, care must be taken to prevent peripheral vasoconstriction due to hypovolemia, decreased core body temperature, or metabolic acidosis. Therefore, it is important to use generous volume replacement with blood or plasma expanders, to maintain a warm ambient operating room temperature, and to monitor the pH of the arterial blood regularly throughout the procedure. When epidural anesthesia is used, maintenance

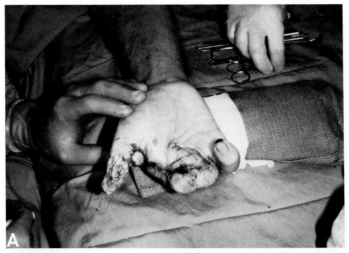

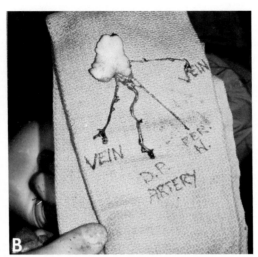

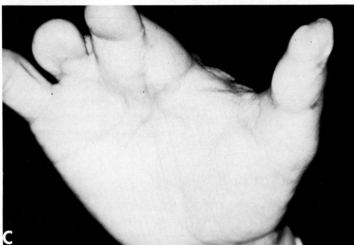

FIGURE 78-8. (*A*) Soft tissue loss, with digital nerve and flexor tendon loss of palmar aspect of thumb. Simultaneous amputation of index, long, and ring fingers. (*B*) Isolated first webspace flap of foot with cutaneous nerves. (*C*) One year after operation. There was two-point discrimination of 8 mm and satisfactory thumb function.

of a continuous infusion for 2 to 3 days after the operation will provide a sustained sympathetic blockade and analgesia to the operative site. It also may be effectively "topped off" a few days later if secondary surgical intervention for flap revision, insetting, or skin grafting is required.

The choice of donor site for the flap is chiefly predicated on the geometry of the soft-tissue defect, the need for a compound flap containing bone, the ease of patient positioning on the operating table, and surgeon or patient preference. Defects needing both bone and soft-tissue reconstruction frequently require a compound osteocutaneous flap, usually from the fibula or iliac crest region. Defects involving only soft tissue or with bone defects amenable to standard bone grafting techniques may be effectively managed by a wide variety of flaps. Although cutaneous and myocutaneous flaps may be used, muscle flaps covered by a split-thickness skin graft are preferred for most orthopaedic soft-tissue reconstructive problems. A muscle flap usually can be obtained with a direct, tension-free skin closure of the donor site, thus minimizing the broad, irregular scar so characteristic of donor site incisions closed under tension. Furthermore, and of particular relevance about the ankle and foot, a muscle flap covered by skin graft will atrophy to a remarkable degree, leaving a minimum of

undesirable bulk (see Fig. 78-6*C*). A cutaneous or myocutaneous flap, however, includes an obligatory amount of adipose subcutaneous tissue, which may require a secondary debulking if the flap is functionally or esthetically objectionable.

Many different muscle flaps are available, including the tensor fascia femoris, gracilis, gastrocnemius, pectoralis major, and serratus anterior. However, the most widely used donor muscle is either the latissimus dorsi or the rectus abdominis. Both of these muscles will supply a flat sheet that easily conforms to a deep, irregular soft-tissue or bone cavity. The rectus abdominis offers less surface area than the latissimus dorsi but is adequate for most patients who require a free flap. Generally, the choice of latissimus dorsi or rectus abdominis is directed by the ease of patient positioning. When access to the recipient site is facilitated by the lateral or prone position, the latissimus dorsi is preferred. Conversely, when a recumbent position is best suited, the rectus abdominis is most easily accessible. When the choice is equivocal, the rectus abdominis is preferred over the latissimus dorsi for lower extremity reconstruction because the patient experiences less discomfort at the donor site when crutches are used during the immediate postoperative period, and seroma problems at the donor site are also less.

With the exception of one-vessel limbs, most free tissue transfers will require the surgeon to choose the most appropriate recipient site vessels for anastomosis. The use of a heavily scarred or previously occluded vessel should be avoided. When perivascular scarring is not a problem, we select the posterior tibial vessels about the distal tibia or ankle, the popliteal vessels about the knee, and the superficial femoral vessels about the thigh. If the patient is extremely scarred, and particularly if the patient has a prior major vascular injury, vascular exposure should be avoided near the site of reconstruction. In such patients, long venous grafts may be coapted to healthy proximal vessels and channeled subcutaneously to the flap (Fig. 78-9).

The vascular anastomoses themselves should be carefully executed with uncompromising precision. With few exceptions, end-to-side arterial anastomoses are preferred. This preference is particularly true for free tissue transfers to the lower extremity. End-to-side arterial coaptation minimizes more distal vascular insult to the limb, permits free tissue transfer in a limb that has only a single patent major vessel, obviates the technical problems associated with end-to-end repair of disparate-sized vessels, and may minimize vessel spasm problems associated with vessel retraction consequent to complete transsection.

During preparation of the recipient site artery for end-to-side coaptation, select the largest caliber, most pristine major artery in the region. Isolate a segment at least 3 cm long and free of any tethering side branches to permit exposure for microvascular clamp application and to allow vessel manipulation to facilitate repair of the back wall. Take care to place the side-wall arteriotomy in a position such that the free flap artery exits at 90° from the recipient site artery and courses directly to the flap without kinks or turns. The side-wall arteriotomy itself should resect a full-thickness elipse of vessel, permitting clear identification of the lumen of the recipient site vessel and the cut edge of the intima about the arteriotomy. If the vessel is arteriosclerotic, place the arteriotomy as remotely as possible from visible or palpable plaques.

I place interrupted monofilament nylon sutures through the

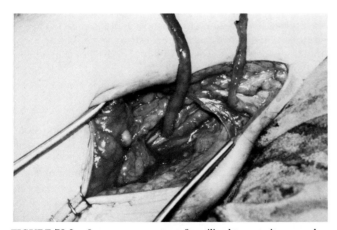

FIGURE 78-9. Long venous autografts utilized to permit revascularization of free muscle flap in a patient in whom regional vessels near the defect were damaged. Note that polarity of the vein graft is reversed for arterial graft but not for venous graft.

full thickness of the walls of both recipient and donor vessels. The size of suture depends on the size of the smallest artery and varies from 10-0 (a vessel diameter of 1.5 mm or less) to 8-0 (a vessel diameter of 3 mm or more). With few exceptions, end-to-end venous anastomosis is preferred. Select a recipient site vein of similar caliber to that exiting the flap. Whenever possible, two venous anastomoses are desirable, especially if venous hypertension is present at the recipient site. If only a single vein is present in the flap pedicle, two recipient site veins can provide drainage by coapting one end-to-end and the second end-to-side approximately 1 cm more distally along the pedicle vein.

Once completed, inspect all anastomoses for patency. Usually this can be accomplished visually, but if not, an atraumatic "milking test" can be performed. Active bleeding should be visible from the cut edges of the flap, and if the flap is cutaneous, visible capillary refill should be present. If any doubt exists regarding the adequacy of flap perfusion, a careful search for the cause of the problem is required. The most common causes of inadequate flow usually are arterial spasm of the recipient site vessels proximal to the anastomosis, thrombosis at the site of anastomosis, and kinking or excessive tension on the flap pedicle. Arterial vasospasm proximal to the site of anastomosis is best managed initially by topical application of spasmolytic drugs, including local anesthetics, papeverine, or calcium channel blockers. Additionally, bathing the vessel with warm Ringer's lactate solution may be helpful. If vasospasm is particularly difficult to overcome, intraluminal mechanical dilation with a Fogarty balloon catheter can be used. This maneuver requires extreme caution, however, to avoid laceration of the intima or even vessel rupture, particularly when the artery is sclerotic or scarred. Thrombosis of the anastomosis requires revision and a careful search for the cause of the thrombosis. When a thrombosed site is being repaired, remove all platelet aggregates, taking care to avoid embolization into the flap. Problems related to excessive pedicle tension or kinking are remedied by revising the position of the pedicle. Revision may require either shortening the pedicle and repeat anastomosis or lengthening the pedicle using an interposed vein graft segment.

The final surgical step of free tissue transfer, after confirmation of adequate flap flow, is insetting and closure. Generally, complete flap insetting should be delayed for a few days to allow for swelling or hematoma collection deep to the flap. Thus, approximately half the flap circumference is inset at the time of the initial flap transfer (Fig. 78-10). Two to three days later, the patient is returned to the operating room, any hematoma or drainage deep to the flap is evacuated, and the insetting is completed. If a muscle flap is used, skin grafting is done at the completion of flap insetting. If any active suppuration is encountered, flap insetting will be further delayed until sepsis is controlled. In a few instances, control has required as long as 2 weeks. Generally, flap failure is not a result of delaying insetting.

At the initial procedure, as well as at flap insetting, the application of dressing should be a meticuluous ritual. The dressing should ideally immobilize the limb, avoid strangulation of the flap, allow for drainage and bleeding, and permit safe patient transfer and positioning in bed. There should be some access through the dressing to inspect the flap during the postoperative period. This access may simply be a small edge of

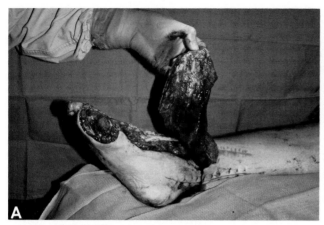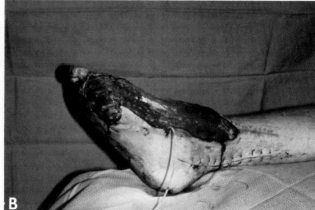

FIGURE 78-10. (*A*) Partial insetting of muscle flap at time of flap transfer. (*B*) Two days later, hematoma under the flap is evacuated, the wound is irrigated, and complete flap insetting is performed.

a muscle flap protruding through the dressing or an observation window through the dressing for a cutaneous flap.

Postoperative Management

Postoperative treatment will vary somewhat with the clinical indication requiring free tissue transfer. However, the postoperative care common to all of these procedures should be guided by factors that enhance wound healing, maintain patency of the microvascular anastomoses, and promote regional tissue equilibrium. Usually, elevation of the limb is important during the immediate postoperative period. Elevation is particularly helpful for lower extremity reconstruction and in patients with venous hypertension. For this purpose, it is desirable to use a lymphedema sling or balanced suspension frame (Thomas-Pearson, Hodgins, and so forth).

Any condition known to induce vasospasm or peripheral vasoconstriction should be avoided or minimized during the early postoperative period. This includes smoking or the use of smokeless nicotine, anxiety, or a cool ambient temperature. The use of antiplatelet drugs is continued for 2 to 4 weeks after operation, if there are no undesirable side effects. The frequency of dressing changes will vary with the particular flap used, the amount of wound drainage, and the timing of flap insetting or skin grafting. In general, however, after the first few postoperative days, a dressing that provides gentle and even compression over the flap to minimize edema is utilized. Because vascular thrombosis is rare after the first 48 to 72 hours, continuous flap observation is unnecessary after this period. Continuous gentle compression of the flap by a cast or elastic wrap is most often continued for 6 weeks after operation. For free tissue transfers about the foot or ankle, weight-bearing is not permitted for this 6-week period. In most patients, a support stocking that applies an even compression about the foot and ankle is made at 6 weeks and is used for several months or until flap-dependent edema ceases to be a problem.

Whenever possible, secondary operative interventions involving elevation of the flap should be deferred until tissue equilibrium is achieved. This period usually will range between 3 and 6 months. Any secondary intervention should attempt to avoid damage to the flap's vascular pedicle. Avoiding such damage is particularly important for muscle flaps, because late failure from trauma to the vascular pedicle has been reported. Decisions regarding flap debulking should be deferred until 6 months after operation. If required, debulking is best done in two or more stages.

TISSUE DONOR SITES

Selection of the optimal donor site depends on the geometry of the defect, reconstructive goal, surgeon's preference, and other factors. A detailed description of the technique of flap harvest and the spectrum of anatomic variations is beyond the scope of this chapter. The reader should refer to available atlases[13] or the present references before utilizing any of the following flaps.

Muscle Flaps

Muscle provides a well-vascularized, readily contoured mass of tissue that reliably supports a split-thickness skin graft and can be expected to atrophy with time. In general, muscle flaps are useful for most orthopaedic reconstructive problems, except those in which cutaneous sensibility is desired or maintenance of flap bulk is required.

Latissimus Dorsi

The latissimus dorsi is the most readily available and widely used muscle flap for free soft-tissue transfer in orthopaedic reconstruction.[14] With rare exceptions in an otherwise normal patient, loss of this muscle entails a negligible functional deficit. The latissimus dorsi can provide an area of coverage approximating 20 by 40 cm. The flap is based on the thoracodorsal vessels, which provide a pedicle length of 8 to 14 cm (Fig. 78-11). The thoracodorsal artery is 1.5 to 3.0 mm in diameter. One or more veins accompany the artery and usually are of larger caliber than the artery. Access to the muscle is easiest

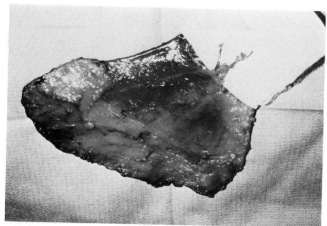

FIGURE 78-11. Isolated latissimus dorsi muscle. Note position of vascular pedicle.

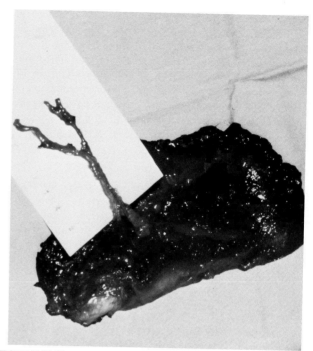

FIGURE 78-12. Isolated rectus abdominis muscle. Note flat contour and length of vascular pedicle.

when the patient is positioned laterally. A linear incision 2 to 3 cm posterior to the anterior margin of the muscle from axilla to posterior iliac crest is adequate for exposure. The most frequent donor site problem is wound seroma. Therefore, meticulous hemostasis before closure and an extended period of suction drainage, deep to the skin flaps, are recommended.

Rectus Abdominis

The rectus abdominis provides an adequate mass of tissue for most clinical situations.[17,18] It shares many of the desirable features of the latissimus dorsi, including expendability, a flat, rectangular shape, and a long vascular pedicle. The rectus abdominis offers distinct advantages over the latissimus dorsi, including easier positioning of the patient in the supine position and fewer problems for crutch utilization during the postoperative period. The rectus abdominis provides an area of coverage of about 10 by 15 cm. It is based on the deep inferior epigastric vessels, which provide a pedicle length of 7 to 8 cm, and enters the muscle on its deep lateral surface 8 to 10 cm proximal to the pubis (Fig. 78-12). The diameter of the inferior epigastric artery is similar to that of the thoracodorsal artery and ranges from 2.0 to 2.5 mm. One or two veins of larger caliber accompany the artery.

Unlike the latissimus dorsi, the rectus abdominis receives a segmental motor innervation. Thus, it cannot be used as a functioning muscle transfer. Access to the rectus abdominis may be gained with the patient in either a recumbent or a lateral position through a midline, paramedian, or transverse abdominoplasty incision. Donor site problems have been rare. We have encountered one instance of an abdominal hernia in a series of more than 60 such flaps.

Gracilis

Although the gracilis may be used for soft tissue coverage, the most notable indication for the use of this muscle is as a functioning muscle for finger flexion.[11] Structurally, the gracilis is a long, narrow muscle with a well-defined tendon of origin and

insertion. It is supplied by one or two vascular pedicles and has the major pedicle entering the undersurface of the muscle in its upper third.[10] Although the dominant artery is of large caliber (1.5–2.5 mm), the vascular pedicle is relatively short. Two venae comitantes accompany the artery.

Tensor Fascia Femoris

The tensor fascia femoris probably is used less frequently because of the increasing popularity of the latissimus dorsi and rectus abdominis flaps. Nonetheless, the tensor fascia muscle may be ideal for transfer in certain situations. Structurally, this muscle is somewhat thick and long, measuring up to 10 by 30 cm.[6,10,21] It is supplied by the lateral femoral circumflex vessels,

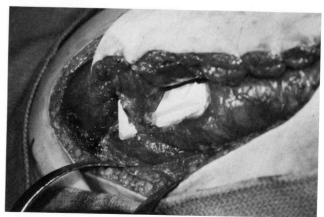

FIGURE 78-13. Isolated tensor fascia of femoris muscle. Note lateral femoral circumflex vascular pedicle.

which provide a pedicle length of 6 to 8 cm and an arterial diameter of 1.5 to 2.5 mm (Fig. 78-13). The tensor fascia femoris can be safely contoured to a cuboidal shape, making it ideal for obliterating dead spaces of rectangular dimensions. It also has the advantage of being readily available in the lower extremity, thus often facilitating patient positioning and anesthetic considerations. Donor site problems have not been reported, although in some patients the lateral cutaneous nerve of the thigh has been sacrificed.

Other Muscle Flaps

Virtually any muscle with a defined vascular pedicle can be utilized as a free tissue transfer. There are few, if any, reconstructive situations that cannot be managed by one of the muscles previously mentioned. However, free transfer of the pectoralis major,[12] gastrocnemius,[2] serratus anterior, brachioradialis, rectus femoris, and gluteus maximus has been performed.

Myocutaneous Flaps

Most of the muscle flaps described here may be isolated as myocutaneous flaps by inclusion of a skin island over the muscle. The musculocutaneous perforators between the skin and muscle must be meticulously preserved. The chief drawbacks to musculocutaneous free tissue transfers are difficult skin closure of the donor sites under tension and the bulkiness of the flap.

Cutaneous Flaps

Cutaneous flaps have the distinct benefit of providing skin coverage without requiring a separate skin grafting procedure to achieve definitive wound closure. Moreover, in contrast to a muscle flap, a cutaneous flap may be readily monitored for patency of the nutrient vessels by color, capillary refill, and various temperature, Doppler, or oxygen tension recording systems. Select cutaneous flaps with a defined sensory nerve may be useful for sensate skin coverage. Management of the donor site defect of a cutaneous flap, however, usually requires a skin graft or closure under tension. Therefore, a less predictable and esthetically less pleasing donor site scar may result (Fig. 78-14). In addition, these flaps require an obligatory quantity of subcutaneous tissue, which often results in an excessively bulky flap.

Groin Flap

The groin flap, based on the superficial circumflex iliac artery and vein, was the first free skin flap to be successfully transferred.[20,23,25] This flap still has clinical application, particularly in thin patients. A flap of 20 by 30 cm can be readily obtained with primary donor site closure. The donor site scar, although characteristically spread out, is generally well concealed in the groin crease. The major drawback to the groin flap is its short vascular pedicle (2–4 cm) (Fig. 78-15) and variable caliber of artery (0.8–2.0 mm in diameter). Additionally, a modified groin flap may be based on the deep circumflex iliac vessels. This flap, however, is most helpful when used as a compound osteocutaneous flap.

Scapular Flap

The scapular flap has gained widespread acceptance as one of the contemporary cutaneous flaps of choice.[5,26] It can furnish a limited area of skin up to 10 by 24 cm but usually has relatively little accompanying subcutaneous fat (Fig. 78-16). Unlike the groin flap, the scapular flap has a long pedicle based on the circumflex scapular vessels, the pedicle being between 4 and 9 cm and of large caliber, ranging between 1.2 and 3.5 mm. The donor site scar is less than ideal, being broad and somewhat conspicuous (see Fig. 78-14). A variation of the scapular flap is the parascapular flap.[19] The latter flap has similar dimensions

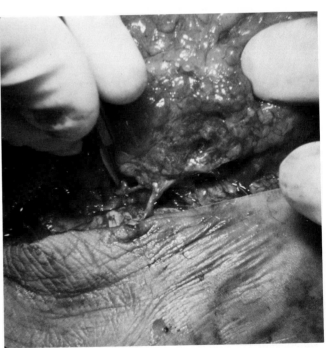

FIGURE 78-15. Isolated groin flap. Note short vascular pedicle.

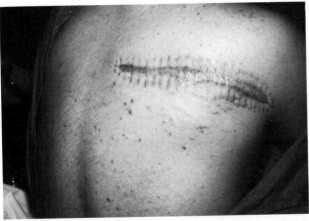

FIGURE 78-14. Residual donor site scar of scapular free flap 10 months after operation. Note broadly spread appearance.

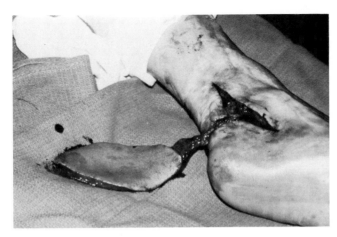

FIGURE 78-16.   Isolated scapular flap. Note minimal accompanying subcutaneous fat.

and anatomy, but the donor site scar has a more favorable appearance.

Radial Forearm Flap

The radial forearm flap is based on the radial artery and fasciocutaneous perforating vessels.[9,24] Although the major role for this flap may be as a vascular island pedicle (see Fig. 78-4A), the flap has been used for free tissue transfer. It can provide a large area of skin, up to 12 by 25 cm, with a defined cutaneous sensory nerve (lateral antebrachial cutaneous nerve). Thus, it has found important applications for providing sensate skin coverage (Fig. 78-17). The pedicle may have an impressive length (10–12 cm) and caliber (2.5–3.5 mm). This flap, however, has significant drawbacks, which most notably include sacrifice of a major upper limb artery and an obvious donor site scar that requires a skin graft for closure (see Fig. 78-4B). The latter disadvantage largely excludes the use of the radial forearm flap in women.

Foot First Web Flap

The first webspace of the foot provides a flap of very limited dimensions, usually being only about 4 by 8 cm (see Fig. 78-8B). Despite its small size, however, this webspace provides a densely innervated flap with a well-defined sensory nerve supply (deep peroneal nerve, first web common digital nerve). The flap is based on the dorsalis pedis artery or the first dorsal metatarsal artery.[3,4] Its pedicle is 5 to 10 cm long and has an arterial caliber of 1.5 to 2.5 mm. The donor defect requires a skin graft for closure. The flap is most useful for digit tip resurfacing where a limited quantity of thin sensate skin is required (see Fig. 78-8).

Lateral Arm Flap

The lateral arm flap is based on the posterior radial collateral vessels and may provide a skin flap of up to 10 by 15 cm. A

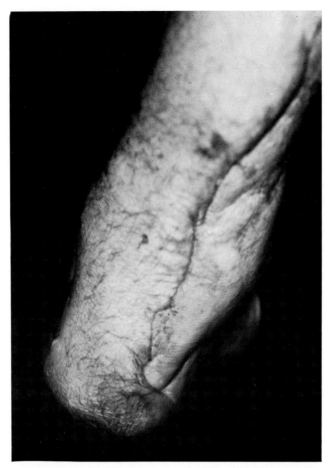

FIGURE 78-17.   Healed innervated radial forearm flap to provide coverage over Achilles tendon and posterior aspect of heel.

pedicle length of 6 cm and an arterial diameter ranging between 1.0 and 3.0 mm may be obtained.[8] The lateral arm flap has been used mainly for upper limb free skin flap transfer because of the convenient proximity of the donor site. The donor scar is less than ideal.

Dorsalis Pedis Flap

Although still used occasionally, the dorsalis pedis flap has largely been discarded because of donor site problems that require a skin graft for closure (Fig. 78-18). The vascular anatomy is the same as for the foot first webspace. The dorsalis pedis flap can be a sensate flap supplied primarily by the superficial peroneal nerve.[15,22]

Other Cutaneous Flaps

Other cutaneous flaps have been described, including the deltopectoral, axillary, deltoid, saphenous,[1] intercostal, lateral thigh, and perineal flaps. Although each of these flaps has its advocates, the usefulness of these flaps beyond that of the flaps described is doubtful.

Other Soft Tissue Flaps

Omentum

Perhaps the earliest free soft-tissue flap transfers for cutaneous reconstruction used omentum.[7,16] The omentum supplied by the right and left gastroepiploic vessels provides a richly vascularized tissue mass of extremely large dimensions. The omentum is particularly ideal for obliteration of irregular dead space cavities and thus has been effectively utilized in providing coverage after saucerization for chronic osteomyelitis. The major drawbacks to the use of omentum is that a laparotomy is required for its harvest. Moreover, the gastroepiploic vessels may be surprisingly small (1.0–1.5 mm) and thin-walled.

Temporalis Fascia

The temporalis fascia based on the superficial temporal vessels and covered by a skin graft has been effectively used for extremely thin vascularized tissue coverage (Fig. 78-19). It is recommended for soft-tissue cover over the extensor tendons on the dorsum of the hand as well as over the Achilles tendon. In both of these locations, other available flaps are usually excessively thick and bulky. Donor site problems have been relatively minimal, but areas of alopecia along the incision line of the scalp have been reported. Because the temporalis fascia flap requires a scalp incision and the specific clinical indications for this flap are limited, it is unlikely to gain widespread popularity for orthopaedic reconstruction.

Damaged or Useless Parts

Although they are used infrequently, damaged or useless parts should be considered as donor sites for free soft-tissue transfer. At times, a filleted unsatisfactory finger or a portion of a paralyzed or congenitally malformed extremity may provide a logical source of vascularized skin, muscle, bone, or fascia for free tissue reconstruction (Fig. 78-20).

PITFALLS AND COMPLICATIONS

Perhaps the most common, but rarely recognized, pitfall of free tissue transfer, is an unrealistically zealous expectation of what can be achieved by these procedures. This can be true for patient and surgeon alike. Errors may include an attempt to proceed with reconstruction before the patient or the wound has stabilized or to reconstruct in a single sitting an injury that would be better managed by a multistaged approach. The recognition that certain injuries or limbs may be better served by amputation is of paramount importance.

Ultimately, the most dramatic and obvious determinant of the success of this procedure is the sustained patency of the microvascular anastomosis. The improper selection of recipient site vessel, failure to recognize an imperfect anastomosis, or improper positioning of the vascular pedicle all carry a high penalty. If there is doubt about any of these factors, revision of the anastomosis is probably necessary.

Finally, with focus on the reconstruction of the recipient site, proper management of the donor site occasionally may escape scrutiny. Generally, donor site problems are prevent-

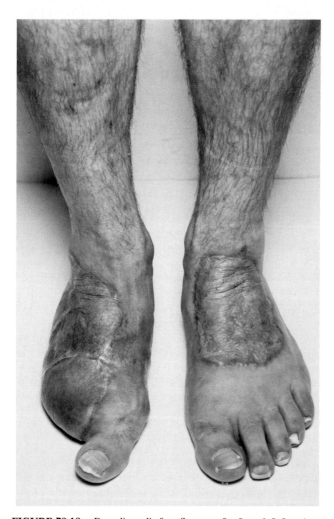

FIGURE 78-18. Dorsalis pedis free flap transfer from left foot (note donor site defect covered by skin graft) to amputation stump of right foot 7 months after operation.

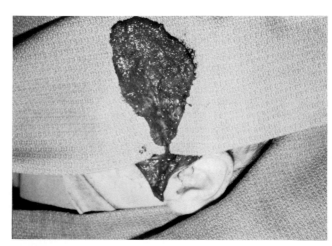

FIGURE 78-19. Isolated temporalis fascia flap. Note extreme thinness of flap tissue and pedicle.

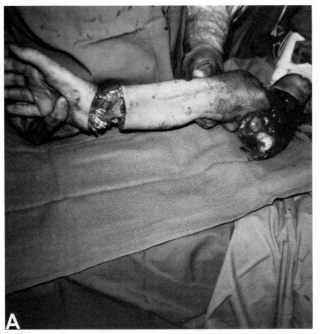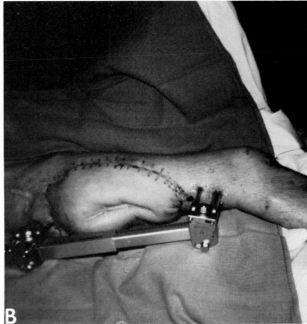

FIGURE 78-20. (*A*) Entire forearm isolated as an osteomusculocutaneous flap for reconstruction of a soft tissue defect in the thigh, with loss of femur segment in a patient with an old flail anesthetic limb from trauma to the brachial plexus. (*B*) Flap transferred and inset with reconstruction of femur using radius and ulna. Subsequent healing and bone union was uneventful. (*A*, Wood, M.B., and Cooney, W.P., III: Vascularized Bone Segment Transfers for Management of Chronic Osteomyelitis. Orthop. Clin. N. Amer. **15**:461–472, 1984.)

able, although they do occur. Meticulous hemostasis, careful fascial closures, adequate wound drainage, and esthetically pleasing skin closures should be routine.

REFERENCES

1. Acland, R.D., Schusterman, M., Godina, M., Eder, E., Taylor, G.I., and Carlisle, I.: The Saphenous Neurovascular Free Flap. Plast. Reconstr. Surg. **67**:763–774, 1981.
2. Arnold, P.G., and Mixter, R.C.: Making the Most of the Gastrocnemius Muscles. Plast. Reconstr. Surg. **72**:38–48, 1983.
3. Caffee, H.H., and Hoefflin, S.M.: The Extended *Dorsalis Pedis* Flap. Plast. Reconstr. Surg. **64**:807–810, 1979.
4. Gilbert, A.: Composite Tissue Transfers from the Foot: Anatomic Basis and Surgical Technique. In Daniller, A.I., and Strauch, B. (eds.): Symposium on Microsurgery. St. Louis, C.V. Mosby, 1976, pp 230–242.
5. Gilbert, A., and Teot, L.: The Free Scapular Flap. Plast. Reconstr. Surg. **69**:601–604, 1982.
6. Hill, H.L., Nahai, F., and Vasconez, L.O.: The Tensor Fascia Lata Myocutaneous Free Flap. Plast. Reconstr. Surg. **61**:517–522, 1978.
7. Irons, G.B., Witzke, D.J., Arnold, P.G., and Wood, M.B.: Use of the Omental Free Flap for Soft-Tissue Reconstruction. Ann. Plast. Surg. **11**:501–507, 1983.
8. Katsaros, J., Schusterman, M., Beppu, M., Banis, J.C., Jr., and Acland, R.D.: The Lateral Upper Arm Flap: Anatomy and Clinical Applications. Ann. Plast. Surg. **12**:489–500, 1984.
9. Lamberty, B.G.H., and Cormack, G.C.: The Forearm Angiotomes. Br. J. Plast. Surg. **35**:420–429, 1982.
10. LaRossa, D., Mellissinos, E., Matthews, D., and Hamilton, R.: The Use of Microvascular Free Skin-Muscle Flaps in Management of Avulsion Injuries of the Lower Leg. J. Trauma **20**:545–550, 1980.
11. Manktelow, R.T., and McKee, N.H.: Free Muscle Transplantation to Provide Active Finger Flexion. J. Hand Surg. **3**:416–426, 1978.
12. Manktelow, R.T., McKee, N.H., and Vettese, T.: An Anatomical Study of the Pectoralis Major Muscle as Related to Functioning Free Muscle Transplantation. Plast. Reconstr. Surg. **65**:610–615, 1980.
13. Mathes, S.J., and Nahai, F.: Clinical Applications for Muscle and Musculocutaneous Flaps. St. Louis, C.V. Mosby, 1982.
14. Maxwell, G.P., Stueber, K., and Hoopes, J.E.: A Free *Latissimus Dorsi* Myocutaneous Flap: Case Report. Plast. Reconstr. Surg. **62**:462–466, 1978.
15. McCraw, J.B., and Furlow, L.T., Jr.: The *Dorsalis Pedis* Arterialized Flap: A Clinical Study. Plast. Reconstr. Surg. **55**:177–185, 1975.
16. McLean, D.H., and Buncke, H.J., Jr.: Autotransplant of Omentum to a Large Scalp Defect, with Microsurgical Revascularization. Plast. Reconstr. Surg. **49**:268–274, 1972.
17. McVay, C.B., and Anson, B.J.: Composition of the Rectus Sheath. Anat. Rec. **77**:213–225, 1940.
18. Milloy, F.J., Anson, B.J., and McAfee, D.K.: The Rectus Abdominis Muscle and the Epigastric Arteries. Surg. Gynecol. Obstet. **110**:293–302, 1960.
19. Nassif, T.M., Vidal, L., Bovet, J.L., and Baudet, J.: The Parascapular Flap: A New Cutaneous Microsurgical Free Flap. Plast. Reconstr. Surg. **69**:591–600, 1982.
20. O'Brien, B.M., MacLeod, A.M., Hayhurst, J.W., and Morrison, W.A.: Successful Transfer of a Large Island Flap from the Groin to the Foot by Microvascular Anastomoses. Plast. Reconstr. Surg. **52**:271–278, 1973.
21. O'Hare, P.M., Leonard, A.G., and Brennen, M.D.: Experience

with the Tensor Fasciae Latae Free Flap. Br. J. Plast. Surg. **36:**98–104, 1983.

22. Ohmori, K., and Harii, K.: Free *Dorsalis Pedis* Sensory Flap to the Hand, with Microneurovascular Anastomoses. Plast. Reconstr. Surg. **58:**546–554, 1976.

23. Smith, P.J., Foley, B., McGregor, I.A., and Jackson, I.T.: The Anatomical Basis of the Groin Flap. Plast. Reconstr. Surg. **49:**41–47, 1972.

24. Song, R.Y., Gao, Y.Z., Song, Y.G., Yu, Y.S., and Song, Y.L.: The Forearm Flap. Clin. Plast. Surg. **9:**21–26, 1982.

25. Taylor, G.I., and Daniel, R.K.: The Anatomy of Several Free Flap Donor Sites. Plast. Reconstr. Surg. **56:**243–253, 1975.

26. Urbaniak, J.R., Koman, L.A., Goldner, R.D., Armstrong, N.B., and Nunley, J.A.: The Vascularized Cutaneous Scapular Flap. Plast. Reconstr. Surg. **69:**772–778, 1982.

27. Weiland, A.J., Moore, J.R., and Daniel, R.K.: The Efficacy of Free Tissue Transfer in the Treatment of Osteomyelitis. J. Bone. Joint. Surg. **66-A:**181–193, 1984.

28. Wood, M.B., Cooney, W.P., and Irons, G.B.: Lower Extremity Salvage and Reconstruction by Free-Tissue Transfer: Analysis of Results. Clin. Orthop. **201:**151–161, 1985.

29. Wood, M.B., and Irons, G.B.: Upper-Extremity Free Skin Flap Transfer: Results and Utility as Compared with Conventional Distant Pedicle Skin Flaps. Ann. Plast. Surg. **11:**523–526, 1983.

30. Wood, M.B., Irons, G.B., and Cooney, W.P. III: Foot Reconstruction by Free Flap Transfer. Foot Ankle **4:**2–7, 1983.

CHAPTER 79

Vascularized Bone Grafts

J. RUSSELL MOORE and
ANDREW J. WEILAND

Graft Donor Sites
Clinical Indications
Case Examples
Operative Technique
   Vascularized Fibular Grafting

The concept of a bone graft with an intact blood supply is attractive because it circumvents the time needed for bone resorption and replacement by creeping substitution and because the graft may participate directly in bony healing. The free vascularized bone graft offers the advantage over pedicle grafting of not being limited by the length of the vascular pedicle, allowing the surgeon the potential to transfer bone to nearly any segment of the body with an adequate recipient blood supply. Reported clinical use of the vascularized bone graft demonstrates union of the vascularized graft and recipient bone in about 3 to 5 months, and signs of hypertrophy of the graft at about 15 months. This compares favorably with nonvascularized bone grafts of large segmental defects, which may take 8 to 15 months for bony incorporation and healing to occur.[44]

GRAFT DONOR SITES

The most popular sites for harvest of the vascularized bone graft have been the fibula, iliac crest, scapula, and rib. The vascularized rib graft based on the intercostal vessels was initially extremely popular for reconstruction of complex mandibular tumor resections. For orthopaedic reconstruction, the vascularized rib graft has been employed as a pedicle graft for use in spinal fusion; however, it does not enjoy common usage.[12,14,35,39,42] Swartz has described the use of the osteocutaneous scapular flap for use in maxillofacial and hand surgery.[38] The iliac crest based on the deep circumflex iliac artery may be taken either as a composite graft with overlying subcutaneous tissue and skin or merely as a vascularized bone graft. Anatomic considerations make it difficult to reconstruct bone defects greater than 8 cm with an iliac crest graft, and the attendant donor site morbidity may be somewhat greater than in other types of vascular bone grafts.

The vascularized fibular graft based on the peroneal artery and its venae comitantes has been the graft of choice of most extremity surgeons who deal with large segmental bone defects. The fibula has been shown to be especially well suited for large segmental cortical bone defects, and bone segments ranging from 6 to 22 cm may be bridged. The ease of harvest, lack of donor site morbidity, lack of interference with ambulation, and near invisibility of the donor site scar make the fibular graft attractive as a source for donor bone. Furthermore, the size of the fibula is suitable for reconstructing both large tibial defects and defects in the upper extremity as well.

CLINICAL INDICATIONS

The surgical decision as to which type of bone graft is most appropriate depends on a host of factors, including the age of the patient, availability of donor bone, length and type of defect, and, most importantly, the condition of the soft-tissue bed. In a well-vascularized soft-tissue bed free of infection and protected by adequate skin coverage, a variety of grafting techniques should yield successful results. When defects in bone of greater than 6 cm to 8 cm need to be bridged, unusual demands are placed upon conventional bone graft mechanisms. In fact, massive autogenous grafts have displayed a high degree of failure characterized by nonunion, fatigue fracture, and lengthy immobilization required for eventual healing. In a previously traumatized, irradiated, or infected limb, significant scarring and lack of vascularity too often are harbingers of poor grafting results. The vascularized bone graft is not independent of a bad environment but is able to provide increased vascularity to the area being grafted. Osteogenic cells in the vascularized graft survive and contribute to appositional healing rather than remaining as a passive framework in creeping substitution. Clinically, the vascularized graft has been applied most frequently to rectify bone loss following trauma, but it has also demonstrated its usefulness in resections following debridement of osteomyelitis, tumor resection, and treatment of congenital pseudarthrosis of the tibia, radius, and ulna.

CASE EXAMPLES

In many cases of locally aggressive osseous tumors that are amenable to wide excision, one can avoid amputation and restore bony continuity with a vascularized graft. We have used the vascularized fibular graft following reconstruction of bone defects left by resection of giant cell tumors, chondrosarcomas, adamantinomas, irradiated Ewing's sarcomas, and recurrent unicameral bone cysts, as well as fibrosarcomas of bone.[31] The surgical approach for tumor resection will be facilitated if a two-team approach is used. One team can direct its attention to performing adequate tumor resection and preparation of the recipient vessels. The other team, isolated from the primary team and with separate instruments, will perform the fibula dissection. The following representative cases demonstrate the utility of the vascularized fibular graft.

Case 1.   A 20-year-old college athlete presented with pain, swelling, and increased deformity of his wrist and forearm over several months' duration (Fig. 79-1A). A locally aggressive fibromyxoma was treated by *en bloc* resection (Fig. 79-1B) and vascularized fibular grafting (Fig. 79-1C).

Case 2.   A 32-year-old woman presented with a longstanding infected nonunion of the distal femur. The patient had undergone irradiation for a Ewing's sarcoma as a child and subsequently developed a pathologic fracture. She had undergone several operative procedures and, at the time of presentation, had a persistent nonunion in spite of an interlocking nail type of fixation (Fig. 79-2A). A preoperative angiogram displayed a healthy-appearing femoral artery (Fig. 79-2B) with many perforators. A combined medial and lateral operative approach was used to expose the entire length of the femur laterally and the donor vessels medially (Fig. 79-2C). After thorough wound debridement, internal fixation with a condylar blade-plate (Fig. 79-2D) was performed. Medially, a vascularized fibular graft was secured to the distal femur bayonet-fashion (Fig. 79-2E). Cancellous bone graft was also added to the juncture sites. The radiographic appearance 4 months after surgery (Fig. 79-2F) shows bony consolidation at the site of the previous nonunion.

In cases of post-traumatic osteomyelitis, the surgeon is often faced with a more difficult challenge in assessing levels of bone resection than in tumor cases. Often less reliable information is obtained from MRI or CT scans, so experience and judgment must be used in determining the extent of surgical debridement. Patients about to undergo reconstruction for large bone defects left by post-traumatic osteomyelitis resection should be forewarned that a significant complication rate on the order of 25% to 30% can be expected, possibly resulting in graft failure, and amputation may be the only alternative.[43]

Case 3.   In cases of osteomyelitis involving a substantial bone defect, the patient must be prepared for prolonged healing time or repeat surgery in order to obtain an eventual union. An individual sustained a bumper-type injury that resulted in a comminuted compound fracture of the proximal tibia (Fig. 79-3A). Following debridement and application of an external fixator, the patient was left with a 13-cm bone defect (Fig. 79-3B), with interval healing after a vascular latissimus dorsi flap (Fig. 79-3C). A vascularized fibular graft was performed (Fig. 79-3D). However, the patient subsequently fractured at the proximal juncture site and later required an open reduction internal fixation and plating (Fig. 79-3E) before complete healing occurred.

One significant application of the vascularized fibular graft is in the treatment of congenital pseudarthrosis of the tibia, a condition that has remained an enigma for orthopaedic surgeons for many years. Congenital pseudarthrosis usually involves the tibia and fibula; however, it may also involve the radius and ulna. Many articles have described the classification, histology, and etiology of congenital pseudarthrosis of the tibia.[1-3,5,6,8-11,13,15-24,26-30,32-34,36,37,40,41] A failure rate of up to 50% resulting in amputation has been cited.[41] The proper surgical treatment of this lesion should most rationally follow a proper classification of congenital pseudarthrosis.[2,16,32,41] The less severe varieties can be suitably treated with a brace. However, intermediate degrees may need bone grafting or pulse electromagnetic stimulation coupled with immobilization. It has been discovered that, for Type III lesions—characterized by a bony gap greater than 5 mm, atrophic spindled bone ends, fibular involvement, and anterolateral bowing—conventional techniques had a success rate of only 20%.[25] Therefore, we consider that a Type III (more severe) lesion is best managed with a vascularized fibula graft. A vascularized graft may be successfully performed as early as 1.5 to 2 years of age, once the surgeon is convinced more conventional treatment is unlikely to succeed.

In congenital pseudarthrosis, the surgical approach is similar to the one employed in tumor resection, and an extraperiosteal dissection of the bone and pseudarthrosis is meticulously carried out with protection of the neurovascular bundles. The fibula pseudarthrosis should be resected as well, and the fibula appropriately immobilized and bone grafted if necessary. In most instances, it is useful to dowel the fibula into the medullary canal of the tibia distally as well as proximally. If this is not technically possible, however, bayonet apposition is satisfactory. The choice of optimal fixation may challenge the surgeon's repertoire. AO one-third tubular plates have been successful in small children, as have standard plates for older patients. If intramedullary fixation is chosen, one should avoid passing the device through the graft (Fig. 79-4).

Case 4.   An 11-year-old boy with Von Recklinghausen's disease presented with a congenital pseudarthrosis of the right

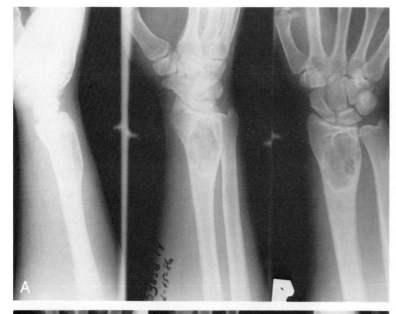

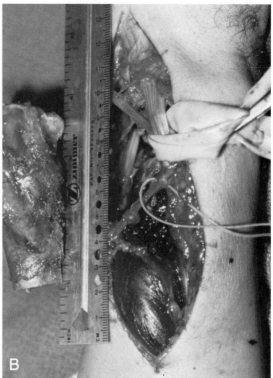

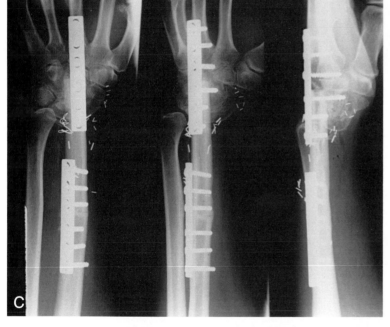

FIGURE 79-1. (*A*) Radiographs of a 20-year-old man demonstrate a lytic lesion in the distal radius that has thinned and expanded the cortex. (*B*) Intraoperative photograph demonstrating a 7-cm *en bloc* resection of the distal radius from a dorsal approach. (*C*) Four-month postoperative radiograph demonstrates sound union proximally and distally.

tibia and fibula that had defied several previous attempts at bone grafting and immobilization (Figs. 79-5*A* and *B*). An extraperiosteal dissection and excision of the pseudarthrosis of the tibia and fibula were performed (Fig. 79-5*C*), resulting in an 8-cm tibial defect (Fig. 79-5*D*). A buttress plate was used to secure the graft to the tibia proximally and distally (Fig. 79-5*E*). Six months postoperatively there is good incorporation of the fibula graft proximally as well as distally (Fig. 79-5*F*). This patient subsequently required a contralateral epiphysiodesis to equalize a leg-length discrepancy and an osteotomy of the tibia due to valgus bowing.

Case 5. A very rare form of congenital pseudarthrosis in the forearm with radius and ulna involvement may also occur (Fig.

79-6*A* and *B*). The pseudarthrosis was exposed through a volar distal forearm incision (Fig. 79-6*C*). After neurovascular identification, the pseudarthroses of both the radius and ulna were excised with an extraperiosteal dissection. The vascularized fibula graft was then fixed to the radius proximally and distally with small AO plates (Fig. 79-6*D*).

As mentioned previously, care should be taken to preserve an intact ankle mortise, and the distal fibula should be synostosed to the adjacent tibia in order to prevent progressive ankle valgus during growth. Screw fixation and cancellous grafting are usually sufficient. Postoperatively, patients are immobilized in bilateral hip spica casts and are carefully braced for the first year after surgery. Parents should be counseled that there is a great likelihood that future surgery will be necessary to remove

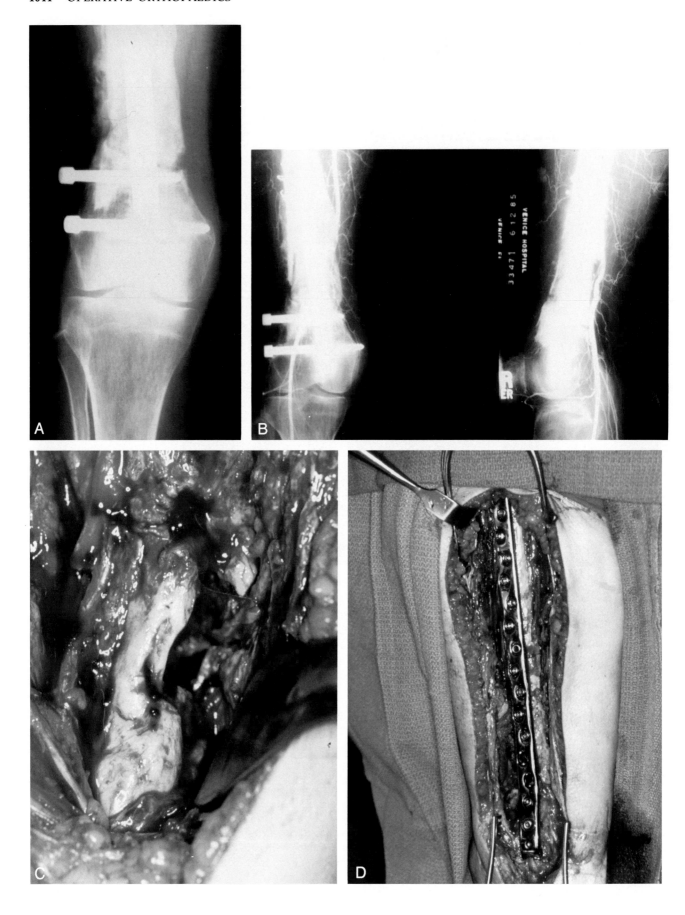

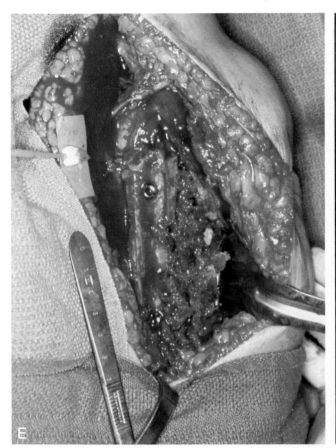
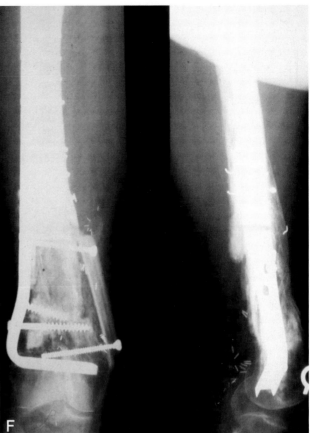

FIGURE 79-2. (*A*) Anteroposterior radiograph of a 32-year-old woman who developed a chronic infected nonunion as the result of a stress fracture following radiotherapy for a Ewing's sarcoma as a child. (*B*) Preoperative angiogram demonstrates a healthy-appearing femoral artery with numerous perforators. (*C*) Medial approach to the distal femur demonstrates the scalloped cavitary lesion of the bone. (*D*) Lateral approach displays the condylar blade plate used in reconstruction. (*E*) The vascularized fibular graft which was fixed to the femur in a bayonet type fashion. Cancellous bone chips were packed in and about the graft site. (*F*) Four-month postoperative radiograph demonstrates solid union and incorporation of the vascularized fibular graft.

internal fixation, to correct leg-length inequality, and perhaps to perform realignment osteotomy at some phase during a child's growth.

OPERATIVE TECHNIQUE

Vascularized Fibular Grafting

In most instances, the fibula receives its nutrient blood supply from perforators off the peroneal artery, which is intimately related to the undersurface of the bone. Preoperative arteriography is important in identifying the particular variations in circulatory anatomy that may be present in the donor site and also may provide information about the extent of disease in the arterial tree in the recipient site. Most commonly, a nontraumatized donor leg angiogram will exhibit a proximal anterior tibial artery takeoff followed by a bifurcation of posterior tibial and peroneal arteries (Fig. 79-7). Occasionally, a separate peroneal artery does not exist, which may preclude use of the fibula

as a donor (Fig. 79-7). Another contraindication to use of the fibula as a donor bone is seen in (Fig. 79-8). The fibula is clearly hypertrophied and significantly contributes to stability in a leg that has had a severe distal tibial fracture.

Venography may also be useful in the assessment of the deep or superficial system of the recipient extremity in cases of microvascular reconstruction (Fig. 79-9). In recent years, patient morbidity has been decreased by the improved imaging techniques. With digital subtraction angiography, high resolution may be obtained even with much lower concentrations of contrast material, which cause considerably less pain for the patient and less potential damage to the intima. It should be recognized that the arteriogram displays anatomy but does not give information about blood flow. Frequently, patients who have had a seemingly normal arteriogram may have diseased blood vessels that are severely scarred or prone to spasm.

Although not essential, a two-team approach may be expected to save considerable operative time. The surgical technique for the donor fibula is rather constant, with the patient supine and the hip and the knee flexed. A lateral approach to

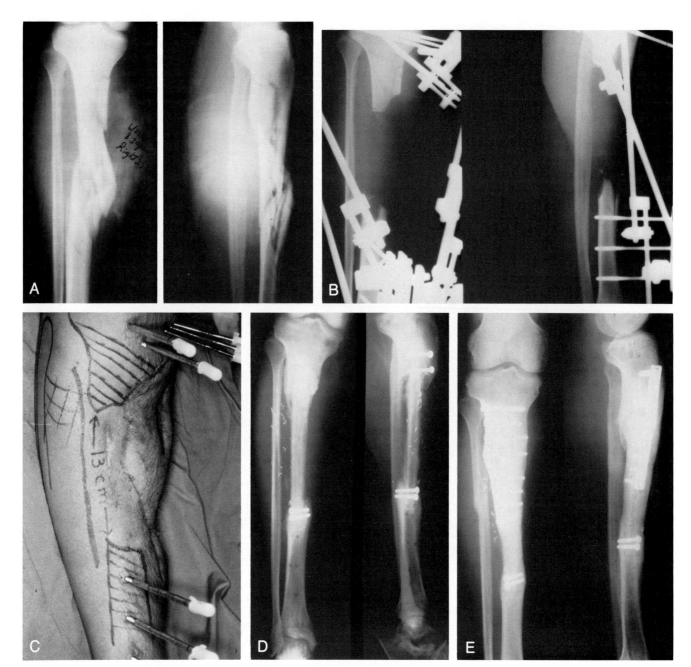

FIGURE 79-3. (*A*) Radiograph of an individual who sustained a bumper-type injury, which resulted in a comminuted compound fracture of the proximal tibia. (*B*) Radiographic appearance following radical debridement demonstrates a 13-cm bone defect. (*C*) Clinical appearance of leg following free soft tissue transfer and coverage. (*D*) Six-month postoperative radiograph demonstrates sound union of vascularized fibular graft proximally and distally. (*E*) Radiograph of patient 3 months following a repeated internal fixation performed because of a stress fracture of the proximal juncture site.

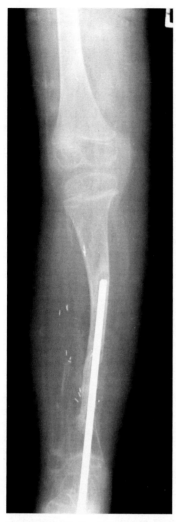

FIGURE 79-4. A 4-month postoperative radiograph of a child who underwent a vascularized fibular graft for congenital pseudarthrosis of the tibia. Intramedullary fixation with a Steinmann pin was chosen to stabilize the proximal and distal fragments in this child with extremely soft metaphyseal bone. Note, however, that the vascularized fibular graft was positioned in a bayonet fashion and that the internal fixation device does not pass through the intramedullary canal of the graft.

the fibula is used, extending from the neck of the fibula in a distal direction. Identify the interval between the peroneus longus and the soleus muscles (Fig. 79-10), and incise the deep fascia the entire length of the incision. Next, expose the lateral border of the fibula (Fig. 79-11). Approach the fibula in a proximal-to-distal fashion, and elevate an extraperiosteal dissection of the peroneus longus and brevis off the anterior border of the fibula. Next, divide the anterior crural septum along the length of the graft, and identify and protect the deep peroneal nerve and anterior tibial artery and vein as the extensor group of muscles is dissected off the interosseous membrane.

Divide the posterior crural membrane the entire length of the graft, and reflect the soleus as well as flexor hallucis muscles off the posterior border of the fibula. It is important to preserve the nerve origin to the flexor hallucis longus while performing this dissection. Continue this dissection until the peroneal vessels are encountered. Measure the length of the fibular graft needed, and mark it, taking care to preserve at least the distal 6 cm of fibula in order to maintain stability of the ankle mortise. In children less than 10 years of age, we perform a synostosis between the fibula and tibia in order to prevent proximal migration of the distal fibula and resultant valgus ankle deformity.

Perform the proximal and distal osteotomies, taking care to place the bone retractor between the peroneal vessels and the fibula. Retract the bone graft posteriorly and laterally, and divide the interosseous membrane along the entire length of the bone graft. Next, retract the graft anteriorly. The tibialis anterior muscle may be dissected off the posterior aspect of the middle third of the fibula. At this point, the fibula graft will be isolated on the peroneal neurovascular bundle. Dissect the pedicle proximally until the bifurcation of the posterior tibial artery and peroneal artery is identified. Prior to division of the pedicle, deflate the tourniquet and allow circulation to the fibula for 10 to 15 minutes.

The technique for preparation of the recipient site varies, depending on the clinical condition being treated. In post-traumatic cases, initial attention is focused at neurovascular identification and protection. Failure to isolate a healthy level of recipient vessel is the most frequent cause for failure of free tissue transfer. The zone of injury frequently far exceeds the limits of the bone defect in post-traumatic and infected cases.

Resect necrotic or nonviable bone ends. Next, rigidly fix the fibular graft into the defect. A variety of techniques may be used, including doweling of the end of the fibula inside the tibia, end-to-end apposition, or bayonet-type fixation. Regardless of the position of the fibular graft, rigid fixation is needed, and may be provided with either external or internal fixation. Do not use intramedullary fixation through the vascularized fibular graft in order to avoid disrupting its vascularity. In most instances, cancellous bone graft is packed in and around the juncture points of the recipient and donor bone in order to promote more rapid union.

Next, perform the microvascular anastomoses. Most frequently, one artery and one vein are anastomosed. Whenever possible, an end-to-side arterial anastomosis is performed so as not to compromise distal circulation to the extremity. End-to-end vein anastomosis is chosen. It is important that the caliber of the recipient vein be equal or larger than that of the peroneal vein so that venous hypertension will not ensue. The recipient vein may be from either the superficial venous system or venae comitantes, as long as it is of sufficient caliber and free of scar. The fibular graft, being devoid of large amounts of soft tissue or muscle, seems particularly tolerant of ischemia of up to several hours, and one should not rush attempts at achieving secure bony fixation to limit ischemia time. Adequate circulation is assessed by a patent and functioning venous anastomosis as well as bleeding of the edges of the muscle cuff on the fibular graft. Prior to wound closure, ascertain that the vascular pedicle is not redundant, twisted, or kinked. It is preferable to resect and tailor a functioning anastomosis that is looped or kinked because of the potential danger of thrombosis. Although there is no universal agreement on the use of anticoagulants, some find it helpful to administer intraoperative heparin before applying clamps to large lower extremity vessels.

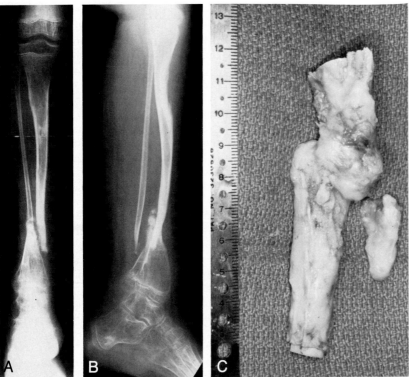

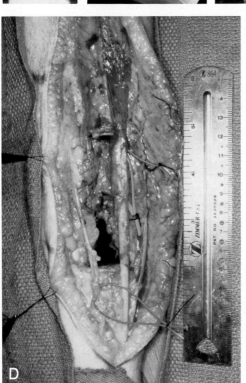

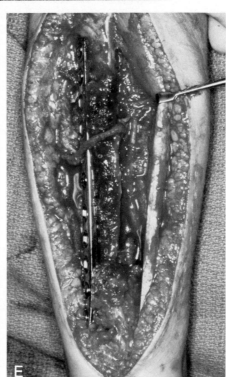

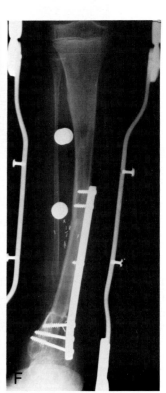

FIGURE 79-5. (*A*) Anteroposterior radiograph of an 11-year-old boy with Von Recklinghausen's disease and congenital pseudarthrosis of the tibia. (*B*) Lateral radiograph demonstrating a proximally as well as distally bowed tibia along with marked osteoporosis of the distal tibia and foot. (*C*) Intraoperative photograph of resected specimen, including tibial and fibular pseudarthrosis. (*D*) Intraoperative photograph demonstrating bony defect. Vessel loops are noted around the anterior neurovascular bundle as well as the saphenous vein. (*E*) Intraoperative photograph demonstrating buttress plate. The vascular pedicle can be seen transversing the proximal portion of the plate into the graft. (*F*) Radiograph of leg 6 months postoperatively, demonstrating sound union of vascularized graft. However, tibial bowing was noted.

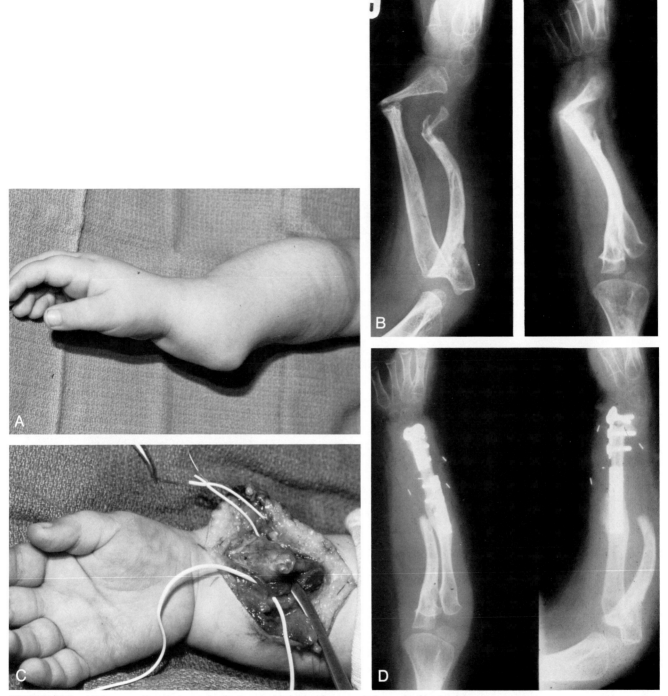

FIGURE 79-6. (*A*) Preoperative photograph of a 4-year-old child with congenital pseudarthrosis of the radius and ulna. (*B*) Preoperative radiograph demonstrating severe angulation and deformity associated with the congenital pseudarthrosis. (*C*) Intraoperative photograph demonstrating the exposed pseudarthrosis of the radius through a volar approach. (*D*) Four-month postoperative radiograph demonstrating sound healing of the fibular graft proximally and distally.

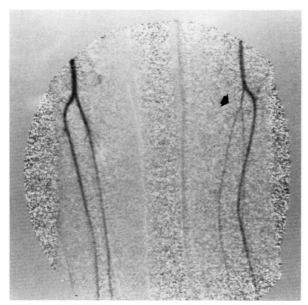

FIGURE 79-7. Digital subtraction angiography of the bilateral lower extremities of a child with congenital pseudarthrosis of the tibia exhibits a normal-appearing proximal takeoff of the anterior tibial artery and then a bifurcation of the peroneal and posterior tibial vessels (*arrow*). Note that on the contralateral extremity, however, there is no separate peroneal and posterior tibial artery.

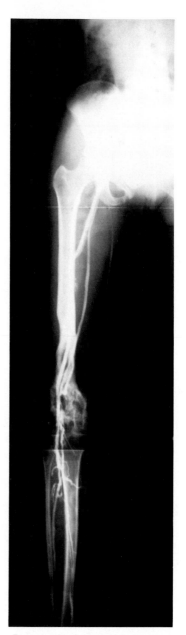

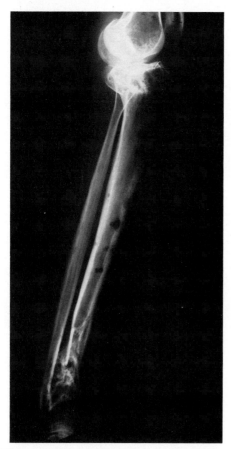

FIGURE 79-9. Preoperative lower extremity venogram of a patient with a chronic osteomyelitis of the distal femur.

FIGURE 79-8. Lateral radiograph of the fibula and tibia in a patient with bilateral distal tibia fractures. The fibula is clearly hypertrophied and undoubtedly played a significant role in the stabilization and support of this extremity, which had a precarious union of the distal tibia. For this reason, it was felt that this fibula could not be used to help reconstruct a defect in the contralateral tibia.

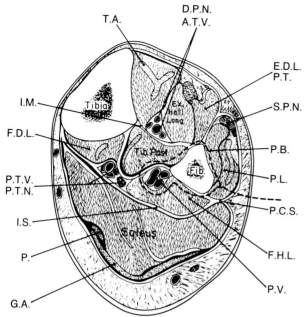

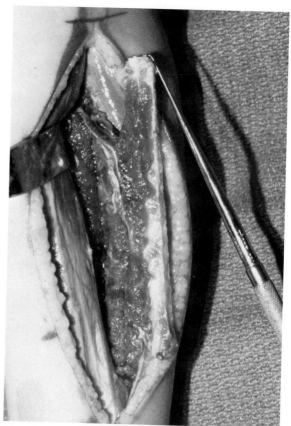

FIGURE 79-10. Cross section of the middle third of the lower extremity which outlines the lateral approach for harvest of the fibula (*dotted line*). *T.A.,* tibialis anterior; *D.P.N.,* deep peroneal nerve; *A.T.V.,* anterior tibialis vessels; *E.D.L.,* extensor digitorum longus; *P.T.,* peroneus tertius, *S.P.N.,* superficial peroneal nerve; *P.B.,* peroneus brevis; *P.L.,* peroneus longus; *P.C.S.,* posterior crural septum; *F.H.L.,* flexor hallucis longus; *P.V.,* peroneal vessels; *G.A.,* gastrocnemius aponeurosis; *P.,* plantaris; *I.S.,* intermuscular septum; *P.T.V.,* posterior tibial vessels, *P.T.N.,* posterior tibial nerve; *F.D.L.,* flexor digitorium longus; *I.M.,* interosseous membrane. (Weiland, A.J.: Vascularized bone transfers. In Murray, J.A. (ed.): AAOS Instructional Course Lectures, Vol 33., St. Louis, C.V. Mosby, 1984, p. 448.)

FIGURE 79-11. The osteotomized fibula after the interosseous membrane has been divided. The vascular pedicle of the peroneal artery and vein are clearly visible in the proximal extent of the wound.

Pack cancellous bone chips harvested from the iliac crest about the proximal and distal juncture sites, insert deep drains, and close the skin. Postoperatively, low-dose aspirin therapy is continued and patients are instructed not to smoke.

At present, there are no 100% reliable techniques for monitoring the vascularity to the bone graft in a noninvasive fashion. Overlying skin islands may be taken with the fibula; however, the presence or absence of the cutaneous circulation may not accurately reflect the osseous circulation. Bone scans have been used in the laboratory[4,7] as well as clinically; however, these are only useful for the first week after surgery and are not practical for a sequential monitoring system. Internal probes are difficult and time consuming to insert safely and may be confusing to interpret. Undoubtedly, technical advances will soon offer suitable solutions. MRI may soon be defined to make it possible to monitor osseous circulation by noninvasive techniques.

The grafted bone segment is immobilized and protected from weight-bearing for at least 2.5 months or until incorporation and callus around the juncture sites are seen. In the adult, lower extremity graft incorporation usually occurs in 4 to 6 months. However, keep patients ambulating with an orthosis throughout the first year.

Even an experienced microsurgeon, if a novice at vascularized fibular grafting, should perform cadaveric dissections to properly appreciate the relationships of neurovascular struc-

tures to the interosseous membranes. With attention to good technique, a very low incidence of donor site morbidity can be expected.

REFERENCES

1. Anderson, K.S.: Congenital Angulation of the Lower Leg and Congenital Pseudarthrosis of the Tibia in Denmark. Acta Orthop. Scand. **43:**539–549, 1972.
2. Anderson, K.S.: Radiologic Classification of Congenital Pseudarthrosis of the Tibia. Acta Orthop. Scand. **44:**719–727, 1973.
3. Bassett, C.A.L., Pilla, A.A., and Pawluk, R.J.: A Non-Operative Salvage of Surgically-Resistant Pseudarthrosis and Non-Unions by Pulsing Electromagnetic Fields: A Preliminary Report. Clin. Orthop. **124:**128–143, 1977.
4. Berggren, A., Weiland, A.J., and Ostrup, L.T.: Bone Scintigraphy in Evaluating the Viability of Composite Bone Grafts Revascularized by Microvascular Anastomoses, Conventional Autogenous Bone Grafts, and Free NonVascularized Periosteal Grafts. J. Bone Joint Surg. **64-A:**799, 1982.
5. Berk, L., and Mankin, H.J.: Spontaneous Pseudarthrosis of the Tibia Occurring in a Patient with Neurofibromatosis. J. Bone Joint Surg. **46-A:**619, 1964.
6. Berkshire, S.B., Jr., Maxwell, E.N., and Sams, B.F.: Bilateral Symmetrical Pseudarthrosis in a Newborn. Radiology **97:**389–390, 1970.
7. Bos, K.E.: Bone Scintigraphy of Experimental Composite Bone

Grafts Revascularized by Microvascular Anastomoses. Plast. Reconstr. Surg. **64:**353, 1979.

8. Boyd, H.B.: Congenital Pseudarthrosis: Treatment by Dual Bone Grafts. J. Bone Joint Surg. **23:**497, 1941.

9. Brighton, C.T., et al.: Direct Current Stimulation of Nonunions and Congenital Pseudarthrosis. J. Bone Joint Surg. **57-A:**368, 1975.

10. Briner, J., and Yunis, E.: Ultrastructure of Congenital Pseudarthrosis of the Tibia. Arch. Pathol. **95:**97, 1973.

11. Brown, G.A., Osebold, W.R., and Ponseti, I.V.: Congenital Pseudarthrosis of Long Bones: A Clinical, Radiographic, Histologic, and Ultrastructural Study. Clin. Orthop. **128:**228–242, 1977.

12. Buncke, H.J., Furnas, D.W., Gordon, L., and Achauer, B.M.: Free Osteocutaneous Flap from a Rib to the Tibia. Plast. Reconstr. Surg. **59:**799–805, 1977.

13. Charnley, J.: Congenital Pseudarthrosis of the Tibia Treated by the Intramedullary Nail. J. Bone Joint Surg. **38-A:**283–290, 1956.

14. Daniel, R.K.: Free Rib Transfer by Microvascular Anastomoses. Plast. Reconstr. Surg. **59:**737, 1977.

15. Ducroquet, R.: A Propos des Pseudarthroses et Inflexions Congenitales du Tibia. Mem. Acad. Chir. **63:**863, 1937.

16. Edvarsen, P.: Resection Osteosynthesis and Boyd Amputation for Congenital Pseudarthrosis. J. Bone Joint Surg. **55-B:**179–182, 1973.

17. Eyre-Brook, A.L., Baily, R.A.J., and Price, C.H.G.: Infantile Pseudarthrosis of the Tibia. J. Bone Joint Surg. **51-B:**604–613, 1969.

18. Gordon, E.J.: Solitary Intraosseous Neurilemmoma of the Tibia. Clin. Orthop. **117:**271, 1976.

19. Green, W.T., and Rudo, N.: Pseudarthrosis and Neurofibromatosis. Arch. Surg. **46:**639, 1943.

20. Hardings, K.: Congenital Anterior Bowing of the Tibia: The Significance of the Different Types in Relation to Pseudarthrosis. Ann. R. Coll. Surg. Engl. **51:**17–30, 1972.

21. Hart, M.S., and Basom, W.C.: Neurilemmoma Involving Bone. J. Bone Joint Surg. **40-A:**465, 1958.

22. Hatzoecher, cited by Boyd, H.B., and Sage, F.P.: Congenital Pseudarthrosis of the Tibia. J. Bone Joint Surg. **40-A:**1245–1270, 1958.

23. Jacobs, J.E., Kimmelstiel, P., and Thompson, K.R., Jr.: Neurofibromatosis and Pseudarthrosis. Arch. Surg. **59:**232, 1949.

24. Jaffe, H.L.: Tumours and Tumorous Conditions of Bones and Joints. Philadelphia, Lea and Febiger, 1958, pp. 117, 140.

25. Kort, J.S., Schink, N.M., Mitchell, S.N., and Bassett, C.A.L.: Congenital Pseudarthrosis of the Tibia: Treatment with Pulsing Electromagnetic Fields. Clin. Orthop. **165:**124, 1982.

26. Lloyd-Roberts, G.C., and Shaw, N.E.: The Prevention of Pseudarthrosis in Congenital Kyphosis of the Tibia. J. Bone Joint Surg. **51-B:**100–105, 1969.

27. Masserman, R.L., Peterson, H.A., and Bianco, A.J.: Congenital Pseudarthrosis of the Tibia: A Review of the Literature and 52 Cases from the Mayo Clinic. Clin. Orthop. **99:**140–145, 1974.

28. McCarroll, H.R.: Clinical Manifestations of Congenital Neurofibromatosis. J. Bone Joint Surg. **32-A:**601, 1950.

29. McFarland, B.: Pseudarthrosis of the Tibia in Childhood. J. Bone Joint Surg. **33-B:**36, 1951.

30. Moore, J.R.: Congenital Pseudarthrosis of the Tibia. American Academy of Orthopaedic Surgeons Instructional Course Lectures **14:**222–237, 1957.

31. Moore, J.R., Weiland, A.J., and Daniel, R.K.: Use of Free Vascularized Bone Grafts in the Treatment of Bone Tumors. Clin. Orthop. **175:**37–44, 1983.

32. Rathgeb, J.M., Ramsey, P.L., and Cowell, H.R.: Congenital Kyphoscoliosis of the Tibia. Clin. Orthop. **103:**173–190, 1974.

33. Samter, T.G., Vellios, F., and Shafer, W.G.: Neurilemmoma of Bone. Radiology **75:**215, 1960.

34. Sane, S., Yunis, E., and Greer, R.: Subperiosteal or Cortical Cyst and Intramedullary Neurofibromatosis. J. Bone Joint Surg. **53-A:**1194, 1971.

35. Serafin, D., Villarreal-Rios, A., and Georgiade, N.G.: A Rib-Containing Free Flap to Reconstruct Mandibular Defects. Br. J. Plast. Surg. **30:**263–266, 1977.

36. Sofield, H.A.: Congenital Pseudarthrosis of the Tibia. Clin. Orthop. **76:**33–42, 1971.

37. Sofield, H.A., and Miller, E.A.: Fragmentation, Realignment, and Intramedullary Rod Fixation of Deformities of Long Bones in Children: A Ten-Year Appraisal. J. Bone Joint Surg. **41-A:**1371, 1959.

38. Swartz, W.M., Banis, J.C., and Newton, E.D.: The Scapular Osteocutaneous Flap. J. Reconstr. Microsurg. **2:**60, 1985.

39. Tschopp, J.H.: Microsurgical Neuro-Vascular Anastomoses for Transplantation of Composite Bone and Muscle Grafts—An Experimental Study. New York, Springer-Verlag, 1976.

40. Vilkki, P.: Preventive Treatment of Congenital Pseudarthrosis of Tibia. J. Pediatr. Surg. **12:**91–94, 1977.

41. Weiland, A.J., and Daniel, R.K.: Congenital Pseudarthrosis of the Tibia: Treatment with Vascularized Autogenous Fibular Grafts. A Preliminary Report. Johns Hopkins Med. J. **147:**89–95, 1980.

42. Weiland, A.J., Kleinert, H.E., Kutz, J.E., and Daniel, R.K.: Free Vascularized Bone Grafts in Surgery of the Upper Extremity. J. Hand Surg. **4:**129–144, 1979.

43. Weiland, A.J., Moore, J.R., and Daniel, R.K.: The Efficacy of Free Tissue Transfer in the Treatment of Osteomyelitis. J. Bone Joint Surg. **66-A:**181–193, 1984.

44. Weiland, A.J., Moore, J.R., and Daniel, R.K.: Vascularized Bone Autografts. Experience with 41 Cases. Clin. Orthop. **174:**87–95, 1983.

PART X

Hand

CHAPTER 80

Surgery of the Hand: Basic Principles

PAUL R. LIPSCOMB

Sterling Bunnell (1882–1957), father of modern surgery of the hand, once stated, "Next to the brain, the hand is man's greatest asset and to it is due the development of man's handiwork. The hand begins in the opposite cerebral cortex and extends from there to the tips of the nails."[4,5] He emphasized the importance of a detailed knowledge of structural and functional anatomy of the hand and a basic comprehension of that of the entire upper extremity.[9] He also stressed the importance of atraumatic surgical technique for those who perform reconstructive hand surgery. Furthermore, it must be recognized that reconstruction of the hand is often a composite problem, requiring the correlation and knowledge of orthopaedic, plastic, and neuroloic surgical techniques. The hand surgeon must be educated and trained to handle all of the tissues in the extremity.

Surgical reconstruction of the hand requires careful technique to minimize the formation of the adhesions, which tend to bind together the nicely adjusted, movable parts. Although cosmesis is important, the primary purpose of surgical reconstruction is to restore enough function to allow the patient to be self-sufficient.[1,4–7,9–14]

PREOPERATIVE PLAN FOR SURGICAL PROCEDURES

Even in emergency surgical operations involving the hand, the surgeon usually has the opportunity and time to examine carefully the extremity to determine the severity of involvement of the skin, vessels, nerves, tendons, and skeleton. He or she can thereby plan for the anticipated surgical procedure which, following cleansing and debridement, might call for a skin graft or repair of lacerated radial, ulnar, and digital arteries and nerves. By clinical examination and radiographs, the physician can evaluate the skeletal structures and plan for reduction and internal fixation of subluxations, dislocations, and fractures.

For severe injuries, paralytic conditions, and some disease entities, staged surgical repair and reconstructive procedures may be indicated. In these cases, a chronologic sequence of surgical procedures can be planned, and in most cases, can be discussed with the patient and relatives before surgery.

The primary requirement in hand surgery is the restoration of the position of function, nutrition, sensibility, motion, and good skin cover. The ends of the digits should have noncicatricial touch surfaces. The thumb should oppose the fingers, and the hand should open and close for the functions of pinch, hook, and grasp. The wrist should usually be in an extended position, or occasionally in a straight position, and the fingers should be flexed partially at the metacarpophalangeal, proximal interphalangeal, and distal interphalangeal joints. The order of priorities of reconstruction is as follows:[1]

1. Artery
2. Skin
3. Bone and nerve
4. Tendon

When an operation is indicated for emergency or reconstructive procedures, both careful surgical technique and meticulous planning are essential to obtain the best possible results.

POSITION OF THE PATIENT, OPERATING TABLE, ARM BOARD, LIGHTS, EXTREMITY, SURGEON, AND ASSISTANT

A standard operating table is positioned so that a hand board can be attached to it or placed beneath the patient so that its proximal end is anchored firmly. The distal end should have a stable, perpendicular appendage that extends to the floor and is connected to the hand board by a stable hinge. The board should be approximately 15 to 18 inches wide and 48 inches long. With the patient in a comfortable, supine position, the extremity is usually abducted 90° and placed on the arm board. The table and board are arranged so that one of the overhead lights can be positioned above the surgeon's left shoulder and easily focused on the operative field. The stools on which the surgeon and the assistant sit opposite from each other should be firm and stable. Both must be comfortably erect with their forearms resting on the hand board. The assistant positions the hand, holds it stable, and helps as necessary throughout the procedure.[6]

TOURNIQUETS

Use of a tourniquet is mandatory for almost all hand surgery. As Bunnell maintained "A jeweler can't repair a watch in a bottle of ink and neither can we repair a hand in a pool of blood."[5] A bloodless field allows very small vessels and nerves to be seen and to be dissected with accuracy and minimal trauma.

Formerly, Esmarch bandages were used as tourniquets, and tourniquet palsy was not uncommon. Likewise, with the use of blood pressure cuffs that were not monitored by a mercury manometer or equipped with protective safety devices, false pressure readings, which sometimes masked extremely high pressures, remained undetected. The tourniquet gauge should, therefore, be checked and calibrated at least daily, and the figures recorded.[18] Until a time of 2 hr was established by Wilgis as a safe period for a tourniquet to remain in place, tourniquet palsy was common.[19] I have not personally seen or heard of a case of tourniquet palsy in the last 15 years.

Application of Upper Arm Tourniquet

After the patient and the extremity to be operated upon are properly positioned on the table and arm board, respectively, smoothly wrap several layers of sheet wadding or Webril-type soft cast padding around the upper arm and into the lower axilla. Then apply the pneumatic cuff snugly and as high as is comfortably possible over the padding. Securely attach the cuff to the tubing that leads from a storage tank containing nitrogen, and inflate the tourniquet briefly to ensure that the system is operating properly.

During skin preparation, take care to avoid seepage of solutions onto the cast padding and tourniquet cuff. After preparation and draping, the skin may be marked with methylene blue to outline proposed incisions. Then elevate and exsanguinate the extremity with a snugly wrapped, 4-inch-wide, rubber or Ace bandage. In most adults, the tourniquet is then inflated to a pressure of 250 mm Hg; occasionally, in patients with heavily muscled arms or significant hypertension, the tourniquet is inflated to 300 mm Hg. In children, the pressure generally need not exceed 200 mm Hg. Exsanguination is contraindicated in patients with infections or tumors. However, in these patients, elevate the extremity for a couple of minutes before inflating the tourniquet.

In most surgical procedures requiring more than 2 hr of operating time, I deflate the tourniquet for 10 to 15 min at the end of the first 1 to 1.5 hr. During this period, apply pressure to the wound with a soft pad for the first 5 min. Then gently remove the pad and secure hemostasis with the electrocautery unit and ligatures. After 10 to 15 min, elevate the extremity again and reinflate the tourniquet. For more details on use of the tourniquet see chapter 5.

Following application of the dressing, splint, or cast (if such is required), immediately remove the tourniquet and underlying padding. Gently elevate the extremity on one or two pillows to avoid venous congestion.

Finger Tourniquets

A relatively minor procedure, such as excision of a mucous cyst, can be performed safely using digital block anesthesia. Inject the anesthetic agent at the level of the metacarpophalangeal joint. Then apply an encircling rubber tourniquet at the base of the digit. I prefer to use a Penrose drain with a diameter of 12.5 mm (0.5 inch). Wrap the drain once around the base of the digit without tension; then mark and clamp with a hemostat the points at which the surfaces of the drain meet on the circumference. Remove the loop. Shorten the distance between the two marks by 20 mm. Reposition the Penrose drain around the base of the digit. As the assistant elevates and compresses the finger, stretch the drain around the finger so that the length is shortened by 20 mm. Then clamp the drain with the hemostat. The pressure thus generated will produce a bloodless field; the risk of digital nerve and arterial damage secondary to this pressure is minimal.

As an alternative, Salem described a method of simultaneous exsanguination of the finger and application of a digital tourniquet.[16] A finger is cut from a sterile rubber glove and rolled onto the finger. The tip is cut from it and the remaining portion is then rolled proximally to form a rubber ring at the base of the finger. This technique is contraindicated in the presence of infection or tumors.

SELECTION OF ANESTHESIA

The ultimate choice of anesthesia for each procedure, other than a local block, is decided by the anesthesiologist.[15,17] It is important to discuss with the anesthesiologist the patient's concerns and wishes, the estimated length of the operation, and the length of time the tourniquet will be in place. For most children, for apprehensive adults, and for extensive procedures and cases requiring surgery elsewhere on the body, general anesthesia is usually preferable. A general anesthetic may also be necessary because infection or neoplasm may contraindicate regional anesthesia.

Regional anesthesia in the form of supraclavicular, axillary, brachial, and peripheral nerve blocks is very satisfactory for many procedures involving the upper extremity. Preoperative and, if necessary, intraoperative sedation may be used to keep the patient from moving and to lessen discomfort from the tourniquet.

Intravenous anesthesia using 1% lidocaine solution and two tourniquets on the arm, when administered by a competent anesthesiologist, is satisfactory for many surgical procedures on the hand.

Occasionally, when active movement of the patient's fingers is desirable during surgery, a block of the superficial branch of the radial nerve above the styloid process of the radius, as well as of the ulnar and median nerves on the palmar aspect of the wrist, is indicated. With proper preoperative sedation and, if necessary, intravenous augmentation, the tourniquet is generally tolerated well for half an hour or longer.

INSTRUMENTS

Just as the jeweler cannot use the same instruments to repair a watch as does the automobile mechanic to repair a car, the hand surgeon requires special instruments that are often smaller than those required for most other surgical procedures.[6] Small knife blades, such as Bard Parker Nos. 15 and 11; small Adson forceps; pointed, curved, and straight scissors; osteotomes and chisels; ronguers and small bone cutters; probes; hemostats; curettes; gouges; tendon strippers; sharp hook and blade retractors; needles; sutures; and ligatures are indispensable for surgery of the hand. Other special instruments; various hand holders, including those made of malleable lead; as well as hand and motorized drills; special sutures; and small needles are available from several manufacturers. Special sterilized sets of hand instruments should be available in every operating suite.

MAGNIFICATION

Many hand surgeons routinely use 2.5- to 4-power magnifying glasses or loupes when dissecting. With magnification, the planes between diseased and normal tissue are immediately apparent. Likewise, the small branches of the digital nerves and arteries are seen and protected easily. Moreover, routine repair of lacerated digital nerves is facilitated. For those who perform microvascular surgery, a variety of microsurgical instruments, as well as a triple- or double-headed binocular microscope with electric foot controls that allows 6- to 15-power magnification, are necessary. It must be emphasized that the surgeon should learn, practice, and develop the technical skills of operating with microscopic magnification in the microsurgery laboratory. Only after this experience may the surgeon apply this skill to patients.

SKIN PREPARATION AND DRAPING

Each hand surgeon and operating facility should establish a standardized routine for preparation of the skin and draping, thereby ensuring that each patient receives the same careful attention to detail that is necessary for successful hand surgery. If the surgical procedure is an elective one, the patient is cautioned at the time of scheduling about the importance of avoiding scratches and abrasions to the hand and entire extremity for 1 to 2 weeks before the operation. Patients who are manual laborers and who are accustomed to having grease and dirt on their hands are advised to scrub their hands with a detergent solution twice daily for several days prior to surgery.

Formerly, it was customary to shave the entire extremity to be operated on, but it has been shown that this is unnecessary and, in fact, may do more harm than good. In recent years, shaving has been limited to the site of the proposed incisions and is done in the operating room before final skin preparation. The nails should be cleansed and trimmed, and polish should be removed before the patient enters the operating room.

After the patient and the extremity are properly positioned on the operating table and arm board, respectively, scrub the hand and forearm for 10 min with a sterile povidone-iodine solution from the tips of the nails to the upper arm where the pneumatic tourniquet is in position. Then dry the extremity with sterile towels and paint it with povidone-iodine. Next, apply sterile drapes and stockinette to the hand and forearm. Then, exsanguinate or elevate the extremity, requesting that the tourniquet be inflated. Take a seat, usually on the axillary side of the patient, and cut the stockinette to expose the hand. The assistant, who is stationed across from the surgeon, holds the patient's hand firm and motionless as the operation proceeds.

BASIC SURGICAL TECHNIQUE

The basic aim of hand surgery is to restore function and cosmesis to the greatest extent possible within the shortest, safest period of time. In acute injuries, this can often be accomplished by thorough cleansing and debridement of the wound, followed by primary repair of nerve, bone, and tendon injuries. However, it must be remembered that, in some cases of severe and mutilating injuries, the primary object of treatment is to obtain healing of the skin and subcutaneous tissues without intercurrent wound infection. These injuries often mandate delayed wound closure and a further delay in the repair of tendons and nerves. For each injury or reconstructive procedure, a basic plan, which may consist of one or more stages, should be formulated.[11,12]

The time required for subsidence of the induration of tissues which follows each injury and surgical procedure is variable, and must be anticipated. It is best to wait until all inflammatory signs have subsided, the danger of infection is past, the tissues are soft and supple, and the joints are flexible. During this waiting period, proper positioning, encouragement of active motion, and the use of corrective splinting help to prevent permanent stiffness.

Surgical incisions are made so that they offer the best possible exposure, protection of important structures, and healing with minimal scar. For some conditions, they should parallel the flexion creases in the fingers, palm, and wrist. Frequently, zigzag incisions, as described by Bruner, or the traditional Bunnell incision in a midlateral location are most appropriate.[3,5] On the dorsum, curved and S-shaped incisions are frequently appropriate for the fingers, metacarpal area, and wrist. Often, transverse incisions are used at the level of the wrist. (See chapter 2 for surgical exposures).

Sharp dissection with the aid of loupes or magnifying glasses, Bard Parker Nos. 15 and 11 blades, and small curved Mayo scissors is essential for the atraumatic technique that has been championed by Bunnell and his disciples.

Maintain hemostasis with small hemostats and a bipolar cautery unit, both during the surgical procedure and just before wound closure when the tourniquet is deflated for a few minutes. Then, irrigate the wound with Ringer's or normal saline solution and elevate the extremity while the tourniquet is reinflated and the skin is closed.

Primary skin closure is appropriate for most surgical procedures and some sharp traumatic wounds. Interrupted 5-0 or 6-0 nylon sutures are usually used for closure of surgical wounds of the hand. An occasional subcutaneous absorbable suture of 5-0 chromic catgut allows removal of the skin sutures at the end of 1 week. If necessary, Steri-strips can then be applied, thereby eliminating cross-hatch suture scars. For children, I frequently use 5-0 chromic catgut subcuticular suture and small Steri-strips to obviate the need for suture removal.

POSTOPERATIVE CARE

Dressings

After most surgical procedures, the hand can be placed in the position of function in a large, soft, Bunnell-type dressing. A sterile pad of medium-coarse steel wool is incorporated for compression. I prefer this because steel wool does not lose its sponginess as do other materials, including the sea sponge. Plaster of Paris, fiberglass, or thermoplastic material is incorporated in the well-padded dressing, which usually extends from the proximal level of the nails to the upper forearm. If flexor tendons or nerves are repaired, the wrist and involved digit are immobilized in a semi-flexed position to remove tension, but are never positioned in full flexion. In extensor tendon injuries, the wrist is immobilized in extension, as is the involved digit. In most cases, the dressing and splints should be applied with the forearm in supination. This is especially important if the splints or cast extend above the elbow. Of course, there are times when the forearm should be in a mid position. Rarely should it be immobilized in pronation.

General Care

Upon removal of the drapes and tourniquet, evaluate and record the status of circulation in the exposed finger tips. Keep the hand elevated on pillows that are appreciably higher than the shoulder. Evaluate the status of circulation hourly if the procedure was extensive enough to warrant hospitalization. If there is any question about adequacy of circulation, loosen the bandages and splints; if a cast has been applied, it should be split and spread along its full length.

When the patient becomes ambulatory, the extremity should be held in an elevated position at shoulder level or above. This position is often easiest to maintain if patients are advised to place the operated hand on the opposite shoulder. They are cautioned not to place the hand in a dependent posi-

tion. Formerly, the extremity was always placed in a sling. However, this practice results in much more dependent edema and postoperative stiffness than occurs when cooperative patients keep the extremity elevated by use of their own muscles.

Upon dismissal from the hospital or outpatient facility, patients and their relatives are instructed to check circulation in the fingertips by the blanch test. Patients are advised to return immediately should there be any concern about the adequacy of circulation.

Splinting

The correct use of splints is an important aspect of surgery of the hand. Splinting is used to prevent deformity, immobilize the operated part, protect joints and tendons, change or correct the position of joints, substitute for paralyzed muscles, and move joints passively.

The wrist is the key joint in the mechanics and function of the hand, whereas the metacarpophalangeal joint is of primary importance in the mechanical balance of a finger. Splinting the wrist in extension and the metacarpophalangeal in flexion is of fundamental importance unless specifically contraindicated.

Temporary splinting or immobilization is used before, as well as after, many injuries and surgical procedures. Splints may be made with plaster of Paris, fiberglass, plastics, or malleable metals. They are usually padded with sheet wadding, cotton, or felt, and are fastened to the extremity with web straps and buckles or Velcro fasteners.

Immobilization is used for treating infection, holding fractured bones in place, and facilitating healing after trauma or surgery. A limb is held in a certain position to protect against breaking newly repaired tissues, such as tendons, nerves, ligaments, and arteries; to keep paralyzed muscles in a relaxed position; and, in some cases, to allow tissues to grow until they adapt to the desired position. Joints are gradually pulled into increased flexion or extension to correct deformities, to place the limb in the position of function, or to produce more motion in a joint.

Splints should not only maintain the position of function, but should also allow function of all uninjured parts. Only injured joints are splinted. Dynamic splinting is used to draw joints into flexion or extension gradually, as in changing the position from one of nonfunction to that of function. Rubber bands, spring wire, or flat blue spring steel produce tension that is controllable yet insufficient to injure the joints or to cause ischemia. In recent years, active splinting, with the aid of electrical appliances, has also been used to produce continuous passive motion.

Internal splinting, using Kirschner wires, pins, screws, or plates, is used to pin and immobilize fractured bones or joints. Special, internal, removable sutures can be used to pull the proximal ends of severed tendons distally, thereby eliminating or diminishing tension at the site of repair where individual sutures are used.[2,8]

Numerous and various hand splints, fabricated for different purposes, are advertised in orthopaedic periodicals and can be obtained from surgical supply houses or manufacturers. It is advisable for hospitals and outpatient facilities to maintain a supply of commonly used hand splints in several sizes to permit ready access by physicians who care for injuries and deformities of the hand.

CONCLUSION

The following article, entitled "Who Should Do Surgery of the Hand?", which was published as an editorial 27 years ago, is as applicable to hand surgery today as it was then:[10]*

Approximately one-third of all injuries requiring the services of a physician or a surgeon, whether in the emergency department of a metropolitan hospital or the office of a rural practitioner, involve the hand. The physician administering the primary treatment for such injuries has a great responsibility, since his treatment determines, to a large extent, the final outcome.

All physicians must be taught the basic principles that should govern the treatment of an injury to the hand. They must know that it is important to protect wounds from contamination and infection and that adequate help, facilities, and proper instruments must be available before one starts to care for the injured hand. The traumatized hand must be cleansed thoroughly but gently. When compared with injuries of the arm, leg, or abdomen, the involved tissue of the hand should be sparingly debrided. Whereas many wounds of the arms and legs should be treated by delayed closure, almost all wounds of the hand should be closed primarily and this closure must be without tension. In some instances, the use of skin grafts is necessary to avoid tension. When possible, fractures should be reduced and immobilized at the time of the primary treatment. However, if the physician is not trained to care adequately for the bone injury, less harm will be done if the skin is closed, the hand is placed in a position of moderate dorsiflexion of the wrist, moderate flexion of the fingers, and moderate abduction and opposition of the thumb, and a bulky dressing is applied to prevent edema. In such selected instances, the fractures can be dealt with after the cutaneous wound has healed. Even more important is the necessity to realize that severed nerves and tendons do not require primary repair; less harm will be done under unfavorable conditions by secondary repair of nerves and tendons after the initial wound has healed. A surgeon who attempts primary suture of a flexor tendon in its digital sheath should have had considerable education, training, and experience in reconstructive surgical treatment of the hand and should be capable of performing a tendon graft.

Extensive, reparative, restorative, reconstructive, and rehabilitative surgery of the hand should be carried out in hospitals by surgeons well qualified and dedicated to this field of surgery. The surgeon interested in treatment of the severely injured hand must be educated to work in orthopedic surgery, plastic surgery, and neurosurgery. He should have knowledge of dermatologic, circulatory, paralytic and arthritic diseases which are prone to affect the hand. He must be well versed in the most minute details of the surgical and functional anatomy of the entire upper extremity. He

must be versed in rehabilitative procedures and trained in splinting and bracing. He must be capable of teaching the patient how to prevent and overcome stiffness of joints and how to co-ordinate muscles which formerly had one function but after a tendon transfer have another function.

Above all, the surgeon who devotes much of his time to surgery of the hand must teach medical students, interns, and residents how to care properly for injuries which affect the hand. Many of the principles established by such pioneers as Allen Kanavel, Sterling Bunnell, and Sumner Koch are still basic and pertinent. It is important that these principles be learned if crippling of the hand is to be minimized.

REFERENCES

1. Boyes, J.H.: Bunnell's Surgery of the Hand, 4th ed. Philadelphia, J.B. Lippincott, 1964.
2. Brown, C.P., and McGrouther, D.A.: Excursion of the Tendon of Flexor Pollicus Longus and Its Relation to Dynamic Splintage. J. Hand Surg. **9-A:**787, 1984.
3. Bruner, J.M.: The Zigzag Volar-digital Incision for Flexor Tendon Surgery. Plast. Reconstr. Surg. **40:**571, 1967.
4. Bunnell, Sterling: Splinting the Hand. *In* Instructional Course Lectures, American Academy of Orthopaedic Surgeons. **9:**233, 1952.
5. Bunnell, Sterling: Surgery of the Hand, 3rd ed. Philadelphia, J.B. Lippincott, 1948.
6. Bunnell, Sterling: Personal Communication, 1953.
7. Green, D.P.: General Principles in Operative Hand Surgery. *In* Operative Hand Surgery. New York, Churchill Livingstone, 1982, pp. 1–21.
8. Hester, R.T., Jr., and Foad, N.: Early Mobilization of Repaired Flexor Tendons Within Digital Sheath Using an Internal Profundus Splint: Experimental and Clinical Data. Ann. Plastic Surg. **12:**187, 1984.
9. Kaplan, Emanuel B.: Anatomy and Kinesiology of the Hand. *In* Flynn, J.E. (ed.): Hand Surgery, 3rd ed. Baltimore, Williams & Wilkins, 1982, pp. 33–44.
10. Lipscomb, P.R.: Who Should Do Surgery of the Hand? Surg. Gynecol. Obstet. **113:**233, 1961.
11. Lipscomb, P.R.: Treatment of Acute Injuries of the Hand. South Dakota J. Med. Pharmacol. **11:**447, 1958.
12. Lipscomb, P.R.: Management of Recent Injuries of the Hand. Minn. Med. **38:**299, 1955.
13. Lynch, A.C., and Lipscomb, P.R.: Management of Fractures of the Hand. Am. Surg. **29:**277, 1963.
14. Milford, Lee: The Hand. *In* Allen S. Edmonson, M.D. and A.H. Crenshaw, M.D. (eds.): Campbell's Operative Orthopaedics, 6th ed. St. Louis, Mosby, 1980, pp. 110–417.
15. Ramamurthy, S.: Anesthesia. *In* Green, D.P. (ed.): Operative Hand Surgery. New York, Churchill Livingston, 1982, pp. 23–54.
16. Salem, M.Z.A.: Simple Finger Tourniquet. Br. Med. J. **1:**779, 1973.
17. Vandam, L.D.: Anesthesia for Hand Surgery. *In* Flynn, J.E. (ed.): Hand Surgery, 3rd ed. Baltimore, Williams & Wilkins, 1982, pp. 74–84.
18. Wheeler, D.K., and Lipscomb, P.R.: A Safety Device for a Pneumatic Tourniquet. J. Bone Joint Surg. **46-A:**870, 1964.
19. Wilgis, E.F.S.: Observations on the Effects of Tourniquet Ischemia. J. Bone Joint Surg. **53-A:**1343, 1971.

* Reprinted by permission of *Surgery, Gynecology & Obstetrics.*

CHAPTER 81

Injuries of the Fingernails

JAMES A. LILLA

Injuries of the fingertips are the most common hand injuries, and they often include or are limited to injuries of the fingernails. The best results in patients with nail injuries are achieved by optimal initial treatment; revision or reconstructive surgery is generally less rewarding.

NAIL NOMENCLATURE, ANATOMY, AND PHYSIOLOGY

The nail complex comprises four components. These include the nail plate, the nail bed or matrix, the perinail soft tissues, and the underlying bone and ligamentous support.

The nail plate provides support and stability to the soft tissues of the distal finger and also provides a firm, sharp edge to aid in grasping and in picking up small objects. It is a cornified, epithelial structure and is inert insofar as repair is concerned. Though not directly innervated, the nail plate provides tactile feedback through its attachments to the richly innervated nail bed. The nail plate is produced by the underlying matrix or bed, with about 90% of the plate being formed by the germinal tissues that are within and just distal to the proximal nail fold. As the growing nail is pushed out from within the proximal fold, it is held to and slightly thickened by the specialized cells of the more distal nail bed. According to Zaias[24] and Norton,[16] the basal cells of the proximal nail bed stream distally with the nail plate as it advances. The cells on the undersurface of the roof over the proximal nail fold adhere to the nail plate; although these cells create the finished surface of the nail plate, they contribute very little to its bulk.

The nail plate and underlying bed are supported by the distal phalanx and associated ligaments (Figs. 81-1 and 81-2). The bed is bound to the periosteum on the dorsum of the distal phalanx. The lateral margins of the nail plate are anchored through the bed to the lateral interosseous ligaments of the distal segment and to the tuft and lateral tubercle of the distal and proximal portions of the distal phalanx, respectively (see Fig. 81-2). The rich blood supply and innervation of the nail bed stem from the palmar neurovascular bundles to the dorsum of the tip and are at least partially protected by the lateral interosseous ligament.[9,20] The insertion of the extensor tendon of the distal phalanx extends across the dorsal lip of the distal phalanx to the proximal margin of the nail matrix.

The nomenclature used to describe the tissues that form and hold the nail varies.[1,10,12,16,24,27] I will use the term nail bed to describe the nail-forming and nail-holding tissues as a unit; the term germinal matrix will be used to describe the proximal ventral tissue that generates the main nail plate (from the proximal nail fold), whereas sterile matrix will be the term used to designate the more distal tissue of the nail bed that holds down the nail plate (see Fig. 81-1).

Other soft tissues surrounding the nail include the following:

1. Hyponychium—the tissue beneath the free distal margin of the nail plate that serves as a transitional area to the normal glabrous skin of the fingertip
2. Eponychium—the transitional area at the distal margin of the proximal nail fold where the epithelium of the dorsal skin adheres to the advancing nail plate

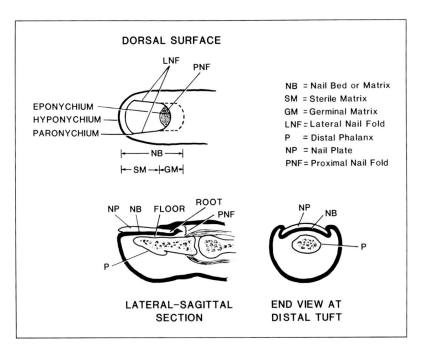

FIGURE 81-1.   Anatomy of and terminology for the distal segment of the fingernail.

3. Peronychium—the skin at the nail margin at the lateral nail folds
4. Perionychium—all of the soft tissues that surround the nail at its margin in a composite manner
5. Lunula—the white half-moon beneath the proximal nail plate just distal to the proximal nail fold; the lunula corresponds to an area of thin, more loosely adherent nail plate at the distal margin of the germinal matrix.[10]

Nail growth rates may vary as a result of many factors, including age, injury, metabolic or systemic illness, and the digit involved. There may be seasonal or familial factors involved as well. In general, fingernails grow about 0.1 mm/day so that it takes approximately 3 months or 100 days to replace a nail. Fingernails tend to grow faster than toenails, and the rate of nail growth tends to decline with age.[24,25]

The growth of a nail can often be monitored by observing the advancement of the transverse ridges that may form under certain circumstances. If the distal segment of a digit is traumatized, even without loss of the nail, or if there has been some systemic illness or metabolic disturbance, there may be a lag period followed by a period of accelerated nail growth during which a transverse ridge may form across the nail plate. This ridge may cause concern for the patient, but it usually advances off the end of the digit with continuing nail growth. When a nail plate has been removed, the advancing edge of the new nail plate often has a ventrally curved mound at its leading edge, giving it the appearance of an ingrowing nail. Unless there is a discontinuity in the bed, such as from scar, this edge is not likely to grow inward; rather, it usually pushes the debris of the distal portions of the nail bed as it advances, gradually lifting off, leaving a typical free margin of nail plate.

ACUTE INJURIES

Nail injuries may include a loose nail plate, a laceration, a loss of tissue, or an associated bone injury. Frequently, the injury is a combination of these.[26]

A sharp laceration may create a simple linear wound, the edges of which may lie in excellent apposition without suturing. However, it is much more common for the nail bed wound to be stellate, with irregular margins. The goal of repair or reconstruction is to provide a functional and esthetic fingernail. This requires conservation of parts and minimization of scar within the nail bed.

A longitudinal scar within the nail bed can produce a longitudinal split-nail deformity, whereas a transverse scar in the

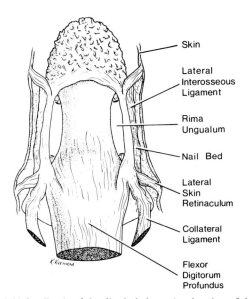

FIGURE 81-2.   Fascia of the distal phalanx. A volar view of the deep dissection of the distal phalanx with the various fibrous attachments to the lateral tubercle and distal tuft. Note the nail bed attachment to the lateral interosseous ligament. (Shrewsbury, M., and Johnson, R. K.: The fascia of the distal phalanx. J. Bone Joint Surg. **57-A:**784, 1975.)

bed may cause the nail plate to "lift off" prematurely. Another type of split-nail deformity occurs when there is a transverse scar at the proximal nail bed; this sometimes causes a second, small, thin nail plate to be created by the distal bed. This secondary plate may then emerge beneath the free margin of the proximally generated plate. If any portion of the nail bed does not participate in nail plate production, it will produce keratinous debris. If there is a deficiency of the soft tissues surrounding the nail bed or a lack of underlying support, there may be distortion of the advancing nail plate, the most common example of which is the "beak" nail, which curves in a palmar direction over the tip of an amputated digit.[2]

Portions of the nail matrix that are trapped beneath the surface after injury may produce epidermal inclusion cysts. These cysts may occur within the soft tissues, or they may involve bone by external pressure or by being trapped within a previous fracture line. These inclusion cysts may also form from residual remnants of the nail bed following amputations through the proximal nail bed or after attempts at surgical ablation of the nail. Often, these cysts are not clinically evident for 6 months or longer after the surgery, but they may be a cause of continuing discomfort or inflammation of an injured fingertip.

Principles and Technique of Preoperative, Operative, and Postoperative Care

The following general principles apply to the evaluation of and planning for repair of nail bed injuries:

Inspect the nail bed for reparable injury if the nail plate is loose.
Avoid disturbing the intact nail bed whenever possible.
Leave any intact, adherent nail plate in place.
Retain the attached flaps of nail bed tissue for repair.
Restore underlying bone support.
Retain distal phalanx length beneath the nail bed.
Provide appropriate perinail supportive tissue, especially at the fingertip.
Repair the nail bed and perinail tissue with meticulous technique.
Replace the nail plate or similar "spacer" beneath the proximal nail fold if there is any injury at that level.
Monitor the postoperative course closely.

The remainder of this section describes the techniques used to apply these principles to each clinical situation.

Radiography

In most nail injuries other than nail plate avulsion, there will be associated trauma to the fingertip. Knowledge of the status of the distal phalanx, as determined by radiographic evaluation, facilitates assessment and treatment. This is especially important if there is a history of a crush or penetrating injury, as nail bed tissue can easily be trapped within a fracture.

Anesthesia

A digital block is usually adequate for evaluation and repair of nail bed injuries. A wider anesthetic might be dictated by associated injuries.

Wound Preparation

The wound is cleansed and irrigated, after which an initial assessment of the injury is made. Adherent nail indicates an intact, uninjured nail bed. Any nail plate that is not attached to its bed, as evidenced by the appearance of air or hematoma beneath the nail plate, should be considered for removal. An exception to this rule is when a very small area (less than 25% of the nail area) shows evidence of hematoma but no lacerations of the perinail tissues and no underlying fracture.

Removal of the Nail Plate

Separate the proximal portion of the nail plate at the germinal matrix from its bed by blunt dissection from a free margin. Remove the more distal nail plate by blunt transverse dissection, just under the plate, with fine tenotomy scissors or periosteal elevator. Remove the nail plate in one piece, if possible, especially at the proximal portions, so that it may be used as a stent at the conclusion of the repair.

If the nail plate is in one piece and is adherent at its margins but obviously loose and undermined by hematoma, remove it for inspection of the nail bed. Replace the nail as a splint once appropriate inspection and repair are completed. In the past, it was suggested that the nail be left in place to act as a splint in such instances. However, that practice may cause a significant nail bed injury or entrapment of soft tissue in a fracture to remain hidden, and trapped hematoma may serve as a substrate for infection. Replace the nail as a splint once inspection and repair are completed.

Tourniquet

Hemostasis is necessary for appropriate evaluation and repair of the nail bed. Use a digital or limb tourniquet, as preferred, during the repair, but remove it before applying the dressing.

Debridement

After careful inspection and with the aid of loupe magnification, remove contaminated or devitalized tissue, preserving as much of the original tissues as possible. There is considerable resistance to infection and good healing potential in this area because of the blood supply, so retain any potentially viable tissue for repair. Gently scrub and extensively irrigate the area with sterile saline solutions to minimize the risk of infection. It is difficult to compensate for gaps in the nail bed by advancing local tissues unless there has been shortening of the bone, so keep debridement to the minimal level that is compatible with good overall wound management. Occasionally, definitive repair should be delayed for a few days to allow tissue demarcation.

Surgical Repair

Repair injured tissues around the nail first. Then repair the nail bed using fine, absorbable suture material (6-0 or 7-0 chromic or plain gut) and atraumatic needles with accurate edge-to-edge approximation (Fig. 81-3). If nonabsorbable sutures are used, remove them within 5 to 7 days to prevent their incorporation in the healing epithelium and developing nail plate.

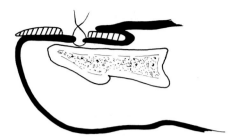

FIGURE 81-3. Suture placement, lateral view. The adherent nail plate is left in place.

The nail bed is quite soft and the suture or needle can easily cut through the free edge that is being sewn. At times, it may be more difficult to place the sutures when the edges of the wound are approximated than when they are apart. In this instance, it may be advantageous to place all of the sutures without tying them until the last one is placed, while leaving adequate length for tying. The wound edges can then be approximated and the sutures gently tied.

Carry the repair into the sulci along the lateral nail folds and beneath the proximal nail fold if the wound extends into those areas. It may be necessary to elevate the roof of the proximal nail bed with incisions at the proximal corners (Fig. 81-4) in order to gain access. Use corner incisions to minimize scarring of the roof that might otherwise blemish the surface of the new nail or cause synechiae with the germinal matrix below.

When there is an associated fracture of the physis or metaphysis of the distal phalanx, it may be necessary to elevate the proximal nail fold for reduction of the bone and dislocated nail matrix; the fracture can then be irrigated and reduced under direct vision and the nail matrix returned beneath the proximal nail fold. Half-buried horizontal mattress sutures extending from the base of the nail bed or nail plate, passing through the sulcus to the dorsum of the finger, and tied over small bolsters provide appropriate anchorage to the nail bed. When combined with an appropriate postoperative splint, these sutures may be adequate to stabilize the fracture (Fig. 81-5).

If a laceration is immediately adjacent to an area with an adherent nail plate, I prefer to remove only a 2-mm strip of nail

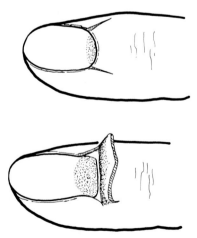

FIGURE 81-4. The proximal nail fold may be elevated to gain access to the proximal nail bed.

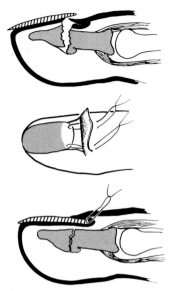

FIGURE 81-5. Use of half-buried horizontal mattress sutures, in conjunction with nail roof elevation, to anchor a displaced nail plate or nail bed, or both, into the proximal nail fold.

plate at that margin in order to gain access to the underlying nail bed (see Fig. 81-3). Although it is possible to pass some needles through intact nail, these needles are larger than those needed for the repair. Moreover, and more importantly, one cannot achieve accurate approximation of the nail bed if the suture encompasses the overlying nail plate as well.

Some surgeons advocate removal of the entire nail plate if a repair is necessary. This practice eliminates the need to work around the residual nail plate, and does not seem to detract from the ultimate result. However, it is more comfortable for the patient not to have uninvolved nail plate removed, and the possibility for iatrogenic injury to the bed is thereby decreased. No interference in nail growth occurs as a result of residual, distally situated, attached nail plate; it is simply loosened and pushed off by the advance of the new nail growth.

Application of the Dressing and Stenting

After release of the tourniquet and establishment of hemostasis by gentle compression over the nail bed (with or without the use of topical hemostatic agents), cover the repaired nail bed with a nonadherent dressing, such as Adaptic or Xeroform. Porcine xenograft has also been used as a temporary nail bed cover.[8] If a stent is to be placed beneath the proximal nail fold, there is not enough room for any further dressing in the fold. A stent serves as a splint for the repaired nail bed and as a spacer to keep the roof of the nail bed from healing directly to the underlying germinal matrix. In any but the most innocuous nail plate avulsions, a wound in the matrix can form an adhesion between the floor and the roof of the nail fold, thereby dividing the components of the germinal matrix and separating the developing nail plate. These adhesions or synechiae can be minimized by using a stent composed of the old nail plate or a thin (0.020-inch), nonreactive, synthetic sheeting, such as Silastic. Commercial stents are also available. Suture the stent to the nail margin with fine, nonabsorbable sutures to prevent it from dislodging easily. The stent must allow for drainage at its margins for good wound hygiene (Fig. 81-6). Complete the dressing with gentle compression using sterile gauze.

Postoperative Care

The use of antibiotics is dictated by the nature of the wound, but is usually not mandated by nail bed injury alone. The wound should be inspected and cleansed every few days, especially if a stent is used, in order to prevent accumulation of drainage material beneath the stent which might otherwise provide a substrate for infection. If the gauze dressing is partially adherent, it may be loosened gently by soaking in a sterile, nontoxic solution, such as a 1:1 saline/hydrogen peroxide mix. If a thin layer of adherent gauze becomes incorporated into the crust without evidence of drainage beneath it, the gauze can be left in place. It will be sloughed as underlying epithelialization is completed, much as occurs in a split-thickness skin graft donor site. Stents are usually removed within 2 weeks or when the wounds appear to be epithelialized beneath the proximal nail fold.

Subungual Hematoma

Frequently, fairly minor, nonpenetrating trauma of the distal segment will result in the separation of the nail plate from its bed without major disruption of the bed. The space that results from this separation will fill with blood, and this entrapped hematoma may exert sufficient pressure on the nail bed to cause considerable pain for the patient. When there is evidence of enough trauma to have caused a reparable laceration of the bed, remove the involved nail plate and inspect the nail bed for possible repair. If there is a small, subungual hematoma that does not cause much discomfort for the patient, no further treatment may be necessary. However, hematomas that cause considerable pain should be treated with drainage. The potentially adverse effects of such drainage include further nail bed injury secondary to overpenetration into the nail bed or an increased possibility of infection as a result of the conversion from a sealed to an open wound.

To drain a subungual hematoma, perforate the nail plate over the hematoma. This perforation may be made with any sharp, sterile object, such as a heavy needle, a No. 11 scalpel blade, or a small drill bit. Alternatively, a small hole may be burned through the nail plate with a thermal cautery device or

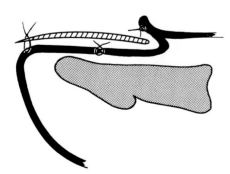

FIGURE 81-6. The stent is positioned in the proximal nail fold to prevent adhesions. Note the anchoring suture at the distal nail bed.

a heated, blunt paper clip. Whatever technique is used, the hole should be large enough to allow continuous drainage and to minimize fluid retention beneath the plate. Typically, there is a small eruption of seroma as the pressure beneath the plate is relieved, and the patient experiences almost immediate relief. The fingertip is dressed for the first few days to minimize the potential for infection, and the patient is asked to keep the fingertip clean and dry. Occasionally, it may be necessary to repeat the drainage procedure a day or two later if there is a recurrence of the throbbing pain and the original hole appears to be sealed. Nail plate perforation is also used to enhance drainage from beneath a nail if the nail is to be replaced as a stent after nail bed repair.

Tissue Loss

As long as the nail bed tissues are present and attached, a meticulous repair is indicated. Occasionally, there will be loss of tissue with a commensurate loss of underlying distal phalanx, such as might occur from a transverse or slightly oblique power-saw injury across the dorsum. In such cases, the surgeon may find that the nail bed can be trimmed back to a level that permits direct approximation and repair after the gap in the bone has been closed.

Longitudinal defects in the nail bed, with or without central bone loss, may be closed by undermining the lateral remnants of nail bed, but a split-nail deformity is still likely to occur later. The fibrous attachments of the lateral portions of the nail bed will limit the degree to which these tissues can be moved, particularly at the proximal nail bed.

If there is a partial- or full-thickness nail bed loss, salvage the detached tissues from the avulsed nail plate and use them as skin grafts to resurface the nail bed. Cleanse the avulsed tissues, gently dissect them off the nail plate or other tissues, and suture them into place where needed, usually into their original location.

When the missing tissues are not recoverable or usable, the surgeon may apply a split-thickness skin graft or choose to allow the area of the defect to heal by secondary intention.[19,25] Split-thickness nail bed grafting with the toe as a donor site has produced good results (Fig. 81-7). Skin grafting from other non-nail donor areas generally provides wound coverage, but such grafts will not participate in nail regeneration or adherence. In many instances, satisfactory nail regeneration and adherence will occur if a partial-thickness loss of the distal nail bed is allowed to heal by secondary intention. Zaias has shown that the epithelial cells of the proximal matrix will advance with the nail plate, and that the cells of the lateral nail bed will repopulate the central portions of the nail bed.[24] The prognosis is worse the more proximal the injury where nail matrix responsible for the nail plate formation is located. The proximal nail bed is also the most difficult area to replace, although free full-thickness grafts of partial or complete nail beds have been successful.[14,17,18,21] Donor digit morbidity must be considered when full-thickness nail bed grafting is contemplated. Most often, full-thickness nail bed grafting is reserved for secondary reconstruction unless the tissue becomes available as the result of the initial injury (i.e., if it is salvaged from another irreparable digit). Reversed dermal grafts have also been used as donor tissue.[3]

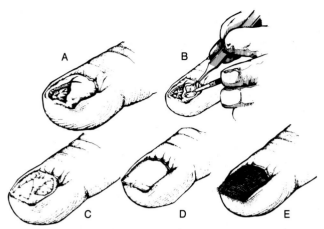

FIGURE 81-7. Split-thickness skin graft to the nail bed. (*A*) Diagram of a full-thickness nail bed avulsion. (*B*) Technique for removing a split-thickness nail bed graft. Magnification is used. (*C*) A split-thickness nail bed graft is sutured over the defect with 7-0 chromic catgut. (*D*) The nail, when available, is replaced over the defect and a pressure dressing is applied. (*E*) When the nail is not available, a single thickness of Betadine gauze (Purdue Frederick Co., Norwalk, CT) is placed over the defect with the proximal portion slipped under the proximal nail fold. (Shepard, G.H.: Treatment of nail bed avulsions with split-thickness nail bed graft. J. Hand Surg. 8:49, 1983.)

Extensive loss of nail bed is often accompanied by a loss of underlying bone as well. In such cases, the distal segment of a digit can be shortened to allow direct closure of the soft tissues. Immediate or delayed reconstruction of extensive defects with composite vascularized tissue transfer, usually from a toe donor site, is possible using microscopic techniques.[15]

RECONSTRUCTION

Split-Nail Deformity

When a nail grows out with more than one plate portion, the patient may either accept the deformity and keep the edges well-trimmed and smooth, or consider a reconstructive procedure. The surgeon undertaking reconstruction has several op-

tions. An attempt can be made to reconstruct a smooth bed by excising scar and realigning the nail bed (ideally, leaving less scar and creating a fused nail plate). Alternatively, the smaller nail part may be ablated, thereby leaving a nail of reduced size, or the entire nail may be ablated. Finally, complete nail bed grafting may be attempted.

Secondary nail bed reconstruction is challenging. Portions of the bed are mobilized to bring the parts into approximation after scar excision, and underlying bone malposition is corrected (Fig. 81-8).[3,11]

I prefer partial nail bed ablation for most split-nail deformities, regardless of whether they are longitudinally or transversely oriented. A slightly shortened nail bed is usually preferable to a nonadherent nail at the tip; moreover, a slightly narrow but otherwise one-piece, full-length nail is both functional and usually esthetic.

Partial or Complete Nail Ablation

For any nail ablation, first elevate the proximal nail fold with incisions at one or both corners (see Fig. 81-4) to remove the involved nail matrix. Include the nail-producing elements of the roof of the nail bed beneath the proximal nail fold in the excision, leaving a flap of dorsal skin to cover the denuded proximal bed. If the central portions of the germinal matrix are ablated, take care to avoid detaching the insertion of the extensor tendon at the base of the distal phalanx. Any remnant of matrix may subsequently produce a symptomatic epidermal cyst. Advise the patient that a secondary operation may be needed to remove such a cyst. Epidermal cysts should be excised intact in order to ensure inclusion of all germinal elements.

Allow the ablated area to heal by secondary intention or obtain coverage by mobilizing surrounding tissue or grafting skin directly onto the exposed bone. Flap coverage is usually unnecessary. If a complete nail ablation is performed, a full-thickness skin graft, set as a unit into the nail bed defect, will have a slightly different color than the surrounding skin, but will yield an acceptable esthetic result. Nail-pouch reconstruction for placement of artificial nails has also been described.[6,7]

Another method of nail ablation may be useful when there is adequate skin coverage of the distal nail bed, but when nail

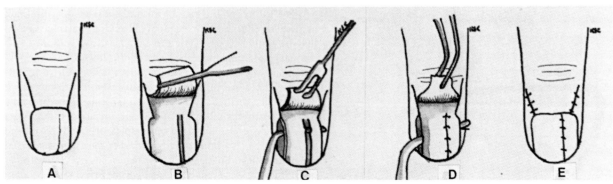

FIGURE 81-8. Split-nail reconstruction. (*A*) Corner incisions are made to permit access to the nail matrix. (*B* and *C*) The scar is excised and the nail bed is elevated. (*D*) The central wound is closed after "relaxing" the lateral tissues. (*E*) Proximal closure. (Note: The author recommends a stent dressing be placed in the proximal nail fold.) (Johnson, R.K.: Nail plasty. Plast. Reconstr. Surg. 47:275, 1971.)

spurs are formed by the germinal matrix remnants proximally. Excise the proximal nail-producing elements, leaving the distal bed in place. Because the proximal matrix creates the bulk of the nail plate, the nail spurs are thereby eliminated, the dorsal skin flap can be used for coverage of the proximal bed, and the remaining distal bed can be expected to create either a very thin or no residual nail plate (Fig. 81-9).[23]

Creating a "Roll" at the Lateral Nail Margin

One of the problems in achieving an esthetic result with nail and perinail reconstruction is the creation of a satisfactory "roll" to the tissues of the lateral nail margins when this tissue has been lost or resected. It is generally not possible to create such a fine curve by direct suture, but one can take advantage of wound contracture to tubulate tissue along the nail margin. Whether advancing lateral flap tissue slightly dorsally or resurfacing the lateral margin of the digit with a distant flap or full-thickness skin graft, the general principle is to allow the free edge of the tissue to override the nail margin by 1 to 2 mm rather than to suture it to the nail bed margin (Fig. 81-10). The overriding tissue will tend to contract with healing, tubulating the lateral tissues into a slight mound or roll.

Creating a Proximal Nail Fold

It is difficult to reconstruct a proximal nail fold because of the thin, tapered edge of the fold and the fact that the undersurface of the fold lies on the proximal nail plate. A small notch on one side of the fold can be repaired by sliding in lateral tissues as a proximally based rotation flap to close the notch, by excising a portion of the remaining fold to smooth the line by making the notch uniform, or by inserting a full-thickness skin graft into the notch (Fig. 81-11). If there is a healthy rim of tissue adjacent to the notch, the skin graft may achieve cover-

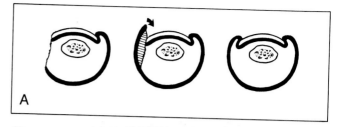
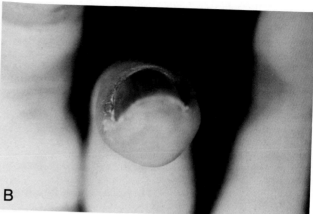

FIGURE 81-10. Creating a "roll" at the nail margin. (*A*) The defect is covered by tissue with free margin which tubulates as it heals. (*B*) End-on view of the result where digit with a skin defect at the nail bed margin is covered with a full-thickness graft which healed by this technique. (Courtesy of John M. Markley, Jr., M.D.)

age by a phenomenon known as bridging, even though the central portions of the graft may be situated directly on avascular nail plate. A small full-thickness skin graft (less than 1 cm in diameter), when sutured with excellent apposition to the edges of the defect, can establish sufficient intradermal circulation from its attachments at the vascularized margin to survive over the nail plate.

When there is a major defect, distally based flaps from one or both sides of the digit may be created in a staged manner. These are then rotated across the dorsum to cover the proximal nail (Fig. 81-12).[5]

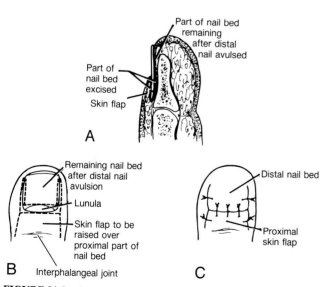

FIGURE 81-9. Nail ablation by excision of the germinal matrix to the level of the lunula, leaving the distal nail bed intact. (Zadik, F.R.: Obliteration of the nail bed of the great toe without shortening the terminal phalanx. J. Bone Joint Surg. **32-B:**66, 1950.)

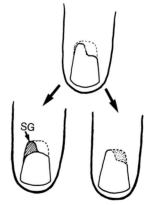

FIGURE 81-11. A notch in the proximal nail fold that is treated by a full-thickness skin graft (SG) to the defect or by excision of a portion of the remaining tissue to in order smooth the contour. (See text for further details.)

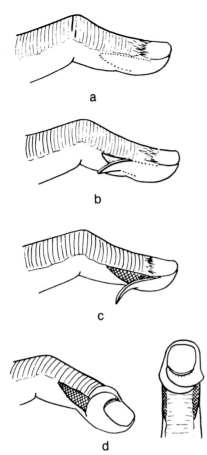

FIGURE 81-12. Proximal nail fold reconstruction utilizing distal flaps of mid-lateral tissue. The procedure is staged to enhance the probability of success. After the initial flap incision is made (a), half of the flap is undermined at 10 days (b). Final elevation and transfer (c and d) are completed after another 10 days. The donor area is covered with a split-thickness skin graft. (Barfod, B.: Reconstruction of the nail fold. *In* Pierre, M. (ed.): The Nail (GEM Monograph). New York, Churchill Livingstone, 1981.)

Hook-Nail Deformity at the Fingertip

A problem that commonly occurs with fingertip amputation is the formation of a beaked, hooked, or drooped nail that curves in a palmar direction across the tip. It is caused by inadequate bone or soft tissue support at the fingertip. Fingertip amputations that are allowed to heal by secondary wound contracture tend to deform the distal nail unless there is excellent phalangeal support; even then, there may be some pinching of the nail at the tip (Fig. 81-13, *A–C*).

In secondary reconstruction of a hook-nail deformity, the nail bed is usually shortened to the level of bone support. Soft tissue reconstruction at the tip is then undertaken. Successful osteoplastic lengthening of the distal phalanx has also been reported;[22] this may be worth considering in selected cases in which there is a considerable amount of nail bed available with very little phalangeal support. Bone grafting to the tip of a digit is not always successful, however, as resorption of the graft is common.[13]

Once the nail bed has been elevated and appropriately supported, supplement the pulp tissues either by filling in the gap

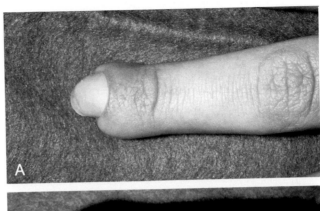

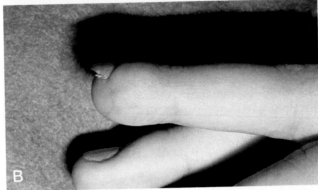

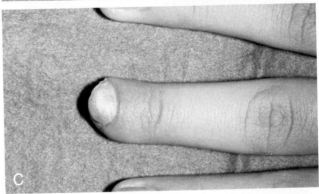

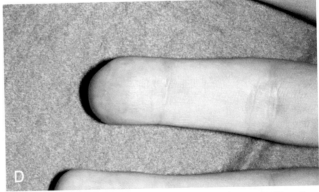

FIGURE 81-13. (*A*) Moderate beak-nail deformity on a patient whose fingertip amputation healed by secondary intention. (*B–D*) Appearance after elevation of nail bed and inset of thenar flap to support tip.

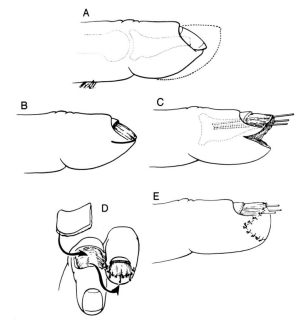

FIGURE 81-14.   The "antenna" procedure for repair of a hook-nail deformity. (*A*) Hook-nail deformity and normal contour of fingertip (dotted line). (*B*) Removal of the nail plate and marking of the skin. (*C*) Reflection of pulp, elevation of full thickness of nail matrix and splinting of it with three small Kirschner wires resembling antennae. (*D*) Coverage of the defect with a cross-finger flap. (*E*) Appearance after division of the flap (2 weeks after operation). (Atasoy E., Godfrey, A., and Kalisman, M.: The "Antenna" Procedure for the Hook-Nail deformity. J. Hand Surg. **8:**55, 1983.)

at the tip or by advancing the volar tissues. Atasoy has described a method of support for a hooked nail that utilizes an "antenna" of Kirschner wires beneath the nail bed, with soft tissue (cross-finger flap) interposed beneath (Fig. 81-14).[4] Other means of filling in the gap at the tip include a full-thickness skin graft, a composite graft of skin and fat (possibly from a toe), or a distant flap from the palm or an adjacent digit (Fig. 81-13, *D–F*). Palmar soft tissue advancement is also possible, usually in a V-Y fashion or from mid-lateral line to mid-lateral line, as will be outlined in Chapter 82 as a means of primary coverage of an amputated fingertip.

REFERENCES

1. Achten, G.: Histopathology of the Nail. *In* Pierre, M. (ed.): The Nail (GEM Monograph). New York, Churchill Livingstone, 1981.
2. Allen, M.J.: Conservative Management of Fingertip Injuries in Adults. Hand **12:**257, 1980.
3. Ashbell, T.S., Kleinert, H.K., Putcha, S., and Kutz, J.E.: The De-formed Fingernail: A Frequent Result of Failure to Repair Nail Bed Injuries. J. Trauma **7:**177, 1967.
4. Atasoy, E., Godfrey, A., and Kalisman, M.: The "Antenna" Procedure for the "Hook-nail" Deformity. J. Hand Surg. **8:**55, 1983.
5. Barfod, B.: Reconstruction of the Nail Fold. *In* Pierre, M. (ed.): The Nail (GEM Monograph). New York, Churchill Livingstone, 1981.
6. Buncke, H.J., and Gonzalez, R.J.: Fingernail Reconstruction. Plast. Reconstr. Surg. **30:**452, 1962.
7. Dufourmentel, C.: Nail Prostheses. *In* Pierre, M. (ed.): The Nail (GEM Monograph). New York, Churchill Livingstone, 1981.
8. Ersek, R.A., Gadaria, U., and Denton, D.: Nail Bed Avulsions Treated with Porcine Xenografts. J. Hand Surg. **10-A:**152, 1985.
9. Flint, M.H.: Some Observations on the Vascular Supply of the Nail Bed and Terminal Segments of the Finger. Br. J. Plast. Surg. **8:**186, 1956.
10. Harty, M.: The Dermal Papillae in the Fingertip. Plast. Reconstr. Surg. **45:**141, 1970.
11. Johnson, R.K.: Nail Plasty. Plast. Reconstr. Surg. **47:**275, 1971.
12. Lewis, B.L.: Microscopic Studies of Fetal and Mature Nail and Surrounding Soft Tissue. Arch. Derm. Syph. **70:**732, 1954.
13. McCash, C.R.: Treatment of Fingernail Deformities. *In* Transactions of the Third International Congress of Plastic Surgeons, Washington, D.C. Amsterdam, Excerpta Medica, 1964, pp. 976–983.
14. McCash, C.R.: Free Nail Grafting. Br. J. Plast. Surg. **8:**19, 1956.
15. Morrison, W.A.: Reconstruction of the Fingernail By Microvascular Transfer from the Toes. *In* Pierre, M. (ed.): The Nail (GEM Monograph). New York, Churchill Livingstone, 1981.
16. Norton, L.A.: Incorporation of Thymidine-Methyl-H3 and Glycine-2-H3 in the Nail Matrix and Bed of Humans. J. Invest. Derm. **56:**61, 1971.
17. Saito, H., Suzuki, Y., Fujino, K., and Tajima, T.: Free Nail Bed Graft for Treatment of Nail Bed Injuries of the Hand. J. Hand Surg. **8:**171, 1983.
18. Schiller, C.: Nail Replacement in Fingertip Injuries. Plast. Reconstr. Surg. **19:**521, 1967.
19. Shepard, G.H.: Treatment of Nail Bed Avulsions with Split-thickness Nail Bed Grafts. J. Hand Surg. **8:**49, 1983.
20. Shrewsbury, M., and Johnson, R.K.: The Fascia of the Distal Phalanx. J. Bone Joint Surg. **57-A:**784, 1975.
21. Swanker, W.A.: Reconstructive Surgery of the Injured Nail. Am. J. Surg. **74:**341, 1947.
22. Verdan, C.: Plastic Surgery and the Claw Nail. *In* Pierre, M. (ed.): The Nail (GEM Monograph). New York, Churchill Livingstone, 1981.
23. Zadik, F.R.: Obliteration of the Nail Bed of the Great Toe Without Shortening the Terminal Phalanx. J. Bone Joint Surg. **32-B:**66, 1950.
24. Zaias, Nardo: The Nail in Health and Disease. New York, S. P. Medical & Scientific Books, Spectrum Publications, 1980.
25. Zook, E.G.: Nail Bed Injuries. Hand Clin. **1:**701, 1985.
26. Zook, E.G., Guy, R.J., and Russell, R.C.: A Study of Nail Bed Injuries: Causes, Treatment, and Prognosis. J. Hand Surg. **9-A:**247, 1984.
27. Zook, E.G., Van Beek, A.L., Russell, R.C., and Beatty, M.E.: Anatomy and Physiology of the Perionychium: A Review of the Literature and Anatomic Study. J. Hand Surg. **5:**528, 1980.

CHAPTER 82

Fingertip Injuries

HOWARD W. KLEIN

Primary Repair
Secondary Intention, or Open Treatment
Skin Grafting
Local Flaps
   V-Y Advancement Flap
   Bilateral V-Y "Kutler" Flaps
   Palmar Advancement (Moberg) Flap
Regional Flaps
   Thenar Flaps
   Cross-Finger Flaps
Neurovascular Flaps
Distant Flaps
Amputation Revision

The fingertip has a crucial role as the primary organ of touch. After injury, restoration of sensibility, stable skin coverage, and adequate padding are the goals of reconstruction. No single technique is satisfactory for all situations, but careful examination of the fingertip, along with information regarding the patient's labor history, avocations, and the mechanism of injury, invariably suggests the appropriate solution.

Examination and classification of fingertip injuries are the first and most important steps in arriving at a surgical plan. There are three major considerations:

1. *Associated nailbed injury:* Support for the nailplate is essential in avoiding troublesome secondary deformities such as a "hooked" nail. If the nailbed is intact but the underlying phalanx is fractured, the small fragments may be held in place with the use of a small Kirchner wire. If nailbed or germinal matrix tissue is missing, dermal grafting or ablation should be considered.
2. *Bone exposure:* If no bone is exposed, then free skin grafting with either split- or full-thickness skin can be used. However, skin grafts will not be successful if bone is exposed, and a flap is needed if length is to be maintained.
3. *Angle of injury* (Fig. 82-1): If dorsal angulation is present, then a local flap, such as the V-Y advancement, may be used reliably. If the angle is reversed, that is with a predominant loss of palmar tissue, then other flaps or amputation revision is necessary.

Figure 82-2 summarizes a general approach to managing patients with fingertip injuries.

PRIMARY REPAIR

Some crushing injuries involve essentially no tissue loss. These wounds must be carefully inspected and then copiously irrigated. Associated nailbed injury should be repaired by removal of the nail plate and reapproximation of the damaged tissue with fine (7-0) catgut. Devascularized pulp fat should be excised and reapproximation of pulp skin carried out with nonabsorbable 6-0 suture. Such crushing injuries are frequently associated with underlying distal phalanx fractures. If the soft-tissue envelope is intact and the fracture does not involve the articular surface, then no specific fracture treatment is necessary after the soft tissue has been repaired.

SECONDARY INTENTION, OR OPEN TREATMENT

This method relies on the processes of epithelialization and contraction to provide wound closure. This option is best reserved for small defects (6–8 mm) without exposed bone and with minimal loss of pulp tissue. Because the missing tissue is replaced by scar, a tender fingertip may result. Therefore, it is important that an occupational history be obtained when this method is being considered. A patient who uses his fingertip to push or hammer repetitively would be a poor candidate for this procedure.

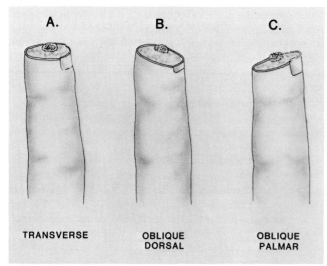

FIGURE 82-1. Angles of injury. (*A*) Transverse. (*B*) Dorsal oblique. (*C*) Palmar oblique.

Many surgeons use healing by secondary intention as the preferred method of treatment. In a review of 110 patients, Bojsen-Moller and co-workers compared patients treated conservatively with those treated by amputation revision or skin grafting.[4] They observed that conservative treatment was almost always uncomplicated and that patients were away from work no longer than those treated by other methods.

In children conservative treatment is probably the method of choice. In 1974 Illingworth reported a follow-up study of children treated by conservative methods and clearly showed this to be the best alternative.[7]

If one does elect to allow healing by secondary intention, it is important to clean the wound thoroughly after digital block has been performed. This allows healing to begin in a wound in which bacterial contamination is low. The patient is instructed to begin twice-daily soaks until healing has occurred, usually in 2 to 4 weeks. Under ideal conditions, open treatment minimizes joint contractures because of early mobilization. The force of contraction provides stable, color-matched skin of like sensibility.

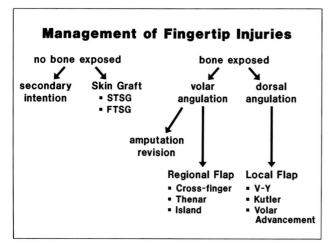

FIGURE 82-2.

It seems that cold intolerance may be a troublesome consequence of therapy, occurring in almost 40% of patients who heal by secondary intention.

SKIN GRAFTING

When larger areas of only skin has been lost, skin grafting is indicated. Although the likelihood of a "take" with split-thickness skin is higher, a full-thickness skin graft is generally preferred, since it gives a better cosmetic result, better sensory return, and better durability. Many donor sites are available for full-thickness skin grafts, but use of local or regional skin will avoid hyperpigmentation. The palmar wrist crease is easily accessible and usually prepped in the surgical field; this area will provide grafts of 2 cm by 6 cm. If more skin than this is needed, the hairless area of the inguinal crease may be used. Donor areas should be closed primarily and meticulously with a running intradermal suture. Some authors have suggested using the hypothenar area as a donor site, but we have found that this donor site often leaves an unsightly, tender scar and frequently has to be closed under excessive tension.

Wound closure by composite grafts from the toe or earlobe have been recommended in the past.[6] These areas are limited both by the amount of tissue available and certainly by the potential unsightly and painful complications of the donor site.

Since success in skin grafting requires a good bed and immobilization, meticulous debridement and absolute hemostasis must be achieved before graft placement. The graft should be secured with a bolus "stent" type of dressing and left undisturbed for 10 to 14 days, unless there is a clinical reason to suspect a problem.

After removal of the stent, the patient is begun on active range-of-motion exercises and soaks. A patient who has an uncomplicated skin-grafted fingertip injury can expect to be absent from a job requiring manual skills for 3 to 4 weeks. We feel that patients who injure their dominant hands with no bone exposed, and who require fine sensibility of fingertips, are best treated with full-thickness skin grafts. The better sensory recovery and decreased cold sensibility are good trade-offs for perhaps a slightly longer time off work.

The complications of skin grafting are basically those of hematoma, infection, and donor site complications.[3] With attention to meticulous wound preparation and technique, these may all be minimized.

LOCAL FLAPS

For major pulp loss, a flap is indicated. If the injury preserves the lunula and the germinal matrix is intact, a stable nail can be expected. In these cases, a local flap is ideal to restore a well-padded fingertip and to avoid a "hooked" or "claw" nail. Local flaps also acquire better sensitivity than grafts and do not contract.

V-Y Advancement Flap

Popularized by Atasoy and colleagues, the V-Y flap is most useful in patients who have sustained a dorsally angulated amputation (Fig. 82-3).[2] This technique is difficult to use in the transverse and contraindicated in the palmar oblique type of amputation. It can be used for primary repair in patients of all ages and replaces missing tissue with like tissue.

Proper design of the flap is crucial in providing adequate coverage. The apex of the V is designed in the midpalmar distal interphalangeal joint skin crease, and the ends of the V should lie at the widest part of the amputation wound. After incising the skin, it is important to release the fibrous septa that anchor the palmar pad to the distal phalanx. Do this while placing traction distally with a skin hook. Since this flap is based on a subcutaneous pedicle, divide only these fibrous ligaments (at the level of the phalanx) to avoid damage to the subcutaneous tissue. Take care not to undermine excessively, since this might compromise the delicate innervation by the terminal branches of the digital nerves and the subdermal vascular plexus. This flap provides like tissue with good color and sensory characteristics and does not require immobilization. The scar is inconspicuous and restores relatively normal fingertip contour in a single stage.

While the pitfalls in elevating this flap are described above, the most common complication is partial or complete flap loss. When this occurs, the patient should be treated conservatively with frequent wet-to-dry dressing changes and twice-a-day soaks.

Bilateral V-Y "Kutler" Flaps

The bilateral V-Y "Kutler" flaps are similar in concept to the Atasoy V-Y flap in that two V-shaped flaps are mobilized, but from the lateral portion of the fingertip (Fig. 82-4).[9] This can be most useful for patients with transverse amputations, but we

have generally been disappointed with the limited advancement and excessive scarring that occurs with these flaps.

Our perception is in agreement with other studies, including that of Freiberg and Manktelow, who found that one-third of their patients complained of hypersensitivity and another one-third of numbness.[5] For these reasons we seldom use this reconstruction.

Palmar Advancement (Moberg) Flap

Although the palmar advancement flap is most useful for pulp loss in the thumb up to 1 cm, some physicians have extended this flap's use to other fingers (Fig. 82-5).[12] It has the advantage of providing stable coverage with innervated like skin, but can cause secondary problems with joint contracture if the patient needs this interphalangeal joint splinted in flexion for several weeks.

First described by Moberg in 1964, the palmar advancement flap requires extensive mobilization of the palmar soft tissue through midaxial incisions to provide coverage in palmar oblique or guillotine-type amputations. The bilateral midaxial incisions extend usually to 1 cm proximal to the proximal interphalangeal joint and carefully preserve the dorsal branch of the neurovascular bundle.

Most authors agree that this method is more useful for thumb resurfacing than in the fingers. The main disadvantage to use of this flap in the fingers is flexion contracture secondary to splinting in the hyperflexed position at the interphalangeal joints. In the thumb, where the tissue tends to be more mobile, fixed flexion deformity seems to be less common. An additional drawback to using this flap is the theoretical disruption of the vasculature to the flexor tendon sheath.[1] If the dorsal branch

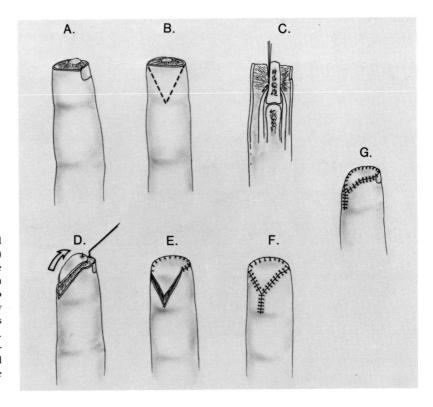

FIGURE 82-3. V-Y advancement flap, most useful in patients with a dorsal oblique type of injury (*A*). (*B*) Plan the incision with the apex of the triangle at the level of the midpalmar distal interphalangeal flexion crease. (*C*) After making the incision, carry it down to the level of the fibrous septal attachments at the bony phalanx. (*D*) Release these septae as needed at this level while placing traction distally with a skin hook. (*E*) Release all tension so that suturing the distal margin of the flap is done without blanching (use small monofilament suture, 6-0 or 7-0). (*F*) Complete the closure.

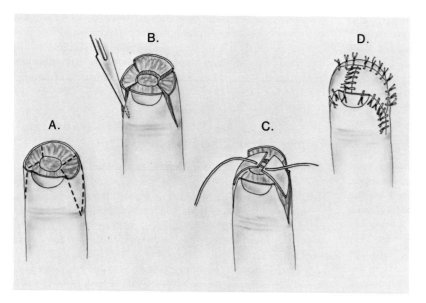

FIGURE 82-4. Kutler flaps. (*A*) Most useful for transverse amputations, bilateral flaps are designed with the apex of the triangles in the midlateral line of the distal interphalangeal flexion crease. (*B*) Make the incisions to the level of the fibrous septal attachments at the bony phalanx, using traction distally with a skin hook to release proximal septa so flaps advance to the midline. (*C*) Begin tension-free closure with small (6-0 or 7-0) nonabsorbable monofilament suture. (*D*) Complete closure with several interrupted absorbable sutures at the amputated nailbed margin.

of the neurovascular bundle is injured, dorsal necrosis may result. Snow has managed to avoid this complication in a series of 75 patients by carrying the incision no further than 1 cm proximal to the proximal interphalangeal joint.[16]

When primary healing occurs with this method, time off from work is only 2 weeks. However, if the patient had to be aggressively flexed at the interphalangeal joints, another several weeks of intensive physical therapy may be necessary.

We tend to use this flap only in the thumb and only for defects of up to, but not exceeding, 1 cm.

REGIONAL FLAPS

Thenar Flaps

The thenar flap is useful mainly for palmar oblique and transverse amputations of the fingers (Fig. 82-6).

Because of the need to splint the recipient finger in flexion, the possible development of flexion contracture should be considered. For this reason, thenar flaps should be avoided in patients older than 50 years of age and in patients with conditions that predispose them to small-joint stiffness (e.g., rheumatoid arthritis, Dupuytren's contracture). Consideration should be given to using this flap when preservation of length is important for occupational or aesthetic reasons. Because of the staged nature of the procedure, patients may expect to be away from work for 6 to 8 weeks. Although this seems a long time, the improved sensory recovery associated with flaps as compared with grafts is desirable in some patients.[15]

This flap may be based in any direction (proximal, distal, lateral) and should be as high on the thenar eminence as possible. There are several important technical points that should be observed during elevation of this flap. The radial digital nerve to the thumb is at significant risk for injury, since it is frequently exposed; it should be identified and protected. To

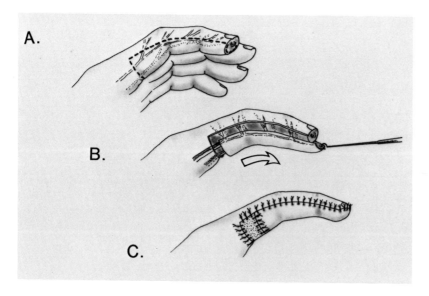

FIGURE 82-5. Palmar advancement flap. (*A*) Design bilateral midaxial incisions to 1 cm proximal to the proximal interphalangeal joint, preserving dorsal neurovascular branches. (*B*) Use a skin hook to provide traction when advancing the entire palmar soft tissue. (*C*) Suture into place distally, using small (6-0 or 7-0) monofilament suture without tension. It may be necessary to flex the interphalangeal joint(s) to achieve tension-free closure. Place a full-thickness skin graft over the donor defect.

minimize recipient finger proximal interphalangeal flexion, the finger should have full metacarpophalangeal and distal interphalangeal flexion while the thumb is placed in palmar abduction. This will minimize the need to flex the proximal interphalangeal joint.

The thumb donor site may be closed directly if it is small, but in larger flaps full-thickness skin grafting is indicated. This skin can conveniently be taken from the palmar wrist crease.

Ten to 14 days after application of the pedicle, the base may be severed and active motion begun. After division, the wounds are not closed directly, but rather allowed to heal by secondary intention. Experience has shown that tailoring and insetting these flaps immediately is associated with a high rate of significant skin necrosis and other wound complications. With frequent soaks and dressing changes, complete healing usually occurs quite rapidly.

Cross-Finger Flaps

Dorsal Cross-Finger Flap

Dorsal cross-finger flaps are primarily indicated for repair of palmar fingertip defects (Fig. 82-7). The procedure is contraindicated in hands that have sustained multiple injuries because of a greater than normal risk of stiffness. Buerger's disease, Raynaud's phenomenon, and any vasospastic or primary small-vessel disease (e.g., diabetes mellitus) are conditions in which this flap should not be used. Furthermore, patients who are prone to small-joint stiffness (e.g., those with rheumatoid arthritis, those who are over 50 years of age) should not be treated with this flap. The dorsal skin used for resurfacing is quite thin and cannot restore the completely lost palmar fingertip pad. Additionally, the dorsal scar may be unacceptable.

The dorsal flap is based on the palmar longitudinal neurovascular bundle and its dorsal branches. The flap is elevated in the plane just above the extensor paratenon over the middle or proximal phalanx on a finger adjacent to the injured digit. The procedure is very reliable and, because it is a flap, provides

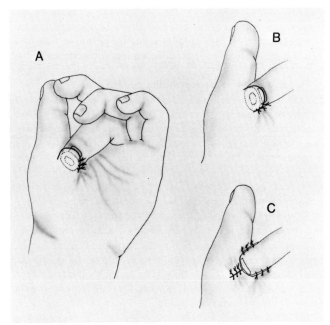

FIGURE 82-6. Thenar flap. (*A*) Base the thenar superiorly, inferiorly, ulnarward, or radialward as appropriate. It should lie with its midpoint high on thenar mass, preferably at the palmar metacarpophalangeal crease. (*B*) After identifying the radial digital nerve, suture the flap into the defect. (*C*) Close the donor site in a linear fashion with interrupted monofilament sutures.

better sensation than healing by secondary intention or skin grafting. However, its use in children is difficult because of the need to immobilize the donor finger flap attachment. The donor defect over the middle or proximal phalanx is skin grafted, preferably with full-thickness skin. This graft can conveniently be taken from the hairless area of the groin and so provides an inconspicuous donor scar. In black patients, however, hyperpigmented groin skin may be cosmetically objectionable on the palmar surface of the fingers, in which case an

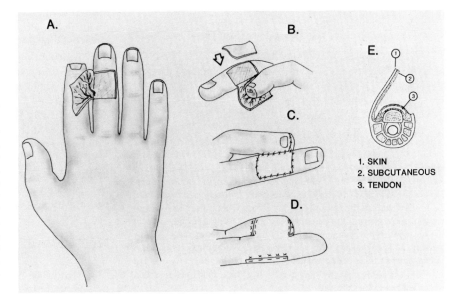

FIGURE 82-7. Dorsal cross-finger flap. (*A*) Design the flap over the middle phalanx of an adjacent finger extending from the midaxial line to the midaxial line of the donor finger. Elevate the flap just above the extensor paratenon, ligating the dorsal veins at proximal and distal flap margins. (*B*) After removing the digital tourniquets to confirm flap viability, fold the flap over to cover the fingertip defect. Suture a full-thickness skin graft into place over the paratenon in the adjacent finger, and apply a bolus dressing. (*C*) Suture the flap onto the recipient finger defect, using interrupted half-buried mattress monofilament suture (6-0 or 7-0). (*D*) Palmar view of completed repair. (*E*) Schematic cross section of the donor finger illustrating the proper plane of flap elevation.

1. SKIN
2. SUBCUTANEOUS
3. TENDON

available palmar donor site should be used. Because of the tendency of full-thickness grafts to hyperpigment, a patient who is sensitive to appearance might be better served by a thenar flap, which is associated with a less conspicuous donor scar.

The adjacent fingers may be immobilized in several ways. The most common method in the cooperative adult patient is to use a bulky dressing with a plaster splint. We have recently used a small external fixator to align the fingers more accurately. This method is especially useful in uncooperative patients and in patients with spastic conditions. K-wires may also be used between digits, but they tend to bend and lose shape with finger movement. Ten to 14 days after application, the flap is divided without insetting and motion begun immediately.

As already indicated, the sensory recovery of flaps is excellent. In a recent review of 23 patients, Kappel and Burech reported an average two-point discrimination of 8.25 mm, which is superior to that associated with the dorsal donor site skin.[8] Dexterity testing was only 17% slower than normal, and pinch testing was over 80% of normal. Overall, patients usually report a pain-free, durable result.

Reverse Cross-Finger Flap

A modification of the dorsal cross-finger flap, the reverse cross-finger flap is most suitable for dorsal defects (Fig. 82-8). The main difference between this flap and the conventional dorsal cross-finger flap is that the dorsal skin is reflected and the flap consists mainly of the subcutaneous tissue reflected onto the recipient finger. The native skin is then laid back onto the phalanx over the donor finger. The flap of reflected subcutaneous tissue is then skin-grafted. The main advantage of this procedure over a conventional cross-finger flap is that the donor finger has a more acceptable appearance.

Flag Flap

The flag flap is another modification of the dorsal cross-finger flap.[17] The "flagpole" is the dorsal branch of the neurovascular bundle, which measures approximately 1 mm in diameter and originates approximately 1 cm proximal to the proximal interphalangeal joint. This is, in fact, an axial pattern flap and quite reliable. The narrow pedicle increases flap mobility and can be used to cover palmar defects of the donor digit as well as palmar and dorsal defects of adjacent digits; it may also be rotated to cover defects over the metacarpophalangeal joints of donor or adjacent digits. Many hand surgeons use this flag flap to resurface palmar defects of the thumb tip. With careful dissection, a vascularized flap of 10 cm^2 may be elevated in the adult hand.[10]

There are several pitfalls to avoid when using this flap. First, be sure that the vascular pedicle (the dorsal branch of the neurovascular bundle) has not been damaged from the primary injury. Second, since this flap tends to be quite sensitive to tension, take care to see that it does not become partially or completely avascular when sutured into place. Removing a suture or incising the skin (*not* the subcutaneous tissue or deeper structures) in a back-cut may help relieve this problem.

Palmar Cross-Finger Flap

The palmar cross-finger flap employs a similar technique in elevation but is based on the palmar surface of the middle or proximal phalanx (Fig. 82-9).[3] This technique is especially applicable for injuries involving distal thumb amputations. The donor site is the middle or proximal phalanx of the middle finger when used for the thumb, or the finger adjacent to the injured digit. The "hidden" palmar donor scar may represent an attractive alternative in patients sensitive to their appearance. One must take care not to dissect the flap away from the neurovascular bundle during elevation, since ischemia is inevitable due to the vertical blood supply. This is in contrast to the dorsal cross-finger flap, in which the blood supply is longitudinal. Extreme care must be taken when dividing the flap to avoid damaging the donor neurovascular bundle. This flap is also allowed to heal by secondary intention after division to avoid necrosis from insetting.

The palmar cross-finger flap provides skin of perfect texture and color, and the sensory return is good. The donor scar is inconspicuous and positioning of the donor finger tends to be easier, with less chance of stiffness, than with dorsal flaps.

NEUROVASCULAR FLAPS

The island flap is rarely used for fingertip injury and should only be undertaken by those familiar with detailed hand anat-

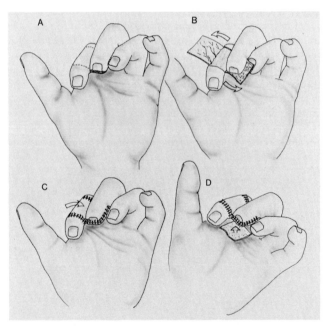

FIGURE 82-8. Reverse cross-finger flap. (*A*) Design the flap with its base at the midaxial line of the middle phalanx of the donor finger. Elevate the skin as a full thickness skin graft, and reflect it away from the injured digit to the opposite midaxial line. Then raise the subcutaneous tissue overlying the extenor paratenon, basing it in the midaxial line adjacent to the recipient digit. (*B*) Flip the subcutaneous flap over onto the adjacent finger. (*C*) Suture the elevated donor skin back into place over the donor middle phalanx. (*D*) Suture the subcutaneous flap onto the recipient digit and cover it with a thick split-thickness skin graft. Apply a bolus dressing.

FIGURE 82-9. Palmar cross-finger flap. (*A*) Design the flap on the palmar surface of the middle phalanx. Its base should lie along the ulnar border in the midaxial line. (*B*) Elevate the flap just superficial to the flexor sheath, taking care to preserve the ulnar neurovascular bundle and to not separate the flap from the radial neurovascular bundle. (*C*) Suture the flap into place with fine monofilament suture, and suture a full-thickness skin graft over the donor middle phalanx. Apply a bolus dressing. (*D*) Complete the repair. (*E*) Schematic cross section of the donor finger illustrating the proper plane of dissection.

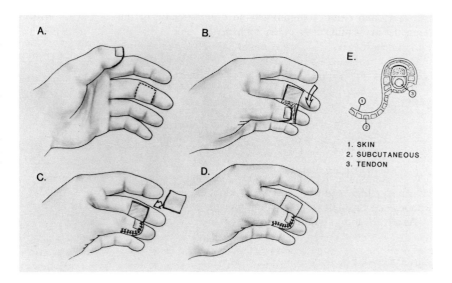

omy who have an in-depth knowledge of the techniques of hand surgery (Fig. 82-10).[11] Basically, a block of tissue from a relatively unimportant area (e.g., ulnar border of the ring finger) is transferred on its neurovascular bundle to a more crucial area (e.g., thumb). Most surgeons use this flap only for isolated thumb pulp injury in a clean wound.

Loupe magnification is essential. A generous cuff of perivascular fat should be left around the neurovascular pedicle and care taken to assure that there is no kinking or compression when the island is transferred. An extensive zig-zag incision is used to mobilize the leash of vessels to its midpalmar origin. The flap should always begin at the tip of the finger because of the greater sensibility there. Generally, the proximal border is in the region of the proximal interphalangeal joint.

Pitfalls in the use of this flap are related mostly to injury of the neurovascular pedicle from compression, kinking, or he-

matoma. Because of cortical representation, patients continue to perceive the transferred skin as another part of the hand. Reorientation may take several years. Although no study of moving two-point discrimination has been published, the results of static two-point discrimination studies have ranged from a low of 2 mm to 10 mm to a high of greater than 15 mm to 20 mm.[13,14]

DISTANT FLAPS

Distant flaps are infrequently used for fingertip injury. Generally they provide thick, fatty coverage with poor sensibility. When there is a total loss of palmar tissue with the nail and dorsal tissue undamaged, consideration may be given to this method. The cross-arm or lateral thoracic flaps are best for

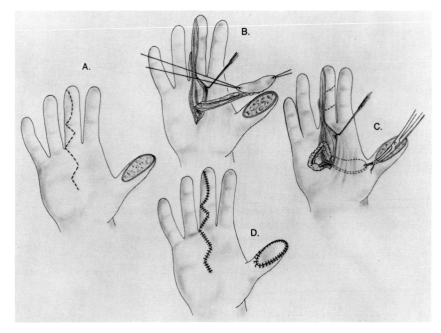

FIGURE 82-10. Island flap. (*A*) Design the flap over the ulnar border of the long finger. It should be of the size necessary to match the recipient defect. Take care not to detach the neurovascular bundle from the undersurface of the flap. Use Bruner incisions to mobilize the donor vessels back to the palmar arch. (*B*) Use sutures for traction as flap elevation and mobilization proceed. (*C*) Make a generous tunnel beneath the palmar skin to allow the tension-free passage of the flap into the recipient defect. (*D*) Complete the repair with a full-thickness skin graft placed onto the donor defect. Apply a bolus dressing.

providing thin tissue, minimizing elbow and shoulder problems, and avoiding extensive donor scars.

AMPUTATION REVISION

When all other approaches have been found to be inappropriate, amputation revision provides a sensate, durable stump. Sacrifice of length should never be employed for thumb injury. Resecting the neurovascular bundles well back from the site of injury will help avoid neuroma problems. It is contraindicated to suture the flexor tendon to the extensor tendon to provide "extra padding"; this will cause flexion deformity at the metacarpophalangeal joint level and further interfere with function.

REFERENCES

1. Armenta, G., and Lehrman, A.: The vincula to the flexor tendons of the hand. J. Hand Surg. **5:**127, 1980.
2. Atasoy, E., Ioakimudis, E., Kasdan, M.L., et al.: Reconstruction of the amputated fingertip with a triangular volar flap. J. Bone Joint Surg. **52-A:**698, 1970.
3. Beasley, R.W.: Hand Injuries. Philadelphia, W.B. Saunders, 1981.
4. Bojsen-Moller, J., Pers, M., and Schmidt, A.: Fingertip injuries: Late results. Acta Chir. Scand. **122:**177, 1961.
5. Freiberg, A., and Manktelow, R.: The Kutler repair of fingertip amputations. Plast. Reconst. Surg. **50:**371, 1972.
6. Gurdin, M., and Pangman, W.J.: The repair of surface defects of fingers by transdigital flaps. Plast. Reconst. Surg. **5:**368, 1950.
7. Illingworth, C.M.: Trapped fingers and amputated fingertips in children. J. Pediatr. Surg. **9:**853, 1974.
8. Kappel, D., and Burech, J.: The cross-finger flap: An established reconstructive procedure. Hand Clin. **1**(4), 1985.
9. Kutler, W.: A new method for fingertip amputation. JAMA **133:**29, 1947.
10. Lister, G.: The theory of the transposition flap and its practical application in the hand. Plast. Surg. Clin. **8**(1):115, 1981.
11. Littler, J.W.: Neurovascular pedicle transfer of tissue in reconstructive surgery of the hand. J. Bone Joint Surg. **38-A:**917, 1956.
12. Macht, S.D., and Watson, H.K.: The Moberg volar advancement flap for digital reconstruction. J. Hand Surg. **5:**372, 1980.
13. Markley, J.M., Jr.: The preservation of close two-point discrimination in the interdigital transfer of neurovascular island flaps. Plast. Reconst. Surg. **59:**813, 1977.
14. McGregor, I.A.: Less than satisfactory experiences with neurovascular island flaps. Hand **1:**21, 1969.
15. Porter, R.W.: Functional assessment of transplanted skin in volar defects of the digits. A comparison between free grafts and flaps. J. Bone Joint Surg. **50-A:**955, 1968.
16. Snow, J.: Volar advancement skin flap to the fingertip. Hand Clin. **1**(4), 1985.
17. Vilain, R., and Dupuis, J.F.: Use of the flag flap for coverage of a small area on a finger or the palm. Plast. Reconst. Surg. **51:**397, 1973.

CHAPTER 83

Amputations of the Hand

TERRY R. LIGHT

PRINCIPLES AND GOALS

Amputation of a portion of the hand is not a pleasant event for either the patient or the surgeon. Nonetheless, a carefully planned and skillfully executed surgical procedure is essential if the patient is to experience early restoration of pain-free, useful hand function. The ultimate goal of surgery is the restoration of a hand of acceptable appearance capable of the highest degree of function consistent with its remaining musculoskeletal elements.[1]

In general, optimal hand function is achieved through prompt wound healing with digits of maximal length and joint mobility. It is essential that sensibility be preserved in retained elements and that care be taken to avoid painful neuromas.

Because the thumb is essential for both power and precision prehension, thumb preservation or restoration is of paramount importance. When the radial fingers are compromised, precision prehension is impaired, while loss of the ulnar digits reduces effective power grip.[6] Preservation of length and sensibility is vital to radial digits, whereas preservation of joint mobility is more important to ulnar digits.

INDICATIONS

Partial hand amputation procedures may be carried out as either primary or secondary procedures. Trauma continues to be the most common indication for deleting portions of the hand. The management of acute traumatic amputation requires considerable judgment. The surgeon must often decide which parts should be retained by revascularization or replantation, which should be managed with direct wound closure, and which should be primarily managed by more proximal amputation.

In severe trauma affecting several digits, it is usually decided to preserve all viable tissue that might be useful in the secondary reconstruction of remaining viable digits. Otherwise useless digits may be converted to filet flaps for soft-tissue coverage, while digital nerve and bone may be harvested as graft. Though this approach is by design "conservative," it may prove counterproductive if the decision to delete functionless digits is repeatedly postponed. Retained stiff, insensate, or unstable digits will make rehabilitation of the remaining, less severely affected portions of the hand more difficult. Also, the original decision to delete the irreparably compromised digit may be questioned and additional futile surgeries performed in an attempt to avoid amputation.

Digits may become ischemic and nonviable as a result of microvascular disease or macrovascular disease or a combination of the two. Microvascular disease, seen commonly in conditions such as scleroderma and diabetes mellitus, may result in digital ischemia. Irreversible digital ischemia may also result from macrovascular injury to the brachial artery after cardiac catheterization in the presence of systemic atherosclerotic macrovascular and microvascular disease.

Infection within the hand may necessitate partial hand amputation. The aim may be either to eliminate a refractory focus of infection, usually osteomyelitis, or to remove a part whose function has been irreparably compromised by infection. A painful, swollen finger rendered immobile after flexor sheath infection may occasionally be so impaired that the surgeon and patient elect digital amputation.

Malignant tumor may necessitate partial hand amputation. The histologic character of the tumor and its anatomic location should be the primary determinants of the level of amputation. The desire to preserve functional capability must be subservient to the need for appropriate tumor wound margins. Amputation may be confined to a single digit, a ray, or a more major segment of the hand—radial, central, or ulnar.

Congenitally anomalous hands may occasionally be improved functionally or aesthetically by the amputation of rudimentary digits. Small, floppy nubbins may be excised when they are insufficient for reconstruction. In cases of polydactyly, amputation must be carefully integrated with reconstruction of the remaining digits.

Various forms of thermal injury may lead to amputation. Frostbite injury characteristically affects the distal portions of the fingers (but rarely the thumb), with the extent of remaining viable tissue uncertain for a number of days. Heat may cause burns that primarily affect the dorsal structures, skin, and extensor mechanism without necessitating amputation. Electrical injury, in contrast, may have a more profound effect on deep tissues than upon skin. Residual functional impairment after electrical injury may lead to secondary amputation.

Finally, it is occasionally wise to abandon local reconstructive surgical procedures in favor of prosthetic management. When a hand is painful, deformed, and without function, amputation may be the most effective reconstructive procedure.[2]

THUMB AMPUTATIONS

It is principally the attributes of position, stability, strength, and length that allow the thumb to carry out its unique range of activities.[7] Motion, sensibility, and appearance are important, though less vital, attributes of normal thumb function.

Because of the thumb's unique position and essential role in prehension, the preservation of thumb length is a priority in the treatment of traumatic thumb injuries. A well-motored stiff thumb with basilar mobility of normal length effectively participates in most hand functions.

Acute Management

When amputation of the thumb occurs through the distal phalanx, local flap closure may be required. With disproportionate palmar skin loss, the Moberg palmar advancement flap allows preservation of thumb length with advancement of sensate skin distally.[4] The radial nerve–innervated cross-finger flap from the dorsum of the index finger also brings sensate skin to the distal phalanx.

When thumb amputation occurs through the midproximal phalanx or beyond, satisfactory function may be achieved if maximal length is preserved with local advancement flaps.

When amputation occurs more proximally, prehension is severely compromised. Though thumb length may be sufficient for the buttressing of objects in the palm in power grip, it is insufficient to reach the tips of adjacent fingers in precision prehensile activities. Secondary surgical reconstruction is usually advantageous when amputation occurs at this level. In

such situations the sacrifice of a few millimeters of skeletal length to allow direct soft-tissue closure over bone is usually preferable to extensive primary soft-tissue flap procedures. Once healing of the amputation has been achieved, reconstruction will be required to restore at least a portion of the lost thumb length.

Late Thumb Reconstruction

Late reconstruction procedures to improve the function of a thumb that has sustained amputation injury include phalangization, distraction lengthening, and pollicization, as well as toe-to-hand and wraparound flap microvascular transfers (see Chapter 78).

Phalangization

When all other digits that could achieve pulp-to-pulp contact with the thumb are simultaneously shortened by ischemia or injury, it makes little sense to lengthen the thumb beyond the arc of the remaining fingers. Phalangization restores primitive prehension to the hand but requires supple dorsal skin, normal thenar musculature, and a mobile, normal thumb carpometacarpal joint.[14]

Procedure. A Z-shaped incision provides generous web space exposure and allows flap transposition, which shifts the web space skin margin proximally (Fig. 83-1). Define the adductor pollicis and first dorsal interosseous muscles, and incise and release their investing fascia. Resect the index metacarpal, taking care to preserve the proximal attachment of extensor carpi radialis longus. Excise the first dorsal and first palmar interosseous muscles. Release the adductor pollicis insertion from the sesamoid at the metacarpophalangeal joint level and reinsert it more proximally on the thumb metacarpal. Transpose skin flaps.

A three-digit prehension pattern may be recreated by the additional removal of the ring metacarpal. This procedure increases the mobility and independence of the little-finger metacarpal. Flexion and radial deviation closing-wedge osteotomy of the base of the little-finger metacarpal may allow it to pinch toward the thumb metacarpal.[5]

Thumb Lengthening

When at least two-thirds of the thumb metacarpal remain with good soft-tissue coverage, distraction lengthening is an effective technique for regaining useful thumb length.[8] If proximal joint mobility and thenar musculature is preserved, the patient should be able to use the lengthened thumb effectively for prehensile activity.

Procedure. Make a longitudinal skin incision to expose the middle third of the thumb metacarpal (Fig. 83-2). Incise the periosteum. The skin should be "bunched up" between pin insertion sites such that distraction will not put undue pressure on the skin–pin interface. Insert two parallel groups of pins transversely through the collapsed distraction apparatus in close proximity to the intended osteotomy site. Make a transverse osteotomy through the middle third of the metacarpal.

FIGURE 83-1. Phalangization procedure. (*A*) Resection of the index metacarpal is achieved through the dorsal portion of the Z-plasty incision. (*B*) Z-plasty flap transposition increases the exposed prehensile surface of the thumb.

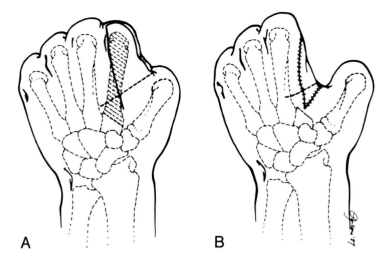

A longitudinal pin may be placed through the proximal and distal metacarpal segments and across the carpometacarpal joint. By transfixing the metacarpal to the trapezium, this pin provides resistance to the tendency of distraction to tighten the adductor and produce secondary adduction contracture. The longitudinal pin also prevents subluxation of the base of the thumb metacarpal on the trapezium with distraction. Circumferentially incise the periosteum at the level of the osteotomy.

Turn the screws on the distraction device to create at least 5 mm of immediate distraction at the osteotomy site. Then close the skin. The digit is gradually lengthened over the ensuing 4 to 5 weeks by turning of the distraction device approximately 1 rotation per day. Soft tissues are gradually stretched as the osteotomy gap is widened. Distraction takes place along the axis provided by the longitudinal pin. It is often possible to gain up to 3 cm to 4 cm of additional thumb length with this technique.

Though bone consolidation may occur spontaneously in young patients, it is our custom to electively add iliac crest bone graft to span the gap between the proximal and distal metacarpal segments. The device remains in place until graft incorporation is radiographically visible. Secondary web space deepening as described in the section on phalangization is occasionally helpful as a secondary procedure.

Pollicization

Because pollicization allows restoration of both digital length and mobility, it is often recommended when traumatic thumb amputation results in basilar joint destruction.[3,7] The index finger is usually the digit selected for pollicization. When the extent of trauma to the thumb has been severe enough to warrant pollicization, the adjacent index finger is often also compromised. This is not necessarily a contraindication to pollicization. An injured digit with limited mobility may be a liability in the index position but may substantially enhance function when transposed to the thumb position.

Reconstruction of posttraumatic thumb injuries is similar to that of pollicization for the congenitally absent or hypoplastic thumb with individual modification. If there is extensive scarring and soft-tissue loss over the radial border of the hand, preliminary groin flap coverage may be required.

Procedure. Skin incisions need to be individualized when skin along the radial border of the hand is scarred (Fig. 83-3). Design skin flaps to bring the best skin—palmar, dorsal, or a combination of palmar and dorsal—into the web space created between the pollicized digit and the middle finger at the time of closure. Skin graft is often necessary dorsally and radially but should be avoided if possible in the web space.

Evaluate digital artery integrity of the index and middle fingers preoperatively by arteriography when there has been proximal injury. Preserve the digital nerves by splitting the common digital nerve to the index and middle fingers.

In adult pollicization, reestablish skeletal length by combining remaining thumb and index parts. The goal is to achieve a reconstructed thumb whose tip extends approximately 60% of

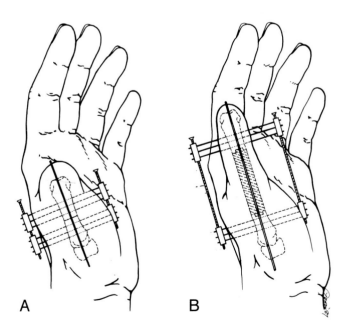

FIGURE 83-2. Thumb distraction lengthening. (*A*) Pin groups are placed adjacent to the mid-diaphyseal osteotomy site. (*B*) Once the desired distraction has been achieved, the bone graft is locked into the medullary canal of the distracted proximal and distal segments.

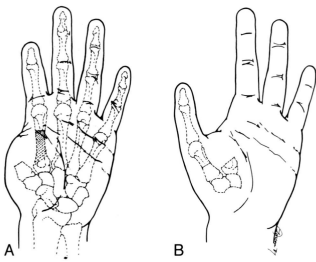

FIGURE 83-3. Index pollicization. (*A*) The extent of index metacarpal resection is dependent on the residual length of both the thumb metacarpal and the index finger. (*B*) The transposed index metacarpal is fixed to the proximal thumb metacarpal remnant.

the length of the proximal phalanx of the middle finger. If the index is of normal length and the basilar joint is absent, then use of the index metacarpal head as a trapezium will prove most satisfactory. When the trapezium and a portion of the metacarpal remain, resect the entire metacarpal and an appropriate portion of the proximal phalanx. The proximal phalanx may be directly set on top of the metacarpal remnant. When the distal portion of the index has been damaged, retain an appropriate metacarpal length to achieve a composite digit of proper length.

When the basilar joint and thenar musculature are absent, carry out a musculotendinous rearrangement as in pollicization for thumb aplasia. Advance the first dorsal and first palmar interossei insertions distally on the hood and shorten the extensor tendons. If the first dorsal interosseous muscle has been damaged, consider simultaneous opponesplasty tendon transfer. When the index digit is damaged distally and is merely being moved radialward without skeletal shortening, extensor tendon shortening may not be required.

DIGITAL AMPUTATION

Fingertip and distal phalangeal injuries have been discussed in Chapter 82. When amputation occurs at or proximal to the distal interphalangeal joint, distal flap coverage is rarely indicated. Modest bone shortening and contouring is usually preferable, unless the potentially sacrificed bone length is judged critical to preservation of the functional integrity of the affected finger. In general, any digit that retains its superficialis insertion will continue to contribute effectively to grasp activity. When amputation occurs more proximally (e.g., proximal middle phalanx, proximal phalanx), the digit will have only limited value in the little-finger position and will probably be a nuisance in the index position. When amputation occurs proximal to the superficialis but distal to the midproximal phalanx, preservation of the digit in the middle or ring position may help

prevent small objects from falling through the hand, though only limited metacarpophalangeal joint flexion will occur through the pull of the intrinsic muscles.

When multiple digits have been compromised by amputation or other severe mutilating injury, it is best to preserve all available bone length. In multi-digit degloving injuries, distant flap coverage may be indicated.

Procedure

Amputation through an interphalangeal joint requires attention to bone as well as soft tissue to avoid a bulbous distal contour (Fig. 83-4). Create palmar and dorsal tongue-shaped flaps by bilateral midlateral incisions. The palmar flap should be slightly longer, if possible, so that the ultimate scar will be dorsal. Pull tendons and digital nerves distally and divide them sharply. Gently divide digital nerves and allow them to retract. Ligate digital arteries. Identify the palmar plate and excise it. Remove the cartilage from the exposed phalangeal articular surface to facilitate bone contouring. Resect the palmar condylar prominences in line with the palmar cortex of the diaphysis. Shape the remaining flat condylar surface with rongeur and rasp to resemble a paddle. Palpate the bone through the overlying skin to ensure that all prominences have been relieved. Skin closure is accomplished with interrupted sutures. Extensive contouring of skin margins is not necessary, since the skin contour will gradually model to the underlying bony contour.

Diaphyseal phalangeal amputations are handled in a similar fashion.

INDEX FINGER AMPUTATIONS

The normal index finger is ideally situated to pinch and manipulate a myriad of objects. Imperfections of the index finger are, however, poorly tolerated. When the index finger of an otherwise normal hand is compromised by loss of length, altered sensibility, or pain, many patients spontaneously shift to a prehension pattern that ignores the index finger in preference to a normal middle finger. The greater length of the middle finger allows it to easily meet the thumb for precision activity. When a short index finger is being ignored, it is often held in a hyperextended posture. Amputation of a short index finger is advised when patterns of disuse become fixed.

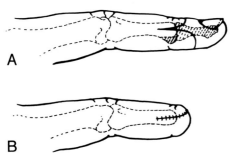

FIGURE 83-4. Interphalangeal joint disarticulation amputation. (*A*) Palmar condylar prominences are removed. (*B*) The greater length of the volar flap brings the suture line away from the contact surface.

Amputation of the index finger may be accomplished by either metacarpophalangeal joint disarticulation or index ray resection. Metacarpophalangeal joint disarticulation preserves the breadth of the palm, which is helpful in stabilizing objects held with a cylindrical grip[9] but presents an obtrusive prominence in the web space. Ray resection narrows the palm and improves the appearance of the hand by achieving a smooth web space contour.

Procedure for Ray Resection

Skin incisions are designed to facilitate exposure and to provide a supple web space that will allow thumb mobility (Fig. 83-5). If an overly large wedge of skin is removed, the distance from thumb to middle metacarpal will be diminished and thumb abduction may be limited.

Dissect skin flaps from the index digit, taking care to preserve flap innervation. Divide the extensor indicis proprius tendon from its insertion ulnar to the index communis tendon and tag it. Osteotomize the index metacarpal obliquely through the proximal metaphysis, preserving extensor carpi radialis longus and flexor carpi radialis tendon insertions.

Although some authors advocate suturing the first dorsal interosseous tendon into the second dorsal interosseous insertion on the middle metacarpal to enhance the strength of lateral pinch, this transfer is occasionally too strong and may result in a fixed radial deviation posture of the middle finger.

Divide the deep transverse metacarpal ligament adjacent to the middle finger. Identify the flexor tendons, pull them distally, divide them, and allow them to retract proximally. Take care in dealing with the digital nerves. The radial nerve to the index must not be extensively mobilized. Sharply divide digital nerves and allow them to retract into the soft tissue without tension. It is essential that the ultimate neuroma end of the nerves be distanced from further trauma. Remove the index

finger. Sew the extensor indicis proprius into the extensor digitorum communis tendon at the level of its insertion to enhance independence of middle-finger extension. Trim the first dorsal and first palmar interosseous muscles as necessary to ensure a smooth web space contour. Close the skin flaps with the thumb in palmar and radial abduction.

CENTRAL RAY RESECTION

When amputation of the middle or ring fingers is carried out at the metacarpophalangeal joint level, an awkward space is left between the remaining digits. This defect makes it difficult to hold or cup small objects in the palm of the hand because of the tendency of such objects to "escape" from the grasp when the hand is in a dependent supinated posture (Fig. 83-6).[3] Ray resection and reconstruction by either soft-tissue coaptation or ray transfer closes this gap and improves the aesthetic appearance of the hand.[12,13] Both procedures narrow the palm and thus predictably weaken grasp and cylindrical grip palmar stabilization.

Soft-tissue coaptation, clearly the simpler procedure, effectively brings the relatively mobile little-finger ray into close approximation to the middle finger but is somewhat less successful in bringing the relatively fixed index metacarpal alongside the ring metacarpal.[13]

Procedure

Ray Resection and Soft-Tissue Coaptation Sling (Fig. 83-7)

Make parallel zigzag incisions on the palmar surface overlying the metacarpal that is to be resected. Remove a generous

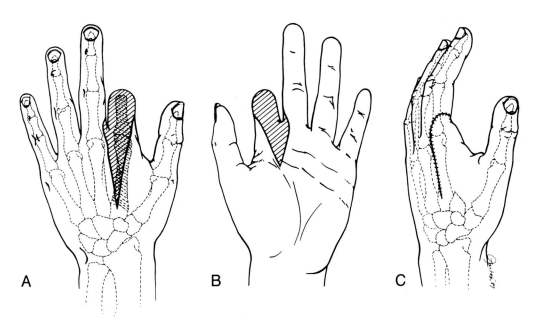

FIGURE 83-5.   Index ray resection. (*A*) Dorsal view. (*B*) Palmar skin resection. (*C*) Wound closure preserves sensate skin throughout the widened web space.

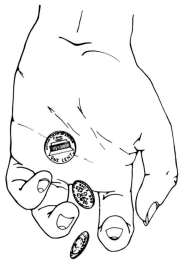

FIGURE 83-6. Absence of either the middle or the ring finger impairs the ability to retain small objects in the palm.

wedge of dorsal skin. The dorsal skin resection will provide a dermodesis, which will stabilize the digit and prevent its rotating into a position in which the fingers will scissor over one another in flexion. Resect the metacarpal subperiosteally. If the middle metacarpal is excised, preserve the proximal insertion of extensor carpi radialis brevis, and take care to preserve the origin of the adductor pollicis muscle. When the ring metacarpal is resected, the entire metacarpal base may be removed, allowing radial shift of the little metacarpal on the hamate. Identify and ligate the proper digital arteries. Sharply divide the proper digital nerves distal to the common digital nerve

bifurcation. Pull flexor and extensor tendons distally, divide them, and allow them to retract proximally. Divide the interosseous and lumbrical tendons.

A single continuous soft-tissue band is retained consisting of the palmar plate and the two adjacent deep transverse metacarpal ligaments, each of which is firmly attached to adjacent digits. Press the metacarpal heads together manually. Tightly secure the digits adjacent to the resected metacarpal to one another by dividing the ligament–palmar plate complex and weaving the two segments together. Then securely suture the shortened ligament–palmar plate complex with interrupted sutures.

Close the palmar skin incision first. Observe the fingers with the wrist in both flexion and extension. Assess the extent of digital scissoring, if any, as the dorsal skin is reapproximated. If residual scissoring persists, excise further dorsal skin. Circumferential dressings and splinting maintain lateral metacarpal pressure and protect the ligament repair during the first 3 weeks following reconstruction.

Central Ray Resection and Ray Transposition (Fig. 83-8)

Recreation of a normal web space contour between the retained digits will be facilitated if the skin of a single web space is preserved and shifted intact to the new web space. If possible, the web space flap should be based on the digit that is not being transposed. For example, if the middle finger is being resected and the index finger is being transposed to the middle-finger position, the web space skin of the middle–ring interval is retained based upon the ring finger and is ultimately sewn to the ulnar border of the index finger. Create palmar zig-zag incisions that converge over the middle third of the metacarpal

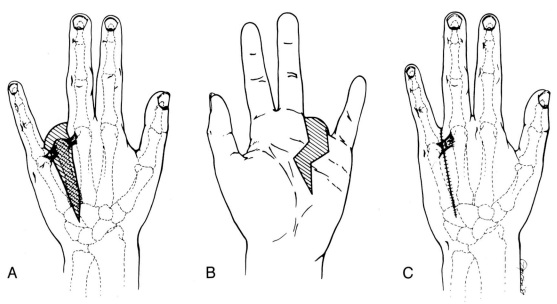

A   B   C

FIGURE 83-7. Ring ray resection with a soft-tissue coaptation sling. (A) Transverse intermetacarpal ligament and palmar plate continuity is preserved as the ring metacarpal is excised through a dorsal exposure. (B) A palmar chevron incision allows resection of redundant palmar skin. (C) Interweaving of the transverse intermetacarpal ligaments brings the little metacarpal head toward the middle metacarpal while dorsal skin closure stabilizes rotational alignment.

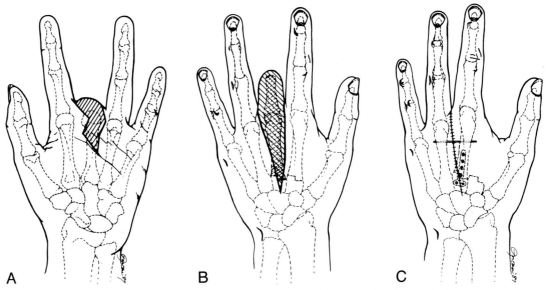

FIGURE 83-8. Middle ray resection and index ray transposition. (*A*) Converging chevron incisions reduce palmar skin and soft-tissue redundancy. (*B*) Corresponding step-cut osteotomies are fashioned in both the index and middle metacarpal proximal metaphyses. (*C*) The transposed index finger is fixed to the middle finger with a plate and is further stabilized with Kirschner wire into the ring metacarpal.

that is being resected. Resect a dorsal wedge of skin with its apex over the proximal third of the metacarpal.

Identify the digital neurovascular structures. Sharply section the proper digital nerves, and ligate the proper digital arteries. Pull flexor and extensor tendons distally and divide them. Define the interosseous muscles inserting on the resected digit distally, dissect them free proximally, isolate them, and excise them. Divide the lumbrical tendon along the radial aspect of the digit being resected. When the middle metacarpal is resected, preserve the origin of the adductor pollicis on the middle metacarpal by subperiosteal dissection.

Because nonunion of the bone-to-bone junction between transferred and recipient rays is a frequent complication of this procedure, careful planning of the bony osteotomy and secure fixation are essential. Osteotomy through the proximal metaphysis rather than diaphysis provides maximal cancellous surface area. Corresponding step-cut osteotomies fashioned in the transferred and recipient metacarpals enhance rotational stability.

Mobilize the transferred ray to allow transfer without tension. The interosseous muscle origins may need to be released. Suture the adductor pollicis origin to the ring metacarpal when the index ray is transposed to the middle position. Precisely fit the transferred ray into the step-cut recipient base. Approximate the deep transverse metacarpal ligaments distally. Ensure that the digit is straight and that the fingers do not overlap in flexion. Secure internal fixation is achieved proximally with multiple Kirschner wires or with a minifragment plate and screws. Transversely placed temporary Kirschner wires distally are helpful in further stabilizing the transferred digit during the first few weeks following surgery.

When the little-finger metacarpal is transposed to the ring position, the ultimate length discrepancy between the little and middle fingers may be minimized if the osteotomy is performed

more proximally in the middle-finger than in the little-finger metacarpal. This technique adds up to 1.5 cm in length to the shifted little-finger ray.

LITTLE-FINGER RAY RESECTION

When amputation of the little finger at the metacarpophalangeal joint level is required, ray resection may be considered. The hand that has undergone little-finger ray resection has an excellent cosmetic appearance and acceptance. For this reason, ray resection is recommended in women or sedentary men. In persons who depend on the breadth of their palm to stabilize a hammer, tennis racket, or other object with a cylindrical grip, removal of the little-finger metacarpal will result in a loss of strength.

Procedure (Fig. 83-9)

Make a dorsoulnar incision to expose the little-finger metacarpal. Isolate and divide the extensor communis and extensor digiti tendons. Because the flexor carpi ulnaris and extensor carpi ulnaris insert on the base of the little-finger metacarpal, disarticulation of the carpometacarpal joint should be avoided. Rather, the metacarpal should be divided obliquely through the tapering metaphysis. Divide the flexor tendons as well as the third palmar interosseous, lumbrical, and hypothenar muscle tendons. Trim the hypothenar muscles as necessary to create a smooth contour along the ulnar border of the hand.

A third alternative, a compromise between metacarpophalangeal disarticulation and ray resection, involves amputating the metacarpal head and neck and obliquely contouring the metacarpal through the distal diaphysis. Though this procedure improves the appearance of the hand and preserves most

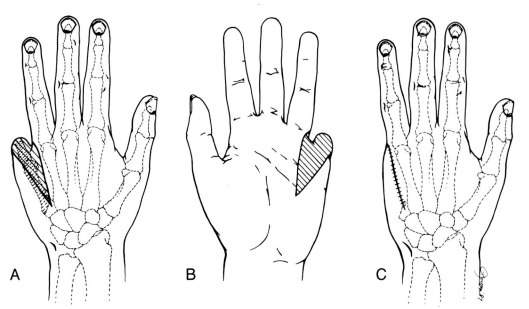

FIGURE 83-9. Little-finger ray resection. (*A*) The extensor carpi ulnaris insertion into the proximal metacarpal is preserved. (*B*) Palmar skin excision. (*C*) Skin closure.

of the width of the palm, it eliminates the firm stabilizing contact surface over the palmar aspect of the little metacarpal head.

WRIST DISARTICULATION

When only the carpal bones remain, it is wisest to carry out wrist disarticulation by removal of the carpal bones. When the entire length of the radius and ulna is preserved, forearm rotation is maximized within a prosthesis. Though fitting of a prosthesis is somewhat simpler with diaphyseal forearm amputations, this advantage is modest and is outweighed by the advantage of preservation of the integrity of the distal radioulnar articulation.

POSTOPERATIVE CARE

The goal of partial hand amputation is the restitution of pain-free, useful hand function. This goal is usually best accomplished by early active movement of the injured hand. When internal fixation is employed, a firm construct should be designed that will permit digital motion at the earliest time. The hand therapist may help guide the patient with a recent partial hand amputation to regain useful hand function. Emotional support should be provided by both the physician and the therapist to help the patient adapt to the alterations in body image occasioned by the amputation.

PITFALLS AND COMPLICATIONS

Quadriga or flexor digitorum profundus blockage[10] occurs when the free distal end of a transected profundus tendon becomes fixed distally and is unable to move to the proximal

extent of its normal excursion. Because of the extensive side-to-side interconnections between the profundus tendons at the wrist and distal forearm level, limitation of motion of a single tendon may have an adverse effect on the motion of adjacent uninjured digits. Patients who have sustained amputation may experience limitation of active distal joint flexion in adjacent digits and may complain of anterior forearm pain with attempted forceful flexion. The condition will be provoked by sewing of the profundus tendon over the end of a digital amputation stump. It is best avoided by early active motion of both amputated and adjacent digits. When quadriga is diagnosed, release of the adherent profundus tendon in the palm proximal to the lumbrical origin will predictably relieve this condition.

The lumbrical-plus phenomena may also be precipitated by digital amputation.[11] When amputation occurs through a finger proximal to the insertion of the profundus but distal to the proximal interphalangeal joint, the proximal pull of the profundus may be transmitted through the lumbrical into the dorsal hood apparatus, where the force of proximal interphalangeal joint extension is augmented. As the individual tries to grip with force, the movement of the profundus results in a posture of proximal interphalangeal joint extension. This paradoxic digital motion may be eliminated either by sectioning of the profundus proximal to the lumbrical origin or by release of the radial lateral band.

Because amputation implies the removal of innervated skin, all amputations inevitably require transection of sensory nerve branches. Neuromas occur whenever a nerve is transected and thus are an inevitable consequence of amputation. With proper surgical and postoperative management, however, neuromas need not be tender or painful. When a neuroma is caught in overlying scar or is adherent to a fixed structure, it often becomes symptomatic. The best approach is prevention. Many initially tender neuromas improve with local massage and desensitization activity under the guidance of a therapist. Surgical revision of tender neuromas should not be considered until the wound has become supple and the skin is no longer adherent to underlying soft tissue and bone.

Other neuromas become symptomatic when they are fixed distally and tethered by proximal joint motion. In such situations the nerve must be freed distally and allowed to migrate proximally. The digit is splinted and early motion encouraged.

REFERENCES

1. Beasley, R.W.: Surgery of hand and finger amputations. Orthop. Clin. North Am. **12**(4):763, 1981.
2. Brown, P.W.: Sacrifice of the unsatisfactory hand. J. Hand Surg. **4**(5):417, 1979.
3. Chase, R.A.: Atlas of Hand Surgery. Philadelphia, W.B. Saunders, 1973.
4. Chase, R.A.: Atlas of Hand Surgery, Vol. 2. Philadelphia, W.B. Saunders, 1984.
5. Campbell Reid, D.A., and Gosset, J. (eds.): Mutilating Injuries of the Hand. Edinburgh, Churchill Livingstone, 1979.
6. Light, T.R.: Kinesiology of the upper limb. In AAOS: Atlas of Orthotics, 2nd ed., pp. 126–138. St. Louis, C.V. Mosby, 1985.
7. Lister, G.: The choice of procedure following thumb amputation. Clin. Orthop. **195**:45, 1985.
8. Matev, I.B.: Thumb lengthening through metacarpal bone lengthening. J. Hand Surg. **5**(5):482, 1980.
9. Murray, J.F., Carman, W., and MacKenzie, J.K.: Transmetacarpal amputation of the index finger: A clinical assessment of hand strength and complications. J. Hand Surg. **2**:471, 1977.
10. Neu, B.R., Murray, J.F., and MacKenzie, J.K.: Profundus tendon blockage: Quadriga in finger amputations. J. Hand Surg. **10-A**(6):882, 1985.
11. Parkes, A.: The "lumbrical plus" finger. J. Bone Joint Surg. **53-B**(2):236, 1971.
12. Posner, M.A.: Ray transposition for central digital loss. J. Hand Surg. **4**(3):242, 1979.
13. Steichen, J.B., and Idler, R.S.: Results of central ray resection without bony transposition. J. Hand Surg. **11-A**(4):466, 1986.
14. Tubiana, R., and Roux, J.P.: Phalangization of the first and fifth metacarpals: Indications, operative technique and results. J. Bone Joint Surg. **56-A**:447, 1974.

CHAPTER 84

Dupuytren's Disease

JAMES W. STRICKLAND

Although the condition had been previously described and treated by others, the Baron Guillaume Dupuytren of France was the first to provide a thorough discussion of the etiology, anatomy, and treatment of the diseased palmar aponeurosis.[5,6] Unfortunately, the pathology responsible for this condition is still poorly understood, and its surgical management has been frustrating. Although the English literature has for many years referred to the condition as Dupuytren's contracture, it is now recognized that the affliction may be present without concomitant finger deformity, and so the term Dupuytren's disease is more appropriate.[37]

Dupuytren's disease is a condition without any obvious etiology. Apparently, a genetic predisposition or diathesis must exist,[17] and the disease may then be triggered by systemic or mechanical factors. The site of its development will depend on hand anatomy and biomechanics and the effects of external forces or injury.[34] The rate of progression of the process is influenced by age, collagen metabolism, neurovascular factors, the use of the hand, and the patient's psychological makeup.[34]

PATHOLOGIC ANATOMY

The normal and pathologic palmar and digital fascia, described by numerous authors,[9,10,23,30,31,34–36,39,40–44,47,48] are beyond the scope of this chapter. However, it is important for the surgeon to have a basic understanding of the anatomy of the disease so that it can be surgically managed in the most expeditious manner without endangering the adjacent flexor tendon system or the neurovascular structures. In this description of the pathologic anatomy of Dupuytren's disease, we will refer to normal fascial tissues as bands and diseased tissue as cords, as suggested by Luck.[25]

The palmar fascia arises proximally in the hand from the terminal divisions of the palmaris longus tendon or from the deep transverse carpal ligament (Fig. 84-1). Longitudinal fibers then fan over the palm as four pretendinous bands that terminate superficially in the skin just distal to the metacarpophalangeal joint. Extensions of the pretendinous bands then divide distally into two oblique strips that twist around, plunge inward, and run close to the lateral aspect of the metacarpophalangeal joint capsule, as described by Gossett.[9,10] Just proximal to the skin insertions of the pretendinous bands, a deeper layer, known as the superficial transverse ligament, crosses the palm from the thenar to the hypothenar fascia. Usually, it is not involved in disease,[40,41] although it may be a cause of thumb web contracture.[29–32]

In the distal palm, the natatory ligaments consist of a band of fascia in the web spaces that extend from the proximal thenar crease to the hypothenar fascia with attachments to the flexor sheaths and the lateral digital fascia. When contracted by a pathologic process, they are thought to produce digital adduction and flexion deformities. The spiral bands described by McFarlane are composed of the deep distal extensions of the pretendinous bands and the vertical septae of Legueu and Juvara, as well as the fascia of the intrinsic muscles. They cross obliquely beneath the neurovascular bundle and insert into the natatory ligaments and lateral digital sheets. The hypothenar fascia is a condensation along the ulnar border of the palm that extends between the digital fascia of the proximal phalanx and

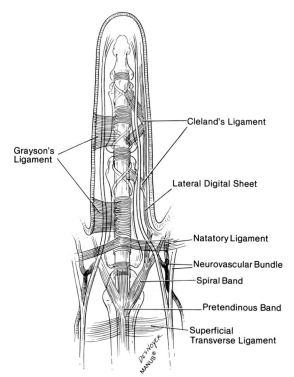

FIGURE 84-1. Normal palmar-digital fascial anatomy. (Modified from McFarlane, R.M.: Patterns of the Diseased Fascia in the Fingers in Dupuytren's Contracture: Displacement of the Neurovascular Bundle. Plast. Reconstr. Surg. **54:**31, 1974, with permission.)

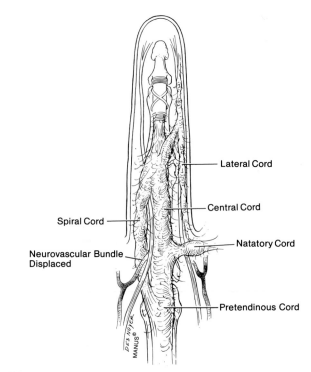

FIGURE 84-2. Artist's representation of the pathologic cords found in Dupuytren's disease. (Modified from McFarlane, R.M.: Patterns of the Diseased Fascia in the Fingers in Dupuytren's Contracture: Displacement of the Neurovascular Bundle. Plast. Reconstr. Surg. **54:**31, 1974, with permission.)

the hypothenar aponeurosis and that is frequently implicated in contractures of the small finger.

McFarlane[29–32] favors the concept that Dupuytren's disease results from pathologic changes in pre-existing normal fascia. This is in contrast to the theory of McCallum and Hueston[26] which states that the disease arises *de novo* in the subdermal tissues and attaches and grows on the underlying fascial bands. According to McFarlane, normal anatomic bands and sheaths become diseased and contract into cords; they can be classified as one of the following (Fig. 84-2):

Pretendinous cords
Central cords
Spiral cords
Natatory cords
Lateral cords
Retrovascular cords

Although many of these cords are a combination of both the palmar and digital fasciae (Fig. 84-3), isolated digital cords have also been described without palmar attachments (Fig. 84-4).[46]

Pretendinous cords are described as diseased pretendinous bands that produce metacarpophalangeal joint flexion via their deep attachments to the volar plate in continuity with the extensions of the septae of Legueu and Juvara. The *central cord* is a distal extension of the pretendinous cord. The central cord is the subject of considerable controversy because it arises in an area of superficial fibrofatty tissue on the palmar surface of the digit with no known fascial precursor. It inserts near the mid-

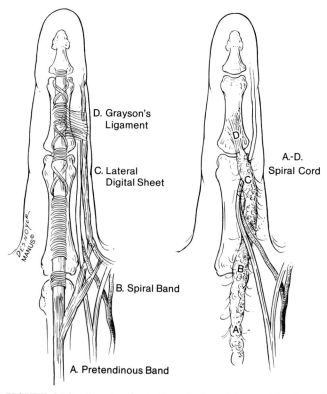

FIGURE 84-3. Development of a spiral cord by combination of pathologic changes in the pretendinous band (*A*), spiral band (*B*), lateral-digital sheet (*C*), and Grayson's ligament (*D*).

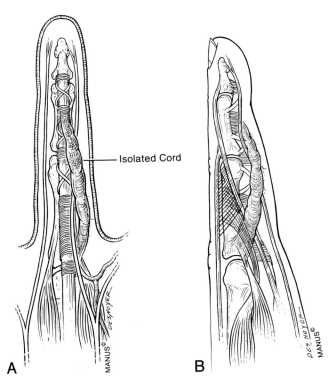

FIGURE 84-4. (A) An isolated digital cord originating from the base of the proximal phalanx, crossing the neurovascular bundle, and inserting centrally into the flexor tendon sheath and periosteum of the middle phalanx. (B) Lateral view of the same cord demonstrating its origin from the periosteum and intrinsic tendon insertions at the base of the proximal phalanx. It displaces the neurovascular bundle to the midline and crosses it near the distal portion of the proximal phalanx.

line of the middle phalanx on the bone, tendon sheath, and skin. *Spiral cords* arise from either the pretendinous cords or the intrinsic muscle-tendons, extending deep via the spiral band to the neurovascular bundle and displacing it superficially and medially, rendering it vulnerable to surgical dissection (Fig. 84-5). Along with possible attachments to the natatory cord, the spiral cords insert on the lateral digital cord and then proceed to insert on the flexor fascia of the middle phalanx in the area of Grayson's ligaments. *Natatory cords* are primarily associated with web space contracture, sometimes participating with other cords in the development of proximal interphalangeal flexion deformities. The *lateral cord* is intimately adherent to the skin and may also be attached to the flexor sheath at the area of the proximal interphalangeal joint, as described by Gossett.[9,10] These fibers are thought to arise from the superficial fascia that surrounds the finger and from the natatory ligaments. They result in contracture at the proximal interphalangeal joint and occasionally, at the distal interphalangeal joint level. The dorsal portion of the lateral fascia corresponds to the *retrovascular cord* of Thomine and extends along the digit in the area of Cleland's ligaments. The fascia in this area is thought to be a cause of recurrent contracture.

Strickland and Bassett[46] describe the occurrence of isolated Dupuytren's fascial cords within digits without proximal palmar connections (Fig. 84-6). These fibers are either single or double and originate from the periosteum at the base of the

proximal phalanx in conjunction with adjacent ligaments and intrinsic tendons. They proceed in an oblique direction to displace and cross the neurovascular bundles before inserting on the bone or flexor tendon sheath of the middle phalanx. They are associated with significant proximal interphalangeal joint flexion deformities.

SURGICAL MANAGEMENT OF DUPUYTREN'S DISEASE

To date, no nonsurgical treatment has been effective in the management of Dupuytren's disease. Numerous surgical procedures designed to arrest, ablate, or palliate the disease have been described; however, none of them is universally applicable to patients with this condition. Moreover, no one method of treating Dupuytren's disease has been shown to be superior to any other established method. The type of surgical treatment remains a decision unique to each surgeon; based on training, technical skill, and concept of the disease process.[30]

General Considerations

Regardless of the procedures selected, patients undergoing surgery for Dupuytren's disease should be counseled carefully with regard to the nature of the disease process and the prognosis for additional contracture and functional impairment should they not elect to proceed with surgery. The intricacies of the operative procedure should also be discussed, including the possibility of complications and the need to commence early postoperative digital motion in order to minimize stiffness or recurrent contracture. The surgeon should attempt to identify patients who may develop a postoperative sympathetic "flare." It has been said that a moist, sweaty hand is a bad prognostic sign, as is the thickened hand of a laborer.[34-36] Alcoholics, epileptics, and patients with Dupuytren's diatheses (strong family history, early onset of the disease, multiple areas of fibromatosis) may not be expected to do as well with surgery. Nonetheless, the indications for surgery in these individuals is the same as for others.

Indications for Surgery

Howard perhaps stated it best when he wrote that surgery was indicated for the release of "bothersome contractures."[11] It should be emphasized that a painful or annoying palmar nodule is rarely an indication for surgery because the potential complications of the procedure outweigh the "nuisance value" of the lesion. Progressive flexion contractures of the metacarpophalangeal joint or proximal interphalangeal joints may be indications for surgery, and because one can almost always correct metacarpophalangeal joint deformity, surgery at this level is less urgent than that undertaken to correct developing contractures at the proximal interphalangeal joint. At about 30°, an isolated metacarpophalangeal joint contracture begins to become annoying to many patients, and surgery may be appropriate. Proximal interphalangeal joint contractures secondary to Dupuytren's disease are much more difficult to correct. Indeed, the greater the magnitude of the presenting con-

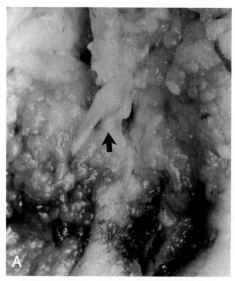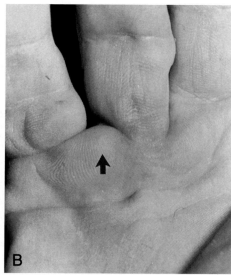

FIGURE 84-5. Pathologic features of a spiral cord. (*A*) A firm, nodular enlargement at the ulnar base of the ring finger with a small distal depression is thought to represent a spiral fascial cord. (*B*) The appearance of a spiral cord passing underneath the ulnar digital nerve and displacing it superficially and medially. Both nerve and artery are vulnerable to surgical dissection at this point.

tracture, the less likely it is that significant, long-term improvement can be achieved by surgery.[49] For that reason, it is recommended that surgery be considered before proximal interphalangeal joint contractures exceed 30°.[29,49]

SURGICAL TECHNIQUES

The surgical procedures available for Dupuytren's contracture include the following:

> Local excision
> Fasciotomy
> Fasciotomy and full-thickness skin grafting
> Radical fasciectomy
> Limited fasciectomy
> Dermal fasciectomy and full-thickness skin grafting
> Open palm technique

Each of these procedures will be considered separately.

Local Excision

Local excision of a palmar nodule, as recommended by Luck,[25] is generally not advised. Although it may be appropriate for those few individuals who are so annoyed or obsessed by the nodule that they demand its excision, they must understand that, because of the diffuse nature of the underlying pathologic process, the procedure will not prevent the progression of the disease or the development of joint deformity.[30]

Fasciotomy

Fasciotomy, or simple division of the offending fascial cords, was advocated by Dupuytren in 1932.[34] Although generally scorned by many surgeons as incomplete and palliative, the operation is simple and effective for those patients in whom a more extensive surgical ablation of the fascia is contraindicated. The procedure is best suited for individuals with thin

palmar fascial cords and contractures that primarily involve the metacarpophalangeal joint. It is particularly useful in elderly chronically ill patients, and in some instances, it may be used as a preparation for fasciectomy in order to extend the digit partially and to facilitate skin incisions and dissection.

The procedure, as described by Coville,[4] is performed after administration of a local anesthetic (Fig. 84-7). Following routine preparation of the hand, insert a No. 15 surgical blade subcutaneously and delicately free the distal skin from the underlying cord. Then turn the blade perpendicular to the cord and passively extend the involved finger to deliver the fascia against the knife edge. Apply gentle downward pressure. The cord can be felt to divide and elongate, and the metacarpophalangeal contracture will partially or completely be released.

It is important that fasciotomy be performed at or proximal to the distal palmar crease where the neurovascular bundles are mobile and well protected. Fasciotomy at the base of the digit is contraindicated because of the vulnerability of neurovascular structures, particularly when spiral cords are present. McFarlane believes that fasciotomy is best performed with direct exposure so as to minimize the possibility of nerve damage.[30] In either case, the resulting palmar wounds are left open, and small compressive dressings are applied. Digital motion is permitted immediately, and extension splinting is used intermittently for several months. Although most authors report that the recurrence rate is high following this simple surgical procedure, it is often of considerable long-term benefit in many situations.

Fasciotomy and Full-Thickness Skin Grafting

Gonzalez[7,8] has advocated transection of contracting skin and fascial cords at points of maximal tension, together with the insertion of full-thickness skin grafts in an effort to interrupt the continuity of the cord. Dissection and undermining are minimized and no effort is made to excise the offending fascia. After surgery, the digits are splinted in extension, and motion is commenced within 10 to 14 days. Gonzalez indicates that the

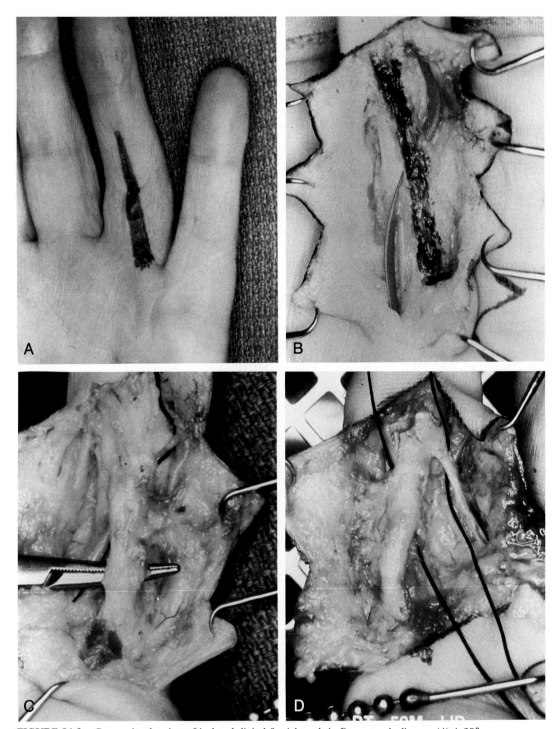

FIGURE 84-6. Composite drawing of isolated digital fascial cords in Dupuytren's disease. (*A*) A 35° flexion deformity of the proximal interphalangeal joint of the ring finger produced an isolated fascial cord (marked in black) that was barely palpable and had no proximal palmar connections. (*B*) The appearance of the cord (stained with methylene blue); the course of the digital artery and nerve is indicated by the rubber marker. Note the medial displacement of the neurovascular structures which are then crossed by the cord in the distal portion of the proximal phalanx. (*C*) An isolated hypothenar cord on the ulnar aspect of the fifth finger. (*D*) Double isolated digital cords in an index finger with a large radial and small ulnar component. The black threads indicate the course of the neurovascular bundles.

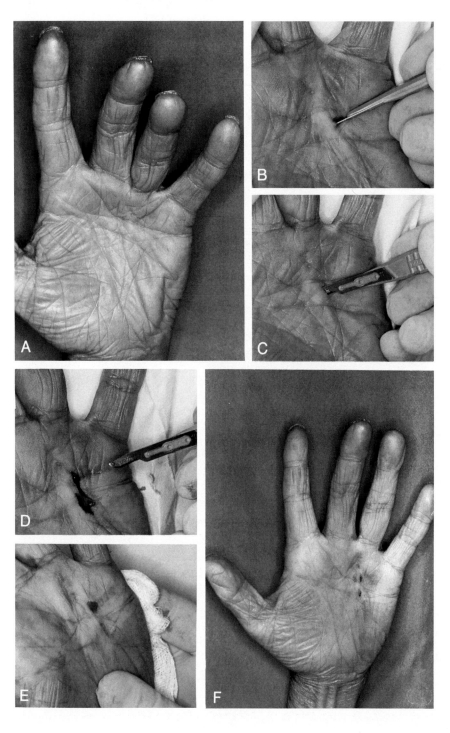

FIGURE 84-7. Technique for subcutaneous fasciotomy. (*A*) Appearance of the hand of an elderly patient with a 40° flexion contracture of the metacarpophalangeal joint of the ring finger secondary to a linear fascial cord. (*B*) Following the administration of a local anesthetic, a No. 15 blade is introduced beneath the skin and directly over the fascial cord. (*C*) The cutting edge of the blade is turned perpendicular to the cord, and gentle, downward pressure is applied as the digit is passively extended. (*D*) The procedure is repeated at a level just distal to the distal palmar crease, and the knife is withdrawn. (*E*) Passive extension of the digit completes the release of the fascial cord in the palm. (*F*) Appearance of the palm and digit following fasciotomy. The metacarpophalangeal joint contracture has been released completely.

procedure results in minimal morbidity and a low recurrence rate. McGregor[33] has also utilized a surgical technique involving fasciotomy and the interposition of skin grafts to separate cords and to release tension. He emphasizes the need to divide all fascial fibers to ensure release of the continuity of the offending cord. Although these procedures have not gained wide acceptance among hand surgeons, those who have used them report that they are effective and are associated with few complications. Perhaps it is the surgeon's compulsion to excise all pathologic tissue that impedes the popularity of these methods.

Radical Fasciectomy

There has been some debate regarding the amount of palmar fascia that should be excised at the time of surgery for Dupuytren's disease. McIndoe[37] advocated a transverse incision in the palm through which one could excise all of the palmar aponeurosis. This procedure was referred to as radical palmar fasciectomy and, when necessary, was combined with Z-plasty incisions in the digits. Although the procedure successfully removed almost all of the palmar fascia, it was not always successful in correcting contracture at the proximal interphalangeal joint,[30] and complications, including hematoma in the palm, were not uncommon. The procedure failed to take into account the various layers and individual ligamentous structures within the palmar fascia,[34] and skin necrosis and joint stiffness were additional postoperative problems. Furthermore, there was no evidence that radical excision of the palmar fascia prevented subsequent development of contracture in unoperated fingers, or recurrence of disease in operated digits. Use of this procedure has declined significantly.

Limited Fasciectomy

Surgery for contractures involving the palm and fascia of one or more digits is now managed by operative procedures designed to remove only the fascia that is responsible for joint contracture.[3,14,30,41] Hueston[12] has applied the term regional fasciectomy to this procedure, and has defined it as the removal of diseased fascia within the area. He has stated that "the only difference between a radical and conservative operation is the extent of the palmar dissection. Digital dissection will be required for interphalangeal joint deformity in any case."[14]

Skoog[40] believes that the transverse palmar fibers are never involved and that they should not be excised. His surgical technique advocates preservation of the deep transverse fibers, excision of involved longitudinal fascia, preservation of the covering of the neurovascular bundles proximal to the distal palmar crease, as well as removal of only the involved fascia, with preservation of fat whenever possible.

Limited fasciectomy requires wide surgical exposure of the offending fascia. One should strive to release contractures at both the metacarpophalangeal and proximal interphalangeal joints. Incisional options (Fig. 84-8) include the use of a continuous Z-plasty; multiple, long, zigzag incisions, as described by Bruner;[1] or shorter, Y-shaped incisions that are converted to V-shaped incisions in order to bring additional skin to the midline. The zigzag incision with Y-V closure, as advocated by King and associates,[21] has the advantage of allowing mobilization of considerable skin to the longitudinal axis of the palm and digit. As a result, there is rarely a need for skin grafting following correction of the deformity, and parallel incisions may be made in the adjacent palm or digits. Because limited palmar fasciectomy utilizing the Y-V–plasty incisions is the author's preferred method for the surgical management of Dupuytren's disease, this technique will be described in detail.

The procedure is now usually performed on an outpatient basis, and patients are usually quite comfortable following administration of regional or general anesthesia. Patients and their families should be prepared in advance for the need to elevate the hand and to remove a small drain after surgery.

Center incisions directly over the involved fascia, beginning at the proximal palm and extending to a level distal to the terminal fibers of the diseased cord (Fig. 84-9). If several digits are involved, carefully planned, parallel incisions may be made contiguously in the palm and digit. Following exsanguination of the hand with an Esmarch bandage and elevation of the tourniquet, begin dissection. Although many surgeons prefer the use of a magnifying loupe, magnification of greater than 2× may hinder dissection by limiting one's field of vision.

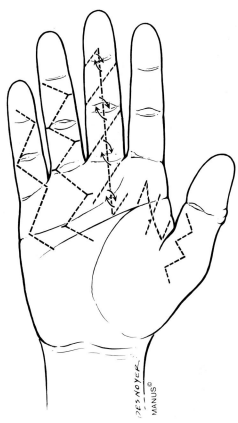

FIGURE 84-8. Incisional options for the treatment of Dupuytren's disease. The small finger depicts multiple, long, zigzag incisions, as advocated by Bruner.[1] The ring finger depicts multiple, shorter, Y-shaped incisions that are subsequently converted to a V-shaped configuration at the time of closure.[21] The long finger depicts multiple, continuous, Z-plasty incisions; the rotation and interdigitation of flaps is indicated by the arrows. Incisional options for the thumb web and thumb are also shown.

Throughout the dissection, immediately cauterize small blood vessels in an effort to minimize bleeding at the time of tourniquet release. Carefully dissect skin flaps off of the underlying diseased area; despite the intimate relationship between the fascia and its overlying skin, a satisfactory plane can almost always be identified. Sharp dissection utilizing a No. 15 blade is recommended, and flaps are mobilized until the entire diseased cord has been exposed.

Expose neurovascular bundles from the distal palm to the distal digital level on both the radial and ulnar sides of the cord. Take particular care to identify spiral cords and to protect the vulnerable neurovascular bundles that are delivered in a superficial and medial direction by these fascial projections. It is usually preferable to remove the fascia *en bloc* in a proximal-to-distal fashion once the neurovascular bundles have been identified and protected. However, in some cases in which the nerve and artery are intricately involved with digital disease, it is best to remove the fascia in a piecemeal fashion to ensure the protection of these structures. Preserve as much fatty tissue as possible in order to provide a well-padded bed for the neurovascular bundles. Divide vertical septae just deep to the plane of the fascia; make no effort to remove them at a deeper level,

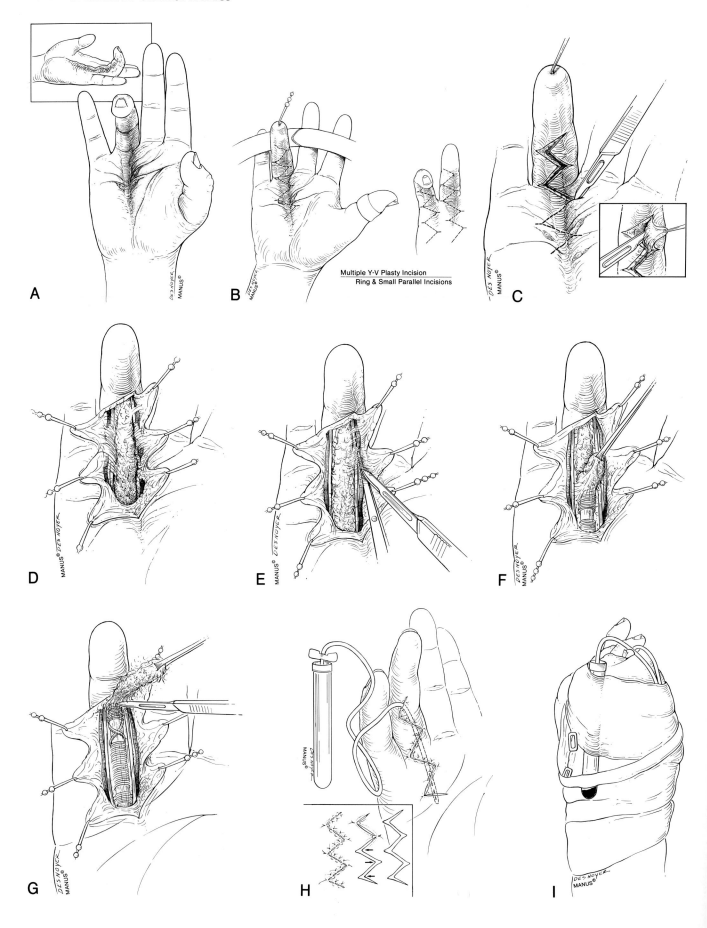

A

B

Multiple Y-V Plasty Incision
Ring & Small Parallel Incisions

C

D

E

F

G

H

I

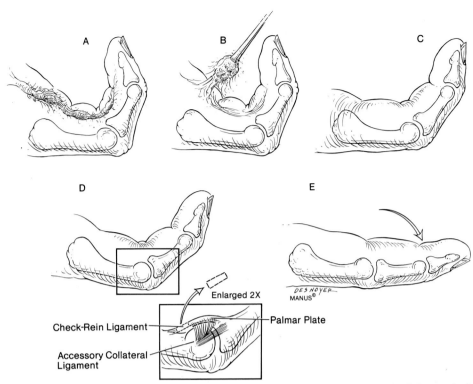

FIGURE 84-10. Restoration of digital extension by fasciectomy and capsulectomy. (*A–C*) Removal of the offending fascia from a contracted digit; improvement, but not correction, is evident at the proximal interphalangeal joint level. (*D*) (*Inset*) The excision of the paired "check-rein" extensions of the palmar plate and division of the palmar fibers of the collateral ligaments. (*E*) Full extension at the proximal interphalangeal joint.

as they are neither diseased nor a cause of contracture.[30] Perform similar dissection in the adjacent palmar-digital areas; when all diseased fascia has been excised, determine whether or not full joint extension has been achieved.

Persisting proximal interphalangeal joint contractures may then require capsulectomy; the technique of Watson and colleagues[51] is recommended (Fig. 84-10). In this procedure, the flexor sheath is opened just proximal to the A_3 pulley and with the flexor tendons alternately retracted to the radial and ulnar sides of the digit. The "check-rein" proximal extensions of the palmar plate are then excised. If necessary, the fibers of the collateral ligaments that are most palmar are also released. Failure to achieve full extension may require additional explo-

ration and release of portions of the lateral digital sheet, or further Y-V extension of the skin incisions.

In the small finger, one should always expose the ulnar aspect of the digit to determine if a hypothenar cord is present. If so, it should be excised, as it may represent the most likely cause of recurrence of deformity in that digit. In instances in which there is an isolated digital cord without palmar connections, a zigzag incision, centered directly over the cord, usually provides adequate exposure for cord excision. Associated proximal interphalangeal joint contractures are dealt with in a manner identical to that indicated for palmar digital fasciectomy. Zigzag or Z-plasty incisions are best utilized in order to avoid the contracting influence of linear scars.

FIGURE 84-9. Technique for limited fasciectomy for Dupuytren's disease. (*A*) A ring finger with contracted interdigital joints secondary to palmar-digital fascial disease. (*B*) Multiple Y-V incisions over the offending cord are shown. Optional parallel incisions for the small finger are also depicted; these are used when the disease extends into that digit. (*C*) Completion of the surgical incisions. The method for careful dissection to separate the skin flaps from the underlying fascia is shown in the inset. (*D*) With all flaps reflected, the pathologic fascial cord is visualized. (*E*) Careful dissection in the distal palm and digit is performed to expose and protect the neurovascular bundles on both the radial and ulnar sides of the digit. (*F*) With direct observation of the neurovascular bundles, the offending fascial cord is excised from proximal to distal. (*G*) Completion of the dissection and removal of the cord. (*H*) A small butterfly catheter drain (scalp vein set) and Vacutainer tube are used for low-suction drainage. Wound closure utilizing the Y-V technique is also shown in the inset. (*I*) At the conclusion of the procedure, a large compressive dressing is applied; a Vacutainer tube is incorporated into the dressing for 24 hours.

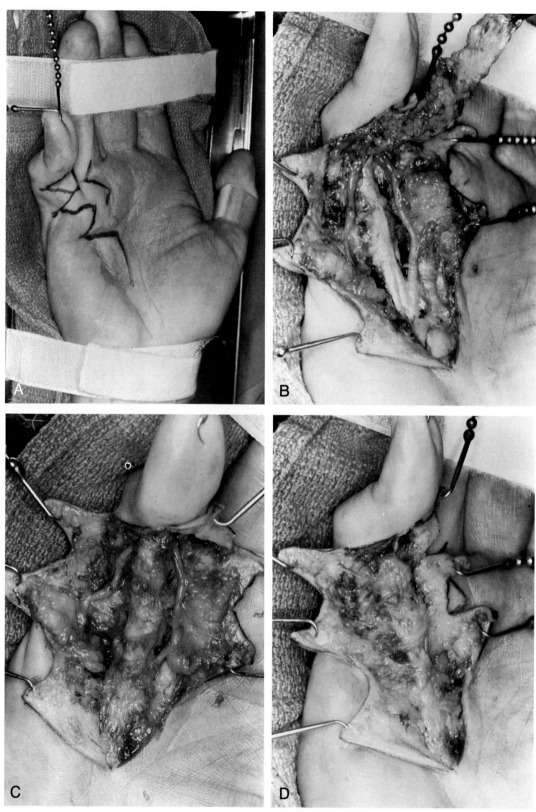

FIGURE 84-11. Surgical photographs of a limited fasciectomy procedure performed in a patient with severe contracture of the proximal interphalangeal joint of the small finger and limited fascial involvement of the ring finger. (*A*) Y-V surgical incisions over the fascial cords of the small finger and a small, zigzag incision at the base of the ring finger. (*B*) Appearance of the diffuse fascial cord of the small finger following reflection of the skin flaps. (*C*) Neurovascular bundles are exposed on both the radial and ulnar sides of the digit, and are mobilized well away from the offending cord. (*D*) The pathologic fascia is excised in a proximal-to-distal fashion and is then excised distally, with careful protection of the neurovascular bundles.

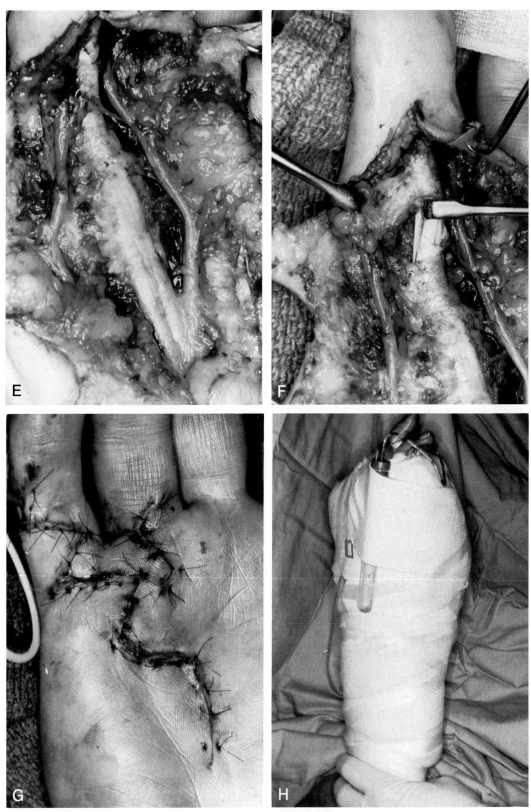

(*E*) The flexor tendon sheath and neurovascular bundles following complete excision of the fascial mass. (*F*) An incision is made into the flexor tendon sheath at the level of the proximal phalangeal joint; the flexor tendons are then retracted to expose the palmar plate so that capsulectomy may be completed by excising the "check-rein" extensions of the palmar plate and incising the collateral ligaments. (*G*) The appearance of the wounds at the time of closure. The tubing of a pediatric scalp vein set is placed beneath the small finger wound. (*H*) A compressive dressing is applied at the conclusion of the procedure. Note the connection of the scalp vein needle to the Vacutainer tube for continuous low-suction drainage.

At the conclusion of the fascial excision, release the tourniquet and apply compression to the hand for 10 minutes to control the resulting wound hyperemia. Cauterize all brisk bleeders, either leaving the tourniquet deflated or reinflating it, depending on the amount of vascular "ooze" that persists. Close the wound with 5-0 nonabsorbable sutures; approximately two-thirds the normal number of skin sutures are utilized to effect a loose closure. Introduce the tubing of a pediatric scalp vein set into each wound in a distal-to-proximal fashion after several small holes have been placed along the length of the tube.

Apply a bulky compressive dressing in such a manner as to produce anteroposterior compression of the hand. Splint the fingers in nearly full extension using a palmar plaster slab. Introduce the scalp vein needle, which has been excluded from the distal aspect of the dressing, into the rubber stopper of a suction collection tube and release the tourniquet if it has been reinflated. Incorporate the drainage tube into the dressing and place an additional tube close by in case the first tube fills with blood (Fig. 84-11).

At the time of release from the hospital, patients and/or their families are instructed to remove the drain from the digit on the following day. Patients are scheduled for a follow-up appointment within 3 to 5 days of surgery for the removal of the bulky dressing and the initiation of vigorous digital motion. Continuous extension splinting of the involved digits is maintained for several weeks, although the splint is removed frequently for gentle active and passive exercises. Two weeks after operation, skin sutures are removed, and formal therapy is instituted for those patients who have difficulty with active flexion. Night extension splinting of the involved digits is continued for 6 to 12 months to minimize the possibility of recurrent contractures.

Dermal Fasciectomy and Full-Thickness Skin Grafting

Hueston[16,17] has advocated *en bloc* excision of the fascia and overlying skin for recurrences of Dupuytren's contracture. He contends that recurrence never occurs deep to free skin grafting; if that is true, the procedure may be of considerable value. McFarlane[30] objects to the procedure on the grounds that the diseased fascia can almost always be separated from the overlying skin, that the procedure does not involve the spiral or retrovascular cords, and that it results in the exposure of the flexor tendon sheaths, creating an unfavorable bed for skin grafting. A review of his series of patients did not reveal a high incidence of Dupuytren's diathesis or a significant incidence of recurrence following the use of conventional fasciectomy techniques.

This procedure requires the excision of all of the skin and fascia of the involved ray from the distal palmar crease of the proximal interphalangeal joint crease to each mid-axial line. The areas are resurfaced by full-thickness or split-thickness skin grafts. With this procedure, there is an obligatory lengthening

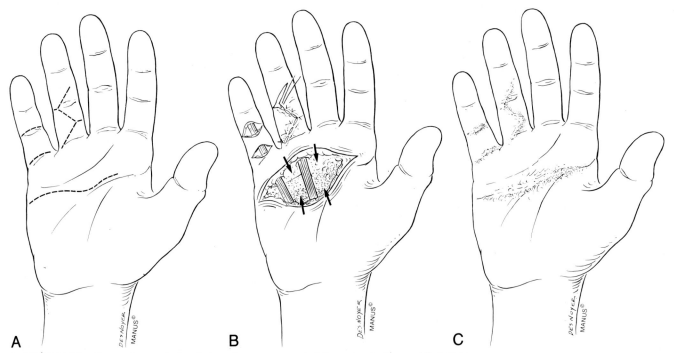

FIGURE 84-12. Open palm surgical technique for management of Dupuytren's disease. (*A*) A transverse incision is made in the palm; it must be long enough to allow extensive undermining and surgical dissection. Transverse finger incisions may also be used if the digital wound is to remain open. Alternative zigzag or Y-V incisions may also be made in the digits; these are closed at the conclusion of the procedure. (*B*) Appearance of the wounds at the conclusion of fascial excision. Wound closure by contraction is indicated by the arrows. (*C*) Palmar and digital wounds following skin healing and maturation.

of the interval between surgery and the initiation of digital motion.[34] Nonetheless, the method is particularly appropriate for the treatment of recurrent Dupuytren's disease when the skin is scarred and of poor quality.[12–19,50]

Open Palm Technique

McCash[27,28] has long advocated the open palm technique for the surgical management of Dupuytren's disease, emphasizing that the method eliminates the possibility of hematoma and reduces morbidity following extensive palmar dissection (Fig. 84-12). Postoperative swelling is minimal and joint stiffness is thought to be less difficult to manage with this procedure. The palm will usually heal by wound contracture in 3 to 6 weeks, at which time the patient should have regained full digital joint motion. The resulting transverse palmar scar is surprisingly small. Many surgeons strongly believe that this method is the best technique for the management of Dupuytren's disease.[2,22,24,28,38] McCash recommends the closure of digital wounds, whereas some surgeons advocate leaving both the palm and digital wounds open.

Following routine preparation, exsanguination of the extremity, and inflation of a pneumatic tourniquet, the procedure is begun. Make a transverse incision across the palm at a level just distal to the distal palmar crease. Mobilize skin flaps proximally and distally off of the underlying pathologic fascia,

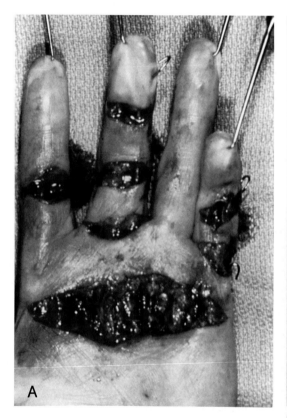

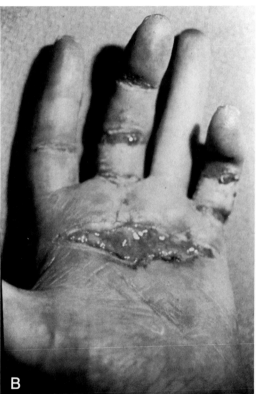

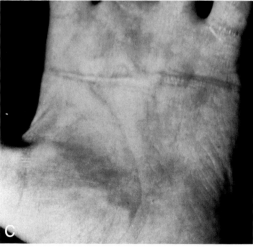

FIGURE 84-13. Appearance of the palmar and digital wounds in a patient with severe Dupuytren's disease involving multiple digits. Transverse incisions were used in the digits and all wounds were left open. Several Kirschner wires were used to maintain extension following the release of severe digital flexion deformities. (*B*) Appearance of the granulating palmar and digital wounds 2½ weeks after surgery. (*C*) Appearance 3 months after the procedure.

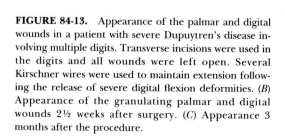

taking care to identify and protect the neurovascular structures. Transverse incisions are also utilized in the digits, although if one intends to use the open wound technique in these areas, one may prefer a zigzag incision in the digits in a manner identical to that described for subtotal palmar fasciectomy.

Following excision of the offending fascia from the palm and digits, release the tourniquet and cauterize all brisk bleeders. Apply fine-mesh gauze to all wounds, and use a bulky compressive dressing with a palmar plaster splint to maintain the digits in nearly full extension (Fig. 84-13).

The open palm technique, as advocated by McCash, involves changing the dressing 7 days after operation, with daily dressing changes thereafter until the wound has healed. Active and passive range of motion exercises are encouraged throughout the healing process. Weekly observation of the wound is also recommended.

COMPLICATIONS OF SURGERY

The immediate potential complications of surgery for Dupuytren's contracture include palmar hematoma and skin necrosis (Fig. 84-14). The use of low-suction drainage should minimize the likelihood of hematoma; when it does occur, prompt evacuation is recommended. Skin necrosis may be managed by careful observation if the area involved is no greater than 1 cm in diameter; larger areas must be excised as soon as possible. The defect that results from excision of necrotic skin may be left open, or it may be closed by the use of a free graft.

A postoperative sympathetic disturbance or "flare" is probably the most severe complication that may occur following surgery for Dupuytren's contracture. This condition is thought to be secondary to an over-response of the sympathetic nervous system or to Sudeck's atrophy, and may be very difficult to manage. Pain, swelling, and stiffness may involve not only the operated digits, but also the unoperated fingers, the hand, and to some extent, the entire extremity. Wounds may be inordinately reddened and firm, and the hand may sweat excessively. The onset of this unfortunate complication must be suspected when the degree of pain, edema, and stiffness experienced by the patient exceeds that which is normally seen during the early stages of surgical recovery.

Treatment of severe "flare" usually consists of a gentle but vigorous therapeutic program that includes active and passive range of motion exercises, dynamic splinting, continuous passive motion devices, transcutaneous nerve stimulation, and administration of anti-inflammatory medications or steroids. Oral steroids may be of considerable value in patients with particularly severe dystrophy characterized by marked inflammation and stiffness. Carpal tunnel decompression has been shown to be of value when the median nerve is involved in the process.[38,45] Occasionally, one or more stellate ganglion blocks may help to reverse this phenomenon.

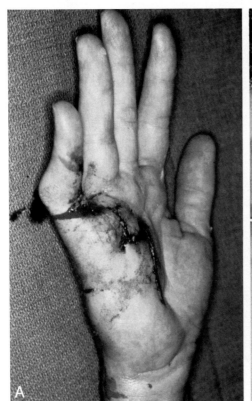 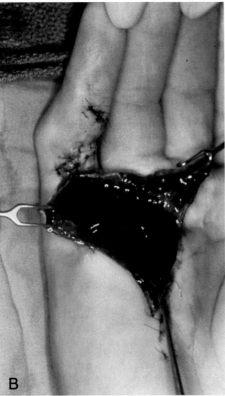 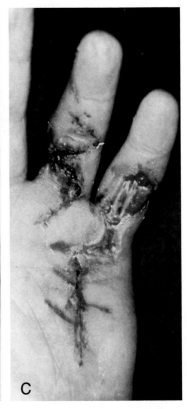

FIGURE 84-14.   Early complications of surgery for Dupuytren's disease. (*A*) Swollen palm following limited fasciectomy for Dupuytren's disease. (*B*) Same hand at the time of surgical evacuation of a large palmar hematoma. (*D*) Fasciectomy of a fifth finger was complicated by skin slough over the entire proximal digit exposing a flexor tendon.

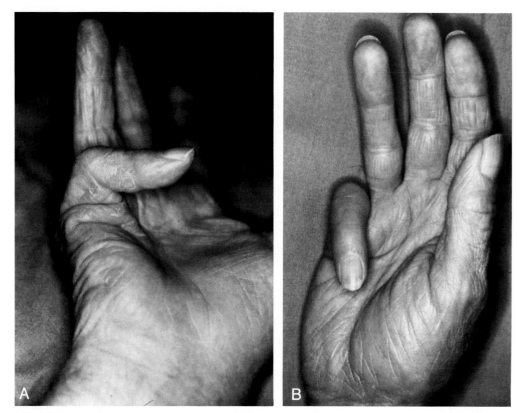

FIGURE 84-15. (*A* and *B*) Appearance of a small finger with severe, recurrent contracture following previous limited fasciectomy.

When postoperative "flare" or dystrophy occurs, patients must be advised that their recovery will be considerably slower than that originally expected, and that a great deal of patience and effort will be required to maximize eventual recovery. Failure to comply with the vigorous therapeutic program may result in permanent and severe stiffness of the digital joints of the involved digit, and sometimes, of the uninvolved digits of the operated hand.

RECURRENCE

Recurrent Dupuytren's disease is common and almost always involves the proximal interphalangeal joint (Fig. 84-15). Because of the added difficulty in correcting recurrent contractures, the indications for additional surgery are somewhat different than those governing the original procedure. If the degree of contracture is not great and the condition appears to be reasonably stable, one may elect to accept the results of the initial operation rather than to attempt surgical correction once again. If, however, the contracture is severe and progressive, additional efforts at ablation of the offending tissue may be indicated. It must be recognized, however, that reoperation is much more difficult because the diseased fascia is intertwined with scar secondary to the previous surgery. As with the original fasciectomy, complete exposure of the neurovascular bundles is required; however, protection of those structures may be considerably more difficult than it was at the time of the

initial procedure. Digital joint capsulectomy is almost always required when dealing with recurrent contracture; if the skin is of good quality, it may be retained and closed. Poor quality skin should probably be excised and replaced by full-thickness skin grafts, as advocated by Hueston.[14] Local rotation flaps or cross-finger flaps have also been employed occasionally to

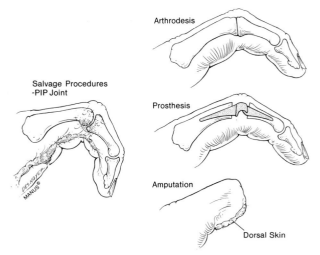

FIGURE 84-16. Salvage options for severe recurrent contractures of the proximal interphalangeal (PIP) joint include arthrodesis, skeletal shortening and the interposition of a silicone spacer, and amputation.

cover complex defects resulting from skin and fascial excision for recurrent contracture.

Salvage Procedures

When irreparable contracture exists at the proximal interphalangeal joint, several salvage options are available (Fig. 84-16). Skeletal shortening at the proximal interphalangeal joint level, together with silicone rubber implant arthroplasty, may be applicable in some instances when the preservation of joint motion is important.[20] In most instances, however, it is preferable to achieve improved extension and joint stability by arthrodesis. A sufficient wedge of dorsal bone is removed to allow the digit to be brought into approximately 40° of extension; Kirschner wire fixation or tension band wiring is usually appropriate for fixation. Given the fact that metacarpophalangeal joint function is usually normal, a good grasping digit can be preserved in this manner. When severe deformities (greater than 90°) are present, or for those individuals who request amputation because of occupational concerns or disdain for the digit, amputation either through the proximal phalanx or by ray excision may be indicated.

REFERENCES

1. Bruner, J.M.: Incisions for Plastic and Reconstructive (Non-septic) Surgery of the Hand. Br. J. Plast. Surg. 4:48, 1951.
2. Carroll, R.E., and Connolly, W.B.: Open Wound Technique for Dupuytren's Contracture. J. Bone Joint Surg. 52-A:1068, 1970.
3. Clarkson, P.: The Radical Fasciectomy Operation for Dupuytren's Disease: A Condemnation. Br. J. Plast. Surg. 16:273, 1963.
4. Coville, J.: Dupuytren's Contracture—The Role of Fasciotomy. Hand, 15:162, 1983.
5. Dupuytren, G.: Permanent Retraction of the Fingers Produced by an Affection of the Palmar Fascia. Lancet 2:222, 1934.
6. Dupuytren, G.: Lecons Orales de Clinique de Chirurgicale, vol. 1. Paris, G. Balliere, 1832.
7. Gonzalez, R.I.: Open Fasciotomy and Full Thickness Skin Graft in the Correction of Digital Flexion Deformity. In Hueston, J.T., and Tubiana, R. (eds.): Dupuytren's Disease. New York, Churchill Livingstone, 1985.
8. Gonzalez, R.I.: Dupuytren's Contracture of the Fingers: A Simplified Approach to the Surgical Treatment. Calif. Med. 115:25, 1971.
9. Gossett, J.: Dupuytren's Disease and the Anatomy of the Palmodigital Aponeuroses. In Hueston, J.T., and Tubiana, R. (eds.): Dupuytren's Disease. London, Churchill Livingstone, 1985.
10. Gossett, J.: Dupuytren's Disease and the Anatomy of the Palmodigital Aponeuroses. In Hueston, J.T., and Tubiana, R. (eds.): Dupuytren's Disease. London, Churchill Livingstone, 1974.
11. Howard, L.D.: Dupuytren's Contracture, A Challenge—Not a Blessing. AAOS Instructed Course Lecture Handbook (unpublished), 1965.
12. Hueston, J.T.: Dupuytren's Disease in Hand Surgery. In Flynn, J.E. (ed.): Baltimore, Williams and Wilkins, 1982, pp. 797–822.
13. Hueston, J.T.: Dupuytren's Contracture and Specific Injury. Med. J. Aust. 1:1084, 1968.
14. Hueston, J.T.: Dupuytren's Contracture: The Trend to Conservatism. Ann. R. Coll. Surg. Engl. 36:134, 1965.
15. Hueston, J.T.: Dupuytren's Contracture. Edinburgh, E & S Livingstone, 1963.
16. Hueston, J.T.: Digital Wolfe Grafts in Recurrent Dupuytren's Contracture. Plast. Reconstr. Surg. 29:342, 1962.
17. Hueston, J.T.: Dupuytren's Contracture. Edinburgh, E & S Livingstone, 1962.
18. Hueston, J.T.: Limited Fasciectomy for Dupuytren's Contracture. Plast. Reconstr. Surg. 22:569, 1961.
19. Iselin, F.: Dermofasciectomy for Recurrent Dupuytren's Disease. In Hueston, J.T., and Tubiana, R. (eds.): Dupuytren's Disease. New York, Churchill Livingstone, 1985.
20. Kates, J.L., Burkhalter, W., and Mann, R.J.: Open Palm Open Digit Technique for Dupuytren's Contracture. Orthop. Trans. 3:331, 1979.
21. King, E.W., Exeter, N.H., Bass, D.M., and Watson, H.K.: The Treatment of Dupuytren's Contracture by Extensive Fasciectomy Through Multiple Y-V-plasty Incisions. J. Hand Surg. 4:234, 1979.
22. Kleinman, W.B.: Dupuytren's Contracture: Treatment by the Open Palm Technique. In Strickland, J.W., and Steichen, J.B. (eds.): Difficult Problems in Hand Surgery. St. Louis, C.V. Mosby, 1982.
23. Landsmeer, J.M.F.: The anatomy of the dorsal aponeurosis of the human finger and its functional significance. Anat. Rec. 104:35, 1948.
24. Lubahn, J.D., Lister, G.D., and Wolfe, T.: Fasciectomy and Dupuytren's Disease: A Comparison Between the Open-palm Technique and Wound Closure. J. Hand Surg. 9:53, 1984.
25. Luck, J.V.: Dupuytren's Contracture: A New Concept of the Pathogenesis Correlated with Surgical Management. J. Bone Joint Surg. 41-A:635, 1959.
26. MacCallum, P., and Hueston, J.T.: The Pathology of Dupuytren's Contracture. Aust. N. Z. J. Surg. 31:241, 1962.
27. McCash, C.R.: The Open Palm Technique in Dupuytren's Disease. In Hueston, J.T., and Tubiana, R. (eds.): Dupuytren's Disease. New York, Churchill Livingstone, 1985.
28. McCash, C.R.: The Open Palm Technique in Dupuytren's Contracture. Br. J. Plast. Surg. 17:271, 1964.
29. McFarlane, R.M.: The Current Status of Dupuytren's Disease. J. Hand Surg. 8:703, 1983.
30. McFarlane, R.M.: Dupuytren's Contracture. In Green, D.P. (ed.): Operative Hand Surgery. New York, Churchill Livingstone, 1983.
31. McFarlane, R.M.: Patterns of the Diseased Fascia in the Fingers in Dupuytren's Contracture: Displacement of the Neurovascular Bundle. Plast. Reconstr. Surg. 54:31, 1974.
32. McFarlane, R.M., and Jamieson, W.B.: Dupuytren's Contracture: The Management of One Hundred Patients. J. Bone Joint Surg. 48-A:1095, 1966.
33. McGregor, I.A.: Fasciotomy and Split Skin Grafting in Dupuytren's Disease. In Hueston, J.T., and Tubiana, R. (eds.): Dupuytren's Disease, 2nd ed. London, Churchill Livingstone, 1986.
34. McGrouther, D.A.: Dupuytren's Disease. In Watson, N., and Smith, R.J. (eds.): Methods and Concepts in Hand Surgery. Scarborough, Ont., Butterworth and Co., 1986, pp. 75–96.
35. McGrouther, D.A.: The Microanatomy of Dupuytren's Disease. In Hueston, J.T., and Tubiana, R. (eds.): Dupuytren's Disease. London, Churchill Livingstone, 1985.
36. McGrouther, D.A.: The Microanatomy of Dupuytren's Contracture. Hand, 14:215, 1982.
37. McIndoe, A., and Beare, R.L.B.: The Surgical Management of Dupuytren's Contracture. Am. J. Surg. 95:197, 1958.
38. Michon, J.: Operative Difficulties and Postoperative Complications in the Surgery of Dupuytren's Disease. In Hueston, J.T., and Tubiana, R. (eds.): Dupuytren's Disease. London, Churchill Livingstone, 1985.

39. Milford, L.: Retaining Ligaments of the Digits of the Hand. Philadelphia, W.B. Saunders, 1968.

40. Skoog, T.: The Superficial Transverse Fibers of the Palmar Apoeneurosis and Their Significance in Dupuytren's Contracture. Surg. Clin. North Am. **47**:433, 1967.

41. Skoog, T.: The Transverse Elements of the Palmar Aponeurosis in Dupuytren's Contracture. Scand. J. Plast. Surg. **1**:51, 1967.

42. Skoog, T.: Dupuytren's Contracture. Acta Chir. Scand. **96**(suppl. 139):1, 1948.

43. Stack, H.G.: The Palmar Fascia and the Development of Deformities and Displacements in Dupuytren's Disease. *In* Hueston, J.T., and Tubiana, R. (eds.): Dupuytren's Disease. London, Churchill Livingstone, 1985.

44. Stack, H.G.: The Palmar Fascia. London, Churchill Livingstone, 1973.

45. Stein, A.M.H., Jr.: The Relation of Median Nerve Compression to Sudeck's Syndrome. Surg. Gynecol. Obstet. **115**:713, 1962.

46. Strickland, J.W., and Bassett, R.L.: The Isolated Digital Cord in Dupuytren's Contracture: Anatomy and Clinical Significance. J. Hand Surg. **10-A**(1):118, 1985.

47. Thomine, J.M.: The Development and Anatomy of the Digital Fascia. *In* Hueston, J.T., and Tubiana, R. (eds.): Dupuytren's Disease. London, Churchill Livingstone, 1985.

48. Thomine, J.M.: The Development and Anatomy of the Digital Fascia. *In* Hueston, J.T., and Tubiana, R. (eds.): Dupuytren's Disease. London, Churchill Livingstone, 1974.

49. Torstrick, R.F., Hartwig, R.H., and Strickland, J.W.: Long-term Results of Regional Fasciectomy of Dupuytren's Contracture of the Proximal Interphalangeal Joint. J. Hand Surg. **6**(3):297, 1981.

50. Varian, J.P.W.: Full Thickness Skin Grafting in the Management of Recurrent Dupuytren's Disease. *In* Hueston, J.T., and Tubiana, R. (eds.): Dupuytren's Disease. London, Churchill Livingstone, 1985.

51. Watson, H.K., Light, T.R., and Johnson, T.R.: Check-rein Resection for Flexion Contracture of the Middle Joint. J. Hand Surg. **4**(1):67, 1979.

CHAPTER 85

Intrinsic Muscle Contractures

CLAYTON A. PEIMER

A balanced interaction of the intrinsic and extrinsic muscles provides the normal dexterity and power of the hand. If an injury or other pathologic condition affects one set of these muscles, the hand may become dysfunctional. Intrinsic muscle dysfunction may be attributable to weakness, paralysis, loss of compliance, stiffness, and/or contracture. Contracture or stiffness of the hypothenar, lumbrical, or interosseous muscles leads to digital imbalance which disables the hand. This chapter focuses on the correction of hand problems caused by contracture of the intrinsic muscles. An understanding of the anatomy, as well as of the specific pathophysiology, is essential if the operating surgeon is to correct these problems. Although the causes of intrinsic contractures may vary, there are a number of typical pathologic patterns based on the common mechanisms of trauma, spasticity, and connective tissue diseases.

ANATOMY

The mid axis of the hand, as viewed from the dorsum, is defined as the central axis of the third metacarpal. The dorsal interosseous muscles abduct the fingers from this axis, whereas the palmar interosseous muscles adduct them. There are four dorsal and three palmar interosseous muscles. In addition, there are three hypothenar muscles that function like dorsal interosseous muscles. Dorsal interosseous muscles arise from the metacarpal shafts and insert so as to achieve digital abduction; the designation of first dorsal interosseous muscle thus belongs to that muscle on the radial side of the index, and so on, in an ulnar direction. The little finger is actually abducted by the abductor digiti quinti; the middle finger is abducted in both a radial and ulnar direction and, therefore, has two dorsal interosseous muscles.[1,2,4]

Except for the third, the other dorsal interosseous muscles have two muscle bellies and, therefore, two (tendon) insertions —one into the base of the proximal phalanx and the other via the dorsal (tendon) mechanism (Fig. 85-1). The bony insertion deviates the digit and has a mild effect on proximal phalangeal (metacarpophalangeal joint) flexion. The tendon insertion produces metacarpophalangeal joint flexion via the transverse fibers over the dorsum of the proximal phalanx. The tendon insertion also assists with proximal interphalangeal and distal interphalangeal extension via the oblique fibers that continue distally to join the lateral slips of the extensor tendon, forming the conjoined lateral band. The (radial and ulnar) lateral bands unite over the dorsum of the middle phalanx to become the terminal tendon. The abductor digiti quinti inserts into bone on the ulnar side of the proximal phalanx of the little finger, and the flexor digiti quinti brevis forms the ulnar lateral band in the little finger. The palmar interosseous muscles also arise from the metacarpal shafts, but each has only one muscle belly. None has a bone insertion into the proximal phalanx, but each functions as do the lateral bands from the dorsal interossei (via the transverse fibers, conjoined lateral band, and terminal tendon). The opponens digiti quinti, the most dorsal of the three hypothenar muscles, has an unusual insertion into the ulnopalmar shaft of the fifth metacarpal, producing carpometacarpal flexion and supination when it contracts.

The lumbricals extend the proximal interphalangeal and distal interphalangeal joints but also assist in flexing the meta-

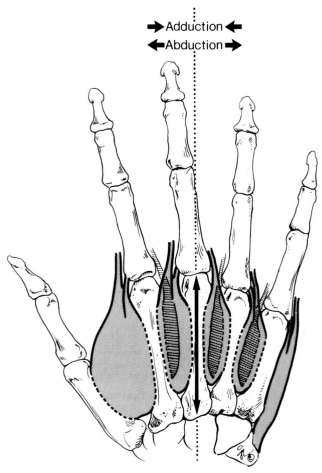

→Adduction←
←Abduction→

FIGURE 85-1. Dorsal view of the anatomy of the interossei muscles. Except for the third, all dorsal interossei have two muscle bellies and two tendon insertions. The dorsal interossei act as digital abductors. The hypothenar muscles function as dorsal interossei. Without exception, the palmar interossei muscles, which have only one muscle belly, insert into the lateral band and oblique fibers.

carpophalangeal joints. The lumbricals are unique in that they arise on their antagonist, originating from the tendons of the flexor digitorum profundus in the mid palm (Fig. 85-2). Lumbricals of the index and middle fingers originate from the radial side of the respective flexor digitorum profundus tendons. Lumbricals of the ring and little fingers originate from bipennate muscle bellies on the adjacent surfaces of the flexor digitorum profundus tendons. Lumbrical tendons course distally palmar to the deep transverse intermetacarpal ligaments, becoming part of the radial lateral bands at the mid portion of the proximal phalanges. When the lumbrical muscles contract, they pull the flexor digitorum profundus tendon distally, decreasing its flexion effect (relaxing the antagonist), as well as pulling proximally on the lateral band and terminal tendon, thereby extending the proximal interphalangeal and distal interphalangeal joints.

The extrinsic extensor tendons are the only extensors of the proximal phalanges (metacarpophalangeal joints), lying in the dorsal midline and inserting via the sagittal bands (Fig. 85-3). These aponeuroses pass in a palmar direction, attaching into the palmar plate and base of the proximal phalanges. The sagittal bands (extrinsic extensor fibers) are proximal and medial to

the transverse fibers (intrinsic flexor fibers). It is important not to confuse the sagittal bands with the transverse fibers, since the sagittal bands arise from the extensor tendon, pass in a palmar direction, and extend the finger, whereas the more distal transverse fibers arise from the lateral band and pass dorsally, insert into the dorsal tendon mechanism (not bone) and flex the proximal phalanx (Fig. 85-4).[15]

DIAGNOSIS OF CONTRACTURE

Intrinsic muscles flex the metacarpophalangeal joints, extend the interphalangeal joints, and deviate the fingers. Therefore, intrinsic contractures, with concomitant loss of compliance or elasticity, would be expected to interfere with interphalangeal joint flexion and metacarpophalangeal joint extension. Less severe contractures tend to affect the interphalangeal joints, whereas more severe contractures produce deformity at both levels.

Intrinsic muscle tightness, or an intrinsic contracture, should be suspected when active proximal interphalangeal flexion is limited (Fig. 85-5). A simple physical test will usually confirm the diagnosis. Passive proximal interphalangeal flexion is tested by the examiner while the metacarpophalangeal joint is held flexed; it is then tested again while the metacarpophalangeal joint is held extended. A test of intrinsic tightness is positive if there is significantly less passive proximal interphalangeal flexion with the metacarpophalangeal joint extended than with it flexed. Many authors have described this test, and it is often (confusingly) described eponymically.[5,8,16] In contrast, extrinsic tightness (contracture of the extensor tendons) is present if passive proximal interphalangeal flexion is more limited when the metacarpophalangeal joint is flexed than when it is held in extension. It may not be possible to perform these tests effectively if there are contractures in the metacarpophalangeal or proximal interphalangeal joints (or if a joint is dislocated). If there are both intrinsic and extrinsic contractures simultaneously, one may obscure the other.

The most frequent presentation of a functionally significant intrinsic contracture follows trauma, probably caused by muscle changes as a consequence of edema, anoxia, and immobilization. For example, a patient may complain that he or she is unable to grasp objects; sometimes, patients present for weakness. A careful history and examination will reveal the intrinsic muscle pathology. When examined in the office, the patient may be almost able or fully able to make a fist with unrestricted simultaneous metacarpophalangeal and proximal interphalangeal flexion. In attempting to grasp a hammer, however, the flexion of the metacarpophalangeal joints is blocked (by the hammer), and active flexion of the proximal interphalangeal joints is decreased. This activity is a functional test of intrinsic tightness.

MILD INTRINSIC CONTRACTURE

Nonsurgical Treatment Immediately after Injury

If a diagnosis of mild intrinsic tightness or of contracture is made soon after injury (after a Colles' fracture, for example),

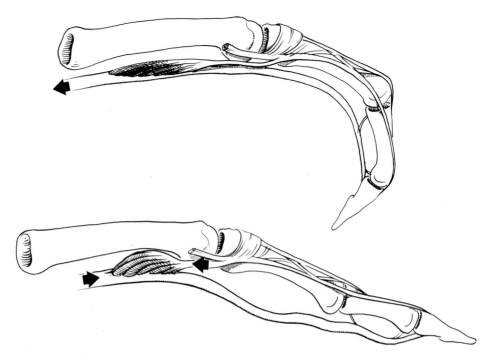

FIGURE 85-2. Lumbrical anatomy. The lumbrical is unique in that it both arises and inserts into a tendon, relaxing its antagonist when functioning. Normal lumbrical contraction tightens the lateral band (interphalangeal extensor fibers); it also pulls the flexor digitorum profundus tendon distally, diminishing flexor tone.

significant dysfunction may be avoided. Treatment can be designed to reduce swelling, mobilize the intrinsic muscles, and stretch the muscle bellies. Elevation, fluid-flushing massage, and intrinsic muscle stretching exercises should be instituted. The intrinsic muscles are stretched by gradually and repetitively performing an intrinsic tightness test, which involves simultaneous passive extension of the metacarpophalangeal joints and passive flexion of the proximal interphalangeal joints. This home and supervised outpatient therapy program needs to be continued for several weeks to be fully effective.

Acute Post-traumatic Edema: Fascial Release

During the immediate post-traumatic phase, if the hand is severely swollen, pressure of the intrinsic muscle compartments should be measured. (See Chapters 16 and 104 for information

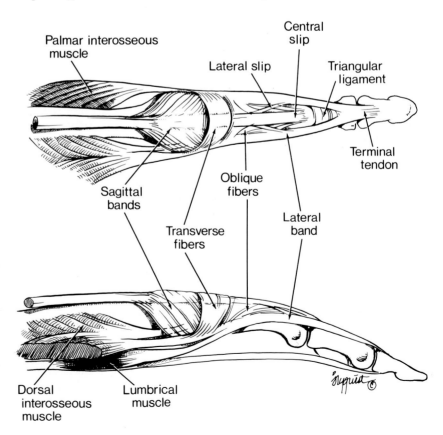

FIGURE 85-3. Anatomy of the extrinsic extensor tendons. The dorsal tendon mechanism at the metacarpophalangeal and proximal interphalangeal joints is composed of metacarpophalangeal joint extensor fibers from the sagittal bands and intrinsic flexor fibers via the transverse fibers. More distally, the interphalangeal extensor tendons are formed from both the intrinsic and extrinsic tendons.

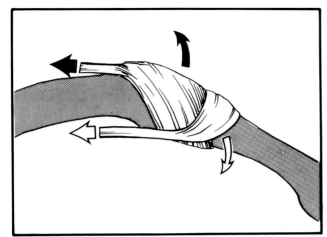

◀ Extrinsics = MP Joint extension

◁⌐ Intrinsics = MP joint flexion

FIGURE 85-4. Functional slings. At the metacarpophalangeal (MP) joint, the more proximal extrinsic extensor tendon extends the joint via the sagittal fibers which course distally and in a palmar direction to insert on the palmar plate and flexor sheath. The intrinsic tendons act as flexors via the transverse fibers, coursing distally and dorsally over the base of the proximal phalanx.

on compartment syndromes.) In acute cases, surgical release of the fascial envelope about the intrinsic muscles, in addition to the adductor pollicis and the carpal tunnel, may be required.

Approach the intrinsic compartments of the swollen hand, to which a tourniquet has been applied, through longitudinal incisions that are approximately 5 cm in length and are centered over the mid shafts of the second and fourth metacarpals, avoiding injury to the dorsal veins and sensory nerves. Retract the extensor tendons and incise the interosseous fascia longitudinally at each intermetacarpal space. If the second metacarpal incision does not afford adequate access to the adductor pollicis in the first web, once the first dorsal interosseous muscle fascia has been released, make an additional, 3-cm longitudinal incision just ulnar to the thumb metacarpophalangeal joint, extending it proximally. Incise the fascia dorsal and palmar to the adductor. In the case of severe injuries, hypothenar muscle decompression via a longitudinal, 3-cm incision at the ulnopalmar aspect of the hand and one over the thenar muscles, as well as a carpal tunnel release, may be necessary.

Pin the metacarpophalangeal joints of severely swollen hands at approximately 70° of flexion with smooth, 0.045-inch Kirschner wires; pin the thumb metacarpal in wide palmar abduction and pronation. Do not close these (longitudinal) wounds while the hand remains swollen; they may be closed secondarily after several days, or by skin grafting.

The hand is kept elevated, and circulation is observed closely. Hand therapy may begin with bedside visits to encourage tendon gliding and small joint motion (except in those joints that are transfixed).

Active exercises will continue during the period of healing and maturation of skin grafts, if grafting has been required. Dynamic splints and closely supervised active exercises may be necessary. The transfixion Kirschner wires are removed when

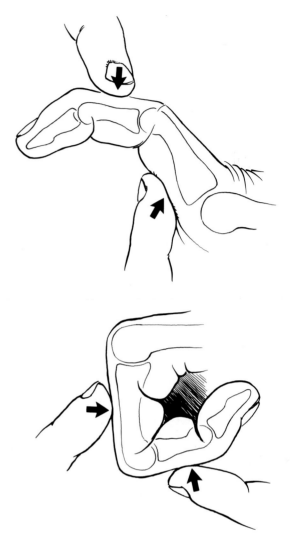

FIGURE 85-5. Intrinsic muscle tightness is tested by passively flexing the proximal interphalangeal joint while the metacarpophalangeal joint is held flexed; it is then tested again while the metacarpophalangeal joint is held extended. The intrinsic tightness test is positive if there is significantly less passive proximal interphalangeal flexion with the metacarpophalangeal joint extended than with it flexed.

the swelling has subsided adequately; in any event they should be removed within 21 to 28 days following insertion.

MODERATE INTRINSIC CONTRACTURE: DISTAL INTRINSIC RELEASE

Presenting Signs and Symptoms

Following traumatic injury, the moderately edematous hand is likely to develop intrinsic tightness that affects the proximal interphalangeal joints exclusively. In unprotected, swollen, metacarpophalangeal joints, flexion becomes difficult. The intrinsic muscles, however, are able to achieve relatively unresisted proximal interphalangeal extension because the capsule and collateral ligaments are initially more lax in that position.

Continued proximal interphalangeal extension via tight intrinsic muscles results in limited proximal interphalangeal flexion; in severe cases, it may be associated with actual capsular tightness at the proximal interphalangeal level. The intrinsic tightness test is positive in such cases.

Surgical Technique

In order to relieve the tightness (assuming that a program of intrinsic stretching exercises has failed), it is necessary to perform a distal intrinsic release. The entire intrinsic mechanism need not be sacrificed, since only proximal interphalangeal flexion is impaired. This operation—release of the oblique fibers of the lateral bands—is known as a distal intrinsic release (i.e., distal to the transverse fibers).[8]

Approach the lateral bands in the affected fingers through a dorsal, longitudinal incision that is 2 to 3 cm long and is situated over the middle third of the proximal phalanx. Carry the incision down to the dorsal mechanism; then elevate the skin flaps, first to the radial side and then to the ulnar side, exposing the lateral bands, the oblique fibers, and the central and lateral slips of the tendon mechanism. Divide the lateral bands and their oblique fibers near the distal edge of the wound as they insert into the central slip of the extensor mechanism (Fig. 85-6). Do not divide the lateral slip nor the central slip of the extensor tendon; preserve the transverse fibers of the intrinsic tendon, as well. Resect a 1-cm piece of the lateral band and its oblique fibers to correct the contracture completely.

Repeat the intrinsic tightness test after both the radial and ulnar lateral bands have been resected to verify the completeness of the surgical procedure (Fig. 85-7, A–H). Close the wounds and splint the metacarpophalangeal joints in extension, taping the proximal interphalangeal joints into flexion. Active and passive proximal interphalangeal flexion exercises must begin within a day or two of surgery. The metacarpophalangeal flexion-block splint can generally be discontinued after 14 days, although intrinsic stretching and exercises should be continued for several weeks.

SEVERE POST-TRAUMATIC INTRINSIC CONTRACTURE: PROXIMAL INTRINSIC RELEASE

Presenting Signs and Symptoms

An extended anoxic injury, severe swelling, and prolonged elevated compartment pressure will produce intrinsic myonecrosis, with secondary fibrosis causing deformities at both the metacarpophalangeal and interphalangeal joints.[1,2,16] These metacarpophalangeal flexion contractures result only from marked and severe intrinsic fibrosis, as evidenced by the fact that the majority of significant post-traumatic metacarpophalangeal joint deformities are extension contractures resulting from tight collateral ligaments and secondary capsular scarring. The swollen metacarpophalangeal joints strongly resist being flexed, and only in the presence of marked intrinsic muscle scarring will a contracture be severe enough to force the already tight, extended metacarpophalangeal joints into a flexed position. Severe proximal interphalangeal extension or hyperextension may also be a part of this often static deformity. Secondary changes at both joints, with pericapsular fibrosis in the deformed position, are not uncommon. Often, the first web is limited because of contracture of the adductor pollicis and the first dorsal interosseous muscles. A significant degree of hand dysfunction results from these contractures.

Surgical Technique

Correction of severe contracture requires release, not only of the distal intrinsic fibers, but also of the transverse fibers of the dorsal tendon mechanism that normally flex the metacarpophalangeal joints (Fig. 85-8). It is unlikely that these scarred intrinsic muscles will be functional to any extent; therefore, they are best handled by removing the tendons altogether, thus eliminating the deforming force. Overcorrection is rarely a problem, even with an aggressive and complete release. Indeed, full correction may be difficult to achieve.

Make a dorsal transverse incision that extends from the radial mid axis of the second metacarpal to the ulnar mid axis of the fifth, just proximal to the metacarpophalangeal joints at the metaphyseal flare of the metacarpals. Divide the tendons of all interossei and of the abductor digiti quinti muscles at the metacarpophalangeal joints. If metacarpophalangeal flexion persists even after the tendons have been removed, free the accessory collateral ligaments and palmar plate from their attachments to the base of the proximal phalanx, and, with a dental probe, release any scarring between the plate and the metacarpal head. Verify relief of the combined metacarpophalangeal flexion and proximal interphalangeal extension contractures by repeating the intrinsic tightness test.

When residual capsular inelasticity hinders positioning of the metacarpophalangeal joints in extension, it may be necessary to pin them in that position with oblique, smooth, Kirschner wires for about 2 weeks. To correct proximal interphalangeal extension, it may also be essential to release the lateral bands separately—in much the same manner as the distal intrinsic release was performed—at the time of the proximal intrinsic release. In such cases, individual dorsal incisions may also be required to relieve the proximal interphalangeal contractures completely. Postoperative care is essentially the same as it is for a distal intrinsic release, as described earlier.

With severe contractures, a release of the adductor pollicis

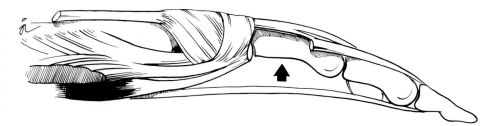

FIGURE 85-6. Distal intrinsic release. For moderate intrinsic contracture that limits proximal interphalangeal flexion, resection of the oblique fibers and contiguous lateral bands is performed on both the radial and ulnar sides of the finger through a dorsal incision. (See also Fig. 85-7E.)

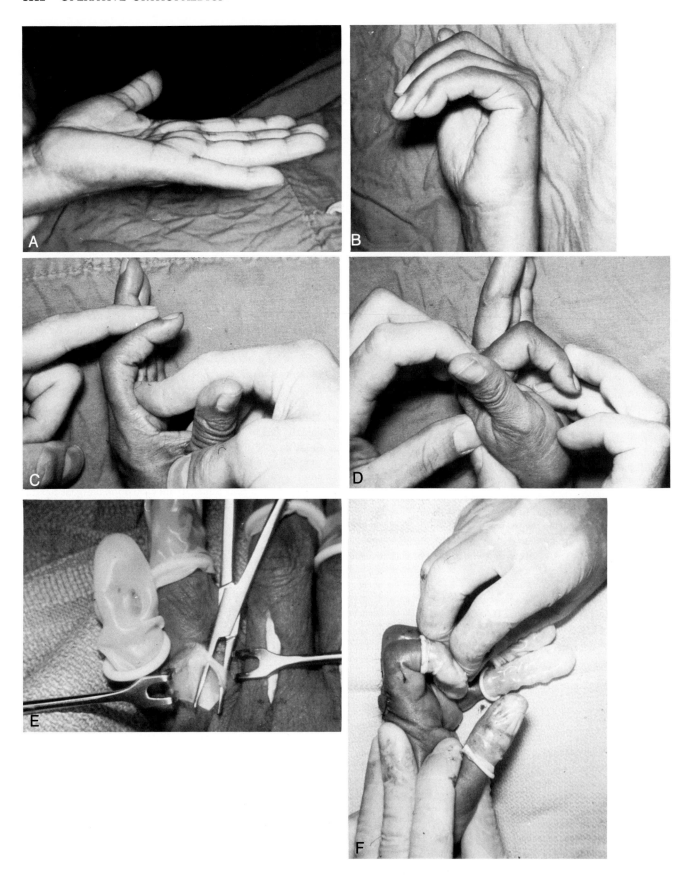

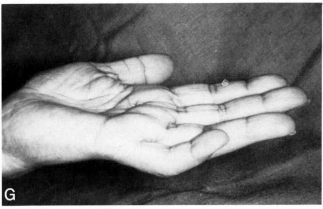
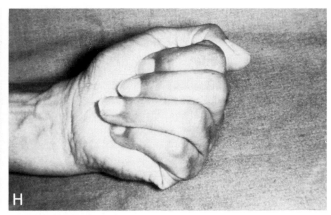

FIGURE 85-7. (*A* and *B*) A 56-year-old woman had limited active proximal interphalangeal flexion 6 months after a Colles' wrist fracture. (*C* and *D*) The intrinsic tightness test was positive. (*E*) A distal intrinsic release was performed. (*F*) Immediately following the surgical release of the intrinsic, the tightness test was negative. (*G* and *H*) Two years after surgery, marked improvement in active proximal interphalangeal flexion continues, although motion is still imperfect.

muscle is also necessary. Since the skin is often tight, we have found that the most dependable way to relieve the first web contracture is by approaching the adductor via a standard Z-plasty or a Wolff four-flap Z-plasty in which the dorsal longitudinal limb can be extended as far proximally as necessary.[6] The dorsal approach prevents injury to the palmar neurovascular and tendon structures. Use a small chisel or elevator to free the adductor from its third metacarpal origin. If necessary, pin the first metacarpal in wide palmar abduction and pronation for up to 3 weeks, depending on the ease of maintaining the corrected position with splints and dressings alone.

SPASTIC CONTRACTURE

Presenting Signs and Symptoms

Intrinsic spasticity may cause dysfunctional deformities in patients with cerebral palsy; it may also occur following cerebrovascular accidents, and it may also affect patients with central nervous system diseases.[12,13] At times, the intrinsic spasticity is not clinically evident until after the (tighter and stronger) finger and wrist flexors have been released surgically. Weeks or

months following a flexor release or slide, the previously corrected digits may begin to assume an intrinsic plus posture, with combined metacarpophalangeal flexion and proximal interphalangeal extension or hyperextension, often unexpectedly. Although this deformity is similar to that associated with severe post-traumatic contracture, the cause and treatment are different. This condition is attributable to overactive muscles, not scarred and necrotic tissue. The purpose of a surgical release is (ideally) to decrease the spasticity or (practically) to lengthen the intrinsic muscle–tendon unit in order to correct the deformity and preserve function. Strictly speaking, the intrinsic muscle cannot be lengthened; however, such an effect is attainable by means of a muscle slide.[14,15]

Surgical Technique

The surgical approach, like that for the acutely edematous hand, employs longitudinal incisions. Generally, incisions over the second and fourth metacarpals are sufficient. Take care to avoid injury to sensory nerves, dorsal veins, and extensor tendons. After incising the interosseous fascia longitudinally, completely release the metacarpal origins of the interossei subperiosteally with an elevator. Place the fingers in the intrinsic minus

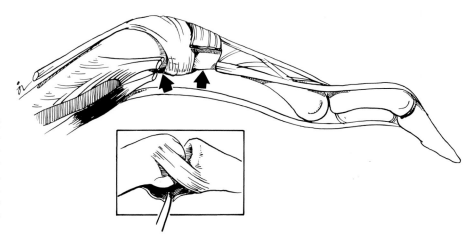

FIGURE 85-8. Proximal intrinsic release. For severe intrinsic contracture causing fixed metacarpophalangeal flexion and proximal interphalangeal extension deformities, transverse fibers of the dorsal mechanism, intrinsic insertions into bone, and contiguous oblique fibers are resected on both sides of the affected digits. Metacarpophalangeal joint release may also be needed.

(claw) position, and slide the released muscles distally (Fig. 85-9). Make separate incisions over the ulnar portion of the first metacarpal for the superficial head of the first dorsal interosseous (avoiding trauma to the princeps pollicis artery) and at the ulnar aspect of the little finger metacarpophalangeal joint to transect the tendons of the flexor digiti quinti. Transection of the abductor digiti quinti may also be necessary. In this situation, splinting in the intrinsic minus (claw) position of combined metacarpophalangeal extension and proximal interphalangeal flexion is best maintained for 2 to 3 weeks before initiation of therapy and exercises so as to encourage the released muscles to reattach more distally.

Certain spastic deformities are so severe that reasonable salvage by intrinsic muscle slide is precluded. Individuals with such deformities may have mild associated contractures or proximal interphalangeal hyperextension. The best operation in these cases is an ulnar motor neurectomy.

Make a curvilinear, longitudinal, ulnopalmar incision extending distally from just proximal and radial to the pisiform and ending in a position that is distal and radial to the hamulus (hook) of the hamate. Identify the (deep) motor branch of the ulnar nerve as it courses dorsally and in a radial direction around (distal to) the hamulus. Excise a 1-cm segment of nerve. Do not cut the sensory branches of the nerve. Contractures, if present, may be addressed appropriately at the same time.

Secondary small joint deformities necessitating ligament reconstruction or replacement may occur in the chronically spastic hand. For a discussion of the sublimis tenodesis and other similar procedures, the reader is referred to Chapter 113.

CONTRACTURE FOLLOWING TERMINAL TENDON INJURY: MALLET FINGER

When the terminal extensor tendon is divided or avulsed, the proximal portion of the terminal tendon and contiguous conjoined lateral bands retract proximally, unbalancing the extensor forces at the proximal interphalangeal joint. A hyperextension deformity of the proximal interphalangeal joint may gradually develop, or the joint may merely become more difficult to flex actively.[9,12] The intrinsic tightness test is typically positive.

Repair of the terminal tendon, as well as intrinsic stretching exercises may be required to correct the problem. Digital rebalancing may have to be undertaken in resistant cases. The need is determined by a careful assessment of the combined effects of the intrinsic and extrinsic tendon contributions to the proximal interphalangeal overpull.

LUMBRICAL CONTRACTURE

Presenting Signs and Symptoms

The lumbrical is a unique muscle that both arises and inserts into a tendon, relaxing its antagonist when functioning. Normal proximal interphalangeal flexion depends on balanced flexor digitorum profundus contraction and lumbrical relaxation. Lumbrical scarring (shortening) and loss of elasticity cause transmission of flexor digitorum profundus traction into the lumbrical tendon, to which it has become tethered, rather than through the more distal portion of the flexor digitorum profundus tendon (Fig. 85-10A). Active pull on the flexor digitorum profundus tendon then causes proximal interphalangeal and distal interphalangeal extension (via the contracted lumbrical) rather than flexion, a situation Parkes termed the "paradoxical lumbrical plus finger."[11]

Paradoxical lumbrical transmission of flexor forces may also be seen when the normal flexor digitorum profundus insertion is lost, as may occur in untreated distal tendon lacerations or distal joint amputations (Fig. 85-10B). The then lax profundus tendon retracts proximally, and contraction of the flexor digitorum profundus muscle is transmitted to the dorsum of the proximal interphalangeal joint via the lumbrical, producing paradoxical extension or limited active flexion. A loosely inserted tendon graft would have the same effect. The intrinsic tightness test is positive in such cases.

Surgical Technique

Resection of the radial lateral band will cure the problem. Indeed, we are careful to test patients with distal interphalangeal amputations for intrinsic tightness, and we often perform an acute radial lateral band release. Intrinsic stretching exercises become a regular part of the rehabilitation program.

INTRINSIC CONTRACTURE AND CONNECTIVE TISSUE DISEASE

Presenting Signs and Symptoms

Interosseous contracture is common in the rheumatoid. Unlike post-traumatic deformities, contracture may be associated with painful synovitis, ulnar digital drift, joint subluxation, and joint destruction. Secondary deformities are common, and may require the combination of joint and tendon reconstruction and releases.[3,7,17,18] It is beyond the scope of this chapter to discuss

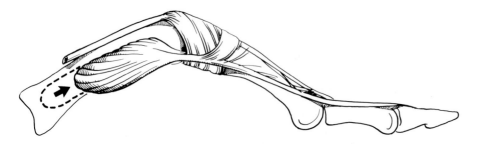

FIGURE 85-9. Intrinsic muscle slide. The metacarpal origins of the interossei are completely released subperiosteally with an elevator. Placing the fingers in an intrinsic minus (claw) position causes the released muscles to slide distally.

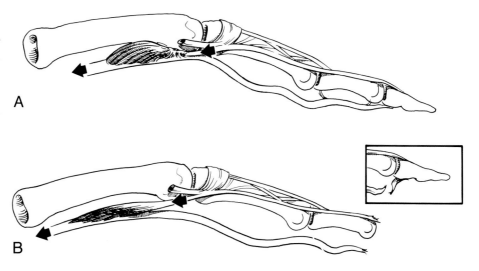

FIGURE 85-10. Lumbrical contracture. (*A*) Lumbrical scarring to the flexor digitorum profundus causes transmission of flexor force into the lumbrical tendon rather than through the more distal portion of the flexor digitorum profundus tendon. (*B*) When the normal flexor digitorum profundus insertion is lost (as in an untreated flexor digitorum profundus laceration or distal joint amputation), contraction of the flexor digitorum profundus muscle is transmitted distally only via the intact lumbrical, thereby producing a paradoxical extensor effect.

correction of rheumatoid ulnar drift, swan neck deformities, intrinsic tenodesis, and spiral oblique retinacular ligament reconstruction. The reader is referred to Chapter 117.

PITFALLS AND PROBLEMS

The most common problem accompanying intrinsic tightness and contractures is failure to recognize the underlying cause of limited proximal interphalangeal motion following injury. Intrinsic contractures are far more common than is generally appreciated. Adequate correction requires accurate diagnosis. When active proximal interphalangeal flexion is limited as a result of post-traumatic hand edema, intrinsic tightness and impending contractures should be suspected. An intrinsic tightness test should be performed. Prompt institution of intrinsic muscle stretching exercises and regular supervised therapy will often prevent the development of deformity and fixed contractures.

Surgical release of the intrinsic muscles, when required, should not be considered an end in itself, but rather a means to an end—a second chance at therapy. Intrinsic contracture destroys the delicate balance of the hand. Intrinsic release will not achieve functional improvement unless these very demanding and unforgiving small joints and tendons are made to glide in order to regain the full range of motion in the postoperative interval. Patients should be selected carefully, and every effort must be made to help them understand the crucial role they will play in their own recovery. Those individuals who are not intellectually and emotionally committed to a recovery that requires regular participation in tediously repetitive therapeutic exercises, including frequent hand therapy and office visits, should not undergo the procedure.

REFERENCES

1. Bunnell, S.: Ischemic Contracture, Local, in the Hand. J. Bone Joint Surg. **35-A:**88, 1953.

2. Bunnell, S., Doherty, E.W., and Curtis, R.M.: Ischemic Contracture, Local, in the Hand. Plast. Reconstr. Surg. **3:**424, 1948.

3. Ellison, M.R., Flatt, A.E., and Kelly, R.J.: Ulnar Drift of the Fingers in Rheumatoid Disease. J. Bone Joint Surg. **53-A:**1061, 1971.

4. Eyler, D.L., and Markee, J.E.: The Anatomy and Function of the Intrinsic Musculature of the Fingers. J. Bone Joint Surg. **36-A:**1, 1954.

5. Finocohietto, R.: Retraccion de Volkmann de los Musculos Intrinsicos de las Manos. Bol. Trab. Soc. Chir. **4:**31, 1920.

6. Flatt, A.E.: The Care of Congenital Hand Anomalies. St. Louis, C.V. Mosby, 1977, pp. 64–65.

7. Flatt, A.E.: Some Pathomechanics of Ulnar Drift. Plast. Reconstr. Surg. **37:**295, 1966.

8. Harris, C., Jr., and Riordan, D.C.: Intrinsic Contracture in the Hand and its Surgical Treatment. J. Bone Joint Surg. **36-A:**10, 1954.

9. Kaplan, E.B.: Anatomy, Injuries and Treatment of the Extensor Apparatus of the Hands and the Digits. Clin. Orthop. **13:**24, 1959.

10. Kaplan, E.B., and Smith, R.J.: Kinesiology of the Hand and Wrist and Muscular Variations of the Hand and Forearm. *In* Spinner, M.B. (ed.): Kaplan's Functional and Surgical Anatomy of the Hand, 3rd ed. Philadelphia, J.B. Lippincott, 1984, pp. 283–349.

11. Parkes, A.: The "Lumbrical-plus" Finger. J. Bone Joint Surg. **53-B:**236, 1971.

12. Pratt, D.R., Bunnell, S., and Howard, L.D., Jr.: Mallet Finger. Classification and Methods of Treatment. Am. J. Surg. **93:**573, 1957.

13. Smith, R.J.: Surgery of the Hand in Cerebral Palsy. *In* Pulvertaft, R.G. (ed.): Operative Surgery, The Hand, 3rd ed. London, Butterworth, 1977, p. 215.

14. Smith, R.J.: Intrinsic Muscles of the Fingers: Function, Dysfunction and Surgical Reconstruction. AAOS Instructional Course Lectures, vol. 24. St. Louis, C.V. Mosby, 1975, p. 200.

15. Smith, R.J.: Balance and Kinetics of the Fingers under Normal and Pathological Conditions. Clin. Orthop. **104:**92, 1974.

16. Smith, R.J.: Non-ischaemic Contractures of the Intrinsic Muscles of the Hand. J. Bone Joint Surg. **53-A:**1313, 1971.

17. Smith, R.J., and Kaplan, E.B.: Rheumatoid Deformities at the Metacarpophalangeal Joints of the Fingers. A Correlated Study of Anatomy and Pathology. J. Bone Joint Surg. **49-A:**31, 1967.

18. Thompson, J.S., Littler, J.W., and Upton, J.: The Spiral Oblique Retinacular Ligament (SORL). J. Hand Surg. **3:**482, 1978.

CHAPTER 86

Burn Contractures

PETER J. STERN

Burns remain a major health hazard, being second only to motor vehicle accidents as the leading cause of accidental death in the United States.[5] Despite more aggressive techniques of acute burn wound management, crippling hand deformities still occur. In a severe burn, the hand, which accounts for 5% of the total body surface area, is often neglected while attention is focused on survival of the burn victim. By the time survival has been assured, fixed contractures which are functionally disabling and aesthetically displeasing often have developed, and surgical reconstruction may be indicated.[6,13,15,16]

First and superficial second degree burns will heal satisfactorily without tissue replacement; however, deep second (partial skin thickness), third (full skin thickness), and fourth (tendon, bone, nerve, or joint) degree burns which are not debrided and covered with skin grafts or flaps will heal by granulation tissue, producing scar and hence, contractures. Prevention of contractures during the acute burn period by early wound closure and splinting is paramount in minimizing the necessity for secondary reconstruction. Beasley has pointed out that the triad of edema, inflammation, and especially immobility, is responsible for the deformities produced by thermal injuries.[3] He further notes that the severity of the deformities is directly proportional to the amount of time a wound remains open.

Before upper extremity burn reconstruction is undertaken, there are several factors that require special consideration. First and foremost, the surgeon must assess the functional needs of the patient. There is no reason to launch into a series of reconstructive procedures if a patient has fully adjusted to his or her condition and is able to carry out the activities of daily living as easily as before the burn. Having decided to proceed with reconstruction, it must be remembered that other priority areas, particularly the head and neck, may require surgical correction, and if a large total body surface area has been burned, unscarred skin may be at a premium. Therefore, one must plan ahead for the appropriate allocation of skin. Preoperative radiographs are mandatory prior to any procedure involving the mobilization of joints. Complete restoration of joint motion may not be possible with a soft tissue release because the articular surfaces may be incongruous or immobile secondary to sepsis, dislocation, or heterotopic ossification.

Often, both extremities are burned and require reconstruction. Because of limited skin availability, it may be feasible to reconstruct only one extremity, leaving the other as an assistive appendage. If the entire extremity including the axilla is burned, reconstruction should proceed in a proximal to distal fashion; that is, shoulder and elbow mobility should be restored appropriately before hand procedures are performed. Reconstructive procedures should preferably not be performed through scar that is hypertrophic and red; rather, one should wait until the scar has matured, a process that can be accelerated with the use of elastic pressure garments.

GENERAL CONSIDERATIONS: SOFT TISSUE COVERAGE

Certain principles of soft tissue coverage must be understood before reconstruction of specific anatomic locations can be accomplished (Fig. 86-1). Burn contractures are corrected by

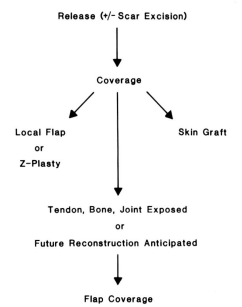

FIGURE 86-1. Outline of the surgical treatment for burn contractures.

scar incision, excision, or a combination of both procedures. Once this has been done, a soft tissue defect exists.

Most defects in the hand can be covered by a skin graft, a local flap, or a combination of the two. After burn releases, local flaps, such as Z-plasties, have limited application and should only be considered for coverage if the flap consists of pliable, unburned skin (see Fig. 86-5). Scarred skin will usually not tolerate the stress of being rotated as a local flap, and invariably, a significant portion of the flap will become necrotic. When indicated, local flaps have the advantages of providing a good color match and the need for a skin graft is usually obviated.

Skin grafting is the mainstay of treatment after contracture release or excision. It must be remembered that skin grafts will only adhere to a well-vascularized surface. A tendon denuded of paratenon, bone denuded of periosteum, or articular cartilage will not accept a skin graft; they require coverage with either a local or distant flap. If simultaneous or future bone, nerve, or tendon reconstruction is being considered, a skin graft alone will not provide adequate coverage.

Having decided to use a skin graft, several additional decisions must be made, and these depend on the size and location of the defect, as well as the availability of unburned donor skin. A donor site should be inconspicuous and should match the recipient defect as closely as possible. For example, a defect on the palm would ideally be covered with adjacent, unscarred palmar skin; however, this is rarely possible because of the limited availability of palmar skin. In practicality, there is usually unscarred skin available from the lateral, non–hair-bearing portion of the groin or from the buttocks. Having selected a donor site, one must next choose between a split-thickness skin graft and a full-thickness skin graft.

A full-thickness skin graft has several advantages in burned hand reconstruction. It is durable and is particularly suited for contact areas, such as the palm and the mobile palmar surface of the fingers. In addition, a full-thickness skin graft contracts less than does a split-thickness skin graft, so recontracture after grafting is less likely to occur. All skin grafts become hyperpigmented, but a full-thickness skin graft does so less than is a split-thickness skin graft and is, therefore, less conspicuous. Finally, the donor site for a full-thickness skin graft is closed primarily, so there is considerably less postoperative pain than occurs after a split-thickness skin graft in which the reepithelializing donor site may be painful for several days after graft harvesting.

There are two circumstances in burn reconstruction in which a split-thickness skin graft is a more practical choice for coverage than a full-thickness skin graft. First, if the area to be covered is large, a split-thickness skin graft is indicated. The donor site for a split-thickness skin graft does not require primary closure and, hence, more skin is available for grafting. Furthermore, the split-thickness skin graft can be expanded by meshing, although the appearance of meshed skin is aesthetically displeasing and it tends to contract more than a non-meshed split-thickness skin graft. A split-thickness skin graft is also indicated when the recipient bed has poor vascularity. Such circumstances are seen after radiation burns or with burns in which there is residual skin ulceration and low-grade sepsis.

There are certain conditions in which skin grafting is not applicable. Fourth degree burns, particularly when untreated during the acute burn period, tend to leave the extremity in a contracted, fibrotic condition. After the scar has been excised, there is often exposed bone, tendon, or joint, and skin grafting of any kind will not be accepted by these structures. Furthermore, with deep fourth degree burns, it is often necessary to perform reconstructive procedures involving the tendons (tenolysis or tendon graft) or joints (capsulotomy), and coverage with a skin graft is not appropriate because the graft, even if it does take, will tightly adhere to the tendon or joint, limiting mobility. Burn release or scar excision should always be performed prior to elevation of a flap. After burn cicatrix has been excised, the recipient bed may be three to four times larger than it was before scar excision. Knowing the dimensions of the recipient bed, one can better design an appropriately sized flap.

Fortunately, in the majority of cases, skin flaps are unnecessary. Most burns involve injury to the skin alone; and a flap in these circumstances is usually not indicated. Nevertheless, particularly when mobile structures are exposed or when future reconstruction is anticipated, one should not hesitate to apply a flap.

THUMB RECONSTRUCTION

The thumb contributes 40% to 50% of the function of the hand, so its functional restoration is a primary goal in upper extremity reconstruction following burns. For normal thumb function, there must be adequate length, sensibility, mobility, stability, and strength, as well as a satisfactory appearance. The majority of thermal injuries produce skin contractures that limit thumb mobility and use. In severe burns, loss of thumb length is usually secondary to a fourth degree injury in which the distal portion or more of the thumb becomes necrotic, necessitating amputation. In the child, longitudinal growth may be restricted either secondary to a burn contracture or secondary to direct thermal injury to the growth plates.

Adduction Contracture

Adduction contracture of the thumb (when the thumb metacarpal is adducted toward the index finger metacarpal in a plane perpendicular to the palm) is the most common contracture of the burned thumb.[18] In its mildest form, it is produced by dorsal scarring over the thumb–index cleft. In such patients, the palmar skin is usually not burned. Reconstitution of the thumb–index cleft can be accomplished by a variety of techniques.

Z-plasty

The Z-plasty is designed so that the palmar limb generally follows the thenar crease, the middle limb parallels the leading edge of the thumb–index cleft, and the dorsal limb parallels the ulnar aspect of the thumb metacarpal. All limbs should be of equal length. Following incision, elevate the flaps, making them as thick as possible and preserving any blood vessels that penetrate the base of the flap. Be careful to avoid dividing the radial neurovascular bundle to the index finger which lies immediately beneath the palmar flap. After the flaps have been raised, release the previously inflated tourniquet and secure meticulous hemostasis. Rotate the flaps and sew them into position. Be sure that the flaps are pink. A flap that is dark and congested (indicating venous insufficiency) or one that is pale and white (indicating arterial insufficiency) will invariably become necrotic. If this is the case, return the flap to its original position and consider an alternative form of coverage, such as skin grafting.

A Z-plasty is indicated in the correction of mild linear contractures and can only be performed when the skin being rotated is relatively pliable and unburned. If the skin is scarred and fibrotic, alternative techniques of coverage should be sought.

Skin Grafting

If a more severe contracture exists, it is best to divide the contracture band sharply by incising perpendicular to it (Fig. 86-2). Carry the incision down to the fascia overlying the first dorsal interosseous muscle and to the leading edge of the adductor pollicis muscle. Cover the resultant defect, which is elliptical, with a skin graft.

Adductor Release and Trapezial Excision

If the patient has sustained a deep burn, a severe adduction contracture may result. This type of contracture involves more than skin, necessitating release of deep structures.

First, release the dermal contracture, as well as the fascia overlying the first dorsal interosseous and adductor, as outlined above. If the thumb remains tightly adducted, consider releasing the insertion of the adductor pollicis muscle from the base of the thumb proximal phalanx. The adductor muscle in a severe burn is often fibrotic but is rarely nonfunctional; therefore, it is advisable to reinsert the muscle more proximally on the neck or shaft of the thumb metacarpal through a pull-out wire. On rare occasions, even after having released the skin and adductor muscle, an adduction contraction may persist. In these instances, carry the incision down over the trapeziometacarpal joint and release the capsule of this joint. If the contracture still persists, excision of the trapezium is indicated. Usually, it is necessary to pass a temporary Kirschner pin from the thumb metacarpal into the carpus to hold the thumb in its newly released position. Following such an extensive release, coverage with a skin graft is usually inadequate. In these circumstances, plan on using a distant flap, such as one from the non–hair-bearing, inner aspect of the contralateral forearm, to resurface and maintain breadth of the thumb–index cleft.

After release of any adduction contracture, postoperative splinting is mandatory. Although there are several causes of a persistent contracture, including inadequate surgical release, loss of skin graft, or the inappropriate use of burned skin for flap coverage, one of the most common causes is failure to splint the thumb metacarpal midway between palmar and radial abduction. A splint can be fabricated from a thermoplastic material and lined with silicone to maintain satisfactory breadth between the thumb and index finger. The splint should be worn until the wound has matured, a period lasting 3 to 9 months. In addition, it is often helpful to alternate splinting with an elastic compressive glove which also helps the scar mature faster.

Opposition, Extension, and Flexion Contractures

Less commonly, the thumb metacarpal may be drawn into a position of *opposition* (pronation and palmar abduction of the thumb), *extension* (when the thumb is drawn away from the index finger by a scar band between the distal radius and thumb metacarpal), or *flexion* (when scarring over the palmar aspect of the thumb produces flexion of the interphalangeal or metacarpophalangeal joint).[18] As in adduction contractures, all of these contractures require surgical incision (with or without a scar excision), followed by appropriate soft tissue coverage and splinting. It should also be emphasized that, with opposition and extension contractures, severe flexion or hyperextension contractures of the interphalangeal or metacarpophalangeal joint of the thumb often coexist, producing articular incongruity and joint subluxation or dislocation. In such cases, particularly if there is satisfactory mobility of two of the three thumb joints, an arthrodesis of the dislocated joint in a functional position is indicated.

Inadequate Thumb Length

As noted above, severe burn injuries often result in loss of thumb length.[14] Restoration of length can be accomplished by a number of surgical techniques. These include toe-to-hand transfer, osteoplastic reconstruction (involving tube pedicle flap placed around a bone graft followed by neurovascular island transfer for restoration of sensation), metacarpal osteotomy and progressive distraction, or pollicization (movement of

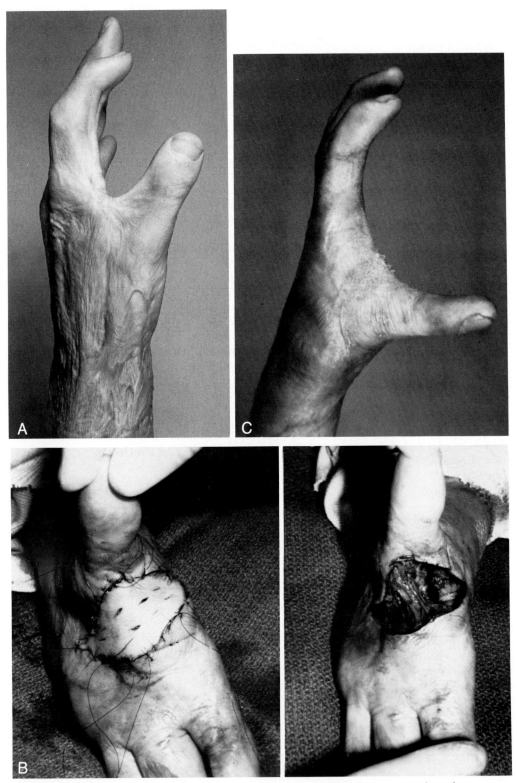

FIGURE 86-2. (*A*) Thumb adduction contracture of moderate severity. (*B*) A transverse release down to the adductor pollicis and first dorsal interosseous muscles (*left*), followed by application of a full-thickness skin graft (*right*). (*C*) The final result 13 months after release. (Stern, P.J., Neale, H.E., Carter, W., and MacMillan, B.G.: Classification and management of burned thumb contractures in children. Burns **11**:168, 1985.)

an adjacent digit, usually the index finger, on its neurovascular pedicle to the thumb position). In addition, if only a small amount of thumb length has been lost, a relative increase in thumb length can be accomplished by phalangization. With this procedure, thumb–index contracture is released, followed by proximal transposition of the adductor muscle to the thumb metacarpal so that the thumb–index cleft is deeper, thereby giving the thumb more apparent length.[19]

Often, the burn is so severe that thumb reconstruction is not feasible. The phalanges may have been amputated and varying lengths of metacarpals may be encased in a cocoon of burned skin. If thenar muscle contraction can be appreciated by manual palpation, a "mitten hand" can be created. This is accomplished by excision of the index finger metacarpal (leaving the base where the wrist flexor and extensor tendons attach), thereby creating a cleft between the thumb and ulnar digits so that a pinch maneuver of a crude side-to-side type can be accomplished (Fig. 86-3).

The pollicization procedure involves placing a digit (usually the index finger) on top of the remains of the thumb.[12,20] Pollicization is more likely to be successful if there is an intact thumb trapeziometacarpal joint, functioning thenar musculature, and relatively good sensibility of the digit to be pollicized.

Prior to performing the procedure, if there is scarring in the thumb–index cleft, it is advisable to excise scarred tissue and replace it with a skin flap from the groin or abdomen. This can later be used to resurface the cleft between the pollicized thumb and remaining ulnar digits. Once flap tissue has been transferred, the pollicization procedure can be performed. It is preferable to transfer the index ray, particularly if it has been damaged and is already short (Fig. 86-4). If it is absent, however, any digit can be transferred.

For conventional pollicization (such as for aplasia of the thumb), design the incisions so that the pollicized digit can be transposed and rotated in such a fashion that skin flaps are available to create a cleft between the thumb and the remainder of the hand. When a burned index finger is pollicized, make the incisions along the border of areas that have previously been scarred so that the index metacarpal shaft, as well as the tip of the thumb, are exposed. Reflect the interosseous muscles from the index metacarpal shaft. They are often fibrotic and are not useful for future motor function, as in conventional pollicizations. Next, ligate the proper digital artery to the radial side of the middle finger and split the common digital nerve to the index and middle finger proximally as far as possible. Osteotomize the index finger metacarpal through its base and remove a segment of metacarpal shaft, being careful to preserve the index metacarpophalangeal joint. Leave the flexor tendons to the index finger intact. If necessary, Z-lengthen the extensor tendons, which often are scarred. Then, rotate the index finger so that it can be put on top of the thumb remnant with the pulp of the pollicized digit directly facing the ulnar digits. Turn the pollicized digit so that it is 120° to 140° from the plane of the palm. It is easiest to stabilize the skeletal structure of the pollicized digit with one or two longitudinal Kirschner pins. Deflate the tourniquet to ensure that the pollicized digit is viable and that its vascular pedicle has not been stretched or twisted. Close the wound, being extremely careful to line the thumb–index cleft with soft, pliable skin. Skeletal pin fixation is maintained for 6 to 8 weeks, and splinting of the thumb in wide palmar abduction is usually maintained for 6 to 9 months.

The most common complications of pollicization are caused by errors in positioning of the transferred digit, inadequate bony fixation, or contracture of the thumb cleft. These can

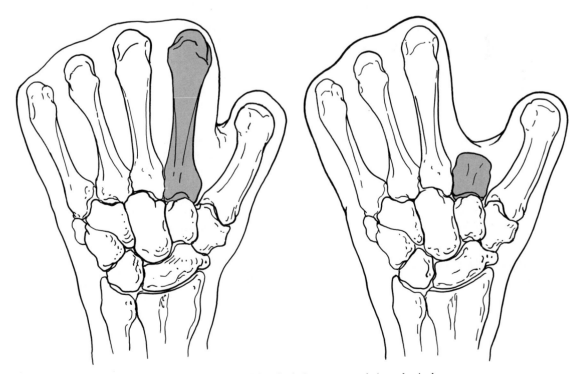

FIGURE 86-3. A "mitten hand" is created by excising the index metacarpal. A crude pinch maneuver is possible if the thenar motors are intact.

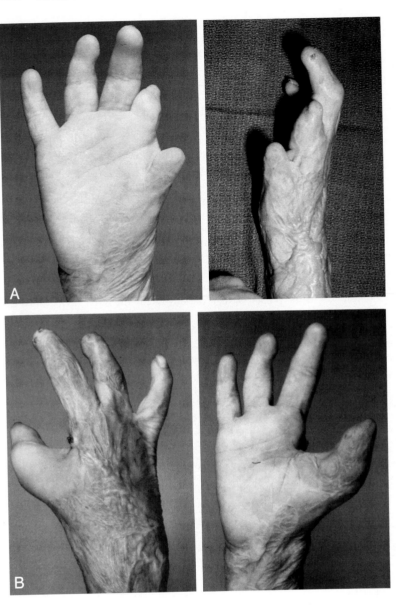

FIGURE 86-4. (A) A preoperative photograph of a hand that is ideally suited for pollicization of the index finger. Neither the thumb nor index remnant are functional. (B) Index pollicization and application of the distant flap have resulted in creation of a useful thumb.

usually be prevented by careful preoperative planning and attention to intraoperative technique.

Pollicization for the severely burned hand has the advantage of being a one-stage procedure that does not require microvascular techniques. In addition, it converts two relatively useless digits into a single, functional, opposable thumb, thereby making activities requiring opposition and prehension possible.

THE PROXIMAL INTERPHALANGEAL JOINT

Burns of the proximal interphalangeal joint can produce either flexion or extension contractures. If surgical intervention is necessary, preoperative radiographs of the proximal interphalangeal joint should be taken to confirm that a cartilaginous space is present and that the joint is not subluxated or dislocated.

Burn flexion contractures may arise from scarring of the palmar skin of the proximal interphalangeal joint; from dorsal burns in which the central tendon over the proximal interphalangeal joint is disrupted, resulting in a so-called "burn boutonnière" deformity; or from a dorsal burn over the metacarpophalangeal joint, producing a metacarpophalangeal hyperextension deformity and a proximal interphalangeal flexion deformity secondary to the tenodesis effect of the tightened flexor tendons. To treat these contractures successfully, one must determine the cause, and then select an appropriate technique for surgical correction.

Mild digital flexion contractures, produced by a linear scar band across the interphalangeal or metacarpophalangeal joints with pliable skin on either side of the band, can be corrected either by a single Z-plasty or a series of Z-plasties (Fig. 86-5). If, however, there is extensive scarring of the palmar skin, incision (and possibly excision) of the scar band will be necessary (Fig. 86-6).

FIGURE 86-5. (*A*) A linear contracture of the index finger (*left*) with pliable skin on each side of the scar band. A series of multiple Z-plasties are designed (*right*). (*B*) The Z-plasties are rotated into position (*left*), and there is full digital extension following surgery.

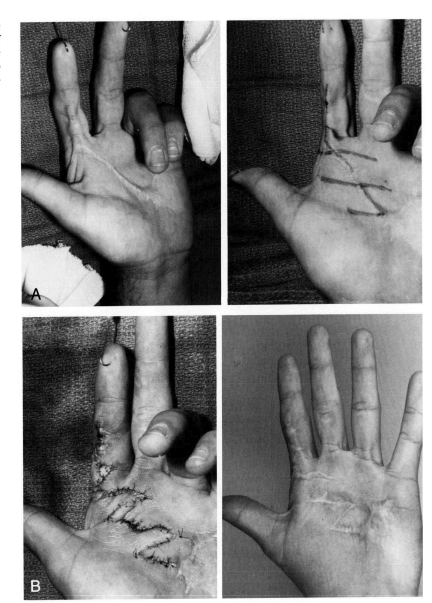

If a contracture of only the proximal interphalangeal joint exists, incise the scar transversely across the anterior aspect of the joint, extending the incision from the radial to the ulnar mid axial line.[2] It is usually unnecessary to excise the contracture band completely. Carry the incision down to the flexor tendon sheath, taking care not to sever the digital nerves that are always deep to the burn scar and that are usually covered by a thin layer of fat.

If a proximal interphalangeal flexion contracture persists after dermal release, one must decide whether a proximal interphalangeal capsular release should be performed. If this is done, the flexor tendons will be exposed and flap coverage, using either an adjacent cross-finger flap or a distant flap, will be necessary to prevent tendon desiccation.[8] If such a flap procedure is not feasible, a capsular release should not be performed and coverage should be accomplished with a skin graft. Regardless of the coverage technique, deflate the tourniquet and secure meticulous hemostasis. Assess the newly ex-

tended finger for vascular integrity, as arterial inflow may be compromised because of the sudden digital extension. If the digit is pale, flex it until it becomes pink and circulation has been restored. Often, temporary proximal interphalangeal joint immobilization with an oblique transarticular Kirschner pin is helpful. Cover the defect with a skin graft that is stented with a tie over a bolus dressing. After graft take has been confirmed, extension splinting at night with a silicone-lined, static splint is recommended until graft maturity.

Flexion deformities secondary to destruction of the central tendon over the dorsum of the proximal interphalangeal joint are difficult to reconstruct. This is because the skin over the dorsum of the joint is scarred, the central tendon has been destroyed, and usually, there is a fixed contracture of the palmar plate and collateral ligaments. Restitution of proximal interphalangeal extension should only be considered if the joint is passively extendable and radiographs show joint congruity. If these requirements are met, the scarred tendon over the prox-

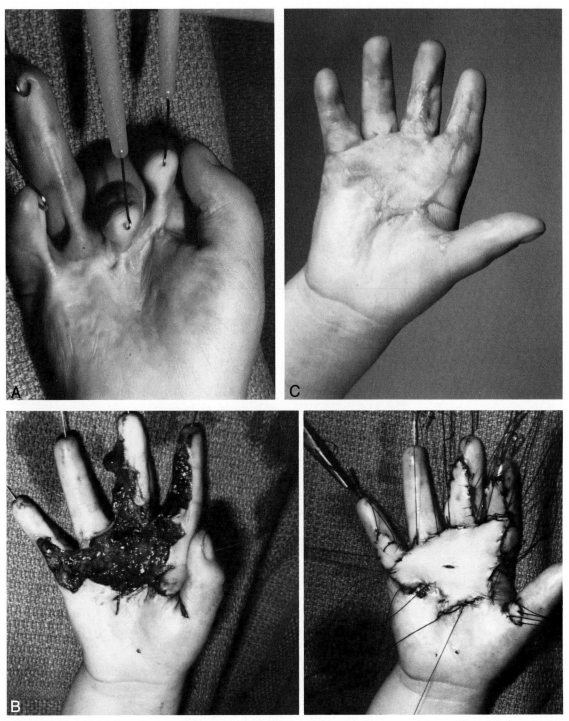

FIGURE 86-6. (*A*) Moderately severe contracture of all digits as a result of a palmar contact burn. (*B*) The burn scar was excised, the digits were pinned temporarily in extension, and a full-thickness autograft was applied. (*C*) After operation, nearly full digital extension is possible.

imal interphalangeal joint is excised, and the more proximal, unscarred, central tendon is advanced into the dorsal base of the middle phalanx. Occasionally, elongation of the central tendon with a graft is necessary. After the central slip has been reconstructed, the proximal interphalangeal joint is pinned in extension for 3 weeks. Following this, active flexion is initiated. The results of such surgery are unpredictable and often unsat-

isfactory. If a fixed flexion contracture exists, arthrodesis of the joint in a functional position will provide a more reliable result.

Like the boutonnière deformity, proximal interphalangeal extension contractures are difficult to treat successfully. They are caused either by skin fibrosis over the dorsum of the joint or by ischemic contractures of the interosseous muscles. When the contracture is secondary to a dorsal skin burn, a simple transverse release of tightened skin and skin graft is adequate. Often, however, it is necessary to mobilize the dorsal apparatus, perform a dorsal capsulotomy, and partially divide the dorsal, cord-like portion of the collateral ligaments. Having done this, the extensor tendon is usually exposed, and coverage with a local flap must be performed.

Extension contractures resulting from intrinsic tightness often can be corrected successfully. The diagnosis is made by passively extending the metacarpophalangeal joint and then passively flexing the proximal interphalangeal joint; shortened, scarred, intrinsic muscles will resist flexion. Conversely, when the metacarpophalangeal joint is passively flexed, the intrinsic muscles, whose axis of motion is palmar to the metacarpophalangeal joint and dorsal to the proximal interphalangeal joint, are relaxed, and passive proximal interphalangeal flexion is unresisted. An intrinsic release can usually be performed by excising the distal fibers of the lateral bands at the level of the neck of the proximal phalanx.

BURN SYNDACTYLY

Dorsal burns often extend into the distally sloping interdigital clefts. During the acute burn period, it may be difficult to gain access to this area, particularly if the metacarpophalangeal joints are immobilized in the "safe" position of metacarpophalangeal flexion. Syndactyly, usually of the dorsal skin, results. The degree of syndactyly varies; in severe cases, it may extend beyond the proximal interphalangeal joint.

Indications for correction of postburn syndactyly vary. Syndactyly of any degree restricts digital abduction, making the grasping of large, cylindrical objects difficult, if not impossible. Often, the syndactylized digits are subjected to a sudden abduction force that can lead to traumatic breakdown of the scar contracture, bleeding, and additional fibrosis. Some patients complain that they are unable to wear gloves, whereas others have problems with hygiene because particles of dirt collect in a pocket formed by dorsally syndactylized skin and the normal distal edge of the palmar skin.

The technique for the release of web syndactyly depend on the severity of the syndactyly and the condition of the adjacent skin.[1,9,11] Mild or moderate syndactyly can be treated either by a Z-plasty or a local rotation flap. The lateral palmar rotation flap is particularly appealing because it allows the surgeon to create a new interdigital cleft with supple, local, full-thickness skin that is unlikely to recontract (Fig. 86-7). The donor defect for rotation flaps can be closed primarily if it is small, or it can be covered with a skin graft.

In severe cases of burn syndactyly, a longitudinal incision of the burn cicatrix is necessary (Fig. 86-8). The incision, both on the palmar and dorsal side, should extend to the bifurcation of the common digital artery. Once the release has been accomplished, it can be covered with a thick split- or full-thickness autograft. Because the graft is placed on a concave surface, great care must be exercised to ensure that there is good contact between the graft and its recipient bed. To ensure contact, the graft should be stented into place. Once success of the graft is certain, night extension splinting with the digits abducted is advised for 6 to 9 months.

EXTENSION CONTRACTURES OF THE WRIST AND METACARPOPHALANGEAL JOINTS

Extension contractures of the wrist and metacarpophalangeal joints often occur simultaneously. These contractures usually are the result of flame burns in which the victim tightly clenches the fist to protect the face from thermal injury. Metacarpophalangeal extension contractures arise either from scarred skin over the dorsum of these joints or from immobilization of the metacarpophalangeal joints in extension during the acute burn period, thus allowing the collateral ligaments and soft tissues around the metacarpophalangeal joints to contract. Contracture severity at the level of the metacarpophalangeal joints is variable. In mild metacarpophalangeal contractures, when the wrist is dorsiflexed (thus relaxing the skin over the dorsum of the hand), full, active, metacarpophalangeal flexion can be accomplished. However, if the wrist is pas-

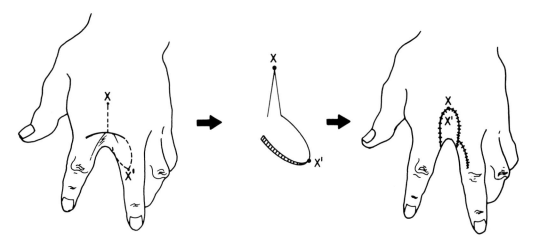

FIGURE 86-7.   A dorsal web syndactyly exists between the index and middle fingers. A lateral volar flap (apex X′) is designed to rotate 180° so that points X and X′ can be opposed. In this example, the donor defect was closed primarily; however, if tension exists, a skin graft should be applied.

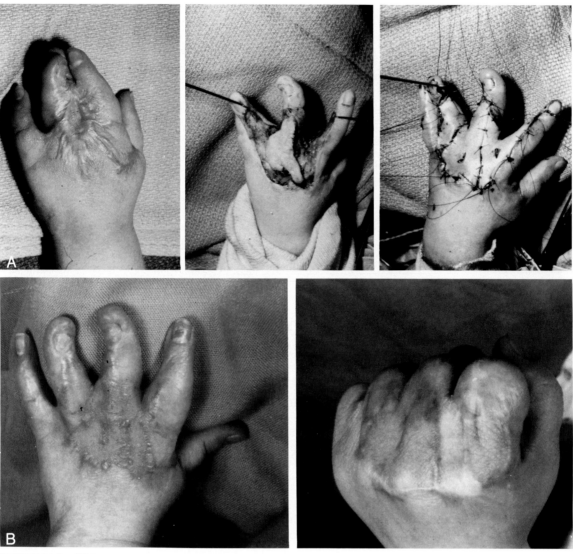

FIGURE 86-8. (*A*) Severe dorsal burn syndactyly (*left*). Scar excision (*center*) is followed by application of a full-thickness skin graft (*right*). (*B*) Postoperative extension (*left*) and flexion (*right*) views.

sively flexed, metacarpophalangeal flexion is limited by tight skin over the dorsum of the wrist and hand. For such contractures, a dorsal transverse incision of the contracted skin at the level of the metacarpal necks is often sufficient to release the contracture. If the scar tissue of the dorsum of the metacarpophalangeal joints is thick or has been previously grafted with meshed autograft, giving the skin a corrugated appearance, one may prefer to excise, rather than incise, the burn scar. In such instances, carry the excision down to the subcutaneous fat, taking care to preserve the dorsal veins that are nearly always deep to the burn scar.

Sometimes metacarpophalangeal extension contractures are produced by linear bands of scar that mimic the extensor tendons. In such cases, the surgeon may make the error of not performing a deep enough release for fear of severing a tendon that is mistakenly thought to be within the burn cicatrix. This is virtually never the case. The extensor tendons lie deep to the scar in a bed of loose, areolar, connective tissue. Once the

release has been accomplished—either by incision, excision, or a combination of both—soft tissue coverage can usually be accomplished with a skin graft.

With a moderate or severe metacarpophalangeal contracture, a more aggressive surgical release is necessary. Under such conditions, the position of the metacarpophalangeal joint is fixed, regardless of wrist position, and the metacarpal heads are prominent in the palm. Metacarpophalangeal hyperextension may be so severe that the dorsal surface of the proximal phalanx may lie on top of the dorsal surface of the metacarpal. In such cases, associated flexion contractures of the proximal interphalangeal joints, caused by the flexor tenodesis effect, occur, as does destruction of the central tendon overlying the proximal interphalangeal joint. Grasping objects of any size is difficult or impossible, and often, only a crude pinch maneuver between the index finger and the thumb is possible.

Release of these fixed extension contractures requires careful preoperative planning (Fig. 86-9). Contractures of the

FIGURE 86-9. (*A*) A dorsal burn caused combined wrist and metacarpophalangeal fixed extension contractures. (*B*) Dorsal view (*left*) with outline of the proposed excision. Note that the linear bands over the metacarpophalangeal joints contain scar, not extensor tendons. After dermal release (*right*), metacarpophalangeal capsulotomies, and temporary pinning in flexion, a large dorsal area requires skin grafting. (*C*) The functional result (both hands), demonstrating excellent metacarpophalangeal flexion.

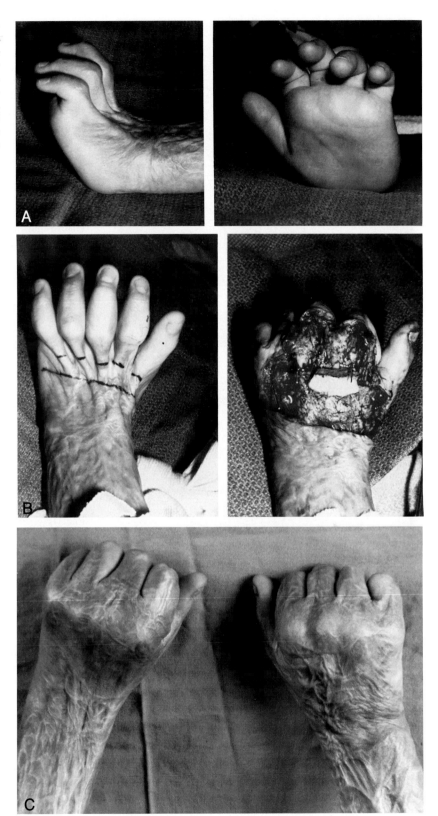

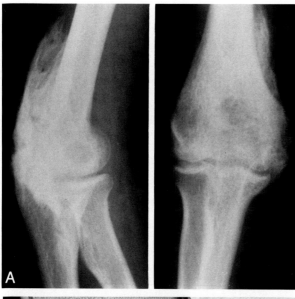

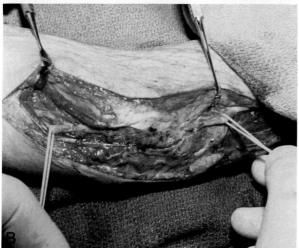

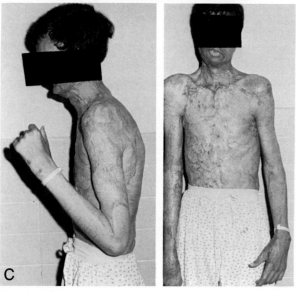

metacarpophalangeal capsule and collateral ligaments are to be expected. Release the metacarpophalangeal capsular contractures by splitting the extensor tendon longitudinally over the joint in its mid portion and incising the dorsal capsule transversely. Release the collateral ligaments by sharply dividing the origin of the ligament from the metacarpal head, preserving the most inferior and proximal fibers so as to prevent lateral joint instability. Once the collateral ligaments and dorsal capsule have been released, position the metacarpophalangeal joints in 70° of flexion by passing a pin from the metacarpal head into the proximal phalanx. Sometimes after metacarpophalangeal capsulotomies, the metacarpophalangeal joints and extensor tendons are exposed, and must be covered with a distant flap. If this is the case, the surgeon must plan ahead to ensure that flap tissue is, in fact, available.

Postoperative range of motion exercises can be initiated once the skin graft has taken. It is important to begin a program of active and passive metacarpophalangeal flexion exercises, as well as night splinting with the metacarpophalangeal joints in flexion, to prevent recontracture.

ELBOW CONTRACTURES

Postburn elbow contractures occur frequently,[17] and surgical correction is often necessary because limited elbow mobility directly affects the efficiency of hand, wrist, and shoulder function. In addition, these contractures are often subjected to the stress of sudden elbow extension, resulting in recurrent tearing of antecubital burn scar, pain, and additional fibrosis. Occasionally, burn scarring forms deep pockets that collect debris and cause hygienic problems.

One of the most devastating problems affecting function in the burn patient is heterotopic ossification[7] bridging the elbow joint (Fig. 86-10). The ossification forms in the acute burn period, is usually associated with a concomitant deep burn to the elbow, and is found in approximately 2% of patients with elbow burns. The first clinical signs of heterotopic ossification appear 4 to 6 weeks after burn injury, and are usually heralded by complaints of increasing elbow pain and a rather rapid decrease in range of motion. Initial radiographs may be unremarkable except for soft tissue swelling, but follow-up radiographs (within 3 months) will show ossification bridging the elbow joint. When heterotopic bone forms bilaterally, functional impairment is severe and the patient will have difficulty performing even simple activities of daily living.

Surgical treatment of heterotopic bone must be timed appropriately. If the bone is excised when it is immature, it will reform more exuberantly, making a second surgical excision even more difficult. Usually, it takes 1.5 to 2 years for the bone to mature. Diagnostic studies used to assess bone maturity include serial technetium phosphate bone scans, as well as measurement of serum alkaline phosphatase levels.

The new bone usually forms posteromedially, and the ulnar

FIGURE 86-10. (*A*) Radiographs demonstrate heterotopic ossification bridging the posteromedial surface of the elbow. The patient's elbow was rigidly fixed in extension. (*B*) An operative photograph shows that the ulnar nerve (marked by vessel loupes) proximal and distal to the elbow joint is encased by heterotopic ossification. It was unroofed and transposed anteriorly. (*C*) After heterotopic bone excision, elbow flexion and extension were restored.

nerve may be encased in it. Therefore, motor and sensory function of the ulnar nerve should be tested before surgery. If function is impaired, an electromyogram and nerve conduction studies are recommended.

Perform surgical excision of the bone through a long, posteromedial elbow incision. First, identify the ulnar nerve, both proximal and distal to the new bone. If bone encases the nerve, it is helpful to unroof and transpose it anteriorly. Once the nerve has been mobilized, it is usually necessary to perform an elbow arthrotomy because there are often intra-articular adhesions that must be lysed. In such cases, detach and reinsert the medial collateral ligament complex. After the skin has been closed, the range of motion should be recorded and the elbow should be splinted for 3 to 5 days in 90° of flexion. Following this, both active and assisted passive range of motion exercises are initiated.

Diphosphonates, which are potent inhibitors of mineralization and bone resorption, have been shown to be of some benefit in the prevention of heterotopic bone formation in patients undergoing total hip arthroplasty. There is, however, no evidence that these compounds are effective in preventing bone from reforming after excision in the burn victim. Other ancillary treatment modalities include low-dose irradiation or oral indomethacin, but it is beyond the scope of this chapter to discuss the merits of such therapy.

AXILLARY CONTRACTURES

Axillary contractures restrict shoulder motion, particularly abduction and forward flexion.[4,10] If surgical procedures are planned for more distal portions of the extremity, correction of an axillary contracture should be performed first, thereby facilitating access to these areas.

The extent of an axillary contracture varies. Most commonly, a band extends anteriorly from the chest to the upper arm parallel to the inferior edge of the pectoralis major. There may also be a posterior band from the chest to the brachium that follows the inferior and lateral edge of the latissimus dorsi. Often, the deep axillary skin in the apex of the axilla is unburned; however, in severe burns, the axillary fossa may be obliterated completely.

Surgical release of an axillary contracture involves the same principles discussed earlier in this chapter. In the majority of cases, the treatment of choice is incision (often combined with excision) of the scar. Carry the dissection down to the axillary fat. It is often helpful to divide the fascia over the latissimus dorsi or pectoralis major muscles. After the release, obtain coverage with a thick split-thickness skin graft.

Sometimes, local skin flaps, in combination with skin grafting, are appropriate. Flaps are particularly useful in patients who have only an anterior axillary contracture; in these cases, a flap can be created from either posterior, unburned skin or from skin in the upper, medial aspect of the arm.

After the flap or skin graft has been applied, the patient should be placed in an abduction brace with the arm abducted 90° to 120°. Splinting should be maintained for approximately 6 months after surgery. Failure to wear an abduction brace often leads to recurrence of the contracture, and may necessitate reoperation.

REFERENCES

1. Alexander, J.W., MacMillan, B.G., and Martel, L.: Correction of Postburn Syndactyly: An Analysis of Children with Introduction of the VM-Plasty and Postoperative Pressure Inserts. Plast. Reconstr. Surg. 70:345, 1982. The VM-plasty, a new operation for correction of postburn digital syndacty is described. In the authors' experience, it is preferable to simple Z-plasties or Y-V–plasties.

2. Alexander, J.W., MacMillan, B.G., Martel, L., and Krummel, R.: Surgical Correction of Postburn Flexion Contractures of the Finger in Children. Plast. Reconstr. Surg. 68:218, 1981. A comprehensive review of treatment techniques for postburn digital flexion contractures is provided, and an analysis of factors affecting the results of surgical correction is outlined.

3. Beasley, R.W.: Secondary Repair of Burned Hands. Clin. Plast. Surg. 8:141, 1981. The pathogenesis of burn contractures is presented, as are the techniques for correction of surface contractures (skin grafting, local and distant flaps), interdigital contractures, and joint contractures.

4. Beasley, R.W.: Burns of the Axilla and Elbow. In Converse, J.M. (ed.): Plastic Reconstructive Surgery, vol. 6. Philadelphia, W.B. Saunders, 1977, pp. 3391–3401. This chapter provides a comprehensive review of the treatment (particularly, the use of local flaps) for correction of axillary and elbow contractures.

5. Demling, R.H.: Burns. N Engl. J. Med. 313:1389, 1985. This article discusses the recent advances in cardiopulmonary resuscitation, metabolic and nutritional supplementation, and wound management that have led to decreased morbidity and mortality from burns in the 1980s.

6. Fleegler, E.J., and Yetman, R.J.: Rehabilitation after Upper Extremity Burns. Orthop. Clin. North Am. 14:699, 1983. A well-illustrated discussion of the surgical treatment of surface contractures is presented.

7. Hoffer, M.M., Brody, G., and Ferlic, F.: Excision of Heterotopic Ossification about Elbows in Patients with Thermal Injury. J. Trauma 18:667, 1978. Eight patients were treated by excision of heterotopic bone around the elbow with generally satisfactory results. Ulnar nerve transposition is recommended.

8. Jackson, I.T., and Brown, G.E.D.: A Method of Treating Chronic Flexion Contractures of the Fingers. Br. J. Plast. Surg. 23:373, 1970. Severe PIP flexion contractures, particularly those that occur after electrical burns, can be successfully treated by excision of scarred skin, release of the flexor tendon sheath and palmar plate, and resurfacing with a cross-finger flap.

9. Krizek, T.J., Robson, M.C., and Flagg, S.V.: Management of Burn Syndactyly. J. Trauma 14:587, 1974. Techniques for burn syndactyly treatment, including Z-plasties, opposing flaps, and skin grafting, are outlined.

10. Law, E.J., Hoefer, R.W., and MacMillan, B.G.: Clinical Experience with Axillary Burns in Children. J. Trauma 12:34, 1972. Types of axillary contractures, techniques of release, and causes of surgical failure are outlined. Postoperative abduction splinting is emphasized.

11. MacDougal, B., Wray, R.C., and Weeks, P.M.: Lateral-Volar Finger Flap for the Treatment of Burn Syndactyly. Plast. Reconstr. Surg. 57:167, 1976. Use of a flap from the lateral and volar aspect of the digit to resurface a web space after surgical release is discussed.

12. May, J.W., Donelan, M.B., Toth, B.A., and Wall, J.: Thumb Reconstruction in the Burned Hand by Advancement Pollicization of the Second Ray Remnant. J. Hand Surg. 9-A:484, 1984. A detailed account of the technique of postburn pollicization, as well as the results obtained with this technique, is presented.

13. Peterson, H.D., and Elton, R.: Reconstruction of the Thermally Injured Upper Extremity. In Salisbury, R.E., and Pruitt, B.A.

(eds.): Burns of the Upper Extremity, vol. 19. Philadelphia, W.B. Saunders Co., 1976, pp. 148–173. A broad outline of the management of upper extremity burn contractures is presented.

14. Pohl, A.L., Larson, D.L., and Lewis, S.R.: Thumb Reconstruction in the Severely Burned Hand. Plast. Reconstr. Surg. **57:**320, 1976. Thumb reconstruction after burns—particularly, techniques for reconstitution of the first web space—is discussed.

15. Salisbury, R.E., and Bevin, A.G.: Atlas of Reconstructive Burn Surgery. Philadelphia, W.B. Saunders Company, 1981, pp. 108–193. This text includes excellent illustrations of the techniques for reconstruction of upper extremity burn contractures; it also emphasizes the areas where pitfalls and complications can occur.

16. Salisbury, R.E., and Dingeldein, G.P.: The Burned Hand and Upper Extremity. *In* Green, D.P. (ed.): Operative Hand Surgery. New York, Churchill Livingstone, 1982, pp. 1523–1551. This chapter provides a broad review of upper extremity burn contractures.

17. Stern, P.J., Law, E.J., Benedict, F.E., and MacMillan, B.G.: Surgical Treatment of Elbow Contractures in Postburn Children. Plast. Reconstr. Surg. **76:**441, 1985. A classification system and treatment outline for the correction of postburn elbow contractures is presented. Marked improvement was noted when severe contractures were treated by a broad release and skin grafting.

18. Stern, P.J., Neale, H.W., Carter, W., and MacMillan, B.G.: Classification and Management of Burned Thumb Contractures in Children. Burns **11:**168, 1985. Thumb contractures are classified as either adduction, opposition, extension, or flexion contractures. Extension contractures and severe adduction contractures demonstrated the poorest results after surgical release, particularly when local flaps were applied.

19. Tubiana, R., and Roux, J.P.: Phalangization of the First and Fifth Metacarpals. J. Bone Joint Surg. **56-A:**447, 1974. A normal carpometacarpal joint, as well as functioning thenar muscles, is necessary for phalangization. Skin coverage is provided by either skin grafts or local or distant flaps.

20. Ward, J.W., Pensler, J.M., and Parry, S.W.: Pollicization for Thumb Reconstruction in Severe Pediatric Hand Burns. Plast. Reconstr. Surg. **76:**927, 1985. The technique for, results of, and complications (malposition of transposed digit and first web contracture) associated with pollicization of the index finger are outlined.

CHAPTER 87

Management of Volkmann's Contracture

RICHARD H. GELBERMAN
and MICHAEL J. BOTTE

HISTORICAL ASPECTS AND PATHOGENESIS

In 1881, Richard von Volkmann described muscle ischemia and extremity paralysis and contracture caused by the application of tight, constricting bandages to an injured limb.[38] In 1914, Murphy described an increase in pressure within a fascia-enclosed muscle space as a result of hemorrhage and edema, and was first to suggest that paralysis and contracture might be prevented by fascial incision.[16] In 1926, Jepson first demonstrated the effects of early fascial decompression on injured muscle.[24] Since then, other authors have provided reports and opinions on the pathogenesis of compartment syndromes and ischemic contracture.[6,13,19] The theory that microcirculatory impairment secondary to sustained increases in intracompartment interstitial pressure is the critical factor in cases of compartment syndrome and Volkmann's ischemic contracture has become widely accepted.[1,2,3,9,10,14–16, 20,21,24,29,31,33]

Muscle, which is highly vulnerable to changes in oxygen tension, undergoes necrosis after ischemia lasting for 4 hours is experimentally produced by application of a tourniquet.[14,15] With prolonged ischemia, large areas of muscle necrosis occur, with subsequent fibroblastic proliferation within the muscle infarct. A variable amount of longitudinal and horizontal contraction of the fibrotic mass may progress over a 6- to 12-month period following the ischemic insult. The necrotic muscle adheres to surrounding structures, fixes muscle position, and reduces mobility. Secondary compression of the surrounding structures may occur. Primary limitation of muscle excursion may lead to loss of joint motion with subsequent joint contracture.

Injury to the forearm muscles that results in ischemic necrosis is most marked in the deep flexor compartment (Figs. 87-1 and 87-2). The flexor digitorum profundus and flexor pollicis longus muscles are most commonly affected. In the mildest contractures, only a portion of the flexor digitorum profundus undergoes necrosis, usually involving the ring and long fingers. In severe contractures, all four digits are involved. The flexor digitorum superficialis and pronator teres are generally less severely affected. In the most severe cases, the wrist flexors and wrist and digital extensors may undergo varying degrees of fibrosis and contracture.

Specific primary involvement of the flexors of the forearm is attributed to their deep location within the forearm compartment, a factor that increases their vulnerability to ischemia.[30] The deepest compartment areas, particularly those regions adjacent to bone, have the highest interstitial pressures.[15] With compression from within, the circulation to the deep portions of the muscle belly are compromised, whereas collateral circulation to the portions of the muscle that are more superficial is retained. When compartment syndromes remain untreated, swelling may resolve, but the damaged muscle becomes fibrotic. The characteristic deformity of ischemic contracture becomes evident in the upper limb with elbow flexion, forearm pronation, wrist flexion, thumb flexion and adduction, digital metacarpophalangeal joint extension, and interphalangeal joint flexion.

The pathomechanics of the Volkmann's clawhand deformity are complex. Although there is an apparent similarity between

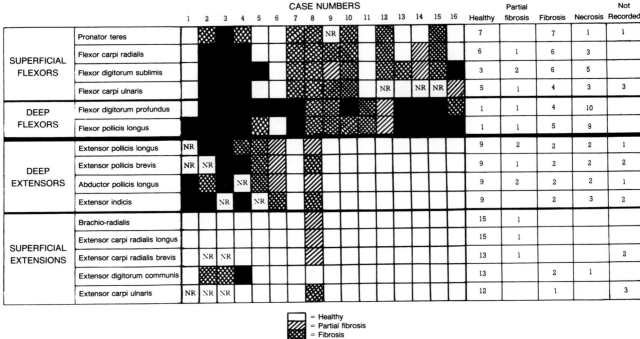

		CASE NUMBERS 1–16	Healthy	Partial fibrosis	Fibrosis	Necrosis	Not Recorded
SUPERFICIAL FLEXORS	Pronator teres		7		7	1	1
	Flexor carpi radialis		6	1	6	3	
	Flexor digitorum sublimis		3	2	6	5	
	Flexor carpi ulnaris		5	1	4	3	3
DEEP FLEXORS	Flexor digitorum profundus		1	1	4	10	
	Flexor pollicis longus		1	1	5	9	
DEEP EXTENSORS	Extensor pollicis longus		9	2	2	2	1
	Extensor pollicis brevis		9	1	2	2	2
	Abductor pollicis longus		9	2	2	2	1
	Extensor indicis		9		2	3	2
SUPERFICIAL EXTENSIONS	Brachio-radialis		15	1			
	Extensor carpi radialis longus		15	1			
	Extensor carpi radialis brevis		13	1			2
	Extensor digitorum communis		13	2	1		
	Extensor carpi ulnaris		12	1			3

= Healthy
= Partial fibrosis
= Fibrosis
= Necrosis
NR = Not recorded

FIGURE 87-1. The muscles affected in 16 cases of Volkmann's contracture of the forearm. (Seddon, H.J.: Volkmann's Contracture: Treatment by Incision of the Infarct. J. Bone Joint Surg. **38-B:**152, 1956.)

Volkmann's contracture and intrinsic muscle contracture, the actual deformities are considerably different. Intrinsic muscle contracture results in an intrinsic-plus deformity, with flexion at the metacarpophalangeal joints and extension at the proximal interphalangeal joints. Volkmann's contracture leads to an intrinsic-minus deformity, with hypertension at the metacarpophalangeal joints and flexion at the interphalangeal joints. Although the two entities are associated and may occur simultaneously, the resultant clawhand deformity is determined by contracture of the more powerful extrinsic finger flexors. A paradoxical situation of a clawhand deformity with intrinsic tightness exists.[32] The intrinsic contracture may not become apparent until the extrinsic flexors have been released by a muscle slide, tendon lengthening, or tenotomy. Only then does intrinsic tightness become evident.

CLASSIFICATION OF CONTRACTURES

Several authors have classified intrinsic contractures according to severity of involvement.[4,20,24,31,37,39] The simplest categories of classification—mild, moderate, and severe—are most useful for determining treatment options.[31,37]

Mild Contractures

A mild or localized contracture is limited to a portion of the deep extrinsic finger flexors, usually involving only two or three fingers. Hand sensibility and strength are normal. The intrinsic muscles are not involved, and fixed joint contractures do not occur. Most mild types of Volkmann's contracture are caused by fractures or crush injuries to the forearm or elbow, and usually occur in young adults.[16,37]

Moderate Contractures

Moderate contracture, the classical type, primarily involves the flexor digitorum profundus and flexor pollicis longus muscles; less frequently, the flexor digitorum superficialis, flexor carpi radialis, and flexor carpi ulnaris are involved. The wrist and thumb become flexed and the hand assumes a clawhand deformity from contracture of the long finger flexors.

Secondary compression neuropathies may develop at specific locations where nerves pass beneath ligaments, fibrous arcades, or through contracted muscles. The median nerve is most frequently compressed, usually at the lacertus fibrosus, pronator teres, or flexor digitorum superficialis, or within the carpal tunnel. The ulnar nerve may be compressed at the elbow between the two heads of the flexor carpi ulnaris. The radial nerve is rarely involved, but may be compressed at the arcade of Frohse or within the supinator muscle.

Most moderate contractures are caused by supracondylar fracture of the humerus. The age at which these fractures occur most commonly is 5 to 10 years.[16,23,24,37]

Severe Contractures

Severe contractures affect forearm extensors, as well as flexors. Complications, including loss of nerve function, malunion or nonunion of forearm fractures, and cutaneous scarring and

A

B

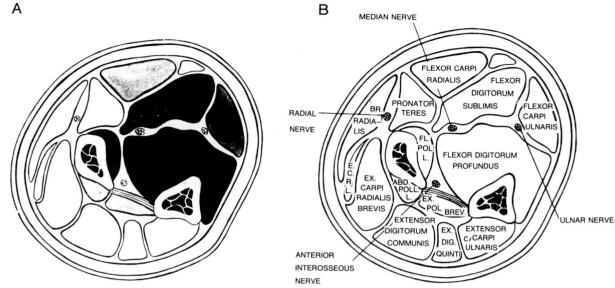

FIGURE 87-2. Cross section of Volkmann's contracture of the forearm. (*A*) The shading represents the degree of involvement of the various muscles. The diagram is based on the data provided in Figure 87-1. (*B*) Key to muscles. The plane of section is through the upper third of the forearm. E and EX, extensor; DIG, digiti, FL, flexor; POL and POLL, pollicis; L, longus; BREV, brevis; BR, brachio; ABD, abductor; C, carpi; R, radialis. (Seddon, H.J.: Volkmann's Contracture: Treatment by Incision of the Infarct. J. Bone Joint Surg. **38-B**:152, 1956.)

contracture, are often encountered. The most common causes of severe contracture are prolonged ischemia secondary to brachial artery injury and prolonged external compression secondary to drug overdose.

TREATMENT

Mild Contractures

The treatment of mild contracture depends on the severity of the deformity and the time interval between injury and initiation of treatment. Contractures of the deep forearm flexors, with normal hand sensibility and strength, may be treated conservatively. Occupational therapy, including passive and dynamic extension splinting, is designed to maintain wrist and interphalangeal joint extension, maintain or improve thumb web space width, and strengthen weak thumb intrinsic muscles. Bivalved pancake plaster casts are alternated with low-profile digital extension and thumb opposition splints. A C-bar may be incorporated into the plaster splint to maintain thumb position. In the early stages, the patient alternates passive and dynamic splints at 2-hr intervals during the day. At night, plaster extension splints are worn. Optimal splinting techniques for Volkmann's contracture have been described in detail by Goldner.[12] A satisfactory outcome can be expected when mild contractures are treated soon after their development using these techniques.

Recommended Technique

Tsuge recommends operative treatment for mild contractures that are encountered late.[37] If the contracture is limited to one or two digits and a cord-like area of induration is palpable, simple excision of the infarcted muscle or lengthening of the involved flexor tendons is recommended.

Infarct Excision

Excision of the infarcted muscle is performed through a curved, longitudinal incision on the palmar forearm. Identify and protect the radial artery, median nerve, and ulnar artery and nerve. Retract the flexor digitorum superficialis and flexor carpi radialis radially and the flexor carpi ulnaris ulnarly to expose the flexor digitorum profundus. Isolate the palpable, cord-like areas of indurated muscle and excise them. The flexor digitorum profundus of the ring and long fingers is most commonly affected. If the contracture is localized to the pronator teres, this muscle may be excised. If the contracture and induration involve three or four digits, flexor tendon lengthening may be required.

Flexor Tendon Lengthening

Z-lengthening of the involved tendons is performed in the distal two-thirds of the forearm. Begin the Z-lengthening incisions proximally, near the musculotendinous junctions, to ensure adequate tendon length for satisfactory correction. Repair the tendons using 4-0 nonabsorbable suture. Following the surgery, immobilize the forearm in supination, the wrist in extension, and the digits in the corrected amount of extension.

Moderate to Severe Contractures

The treatment of moderate to severe Volkmann's contracture may be divided into four phases:[11]

1. Release of secondary nerve compression
2. Treatment of contractures
3. Tendon transfers for substitution and reinforcement
4. Salvage procedures for the severely contracted or neglected forearm

Phase 1: Release of Secondary Nerve Compression

Following muscle infarct, nerves may become compressed within a constricting cicatrix, or at specific anatomic locations where space is minimal. Secondary compressive neuropathies require attention in the earliest stages of treatment. Improvement of nerve function is related to the severity and duration of compression, as nerves may sustain compression for longer periods than muscle and still show some reversibility, particularly in sensory function.[5,30] When continuity is maintained, nerves may show signs of gradual recovery over a 12-month period.[31,34] If both fibrosis and contracture are severe, all three major forearm nerves may become constricted. Careful clinical assessment is essential prior to the first phase of treatment.

Median Nerve. Return of median nerve function is essential for restoring a useful functional extremity. This nerve lies in the center of the constricting cicatrix and may become compressed in four anatomic regions: the lacertus fibrosus, the pronator teres, the proximal arch of the flexor digitorum superficialis, and the carpal tunnel. Sensory and motor loss consistent with median neuropathy warrant aggressive management for decompression.

An incision similar to that used for decompression of an acute forearm compartment syndrome may be used for Median Nerve Decompression (Fig. 87-3). Begin the incision on the palmar aspect of the medial arm, approximately 2 cm proximal to the medial epicondyle; extend it obliquely across the antecubital fossa to the mobile wad. Continue the incision longitudinally, curving slightly ulnarly to reach the palmar distal forearm. Extend the incision into the palm for carpal tunnel release. Locate the distal portion of the incision ulnar to the palmaris longus to avoid injury to the palmar cutaneous branch of the median nerve.

Identify the median nerve in the proximal portion of the incision and trace it distally to the lacertus fibrosus. The lacertus fibrosus is a fascial extension of the biceps tendon and lies anterior to the median nerve at the elbow. Nerve compression occurs frequently in this area in the acute stages of a forearm compartment syndrome, and may also occur in the later stages of contracture. If signs of proximal median nerve compression are present, release the lacertus fibrosus. Incise the fascia of the lacertus fibrosus in a longitudinal fashion along the course of the median nerve to allow complete decompression and exposure of the nerve.

Continuing distally, the median nerve will pass between the two heads of the pronator teres muscle. Nerve compression can occur between these two heads. The ulnar head lies deep to the nerve, and the humeral head is superficial to the nerve. A tendinous band, which often lies along the deep head, may contribute to compression. Completely release the nerve throughout the entire length of its passage through the pronator teres. This requires division of the humeral head, which lies superficial to the muscle, and division of any tendinous bands, deep or superficial, that may impinge on the nerve.

Distal to the pronator teres, the median nerve continues beneath and within the fascia of the flexor digitorum superficialis muscle, passing deep to the arch formed by the ulnar and radial origins. The nerve is most frequently compressed beneath the fibrous origin of this muscle.[27] Decompress the nerve by either incising the investing fascia or by dissecting the flexor digitorum superficialis away from the underlying flexor digitorum profundus. Completely release the nerve from the investing fascia, and transplant it subcutaneously throughout the forearm.[27]

Despite the proximal location of muscle necrosis in Volkmann's contracture, the incidence of median nerve compression in the carpal tunnel is high. The transverse carpal ligament should be incised to the midpalm primarily.

Ulnar Nerve. The incidence of ulnar nerve compression is much lower than that of median nerve compression. Often compressed at the elbow as it passes between the ulnar and humeral heads of the flexor carpi ulnaris, the ulnar nerve should be released if there are signs of ulnar motor and sensory loss.

Radial Nerve. The radial nerve is rarely involved in compression neuropathies following Volkmann's contracture. Occasionally, however, it may require decompression as it passes under the tendinous origin of the supinator muscle (arcade of Frohse) or within the muscle itself. Radial nerve compression is manifested by motor loss of the digital and thumb extensors and the ulnar wrist extensors. Radial wrist extensor strength and radial nerve sensibility remain intact, as these neural branches arise proximal to the area of compression.

To decompress the radial nerve, make a straight, longitudinal incision on the proximal half of the posterior forearm

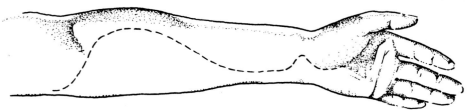

FIGURE 87-3. The incision used for decompression of the median nerve in the forearm and hand. (Gelberman, R.H., et al.: Decompression of Forearm Compartment Syndromes. Clin. Orthop. **134:**225, 1978.)

along an imaginary line extending between the lateral epicondyle and the radial styloid. Develop the interval between the extensor carpi radialis brevis and the extensor digitorum communis. This interval is most easily defined in the distal portion of the incision, and should be developed here first and traced proximally. Retract the extensor carpi radialis brevis radially and the extensor digitorum communis ulnarly. Identify the supinator. Identify the radial nerve proximally where it enters the supinator. The nerve may be found to be compressed by the tendinous bands of the arcade of Frohse, by a vascular leash that crosses the nerve transversely in this region, or by the supinator muscle itself. Carefully divide the appropriate structures to decompress the nerve.

Release of forearm nerve compression should be undertaken as soon as the condition of the patient permits. A nerve stimulator may be helpful for verification of conductivity, especially in heavily scarred areas. An early return of sensibility and a decrease in pain occur when timely decompression is performed. Nerves that are irreparably damaged, or those with loss of continuity, will require secondary excision of damaged nerve segments and repair or reconstruction with microsurgical techniques.

Phase 2: Release of Contracture

Elbow flexion, forearm pronation, wrist flexion, digital clawing, and thumb adduction are fixed deformities that occur over time. The most common procedures utilized to correct established forearm contractures are an infarct incision, a flexor tendon lengthening or excision, or a flexor pronator slide. These operations should be performed at the time of, or subsequent to, nerve decompression.

Infarct Excision. Infarct excision is performed 1 to 6 months after injury (Fig. 87-4).[22,31,37] Seddon recommends at least 6 months of preliminary splinting prior to contracture release.[31] The frequently encountered ellipsoid infarct is excised through a long palmar forearm incision.[31] All functionless muscle and

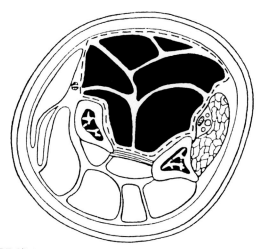

FIGURE 87-4. Excision of an infarct in the forearm, with preservation of the flexor carpi ulnaris and ulnar neurovascular bundle. (Seddon, H.J.: Revue de Chirurgie Orthopedique et Reparatrice de L'Appareil Moteur. **46:**149, 1960.)

contracted scar tissue should be excised. The deep digital flexors and thumb flexor are usually most extensively involved. The pronator teres and pronator quadratus may be released or, if they are fibrotic, excised. The forearm and wrist are gently manipulated into supination and extension, respectively, and are immobilized in that position following surgery.

Flexor Tendon Lengthening. Goldner maintains that infarct excision may be unnecessary, advocating Z-lengthening of the forearm flexors above the wrist.[12] The flexor digitorum profundus, flexor digitorum superficialis, flexor pollicis longus, and pronator teres may be lengthened, and full digital and thumb extension accomplished. If severe forearm fibrosis is encountered and digital contracture is severe, excision of the flexor digitorum superficialis should be performed.

The chief disadvantage of flexor tendon lengthening in the forearm is further weakening of an already weakened muscle. However, contracture release is more important than maintenance of maximal strength. Tendon transfers, if needed, may be performed at a later date.

Flexor Pronator Slide. The flexor pronator slide, first described by Page in 1923, has gained wide acceptance.[10,20,25,37] It has been shown to be more effective than infarct excision alone in obtaining a lasting correction.[10]

Make a skin incision on the medial side of the elbow, 6 cm proximal to the medial humeral condyle and extending to the junction of the middle and distal thirds of the forearm. Separate the subcutaneous tissue from the deep fascia on the ulnar and radial sides of the incision. Isolate the ulnar nerve at the level of the elbow and transpose it anteriorly. Proceed with systematic, complete operative detachment of the origins of the flexor muscles of the forearm. Dissect the muscles subperiosteally, using a scalpel. Release the origins of the pronator teres, flexor carpi radialis, palmaris longus, and the humeral head of the flexor carpi ulnaris, then detach the flexor digitorum superficialis. Detach the ulnar head of the flexor carpi ulnaris and the broad origin of the flexor digitorum profundus from the anterior aspect of the ulna. Carry the dissection across the interosseous membrane and release the origin of the flexor pollicis longus from the anterior aspect of the radius. Take care to avoid injury to the interosseous artery, vein, and nerves when detaching the flexors from the interosseous membrane. Allow the muscles to slide distally 2 to 3 cm. The incision may be extended distally and the palmar wrist capsule and pronator quadratus released. Although excision of the infarct and neural releases may be performed at the time of the flexor pronator slide, tendon transfers are performed secondarily.[37]

After surgery, the extremity is immobilized for 2 to 3 weeks with the elbow at 90°, the forearm supinated, and the wrist and fingers extended.

The flexor pronator slide has been criticized for the unpredictability of correction achieved, the risk of recurrence of deformity with growth, and the resultant decrease in grip strength, particularly at the distal interphalangeal joint.[22,37] Despite these criticisms, the procedure has gained popularity and has been shown to be effective in achieving satisfactory to excellent results in a large group of patients with moderate to severe contractures.[37]

Phase 3: Tendon Transfers for Substitution and Reinforcement

The main goals of tendon transfers in patients with Volkmann's contracture are to augment finger and thumb flexion and to provide thumb opposition. The transfers are usually delayed until nerve recovery has plateaued and the contractures have been corrected maximally with splints or operative releases. In 1947, Phalen and Miller described a series of tendon transfers designed to provide digital flexion and thumb opposition.[28] The extensor carpi radialis longus is transferred to the flexor digitorum profundus, and the extensor carpi ulnaris, lengthened by tendon graft, is transferred to the thumb for opposition.[26,28] The tendons of the flexor digitorum superficialis are excised if they are nonfunctional. The extensor pollicis brevis may be used to reinforce the extensor carpi ulnaris-opponens transfer. Alternative transfers to augment thumb opposition include the abductor digiti quinti opponens-plasty described by Huber,[17,22] and the extensor indicis proprius opponens-plasty described by Zancolli and by Burkhalter.[7,39] To reinforce thumb flexion, the brachioradialis may be transferred to the flexor pollicus longus.[37]

When flexor tendons have been weakened severely by previous Z-plasty lengthening, reinforcement by transfer of the extensor carpi radialis longus to the flexor digitorum profundus, and transfer of the extensor carpi ulnaris to the flexor pollicis longus, can be performed.[12]

Phase 4: Salvage of The Severely Contracted or Neglected Forearm

The procedures of Phase 2 and 3 usually provide satisfactory results, and further procedures are seldom necessary. Occasionally, however, additional measures may be required for satisfactory correction of the severely contracted or neglected forearm. Operations that have proved useful include proximal or distal row carpectomy, radial and ulnar shortening, wrist fusion, and digital joint fusion.

Proximal or distal row carpectomy results in limb shortening that allows wrist extension while maintaining flexibility. In severe deformities, carpectomy may be performed prior to tendon transfer. If adequate muscles for transfer are not available, interphalangeal joint fusion can be performed. The limb can then function as a hook, which is generally superior to a prosthesis, especially if some sensibility is retained.[12] Radial and ulnar shortening and wrist fusion are no longer recommended for the treatment or salvage of Volkmann's contracture.

Reconstruction of Hand Deformities

The hand deformity associated with Volkmann's contracture is complex, requiring a systematic, therapeutic approach. Intrinsic contractures should be addressed only after extrinsic finger flexors have been released. Fixed contractures create a clawhand deformity, with hyperextension of the metacarpophalangeal joints and flexion of the interphalangeal joints. Following extrinsic muscle release, an intrinsic-plus deformity of the hand may occur. The intrinsic-plus contracture is a result of nerve compression in the forearm, not primary intrinsic muscle necrosis in the hand.[32] Complete release of intrinsic contractures

may not be desirable, since retainment of some metacarpophalangeal joint flexion will prevent recurrence of the clawhand deformity. If the intrinsic contracture is severe, the oblique fibers of the extensor hood may be released to permit flexion of the interphalangeal joints.[32]

Thumb-in-palm deformity often accompanies the clawhand in Volkmann's contracture. The deformity may be caused by both intrinsic and extrinsic contractures. Flexion contracture at the interphalangeal joint may be corrected with flexor pollicus longus release or lengthening. Residual deformity is attributable to intrinsic contracture, joint contracture, and/or skin contracture of the first web. Recommended procedures for correction of a severe thumb-in-palm deformity include release of the adductor pollicis, deepening of the thumb web space, fusion of the metacarophalangeal joint or interphalangeal joint, or excision of the trapezium.[12] Thenar origin release and release of the first dorsal interosseous muscle may also be necessary for full correction.

The most significant hand disabilities are not intrinsic, but rather are caused by contractures in the forearm. These include loss of median and ulnar nerve sensibility, intrinsic paralysis secondary to median and ulnar motor nerve paralysis, and interphalangeal joint flexion deformity secondary to contracture of the extrinsic flexors. Proper management of these problems, as described in Phases 1 and 2, should significantly improve hand function.

Free Vascularized Tissue Transfers

Microsurgical advances have allowed free transfer of vascularized skin, nerve, and muscle.[8,18,35] The first use of these techniques for reconstruction in a patient with Volkmann's contracture involved a transfer of the lateral head of the pectoralis major to the flexor forearm by Chien in 1973.[8] Taylor and Daniel reported satisfactory results with a free vascularized superficial radial nerve graft transfer to an irreparably damaged median nerve.[36] Free vascularized tissue transfer has become increasingly commonplace, and reconstruction of forearm muscles using gracilis, rectus femorus, latissimus dorsi, or pectoralis muscles has been described. Although the early results of these procedures are promising, their place in the reconstruction of severe, neglected cases of Volkmann's contracture remains to be determined.

REFERENCES

1. Ashton, H.: The Effect of Increased Tissue Pressure on Blood Flow. Clin. Orthop. **113:**15, 1975.
2. Ashton, H.: Critical Closure in Human Limbs. Br. Med. Bull. **19**(2):149, 1963.
3. Benjamin, A.: The Relief of Traumatic Arterial Spasm in Threatened Volkmann's Contracture. J. Bone Joint Surg. **39-B:**711, 1959.
4. Benkeddache, Y., Gottesman, H., and Hamdani, M.: Proposal of a New Classification for Established Volkmann's Contracture. Ann. Chir. **4**(2):134, 1985.
5. Boyes, J.H.: Bunnell's Surgery of the Hand. Philadelphia, J.B. Lippincott, 1970.
6. Brooks, B.: Pathological Changes in Muscle as a Result of Disturbances of Circulation. An Experimental Study of Volkmann's Ischemic Paralysis. Arch. Surg. **5:**188, 1922.

7. Burkhalter, W.E., Christensen, R.C., and Brown, P.: The Extensor Indicis Proprius Opponensplasty. J. Bone Joint Surg. **55-A:**725, 1973.
8. Chien, C.W., Daniel, R.K., and Terzis, J.K.: Reconstructive Microsurgery. Boston, Little, Brown & Co., 1977.
9. Dann, I., Lassen, A., and Westing, H.: Blood Flow in Human Muscles During External Pressure on Venous Stasis. Clin. Sci. **32:**467, 1967.
10. Eichler, G.R., and Lipscomb, P.R.: The changing treatment of Volkmann's ischemic contractures from 1955 to 1965 at the Mayo Clinic. Clin. Orthop. **50:**215, 1967.
11. Gelberman, R.H.: Volkmann's Contracture of the Upper Extremity: Pathology and Reconstruction. *In* Mubarak, S.J., and Hargens, A.R. (eds.): The Compartment Syndrome and Volkmann's Contracture. Philadelphia, W.B. Saunders 1981.
12. Goldner, J.L.: Volkmann's Ischemic Contracture. *In* Flynn, J.E. (ed.): Hand Surgery. Baltimore, Williams & Wilkins, 1975.
13. Griffiths, D.V.: Volkmann's Ischemic Contracture. Br. J. Surg. **28:**239, 1940.
14. Hargens, A.R., Romine, J.S., Sipe, J.C., et al.: Peripheral Nerve Conduction Block by High Muscle Compartment Pressure. J. Bone Joint Surg. **61-A:**192, 1979.
15. Hargens, A.R., Evans, K.L., Hagen, P.L., et al.: Quantitation of Skeletal-muscle Necrosis in a Model Compartment Syndrome. Orthopedic Research Society, Dallas, TX, Feb., 1978.
16. Holden, C.E.: The Pathology and Prevention of Volkmann's Ischemic Contracture. J. Bone Joint Surg. **61-B:**296, 1979.
17. Huber, E.: Hiltsoperation ber Medianers-lahmung. Dtsch. Z. Chir. **162:**271, 1921.
18. Ikuta, Y., Kubo, T., and Tsuge, K.: Free Muscle Transplantation by Microsurgical Technique to Treat Severe Volkmann's Contracture. Plast. Reconstr. Surg. **58:**407, 1976.
19. Leriche, R.: Surgery of the Sympathetic System. Indicators and Results. Ann. Surg. **88:**449, 1928.
20. Lipscomb, P.R.: The Etiology and Prevention of Volkmann's Ischemic Contracture. Surg. Gynecol. Obstet. **103:**353, 1956.
21. Lister, G.: The Hand: Diagnosis and Indications. Edinburgh, Churchill Livingstone, 1977.
22. Littler, J.W.: The hand and upper extremity. *In* Converse, J.M. (ed.): Reconstructive Plastic Surgery. Philadelphia, W.B. Saunders, 1977.
23. Meyerding, H.W.: Volkmann's Ischemic Contracture Associated with Supracondylar Fracture of Humerus. JAMA **106:**1139, 1936.
24. Mubarak, S.J., and Carroll, N.C.: Volkmann's Contracture in Children: Etiology and Prevention. J. Bone Joint Surg **61-B:**285, 1979.
25. Page, C.M.: An Operation for the Relief of Flexion-Contracture in the Forearm. J. Bone Joint Surg. **5:**233, 1923.
26. Parks, A.: The Treatment of Established Volkmann's Contracture by Tendon Transplantation. J. Bone Joint Surg. **33-B:**359, 1951.
27. Peacock, E.E., Madden, J.W., and Trier, W.C.: Transfer of Median and Ulnar Nerves During Early Treatment of Forearm Ischemia. Ann. Surg. **169:**748, 1969.
28. Phalen, G.S., and Miller, R.C.: The Transfer of Wrist and Extensor Muscles To Restore or Reinforce Flexion Power of the Fingers and Opposition of the Thumb. J. Bone Joint Surg **29:**993, 1947.
29. Rergstad, A., and Hellum, C.: Volkmann's Ischemic Contracture of the Forearm. Injury **12**(2):148, Sept., 1980.
30. Seddon, H.J.: Surgical Disorders of the Peripheral Nerves. Baltimore, Williams & Wilkins, 1973.
31. Seddon, H.J.: Volkmann's Contracture: Treatment by Incision of the Infarct. J. Bone Joint Surg. **38-B:**152, 1956.
32. Smith, R.J.: Intrinsic Muscles of the Fingers: Function, Dysfunction and Surgical Reconstruction. Am. Acad. Ortho. Surg. Instructional Course Lectures 5: 24, 1975.
33. Sorokhan, A.J., and Eaton, R.G.: Volkmann's Ischemia. J. Hand Surg. **8-A:**806, Sept., 1983.
34. Sundoraraj, G.D., and Mani, K.: Pattern of Contracture and Recovery Following Ischemia of the Upper Limb. J. Hand Surg. (Br.) **10**(2):155, June, 1985.
35. Tamai, S., Komatsu, S., Sakamoto, H., Sano, S., Sasaucki, N., Harii, Y., Tatsumi, Y., and Okuda, H.: Free Muscle Transplants in Dogs with Microsurgical, Neurovascular Anastamoses. Plast. Reconstr. Surg. **46:**219, 1970.
36. Taylor, G.I., and Daniel, R.K.: The Free Flap: Composite Tissue Transfer by Vascular Anastamoses. Aust. N.Z. J. Surg. **43:**1, 1973.
37. Tsuge, K.: Treatment of Established Volkmann's Contracture. J. Bone Joint Surg. **57-A:**925, 1975.
38. Volkmann, R. von: Die ischaemischen Muskellahmungen und Kontrakturen. Zentralbl. Chir. **8:**801, 1881.
39. Zancolli, E.: Tendon Transfers after Ischemic Contracture of the Forearm. Classification in Relation to Intrinsic Muscle Disorders. Am. J. Surg. **109:**356, 1965.

CHAPTER 88

Principles of Tendon Repair

PAUL R. MANSKE

The frequency of injury to the functionally important flexor and extensor tendons is well attested to by review of the operative logs of orthopaedic operating rooms and emergency facilities. The specific techniques used in the treatment of lacerated flexor and extensor tendons are reviewed in subsequent chapters. The purpose of this section is to provide a basic set of principles and concepts to use in addressing tendon injuries. Some principles are well accepted, whereas others are still in the developmental stages.

The principles of tendon repair are partially based on traditional practices, partially on clinical experience, and partially on the interpretation of scientific studies in experimental animals. An understanding of the anatomic features of the tendon, the nutrient pathways to the tendon, and the physiology of the healing process is basic to the formulation of a conceptual approach to tendon repair. Flexor and extensor tendons have distinguishing anatomic features and characteristics. Although there has been considerable experimental interest in the flexor tendon, there have been few investigations of the extensor tendon.

TENDON ANATOMY

Flexor Tendons

The anatomic features of the flexor tendon are well known to most surgeons. The flexor tendons pass through several different anatomic environments or zones (Fig. 88-1). Nine flexor tendons pass through the synovium-lined carpal tunnel (zone IV) and enter the palm (zone III), where they are covered by a filmy paratenon. Two flexor tendons proceed to each finger (one to the thumb) and have an intricate arrangement within the digit (zone II) whereby the superficialis tendon divides near the metacarpal phalangeal joint to form a chiasm through which the profundus tendon passes. The superficialis tendon inserts on the palmar surface of the middle phalanx, and the profundus tendon passes out of the digital sheath near its insertion at the distal phalanx (zone I).

The superficialis tendon maintains independent muscle function to each finger (note that the musculotendon unit to the small finger is frequently hypoplastic), whereas the four profundus tendons have a common muscle belly. Consequently, the flexion of any individual distal phalanx by the profundus tendon usually results in movement at the distal joint of the adjacent three digits. This has been referred to as the "quadregia" effect.

Within the digit (zone II), the flexor tendon is in a unique environment in that it passes through a synovium-lined fibro-osseous sheath. Within this digital sheath, the tendon is attached to the periphery solely by two filmy, vascularized, mesenteric vincula (longum and breve), which are located near the mid portion and at the insertion of each tendon, respectively. The vinculum breve is located at the insertion of the superficialis tendon and is intricately associated with the vinculum longum of the profundus tendon (Fig. 88-2); consequently, damage to the superficialis tendon insertion necessarily affects the blood supply to the mid portion of the profundus tendon.

The fibro-osseous sheath consists of a series of fibrous pulleys that are regularly interrupted longitudinally by a filmy

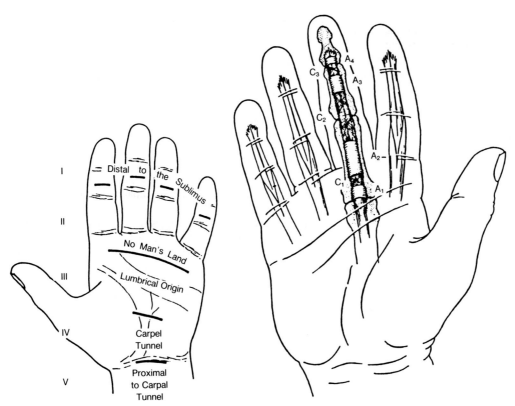

FIGURE 88-1.   Diagram of the flexor tendon zones and the location of the annular and cruciate fibro-osseous pulleys. (Kleinert, H.E., Kutz, J.E., and Cohn, M.: Primary Repair of Zone 2 Flexor Tendon Lacerations. *In* American Academy of Orthopaedic Surgeons: Symposium on Tendon Surgery in the Hand. St. Louis, C.V. Mosby, 1975.)

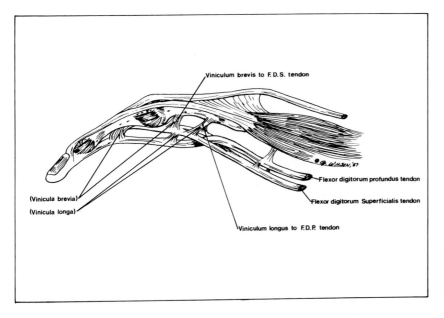

FIGURE 88-2.   Illustration of the common origins of the vinculum breve to the superficialis tendon and the vinculum longus to the profundus tendon.

synovium; together, these form a continuous tunnel through which the tendons pass. The pulleys serve to hold the gliding tendon against the phalanges and to prevent tendon bow-stringing during finger excursion. The pulleys are also thought to have a passive function role in pumping fluid into the tendon during flexion and extension.

Extensor Tendons

The extensor tendons enter the hand through a series of synovium-lined, retinacular compartments on the dorsum of the wrist. In contrast to the flexor tendon, these tendons are attached to the retinacular compartments by long, mesotendinous, synovial sheets rather than by narrow, filamentous vincula. On the dorsum of the hand, the tendons emerge from the retinacular compartments and proceed individually to each digit. The extensor tendons are interconnected by tendinous bands known as juncturae tendinum. Distal to the metacarpophalangeal joint, the extensor mechanism forms an intricate arrangement of fibers that arise from both the extrinsic extensor tendons and from the intrinsic musculotendinous units. This intricately arranged, digital, aponeurotic mechanism is essential to the synchronous movement of the three digital joints.

The microscopic anatomy of the tendon consists of a central core (the *endotenon*) that is composed primarily of acellular, longitudinal, collagenous fibers that are sparsely interspersed with fibroblasts. A thin *epitenon* layer of cells surrounds the central core. The epitenon cells are fibroblasts that may have different functional properties and characteristics from the internal fibroblasts of the endotenon. The epitenon cells are arranged in a matrix that has not been defined specifically, but that is presumed to have a proteoglycan composition.

TENDON NUTRITION

Although vascular perfusion via the mesenteric vincula is an obvious nutrient pathway to the flexor tendon, recent studies have suggested that diffusion of nutrients into the tendon is a more significant pathway within the digital sheath.[14] Synovial fluid produced by the lining cells of the digital sheath is an obvious source of diffusible nutrients.[19] However, corporeal tissue fluid can also effectively diffuse into and maintain the viability of tendons, as shown by experiments in which tendon segments have been placed in an abdominal wall diffusion chamber,[9] as well as in an *in vitro* tissue culture environment.[15]

Proximal to the digital sheath, the tendon in the palm (zone III) is surrounded by filmy paratenon. This vascularized connective tissue is thought to be the source of nutrients to the tendon. Within the carpal tunnel (zone IV), the tendons are surrounded by a synovial mesotenon which arises from the floor of the carpal tunnel. The nutrition of the flexor tendon within the carpal tunnel has not been investigated experimentally.

The *extensor* tendons within the retinacular compartments receive nutrients from the mesotendinous synovial sheets arising from the floor of the compartment, with both diffusion and perfusion serving as nutrient pathways.[16] The filmy paratenon vascularizes the tendons on the dorsum of the hand and digit.

PHYSIOLOGY OF TENDON HEALING

The process by which flexor tendons heal is controversial.[17] The traditional concept of this process is that peripheral fibroblasts from the surrounding connective tissue invade the laceration site and serve as the source of reparative cells; the tendon itself was thought to have no intrinsic capacity for repair. Recent studies,[18] however, have shown that the epitenon cells migrate into and cover the laceration site along a fibrin lattice. Collagenous fibers are subsequently formed by the internal fibroblasts of the endotenon or the epitenon cells, or both, at the laceration site. These studies suggest that the tendon is a viable structure with the intrinsic capacity for participating in the repair process.

Peripheral adhesions are known to attach to the healing tendon, thereby potentially restricting tendon excursion during flexion and extension. It is not known, however, whether the adhesions are essential to the reparative process or whether they are an incidental response of the surrounding tissue to trauma.[6] The concept of the tendon's intrinsic capacity for healing is attractive to surgeons, since this theoretically eliminates the need for peripheral adhesions at the repair site. Nevertheless, restrictive adhesions following tendon repair continue to be the bane of surgeons who perform flexor tendon surgery.

Extensor tendons are thought to heal by invasion of fibroblasts from the periphery. However, experimental studies have not yet defined this process.

BASIC PRINCIPLES

There are basic operative principles that must be followed in caring for flexor or extensor tendon lacerations.

Clinical Examination

The first principle is to diagnose a flexor or extensor tendon laceration by careful clinical examination. The examination begins with a visual inspection of the hand, at which time a disruption of the continuity of the tendon must be suspected by the location of the wound and the resting position of the digit. For example, a skin laceration immediately overlying a flexor tendon on the palm, in association with a digit whose resting position is not as flexed as the adjacent fingers, is strongly indicative of a lacerated flexor tendon. However, the examiner must realize that sharp, stiletto-type, penetrating objects can lacerate tendons through a small, inconspicuous, skin wound at a distance from the tendon.

Visual inspection is then followed by evaluation of the active motion of the joint mobilized by the tendon. The flexor profundus tendon to each digit can easily be examined by asking the patient to flex the distal joint of the involved digit actively (Fig. 88-3); inability to flex the distal interphalangeal joint actively is indicative of a lacerated profundus tendon.

Testing for a lacerated superficialis tendon is not difficult if the profundus tendon is also cut, since the patient will be unable to active flex either the proximal interphalangeal joint or the distal joint actively. However, it is difficult to test for a

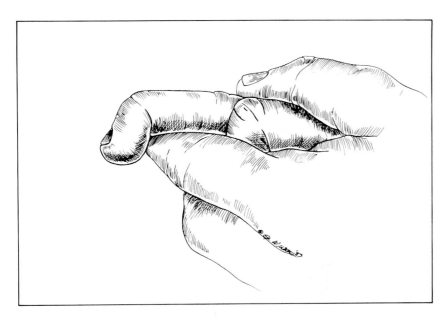

FIGURE 88-3. Examination of an intact flexor profundus tendon.

suspected superficialis tendon laceration when the profundus tendon is intact. One must eliminate the flexion force of the profundus tendon by making use of the quadregia effect (Fig. 88-4). This is accomplished by manually holding the distal joints of the adjacent digits in full extension while the patient attempts to flex the involved finger actively. An inability to flex the involved digit actively at the proximal interphalangeal joint indicates a lacerated superficialis tendon.

The extensor tendons to the fingers can be tested by asking the patient to extend the digit actively. Failure to achieve complete extension indicates a tendon laceration. However, the ability to obtain full extension may be misleading, since this may be accomplished even where there is an extensor tendon laceration via an interconnecting juncturae tendinum from an adjacent tendon. The examiner can avoid this misleading pitfall by testing the comparative strength of digital extension against resistance; A digit that is being extended by an interconnecting juncturae tendinum will have a comparatively weaker extension force than will the adjacent fingers.

Adequate Exposure

A second principle involves adequate exposure of the wound site. In many instances, this is necessary to confirm the diagnosis of tendon laceration when the clinical examination of the tendon is not conclusive, or when the extent of significant injury to adjacent structures is questionable. This occurs frequently in children with tendon injuries who are not fully able to cooperate, in comatose patients, and in those with partial tendon lacerations or complete tendon lacerations in which partial function of the digit is sustained by the adjacent intact

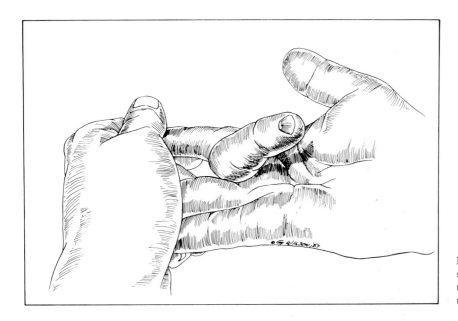

FIGURE 88-4. Examination of an intact flexor superficialis tendon using the quadregia effect to eliminate the flexion force of the profundus tendon.

structures, such as the junctura tendinae or intact vincula. The burden of proof as to whether a flexor or extensor tendon laceration exists rests with the surgeon; if that cannot be determined by clinical examination, surgical exploration of the wound is indicated.

Adequate surgical exposure is also necessary to properly identify and expose the tendon ends. Generally speaking, proximal or distal extension of the original wound is achieved through a zigzag approach, as described by Bruner,[2] incorporating the original skin laceration (Fig. 88-5). Lacerated flexor tendons frequently retract into the palm or forearm unless an intact vinculum or lumbrical muscle prevents this proximal retraction. A second proximal incision may be necessary to retrieve the retracted tendon and pass it into the original wound site. Fortunately, proximal retraction of lacerated extensor tendons occurs infrequently because the tendon is usually held in place by the junctura tendinae or the synovial mesotendon beneath the retinaculum.

When it is necessary to incise the digital sheath in order to expose the flexor tendon ends, the surgeon should avoid cutting the fibro-osseous pulleys, and should limit the incisional area to the intervening synovial portion of the sheath. This is best accomplished by an L-shaped or hockey stick incision[12] which facilitates closure of the digital sheath.

Associated Injuries

The third basic principle in the treatment of tendon injuries is to identify any associated injuries to the adjacent bones, nerves, or blood vessels. Before repairing the lacerated tendon, the injuries to these associated structures must be defined. If possible, the injured structures should all be repaired at the time of initial surgical treatment. The sequence of repair is usually as follows: bone, ligament, tendon, nerve, and finally, blood vessels. One should keep in mind that not all vessels require reanastomosis, and one may choose to perform a delayed repair of crushed or explosion-injured nerves. In replantation surgery, this sequence of repair may be altered in the interest of quickly restoring circulation to the digit.

Atraumatic Technique

Another basic principle related to tendon repair is that the surgeon should handle the tendon in an atraumatic manner, since rough manipulation of the tendon is associated with increased adhesions and the formation of restrictive scar tissue.[3,20] This principle cannot be emphasized enough. When possible, only the exposed, cut end of the tendon should be handled with the forceps, crushing clamps should not be applied to the tendon, and puncture holes made by suture needles or forceps inserted into the tendon substance should be kept to a minimum. Frequently, the surgeon draws the proximal and distal ends of the lacerated tendon into the wound site and holds them in position with fine milliner needles placed transversely through the tendon and the adjacent soft tissue; this allows the repair to be accomplished in the absence of tension, thereby minimizing repeated manipulation of the tendon ends.

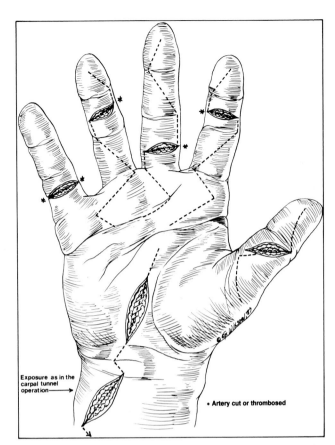

FIGURE 88-5. Proximal and distal incisions extending from the laceration site to obtain exposure.

Suture Technique

The basic objective of tendon surgery is to appose the lacerated tendon ends in order to allow the healing process to reestablish the continuity of the disrupted collagen bundles and the smooth gliding surface of the tendon. The surgeon must restore the tubular form to the tendon, avoiding both gapping or thickened overlapping margins at the repair site. This is particularly true for flexor tendon injuries within the digital sheath (zone II), where repair is most difficult because of the adhesions that may form between the sheath and the tendon, thereby restricting motion. Although tendon repair in zone II was at one time discouraged, clinical experience in recent years has made it an acceptable option for qualified surgeons.

Numerous suture techniques have been described for flexor tendon repair (Fig. 88-6). For the most part, all of them include a "core" suture through the endotenon substance of the tendon (to provide strength and stability to the repair until healing takes place), as well as a circumferential running suture around the laceration site, frequently referred to as an "epitenon" suture. (This is actually a misnomer since the epitenon layer, by itself, is not strong enough to hold the suture, and peripheral collagen fibers are necessarily involved.) The Bunnell[1,11] or Kessler[10] core sutures have been shown to provide the greatest strength at the repair site,[23] and are used by most surgeons (Fig. 88-7). These techniques have been modified to place the knot within the repair site; this modification has the advantage

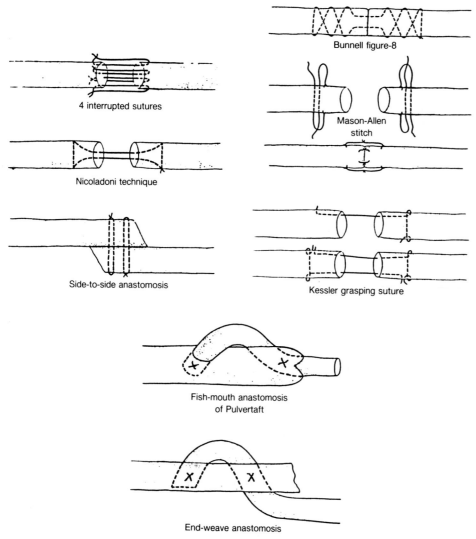

FIGURE 88-6. Various tendon suture techniques. (Urbaniak, J.R., Cahill, J.D., and Mortenson, R.A.: Tendon Suturing Methods: Analysis of Tensile Strength. *In* American Academy of Orthopaedic Surgeons: Symposium on Tendon Surgery in the Hand. St. Louis, C.V. Mosby, 1975.)

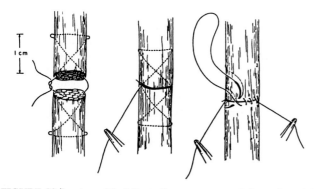

FIGURE 88-7. A modified Bunnell core suture and circumferential running suture. (Kleinert, H.E., Kutz, J.E., and Cohen, M.: Primary Repair of Zone 2 Flexor Tendon Lacerations. *In* American Academy of Orthopaedic Surgeons: Symposium on Tendon Surgery in the Hand. St. Louis, C.V. Mosby, 1975.)

of not leaving suture material exposed within the fibro-osseous digital sheath.

From injection studies, Caplan[4] determined that the internal vasculature of the tendon is concentrated on the dorsal, as opposed to the palmar, cross-sectional area of the tendon. Consequently, it was recommended that the core suture be placed in the palmar portion of the tendon in order to avoid interference with internal vascular perfusion. However, the concept of diffusion as a significant nutrient pathway to the tendon obviates this concept of suture placement, and suggests that the precise placement of the core suture is not that significant. Rather, it is more important that the core suture be placed in such a way as not to strangulate or "bunch up" the tendon end.

The epitenon suture was, at one time, considered to be primarily cosmetic. However, recent studies of tendon healing emphasize the importance of this suture. The initial cellular response to trauma occurs in the epitenon layer, the cells of which proliferate and migrate into the laceration site.[18] Gelberman[8] has shown that the epitenon response is increased and a greater fibrous "callous" is produced when there is a large gap between the tendon ends. Studies from our laboratory suggest that the epitenon cells migrate not only into the laceration site, but can also migrate peripherally into the surrounding tissue. These studies indicate that a properly placed epitenon suture which coapts and invaginates the tendon ends[12] helps to prevent postoperative adhesions.

The suture technique for flexor tendons outside of zone II, as well as for extensor tendons, is not as critical, since the healed tendons do not have to glide in a confined sheath. Nevertheless, the surgeon is encouraged to follow the same careful techniques to minimize postoperative adhesions.

Various suture materials have been advocated. It is important that the suture be strong and nonreactive. Monofilament stainless steel, or nylon, is the strongest and least reactive of the available suture materials, but it is difficult to use without kinking or crimping which potentially weakens the suture at that point and leads to breakage. Most surgeons use one of the several available nonreactive synthetic materials—4-0 or 5-0 for the core suture and 6-0 or 7-0 for the circumferential epitenon suture.

Sheath Repair

There is an ongoing controversy as to whether the digital sheath should be excised or repaired at the time of tendon repair. Recently, repair of the digital sheath at the time of zone II flexor tendon injuries has become popular.[12] The premise that this will enhance tendon nutrition by restoring the synovial environment is contradicted by the experimental studies of Katsumi and Tajima,[9] which showed that tendons healed in an extrasynovial fluid environment (i.e., in an abdominal pouch diffusion chamber). This premise is also refuted by the studies of Peterson,[21] which indicated that the integrity of the digital sheath (i.e., whether the sheath was excised or repaired) did not affect the uptake of nutrients into the tendon. In experiments with animals, Strauch[22] demonstrated that sheath closure resulted in improved tendon gliding, presumably by preventing the attachment of peripheral adhesions to the tendon. However, it is important to realize that sheath closure in the presence of an edematous swollen tendon may produce relative narrowing of the fibro-osseous tunnel, and may restrict, rather than enhance, tendon gliding. If sheath closure is to be accomplished at the time of tendon repair, it should be performed meticulously, taking particular care not to compromise the volume of the fibro-osseous tunnel.

Postoperative Management

The postoperative management of tendon injuries is critical. Logically, one should minimize tension at the repair site by immobilizing the involved digit in order to allow the tendon to heal; in theory, this would prevent rupture of the tendon repair site. In general, this concept has prevailed in the treatment of extensor tendon lacerations. Adhesions that form around the extensor tendons usually become filmy and do not interfere with motion; when the adhesions do interfere with motion, they can be released by surgical tenolysis after the laceration site has healed.

Although this concept is also appropriate in the postoperative management of flexor tendon lacerations, there has been considerable concern that the prescribed 3- to 4-week period of immobilization results in the formation of restrictive adhesions. Consequently, carefully supervised, controlled, passive range of motion[5] or protected active range of motion[11,13] of the tendon at the repair site has been initiated early in the postoperative period with good clinical results. The experimental studies of Gelberman[6,7] indicate that such a program of early motion effectively restores the gliding surface of the tendon and increases the strength at the repair site.

The principles associated with tendon repair have long been in a dynamic state of development. Undoubtedly, this indicates that the underlying concepts regarding tendon repair are not firmly established. Although it is essential that the treatment of any disease proceeds from a strong conceptual base, one should keep in proper perspective the relationship between experimental studies and established clinical practices. Perhaps it is best to regard the principles associated with tendon repair as specific issues that one must continue to address, ponder, consider, and re-think. Only in that way will the objective of restoring the continuity of collagenous fibers and reestablishing the gliding surface of the tendon be realized.

REFERENCES

1. Boyes, J.H.: Tendons. *In* Bunnell's Surgery of the Hand, 5th ed. Philadelphia, J.B. Lippincott, 1970, pp. 393–400.
2. Bruner, J.M.: The Zig-Zag Volar-Digital Incision for Flexor Tendon Surgery. Plast. Reconstr. Surg. **40:**571, 1967.
3. Bunnell, S.: Repair of Tendons in the Fingers and Description of Two New Instruments. Surg. Gynecol. Obstet. **26:**103, 1918.
4. Caplan, H.S., Hunter, J.M., and Merklin, R.J.: Intrinsic Vascularization of Flexor Tendon. *In* American Academy of Orthopaedic Surgeons: Symposium on Tendon Surgery in the Hand. St. Louis, C.V. Mosby, 1975, pp. 48–58.
5. Duran, R.E.: Controlled Passive Motion Following Flexor Tendon Repair in Zones II and III. *In* American Academy of Orthopaedic Surgeons: Symposium on Tendon Surgery in the Hand. St. Louis, C.V. Mosby, 1975, pp. 105–114.
6. Gelberman, R.H., and Manske, P.R.: Factors Influencing Flexor Tendon Adhesions. Hand Clin. North Am. **1:**35, 1985.
7. Gelberman, R.H., Vande Berg, J.S., Lundborg, G.N., and Akeson, W.H.: Flexor Tendon Healing and Restoration of the Gliding Surface. J. Bone Joint Surg. **65-A:**70, 1983.
8. Gelberman, R.H., Vande Berg, J.S., Manske, P.R., and Akeson, W.H.: The Early Stages of Flexor Tendon Healing: A Morphologic Study of the First Fourteen Days. J. Hand Surg. **10:**776, 1986.
9. Katsumi, M., and Tajima, T.: Experimental Investigation of Healing Process of Tendons With or Without Synovial Coverage In or Outside of the Synovial Cavity. J. Niigata Med. Assoc. **95:**532, 1981.
10. Kessler, I.: The "Grasping" Technique for Tendon Repair. Hand, **5:**253, 1973.
11. Kleinert, H.E., Kutz, J.E., and Cohen, M.: Primary Repair of Zone 2 Flexor Tendon Lacerations. *In* American Academy of Orthopae-

dic Surgeons: Symposium on Tendon Surgery in the Hand. St. Louis, C.V. Mosby, 1975, pp. 115–124.

12. Lister, G.D.: Incision and Closure of the Flexor Sheath During Primary Tendon Repair. Hand, **15:**123, 1983.

13. Lister, G.D., Kleinert, H.E., and Kutz, J.E.: Primary Flexor Tendon Repair Followed by Immediate Controlled Mobilization. J. Hand Surg. **2:**441, 1977.

14. Manske, P.R., and Lesker, P.A.: Flexor Tendon Nutrition. Hand Clin. North Am. **1:**13, 1985.

15. Manske, P.R., and Lesker, P.A.: Histological Evidence of Flexor Tendon Repair in Various Experimental Animals. An in vitro study. Clin. Orthop. **182:**353, 1984.

16. Manske, P.R., and Lesker, P.A.: Nutrient Pathways to Extensor Tendons Within the Extensor Retinacular Compartments. Clin. Orthop. **181:**234, 1983.

17. Manske, P.R., Gelberman, R.H., and Lesker, P.A.: Flexor Tendon Healing. Hand Clin. North Am. **1:**25, 1985.

18. Manske, P.R., Gelberman, R.H., Vande Berg, J.S., and Lesker, P.A.: Flexor Tendon Repair: Morphologic Evidence of Intrinsic Healing In Vitro. J. Bone Joint Surg. **66-A:**385, 1984.

19. Matthews, P.: The Fate of Isolated Segments of Flexor Tendons Within the Digital Sheath. Br. J. Plast Surg. **28:**216, 1976.

20. Matthews, P., and Richards, H.: Factors in the Adherence of Flexor Tendons After Repair. An Experimental Study in the Rabbit. J. Bone Joint Surg. **58-B:**230, 1976.

21. Peterson, W.W., Manske, P.R., and Lesker, P.A.: The Effect of Flexor Sheath Integrity on Nutrient Uptake in Chicken Flexor Tendons. Clin. Orthop. **201:**259, 1985.

22. Strauch, B., DeMoura, W., Ferder, M., Hall, C., Sagi, A., and Greenstein, B.: The Fate of Tendon Healing After Restoration of the Integrity of the Tendon Sheath with Autogenous Vein Grafts. J. Hand Surg. **10-A:**790, 1985.

23. Urbaniak, J.R., Cahill, J.D., and Mortenson, R.A.: Tendon Suturing Methods: Analysis of Tensile Strength. *In* American Academy of Orthopaedic Surgeons: Symposium on Tendon Surgery in the Hand. St. Louis, C.V. Mosby, 1975, pp. 70–80.

BIBLIOGRAPHY

Doyle, J.R.: Extensor Tendons—Acute Injuries. *In* Greene, David P. (ed.): Operative Hand Surgery. New York, Churchill Livingstone, 1982, pp. 1441–1464.

Hunter, J.M., and Schneider, L.H. (eds.): American Academy of Orthopaedic Surgeons, Symposium on Tendon Surgery in the Hand. St. Louis, C.V. Mosby Co., 1975.

Leddy, J.P.: Flexor Tendons—Acute Injuries. *In* Greene, David P. (ed.): Operative Hand Surgery. New York, Churchill Livingstone, 1982. pp. 1347–1373.

Strickland, J.W. (ed.): Hand Clin. North Am. **1:** 1985.

CHAPTER 89

Flexor Tendon Injuries: Acute Repair and Late Reconstruction

JOHN S. GOULD
and BETH G. NICHOLSON

Although discussions of the anatomy, physiology, and biomechanics of human flexor tendons are beyond the scope of this chapter, the reader is referred to the recent work of Gelberman,[16,17] Manske,[16–18] and Brand,[3] which form the basis of present approaches to flexor tendon repair technique. Within the past 15 years, this knowledge has changed most of the principles and techniques of flexor tendon surgery, and with the enthusiasm for replantation, the timing. The importance that each surgeon attributes to the blood supply will determine whether a midlateral incision is used for exposure, which, to some extent, decreases blood supply to the tendon from that side (Fig. 89-1); whether a superficialis is excised, which has vascular interconnections with the profundus (Fig. 89-2); and whether "strangulating" criss-cross suture techniques (e.g., Bunnell) are used or sutures are placed more palmarward to avoid disrupting the blood supply entering from and residing in the dorsal aspect of the tendon. If the synovial fluid environment of a closed sheath and intrinsic tendon healing are felt to be of any significance, the surgeon will go to great measures to close or reconstruct the sheath. Finally the effects of motion on tendon healing and strength determine the rehabilitation plan.[8]

Acknowledged principles include the importance of a clean surgical wound and restoration of skeletal stability, sensibility, and circulation. We can appreciate the one wound–one scar concept,[21] the poorer prognosis for function with more damaged structures,[2] and the ideal advantage of the mature wound for tendon repair/reconstruction. Yet, we can also appreciate the opportunity for meticulous repair of all structures with bone fixation techniques that allow immediate motion; the repair of the periosteum or the dorsal portion of the flexor sheath or pulley system as an interposing tissue; the importance of the repair of vessels for proper nerve regeneration; the repair of nerves for ideal rehabilitation; and the repair of tendons to prevent myostatic contracture and to allow rapid restoration of function, utilizing a controlled rehabilitation plan.

TERMINOLOGY

Precise definitions relative to the timing of tendon repair cannot be given, particularly in view of the conflicting opinions of many authorities. *Primary repair* indicates that the tendon repair is carried out acutely, when the wound is initially cleaned and debrided. This also implies that such action is taken within the first few hours of the injury, presumably during the classic "golden period" of 6 hours, when it can be assumed the wound has not been sufficiently colonized with bacteria to prevent closure. In fact, some fresh wounds are so grossly contaminated primarily that there is no "golden period"!

With an older wound (over 6 hours), one might generally hesitate to conduct a definitive repair of flexor tendons, preferring initial debridement only. If one revascularizes or replants a digit six hours after injury, and tendon repair is also carried out, this is also considered primary repair.

On the other hand, if the initial wound is washed and debrided but tendon repair is delayed for 48 hours, 4 days, even 10 to 14 days, and the wound is not yet healed, the repair is referred to as *delayed primary.*

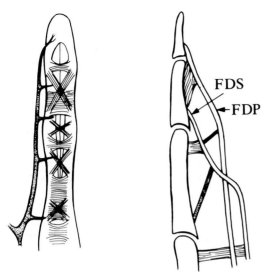

FIGURE 89-1. Segmental blood supply to digital theca. (Modified from Leddy, J.P.: Flexor Tendons—Acute Injuries. *In* Green, D.P. (ed.): Operative Hand Surgery. New York, Churchill Livingstone, 1982, p. 1350.)

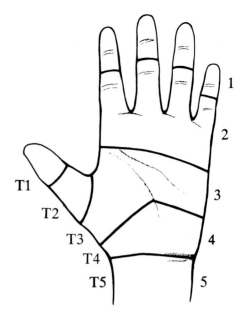

FIGURE 89-3. Verdan's thumb and digital zones (modified).

A repair performed after skin wound healing is considered a *secondary repair* or reconstruction. However, some authors[23] consider repairs between 2 and 6 weeks to be *late delayed primary repair*, because myostatic contracture is not well enough established to prevent "primary" end-to-end repair of the flexor tendon without having to resort to secondary reconstruction (i.e., grafting).

ZONES OF INJURY

Following Bunnell's admonitions about problems with flexor tendon repairs in the pulley area of the digital theca (the "zone of the pulleys" or Bunnell's "no-man's land"),[2] Verdan classified the flexor tendon injury sites into five zones, each with its peculiar anatomy and prognosis[27-29] (Fig. 89-3). The pulley zones of the digit and thumb have been redefined by Doyle (Fig. 89-4), whose classification is currently in general acceptance.[5,6]

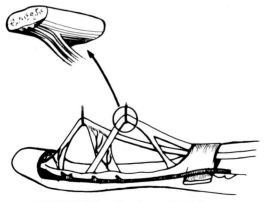

FIGURE 89-2. Vinculae to digital flexors.

Flexor tendons to the digits may be injured in the wrist or forearm proximal to the carpal tunnel, which begins at the distal palmar wrist crease (surface marking) or the proximal edge of the deep transverse carpal ligament, extending from the trapezium to the hook of the hamate. It is important to remember at the outset that the site of the tendon injury is what defines the zone, not the site of the skin lacerations. The tendon injury site is the position of the tendon with the wrist in neutral and the fingers in full extension, although more properly the fingers should be in their resting position of normal muscle tension or digital stance. As the fingers and wrist move into flexion, as the flexor muscles contract, the tendon moves proximally. Therefore, if the injury occurred at the wrist level but the finger or wrist or both were flexed, the tendon injury occurs more distally on the tendon (possibly in the carpal tunnel) when it resumes its neutral or more extended position.

A tendon injury in the wrist or distal forearm is in Verdan's zone 5. The musculotendinous junction area may be involved. Injuries can occur to the two wrist flexors, the palmaris longus, the median and ulnar nerves (and branches), the radial and ulnar arteries, and the nine flexor tendons of the digits and thumb. Multiple tendons and muscles may be injured. The prognosis for function, including individual function, in this area is good. Repairs need not be as meticulous as in other areas, but they still must be done well.

The carpal tunnel, Verdan's zone 4, extends from the distal palmar wrist crease or the proximal end of the deep transverse carpal ligament to its distal margin as noted by the crossing of the proximal superficial palmar arch, formed from the ulnar side by the ulnar artery leaving the canal of Guyon. The surface determination of the distal extent of the tunnel is made by extending a line across the base of the palm from the palmar surface of the maximally extended thumb. In this zone, the nine flexors are tightly packed with the median nerve. Repairs must be meticulous, and results, especially for independent

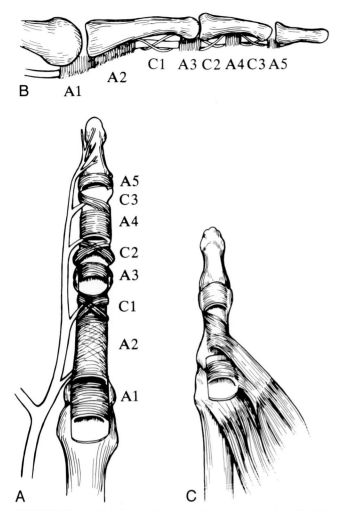

FIGURE 89-4. Digital and thumb pulley systems as described by Doyle and Strauch. (*A* and *B*) Digital. (*C*) Thumb (note annular pulleys at the metacarpophalangeal and just proximal to the interphalangeal joint with oblique pulley over proximal phalanx). (*C*, modified from Doyle, J.R., and Blythe, W.F.: Anatomy of the Flexor Tendon Sheath and Pulleys of the Thumb. J. Hand Surg. **2**:150, 1977.)

function, are more problematic than in any other area except the zone of the pulleys.

Zone 3 extends from the end of the carpal tunnel to the proximal end of the pulleys, which begin at the metacarpophalangeal joints. Surface markings in the palm are the proximal palmar crease for the index, about midway between the proximal and distal crease for the long finger, and the distal palmar crease for the ring and little fingers. In this zone, both the flexor digitorum superficialis and the flexor digitorum profundus are oval tendons, and the lumbrical muscle originates from the flexor digitorum profundus. The lumbrical tendon runs in its own sheath or tunnel radial to the long flexor. Although repairs in zone 3 generally have a good prognosis, secondary reconstructive procedures originating here should allow for problems with intrinsic imbalance and excessive lumbrical action.

Zone 2, the zone of the pulleys, is the area of maximum concern and debate regarding aspects of tendon nutrition,

healing, repair methods, and rehabilitation. Even the extent of the zone is argued. Investigators agree that the zone begins at the metacarpophalangeal level (Bunnell's first pulley, Doyle's first annular [A1]), but the distal extent is not defined. For prognostic purposes, the zone ends at the mid middle phalanx, the site of Doyle's C3 (third cruciate) pulley, but also the distal-most extent of the superficialis slips' insertion (Fig. 89-4). Distal to this point only a one-tendon system, the profundus, exists, but Strauch has described the A5 (fifth annular) pulley at the distal interphalangeal joint level.[24] Zone 2 is peculiar in that actually three tendons (profundus and two slips of the superficialis) exist here in very close proximity; they are surrounded by the dense unyielding cover of a floor (dorsally) of bone, periosteum, and fibrous sheath and by sides and a roof (palmarly) of dense fibrous tissue, thicker even in the condensations of the annular and cruciate pulleys and dorsally at the palmar plates. Within the sheath and pulleys the tendons have an intrinsic blood supply as well as that from the parietal tenosynovium surrounding the tendons. The superficialis tendon in this zone begins to split at the metacarpophalangeal level to allow the profundus to pass through it. It then becomes two flat, slightly concave tendons that lie dorsal to the profundus and hug its sides, and then join just proximal to the proximal interphalangeal joint to form the chiasm of Camper. The flat united tendinous structure then divides after the proximal interphalangeal joint to form two flat slips, which insert along the middle phalanx to almost its midpoint. Good results of surgical repair in this area depend on many of the surgical and rehabilitation techniques discussed in this chapter and are by no means routine.

Zone 1 is the area between the superficialis insertion (distal edge of C3 pulley) and the insertion of the profundus. Excellent technique is also required here, but with good conventional techniques the prognosis for function has been good. Five thumb flexor zones are described, but problems occur less often here with only one tendon of relatively uniform size and no intrinsic. Zone 5 for the thumb flexor is also in the wrist, proximal to the carpal tunnel; Zone 4 is the carpal tunnel; Zone 3 is the relatively inaccessible thenar zone, extending from the distal edge of the tunnel to the metacarpophalangeal joint. Zone 2 is the pulley zone, consisting of an annular ligament at the metacarpophalangeal joint and a long oblique pulley over three-quarters of the proximal phalanx with a second annular pulley distally; and Zone 1 is distal to the pulley, just proximal to the interphalangeal joint, to the insertion of the flexor pollicis longus just distal to the interphalangeal joint.

TECHNIQUES OF DIGITAL FLEXOR TENDON REPAIR

Given the option, I prefer the delayed primary repair of flexor tendons. This implies a thorough wash and debridement of the wound initially, with tendon repair at 48 to 96 hours. Initial care is done on an outpatient basis in an adequate facility, usually the operating room, but it could be an adequate emergency department suite where tourniquet control, anesthesia, and good sterility are all available. The patient is placed on the elective operating schedule in a few days.

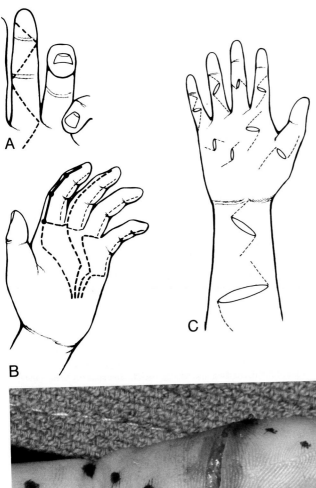

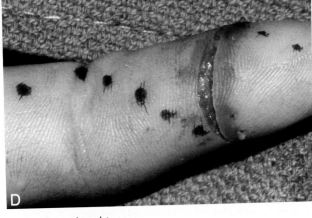

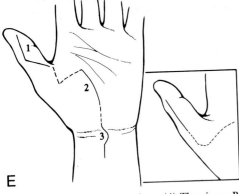

FIGURE 89-5. Incision options. (*A*) The zigzag Bruner incision. (*B*) Midlateral incisions. (*C*) Extensions of lacerations. (*D*) Extension of incision in clinical photo. (*E*) Incision options for the thumb. (*A, B,* modified from Schneider, L.H., and Hunter, J.M.: Flexor Tendons—Late Reconstruction. *In* Green, D.P. (ed.): Operative Hand Surgery. New York, Churchill Livingstone, 1982, p. 1379; *E,* modified from Urbaniak, J.R.: Flexor Pollicis Longus Repair. Hand Clin. **1**:72, 1985.)

Several situations, both medically moderated and socially dictated, preempt this approach. The patient may be unreliable, and so is likely admitted and operated at the next available elective operating time after initial wound care. The patient may be referred from out of town with a day-old injury, in which case surgery is done at the next elective opportunity. Medical conditions indicating acute repair include the zone 5 injury requiring the care of multiple damaged structures, and the repair of muscle and tendons before muscle retraction makes the surgery technically more difficult. Digits with vascular impairment requiring revascularization or replantation are also repaired acutely, as delay may endanger the viability of the digit.

My surgical technique begins with increasing the exposure proximally and distally, converting the original laceration into part of the zigzag Bruner approach[4] (Fig. 89-5). A history of the injury suggests whether the actual site of tendon laceration will be at the skin level or more distally. The carpal tunnel area is opened following the thenar crease, but 1.0 to 2.0 cm distal to the wrist crease; the incision is directed ulnarly to the wrist crease. The direction is then changed sharply and the incision is curved proximally back to the midline. Each zone is managed somewhat differently.

Repairs in Each Zone

In zone 5, after extending the exposure, check each item of the anatomy to verify the findings at physical examination, where each structure was tested for continuity and function. The profundi are aligned at the same level just palmar to the pronator quadratus, with the index profundus frequently independent. The flexor pollicis is more radial yet, and although deeper, just radial to the radial artery. The four superficialis tendons line up, with the long and ring finger tendons lying somewhat more superficially than the index and little finger tendons, which lie to either side and more dorsal. The little finger superficialis is closely associated with the ring finger tendon, although slightly more dorsal. If the profundi and flexor pollicis longus are intact, place an umbilical tape around them to avoid having to recheck their identity repeatedly. Similarly, mark the intact superficialis tendons, and identify the more superficial wrist flexors—the flexor carpi radialis and ulnaris—and tag the median nerve with a vessel loop. While any flexor motor can power any distal tendon, it is best to match the lacerated components, since their lengths when repaired end to end should provide the appropriate tension. This is particularly important for the profundi where, because of their intimate interconnection, tendon length restoration is important to prevent the short tether syndrome, quadriga. Tendons are identified based on their function, location, and appearance—that is, it does what it is supposed to do, lies where it is supposed to lie, and looks as it is supposed to look. This last is an important point—"If it doesn't look like Aunt Minnie, it probably isn't Aunt Minnie!"

The preferred end-to-end tendon repair is the Tajima modification of the four-corner grabbing stitch of Kessler[25] (Fig. 89-6). It is performed with two double-armed 3-0 or 4-0 monofilament polypropylene sutures with pointed tendon needles. Place the suture about 1 cm behind the cut edge, which is minimally trimmed with curved Stephen scissors. Then reinsert each needle just behind the transverse suture and direct it on

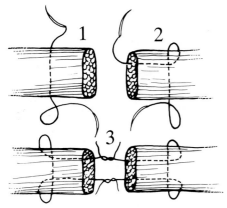

FIGURE 89-6.   The Tajima modification of the Kessler suture technique.

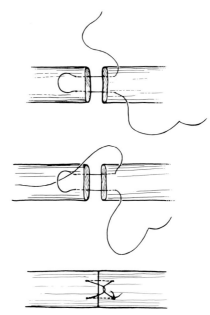

FIGURE 89-7.   The locking horizontal mattress stitch for "flat" tendons.

its side to the open end. Hold the tendon at its cut end with a Beasley-Babcock forceps. This technique is preferred to the conventional or modified Kessler, as the needles are not directed into the cut tendon ends, which seems to create fraying. Use a separate double-ended suture for each end. Once the sutures have been placed, cut the needles off, have the assistant hold tension on the two strands on that side, and tie the sutures on the surgeon's side with a square knot, with a few additional ties. While the assistant holds the tied suture, take up the slack on the untied side, just bringing the ends together, and tie the second side. In zone 5, additional tidying sutures are usually not taken. Occasionally, a horizontal mattress stitch with 6-0 nylon or polypropylene might be used to tuck in an irregular edge.

Muscle repairs are carried out using combinations of horizontal mattress and locking horizontal mattress sutures. In the locking stitch, instead of tying the two ends of the suture in the conventional manner, make one or two throws on the needle end of the suture, then place the needle holder tip through the loop end of the stitch, grasping the loose end on the far side and pull it through the loop (Fig. 89-7). This maneuver not only creates the stitch tension away from the wound edge and everts the edges, but also approximates the edges and prevents excessive eversion. This technique is also applicable in all tendon pairs where a horizontal mattress suture might be used (e.g., superficialis slips, chiasm of Camper) but excessive eversion is undesirable.

In zone 4, more meticulous tendon repair is required. After the Tajima sutures are tied, do not cut the two tied suture ends. Leave them inside the tendon initially. Have the assistant hold the long ends, and place a horizontal mattress or locking horizontal mattress stitch with 6-0 nylon in the outer layer of the tendon. The circumferential running stitch is begun away from the surgeon's side with the tendon flipped over (i.e., on the dorsal or back side). The stitches are taken toward the surgeon, the tendon is then returned to the palmar side and the suturing completed, tying finally to the initial stitch end. Although simple bites, 1 mm or so from the cut edge, are often satisfactory, it is desireable to invert these edges or at least make them even. To invert, take each stitch just behind the cut edge (Fig. 89-8), which rolls in the edge, leaving a repair without pouting edges. Healing is not adversely affected. After the repair of the structures in the carpal tunnel, rehabilitation must be undertaken,

either with the wrist in neutral or dorsiflexion to prevent palmar subluxation of the contents of the tunnel. Since it is preferable to flex the wrist up to 30°, I prefer to repair the transverse carpal ligament. Direct suture is not usually feasible; zigzag cuts on opening risk damage to the palmar cutaneous branch of the median nerve, which may run through the ligament, or to the motor branch of the median nerve. Consequently, I close the tunnel somewhat looser than its original ligament width by lacing it with a strip of tendon like a shoelace (usually using palmaris longus, but occasionally with a sagittal strip of flexor carpi radialis or an accessory tendon).

In zone 3, the repairs are performed in a similar manner. The lumbrical may be repaired, but if it is damaged in its muscle substance, it is probably better to excise it rather than to risk an imbalance due to intrinsic contracture. Repair both the superficialis and profundus if they are lacerated, and also repair a single tendon laceration. Restoration of digital strength and total function requires both tendons.

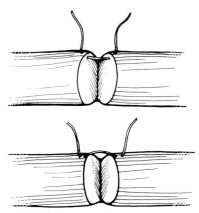

FIGURE 89-8.   Running stitch options at cut edge. The technique, depicted in the lower picture, slightly inverts the ends.

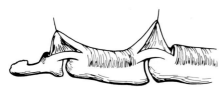

FIGURE 89-9. Lister's technique of opening the sheath to form a funnel.

In zone 2, the technique must be precise. Avoid scratching the tendon to avoid causing adhesions,[22] repair the bed, repair the tendon in a nonbulbous manner, and repair the sheath or pulley system.

Extend the wound into a zigzag or Bruner incision (see Figs. 89-5A and D). Expose the sheath and open it along the side to create a funnel, as described by Lister[14] (Fig. 89-9). The side cut joins the transverse wound in the sheath. If the tendon is sighted proximally, make a second incision more proximally, a mirror image of the first. The distal tendon can usually be easily exposed in this manner and with flexion of the distal joints. If the proximal end is not held by a vincula, or if the profundus alone is cut and not trapped at the metacarpophalangeal level where it passes through the superficialis, it is in the palm, held by the lumbrical. "Fishing" for the proximal end with grasping-type instruments is dangerous to the tendon, the bed, and proximally to blood vessels and nerves. If the proximal end cannot be kneaded and milked into the wound and then grasped with a mosquito hemostat in its cut end, make a proximal incision and find it. Pass a pediatric rubber feeding tube or a silicone-Dacron tendon rod distally to proximally through the sheath, and suture the tendon with a single nylon suture through the cut end to the eyelet in the tubing or to the rod, and draw it back into the distal wound. When both tendons are cut, bring them together distally. Bring the profundus through the superficialis, as the normal anatomic position. If a problem

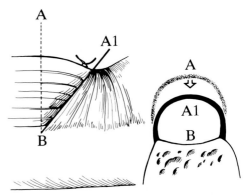

FIGURE 89-11. Buckling of the unrepaired sheath as the tendon attempts to pass through. Note loss of height of pulley (A–B to A1–B).

arises passing through the sheath, open the intervening skin bridge and create another sheath incision. Once the tendon (or tendons) is returned to the distal area, close the sheath opening with 6-0 nylon.

When the tendons are brought into the distal wound, hold them in that position by skewering them with a milliner's needle which passes through the sheath and the tendons proximally. Avoid the neurovascular bundles by placing the needle more palmarly. Keith needles have a cutting edge and are less desirable than the pointed milliner variety.

Except at the open end, where the tendon may be handled with the Beasley-Babcock forceps, handle the tendon with the thumb and index fingers with an interposed moist sponge.

Repair the superficialis slips or chiasm with horizontal mattress sutures or locking stitches, using 4-0 nylon. Collagen suture creates more reaction and is not advocated. Polypropylene is satisfactory; braided polyester sutures do not slide well and have been used but are no longer preferred. Braided nylon has also been satisfactory, but monofilament nylon and polypropylene are preferred.

Repair the profundus tendon with the Tajima technique with 3-0 or 4-0 nylon or polypropylene, with the cut edge repaired with the running stitch. If there has been damage to the periosteum under the tendons, repair it with 6-0 nylon. If it cannot be repaired, a graft of antebrachial fascia may be sutured in place as an interposing membrane. Fractures are repaired prior to tendons, of course, but if neurovascular repairs are indicated, particularly with an intact skeleton, it may be technically easier to retrieve tendons into the wound, and possibly place the Tajima sutures into the tendon but not tie them, initially, in order to perform the neurovascular surgery under the microscope on a flat (unflexed) digit.

When the tendons are repaired, repair the sheath with 6-0 nylon (Fig. 89-10). Leaving a gap in the sheath may result in sagging of the edge of the sheath as the tendon attempts to pass through it, decreasing vertical diameter, trapping the tendon (Fig. 89-11). Simple or horizontal mattress sutures are used to repair the sheath. If a gap remains, fill it by sewing antebrachial fascia to and over the underlying sheath (see Fig. 89-10). If a pulley is missing, reconstruct it, as described later.

In zone 1, the profundus is repaired as described for zone 2. The sheath is also reconstructed. Although there have been "successful" results with flexion "to the palm," and full flexion

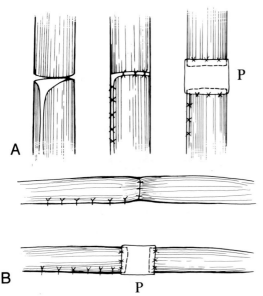

FIGURE 89-10. Closure and reconstruction of the tendon sheath. (A) Anteroposterior view of the sheath demonstrating repair and antebrachial fascial graft (P). (B) Lateral view of repair and graft (P).

FIGURE 89-12. Clinical photograph of a 90% partial tendon laceration.

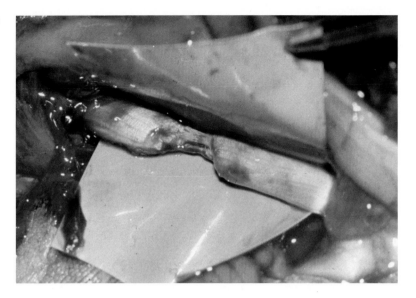

of the distal joint with the proximal interphalangeal joint in extension, full flexion to the distal palmar crease usually requires A5 pulley preservation or reconstruction. When the sheath is cut away, the sagging effect, as tendon moves proximally into the sheath, occurs, blocking full motion. Advancement of the profundus tendon, under the distal stump, for a reinsertion into bone rather than a tendon repair, is not recommended. The short tether or quadriga effect may occur with this maneuver, with loss of full flexion of the adjacent digits.[28] One can usually use this technique safely with the index finger, owing to its usual independence from the other profundi. Advancement still creates slack in the lumbrical, however, which may weaken or unbalance its action. Preferably, if the distal stump is short, take the Tajima stitch proximally, and then pass needles longitudinally through the stump, then adjacent to the sides of the distal phalanx, or through drill holes (with a 0.045-inch pin) in the phalanx from palmar to dorsal, emerging proximal to the germinal matrix of the nail bed, with the sutures tied over a dorsal button. Place horizontal mattress sutures at the cut edge.

Special Circumstances

Partial Lacerations

Three concerns exist with partial lacerations (Fig. 89-12): (1) that the tendon may rupture if it is not repaired; (2) that it will be weakened if sutures are placed in it; and (3) that the unrepaired portion may not fully heal and cause triggering (catching on the edge of the fibrous sheath system [A1]). All of these conditions exist. Based on the available studies, lacerations of

25% or less of the tendon's cross-sectional area in zones 3 and 5 are unrepaired, lacerations of 50% are repaired with horizontal mattress or locking type stitches, and lacerations of 75% or greater have the full repair. In zone 4, lacerations of 25% are tidied up with debridement. In zones 1 and 2, all partial lacerations are repaired; lacerations of 25% are repaired with simple sutures. The "frayed tendon" rehabilitation protocol is used postoperatively.

Segmental Injuries

If a tendon is cut in several locations, as in lawn mower–type injuries, it is similarly repaired in each location. If a segment is missing, it is replaced with a segmental tendon graft (Fig. 89-13). Palmaris or a segment of flexor carpi radialis is used. The length of graft needed is determined by traction on the distal segment to place the digit in its normal stance position (Fig. 89-14). Traction is then applied to the proximal end. Maximum traction determines the extent of the muscle's elasticity. No traction is the zero tension position. Some 50% to 60% of the maximal elasticity is close to the resting tension of

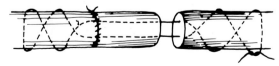

FIGURE 89-13. An intercalary graft repaired with a modified Bunnell suture technique.

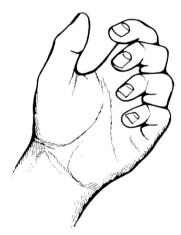

FIGURE 89-14. The normal digital cascade or stance position.

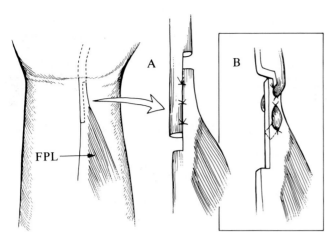

FIGURE 89-15. Lengthening of the flexor pollicis longus at the wrist associated with distal advancement in thumb zone 2. Two methods of repair of the lengthening are depicted. (Modified from Urbaniak, J.R.: Flexor Pollicis Longus Repair. Hand Clin. **1**:73, 1985.)

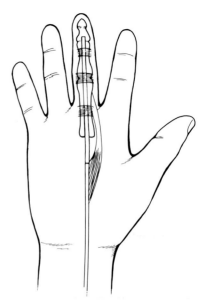

FIGURE 89-16. One-stage tendon grafting from the palm. More extensive pulley preservation is more common than the minimal number depicted. These three (with the proximal one somewhat closer to the metacarpophalangeal joint) are the most critical.

the muscle, which is the desired position. The amount of tendon graft and then a bit more, to achieve the normal stance position, is taken, sutured in tentatively, shortened accordingly, and the suturing completed. This segmental interpositional graft technique, frequently utilized for extensor tendons, is most applicable in zone 5, in zone 4 with longer grafts, and possibly in zone 3. In zones 1 and 2, grafting of the entire distal segment is more appropriate, as discussed subsequently.

Minimal and Maximal Frayed Tendons

Debridement and a special postoperative protocol may be adequate for the minimally frayed tendon that is primarily intact. For severely "chewed up" tendons, replacement is indicated. Segmental grafts are used in zones 3, 4, and 5. In zones 1 and 2, if the tendon is badly damaged and hence irreparable, but the bed is unharmed (not a common occurrence), a one-stage graft is applicable. This may be done primarily or delayed. Options are discussed in the section on grafting. If the bed and tendon are damaged, two-stage grafting is indicated. Placement of a tendon rod in the acute injury is questionable. I prefer to do this in the clean wound at 10 to 14 days.

Muscle Damage

If a profundus muscle is significantly damaged, tendon transfer, using the long or ring superficialis is indicated. When a lone superficialis muscle is injured and is irreparable, no reconstruction is done. For multiple or massive injuries on the flexor side, a transfer from the extensor side may be indicated.

Thumb Flexor Injuries

Lacerations of the flexor pollicis longus may be repaired with direct suture, advancement, or grafting, depending on the zone and preference of the surgeon[26] (see Fig. 89-5C). Direct suture is utilized more often than not, but the usual independence of the muscle-tendon unit (it is occasionally associated

with the profundus of the index) and the lack of lumbrical allow more repair options.

Urbaniak[26] has shown that the flexor pollicis longus may be advanced to the bone insertion when the laceration has occurred within 1.2 cm from the insertion. Between the metacarpophalangeal joint and this point, he advocates advancement with equivalent Z lengthening at the wrist, with and without reinforcing tendon grafting at the wrist (Fig. 89-15). Within the thenar zone, he prefers grafting. I have used these methods successfully, but today, I usually employ direct suture methods.[25] The technique and sheath repair methods are the same as in the digits. While access to the thenar zone is difficult, the injury that exposed and cut the tendon usually makes the access quite easy. If not, the pediatric feeding tube method to retrieve the proximal end and grafting may be necessary. The carpal tunnel frequently must be opened to retrieve the proximal end of the flexor pollicis longus. Direct suture methods have been most successful in achieving full active motion, which is represented by full extension of the thumb into the plane of the digits, and full flexion to the distal palmar crease of the little finger.

LATE RECONSTRUCTION

One-Stage Tendon Grafting

While one-stage tendon grafting was once a common procedure, advocated for all injuries in zone 2, today it has only occasional indications.[2,29] Specifically, it is indicated when the damage to the tendons in zone 1 or 2 is irreparable but the tendon bed is uninjured, or minimally so (Fig. 89-16). Prerequisites include a soft, pliable hand (and digit) with full passive motion of the joints.

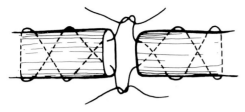

FIGURE 89-17. The modified Bunnell suture, similar to that advocated by Kleinert.

Exposure is generally carried out from the profundus insertion to the palm, using the Bruner or the midlateral incision, extending into the palm as a zigzag or sequential transverse incision (see Fig. 89-5B). Classically, the tendon sheath is partially excised, leaving only the three pulleys of Bunnell. Today, however, most of the pulley and tendon sheath system is preserved, removing only a sufficient amount to obtain access to the remaining portions of tendon. Proximally, the profundus left in the palm is short enough so it will not be drawn into the digital sheath when the digits are in full extension. The lumbrical origin remains, along with about an additional 1 to 2 cm. Distally, a short stump of profundus is preserved. The distal portion of the superficialis is left (the chiasm of Camper), and if it is not already adhered, it is sutured to the sheath proximally as a tenodesis, to prevent hyperextension of the proximal interphalangeal joint.

The usual source of tendon graft is the palmaris longus, taken either through multiple transverse incisions in the forearm, starting just proximal to the distal palmar wrist crease and removed retrograde by passing a small hemostat from the proximal to the distal wound. Alternately, I use the short forearm Brand tendon stripper, which is placed around the tendon distally and then advanced into the forearm while tension is maintained with a hemostat on the distal divided tendon. The device then avulses the tendon at the musculotendinous junction. Whether to remove paratenon or not is a moot question. I remove all muscle and the bulk of the paratenon, but do not compulsively remove all of it.

Distally, just under the profundus stump and distal to the insertion of the palmar plate of the distal interphalangeal joint, drill a hole with a $\frac{5}{64}$-inch drill bit through the palmar cortex of the distal phalanx. This is also distal to the epiphyseal plate in the immature bone. Make two drill holes with an 0.045-inch pin through the dorsal cortex on either side within the palmar cortical hole. Pull the tendon through the digit from the tip to the palm, after suturing it to either a reusable tendon rod or pediatric feeding tube. Make a Bunnell-type weave through a substantial end of the tendon with 3-0 polypropylene on milliner's needles (Fig. 89-17).

Pass the two needles through the bone and through dorsal skin proximal to the germinal matrix of the nail bed, through a rubber button pad, made from medicinal jar stoppers or the disposable irrigating syringe rubber bulb, and through the button. Pull the tendon end into the hole in the distal phalanx and tie the suture over the button (Fig. 89-18). Suture the profundus stump down to the graft with 2 to 4 simple sutures using 4-0 braided polyester suture. Test the integrity of the button by gently attempting to lift it away from the skin (to make certain the "safety sutures" to the stump did not cut the polypropylene). Traction on the proximal tendon graft should flex the digit to the distal palmar crease. If bowstringing

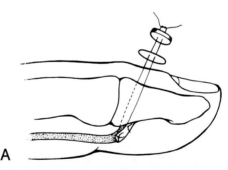

A

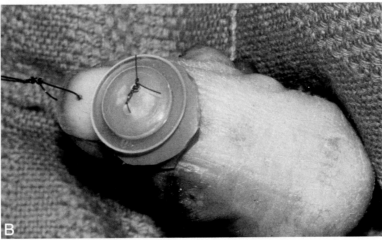

B

FIGURE 89-18. The tendon graft is drawn into the palmar cortex with the suture tied over the dorsal button and button pad. Note that the button suture is placed proximal to the nail and germinal matrix. The graft is sutured to the profundus stump as well. (A) Artist's drawing, lateral view. (B) Clinical photograph of dorsal button. The suture has been placed through the nail for postoperative therapy.

occurs, a pulley may need reconstruction. Then close the skin on the digit.

Although each step is important, this next one is especially critical—setting the proper tension. Make a slit in the distal end of the profundus stump in preparation for the Pulvertaft interweave suture (Fig. 89-19). Pull the motor tendon distally to 60% of its maximum elasticity, and pull the distal tendon graft through until the finger assumes a position slightly more flexed than its normal digital stance. Note that each finger, from radial to ulnar, is slightly more flexed (see Fig. 89-14). Using 4-0 braided polyester, suture the graft and motor tendon together with a simple or horizontal mattress suture. Then withdraw all support, place the wrist in neutral, and observe the stance of the digit. If it assumes the desired posture, the tenodesis effect is noted by flexing and extending the wrist. If the digit moves appropriately with the other fingers and returns to the proper position, the tension is correct; otherwise, it is tightened or loosened. When properly adjusted, make two additional slits at 90° from each other and from the first slit, and complete the weave and suturing. Fold the distal end of the stump around the graft (Fig. 89-19B). Making the slits can be facilitated with a "tendon braiding" forceps. Otherwise, use an 11 blade or a #64 Beaver with a small hemostat placed through the slit to pull through the tendon. Some surgeons wrap the lumbrical muscle around this connection; I prefer not to disturb the lumbrical. Then close the incisions in the palm. By suturing the finger before setting the tension, the zigzag wound is more easily closed, with corner stitches fitting more readily, and the surgeon does not have to assume a contorted position to achieve closure.

Variations in method include other sources of tendon graft: sagittal section of flexor carpi radialis, superficialis of the little finger, the proximal superficialis of the involved digit, and, from the leg, the plantaris or toe extensors. An interesting technique, known as a tenoplasty,[19] involves suturing the cut ends of the proximal profundus and superficialis together at the time of the initial injury. After a month, when this connection is healed, the proximal superficialis is divided in the wrist, drawn into the palm, threaded through the pulley system and attached distally, thus requiring only one connection in the second stage. However, I prefer palmaris or plantaris as grafts, owing to their usual ease of harvesting and lack of bulk. When they are not present, the alternatives are considered. Variations in distal insertions include suture to the profundus stump, through bone and back to tendon, through bone onto nail or tip of finger. When the tendon is brought through the tip of the finger, the tension may be readily set distally, with increased traction until the desired position is achieved. I prefer my own

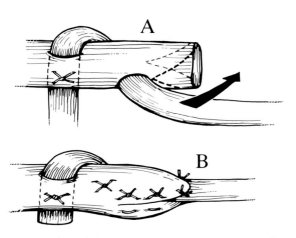

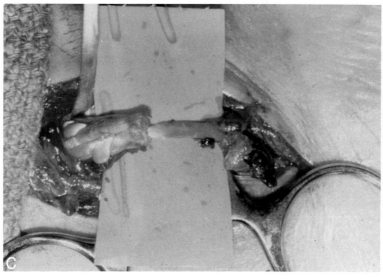

FIGURE 89-19. The Pulvertaft proximal interweave. (*A*) The initial pass of the graft through the motor tendon. (*B*) The motor tendon end is split and sutured around the graft. Two additional passes are usually made through the motor tendon with the openings made 90° to each other. (*C*) Clinical photograph of the proximal interweave. The motor end has not been sewn over. (Modified from Schneider, L.H., and Hunter, J.M.: Flexor Tendons—Late Reconstruction. In Green, D.P. (ed.): Operative Hand Surgery. New York, Churchill Livingston, 1982, p. 1387.)

method, which creates fewer problems with nail growth disturbance or digital pad contour irregularity.

Two-Stage Tendon Grafting

Stage One

Two-stage tendon grafting is a salvage procedure based on the concept that the first stage reconstructs the bed and the pulley system, and the second replaces the tendon.[10,23] The initial step places a silicone tube (Carroll)[1] or silicone or silicone-Dacron rod (Hunter-Swanson or Hunter),[10] shaped like a tendon, into the digit, which results in the formation of a pseudosheath around the rod. The rod is fixed distally and unattached proximally, either at the palm or wrist level. I prefer the silicone-Dacron Hunter rod method and discuss this method below.

The first stage of the procedure is usually performed under brachial plexus block anesthesia. Expose the digit through the extended Bruner incision from the profundus insertion to the palm, and through a curvilinear incision in the wrist.

The exposure in the hand is the same as in one-stage grafting. Preserve the distal profundus stump of about 1.5 cm, as well as the tenodesis effect of the distal end of the superficialis. Preserve or rebuild the pulleys, and carry exposure to the palm. Remove other residual bits of tendon by sharp excision with a Beaver blade (#64). Local scar tissue may be used to fashion a tunnel where the old pulley system was once located (Fig. 89-20). Preserve or create pulleys at the base of the proximal phalanx, over the proximal interphalangeal joint, and in the mid-middle phalanx.

In the wrist, locate the profundus to the involved digit, leave it attached distally to the lumbrical to maintain its resting length, and tag it in the wrist with a colored suture. The superficialis tendon is usually withdrawn into the wrist and excised; sagittal strips of it may be used for pulley reconstruction. Apply distal traction to the profundus at the wrist level to determine its elasticity, which should be equal to the uninvolved adjacent profundus tendons. If it has lost its elasticity due to severe myostatic contracture, the superficialis is left adhered in the palm, tested, and if adequate, tagged as the future motor. If neither is adequate, choose and tag an adjacent superficialis.

Then select an appropriately sized (width) tendon rod. Usually, a size 4 or 5 is correct for the digits, with the wider 5 needed for thumbs, and the 3 for little fingers, smaller people, or children. The rod should fill the proposed sheath but move easily through it. It must also be large enough to create an adequate pseudosheath for the future tendon graft.

The rod is maintained under saline or antibiotic solution in saline until usage, to avoid lint accumulation. It is then handled primarily with smooth instruments or wet gloves. Pass the pointed end of the rod through the digital sheath from distal to proximal to the palm level. Then pass a long hemostat or Kelly clamp just palmar to the profundus and below the superficialis tendons (dorsal to them) through the carpal tunnel (usually on the proposed motor tendon) to the palm to the lumbrical level. Grasp the rod and draw it into the wrist. Place the distal end of the rod snugly under the profundus stump and suture it securely with four simple or horizontal mattress stitches of braided polyester (Fig. 89-21). If a profundus stump is not available, alternatives include suture to periosteum or use of a special rod that has a screw attached that can be fixed to the distal phalanx.

With traction applied to the rod, the finger should flex to the distal palmar crease without bowstringing. Using a large hemostat, open the space palmar to the profundi at the distal forearm. The proximal end of the rod fits into this space (Fig. 89-22). Now, test passive motion of the finger in full flexion and extension to determine if there is any buckling in the digit or the wrist. Extra length of rod in the wrist can be excised. In the palm, a bridge or pulley can be loosened to prevent buckling or a new pulley reconstructed. If buckling persists after skin closure, erosion of the rod through the skin can occur.

Pulley Reconstruction

Reconstruction is frequently required. It may also be needed during acute repair, one-stage grafting, and in tenolysis or after

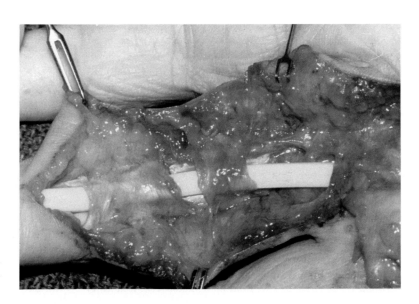

FIGURE 89-20. Clinical photograph of silicone-dacron tendon rod placed through original tendon sheath and pulley system. Tunnelling is also done through healed scar.

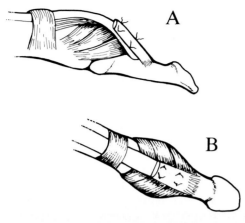

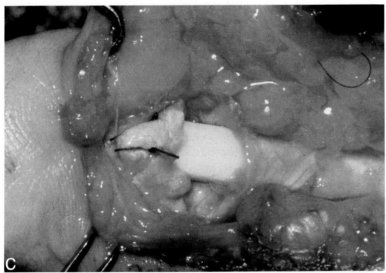

FIGURE 89-21. The tendon rod is sutured under the old profundus stump. (*A*) Lateral view. (*B*) Anteroposterior view. (*C*) Clinical photograph.

tenolysis. My preferred technique is that described by Kleinert and attributed to Weilby.[11] Other methods, for example, that of Lister,[13] can also be employed. The residual base of the annular ligaments and underlying periosteum is employed, along with a long narrow strip of tendon. If superficialis is used, a sagittal strip about one-eighth the width of the tendon is created, several inches in length.

Make a slit through the remnant of the annular ligament on either side of the rod using a #64 Beaver blade or an 11 blade, and place the tips of a cardiovascular hemostat through the slit to grasp the tendon. Draw the tendon over the rod and down through the opposite slit. Make several more pairs of slits distally. Criss-cross the tendon over the rod, through the slits, like a shoelace through eyelets in a shoe. Finally, cinch the lacing (pulley) enough to eliminate bowstringing and yet loose enough to allow passage of the rod during passive range of motion. Pass the tendon ends through themselves or through proximal criss-crosses and suture them.

The technique is effective for immediate utilization without healing, owing to the friction of the interweave and passage through the slits (Fig. 89-23). A simple pulley reconstruction, particularly applicable to the A3 area, over the proximal interphalangeal joint, involves usage of one residual slip of superficialis left attached distally, with the proximal end woven through or sutured to the annular ligament remnant (Fig. 89-24).

Interval Between Stages One and Two

In the interval between stages, the tendon rod is moved back and forth with passive range of motion of the digit. This can be done with passive range using the opposite hand to move the digit through its range, or by trapping the digit using adjacent fingers to draw it into flexion. The intact extensor mechanism extends the digit. If a capsulectomy or use of an artificial joint accompanied placement of the tendon rod, dynamic splinting may be used. This may include a low profile extensor assist splint, alternating with flexor assist rubber band or thread devices or individual spring-loaded assistive joint extensors, flexors, and adjustable static devices. The hand therapist plays a very significant role in helping the patient to achieve a maximum range at this point. It should be appreciated that the maximum attainable range, actively, after the second stage will be no more than that achieved passively at this time.

Ideally, the rod remains in place for about 2 months, possibly 3, to achieve a good pseudosheath, which is also soft, sheer, and flexible. Persistence of the rod beyond this time leads to a thicker, fibrous, less flexible pseudosheath with a poorer end result.

Prior to proceeding with stage two, tendon rod films are taken to determine if the distal end of the rod is in place, if buckling is absent, and if the excursion of the rod is 1 cm or more. If these criteria are not met, stage one may need to be revised. It is not unheard of for the distal end of the rod to break loose and piston into the wrist.[23] Obtain anteroposterior and lateral views of the hand and forearm (fingertips to mid-forearm) in full extension and full passive flexion of the involved digit. To determine excursion, measure the proximal tip of the rod from any fixed bony landmark. Assuming all is well, now proceed to stage two.

The most common problem in stage one is achieving good range of motion. This is essential, however, so do not proceed without it. Occasionally, an inflammatory reaction may occur with the rod. Rest, immobilization, and antibiotics and anti-inflammatories are tried for 10 to 14 days. If the problem quiets down, therapy is resumed. If not, reentry, rod removal, and debridement are indicated. If infection exists, one can utilize suction-irrigation and systemic antibiotics to clear the digit and try again later with rerodding. Most of these attempts are unsuccessful and other approaches to the digit, such as fusions or amputation, may be indicated. If only inflammation occurred, this may have been due to lint contamination and another attempt at rodding is warranted.

Stage Two

The second stage of this procedure is relatively straightforward for the experienced surgeon; the bed is prepared, the pulleys rebuilt, and one needs only add the free tendon graft, connecting it properly at either end. In fact, these steps are identical to those used in one-stage grafting. Unfortunately, there are still pitfalls peculiar to stage two grafting.

The procedure is done under general anesthesia with the arm and a leg prepped (usually the contralateral leg, so a second team can take the graft unencumbered). Prepping is done from digital tips to groin and axilla). Locate the plantaris with a short transverse incision made over the medial edge of the tendo achilles, approximately four finger breadths above the tip of the medial malleolus. If one looks more distally, the tendon may have already fused with the larger tendon or it may

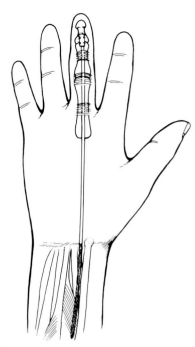

FIGURE 89-22. Tendon rod in first stage of two-stage tendon grafting. The tendon rod is sewn under the profundus stump but lies free in the wrist, under the superficialis and on the profundi. The proximal pulley is drawn somewhat too distally.

be located behind it. It is generally absent or deficient about 14% of the time. Assuming it is present and not hypoplastic, make a second more distal incision, divide the tendon and withdraw it into the proximal wound. Then split the fascia proximally and place the ring of the Brand tendon stripper over the tendon, which is grasped through the ring with a hemostat. With the leg straight and level (usually resting on two folded towels), advance the stripper slowly with a twisting mo-

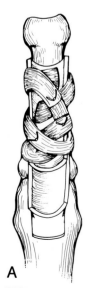
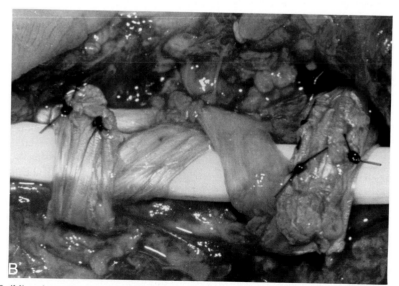

FIGURE 89-23. Building the pulley using the remnant of the old annular ligament system and a strip of tendon; method described by Kleinert and attributed to Weilby. (*A*) Artist's rendition. (*B*) Clinical photograph of pulley built over a tendon rod.

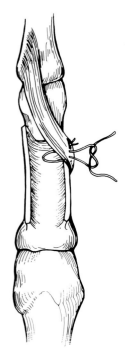

FIGURE 89-24. Pulley built with remaining distal slip of superficialis, placed through and sutured to the remnant of the annular ligament. (Modified from Schneider, L.H., and Hunter, J.M.: Flexor Tendons—Late Reconstruction. In Green, D.P. (ed.): Operative Hand Surgery. New York, Churchill Livingstone, 1982, p. 1425.)

tion of the fingertips while the tendon is held relatively tautly. There is one interval, as the stripper passes between the gastrocnemius and the soleus, where progress is slow and one must be patient so as not to prematurely cut the tendon. Then advance the instrument to the musculotendinous junction, avulse the tendon, and deliver it. Debride muscle and paratenon, but do not remove paratenon compulsively.

If the plantaris is not present or adequate, I prefer to use a toe extensor. If one is grafting for a little finger, only to the superficialis insertion (see the discussion below on Salvage), or to a thumb, a palmaris may be long enough. It is easy enough, in the absence of the plantaris, to take the palmaris, and measure it (on the surface), before proceeding with the toe extensor, which is more difficult to harvest and can result in more morbidity.

The advantage of the toe extensors is that they are always present and are long enough. The short extensor substitutes for the long. The disadvantages are the interconnections between the tendons under the extensor retinaculum and proximally, which make it impossible to harvest a smooth, unblemished tendon, and the time it takes to deliver the specimen. The procedure begins with a transverse incision, just proximal to the level of the metatarsophalangeal joint over the prominent tendon. The fifth is not used, as there is no extensor brevis. I find the third and fourth usually are easiest to harvest. Locate the brevis and suture it to the longus, which is then divided proximally. With traction on the cut end, identify the tendon proximally and make a second transverse incision. With the fascia divided, pass a hemostat distally over the exposed proximal tendon to the distal wound, where the cut end is grasped,

and the tendon delivered retrograde into the proximal wound. Continue proximally until an adequate length is obtained. The maneuver is easy distally, but proximally, the tendon must be separated from its mates. This is done partially by peeling the tendon from the others, and partially with a scissors. Closer interval incisions, proximally, will facilitate this activity. A bulky elastic dressing is used on the leg for about 2 weeks.

On the upper extremity, open the curvilinear incision on the wrist, exposing the tagged motor tendon and the proximal end of the rod. Again test the motor for elasticity. One can still use another motor. Remove the pseudosheath from the end of the rod, and expose the incision over the distal end of the rod. I prefer to open the old zigzag, as a midlateral in a scarred finger, at this point, is more likely to injure digital nerve branches. Note the sutures taken through the profundus stump; locate the proximal extent of the stump, and carefully lift the stump away from the underlying rod as the sutures are cut. At this point, it is important not to damage the pseudosheath under the rod or to damage the palmar plate. A shading differentiation between the white palmar plate and the more opalescent pseudosheath distally over the bone should be apparent. Take the pseudosheath just distal to the plate off the bone with the Beaver #64 blade, and drill a hole with a $5/64$-inch bit through the palmar cortex (as with the one-stage graft). Make two more holes on either side with 0.045-inch pins, from inside the hole through the dorsal cortex, to emerge proximal to the nail and the germinal matrix.

Suture the tendon graft to the rod, proximally, and pull it through the pseudosheath (Fig. 89-25). In the event that the tendon pulls free, it is a simple matter to reinsert the rod through the pseudosheath. Place a hemostat on the proximal tendon and take a weave stitch (usually a Bunnell type) through the distal end with 3-0 polypropylene on milliner's needles, which are then placed through the drill holes to be tied over the dorsal bottom and "button pad" (see Fig. 89-18, One-Stage Graft technique). Draw the tendon snugly into the bone before tying the suture. Secure the graft to the residual profundus stump with safety stitches of 4-0 braided polyester suture. With traction on the proximal tendon, the digit should fully flex, or do so to the extent achieved with passive motion.

Release the motor tendon from its distal attachment at the wrist crease level. Close the incision on the digit and attach the graft to the motor tendon at the proper tension, using the Pulvertaft interweave stitch (see One-Stage Graft technique). Again, this is achieved by making a slit in the motor tendon, which has been pulled up to 60% of its elastic length and by pulling the graft through until the digit assumes a position of flexion slightly greater than the normal stance position relative to the other digits. After the first trial stitch, test the position with the tenodesis maneuver, flexing and extending the wrist. If the digit moves with the other fingers and then, with the wrist in neutral, achieves the proper digital stance, make two additional slits in the motor tendon and complete the interweave. Rehabilitation is described in the final section of the chapter. The position of immobilization in the dressing is with the wrist flexed 30°, the metacarpophalangeals in 75° to 90° of flexion, and the interphalangeals toward extension (the intrinsic plus position). The bulky dressing with a posterior plaster splint is carried above elbow, initially, to enforce elevation.

The potential problems with this stage of the procedure

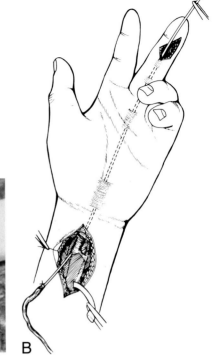

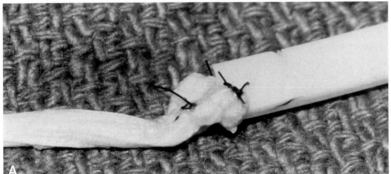

FIGURE 89-25. Stage two tendon grafting. The tendon graft is attached to the rod, which is then drawn out of the hand distally, pulling the tendon through the pseudosheath. (*A*) Clinical photograph of tendon graft sutured to the rod. (*B*) Artist's illustration of graft about to be drawn into the hand.

include detachment of the graft proximally or distally or both, rupture of the graft, adherence of the graft to the sheath, and a flexion contracture of the distal interphalangeal joint. To avoid rupture of the graft or pulling out of the suture distally, take an adequate graft. Do not accept a graft of too small diameter or one with iatrogenic defects. If the graft is damaged or hypoplastic, take the time to harvest the toe extensor. It is not worth the grief that results if this point is not heeded.

To confirm the integrity of the distal polypropylene suture, test that the "safety" stitches have not cut it by gently lifting the button, making sure it is springy, and applying traction to the proximal tendon. If one does not start the polypropylene weave distally more than 1.0 to 1.5 cm from the end of the graft one is usually safe. The proximal attachment is usually safe with a three-slit interweave. If the motor muscle tendon unit is elastic and then has good excursion, the pseudosheath is not thick and fibrous, and the rehabilitation is appropriate, then adhesion in the sheath should not be a problem. If the proximal attachment is in the forearm and not the carpal tunnel, the adhesions at this site can be worked out with activity. A flexion contracture at the distal interphalangeal joint remains an enigma. Avoiding iatrogenic damage to the palmar plate and attending to the problem with therapy are obvious. Pseudosheath contracture may be a factor. Two additional controllable factors may be (1) preserving the A5 pulley, and (2) placing the tendon insertion just distal to the palmar plate, not further distal on the distal phalanx. With attention to all these factors, flexion contracture still occurs in some patients, and although the digit is functional, its appearance is compromised. An ar-

throdesis of the distal interphalangeal joint is the solution in severe cases.

Tendon Grafting for the Flexor Digitorum Profundus with an Intact Flexor Digitorum Superficialis

Ideally, of course, if a profundus is lacerated and the superficialis is intact, one repairs the cut tendon. If, however, the injury is unrecognized or the repair has ruptured, one may be faced with a finger that functions well with full mobility at the metacarpophalangeal and proximal interphalangeal joints, but the tip of which is flail. The dilemma is whether to maintain this full functional proximal interphalangeal motion, sacrificing distal interphalangeal motion, stabilizing the tip in some way, or to risk the excellent motion; that is, compromise the superficialis' full function for the sake of some distal interphalangeal control. Nongrafting measures are tenodesis or arthrodesis of the distal interphalangeal joint.

The goal is to prevent "giving way" or hyperextension of the distal interphalangeal joint during pinch or grasp. In some cases, a tenodesis may already exist from adherence of the distal profundus across the distal interphalangeal joint. It may be accomplished surgically by suturing down the profundus stump to the sheath, residual annular ligament, and periosteum. The joint is pinned for a month and then mobilized. The position of immobilization is in 5° to 10° of flexion for the digits and in 0° or neutral for the interphalangeal joint of the thumb. Theoretically, the digital interphalangeal joints should be increasingly flexed across the hand from radial to ulnar, allowing grip to the distal palmar crease. In reality, this is not necessary for strength if the joint is stable. A flexed or a 'hooked' finger is undesireable functionally and cosmetically. My problem with tenodesis is the "stretching out" of some and the further contraction of others.

With these problems in mind, I prefer arthrodesis. The fusion can be done in a variety of ways.

Grafting is probably most indicated in the small digit where the superficialis is often smaller than normal and may be deficient. It may also rupture if sufficient stress is placed on it (I once observed one rupture 30 years after the profundus injury!). Otherwise, the decision to graft is made after considerable discussion with the patient concerning the potential benefits and risks. Grafting is most applicable in young patients. If the digit is mobile, a one-stage graft is a consideration. A two-stage procedure is more risky for the superficialis, but it is indicated if there is distal bed damage. Goldner has recommended that neither the graft nor the rod should be placed through the split in the superficialis, but rather placed along side in the sheath.[9] Of course, the sheath may have contracted around a single tendon if the profundus has retracted significantly. It is altogether reasonable to suggest to the patient that you may attempt to graft, but if the attempt appears more formidable once the finger is explored, then the distal stabilization will be carried out instead.

Options for the Thumb

When the flexor pollicis longus injury is irreparable, unrecognized, or ruptured, options of one- or two-stage grafting may also be considered. If the muscle has lost its elasticity, a tendon transfer may also be performed, either as one stage, if the bed and pulley system are good, or two stages, through a pseudo-sheath. The usual motor is the superficialis to the ring finger, although the long finger tendon is equally acceptable. If two stages are planned, a large rod, either size 5 or 6, is needed and should be matched for size with the potential motor in the first stage. No graft supplement is needed, as the tendon reaches the distal phalanx easily. Also, with the flexor pollicis brevis, and the adductor and abductor pollicis all acting to flex the metacarpophalangeal joint, arthrodesis of the interphalangeal joint can be considered. The strength and normal function of the thumb are significantly aided by a functioning flexor pollicis longus. The function of the intrinsics is not at significant risk with grafting or transfer, as with an intact superficialis to a digit, so that interphalangeal fusion of the thumbs is far less indicated. It is, however, an option, particularly when there are multiple injuries and transfers and grafts are more important elsewhere.

TENOLYSIS

Tenolysis is indicated when active motion fails to equal the passive range and it is determined that this is due to tendon adhesion or block. The extent of full motion required for functional status depends on the patient's actual requirements and wishes, and a realistic expectation of the results of surgery.

A thumb, for example, that can pinch well to all the digits and particularly to the index and long fingers, but does not flex to the distal palmar crease proximal to the little finger is not disabled by most criteria. However, a digit that does not flex to the palm and defunctionalizes all the others as well (quadriga) is very disabling. The musician, specifically a string player, such as a violinist or cellist, may be significantly more disabled than a keyboard player with the same absent range. Therefore, the decision to perform a tenolysis is individualized.

Timing is also important. It takes time to maximally mobilize a digit and for the tendon to be revascularized. Two negative results of tenolysis are (1) failure to maintain gliding, and (2) rupture. Premature tenolysis may well be the cause of the latter. At least 4 months should elapse before tenolysis to allow adequate revascularization of the tendon so that it can tolerate the procedure. The contraindication to tenolysis, too extensive adhesions, is discussed below.

Tenolysis is a potentially formidable procedure. The results are directly proportional to the extent of the adhesions. If there is a small "spot weld," one might anticipate subsequent full function (to the extent of the passive motion). If the adhesions are extensive and there will be multiple healing or "raw" areas, the likelihood of success is nil. The amount of the initial trauma, particularly the number of tissues injured (bone, sheath, tendon, vessels, etc.) and the extent proximally and distally of damaged structures, determines the density of the adhesions in many cases. However, a simple tendon laceration, with or without infection, may result in multiple adhesions for a considerable distance.

My approach is to tenolyze if the adhesions are limited or if there is a history of infection, and to employ two-stage tendon grafting (insert a rod), if the adhesions are extensive from trauma.

Many surgeons carry out tenolysis under local anesthesia, preferring the patient to begin active mobilization immediately. I prefer to do the procedure under regional block. Therapy may be initiated with the block still in effect, and continuous passive motion (CPM) seems to be helpful, particularly in controlling discomfort. Continuous passive motion is especially indicated if capsulectomy accompanies tenolysis. Leaving an indwelling catheter in the palm around the digital nerves, or around the median or ulnar nerve (if this is adequate), for the injection of a long acting anesthetic is a valuable adjunct postoperatively.

The surgical technique consists of sharply releasing the adherent scar through generous incisions, as needed. The more incisions needed, the more postoperative scarring, of course. As pulleys need to be removed, they must be rebuilt. Classically, tenolysis is carried out, the digit rehabilitated, and then the pulley rebuilt to eliminate the unsightly, uncomfortable bowstringing, in a later operation. Using the surgical technique described earlier for constructing pulleys, immediate construction can be undertaken.

Investigate the site of the initial trauma or surgery first, extending in either direction to open the sheath and determine whether the tendon is free. Remove adherent sheath, done using a Beaver knife blade and Penfield elevators (usually number 4) for the dissection. If the release seems sufficient, particularly if the digit only is involved, make an additional incision in the palm at the lumbrical level and apply traction to pull the tendons proximally. If motion is full with each tendon, apply traction distally to make sure the tendons glide well through the carpal tunnel. At the completion of the procedure, place the indwelling catheter in the hand or wrist to aid with the postoperative care.

POSTOPERATIVE CARE

Obstacles to successful rehabilitation following flexor tendon repair include potential for rupture, adherence of the tendon to surrounding tissues, and joint contractures. Philosophies of postoperative management vary along a continuum from 3 to 4 weeks of complete immobilization, with the intent of minimizing the risk of rupture, to very early protected active mobilization, with emphasis on minimizing tendon adherence and joint contracture. Although controlled clinical studies are few, recent research definitely lends support to the concept of at least early passive mobilization methods of management[7,8,15] (Fig. 89-26).

Many variables must be considered in determining the best method of management for each clinical setting. The degree of trauma and surgical technique will influence the strength of the repair and the degree of scarring. The experience and skill of the therapist are critical factors in the delicate balancing of protection versus mobilization during the early postoperative weeks. The patient's behavior, attitude, and intelligence must be considered in terms of his or her ability to comprehend and implement instructions, degree of motivation, reliability, and availability for follow-up. Consideration of these factors, past experience with joint contractures and well-healed but adherent tendons, and reports from other hand centers have led to

an evolution in our approach over the past 10 years, from 4 weeks of immobilization to an early protected motion program.

Primary Repairs

Although the potential for dense tendon adherence is greater in zones 2 and 4, where there is less yielding adjacent tissue and more confined space, early protected motion management is used for all zones.

Day One

Wrap the wrist in a bulky dressing, and keep it at 30° flexion, with the metacarpophalangeal joints in 70° to 90° flexion, allowing full active interphalangeal extension. Elevate it to control edema.

Elastic traction is attached to a nail suture (provided at time of surgery), and proximally about 8 cm proximal to the palmar wrist crease. Tension should be adequate to maintain the involved digits in a flexed position at rest, yet allow full active interphalangeal extension (Fig. 89-27).

The patient is instructed to actively extend the interphalangeal joint *fully* 5 to 10 times every hour. If extension is difficult or painful, the patient may need to pull the traction distally with the other hand while extending to facilitate full active extension, then release slowly to return the finger passively to the flexed position.

Potential Problems and Variations. Among the problems that may occur are (1) no nail suture; (2) pain or apprehension, limiting full, active interphalangeal extension; (3) inadequate fit of bulky dressing, allowing some metacarpophalangeal extension as the patient attempts to extend the interphalangeals; (4) swelling, relieved by elevation and use of a compression wrap; and (5) interphalangeal flexion contractures.

Days Three to Seven

The bulky dressing is removed, and the hand redressed in a light dressing. It is then placed in a thermoplastic splint with dorsal extension to the fingertips and joint positions are maintained. A palmar piece is added to contour to the palmar arch (to assure stable positioning of the dorsum of the hand in the splint). Otherwise, the splint may have a tendency to slip, and as the patient extends the interphalangeals, the dorsum of the hand may pull away from the splint, resulting in metacarpophalangeal extension, rather than full interphalangeal extension. Two-inch velfoam straps to the forearm and wrist are used with a 1-inch strap across the palmar piece, if necessary. A pulley is attached to the palmar piece. Nylon cord is attached to the nail suture, run through the pulley, and attached to elastic traction. The elastic is attached to a safety pin on the proximal splint strap. The nylon should be of just adequate length so that the elastic does not catch on the pulley during active extension (Fig. 89-28).

Elevation of the hand is continued as are compression wraps for the hand and digits, if necessary, to control edema.

The same exercises are continued, with emphasis on full interphalangeal extension. Early flexion contractures may be

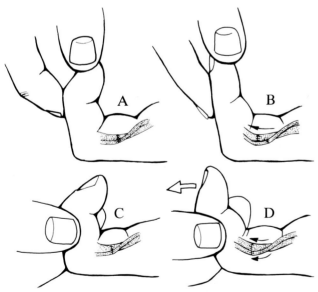

FIGURE 89-26. Postoperative passive motion regimen described by Duran. (*A* and *B*) With proximal interphalangeal joint maintained in a flexed position, the distal interphalangeal joint is flexed (*A*) and fully extended (*B*). (*C* and *D*) With the distal interphalangeal joint maintained in flexed position, the proximal interphalangeal joint is carefully exercised. Both activities create gentle passive motion of tendons, promoting both strong healing, and gliding.

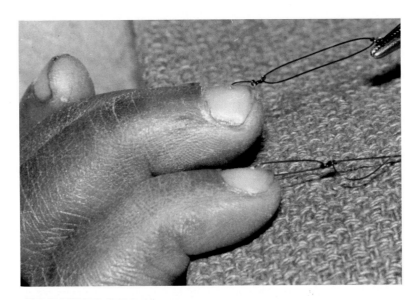

FIGURE 89-27. Suture loops through nails for postoperative controlled passive motion method of Kleinert.

carefully managed with gentle assistive extension of the involved joint with the proximal and distal joints flexed.

The patient is seen twice per week, if possible, to ensure maintenance of positioning and good progress.

Problems and Variations. This stage may be delayed at the discretion of the surgeon if there is excessive trauma or a tenuous repair.

Three Weeks

At 3 weeks, increase the wrist splint position to neutral. Continue traction and exercise program, adding an active flexion hold *after* the digit is passively flexed fully five times per hour. This step requires maximum tendon excursion without maximum tensile loading that results with active flexion from the fully extended position.

Problems and Variations. If impending flexion contractures of the interphalangeal joints are noted, discontinue elastic traction at night and use a static extension strap to dorsal extension of the splint, extending the proximal interphalangeal only. A static aluminum splint may be used for the proximal

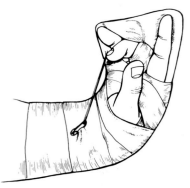

FIGURE 89-28. Postoperative controlled passive motion thermoplastic splint with elastic traction. The splint maintains the metacarpophalangeal joint in flexion, while allowing full extension of proximal interphalangeals against the elastic band.

interphalangeal or distal interphalangeal, but it must be directed to *one* joint only to avoid tendon tension.

If soft tissue contracture appears likely at the metacarpophalangeal, owing to the level of injury, maintain the wrist at 30° flexion and increase metacarpophalangeal extension to 40° to 45°.

The rehabilitation staff is instructed to discuss program changes with the surgeon if any question exists about patient status. Very free joint mobility and tendon excursion may indicate minimal scarring, but the tendon may be more vulnerable to rupture.

Five Weeks

At this time, discontinue the splint, but continue traction to the wrist cuff. Full active wrist and digit motion is allowed, but with protection from full tendon tension via the tenodesis effect. Begin joint blocking with the wrist and metacarpophalangeals in neutral, along with full active flexion from the extended position, ten times per hour. Dynamic flexion splinting can be added, if necessary. Static individual joint extension splinting with the adjacent joints neutral or flexed may be indicated by lack of progress with active and assistive exercise alone.

Problems and Variations. If wrist extension is limited significantly, continue neutral wrist splinting with traction. Remove the splint for exercise.

Six Weeks

Discontinue traction, and continue exercise as at five weeks, but the wrist and digits may be extended simultaneously. Add individual dynamic joint extension splinting, if indicated, with the wrist neutral.

Eight to Twelve Weeks

Full dynamic extension splinting may be added at 8 weeks, if necessary. Graded resistive exercise and activity are added at 10 weeks. By 12 weeks the patient may return to full activity.

Thumb Care

Postoperative management of primary flexor tendon repairs of the thumb is similar to that of the fingers with the following exceptions: the wrist is flexed 30° to 35°; the thumb carpometacarpal joint is held in palmar abduction; the metacarpophalangeal joint is in flexion, with elastic traction attached to the nail via a nylon cord run through the same type of palmar pulley as described for the fingers. When full active flexion is initiated, in addition to joint blocking and opposition exercises, full tendon excursion is encouraged by full active extension of the carpometacarpal, metacarpophalangeal, and interphalangeal, followed by flexion of the thumb toward the base of the little finger.

The patient should be cautioned during the first 5 postoperative weeks against attempted use of the uninvolved digits, as contraction of the flexor digitorum superficialis and flexor digitorum profundus, particularly against resistance, may stress the repaired tendon. Close follow-up is essential for success. If positioning is lost, exercise techniques are incorrect, or adjustments are not made for impending contractures, the results will not be optimal.

Tenolysis

Postoperatively, the primary goal is to maintain the degree of excursion of the lysed tendon achieved at surgery. Consider carefully all factors pertaining to each patient's clinical situation, including (1) the patient's history, (2) previous surgery, (3) preoperative status, (4) the condition of the tendon, and (5) the status of the pulley system. Excessive edema or pain, or diminished vascularity from previous injury or surgery, previous infections, and poor tendon quality and pulley reconstruction are all factors that may require modification of postoperative care in order to achieve the maximum potential without complications.

Twelve to Twenty-Four Hours Postoperative

Remove the bulky dressing and redress the wrist with Xeroform and Kling bandages, using sterile technique. For pain control use TENS, or an in-dwelling catheter with a 0.5% Marcaine injection prior to therapy. Edema is controlled with elevation and a compression wrap, if necessary.

With the wrist in neutral and joint blocking to isolate the flexor digitorum profundus and flexor digitorum superficialis, total flexion and extension are performed ten times each, hourly. With the wrist neutral, passively flex the involved digits, then ask the patient to actively maintain the position. Remove the passive force while the patient continues to hold. This is followed with active extension and the patient repeats the exercise ten times hourly. This requires maximum flexor and extensor excursion while reducing tensile loading of the lysed tendon.

The patient is seen three to five times per week to encourage exercise in spite of pain, with the goal of active range of motion equal to passive. Achievement of this goal within the first two weeks is critical. Joint range of motion, total active range of motion, and total passive motion are measured twice weekly to monitor progress objectively.

Splinting at night and between exercise sessions varies, depending on the tendency toward joint stiffness or the difficulty the patient may find in initiating motion from either a flexed or extended position. Dynamic or static flexion is indicated if there is difficulty regaining preoperative passive flexion, or active flexion is difficult if active extension is easily achieved. Gentle static individual joint extension splinting is helpful in the presence of impending flexion contractures. Discomfort may be minimized by use of a static wrist support in neutral position. Full dynamic extension splints that fully stress the lysed tendon should be delayed until 2 to 6 weeks, depending on tendon status.

Two Weeks

Remove sutures and begin skin debridement and lubrication, as well as scar remodeling techniques. Scar massage and elastomer molds will help to soften and flatten dense elevated or adherent scars. Exercise emphasis is continued, adding joint blocking and full flexion and extension of the digits with the wrist in a dorsiflexed position.

Six to Twelve Weeks

Graded resistive exercise should begin at 6 weeks. By 8 to 12 weeks the patient may return to full activity, including heavy work.

In the presence of a poor quality tendon post-tenolysis, additional protection may be required. The patient is fit with a dorsal protective splint, maintaining the wrist and metacarpophalangeals in flexion to protect the lysed tendon. Elastic traction, as described, with primary tendon repairs may be delayed until 4 weeks postoperatively. Active exercise is limited to passively flexing the involved digits, then asking the patient to actively maintain the position while the passive force is removed. This may be followed with full active extension within the protection of the splint, and will achieve the goal of maximum flexor excursion while reducing the potential risk of rupture.

Continuous passive motion (CPM) devices and protocols, noted earlier, remain investigational. Their use following tenolysis, particularly when capsulectomy was also required, appears beneficial, but active motion with proximal blocking is also necessary, as with the standard technique.

Staged Flexor Tendon Reconstruction

Postoperative Goals

Stage One. The goal is to maximize joint mobility and soft tissue pliability during new sheath formation around the implant.

Stage Two. The goal here is restoration of passive mobility and achievement of a gliding graft within the pseudosheath for optimum active mobility.

Precautions

Stage One. Synovitis may occur, usually within 6 weeks postoperatively, as a result of implant surface contaminants, buckling of the implant, or overzealous therapy. This can usually be avoided with careful handling of the implant and appropriate pulley reconstruction at surgery, and careful postoperative management. Synovitis is characterized by discomfort in the operated digit and swelling with no signs of systemic illness. It is treated with immediate rest and immobilization. Concurrent procedures such as capsulectomy require specific management, but in harmony with the overall plan. Immediate postoperative dynamic splinting may be indicated.

Stage Two.   Complications include (1) adhesions along the graft or at proximal attachment, and (2) rupture of the graft. If it is apparent that adhesions are limiting motion during the first 5 weeks after the second stage (as indicated by the absence of gradual improvement of active motion in the protected position at serial evaluations), earlier active motion and less protective splinting may be indicated.

Absence of a nail suture following stage two may be dealt with by gluing hook Velcro to a nail or by construction of a moleskin sling 3 inches long and ½ inch wide, with an eyelet midway. Tincture of benzoin is applied to the lateral aspects of the finger to facilitate adherence, and the two ends of the sling are attached to the dorsolateral aspect of the distal phalanx. This is then attached to rubberband traction.

Either Stage.   Pulley reconstruction may be a problem. Since stage one involved a passive gliding implant, there is no tension on reconstructed pulleys. Pulley reconstruction at the time of tendon grafting may require protection of the pulleys for 6 weeks postoperatively, with either ½-inch paper tape, or orthoplast rings over the reconstructed pulley. Reconstructions at this center do not require such management unless otherwise indicated.

Flexor Digitorum Superficialis Finger.   Therapy is directed to the proximal interphalangeal joint with appropriate protection of the distal interphalangeal, which will have been either tenodesed or fused.

Stage One Postoperative Management

One to Two Weeks.   Remove the bulky dressing and redress with Xeroform and Kling bandages, using sterile technique. The wrist support is maintained in neutral, if needed, for comfort at night, between exercises. Edema is controlled. Active and assistive range of motion exercises are initiated for the uninvolved joints. Passive range of motion is started for individual involved joints, and total flexion and extension are maintained with the wrist in neutral. Buddy taping is undertaken, as is static splinting for joint contractures.

Two to Six Weeks.   The protective splint and sutures are removed. Soft tissue management includes debridement, lubrication, and scar remodeling techniques. More aggressive range of motion and trapping are initiated, and dynamic or static splinting is added for joint or soft tissue contractures. By eight weeks the implant is gliding without complication. Passive mobility techniques are continued as indicated. The patient may return to work until stage two if the wrist is doing well.

Stage Two Postoperative Management

Options include immobilization for 3 to 4 weeks, followed by protected active and passive flexion and extension until 6 weeks; then dynamic extension is allowed at 6 to 8 weeks, and resistive exercise at 8 to 12 weeks. Early controlled passive motion can be initiated, as for primary flexor tendon repair.

PITFALLS AND COMPLICATIONS

Muscle-tendon units exist to move joints through their full range of motion. If, after injury and repair or reconstruction, this basic function is not restored, one must determine the source of the problem. Simply enough, the muscle must function, the unit must be intact, and the tendon must glide. At times, loss of the normal mechanical advantage is a potential problem, as in the rheumatoid with extensor tendon subluxation; or a pulley may be lost, lessening the effective motion.

Certainly, loss of muscle function may occur from denervation at the time of injury, or from loss of vascularity leading to fibrosis and ischemic contracture. Myostatic contracture and atrophy of disuse may also occur. Surface palpation of muscle contracture, elasticity of the muscle-tendon unit, and electrical studies (EMG) will help in these determinations.

In most cases, however, failure of functional gliding is due to either adhesion formation, disruption of the repair, or both. The intact gliding tendon can be demonstrated with the tenodesis effect (flexing and extending the wrist, which produces the reciprocal motion in the digits) or with the forearm squeeze test to demonstrate digital flexion.

Dehiscence of the repair can occur when excessive muscle contraction is allowed during emergence from anesthesia or early in the postoperative course. All methods of postoperative rehabilitation attempt to avoid this. Even if the suture slips only a little, the resultant gap in a repair may result in flexor lag (the muscle contraction is used up before full motion is achieved and active motion does not equal passive) and in excessive adhesion formation. This situation may be suspected if the resting posture or stance position of the digit is more extended than is appropriate (Fig. 89-29). A complete rupture may actually be in continuity with pseudotendon in the gap. Some active motion is seen and the surgeon is fooled into thinking that the problem is adhesion. After reexploration, an intact, even gliding tendon can be seen, but one can easily fail to note the opalescent appearance of the interposing pseudotendon, and to appreciate that the extended position of the digit represents an old partial rupture with gap formation, active motion remaining insufficient. In one-stage tendon grafting, gapping distal to the lumbrical leads to too long a distal tendon, overpull of the lumbrical, and the "lumbrical syndrome" finger, in which as the digit is flexed at the metacarpophalangeal joints, the interphalangeals extend.

Treatment of the ruptured repair or graft depends on how rapidly the problem is detected and correctly interpreted. With a repair, if the rupture is quickly detected, it is entirely appropriate to reenter the digit and redo the repair. The same is true for the graft. Late recognition of the ruptured tendon repair usually requires a graft, often with two stages, as scarring may be extensive.

FIGURE 89-29. Loss of normal digital stance (little finger) with a tendon repair rupture. Some active motion remained, but the repair was clearly attenuated.

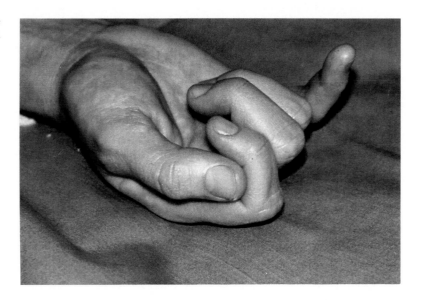

The tendon graft may rupture in midsubstance or pull loose at either end. Proximal disruptions with the interweave are relatively rare and midsubstance ruptures (discussed under the section on two-stage grafting) are often predictable, although uncommon. Pulling out of the insertion is the usual problem. Reinsertion is difficult, as there is no extra tendon to work with. If the pulley-sheath system can be easily reopened, or was never closed, as demonstrated by passing a tendon rod, immediately repeat the second stage with a new graft. A transfer motor, or an entire transfer unit of a superficialis for the thumb or little finger may now be appropriate. If the sheath cannot be readily opened, return to the beginning of stage one. On one occasion, after a patient had suffered two successive distal pullouts, a new insertion technique was devised by drilling transversely across the distal phalanx and inserting the tendon through the bone before suturing it back to itself. This was successful, but is not routinely needed.

Adherence of the tendon is determined by a gliding tendon with insufficient active excursion. This problem was discussed under tenolysis and two-stage grafting. It may be associated with partial rupture, as noted. Adherence of a tendon graft, particularly in two-stage grafting, seems to be more likely with thickened fibrous pseudosheaths after prolonging stage one, but may occur related to inflammation or infection. Tenolysis of grafts, especially two-stage, has not provided good results for us. Redoing the entire two-stage procedure may be worth a try. Grafting only to the superficialis insertion (crossing two digital joints rather than three) has been a salvage maneuver employed by Hunter and Schneider, and by us, and has been successful in such two-stage failures. Apparently, the lesser demands of moving only the proximal interphalangeal joint makes rehabilitation easier and the result better in these cases.

An interesting additional complication of tendon repair in zone 2, observed by us and explained by Gilbert, involved trapping of the profundus dynamically in the superficialis division. When the patient slowly flexed his digit, he could do so to the distal palmar crease. When he attempted full flexion rapidly, the profundus was trapped and the digit fully flexed at the proximal interphalangeal with the distal interphalangeal ex-

tended. Removing one slip of the superficialis solved the problem.

The lumbrical syndrome,[20] secondary to laxity of the one-stage graft or increased lumbrical activity with distal tendon adherence, is resolved by excision of the lumbrical or more simply by the Littler intrinsic release, removing the triangular area of the radial shroud ligament where the condensation of the oblique fibers meets the main portion of the extensor mechanism on the dorsoradial aspect of the digit. This simple maneuver can be done under local anesthesia. If it does not resolve the problem, more anesthesia may be given, if needed, and the tenolysis undertaken.

Infection is truly the most unsolveable complication of tendon surgery. The infection may be cleared, but reconstructive potential is extremely limited. After infection, scarring is extensive. A tendon rod (two-stage reconstruction) is needed, but is contraindicated. Reflaring of the infection is all too common. Options include tenolysis, and we will extend the tolerable limits of the procedure in this circumstance; one- and two-stage grafting; joint (proximal interphalangeal and distal interphalangeal) arthrodesis in functional positions; and amputation. The sequence of attempted reconstruction is in the order cited.

REFERENCES

1. Bassett, A.L. and Carroll, R.E.: Formation of Tendon Sheath by Silicone Rod Implants. J. Bone Joint Surg. **45-A:**884, 1963.
2. Boyes, J.H.: Bunnell's Surgery of the Hand, 5th ed. Philadelphia, J.B. Lippincott, 1970.
3. Brand, P.W.: Clinical Mechanics of the Hand. St. Louis, C.V. Mosby, 1985.
4. Bruner, J.M.: The Zig-zag Volar-Digital Incision for Flexor Tendon Surgery. Plast. Reconstr. Surg. **40:**571, 1967.
5. Doyle, J.R., and Blythe, W.F.: The Finger Flexor Tendon Sheath and Pulleys: Anatomy and Reconstruction. AAOS Symposium on Tendon Surgery in the Hand. St. Louis, C.V. Mosby, 1975.
6. Doyle, J.R., and Blythe, W.F.: Anatomy of the Flexor Tendon Sheath and Pulleys of the Thumb. J. Hand Surg. **2:**149, 1977.

7. Duran, R.J., and Houser, R.G.: Controlled Passive Motion Following Flexor Tendon Repair in Zones Two and Three. AAOS Symposium on Tendon Surgery in the Hand. St. Louis, C.V. Mosby, 1975.

8. Gelberman, R.H., Woo, S.L.-Y., Lothringer, K., et al.: Effects of Early Intermittent Passive Mobilization on Healing Canine Flexor Tendons. J. Hand Surg. **7:**170, 1982.

9. Goldner, J.L., and Coonrad, R.W.: Tendon Grafting of the Flexor Profundus in the Presence of a Completely or Partially Intact Flexor Sublimus. J. Bone Joint Surg. **51-A:**527, 1969.

10. Hunter, J.M., and Salisbury, R.E.: Flexor Tendon Reconstruction in Severely Damaged Hands. A Two Stage Procedure using a Silicone Dacron Reinforced Gliding Prosthesis Prior to Tendon Grafting. J. Bone Joint Surg. **53-A:**829, 1971.

11. Kleinert, H.E., and Bennett, J.B.: Digital Pulley Reconstruction Employing the Always Present Rim of the Previous Pulley. J. Hand Surg. **3:**297, 1978.

12. Kleinert, H.E., Kutz, J.E., Ashbell, T.S., and Martinez, E.: Primary Repair of Lacerated Flexor Tendon in No Man's Land. J. Bone Joint Surg. **49-A:**577, 1967.

13. Lister, G.D.: Reconstruction of Pulleys Employing Extensor Retinaculum. J. Hand Surg. **4:**461, 1979.

14. Lister, G.D.: Incision and Closure of the Flexor Sheath During Primary Tendon Repair. Hand **15:**123, 1983.

15. Lister, G.D., Kleinert, H.E., Kutz, J.E., and Atasoy, E.: Primary Flexor Tendon Repair Followed by Immediate Controlled Mobilization. J. Hand Surg. **2:**441, 1977.

16. Manske, P.R., Gelberman, R.H., and Lesker, P.A.: Flexor Tendon Healing. Hand Clin. **1:**25, 1985.

17. Manske, P.R., Gelberman, R.H., Vande Berg, J., et al.: Flexor Tendon Repair: Morphological Evidence of Intrinsic Healing in Vitro. J. Bone Joint Surg. **66-A:**385, 1984.

18. Manske, P.R., and Lesker, P.A.: Biochemical Evidence of Flexor Tendon Participation in the Repair Process—An in Vitro Study. J. Hand Surg. **9-B:**117, 1984.

19. Paneva-Holevich, E.: Two Stage Tenoplasty in Injury of Flexor Tendons of the Hand. J. Bone Joint Surg. **51-A:**21, 1969.

20. Parkes, A.: The "Lumbrical Plus" Finger. J Bone Joint Surg. **53-B:**236, 1971.

21. Peacock, E.E.: Fundamental Aspect of Wound Healing Relating to the Restoration of Gliding Function after Tendon Repair. Surg. Gynecol. Obstet. **119:**241, 1964.

22. Potenza, A.D.: Tendon Healing within the Flexor Digital Sheath in the Dog. J. Bone Joint Surg. **44-A:**49, 1962.

23. Schneider, L.H.: Staged Tendon Reconstruction. Hand Clin. **1:**109, 1985.

24. Strauch, B., and deMoura, W.: Digital Flexor Tendon Sheath: An Anatomic Study. J. Hand Surg. **10-A:**785, 1985.

25. Urbaniak, J.R.: Repair of the Flexor Pollicis Longus. Hand Clin. **1:**69, 1985.

26. Urbaniak, J.R., and Goldner, J.L.: Laceration of the Flexor Pollicis Longus Tendon: Delayed Repair by Advancement, Free Graft or Direct Suture. A Clinical and Experimental Study. J. Bone Joint Surg. **55-A:**1123, 1973.

27. Verdan, C.E.: Chirurgie Reparatrice et Fonctionnelle des Tendons de la Main. Paris, L'Expansion Scientific Francaise, 1952.

28. Verdan, C.E.: Syndrome of the Quadriga. Surg. Clin. N. Am. **40:**425, 1960.

29. Verdan, C.E.: Half a Century of Flexor Tendon Surgery. J Bone Joint Surg. **54-A:**472, 1972.

CHAPTER 90

"The hand . . . includes exact machinery of much refinement and tissues of great delicacy and specialization."

Sterling Bunnell

Extensor Tendon Injuries: Acute Repair and Late Reconstruction

JAMES S. THOMPSON and
CLAYTON A. PEIMER

The complexity of the extensor mechanism has been appreciated by many anatomists, including Albinus, who presented the first detailed structural description in 1734.[27] Reconstructive surgeons who attempt surgical correction of hand dysfunction resulting from extensor tendon injury or imbalance quickly acquire respect for the awesome negative potential of an impaired extensor system.

With the exception of the possible influence of intrinsic muscle abnormalities, the diagnosis of most extensor lesions (acute and chronic) is relatively simple. Likewise, the surgical exercise of extensor tendon suture is not as technically demanding as that for flexor tendons, because the extensors are extrasynovial throughout most of their length. However, the thin nature of the extensors within the digits, the intimate proximity of the extensor mechanism to bone (to which it readily adheres), and the proximity of the digital extensors to the critical interphalangeal joints[29,30] all contribute to poor functional results following surgical treatment of some extensor lesions.

In the digits, proximal interphalangeal (PIP) and distal interphalangeal (DIP) motion are interdependent, and lack or excess of extension in either joint will reciprocally affect the other. The "swan-neck" or "boutonnière" positions are the classic examples of this interphalangeal reciprocity. The entire mechanism, the total digital deformity, and the lack of motion or abnormal motion at each joint must be considered in planning reconstruction.[10] Eaton[13] has aptly described the extensor mechanism as a "sleeping giant which is not appreciated until it becomes disorderly or out of balance. When out of control it can create great disturbances."

Restoration of a normally functioning extensor mechanism can be more difficult than reconstruction of a flexor system. A surgeon contemplating such a restorative attempt must approach the problem with complete understanding and great care. Failure to appreciate the diverse and complex functional anatomy, proper dressings, splints, and appropriate rehabilitation may contribute to poor results in extensor reconstruction, regardless of the anatomic level or the mechanism of injury.[14]

This chapter is not meant to be a compendium of procedures, but rather describes principles and concepts useful for devising appropriate management for each case. The primary focus of the chapter is the finger extensor mechanism, but the thumb extensor system and the wrist extensors will be discussed briefly.

ABBREVIATIONS AND TERMINOLOGY

Throughout this chapter, several anatomic structures will be referred to using the following abbreviations:

    EIP—extensor indicis proprius
    EDC—extensor digitorum communis
    EDQ—extensor digiti quinti
    EPL—extensor pollicis longus

EPB—extensor pollicis brevis
BR—brachioradialis
ECRL—extensor carpi radialis longus
ECRB—extensor carpi radialis brevis
ECU—extensor carpi ulnaris
APL—abductor pollicis longus
APB—abductor pollicis brevis
FPB—flexor pollicis brevis
AP—adductor pollicis
FDP—flexor digitorum profundus
FDS—flexor digitorum superficialis
MP—metacarpophalangeal
PIP—proximal interphalangeal
DIP—distal interphalangeal
IP—interphalangeal
VP—volar plate
TRL—transverse retinacular ligament
ORL—oblique retinacular ligament

Also, for the sake of clarity, the terms listed below are used throughout the chapter in the context given here:

Juncturae tendinum (conexus intertindineus)—interconnecting oblique tendon fibers on the dorsum of the hand between the four individual tendons of the EDC (see Fig. 90-2)

Sagittal bands—transverse fibers at MP joints centralizing the extrinsic tendon and augmenting active extension through their insertion on the periphery of the MP volar plate (see Figs. 90-1 and 90-3)

Insertional excursion—the excursion of the first (MP sagittal bands) and second (MP capsule/dorsal base of proximal phalanx) extensor insertion points allowing independent IP flexion/extension with the MP joints hyperextended (see Figs. 90-4 and 90-8)

Central slip—the central portion of the extrinsic contribution to digital extension, inserting into the dorsal base of the middle phalanx (see Figs. 90-1, 90-2, and 90-12) after trifurcating and blending into the conjoined lateral bands

Lateral slips—the intrinsic contributions to the extensor mechanism at the proximal phalangeal level, proximal to the trifurcation of the central slip (see Figs. 90-1, 90-2, and 90-9A)

Conjoined lateral bands—the components forming the terminal extensor distal to the PIP joint composed of fibers from the extrinsic and intrinsic extensor contributions (see Figs. 90-1 and 90-2)

Terminal extensor—the extensor tendon formed by the merging of the conjoined lateral bands over the middle phalanx, inserting into the dorsal base of the distal phalanx (see Figs. 90-1, 90-2, and 90-13)

Dynamic interphalangeal tenodesis—augmentation of extension of the DIP joint by the static fixed length ORL which tightens as the PIP joint extends (see Fig. 90-14)

Gliding layer—an integral part of the extensor system; the interpositional layer between the extensor tendon and the phalanges. The gliding layer should be closed, when possible, and extensor tendons should not be repaired in areas of destroyed gliding layer, if feasible. (see under "extensor expendability.")

Extensor expendability—debridement of portions of the extensor mechanism in the proximal and middle phalangeal segments of the fingers if the tendon injury is untidy or the underlying gliding layer is destroyed. If there are undamaged redundant extensor components intact, they will suffice for IP extension.

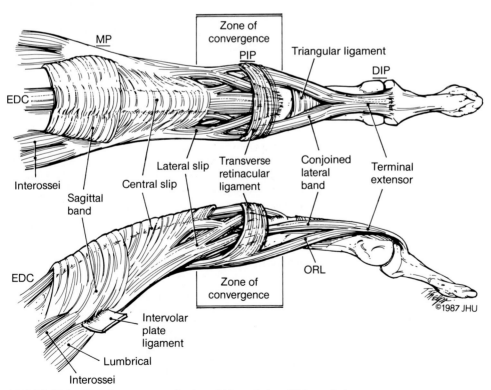

FIGURE 90-1.   Digital extensor mechanism. (A) Dorsal view. (B) Lateral view.

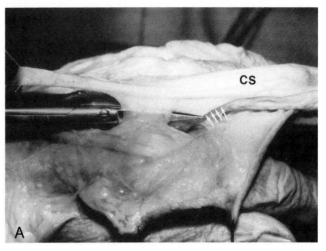

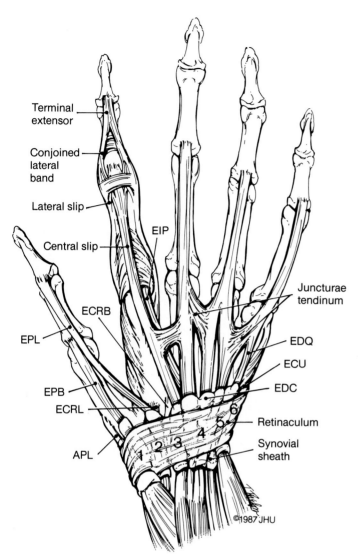

FIGURE 90-2. The extensor mechanism at the wrist and dorsum of the hand. The six extensor compartments at the wrist contain (*1*) the abductor pollicis longus (*APL*) and extensor pollicis brevis (*EPB*); (*2*) the extensor carpi radialis longus (*ECRL*) and extensor carpi radialis brevis (*ECRB*); (*3*) the extensor pollicis longus (*EPL*); (*4*) the extensor digitorum communis (*EDC*) II–V and extensor indicis proprius (*EIP*); (*5*) the extensor digiti quinti (*EDQ*); and (*6*) the extensor carpi ulnaris (*ECU*). An important anatomic detail is the presence of a synovial sheath around each tendon unit within each fibro-osseous canal. These sheaths are frequently involved in rheumatoid disease (see Chap. 117).

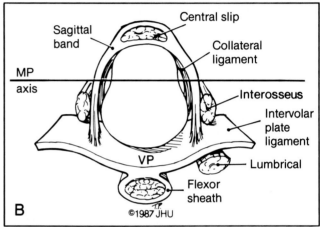

FIGURE 90-3. (A) Radial sagittal band of the middle finger. There is a natural cleavage plane (through which the scissors penetrate) between the transverse fibers of the sagittal band and the oblique fibers from the lateral slip (*arrows*) to the central slip (*CS*). (B) Transaxial view at the MP level of the sagittal bands and their insertion into the periphery of the volar plate (VP) and intervolar plate ligament. Note the relationship of the interossei and lumbrical to the MP axis of rotation and intervolar plate ligament.

FUNCTIONAL ANATOMY

Finger Extensor Mechanism

Anatomically and functionally the digital extensor system is complex, with three joints extended by a single confluent tendinous mechanism (Fig. 90-1). The mechanism itself is formed by the interlinkage of two separate and neurologically independent components: tendons of the extrinsic, radial-nerve–innervated muscles, and tendons of the intrinsic, ulnar/median-nerve–innervated muscles.

The radially innervated extrinsic extensors contributing to the extensor mechanism and their fingers of action are: EDC

—all fingers; EIP—index; and EDQ—little finger (Fig. 90-2). After passing beneath the extensor retinaculum (through synovial sheaths within each extensor compartment), the extrinsic extensor tendons are interconnected by juncturae tendinum on the dorsum of the hand (see Fig. 90-2). Laceration of individual extrinsic extensor tendons proximal to the juncturae may be masked by partial MP extension transmitted through the juncturae by the adjacent tendons. The juncturae tendinum may act as force vectors in the dynamic stabilization of the MP joints during flexion.[1]

At the MP level, the sagittal bands[19] (Figs. 90-1 and 90-3) act to maintain centralization of the extensor tendons and form the most proximal insertion point of the extensor mechanism. The sagittal bands surround the metacarpal heads and insert into the MP volar plate and intervolar plate ligaments (see Fig. 90-3B). The sagittal bands also prevent dorsal migration of the extrinsic extensor tendons during MP hyperextension (Fig. 90-4). Attenuation or injury to the radial aspect of a sagittal band may allow subluxation of the extensor tendon into the

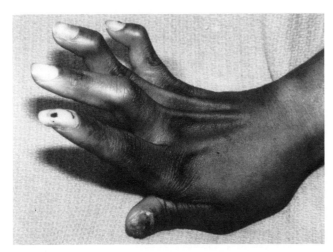

FIGURE 90-4. (A) Hand of a 39-year-old female with systemic lupus erythematosus, treated for 20 years with oral steroids. All five extensor tendons subluxate with digital flexion. With extension, marked MP hyperextension/dorsal prolapse of the EDC tendons is present due to incompetence of the MP sagittal bands.

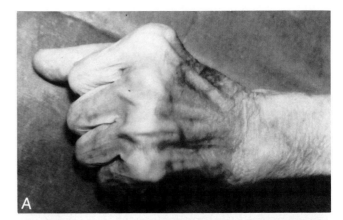

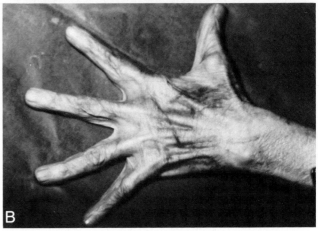

FIGURE 90-5. (A) Ulnar subluxation of the EDC of the middle finger with finger flexion in an elderly patient with extremely atrophic skin. (B) Reduction of the subluxation occurs with finger extension.

ulnar intermetacarpal sulcus with MP flexion. If this subluxation is reducible, the physical finding may simply be painful snapping to and fro of the tendon with MP flexion/extension, as demonstrated in Figure 90-5. However, if the extensor tendon becomes permanently fixed palmar to the MP axis of rotation in the ulnar intermetacarpal sulcus (frequently seen in rheumatoid disease; see Chap. 117), it becomes a strong MP flexor and contributes significantly to ulnar deviation of the fingers.

Because the MP joint is proximal to the zone of convergence (Fig. 90-6) of the intrinsic and extrinsic contributions to the digital extensor mechanism, these two separate and distinct systems act as antagonists at this level. The intrinsics, being palmar to the MP rotational axis, act as MP flexors and the extrinsics, being dorsal, are MP extensors (see Fig. 90-1B). This paradox of action at the MP joint is a primary factor contributing to difficulty in understanding the digital extensor mechanism.[13,24]

An insertion point of the extrinsic extensor is present in the dorsal MP capsule and dorsal base of the proximal phalanx (Figs. 90-7 and 90-8). Although this insertion point has been described as "indifferent"[13] and "variable,"[27] it is consistently present[43] and represents the second of the insertion points of the extensor system—the first being the sagittal bands (see Fig. 90-3). These two insertion points are not firmly fixed bony insertions in the pure sense, as are those at the dorsal base of the middle and distal phalanges. In fact, these insertions have an excursion approximately equal to the amplitude of the central slip at the PIP joint (Table 90-1) and therefore become taut only when the PIP joint is in full extension. This can easily be demonstrated in a normal finger by maintaining the MP joint in maximum hyperextension and actively flexing and extending the IP joints. A fixed insertion of the extrinsic extensor at the MP level would obviate the possibility of this maneuver. If the entire extensor mechanism is lacerated at the proximal phalan-

geal level (rarely the case in an isolated tendon laceration owing to its broad convex shape, but frequently seen in dorsal guillotine-type injuries with transection of the bone), the extensor mechanism will only retract a distance equal to or less than the available insertional excursion.

The intrinsic muscle group contributing to the extensor mechanism is composed of the interossei (all ulnar-innervated), the fourth and fifth lumbricals (ulnar-innervated), and the second and third lumbricals (median-innervated). Along the proximal phalangeal segment, the fibers of the intrinsic tendons (lateral slips) merge, "wing like," into the central slip (see Fig. 90-9A). This observation is the basis for the necessity of the triangular (wing) excision (Fig. 90-9B) in cases of intrinsic muscle contracture proposed by Littler[22] for complete intrinsic release. (See Table 90-3 for description of the intrinsic tightness test.) A smaller excision or simple lateral slip tenotomy will not completely eliminate the influence of abnormal intrinsic muscle tension on the central slip and its attendant limitation of interphalangeal flexion.

At approximately the midportion of the proximal phalanx, the central slip begins its trifurcation. Distal to this level of trifurcation, there is free exchange of fibers from the central slip to the lateral slips and from the lateral slips to the central slip (see Fig. 90-6). Distal to the anatomic zone of convergence,

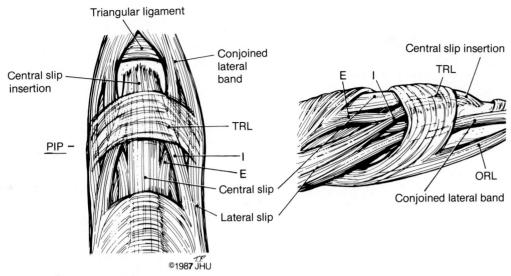

FIGURE 90-6. The zone of convergence of the digital extensor mechanism, which begins at about the midportion of the proximal phalanx and ends at the level of the central slip insertion into the dorsal base of the middle phalanx. Proximal to the zone of convergence the extrinsic and intrinsic components of the extensor mechanism are separate: the central slip is extrinsic, while the lateral slips are intrinsic. Within the zone of convergence there is complete reciprocal crossover of fibers from the central slip and lateral slips. The products of the completed convergence are the central slip insertion and the conjoined lateral bands, both of which have dual muscular activity (intrinsic and extrinsic) for extension of both interphalangeal joints. (*PIP,* proximal interphalangeal joint; *TRL,* transverse retinacular ligament; *ORL,* oblique retinacular ligament; *E,* extrinsic contribution to conjoined lateral bands; *I,* intrinsic contribution to central slip insertion)

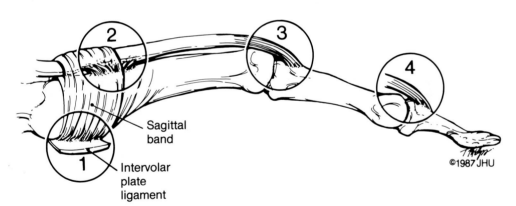

FIGURE 90-7. Lateral aspect of a finger demonstrating the four insertion points of the extensor mechanism. (*1*) Insertion through the sagittal bands into the volar plate and intervolar plate ligament. (*2*) Extensor insertion into the dorsal MP joint capsule and base of the proximal phalanx. This is a loose or indifferent insertion (see Fig. 90-8). (*3*) Central slip insertion into dorsal base of middle phalanx. (*4*) Terminal extensor insertion into dorsal base of distal phalanx.

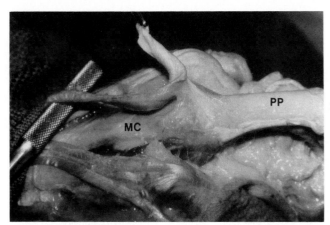

FIGURE 90-8. Extensor insertion into dorsal MP capsule and dorsal base of proximal phalanx. This insertion is filmy, loose and has an excursion equal to the extensor amplitude at the PIP joint. This "insertional excursion" allows PIP and DIP flexion while the MP joint is in maximum hyperextension. With PIP extension, however, this insertion becomes taut and assists extension of the proximal phalanx (*PP*). (*MC*, metacarpal)

the central slip and conjoined lateral bands are truly a dual extensor mechanism with both intrinsic and extrinsic contributions, either (or both) of which is capable of powering active IP extension. This dual nature of the extensor assembly was recognized and presented by Fowler in 1949.[15] Even Bunnell had held a different functional view of the extensor mechanism prior to Fowler's observations.[5,27] * This duality of extensor motor power at the IP joints,[28] plus the mechanical concept of a dynamic interphalangeal tenodesis (ORL),[23,42] form the basis for many procedures involving redistribution of forces in IP joint extensor dysfunction.

At the PIP joint, the transverse retinacular ligaments (TRL) act to gently maintain the conjoined lateral bands within certain limits of dorsopalmar excursion (see Fig. 90-1*B*). This dorsopalmar translation of the conjoined lateral bands (Fig. 90-10) was presented in 1928 by Hauch.[17] Palmar displacement of the conjoined lateral bands occurs normally with PIP flexion, allowing synchronized DIP flexion.[35] Smooth, unrestricted DIP flexion is dependent on normal PIP flexion, which allows relax-

* Riordan, D. C.: Personal communication, 1987.

TABLE 90-1. EXTENSOR TENDON EXCURSION*

Muscles	Amplitude (mm)			
	Wrist	*MP*	*PIP*	*DIP*
Wrist extensors	35			
Finger extensors	50	16	10†	5
Intrinsics		8		

* Measurements in mm are averages and will vary from individual to individual due to skeletal size and, therefore, arc length differences.

† The proximal–distal excursion limit of the MP sagittal bands and the insertional excursion of the extensor insertion at the MP capsule and base of the proximal phalanx equal the extensor amplitude at the PIP joint, allowing full IP flexion/extension with the MP joints held in maximum hyperextension.

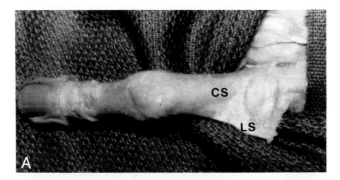

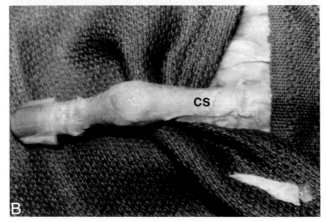

FIGURE 90-9. (A) Anatomic preparation demonstrating wing-like configuration of intrinsic contribution to the digital extensor mechanism. (*CS*, central slip; *LS*, lateral slip) (B) The wing excision of Littler that is necessary for complete elimination of intrinsic influence on the digital extensor mechanism. (*CS*, central slip)

ation of the conjoined lateral bands and oblique retinacular ligament (ORL). Lax PIP volar plates (VP) in some individuals allow DIP flexion while the PIP joint is maintained in extension (usually slight hyperextension). This is possible only in individuals with PIP VP laxity and normal supple intrinsic muscles. Repetition of this "trick" may result in further VP laxity, stretching of the TRL allowing further dorsal migration of the conjoined lateral bands, and development of painful locking of the PIP joint in hyperextension, a dynamic swan-neck deformity (Figs. 90-10 and 90-11). This phenomenon clearly illustrates the participation of the static VP in the normal and abnormal dynamics of extension. The VP as an important adjunct to the dynamic process of normal digital extension has been emphasized by Littler.[30] VP stretching or contracture also contributes to the fixed reciprocal deformities, including the swan-neck deformity (PIP hyperextension and DIP flexion) and the boutonnière (PIP flexion and DIP hyperextension).

The central slip terminates in a broad, strong bony insertion at the dorsal base of the middle phalanx (Fig. 90-12). The conjoined lateral bands merge over the dorsum of the middle phalangeal segment to form the terminal extensor tendon (see Fig. 90-1*A*), which inserts into the dorsal base of the distal phalanx (Fig. 90-13). The triangular ligament[19] is composed of transverse fibers between the conjoined lateral bands distal to the central slip insertion and proximal to the merging of the bands (see Fig. 90-6).

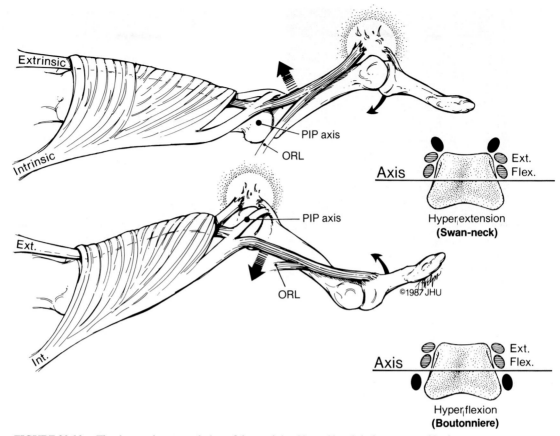

FIGURE 90-10. The dorsopalmar translation of the conjoined lateral bands is demonstrated in the two classic reciprocal digital deformities: "swan-neck" (*top*), and "boutonnière" (*bottom*). The insets are transaxial representations at the condyles of the proximal phalanx, showing the normal positions of the conjoined lateral bands in extension and flexion of the PIP joint. The abnormal positions of the conjoined lateral bands in each deformity are represented in black.

The oblique retinacular ligament (ORL) may play a unique and integral role in the extensor system. The existence and biomechanical significance of the ORL in normal digits is controversial.[38] Weitbrecht[44] illustrated this structure in 1742 and named it the retinaculum tendini longi. The ORL (Fig. 90-14) originates palmar to the PIP axis of rotation from the periosteum of the proximal phalanx and flexor sheath and passes dorsally and distally to join the terminal extensor tendon.[36] Landsmeer subjected the ligament to a sophisticated dynamic analysis[21] and the soundness of the mechanical basis of a "dynamic interphalangeal tenodesis" concept has induced procedures designed to augment DIP extension based on active PIP extension.[20,23,42] ORL tightness (see Table 90-3) may also contribute to pathologic conditions such as fixed DIP hyperextension in the boutonnière deformity and DIP extension contracture in digital Dupuytren's disease (see Chap. 84).

Absolute comprehension of the extensor mechanism is elusive but functional understanding requires only time and assimilation of multiple small bits of information. The complete mechanism (Table 90-2)—extrinsic and intrinsic motors, merging tendons, dynamic and static retaining ligaments, and other contributing components—functioning normally, has been described as "a fugue of motion."*

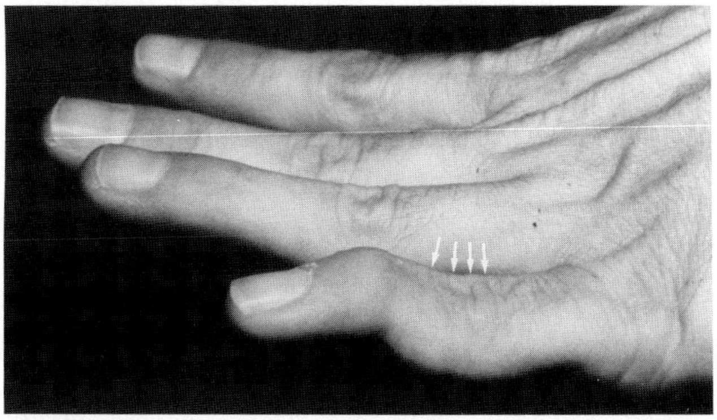

* Littler, J. W.: Personal communication, 1987.

FIGURE 90-11. Dynamic swan-neck deformity in a professional musician with PIP volar plate laxity. The conjoined lateral bands (*arrows*) bowstring dorsally as the transverse retinacular ligament stretches (see Fig. 90-10). The finger is locked in extension at the PIP joint, causing occupational disability. Successful surgical treatment was flexor superficialis tenodesis of the PIP joint blocking PIP hyperextension; this allowed complete DIP extension.

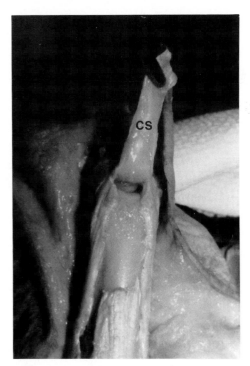

FIGURE 90-12. Broad insertion of central slip into the dorsal base of the middle phalanx. The glistening, gliding layer is seen covering the dorsal aspect of the proximal phalanx. (*CS*, central slip).

Thumb Extensor Mechanism

Extension/abduction of the first metacarpal is provided by the APL inserting on its dorsal base and into the fascia of the thenar intrinsic muscles (see Fig. 90-2). The multiple slips of this muscle tendon unit make it a very useful structure in reconstructive procedures at the base of the thumb.[39]

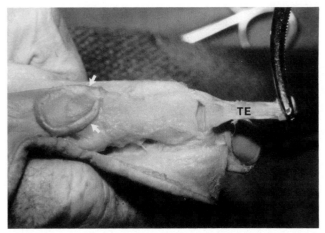

FIGURE 90-13. Bony insertion of the terminal extensor (*TE*) into the dorsal base of the distal phalanx. The proximal ends of the conjoined lateral bands (*arrows*) are visible at the PIP joint level.

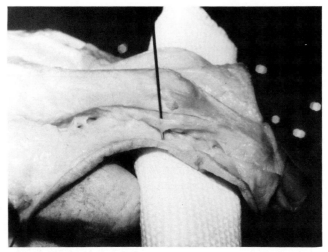

FIGURE 90-14. The oblique retinacular ligament, elevated by the probe, originates along the proximal phalangeal periosteum and flexor sheath, passes volar to the PIP axis of rotation, and joins the terminal extensor tendon. The principle of "dynamic interphalangeal tenodesis" is based on the biomechanical fact that a structure of fixed length extending from the proximal phalanx to the distal phalanx palmar to the PIP axis and dorsal to the DIP axis will relax with PIP flexion and tighten with PIP extension.

The EPB inserts into the dorsal base of the proximal phalanx and the EPL into the dorsal base of the distal phalanx (see Fig. 90-2). These two muscle tendon units exert extensor influence on multiple joints: the EPB on the trapeziometacarpal joint (extension/abduction) and MP joint (extension); and the EPL on the trapeziometacarpal joint (extension/abduction), MP joint (extension), and the IP joint (extension).

The intrinsics of the thumb (APB, FPB, and AP) contribute to IP extension through the extensor hood at the MP joint and frequently confuse the inexperienced examiner in cases of suspected EPL laceration.[29] The intact thenar intrinsics will extend the IP joint to a near neutral position, but the diagnosis of EPL rupture or laceration is obvious if the entire thumb ray is observed, and the uninjured thumb examined for comparison.

TABLE 90-2. COMPONENTS OF THE DIGITAL EXTENSOR SYSTEM

Dynamic Structures*	Static Structures†
Extrinsic muscles (EDC, EIP, EDQ, EPL, EPB, APL)	Retinaculum
	Juncturae
Intrinsic muscles (interossei, lumbricals, thenar intrinsics, hypothenar intrinsics)	Sagittal bands
	Oblique retinacular ligament
	Transverse retinacular ligament
	Triangular ligament
	Gliding layer
	Volar plates

* Directly powered by muscle

† Although static, these structures all have important dynamic functions.

CLINICAL SIGNS

Extensor Laceration or Rupture

A "dropped joint" at the site of extensor muscle tendon action is the simple sign of complete extensor functional deficit. An MP drop is seen with extrinsic extensor laceration or rupture, a PIP drop with complete central slip laceration or rupture, and a DIP drop (mallet) with terminal extensor tendon laceration or rupture.

In the thumb, laceration of the contents of the first extensor compartment (EPB, APL) will present as flexion/adduction of the first metacarpal and a lag in full extension of the MP joint. The EPL will function as both MP and IP extensor in this situation. Isolated laceration of the EPB is rare, and repair of this tendon is optional depending on the functional deficit at the MP joint. This lesion is frequently undiagnosed in the emergency situation due to the presence of MP extension through the intact EPL. However, EPL extension of the MP joint will usually be incomplete when compared to the opposite uninjured side. The magnitude of the MP extensor lag secondary to EPB laceration is variable and it is this factor that determines whether or not EPB repair is warranted. EPL laceration presents in two basic patterns depending on whether the laceration site is proximal or distal to the MP joint. Proximal to the MP joint, the entire thumb ray will be affected and will demonstrate metacarpal adduction, incomplete MP extension, and IP extension lag (some IP extension will remain, effected through intact thumb intrinsics). The EPL will retract significantly when lacerated proximal to the MP extensor hood, and retrieval from the synovial extensor compartment or the distal forearm may be difficult and require a proximal counterincision. EPL laceration distal to the MP joint is a more simple situation, easily diagnosed by consideration of the injury location and loss of IP hyperextension. The tendon cannot retract more than a few millimeters due to its attachment to the MP extensor hood. It should be repaired and treated as a sharply lacerated terminal extensor tendon of a finger, which will be discussed later.

Extensor Component Tenodesis or Contracture

There are several simple maneuvers (Table 90-3) which will establish the location of restriction of gliding (tenodesis) of the extrinsics or contracture/fibrosis of the intrinsic components. The level of extrinsic tenodesis is frequently made obvious by scars. Intrinsic contracture and contracture of the ORL, however, cannot be appreciated without the use of clinical tests.[29]

GENERAL PRINCIPLES OF MANAGEMENT

Bunnell[4] in 1922 was the first surgeon to enumerate the reasons for poor results after tendon surgery. Although his paper was published 65 years ago and Bunnell was primarily discussing flexor tendons, the reasons remain valid and apply equally well to extensor tendons (Table 90-4).

The importance of the integrity of the gliding layer between the extensor mechanism and the phalanges should be emphasized. This layer is frequently described as periosteum, and

TABLE 90-3. CLINICAL TESTS FOR TIGHTNESS OR ENTRAPMENT OF EXTENSOR MECHANISM COMPONENTS

Name of Test	Component Tested	Positive Test	Negative Test	Interpretation of Positive Test
Extrinsic entrapment test	Extrinsic tendon proximal to PIP joint	With MP joint flexed, IP joints cannot flex completely*	With MP joint flexed, IP joints flex completely	Extrinsic mechanism tenodesed by scar or contracted proximal to PIP joint, distal to wrist*
Intrinsic test (Bunnell test)	Intrinsic muscle tendon units	With MP joint extended, IP joints cannot flex completely†	With MP joint extended, IP joints flex completely	Contracture, fibrosis, or adherence of intrinsic muscles reducing their amplitude (see Table 90-1)
ORL tightness test	Oblique retinacular ligament	With PIP joint fully extended, DIP joint cannot flex completely	With PIP joint fully extended, DIP joint can be flexed completely	Shortening contracture or scarring of the ORL, seen post-trauma, in digital Dupuytren's and some connective tissue disorders

* The same test can be done at the wrist; reduction of possible IP flexion by wrist flexion indicates tenodesis by scar or contracture of the extrinsic extensors proximal to the wrist joint.

† Adding radial or ulnar deviation in addition to extension at the MP joint may reveal differential intrinsic tightness (i.e., ulnar intrinsics more contracted than radial, as frequently seen in rheumatoid disease; see Chaps. 85 and 117).

TABLE 90-4. REASONS FOR POOR RESULTS AFTER EXTENSOR TENDON SURGERY*

> Traumatizing technique
> Poor incisions
> Damage to gliding surface
> Too much or too little postoperative movement
> Crude suturing technique

* Modified from Bunnell, S.: Repair of Tendons in Fingers. Surg. Gynecol. Obstet. **35:**88, 1922.

indeed the deep portion of the layer *is* phalangeal periosteum. However, the superficial cellular components of the gliding layer are more areolar in nature and cannot be distinguished from paratenon. Absence of the gliding layer will make adherence to bone much more likely. Repair of a cleanly lacerated gliding layer, when possible, will improve chances for more normal extensor excursion. Preservation of the gliding layer in elective incisional planning for exposure and reconstruction of phalangeal fractures will improve the postoperative range of motion.[11,33] Careful preservation of the gliding layer will improve results after other elective procedures[40] and this specialized tissue should be considered an integral part of the extensor mechanism. Surgical approaches that involve splitting the extensor tendon and gliding layer are unnecessary and should *not* be used. They *do not facilitate* bone reduction but rather *create severe extensor mechanism trauma* resulting in adherence and loss of tendon amplitude. Incisions preserving the entire extensor mechanism allow access and reduction of all phalangeal fractures.[11,32]

The major dualities (Table 90-5) in the digital extensor mechanism should be fixed in the mind of the surgeon, because knowledge of these redundancies in the system will facilitate decision making in both acute repairs and late reconstructions. For instance, an untidy laceration of a lateral slip and portion of the central slip over the proximal phalangeal segment with destruction of the underlying gliding layer and abrasion or cortical chipping of the phalanx (a common power-saw injury), is best treated by debridement of the shredded tendon followed by early motion. Unnecessary repair of tendons in these circumstances is done when the surgeon does not realize that there is sufficient undamaged extensor mechanism to perform IP extension. This can be checked easily after digital anesthesia by asking the patient to straighten the finger. Recognition of the redundancy of the extensor mechanism, and therefore the expendability of certain elements (extensor expendability), should prevent one of the complications of extensor repairs seen by hand surgeons—unnecessary suture of partial lacerations and resultant digits stiffly tenodesed in extension.

TABLE 90-5. EXTENSOR SYSTEM DUALITIES

> Double extrinsic extensors for index finger (EDC, EIP)
> Double extrinsic extensors for little finger (EDC, EDQ)
> Double IP motor power sources (extrinsic, intrinsic)
> Two lateral slips per finger
> Two conjoined lateral bands per finger

TABLE 90-6. SUTURE MATERIALS FOR EXTENSOR TENDON REPAIR*

Tissue	Suture Size
Muscle bellies	2-0, 3-0
Tendons of forearm and wrist	
Core sutures	2-0, 3-0
Outer sutures	3-0, 4-0
Tendons of hand and fingers	
Core sutures	3-0, 4-0
Outer sutures	4-0, 5-0

* Use core sutures of nonabsorbable, synthetic, braided material in areas where the tendons are large enough to allow their use (i.e., dorsum of hand, wrist, forearm). All outer sutures used are synthetic, slowly absorbable, polyglycolic acid, polyglactin, or polydioxanone. Use of nonabsorbable sutures as outer sutures frequently results in irritation at the sites of unburied knots. Use fine, synthetic, absorbable sutures for repair of partial tendon and terminal extensor lacerations in the digits. Proper dressings, splints, patient education and therapy are the keys to successful results.

ACUTE EXTENSOR REPAIR

Forearm and Wrist

Little has been written about the repair of lacerated wrist extensor tendons, and the subject deserves mention. The wrist extensors maintain balanced alignment of the hand and provide stabilization of the hand during grip. They should be repaired when possible. Isolated laceration of a wrist extensor is rare, owing to the intimate anatomic arrangement of the extensor complex in the forearm and wrist. Wrist extensor tendon lacerations are therefore usually associated with laceration of one or more of the digital extensors.

Careful physical examination to rule out associated neurovascular injuries is mandatory (stab wounds in the forearm with small wounds of entry may be very misleading) followed by complete surgical exploration and repair. Dorsal laceration in the proximal forearm frequently involves branches of the radial nerve and these should be explored and repaired if feasible (see Chap. 103). Muscle bellies of the extensor muscles can be opposed with either nonabsorbable or synthetic absorbable sutures (Table 90-6). Fibrous septae within the substance of muscles, when identifiable, afford the most secure purchase for suture placement. Synthetic, slowly absorbed sutures are now preferred for peripheral sutures of muscle and tendon (Table 90-6). The details of extensor repair such as positioning after surgery, proper dressings and splints,[41] patient education, and appropriate type/timing of therapy are more important than the type of suture material used. Because the BR, ECRL, ECRB, ECU, EDC, and EDQ have their origins from the lateral epicondyle, elbow flexion (in addition to wrist extension) may facilitate repair.[12] After surgery a long-arm dressing is used with the elbow at 90° flexion, the forearm in neutral rotation, the wrist extended 45°, and the MP joints flexed approximately 15°. The IP joints are allowed full, unrestricted motion throughout treatment of the injury. At 3 weeks the MP joints are allowed active motion and the elbow is allowed motion at 4 weeks (Table 90-7). At 5 weeks wrist motion is gently instituted under the guidance of a trained hand therapist. A removable

TABLE 90-7. POSTOPERATIVE MANAGEMENT OF EXTENSOR TENDON REPAIRS IN THE FOREARM AND WRIST*

| | | Immobilization | |
Joint	Position	Type	Duration
Elbow	90° flexion; neutral pronation/supination	Cast	4 weeks
Wrist†	45° extension	Cast	4–5 weeks
	Neutral/slight extension	Removable splint‡	3–4 weeks
MP§	15° flexion	Cast/splint	3 weeks
PIP	Allow full ROM	None	
DIP	Allow full ROM	None	

* Include the elbow only in proximal forearm injuries when flexion facilitates repair of muscles originating from the lateral epicondyle, which is proximal to the axis of rotation of the elbow.

† Wrist immobilization alone will retard approximately 60% of extrinsic extensor tendon amplitude.

‡ A removable splint is used for 3 to 4 weeks following the initial 4 to 5 weeks in a static cast at 45° extension.

§ Immobilize the MP joints in slight flexion to maintain the collateral ligaments under tension around the metacarpal heads.

splint maintaining the neutral or slightly extended position is worn between exercise sessions and at night for an addition 3 to 4 weeks. It should be remembered that a minimum of 5 weeks is necessary for the biologic achievement of sufficient tensile strength to allow application of significant stress across the tendon juncture site.[31] However, some motion at the juncture site is beneficial to the return of maximum possible postoperative tendon excursion.

The keys to the best results therefore, are protection that is adequate for the specific repair and some motion that is prompt enough to achieve early tendon gliding. The operating surgeon should determine the immobilization method and mobilization sequence. The juncture can be observed directly prior to wound closure and the effects of passive MP and IP flexion assessed. Because approximately 60% of the digital extensor amplitude occurs at the wrist,[26] immobilization of the wrist in extension affords significant protection for extensor repairs. Graduated institution of range of motion for each of the joints possibly affected by extensor injuries, rather than prolonged immobilization of all joints, contributes to improved results. In addition to individualized mobilization of joints, frequent clinical evaluations by the operating surgeon and close supervision by an informed and experienced hand therapist are necessary to achieve optimum results following extensor repair or reconstruction.

Dorsum of Hand

Laceration of a single tendon of the EDC may be masked by juncturae tendini pull-through. Laceration of the EIP and EDQ will result in loss in independent MP extension of the index or little finger. All of these tendons should be repaired using appropriate core and outer sutures (see Table 90-6).

The method of immobilization (see Table 90-8) is similar to that for lacerations in the forearm and wrist. Involvement of the EDC tendons necessitates inclusion of all fingers in the dressings and splints, but isolated lacerations of the EIP and EDQ may be treated with immobilization of only the involved digit and the wrist (see Table 90-8).

TABLE 90-8. POSTOPERATIVE MANAGEMENT OF EXTENSOR TENDON REPAIRS IN THE DORSUM OF THE HAND

| | | Immobilization | |
Joint	Position	Type	Duration
Wrist*	45° extension	Cast	4–5 weeks
	Neutral/slight extension	Removable splint†	3–4 weeks
Affected MP‡	Neutral	Cast	3 weeks
Other MPs§	15° flexion	Cast	3 weeks
PIP	Allow full ROM	None	
DIP	Allow full ROM	None	

* Wrist immobilization alone will retard approximately 60% of extrinsic extensor tendon amplitude.

† A removable splint is used for 3 to 4 weeks following the initial 4 to 5 weeks in a static cast at 45° extension.

‡ A neutral MP position of the affected digit coupled with MP flexion of digits with intact EDC tendons reduces possible tension at the juncture site.

§ Immobilize the MP joints in slight flexion to maintain collateral ligaments under some tension around the metacarpal heads.

Metacarpophalangeal Joint

Laceration

Delayed repair of a lacerated extensor tendon and MP joint capsule is a prudent course of action. The rationale for wound irrigation, inspection, open wound treatment, splinting, and delayed repair after 5 to 10 days of antibiotic treatment is prevention of primary closure of occult human bites. Primary closure, an inappropriate treatment of a human bite, frequently leads to septic destruction of the MP joint (see Chapter 118). Primary closure of lacerations of the extensor tendon and MP joint should be done only if the surgeon is confident of the history and the wound appears compatible with that history. The method and duration of immobilization are the same as those described for extensor lacerations on the dorsum of the hand (see Table 90-8).

Extensor Subluxation

Closed subluxation of the extensor tendon at the MP joint (see Fig. 90-5) can frequently be managed successfully with extension splinting for 4 to 6 weeks. Acute sharp injuries to the radial sagittal band of the MP joint should be surgically repaired to prevent ulnar extensor tendon subluxation. Chronic subluxation which does not respond to MP extension splinting requires surgical treatment. Release the ulnar sagittal band and, if possible, reef the radial sagittal band. If adequate substance for repair is not present in the radial sagittal band, several surgical reconstructions have been described[7] using juncturae or strips of the tendon secured to soft tissue on the radial side of the joint to prevent the ulnar subluxation.

Proximal Phalanx

Complete laceration of the extensor mechanism at this level is impossible without transection of the proximal phalanx. There-

fore, lacerations over the proximal phalanx are usually partial and affect the tendon only over the convex portion of the phalanx that interrupted the passage of a sharp object through the finger. These tendon injuries do not retract significantly, do not result in loss of extension at the IP joints, and are usually diagnosed only through direct visual inspection of the wound. Repair of the central slip is indicated but lateral slip repair, especially if the gliding layer is disrupted, is optional. Treat untidy injuries of a single lateral slip with debridement of the crushed tendon ends and motion beginning after 10 days of splinting for soft-tissue protection. Remember the dualities of the system and the concept of expendability in crushing and abrading-type injuries. If the central slip is repaired, fine, synthetic, slowly absorbable sutures are preferred. After repair of a partial laceration of the central slip, ask the patient to actively flex and extend the MP and PIP joints. This will provide the surgeon with some idea of whether or not the repair is in jeopardy with early motion. If no tension on the repair is demonstrated with active flexion/extension of the MP or PIP joints, early motion should be considered. If there is significant tension on the repair, the postoperative regimen should follow that for laceration of the extensor tendon at the PIP joint (see Table 90-9).

Proximal Interphalangeal Joint

Untreated laceration of the central slip at the PIP joint will allow development of the button-hole (boutonnière) deformity. The inevitable flexion of the middle phalangeal segment due to unopposed FDS pull encourages herniation of the proximal phalangeal condyles through the central slip defect. As the PIP flexion deformity progresses, the conjoined lateral bands slide palmar to the PIP axis, maintaining and increasing PIP flexion and tightening the terminal extensor, which yields DIP hyperextension (see Fig. 90-10). The boutonnière deformity, when allowed to progress, is one of the most difficult reconstructive challenges to confront a hand surgeon. The key to prevention,

TABLE 90-9. POSTOPERATIVE MANAGEMENT OF EXTENSOR TENDON REPAIRS OF THE PIP JOINT (ACUTE BOUTONNIÈRE DEFORMITY)

| Joint | Position | Immobilization | |
		Type	Duration
MP	Allow ROM	None	
PIP	Full extension	Transarticular Kirschner wire and dorsal splint	5 weeks constant, followed by splint weaning*
	Full extension	Removable thermoplastic splint	3 weeks, night-time only†
DIP	Allow ROM, flexion encouraged‡	None	

* Splint weaning—Remove splint for 1 hour each morning and evening for 3 days, then 2 hours each morning and evening for 3 days. If no PIP extension lag develops and active and passive flexion gradually increase during the 6 days, splinting may be discontinued during the day. If PIP extension lag (>10°) develops, return to constant splinting in full extension for an additional week, then resume the weaning routine.

† Night-time splinting in full PIP extension is recommended for 3 weeks following 5 weeks of constant splint wear. If an extension lag develops during the splint weaning routine, consider prolonging the night splinting period.

‡ Maintain the amplitude of lateral slips and conjoined lateral bands.

TABLE 90-10. TRANSARTICULAR KIRSCHNER-WIRE SIZES*

Joint	Size (mm)
PIP	0.35, 0.45
DIP	0.28, 0.35

* Smooth wires only.

in sharp injuries, is careful exploration of all wounds over the PIP dorsum and extensor tendon repair. If there is a complete PIP extension deficit, the PIP joint should be maintained in full extension with a transarticular Kirschner wire prior to tendon repair. If the PIP extension deficit is not severe (less than 30° to 40°), tendon repair and external splinting will usually suffice. Careful postoperative management (Table 90-9) is necessary for optimum results.

Closed dorsal injury at the PIP level represents the cause of many late-presenting, difficult, fixed boutonnière deformities. Prevention in these cases is simply based on an awareness of the potential problem and a high index of suspicion. Immobilize the PIP joint in extension and observe it with careful follow-up examinations. Unrestricted finger flexion after blunt trauma to the dorsum of the PIP region with central slip contusion/rupture may lead to severe deformity. PIP flexion, therefore, should be instituted gradually and only after follow-up examinations reveal full active PIP extension. If there is significant periarticular swelling and pain with attempted flexion, a prudent assumption is that the injury is a closed boutonnière deformity until proven otherwise and adherence to the regimen presented in Table 90-9 is indicated.

Middle Phalanx and Distal Interphalangeal Joint

The classic "mallet-finger" deformity (dropped distal phalanx) can be separated into at least seven separate groups:

1. Closed rupture of the terminal extensor tendon
2. Intra-articular avulsion fracture of the terminal extensor insertion (dorsal base of the distal phalanx) *without* palmar DIP subluxation
3. Intra-articular avulsion fracture of the terminal extensor insertion (dorsal base of the distal phalanx) *with* palmar DIP subluxation
4. Open laceration of the terminal extensor at the middle phalanx or distal interphalangeal level
5. Dorsal abrasion/degloving-type composite tissue injury with loss of tendon substance
6. Extra-articular fracture at the base of the distal phalanx in adults with marked palmar angulation
7. Transepiphyseal fracture of the distal phalanx in children with marked palmar angulation

The majority of mallet fingers can be included in the first four groups; it is these groups that will form the basis for discussion of mallet fingers within this chapter. Fortunately for the treating surgeon, injuries in the fifth group are relatively rare. When seen, these injuries frequently require flap or graft coverage (see Chap. 120) prior to consideration of extensor tendon reconstruction. The last two groups are fractures usually associated with nail-root avulsions, and are treated relatively easily (see Chap. 81 and 95).

All mallet fingers involving loss of terminal extensor contact with the distal phalanx (groups 1–5) may present with PIP recurvatum (swan neck), the magnitude of which depends on the ability of the PIP VP to resist the increased extensor force (central slip plus conjoined lateral bands) on the middle phalanx (see Fig. 90-10).

Mallet fingers in groups 1 and 2 can be managed satisfactorily by closed means in commercially available ("Stack") splints.[8,38] In group 2, the area of articular surface on the fracture fragment of the distal phalanx is not critical as long as the DIP joint is not palmarly subluxated. Even though anatomic reduction may not be possible in a splint, results are good if joint alignment is maintained. The presence of palmar subluxation of the distal phalanx indicates that enough of the DIP collateral ligament insertion is present on the fracture fragment to allow the unopposed FDP insertion to palmarly displace the distal phalanx. This usually does not occur until 50% or more of the articular surface of the distal phalanx is present on the fracture fragment.

If palmar subluxation of the distal phalanx is present, the injury should be treated surgically with reduction of the DIP joint, transarticular Kirschner-wire fixation (Table 90-10), and open reduction of the fracture fragment. Methods for fragment fixation are diverse and none has a clear advantage. The clear disadvantage of open treatment of any mallet deformity is loss of DIP flexion. A certain amount of flexion loss is the cost of accurate joint and fracture reduction in group 3 mallet deformities and tendon repair in group 4 mallet deformities. A patient who expects this result is usually satisfied with the surgeon's efforts, while the unprepared patient frequently is disappointed. The postoperative management of mallet deformity (Table 90-11) is also used in the treatment of closed mallet injuries.

Open mallet deformities (group 4) are also managed as shown in Table 90-11. Place fine, synthetic, absorbable sutures in the tendon after the DIP joint has been fixed in neutral extension with a transarticular Kirschner wire.

LATE RECONSTRUCTION

Delayed extensor reconstruction is, in itself, an adequate topic for a large volume. Review of hundreds of described procedures may not yield the exact answer for a particular clinical problem. The following are a few simple guidelines divided into general anatomic levels for the management of chronic extensor deficits.

Forearm, Wrist, and Dorsum of Hand

Wrist and MP extension are the functional losses accompanying disruption of wrist extensors and extrinsic digital extensors. Without wrist extensors, grasp function of the hand is disabled. Loss of MP extension eliminates the placement arc of the fingers,[30] while digital encompassment (IP flexion through FDP/FDS and IP extension through intact intrinsic muscula-

TABLE 90-11. POSTOPERATIVE MANAGEMENT OF EXTENSOR TENDON REPAIR OVER THE MIDDLE PHALANX OR AT THE DISTAL INTERPHALANGEAL JOINT (ACUTE MALLET DEFORMITY)*

| Joint | Position | Immobilization | |
		Type	*Duration*
MP	Allow ROM	None	
PIP	Allow ROM†	None	
DIP	Full extension	Transarticular Kirschner wire and plastic splint	5 weeks constant, followed by splint weaning‡
	Full extension	Removable plastic splint	3 weeks, night-time only§

* The same regimen may be used in the treatment of closed mallet injuries.

† A few days of postoperative PIP immobilization is not detrimental, but prolonged PIP immobilization during the treatment of extensor tendon laceration over the middle phalanx or distal interphalangeal joint will result in loss of vital PIP flexion.

‡ Splint Weaning—Remove splint for 1 hour each morning and evening for 3 days, then 2 hours each morning and evening for 3 days. If no DIP extension lag develops and active and passive flexion gradually increase during the 6 days, discontinue splinting during the day. If DIP extension lag (>10°) develops, return to constant splinting in full extension for an additional week, then resume the splint weaning.

§ Night-time splinting in full DIP extension is recommended for 3 weeks following 5 weeks of constant extension splint wear. If an extension lag develops during the splint weaning, prolong night splinting.

ture) is maintained. Loss of either wrist extension or MP extension results in marked disability. Tenodesis and stiffened joints may also contribute to the clinical presentation. Reconstructive goals are independent wrist and/or MP extension through a system with satisfactory power and amplitude to meet functional requirements. Normal amplitude is rarely achieved, but adequate power for extensor function is a reasonable goal, since normal digital extensor strength is 10% of that of all the muscles below the elbow and digital extensor work capacity is less than one-third of that of the digital flexors.[3] Indeed, according to Brand,[3] the FDS and FDP of the middle finger alone are as strong as the extensors of all the other fingers.

The three options available for late reconstruction of extrinsic wrist and digital extensor loss are: (1) attempted delayed repair, (2) interpositional tendon graft, and (3) redistribution of power through tendon transfer. In general, tendon transfers are the most successful. Delayed repair and interpositional tendon graft suffer in comparison owing to the condition of the lacerated muscle tendon unit, which is usually compromised by retraction, adherence, and weakness. There are multiple options for tendon transfers for restoration of wrist and MP extension[37] and these methods are most fully described in treatises dealing with reconstruction following radial nerve palsy (see Chap. 107). If composite tissue loss on the dorsum of the hand or forearm necessitates flap coverage, the use of silicone rods beneath the flap will facilitate later tendon transfer.

Extensor Tenodesis of the Hand and Digits

Post-traumatic tenodesis of the extensor tendons over the metacarpals and phalanges is a relatively common clinical problem, presenting after extensor tendon injuries with or without fractures. The gliding layer has been disrupted in these cases and dense adhesions are present between the bone and exten-

sor tendon. Extensor tendolysis in the hand or digit with or without use of synthetic interpositional material (silicone sheets which eventually require removal) is a worthy surgical attempt to improved functional range of motion. However, the long-term results are highly variable. The gains in range of motion may be dramatically good in some patients and dismally poor in others. Adhesions may extend far beyond the level of injury, and other factors, both objective (e.g., stiffened MP or IP joints, loss of muscle amplitude, altered tendon nutrition) and subjective (e.g., pain perception and tolerance, patient understanding/motivation) are as important as simply lysing tendon from bone. The gains in flexion will be more significant than the reduction in extensor lag, and the necessity for joint capsulotomy will decrease the overall benefit of extensor tendolysis.[9] However, if the joints are supple and a well-motivated patient understands the rigors of maintaining postoperative tendon excursion, tendolysis is an acceptable surgical option.

The PIP joint, which accounts for 85% of final interphalangeal encompassment,[29,30] is most affected by extensor tenodesis of the central slip over the proximal phalanx. The feasibility of separation of the extrinsic and intrinsic contributions to the extensor mechanism at the proximal phalangeal level should be considered. The extrinsics would then be isolated as MP extensors. Excise the area of tenodesis to eliminate the extensor tether of the PIP joint. If the lateral slips are normal and the area of tenodesis is proximal to the "zone of convergence" (see Fig. 90-6), the intrinsic muscles then become the sole IP extensors. When possible, this solution[25,26] to the problem can be very successful.

Few patients complain of loss of DIP flexion after extensor injury followed by tenodesis over the middle phalanx, even though DIP flexion is uniformly decreased after such injuries. Tendolysis at the middle phalangeal level could be considered in a patient with unique occupational demands (e.g., a professional musician, requiring maximum DIP range of motion).

Late Boutonnière Deformity

Reconstruction of the chronic boutonnière deformity is not easily accomplished, and frequently frustrates the most experienced hand surgeons. The fixed or flexible nature of the PIP flexion deformity is extremely important in operative planning (see Chap. 117). All reconstructions in late boutonnière deformities depend on attainment of maximum passive PIP extension followed by appropriate distribution of the available extensor power.[6,10,26,33,34]

Late Swan-Neck and Mallet Deformities

Many innovative reconstructive procedures have been proposed and used in restoration of swan-neck deformity. If the DIP joint assumes the extended position when PIP hyperextension is blocked at neutral or slight flexion, treatment should simply be directed at limiting PIP extension to that neutral or slightly flexed position. A more challenging swan-neck deformity follows rupture of the terminal extensor in patients with lax PIP volar plates. The increased extensor pull on the middle phalanx (see Fig. 90-10) causes progressive PIP hyperextension. In these cases, surgical management can be divided into two basic categories: (1) procedures designed to shift extensor pull from the middle to the distal phalanx, and (2) procedures using the dynamic interphalangeal tenodesis concept to limit PIP hyperextension and augment DIP extension.

The prime example of an extensor shift procedure is the Fowler central slip tenotomy.[2,16] Tenotomy of the central slip reduces extensor tone on the PIP joint and allows proximal shift of the conjoined lateral bands, increasing DIP extensor tone. This procedure is simple and is usually effective in improving DIP extension and reducing PIP hyperextension. However, DIP extension will not be complete in most cases,[40] and PIP extension lag is a potential problem following central slip tenotomy. This procedure should be used exclusively in swan-neck deformities resulting from rupture and separation of the terminal extensor tendon.

Several procedures,[20,23,24,42] all of which represent the creation of a strong, oblique retinacular ligament homologue have been described and reported to be effective. These procedures provide predictable methods for correcting loss of DIP extension and PIP hyperextension.

If the deformity is purely DIP extension loss (mallet finger) with no tendency toward PIP hyperextension, treatment may be directed at reconstituting the terminal extensor tendon by excision of interposed scar and secondary repair, tendon graft, or tenodermadesis.[18]

Thumb

Late extensor deficits in the thumb ray are less common than in the fingers. This is due to the thumb's recessed and palmar abducted position, which provides relative protection from longitudinal and dorsal trauma. (The thumb of the nondominant glove hand in baseball and softball is an exception to this generality. However, athletes tend to sustain fractures and ligament injuries after thumb trauma rather than extensor tendon deficits.) Most late extensor deficits in the thumb occur second-ary to the deformities of rheumatoid disease or attritional rupture of the EPL following a distal radial fracture. Reconstruction of the rheumatoid thumb is discussed in Chapter 117. Tendon transfers[39] provide the most satisfactory solution to late EPL deficit, if the joints are supple. All procedures discussed within this chapter regarding late mallet deformities are applicable, though rarely applied, to the thumb.

REFERENCES

1. Agee, J., and Guidera, M.: The Functional Significance of the Juncturae Tendinae in Dynamic Stabilization of the Metacarpophalangeal Joints of the Fingers. J. Hand Surg. 5:288, 1980.
2. Bowers, W.H., and Hurst, L.C.: Chronic Mallet Finger: The Use of Fowler's Central Slip Release. J. Hand Surg. 3:373, 1978.
3. Brand, P.W.: Clinical Mechanics of the Hand, p. 273. St. Louis, C.V. Mosby, 1985.
4. Bunnell, S.: Repair of Tendons in the Fingers. Surg. Gynecol. Obstet. 35:88, 1922.
5. Bunnell, S.: Surgery of Intrinsic Muscles of the Hand. J. Bone Joint Surg. 24:1, 1942.
6. Burton, R.I.: Extensor Tendons—Late Reconstruction. In Green, D.P. (ed.): Operative Hand Surgery, p. 1465. New York, Churchill Livingstone, 1982.
7. Carroll, C., Moore, J.R., and Weiland, A.J.: Posttraumatic Ulnar Subluxation of the Extensor Tendons: A Reconstructive Technique. J. Hand Surg. 12-A:227, 1987.
8. Crawford, G.P.: The Molded Polythene Splint for Mallet Finger Deformities. J. Hand Surg. 9-A:231, 1984.
9. Creighton, J.J., Jr., and Steichen, J.B.: Retrospective Statistical Analysis of Motion Following Extensor Tenolysis in the Hand and Digit. J. Hand Surg. 11-A:761, 1986.
10. Curtis, R.M., Reid, R.L., and Provost, J.M.: A Staged Technique for Repair of the Traumatic Boutonniere Deformity. J. Hand Surg. 8:167, 1983.
11. Dabezies, E.J., and Schutte, J.P.: Fixation of Metacarpal and Phalangeal Fractures with Miniature Plates and Screws. J. Hand Surg. 11-A:283, 1986.
12. Doyle, J.R.: Extensor Tendons—Acute Injuries. In Green, D.P. (ed.): Operative Hand Surgery, p. 1441. New York, Churchill Livingstone, 1982.
13. Eaton, R.G.: The Extensor Mechanism of the Fingers. Bull. Hosp. Jt. Disease 30:39, 1969.
14. Eversman, W.W.: Complications of Extensor Tendon Injuries. In Boswick, J.A. (ed.): Complications in Hand Surgery, p. 38. Philadelphia, W.B. Saunders, 1986.
15. Fowler, S.B.: Extensor Apparatus of the Digits. J. Bone Joint Surg. 31-B:477, 1949.
16. Grundberg, A.B., and Reagan, D.S.: Central Slip Tenotomy for Chronic Mallet Finger Deformity. J. Hand Surg. 12-A:545, 1987.
17. Hauck, G.: Die Ruptur der Dorsal Aponeurose am ersten Interphalangeal Gelenk, zugleich eim Beitrag zur Anatomie und Physiologie der Dorsal Aponeurose. Arch. Klin. Chir. 123:197, 1923.
18. Iselin, F., Levame, J., and Godoy, J.: A Simplified Technique for Treating Mallet Fingers: Tenodermadesis. J. Hand Surg. 5:214, 1977.
19. Kaplan, E.B.: Functional and Surgical Anatomy of the Hand, 2nd ed. Philadelphia, J.B. Lippincott, 1965.
20. Kleinman, W.B., and Peterson, D.P.: Oblique Retinacular Ligament Reconstruction for Chronic Mallet Finger Deformity. J. Hand Surg. 9-A:399, 1984.
21. Landsmeer, J.M.F.: Anatomy of the Dorsal Aponeurosis of the Human Finger and its Functional Significance. Anat. Rec. 104:31, 1949.

22. Littler, J.W.: Tendon Transfers and Arthrodesis in Combined Median and Ulnar Nerve Paralysis. J. Bone Joint Surg. **31-A:**225, 1949.

23. Littler, J.W.: Restoration of the Oblique Retinacular Ligament for Correcting Hyperextension Deformity of the Proximal Interphalangeal Joint. GEM. L'Expansion Editeur **1:**39, 1966.

24. Littler, J.W.: The Finger Extensor Mechanism. Surg. Clin. North Am. **47:**415, 1967.

25. Littler, J.W.: Principles of Reconstructive Surgery of the Hand. *In* Converse, J.M. (ed.): Reconstructive Plastic Surgery, 2nd ed., vol. VI, p. 3127. Philadelphia, W.B. Saunders, 1977.

26. Littler, J.W.: The Digital Extensor–Flexor System. *In* Converse, J.M. (ed.): Reconstructive Plastic Surgery, 2nd ed., vol. VI, p. 3173. Philadelphia, W.B. Saunders, 1977.

27. Littler, J.W.: The Finger Extensor System. Orthop. Clin. North Am. **17:**483, 1986.

28. Littler, J.W., and Eaton, R.G.: Redistribution of Forces in Correction of Boutonniere Deformity. J. Bone Joint Surg. **49-A:**1267, 1967.

29. Littler, J.W., Herndon, J.H., and Thompson, J.S.: Examination of the Hand. *In* Converse, J.M. (ed.): Reconstructive Plastic Surgery, 2nd ed., vol. VI, p. 2964. Philadelphia, W.B. Saunders, 1977.

30. Littler, J.W., and Thompson, J.S.: Surgical and Functional Anatomy. *In* Bowers, W.H. (ed.): The Interphalangeal Joints, p. 14. New York, Churchill Livingstone, 1987.

31. Mason, M.L., and Shearon, C.G.: The Process of Tendon Repair: An Experimental Study of Tendon Suture and Tendon Graft. Arch. Surg. **25:**615, 1932.

32. Melone, C.P., Jr.: Rigid Fixation of Phalangeal and Metacarpal Fractures. Orthop. Clin. North Am. **17:**421, 1986.

33. Rosenthal, E.A.: Extensor Surface Injuries at the Proximal Interphalangeal Joint. *In* Bowers, W.H. (ed.): The Interphalangeal Joints, p. 94. New York, Churchill Livingstone, 1987.

34. Schneider, L.H.: Reconstruction in Chronic Extensor Tendon Problems. *In* Strickland, J.W., and Steichen, J.B. (eds.): Difficult Problems in Hand Surgery, p. 47. St. Louis, C.V. Mosby, 1982.

35. Schultz, R.J., Furlong, J., and Storace, A.: Detailed Anatomy of the Extensor Mechanism at the Proximal Aspect of the Finger. J. Hand Surg. **6:**493, 1981.

36. Shrewsbury, M.M., and Johnson, R.K.: A Systematic Study of the Oblique Retinacular Ligament of the Human Finger: Its Structure and Function. J. Hand Surg. **2:**194, 1977.

37. Smith, R.J.: Tendon Transfers in the Hand and Forearm. Boston, Little–Brown, 1987.

38. Stack, H.G.: Mallet Finger. Hand **1:**83, 1969.

39. Thompson, J.S.: Surgical Treatment of Trapeziometacarpal Arthrosis. Adv. Orthop. Surg. **10:**105, 1986.

40. Thompson, J.S.: Interphalangeal Arthroplasties. *In* Bowers, W.H. (ed.): The Interphalangeal Joints, p. 156. New York, Churchill Livingstone, 1987.

41. Thompson, J.S., and Littler, J.W.: Dressings and Splints. *In* Converse, J.M. (ed.): Reconstructive Plastic Surgery, 2nd ed., vol. VI, p. 2991. Philadelphia, W.B. Saunders, 1977.

42. Thompson, J.S., Littler, J.W., and Upton, J.: The Spiral Oblique Retinacular Ligament (SORL). J. Hand Surg. **3:**482, 1978.

43. Tubiana, R., and Valentin, P.: Anatomy of the Extensor Apparatus and the Physiology of Finger Extension. Surg. Clin. North Am. **44:**897, 1964.

44. Weitbrecht, J.: Syndesmology (Historia Ligamentum Corporis Humani), 1742. Translated by Kaplan, E.B. Philadelphia, W.B. Saunders, 1969.

CHAPTER 91

Stenosing Tenosynovitis

MARK PRUZANSKY

Normal function of the hand requires the smooth and nearly frictionless gliding of flexor and extensor tendons. Inflammation of the tenosynovium, especially at points where a tendon changes direction, can lead to stenosis of the tendon sheath which interferes with the action of the enclosed tendon. Patients with this condition present with pain and limitation or irregularity of joint motion. Stenosing tenosynovitis may affect any of the flexor or extensor tendons, either alone or in combination.

Causes of stenosing tenosynovitis vary, and may include acute trauma, mild repetitive trauma of occupation or sports, tumor, infection, gout, rheumatoid arthritis, or metabolic disorders. The principles of treatment include cessation or modification of the activities contributing to overuse, use of anti-inflammatory agents, and surgical correction of the impediments to tendon motion.

TRIGGER DIGIT

Trigger digit is usually the result of constriction of the first annular band of the flexor tendon sheath, which causes pain and difficulty in extending the proximal interphalangeal joint.[33,51,71] In the case of trigger thumb, the patient has difficulty extending the interphalangeal joint.[34,75] Repetitive flexion and direct trauma may also cause stenosing tenosynovitis of the flexor tendon of the finger.[6,7,20,50] A painful sensation is felt when the digit is forcibly straightened or flexed. Often, extending the distal interphalangeal joint before straightening the proximal interphalangeal joint avoids the characteristic painful snap. Tenderness on palpation usually occurs just proximal to the metacarpol phalangeal joint on the palmar side.

Traumatic flexor tenosynovitis, a reactive swelling in the flexor digitorum profundus (flexor pollicis longus) tendon which is either proximal or distal to the proximal pulley, or a ganglion within the substance of the first and second annular band may be found in cases of stenosing tenosynovitis of the flexor tendons of the digits.

Interphalangeal joint locking may also be caused by interference with the normal gliding mechanism of the lateral bands, or by irregularities within the interphalangeal joints. Osteophytes and malunions of fractures of the proximal interphalangeal joint can block extensor hood function and the normal motion of the collateral ligaments, whereas joint "mice" can restrict proximal interphalangeal joint mobility.

Trigger digit occurs most commonly in healthy women in their sixth decade.[13,19,39,41,44,50,60,61,71] It is associated with de Quervain's disease and carpal tunnel syndrome, as well as with triggering of any of the other nine digits of the hand.[1,4,5,27,39,41,44,60,61] It occurs more commonly in de Quervain's disease than in carpal tunnel syndrome. The incidence of trigger finger is increased in patients with Dupuytren's disease, rheumatoid arthritis, or diabetes mellitus. It is associated with another type of tenosynovitis in more than two-thirds of all patients, and it is bilateral in 25 percent of them.[60,61] Congenital trigger digit is the most common form of digital flexion contracture in infants.[17] Trigger thumb is sometimes hereditary, and occurs more commonly than does trigger finger.[12,16,17,34,65,70] Surgical correction can be deferred until 1 year of age without permanent loss of motion. Thirty percent of congenital cases will correct spontaneously before 1 year of age.

Splint immobilization and steroid injection in the flexor tendon sheath may be curative. Surgery is warranted if symptoms persist despite conservative management.

Surgical Procedure

Infiltrate the area of the proposed skin incision with local anesthetic. In the case of stenosing tenosynovitis of the index finger, incise the proximal flexor crease of the palm. In treating triggering of the middle, ring, or little fingers, make a 15-mm incision in the distal flexion crease. In the thumb, incise the proximal flexion crease in the area between the two sesamoids (Fig. 91-1). With pneumatic tourniquet control, clear fat from the palmar surface of the flexor tendon sheath by blunt dissection. Use medial and lateral Ragnel retractors to protect the neurovascular bundles (Fig. 91-2). Identify the proximal edge of the first annular band by its thickened transverse collagen bundles, which contrast with the longitudinal striations of the paratenon proximally.

Resect the radial one-half of the proximal pulley, as well as the redundant tenosynovium, from the flexor tendons (Fig. 91-3). The ulnar half of the pulley will prevent ulnar deviation of the fingers. Withdraw both flexors from the wound to examine them for thickening. When tendon nodules are present, resect them with a mid lateral, partial, wedge resection of the tendon substance and primary closure. The reconstruction is evaluated by having the patient move the affected finger. If triggering persists, then partially section the second annular band by gentle pressure with open, blunt, dissecting scissors.

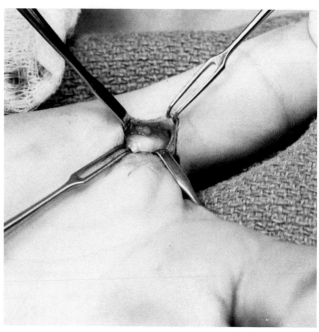

FIGURE 91-2. Exposure of the thickened proximal pulley and trigger thumb.

Fingers caught in extension may have nodular thickening of the flexor digitorum profundus tendon distal to the A2 pulley. Through an oblique incision near the proximal flexion crease of the finger, perform an elliptical resection of tendon substance, followed by primary tendon closure.

Hemostasis is achieved after the tourniquet is released. Close the skin using nonabsorbable, interrupted sutures. A soft compression dressing is applied to maximize finger mobility. Occupational therapy may be necessary to reduce residual soft tissue contractures in chronic cases.

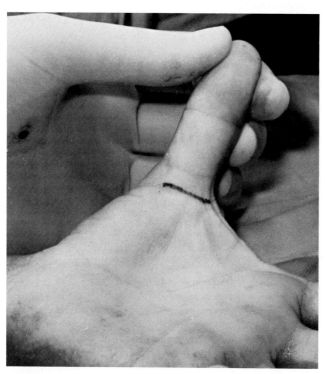

FIGURE 91-1. Skin incision for correction of trigger thumb.

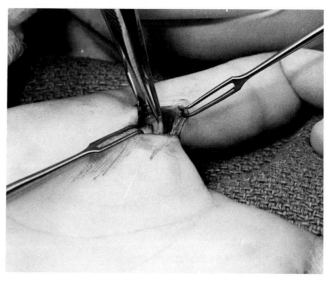

FIGURE 91-3. Resection of the ulnar half of the proximal pulley of the thumb.

Pitfalls and Complications

Patients whose ethnic origins are associated with an increased propensity for Dupuytren's disease (i.e., those of Irish, English, and northern German extraction), may develop localized thickening of the palmar fascia as a complication of surgery for trigger digit. This can partially be prevented by excising the palmar fascia that is visible around the edges of the skin incision. In patients with demonstrable Dupuytren's disease, surgical correction of trigger digit may stimulate progression of fascial thickening; thus, the value of surgery should be weighed carefully against this risk. When neurovascular injury occurs during surgery, immediate microsurgical repair is indicated. Resection of more than 25% of the second annular band must be avoided to prevent reduction of total active range of motion of the digit. First palpating the sesamoids overlying the first metacarpal phalangeal joint will prevent excessive radial placement of the skin incision and potential digital nerve damage.

DE QUERVAIN'S DISEASE

Stenosing tenosynovitis of the abductor pollicis longus and extensor pollicis brevis within the first dorsal compartment of the wrist was described by de Quervain in 1895.[16,22,31] Pain and swelling over the radial styloid, which often radiates up the forearm or down to the thumb, characterize the disorder (Fig. 91-4). Wringing motions of the hand and wrist, as well as repetitive flexion and extension of the thumb, especially the basal joint, magnify the symptoms.[36,57] Finkelstein's maneuver—hyperflexion of the entire first ray with ulnar deviation of the wrist—reproduces the pain during physical examination.[22] Tenderness on palpation of the radial styloid process, and crepitus upon motion of the first ray may be evident.[10,31] The inflammatory process may involve either or both the long abductor and short extensor. Two or more tendons belonging to the abductor pollicis longus are present in 80 percent of patients.[21,47,67] Ganglionic degeneration of the roof of the first extensor compartment is sometimes found.

De Quervain's disease occurs most commonly in healthy women in their sixth decade.[15,38,42,45,53,66,73] An increased incidence of de Quervain's disease has been found in patients with Dupuytren's disease, rheumatoid arthritis, gout, or diabetes mellitus. Most patients with de Quervain's disease will develop

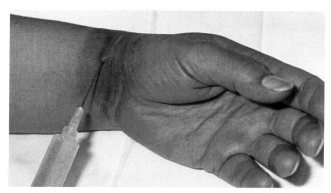

FIGURE 91-5. Infiltration of the skin in surgery for de Quervain's disease.

either trigger finger or carpal tunnel syndrome, or both, although the reverse is not true.[1,20,27,39,41,49,60,61] Thirty percent of patients with de Quervain's disease eventually develop bilateral involvement.[60,61] Osseous malformations, fracture nonunions, and arthritis of the radiocarpal and carpometacarpal joints must be identified prior to treatment. Splint immobilization of the wrist, including the first metacarpal, and glucocorticoid injections of the first dorsal compartment may be curative, although they are less successful in treating de Quervain's disease than they are in other forms of stenosing tenosynovitis. Surgery is indicated if the symptoms persist despite conservative treatment.

Surgical Procedure

Infiltrate the area of the proposed skin incision with local anesthetic before inflating the pneumatic tourniquet (Fig. 91-5). Make the dorsal half of the incision along a transverse extensor crease of the wrist about 10 mm proximal to the tip of the radial styloid (Fig. 91-6). Follow Langer's lines in a palmar direction until a 30-mm incision, centered over the radial styloid, has been made. Radial sensory nerve branches are encountered just deep to the dermis; protect these by gentle retraction (Fig. 91-7). Completely remove the thickened sheath of the first dorsal compartment with a scalpel, both distally and proximally (Fig. 91-8). There may be more than one septum separating the numerous slips of the abductor pollicis longus

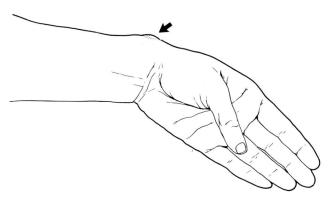

FIGURE 91-4. Schematic drawing of the nodular thickening of the first dorsal compartment in de Quervain's disease.

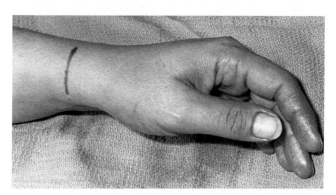

FIGURE 91-6. Skin incision for surgical treatment of de Quervain's disease.

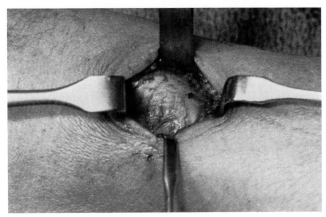

FIGURE 91-7. Exposure of the thickened root of the first dorsal compartment.

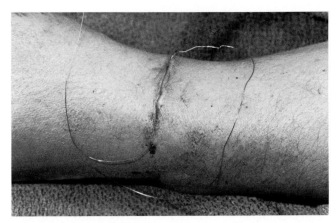

FIGURE 91-9. Running intracuticular 5-0 monofilament steel suture is tied over a 2 × 2 inch gauze dressing.

or the extensor pollicis brevis, so each tendon must be carefully identified. Excise thickened tenosynovium and retinacular ganglia. Examine the floor of the first dorsal compartment for bony, neoplastic, and calcific irregularities, or anomalous tunnels containing aberrant tendons. These, too, must be unroofed. Unimpeded motion may be demonstrated by asking the patient to flex and extend the thumb. After the tourniquet is released, hemostasis is achieved. Close the skin with a nonabsorbable intracuticular suture (Fig. 91-9). In order to prevent palmar subluxation of the tendons, a palmar wrist splint is worn for 2 weeks until the skin suture is removed.

Pitfalls and Complications

Failure to free the extensor pollicis brevis completely from thick adhesions to the abductor pollicis longus, or failure to identify and to incise its separate sheath, may cause symptoms to persist. The abductor pollicis longus may have multiple slips inserting not only into the first metacarpal, but also into the trapezium, carpometacarpal joint capsule, fascia of the opponens or abductor pollicis brevis, or flexor retinaculum. Failure to identify and separate all of the tendons may result in incomplete resolution of symptoms. Laceration of the radial sensory nerve branches warrants immediate microsurgical re-

pair to reduce the likelihood of painful neuroma formation. Compression of the terminal branches of the radial nerve may also produce pain in the area of the first dorsal compartment. Symptoms will include numbness and tingling over the dorsal surface of the thumb and index finger. Paresthesias are accentuated by percussion in this area. The diagnosis of this nerve compression syndrome (Wartenberg's disease) must not be confused with that of de Quervain's disease.

LATERAL EPICONDYLITIS

Lateral epicondylitis is inflammation of the common extensor origin of the elbow. It is often referred to as "tennis elbow."[5,14,25,46,54–56] Usually, there are small tears of the tendon of origin of the extensor carpi radialis brevis, although the extensor digitorum communis may be involved as well.[54,56] The pathology ranges from angiofibroblastic proliferation to complete tendon rupture.[19,55] Pain over the lateral epicondyle and extensor muscle mass when lifting objects palm down and when playing racket sports is characteristic. Throwing and wringing motions may also be painful. Grip strength is decreased as a result of pain on attempts to stabilize the wrist in extension. Tenderness to palpation is noted over the lateral epicondyle of the elbow and radiocapitellar ligament. Wrist extension against resistance causes pain at the lateral epicondyle. X-ray evaluation of the elbow may demonstrate a lateral exostosis, bone chips, or calcific deposits over the lateral epicondyle.

Lateral epicondylitis must be differentiated from radial tunnel syndrome, in which the posterior interosseous nerve is compressed under the fibrous arch of the supinator muscle.[46] Radial tunnel syndrome is characterized by tenderness over the supinator, just distal to the radial head, while pain is reproduced by resisting forearm pronation by the patient, or by resisting middle finger extension with the wrist supported. The two entities may coexist.

Lateral epicondylitis is treated with rest, initial application of ice, and nonsteroidal anti-inflammatory drugs. A 90° long-arm splint with the wrist slightly extended and supinated may be used in recalcitrant cases. Local injections of glucocorticoids are helpful in severe cases; however, limiting their use will help to prevent delayed tendon rupture resulting from their

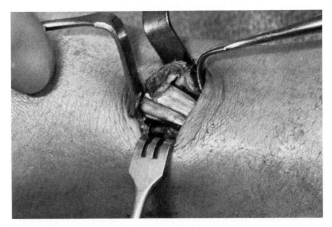

FIGURE 91-8. Elevation of the roof of the first dorsal compartment.

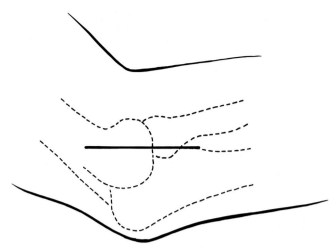

FIGURE 91-10. Skin incision used in the surgical treatment of lateral epicondylitis.

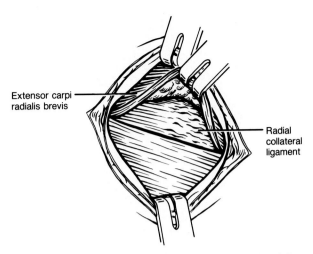

FIGURE 91-12. Partial elevation of the tendon of origin of the extensor carpi radialis brevis, demonstrating tendinous degeneration on its undersurface where it is attached to the lateral epicondyle and radial collateral ligament of the elbow.

catabolic effects. Changing lifting habits to "palm-up" and analyzing sport technique and form are necessary to prevent relapse. A proximal forearm tennis strap may help to prevent relapses. Since the condition is attributable to overuse, wrist curls to strengthen forearm extensors and proper stretching exercises are indicated after the initial recovery is well under way. Surgery is indicated in the few cases that do not respond to conservative therapy.

Surgical Procedure

After administration of regional or general anesthesia make a 6-cm, longitudinal incision that is centered over the radial head (Fig. 91-10). Retract and incise the antebrachial fascia over the extensor carpi radialis brevis and identify the common extensor origin (Fig. 91-11). Gross disruption may be visible at this time. Chronic inflammatory changes may be seen in the proximal margin of the extensor tendon; however, angiofibroblastic changes will become apparent after exposing the deep surface of the tendon of origin. Incise the extensor aponeurosis longi-

tudinally, where the damage will be most accessible. The extensor carpi radialis brevis may or may not need to be elevated completely as a flap (Fig. 91-12). Do not damage the radial collateral ligament or enter the joint. Excise granulation tissue from beneath the extensor carpi radialis tendon (Fig. 91-13) and the extensor digitorum communis, if necessary. Debride degenerated tendon to healthy tissue. The deep surface of the tendon should be free of all granulation tissue (Fig. 91-14). Decorticate the lateral epicondyle to punctate bleeding cortico cancellous bone. Exostoses and calcifications should also be removed at this time. Suture the extensor carpi radialis brevis tendon to the surrounding periosteum and to the extensor digitorum communis tendon (Fig. 91-15). Suture the common extensor aponeurosis closed, and then the skin. The forearm is immobilized in a long-arm splint in neutral rotation with the elbow flexed 90° and the wrist extended 20°. The splint is

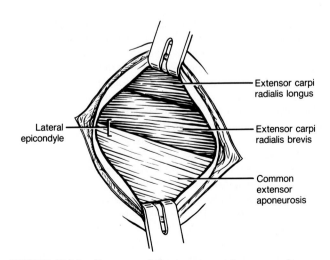

FIGURE 91-11. Exposure of the common extensor muscle group with their tendons of origin after retraction of the antebrachial fascia.

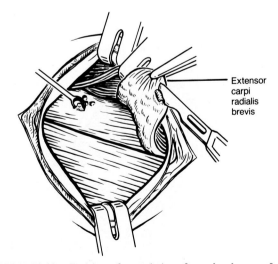

FIGURE 91-13. Excision of granulations from the deep surface of the extensor carpi radialis brevis tendon, and decortication of the lateral epicondyle.

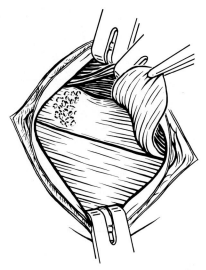

FIGURE 91-14. Well-debrided tendon of origin of the extensor carpi radialis brevis and lateral epicondyle which are decorticated and prepared for tendon reattachment.

removed in 2 to 3 weeks, depending on the degree of extensor tendon repair. Gentle range of motion exercises are permitted, but stress is avoided for a total of 5 weeks. At that time, progressive, resistive exercises are gradually initiated. Vigorous sports are deferred for 6 months in patients with complete tears.

Pitfalls and Complications

Lateral epicondylitis must be differentiated from other causes of lateral elbow pain. Rheumatoid arthritis, gout, radial tunnel nerve syndrome, osteochondritis dissecans, and loose bodies may cause lateral elbow pain alone or in concert with lateral epicondylitis.

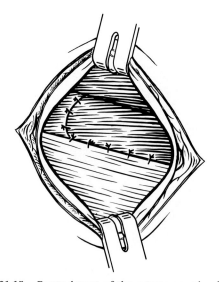

FIGURE 91-15. Reattachment of the extensor carpi radialis brevis tendon of origin to the extensor aponeurosis and periosteum of the lateral epicondyle.

TENDINITIS ABOUT THE WRIST

Finger Flexor Tendinitis in the Carpal Tunnel

Inflammation of the digital flexor tendons can occur in the carpal tunnel. Usually, it is idiopathic in origin, causing compression of the median nerve (see Ch. 104).[2,7,10,45] At other times, it may be attributable to repetitive flexion of the fingers and the wrist, or to direct or indirect trauma.[6,7,9,20,49,50,59] The latter is seen in acute carpal tunnel syndrome.[72] Rheumatoid arthritis; gout; collagen vascular disease; anomalous muscles, tendons, and arteries; as well as tumors, congenital dysplasias, fungus, tubercle bacillus, and atypical microbacteria may precipitate symptomatic digital flexor tenosynovitis at the wrist.[1,2,6,28,30,37,43,44,48,49,52,59,62,74] Splinting the wrist, application of ice, and oral anti-inflammatory agents are usually successful in treating this condition. Occasionally, local steroid injections or even flexor tenosynovectomy are necessary in recalcitrant cases. The treatment of dysplastic, neoplastic, toxic, and metabolic sources of flexor tendinitis usually requires surgical decompression and tenosynovectomy of the flexors of the carpal tunnel, as well as pharmacologic therapy, in order to protect the contents of the carpal tunnel from irreparable damage and to eradicate the underlying disease process.

Surgical Procedure

Digital flexor tenosynovectomy of the wrist can be performed either through a limited incision distal to the transverse flexor crease of the wrist or through a more extensive exposure, involving a 4-cm, zigzag, proximal extension of the original thenar crease incision to include the distal forearm (see Ch. 97).

Pitfalls and Complications

When performing tenosynovectomy of the flexors of the carpal tunnel, laceration of the large, aberrant, sensory branches of the ulnar and median nerves in the subcutaneous fat or penetrating the transverse carpal ligament must be avoided, as must damage to the median nerve. The dorsiflexed wrist is splinted for 2 weeks after surgery to allow a new, loose, retinacular "ligament" to form from granulation tissue, thereby preventing painful recurrent subluxation of the finger flexors from the carpal tunnel during gripping in the flexed wrist position. If subluxing flexor tendinitis occurs at the carpal tunnel, then reconstruction of the transverse retinacular ligament is undertaken using ligamentous remnants or the adjacent fascia. The new ligament is fashioned at the distal margin of the carpal canal so as not to compress the median nerve (Figs. 91-16 and 91-17). Dupuytren's disease or its diathesis is exacerbated by this type of hand surgery; therefore, the pros and cons of surgical management of flexor tendinitis must be weighed carefully in patients with coexistent Dupuytren's disease.

Wrist Flexor Tendinitis

Inflammation of the tendons of the flexor carpi radialis and flexor carpi ulnaris occurs independently, and is usually related to repetitive flexion, direct trauma, or excessive wrist exten-

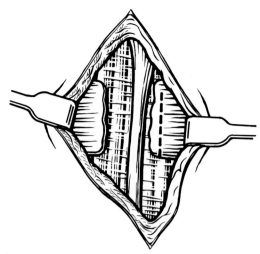

FIGURE 91-16. Formation of a distally based "ligament" that is 5-mm in diameter.

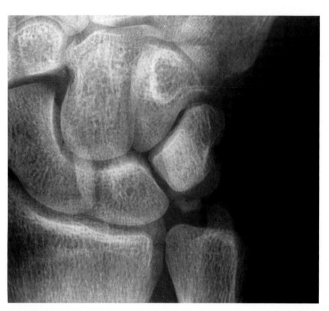

FIGURE 91-18. Calcification of a portion of the tenosynovium of the flexor carpi ulnaris tendon.

sion.[23] Calcifications within the tenosynovium may be present (Fig. 91-18). Rheumatic, metabolic, infectious, and neoplastic diseases may also involve these tendons. Inflammation of the flexor carpi radialis tendon occurs in its fibro-osseous tunnel within the transverse carpal ligament.[23] The flexor carpi ulnaris tendon may become inflamed just proximal to the pisiform.[58] The latter may also be involved in an arthritic process at its articulation with the triquetrum. Ulnar neuritis at Guyon's canal may be secondary to flexor carpi ulnaris tendinitis.[58]

When overuse is the etiology, treatment includes dorsal splinting in 20° palmar flexion, oral anti-inflammatory drugs, and local application of ice. Occasionally, local injections of steroids are also necessary. Surgery is indicated when the patient does not respond to conservative therapy.

Surgical Procedure

Flexor carpi radialis tendinitis is decompressed using a 4-cm zigzag incision that begins at the tuberosity of the scaphoid and

extends proximally. Open the fibro-osseous tunnel of the flexor carpi radialis[23] and perform a Z-lengthening of the tendon. After the skin is closed with interrupted sutures, a dorsal splint in 20° flexion is worn by the patient for 2 weeks. After the sutures are removed, active exercises are begun.

Surgical treatment of chronic flexor carpi ulnaris tendinitis begins with a palmar-ulnar zigzag incision (Fig. 91-19). After sectioning the palmar fascia and abductor digiti minimi muscle, divide the pisohamate ligament, decompressing Guyon's canal (Fig. 91-20). Protect the ulnar nerve and artery proximally and distally, as well as the pisiform metacarpal ligaments. Enucleate

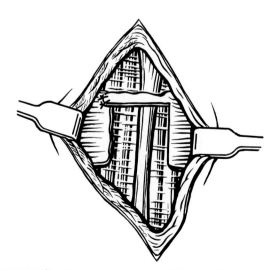

FIGURE 91-17. A new transverse carpal ligament is sutured to the old ligamentous stump on the opposite side of the carpal tunnel.

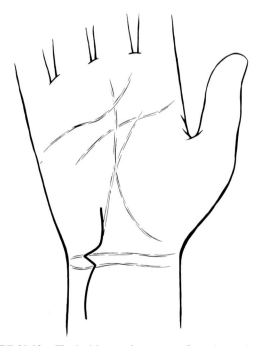

FIGURE 91-19. The incision used to expose Guyon's canal and the distal portion of the flexor carpi ulnaris tendon.

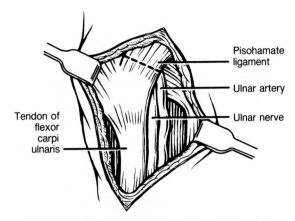

FIGURE 91-20. Incision of the pisohamate ligament.

the pisiform subperiosteally from its capsule through a palmar longitudinal incision[58] (Figs. 91-21 and 91-22). Just proximal to the pisiform, perform a Z-plasty of the flexor carpi ulnaris tendon to allow 5 mm of tendon lengthening[58] (Figs. 91-23 and 91-24). Suture the capsule of the pisiform closed. After the tourniquet is released and hemostasis is achieved, the skin is closed. A dorsal splint in 20° of palmar flexion immobilizes the wrist for 2 weeks until the sutures are removed.

Pitfalls and Complications

The ulnar nerve and artery are in proximity and can be injured by laceration or traction that is too vigorous. The pisiform metacarpal ligament should be maintained intact to avoid weakening palmar-ulnar wrist flexion.

Finger Extensor Tendinitis at the Wrist

Inflammation of the finger extensor tenosynovium can occur over the dorsum of the wrist, distal to and including the extensor retinaculum. Extension of the fingers causes a heaping up of the tenosynovium at the distal margin of the extensor retinaculum (Fig. 91-25). It is usually attributable to repetitive extension of the fingers and wrist, or to direct trauma.[6,7,50] Rheumatoid arthritis, collagen vascular disease, gout, tumors,

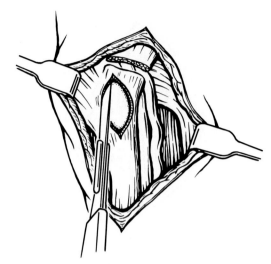

FIGURE 91-22. Removal of the pisiform.

fungus, congenital dysplasias, and typical or atypical microbacteria may also cause symptomatic extensor tenosynovitis of the wrist.[2,3,6,28,30,37,43,44,48,49,52,59,62,74] Palmar splinting of the wrist in 20° extension, local application of ice, and oral anti-inflammatory drugs are usually successful in treating the condition. Occasionally, local injections of steroids around the inflamed tenosynovium, or even extensor tenosynovectomy, may be necessary in severe cases.

Isolated tenosynovitis of the extensor pollicis longus is known as "drummer boy" palsy.[24] It is caused by repetitive flexion and extension of the thumb with ulnar and radial deviation of the wrist. Treatment includes splinting, application of ice, and oral, nonsteroidal, anti-inflammatory drugs. Local instillation of steroid preparations, or even surgery, are occasionally warranted.

Surgical Procedure

After administering regional or general anesthesia, make an oblique incision from the base of the second metacarpal to the

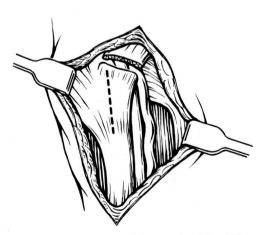

FIGURE 91-21. Incision of the capsule of the pisiform.

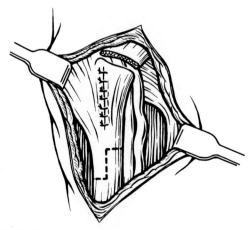

FIGURE 91-23. Incision used to Z-lengthen the flexor carpi ulnaris tendon, with subsequent closure of the capsule of the pisiform.

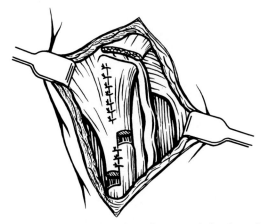

FIGURE 91-24. Lengthening of the flexor carpi ulnaris tendon by 5 mm using a Z-plasty.

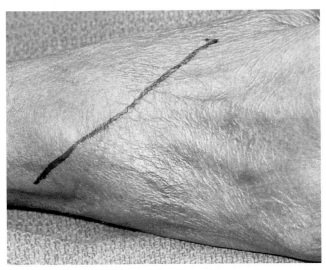

FIGURE 91-26. The incision used to expose the extensor retinaculum.

metaphysis of the distal ulna (Fig. 91-26). Identify and protect the sensory branches of the radial and ulnar nerves. When possible, retract large veins while exposing the tendons in the distal part of the wound (Fig. 91-27). Incise the extensor retinaculum at the septum between the first and second dorsal compartments. Preserve the proximal 20 percent of the extensor retinaculum to prevent bow-stringing of the extensor tendons, and raise the extensor retinaculum as an ulnar-based flap until the sixth compartment is decompressed (Fig. 91-28). Remove Lister's tubercle with a rongeur. Excise the tenosynovium from all of the finger and wrist extensors (Fig. 91-29). Next, pass the flap of extensor retinaculum deep to the finger and wrist extensor, and sew it back to adjacent soft tissues in the area of the first dorsal compartment of the wrist (Fig. 91-30). After the tourniquet is released and hemostasis is achieved, close the wound. Drainage may be continued for 2 days, if necessary. A 20° dorsiflexed palmar splint is worn until the skin sutures are removed, whereupon gentle active range of motion is begun.

Isolated tenosynovitis of the extensor pollicis longus is treated by incising the third dorsal compartment and by removal of Lister's tubercle. This is done through a 2-cm transverse incision that is centered in an ulnar direction from Lister's tubercle. Protect the sensory branches of the radial nerve. Transpose the extensor pollicis longus tendon radially, away from Lister's tubercle, which has been removed. Suture the tendon sheath closed, and then close the skin. A palmar splint is worn for 2 weeks until the skin sutures are removed.

Pitfalls and Complications

The sensory branches of the superficial radial nerve and dorsal cutaneous branch of the ulnar nerve can be lacerated and should, therefore, be avoided. If injured, they should be repaired. The extensor pollicis longus tendon can also be lacer-

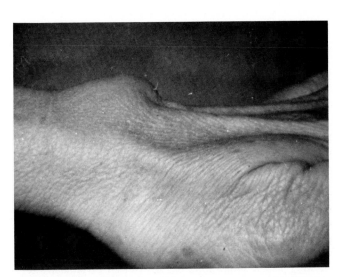

FIGURE 91-25. Heaping up of the extensor tenosynovium distal to the extensor retinaculum during finger extension.

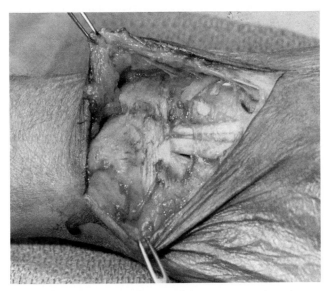

FIGURE 91-27. Tenosynovitis of the extensors at the wrist.

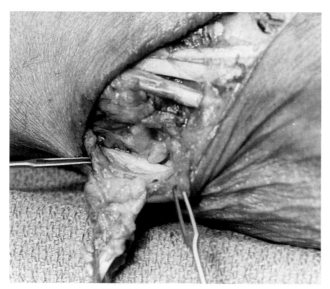

FIGURE 91-28. The extensor retinaculum is raised as an ulnar-based flap.

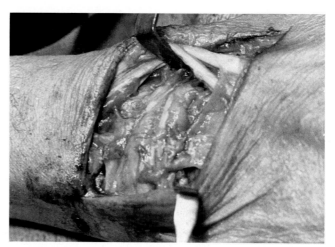

FIGURE 91-30. The extensor retinacular flap is laid deep to the extensor tendons and sewn to the roof of the first dorsal compartment and to the adjacent wrist capsule.

ated as it crosses the radial wrist extensors obliquely. Immediate tenorrhaphy is then performed. Extensor pollicis longus tendinitis can be differentiated from de Quervain's disease on the basis of their differing points of maximum tenderness.

Radial Wrist Extensor Tendinitis (Intersection Syndrome)

Radial wrist extensor tendinitis (intersection syndrome) is caused by inflammation of the tenosynovium of the extensor carpi radialis longus and brevis within the second dorsal extensor compartment of the wrist.[29] Pain and swelling are noted on palpation where the two wrist extensors cross the abductor pollicis longus and extensor pollicis brevis.[4,18,29,32,69] The condition may be attributable to repetitive extension and flexion of the wrist, or to direct trauma. Conservative therapy includes a palmar wrist splint in 20° extension; application of ice; administration of oral, nonsteroidal, anti-inflammatory agents; and

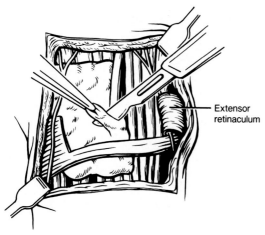

FIGURE 91-29. Extensor tenosynovectomy.

local injections of steroid preparations. Surgery is reserved for recalcitrant cases that are unresponsive to prolonged conservative therapy, including steroid injections around the tendons just proximal to the extensor retinaculum.

Surgical Procedure

Using regional or general anesthesia, make an ulnar-based, chevron incision over the second dorsal compartment, crossing the wrist creases diagonally. Protect the branches of the radial nerve. Incise the second dorsal extensor compartment and remove exuberant tenosynovium from the two radial wrist extensors back to their junction with the tendons of the abductor pollicis longus and extensor pollicis brevis.[29] Examine the latter and remove their tenosynovium. Hemostasis is achieved after the tourniquet is released. Close the skin and apply a palmar splint in 20° dorsiflexion. Skin sutures are removed 2 weeks later, and the splint is discarded.

Pitfalls and Complications

Sensory branches of the radial nerve should be repaired, if lacerated. Intersection syndrome can be differentiated from de Quervain's disease on the basis of their differing points of maximal tenderness.

Ulnar Wrist Extensor Tendinitis (Recurrent Subluxation of the Extensor Carpi Ulnaris Tendon)

Chronic recurrent subluxation of the extensor carpi ulnaris tendon may result in painful tenosynovitis. This condition is usually attributable to a single forceful or repetitive hypersupination motion of the wrist with ulnar deviation.[11] The infratendinous retinaculum of the wrist is stretched or ruptured, allowing palmar subluxation of the extensor carpi ulnaris tendon.[11,26] Conservative management consists of splint immobilization in a dorsiflexed position, pronation, and radial deviation

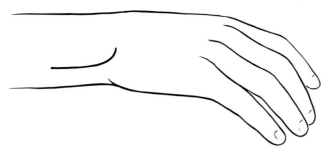

FIGURE 91-31. Incision to reconstruct the sixth dorsal compartment of the wrist.

of the wrist. Oral anti-inflammatory agents, as well as local injections of steroids, may alleviate symptoms. Surgical reconstruction is indicated in selected individuals whose symptoms do not resolve with conservative therapy.

Surgical Procedure

After administration of general or regional anesthesia with the wrist pronated, make a hockey stick incision from the base of the fifth metacarpal, and extend it 2 cm radially and 4 cm proximally (Fig. 91-31). Protect the sensory branches of the ulnar nerve as they cross the distal portion of the wound. As the supratendinous portion of the retinaculum is viewed, identify the sixth dorsal extensor compartment. Make a radially based flap that is about 1 cm wide and about 5 mm proximal to the distal margin of the retinaculum through the supratendinous extensor retinaculum. Be careful to make the window palmar enough to view the extensor carpi ulnaris tendon, which is subluxed into the depths of the wound[8] (Fig. 91-32). Locate the stretched or torn infratendinous retinaculum, which normally creates a medial wall against palmar subluxation of the extensor carpi ulnaris tendon. After assessing the proper dorsal replacement position for the extensor carpi ulnaris tendon, create a second radially based flap, about 1 cm in width, from the proximal portion of the extensor retinaculum. Make it long enough in a palmar-ulnar direction to allow creation of a sling

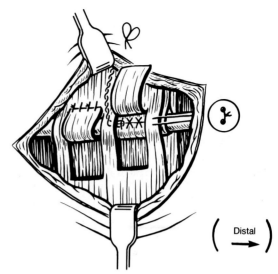

FIGURE 91-33. Creation of an extensor carpi ulnaris sling and repair of the infratendinous retinaculum using a pull-out wire technique.

around the tendon of the extensor carpi ulnaris.[26] After the proximal flap has been wrapped around the extensor carpi ulnaris tendon and sutured to itself with two horizontal mattress sutures, repair the infratendinous retinacular leash around the same tendon, using a pull-out wire suture[11] (Fig. 91-33). If the septal tissues are irreparable, then use the distal flap portion of the extensor retinaculum as a free fascial graft. A portion of the extensor carpi ulnaris tendon proximal to the extensor retinaculum may also be used as a free graft.[11] Close the retinaculum (Fig. 91-34).

After the tourniquet is released, hemostasis is achieved, and the skin is closed. A long-arm splint is worn for 6 weeks with the wrist dorsiflexed at 25° and the forearm in neutral rotation. Active motion is increased in intensity over the next 6 weeks.

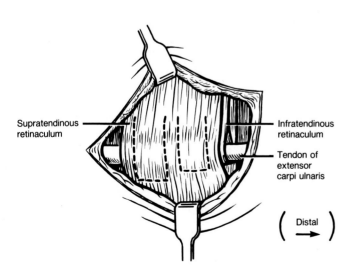

Supratendinous retinaculum

Infratendinous retinaculum

Tendon of extensor carpi ulnaris

Distal

FIGURE 91-32. Preparation of the flaps in the supratendinous portion of the extensor retinaculum.

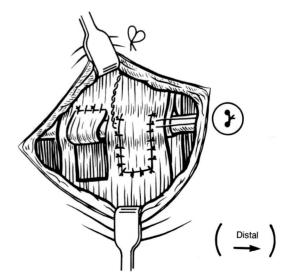

Distal

FIGURE 91-34. Closure of the retinacular window and placement of the pull-out wire.

Pitfalls and Complications

The dorsal cutaneous branch of the ulnar nerve may be lacerated; if it is, it should be repaired microscopically. A free graft must be used, if needed, to repair a deficient infratendinous retinaculum, as swinging a fascial flap toward the deficient medial wall may tether wrist rotation.

REFERENCES

1. Aitken, A.: Stenosing Tendovaginitis at the Radial Styloid Process. N. Engl. J. Med. **232:**105, 1945.
2. Barfred, T., and Ipsa, T.: Congenital Carpal Tunnel Syndrome. J. Hand Surg. **10:**246, 1985.
3. Barfred, T., et al.: Median Artery in Carpal Tunnel Syndrome. J. Hand Surg. **10-A:**854, 1985.
4. Berman, M.: Stenosing Tenovaginitis of the Dorsal and Volar Compartments of the Wrist. AMA Arch. Surg. **55:**752, 1952.
5. Boyd, N.: Tennis Elbow. J. Bone Joint Surg. **55-A:**1183, 1973.
6. Boyes, J. (ed.): Bunnell's Surgery of the Hand, 5th ed. Philadelphia, J.B. Lippincott, 1984.
7. Boyes, J. (ed.): Bunnell's Surgery of the Hand, 4th ed. Philadelphia, J.B. Lippincott, 1970.
8. Broker, A.S.: Extensor Carpi Radialis Tenosynovitis. Orthop. Rev. **6:**99, 1977.
9. Browne, E.Z.: Carpal Tunnel Syndrome Caused by Hand Injuries. Plast. Reconstr. Surg. **56:**41, 1975.
10. Bunnell, S.: Surgery of the Hand. Philadelphia, J.B. Lippincott, 1944.
11. Burkhart, S., et al.: Post-traumatic Recurrent Subluxation of the Extensor Carpi Ulnaris Tendon. J. Hand Surg. **7:**1, 1982.
12. Compere, E.: Bilateral Snappy Thumbs. Am. Surg. **97:**773, 1933.
13. Conklin, J., et al.: Stenosing Tenosynovitis. Surg. Clin. North Am. **40:**531, 1960.
14. Coonrad, R.W.: Tennis Elbow—Its Course, Natural History, Conservative and Surgical Management. J. Bone Joint Surg. **55-A:**1177, 1973.
15. Cotton, F., et al.: De Quervain's Disease. N. Engl. J. Med. **219:**120, 1938.
16. Dellon, A., et al.: Bilateral Inability to Grasp Due to Multiple (Ten) Congenital Trigger Fingers. J. Hand Surg. **5:**470, 1980.
17. Dinham, J., and Maggett, D.: Trigger Thumbs in Children. J. Bone Joint Surg. **56-B:**153, 1974.
18. Dobyns, J., et al.: Sports Stress Syndromes of the Hand and Wrist. Am. J. Sports Med. **6:**236, 1978.
19. Fahey, J., et al.: Trigger Finger in Adults and Children. J. Bone Joint Surg. **36-A:**1200, 1954.
20. Fara, M., et al.: Stenosing Tendovaginitis of the Radial, Dorsal, and Volar Compartments of the Hand. Acta Chir. Scand. **15:**93, 1973.
21. Fenton, R.: Stenosing Tenosynovitis at the Radial Styloid Process Involving an Accessory Tendon Sheath. Bull. Hosp. Joint Dis. **11:**90, 1950.
22. Finkelstein, H.: Stenosing Tendovaginitis of the Radial Styloid Process. J. Bone Joint Surg. **12:**509, 1930.
23. Fitton, J., and Doldie, W.: Lesions of the Flexor Carpi Radialis Tendon and Sheath Causing Pain at the Wrist. J. Bone Joint Surg. **50-B:**359, 1968.
24. Froimson, A.: Stenosing Tenosynovitis. In Green, D. (ed.): Operative Hand Surgery. New York, Churchill Livingstone, 1982.
25. Goldie, I.: Upper Condylitis Lateralis Humeri. Acta Chir. Scand. [Suppl.] **339:**1, 1964.
26. Green, D.: The Sore Wrist Without a Fracture. In American Academy of Orthopedic Surgery: Instructional Course Lectures, no. 34. St. Louis, C.V. Mosby, 1985.
27. Grimes, H.: Stenosing Tenosynovitis. J. Ark. Med. Soc. **77:**499, 1981.
28. Gropper, P., et al.: Flexor Tenosynovitis Caused by Coccydioides immitis. J. Hand Surg. **8:**344, 1983.
29. Grundberg, A., and Reagan, D.: Pathologic Anatomy of the Forearm: Intersection Syndrome. J. Hand Surg. **10-A:**299, 1985.
30. Gumther, S., and Elliot, R.: Mycobacterium kansaii Infection in the Deep Structures of the Hand. J. Bone Joint Surg. **58-A:**140, 1976.
31. Hall, C.L., and Berg, C.: Chronic Stenosing Tenosynovitis of the Wrist. J. Int. Coll. Surg. **12:**509, 1930.
32. Howard, N.: Peritendinitis Crepitans. J. Bone Joint Surg. **19-A:**447, 1976.
33. Hueston, J., et al.: The Etiology of Trigger Finger. Hand **4:**257, 1973.
34. Hueston, J., et al.: Trigger Thumb. Med. J. Aust. **2:**1044, 1973.
35. Jahs, S.A.: Trigger Finger in Children. JAMA **107:**1463, 1936.
36. Janssen, J., et al.: De Quervain's Disease. Wis. Med. J. **69:**95, 1970.
37. Kelly, P.J., et al.: Infections of Tendon Sheaths, Bursae, Joints, and Soft Tissues by Acid-Fast Bacilli and Tubercle Bacilli. J. Bone Joint Surg. **45-A:**326, 1963.
38. Lamphier, T., et al.: De Quervain's Disease. Ann. Surg. **138:**832, 1953.
39. Lapidus, P.: Stenosing Tenovaginitis at the Wrists and Fingers. AMA Arch. Surg. **64:**475, 1952.
40. Lapidus, P., et al.: Stenosing Tendovaginitis of the Wrists and Fingers. Clin. Orthop. **83:**87, 1972.
41. Lapidus, P., et al.: Stenosing Tendovaginitis of the Wrists and Fingers. AMA Arch. Surg. **64:**475, 1952.
42. Leao, L.: De Quervain's Disease: A Clinical and Anatomic Study. J. Bone Joint Surg. **40-A:**1063, 1958.
43. Lee, K.: Tuberculosis Representing a Carpal Tunnel Syndrome. J. Hand Surg. **10-A:**242, 1985.
44. Lipscomb, P.: Tenosynovitis of the Hand and the Wrist: Carpal Tunnel Syndrome, de Quervain's Disease, and Trigger Digit. Clin. Orthop. **13:**164, 1959.
45. Lipscomb, P.: Non-suppurative Tenosynovitis and Paratendinitis. In American Academy of Orthopedic Surgeons: Instructional Course Lecture, no. 7. St. Louis, C.V. Mosby, 1950.
46. Lister, G., et al.: The Radial Tunnel Syndrome. J. Hand Surg. **4:**52, 1959.
47. Loomis, L.: Variations of Stenosing Tenosynovitis of the Radial Styloid Process. J. Bone Joint Surg. **33-A:**220, 1951.
48. Louis, D., et al.: Lipofibromas of the Median Nerve: Long-term Follow-up of 4 Cases. J. Hand Surg. **10-A:**403, 1985.
49. Love, G., and Melchior, E.: Mycobacterium terrae Tenosynovitis. J. Hand Surg. **10-A:**730, 1985.
50. McCue, F., and Miller, G.: Soft tissue injuries in the hand. In American Academy of Orthopedic Surgeons: Symposium on Upper Extremity Injuries in Athletes. St. Louis, C.V. Mosby, 1986.
51. Meachim, G., et al.: The Histopathology of Stenosing Tendovaginitis. J. Pathol. **98:**187, 1969.
52. Moore, J., and Weiland, A: Gouty Tenosynovitis in the Hand. J. Hand Surg. **10-A:**291, 1985.
53. Muckart, R.: Stenosing Tendovaginitis of the Abductor Pollicis Longus and Extensor Pollicis Brevis at the Radial Styloid. Clin. Orthop. **33:**201, 1954.
54. Neviaser, T., et al.: Lateral Epicondylitis: Results of Out-patient Surgery and Immediate Motion. Contemp. Orthop. **22:**43, 1985.
55. Nirschl, R.: Mesenchymal Syndrome. Va. Med. J. **96:**659, 1969.
56. Nirschl, R., and Pettrone, S.: Tennis Elbow: The Surgical Treatment of Lateral Epicondylitis. J. Bone Joint Surg. **61-A:**832, 1979.

57. Oldberg, S.: A New Fact in the Etiology of Chronic Nonspecific Tendovaginitis in the Wrist. Upsala J. Med. Sci. **78:**160, 1973.

58. Palmieri, T.: Pisiform Area Pain Treated by Pisiform Excision. J. Hand Surg. **7:**477, 1982.

59. Phalen, G.: Carpal Tunnel Syndrome. Clin. Orthop. **83:**29, 1972.

60. Pruzansky, M., and Riordan, D.: Trigger Finger, Carpal Tunnel Syndrome, and de Quervain's Disease: Tardive Manifestation of Deficient Connective Tissue. Submitted for publication.

61. Pruzansky, M., and Riordan, D.: The Association of Trigger Finger, Carpal Tunnel Syndrome and de Quervain's Disease with Dupuytren's Disease.

62. Schneider, L.H., and Bush, D.C.: Tuberculosis of the hand and wrist. J. Hand Surg. **9-A:**391, 1984.

63. Seradje, H., and Kleinert, H.: Reduction Flexor Tenoplasty. J. Hand Surg. **6:**543, 1981.

64. Sorensen, V.: Treatment of Trigger Fingers. Acta Orthop. Scand. **41:**428, 1970.

65. Sprecher, E.: Trigger Finger in Infants. J. Bone Joint Surg. **31-A:**672, 1949.

66. Stern, A., et al.: Stenosing Tendovaginitis at the Radial Styloid Process. AMA Arch. Surg. **63:**215, 1951.

67. Strandess, G.: Variations in the Anatomy in Stenosing Tenosynovitis at the Radial Styloid Process. Acta Chir. Scand. **113:**234, 1957.

68. Taleisnik, J., et al.: The Extensor Retinaculum of the Wrist. J. Hand Surg. **9-A:**495, 1984.

69. Thompson, A.R., et al.: Peritendinitis Crepitans and Simple Tenosynovitis: A Clinical Study of 544 cases in industry. Br. J. Ind. Med. **8:**150, 1951.

70. Van Gemechten, F.: Familial Trigger Thumb in Children. Hand **14:**1, 1982.

71. Weildy, A.: Trigger Finger. Acta Orthop. Scand. **41:**419, 1970.

72. Wilgis, E.S.: Compression neuropathies. *In* American Academy of Orthopedic Surgeons: Symposium on Microsurgery. St. Louis, C.V. Mosby, 1979.

73. Younghusband, O., et al.: De Quervain's Disease: Stenosing Tenovaginitis at the Radial Styloid Process. Can. Med. Assoc. J. **89:**508, 1963.

74. Yuan, R.N.: Candida albicans Tenosynovitis of the Hand. J. Hand Surg. **10-A:**719, 1985.

75. Zelle, O., et al.: Snapping Thumb: Tendovaginitis Stenosans. Am. J. Surg. **33:**31, 1936.

CHAPTER 92

Dislocations and Ligamentous Injuries of the Digits

ROBERT J. NEVIASER

Dislocations and ligamentous injuries of the digital joints of the hand are quite common. Fortunately, in the acute phase, most of these injuries can be treated by closed or nonoperative means. This discussion approaches these topics by joint. The fingers are covered as one, except where a specific injury to a specific joint in a specific finger requires individual attention. The joints of the thumb are addressed separately.

ANATOMY

All the interphalangeal and metacarpophalangeal joints of the fingers and thumb are similar in that their stability is provided by a series of ligaments. The volar plate is a fibrocartilaginous structure firmly attached to bone distally with a filmy proximal recess. On the sides of each joint are the collateral ligaments, which blend palmarly with the accessory collateral ligaments. The shape of these collateral ligaments varies from a slightly fanlike shape at the proximal interphalangeal level to very fan shaped at the metacarpophalangeal joint.

The metacarpal head of the fingers is shaped with a proportionately bigger anteroposterior diameter than that of the phalangeal head. In addition the metacarpal origin of the collateral ligament is more dorsal than its counterpart at the proximal interphalangeal joint. These factors dictate that the collateral ligaments of the metacarpophalangeal joint are at their greatest length or most taut in full flexion, while those of the proximal interphalangeal are most taut at only a few degrees of flexion. It is critical to remember this when testing for collateral ligament stability or when determining the tension appropriate for a repaired ligament, both during the repair and after surgery.

GENERAL PRINCIPLES

Most dislocations or ligament injuries can be treated by closed means. Digital block anesthesia can be helpful in evaluating joint stability or reducing dislocations but is often unnecessary.

Dislocations are usually obvious from clinical examination, but good radiographs in at least two planes are valuable. These should include a true lateral view of the digit (not of the hand), both before and after reduction, to assess accurately associated fractures as well as efficacy of treatment. Stress views can be used for ligament injuries if there is a question on clinical testing about whether a ligament is completely ruptured or not. If used, anesthesia (usually a digital block or intra-articular) is helpful to reap the maximum benefit from stress.

If the injury is amenable to closed treatment, the initial immobilization should be in a cast dressing that immobilizes the hand and wrist as well as all the fingers and, if necessary, the thumb. An acutely injured digit can be further harmed by immediately taping it to a digital splint. The ulnar gutter splint does not put the hand at rest, does not reduce the forces acting at the site of injury, rarely keeps the joints in the proper position, and does not control swelling. After surgical intervention a similar cast dressing is applied.

For closed treatment cases the dressing is changed within 5 days, and the appropriate active motion program is begun, with modifications for the specific injury being treated. The same is true for postoperative cases. The goal is to provide joint stability and adequate protection against reinjury or disruption of the repair while gaining maximal motion to prevent tendon adherence or joint stiffness.

FINGERS

Distal Interphalangeal Joint

Dislocations

Dislocations of the distal interphalangeal joint are almost always dorsal and are rare. Closed reduction, with or without digital block anesthesia, is readily accomplished. When the dislocation is chronic or irreducible, open reduction is required.

Technique. Make a straight dorsal midline incision and split the extensor tendon longitudinally in the midline. If the volar plate is interposed between the joint surfaces, excise as much as necessary to displace it palmarly. Strip the collateral ligaments from the middle phalanx subperiosteally with a no. 11 knife. Continue this dissection until the joint can be reduced. When reduction has been achieved, test for stability. If the joint is grossly unstable, transfix it with a 0.035-inch smooth wire for 3 weeks. If the joint is fairly stable, simply close the skin, and immobilize in a cast dressing for a few days for comfort. Then apply a dorsal-block splint and allow active flexion. Remove the splint after 3 weeks. If the joint surface damage is extensive, perform a primary arthrodesis.

Complications. Redislocation occurs if hyperextension is not prevented for at least 3 weeks.

Ligament Injuries

Unless they accompany a dislocation, nearly all ligament injuries of the distal interphalangeal joint are partial tears or sprains at the distal interphalangeal joint level and thus can be treated nonoperatively. Temporary splinting for a few days for comfort should be followed by an early, vigorous active motion program.

Proximal Interphalangeal Joint

Dorsal Dislocations

The direction of the deforming force determines the type of dislocation of the proximal interphalangeal joint, while the amount of force dictates whether the injury is a subluxation or a dislocation. Dorsal dislocations are often accompanied by a longitudinal compressive force; the magnitude of compression influences the complexity of the ultimate injury.

The acute dorsal injury without fracture usually can be reduced by closed means. A digital block is often unnecessary. The volar plate of necessity is ruptured, usually from the prox-

imal phalanx, but the collateral ligaments rarely are ruptured completely from their attachments. The joint usually is stable following reduction, and early active motion—with protection against hyperextension—is encouraged.

Chronic dorsal dislocations are not common; they require open reduction when encountered. An attempt at gentle closed reduction under adequate anesthesia is permissible but is best done in the operating suite; if it is unsuccessful, the joint then can be approached surgically.

Technique. Make a straight dorsal longitudinal incision. Divide the central slip of the extensor mechanism in the midline. Do *not* extend this incision distal to the base of the middle phalanx. The attachments of the central slip to the middle phalanx and triangular ligament must remain intact. If the volar plate is interposed, split the interval between it and each accessory collateral ligament. Mobilize the volar plate, and try to reduce the joint. If this fails release the origins of the collateral ligaments from the proximal phalanx by sharp subperiosteal dissection. This should allow reduction if the joint is hyperextended and the volar plate is pushed palmarward. After reduction test the joint for gross instability; if this is present, transfix the joint with a smooth 0.035-inch wire for 3 weeks. If the joint is fairly stable, close the extensor split and the skin separately with 5-0 nonabsorbable sutures.

Immobilize the hand in a cast dressing with the proximal interphalangeal joints flexed no more than 10° to 20°. After 5 to 7 days, begin active flexion for an additional 2 to 4 weeks, using a dorsal-block splint to prevent hyperextension.

Complications. Redislocation can occur if hyperextension is not prevented for at least 3 weeks. An intraoperative radiograph will help guard against persistent subluxation.

Palmar Dislocations

Palmar proximal interphalangeal dislocations are rare. The importance of this injury is that the head of the proximal phalanx herniates through the extensor mechanism, creating a boutonniere injury[10,12] (Fig. 92-1A and B).

Usually, closed treatment will successfully reduce these dislocations. If so the proximal interphalangeal joint should be splinted in extension for 4 to 6 weeks, either with a smooth pin transfixing the joint or simply with an external splint. The distal interphalangeal and metacarpophalangeal joints should be permitted to move so that the extensor mechanism is less likely to become adherent. If the dislocation is irreducible or chronic, surgery is necessary.

Technique. Make a straight dorsal incision. Mobilize the lateral bands so that the head of the proximal phalanx is no longer caught between them. Reduce the joint, and transfix it in extension with a smooth 0.035-inch wire. Reattach the central slip to the base of the middle phalanx, and repair the interval between each lateral band and the central slip with 5-0 nonabsorbable sutures. Remove the pin after 4 to 6 weeks, having allowed active motion at the metacarpophalangeal and distal interphalangeal joints during that time.

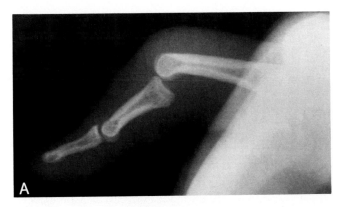

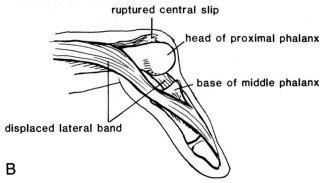

FIGURE 92-1. (*A*) Lateral radiograph of volar proximal interphalangeal dislocation. (*B*) Diagram showing how the boutonniere develops as the head of the proximal phalanx herniates through the extensor mechanism.

Complications. Boutonniere deformity will result if any proximal interphalangeal flexion is allowed during the immobilization period.

Rotary (Irreducible) Dislocations

Irreducible rotary dislocation of the proximal interphalangeal joint is an uncommon injury in which the middle phalanx is displaced laterally and palmarly. On the injured side the collateral ligament is ruptured, and the condyle of the proximal phalanx penetrates through a longitudinal rent between the lateral band and central slip (Fig. 92-2). The lateral band is looped through the joint around the condyle, preventing reduction.

Radiographically, the lateral and palmar dislocation can be improved by closed reduction, but there will be a persistent subluxation and widening of the joint space on the side of injury (Fig. 92-3). The latter problem must be treated surgically.

Technique. Make a midaxial incision on the injured side of the finger. The condyle protruding between the central slip and lateral band will be seen at once (Fig. 92-4). Extricate the lateral band from the joint with a blunt instrument. The joint will promptly reduce. Repair the collateral ligament. If the lateral band is not badly damaged, repair the longitudinal rent in the interval between it and the central slip. If the lateral band

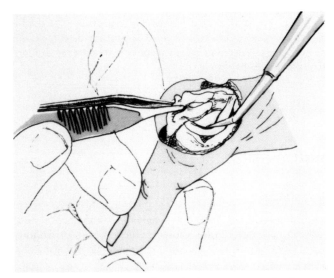

FIGURE 92-2. A longitudinal rent in the extensor mechanism produced by the condyle of the proximal phalanx (*above probe*) splits the central slip (*held by forceps*) from the lateral band (*below probe*); the band then loops around the condyle and through the joint, preventing reduction.

is severely damaged, excise it. The remaining intact central slip and lateral band are sufficient to provide full extension of the finger.[8]

After 5 to 7 days of immobilization in a cast dressing, the patient may start active motion, with the finger strapped to the adjacent finger to protect against reinjury. The finger should be protected for 4 to 6 weeks.

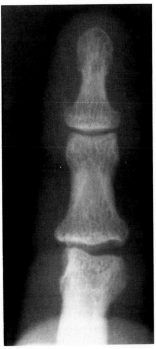

FIGURE 92-3. Anteroposterior radiograph showing persistent subluxation or widening on one side of the proximal interphalangeal joint.

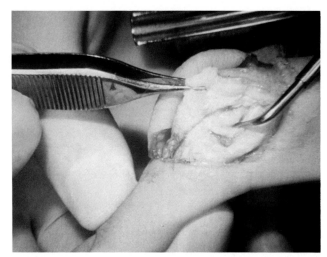

FIGURE 92-4. Clinical photograph corresponding to Figure 92-2.

Complications. Incomplete reduction results from incomplete removal of the lateral band. Joint instability results from inadequate collateral ligament repair.

Fracture–Dislocations

Fracture–dislocation of the proximal interphalangeal joint is probably the most difficult fracture–dislocation to treat in the hand. Many techniques have been reported,[2,13] but none has provided a universal solution to the problem that results from a dorsal dislocation with a significant longitudinal force component. As the middle phalanx displaces proximally and dorsally, the head of the proximal phalanx is driven into the palmar lip of the base of the middle. A comminuted depressed fracture usually results and can involve 70% or more of the articular surface.

Whenever possible this injury should be treated by closed means. The most effective method is the dorsal extension-block splinting technique of McElfresh and co-workers.[7] It should always be tried first, since it yields the best results if applicable (Fig. 92-5A). The key to its usefulness is restoration of the joint alignment, *not* reduction of the fracture. If the fracture reduces also, this is a bonus albeit unnecessary. (Figs. 92-5B, C).

If joint alignment cannot be restored by closed means, extension-block splinting should be abandoned and an open procedure used. Although some surgeons suggest open reduction and internal fixation, the comminution of the palmar lip makes this a demanding and often frustrating technique. Rarely is full motion restored. An alternative that can be used for acute as well as chronic injury is the volar plate arthroplasty described by Eaton.[4]

Technique. Make a palmar zig-zag incision over the proximal interphalangeal joint. Excise the flexor sheath and A3 pulley from the distal edge of the A2 to the proximal edge of the A4 pulley. Protect the digital arteries and nerves at all times. Retract the flexor tendons without damaging the vincula. Mobilize the volar plate and accessory collateral ligaments with the attached palmar lip fragment from the middle phalanx, leaving it attached proximally. Excise (especially in chronic cases) the

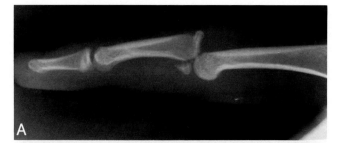

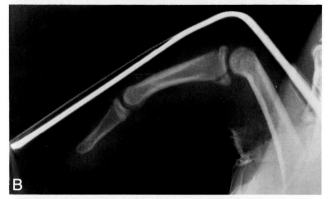

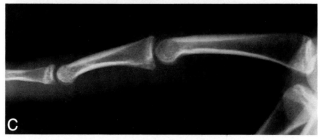

FIGURE 92-5. (*A*) Fracture-dislocation of the proximal interphalangeal joint. (*B*) Joint reduced by flexion of the finger to 60° or more. The fracture reduction—anatomic here—is a bonus, but is not necessary for a good result. (*C*) Healed fracture-dislocation with good joint congruity.

remaining collateral ligaments, connecting the proximal and middle phalanges, and then open the joint by hyperextension (like a shotgun) (Fig. 92-6).

Debride small or loose fragments. If the fragment attached to the volar plate is large, fix it with fine smooth Kirschner wire(s) to the middle phalanx, being careful to establish a smooth articular surface and a congruous joint reduction. Check this on a lateral intraoperative radiograph. More commonly, the volar plate fragment cannot be used. Dissect it free subperiosteally from the volar plate, retaining all possible length of the plate. Mobilize the volar plate as much as possible, leaving its proximal attachment intact, by freeing up any restraining bands in the recess.

Create a transverse trough in the middle phalangeal defect at the dorsalmost part of the cancellous defect, near the palmar margin of the remaining dorsal articular cartilage. The trough will be perpendicular to the long axis of the middle phalanx. Place drill holes at the lateral margins of the trough. Place a criss-cross, 4-0 nonabsorbable suture in the distal volar plate, and pass the ends through the drill holes. Reduce the joint, and pull the volar plate into the trough with the joint flexed no

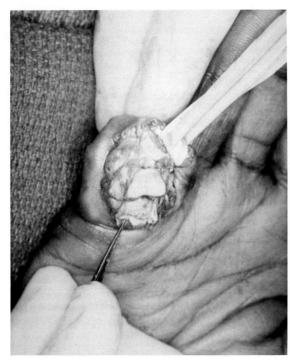

FIGURE 92-6. Proximal interphalangeal joint exposed by opening like a shotgun. From the bottom: fracture fragment with attached volar plate, head of proximal phalanx, base of middle phalanx with defect from compression fracture.

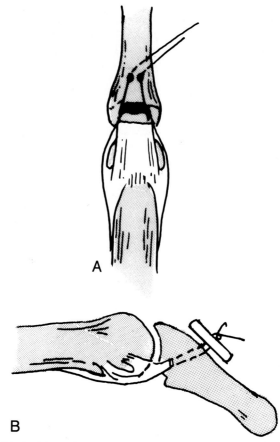

FIGURE 92-7. (*A*) View from palmar side of volar plate arthroplasty as sutures lead the distal edge of the volar plate into trough at base of the middle phalanx. (*B*) Lateral view of volar plate arthroplasty secured with the joint flexed.

more than 30° (Fig.92-7*A* and *B*). Tie the suture over a protected button dorsally. Check the reduction on a lateral intraoperative radiograph. Transfix the joint with a smooth 0.035-inch Kirschner wire.

Immobilize the hand in a cast dressing. Remove the wire at 2 weeks, and encourage active flexion with use of an extension-block splint. Begin active extension at 4 weeks and extension splinting at 5 weeks if full extension is lacking. Motion may continue to improve for several months.

Complications.   Persistent dislocation can occur with closed treatment when the joint hinges instead of reducing congruously. Redislocation results from improper reduction at surgery. Loss of reduction can result from failure of the pull-out suture or improper protection against joint extension.

Collateral Ligament Injuries

Most injuries to the collateral ligaments of the proximal interphalangeal joint are incomplete. These need only to be protected by strapping to an adjacent digit for 3 to 4 weeks. Complete ruptures are uncommon, and their treatment is controversial. In the acute stage most can be dealt with by strapping to an adjacent digit and encouraging full active motion for 3 to 4 weeks. The radial collateral ligament of the index is probably the only ligament that needs early surgery.[35,36]

Technique.   Make a radial midaxial incision. Divide the transverse retinacular ligament and reflect it. Retract the radial lateral band dorsally. Identify the torn collateral ligament, and

repair it to the stump still attached (usually at the middle phalanx) with 4-0 nonabsorbable sutures. If no residual stump is present, roughen the bone and drill parallel holes obliquely across the phalanx. Pass a 4-0 nonabsorbable suture in a modified Bunnell fashion through the torn edge of the ligament; then pass the two ends through the holes in the bone and out through the skin. Tie the suture over a protected button with the joint reduced and the ligament pulled taut. Suture the accompanying partial tear of the volar plate as well. Repair the retinacular ligament, and then close the skin. Splint the digit in no more than 20° of proximal interphalangeal joint flexion for 5 to 7 days. Start active motion with adjacent finger strapping for an additional 2 to 3 weeks.

Chronic collateral ligament injuries are rarely sufficiently symptomatic to require reconstruction. Often, there are degenerative changes in the joint, and ligament reconstruction cannot be expected to alleviate symptoms due to arthritis. Once again, if reconstruction of a chronic proximal interphalangeal collateral ligament rupture is necessary, it is on the radial side of the index finger.

Technique.   Make the same approach as for the acute. Tease out the ligament after identifying and isolating it. Imbricate it in its midportion, or shorten it and suture it with 4-0 nonab-

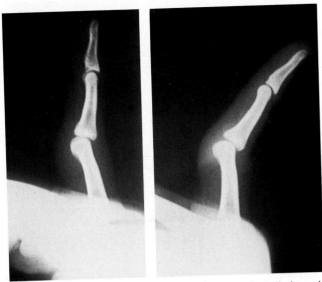

FIGURE 92-8.   Chronic volar plate rupture in a basketball player; it subluxated each time he caught the ball.

sorbable suture at the proper length. If further reinforcement is needed, separate the radial slip of the superficialis, leaving it attached distally and detaching it proximally. Pass it through a drill hole in the head of the proximal phalanx, using a pull-out suture tied over a protected button on the ulnar side. Spread the ligament out dorsally and suture its radial (now dorsal) edge to the remaining fibers of the collateral ligament. Close as previously described. After 10 days of immobilization in no more than 20° of flexion, encourage the patient in active exercise—with strapping to the adjacent long finger—for an additional 4 to 5 weeks.

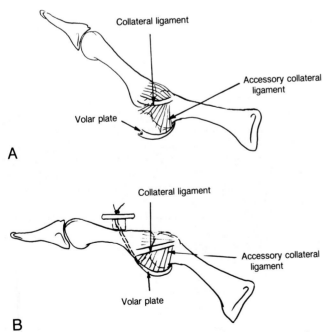

FIGURE 92-9.   (*A*) Volar plate rupture usually occurs distally from the base of the middle phalanx. (*B*) The distal margin of the volar plate is pulled snugly into a trough in the middle phalanx and secured through drill holes in the bone.

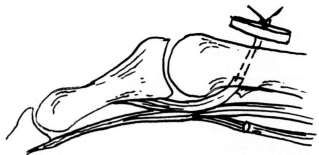

FIGURE 92-10.   One superficialis slip is fixed to the proximal phalanx, creating a tenodesis of the proximal interphalangeal joint.

Complications.   Late reconstruction cannot be expected to produce a perfectly stable joint. Persistent laxity is common.

Volar Plate Ruptures

Volar plate ruptures of the proximal interphalangeal joint can result from a dorsal proximal interphalangeal joint dislocation or hyperextension injury. The plate can detach proximally from the proximal phalanx or distally from the middle phalanx, with or without a piece of bone. If the volar plate ruptures distally with a small fragment of bone (as seen on the lateral radiograph), the joint is inevitably congruous; this injury must be differentiated from the serious proximal interphalangeal joint fracture–dislocation. The minor volar plate fracture should be treated as any other volar plate injury, that is, with protection against hyperextension by either a dorsal-block digital splint or strapping to an adjacent finger for 3 weeks. Full flexion is encouraged.

Chronic volar plate ruptures that are symptomatic (Fig. 92-8) are unusual but can be helped by surgical correction.

Technique.   Make a palmar zig-zag incision, and release the flexor sheath between the A2 and A4 pulleys. Protect the digital vessels and nerves. Retract the flexor tendons, and observe the volar plate. If it has been ruptured in midsubstance and repair is possible, suture the edges directly. More often it will be detached distally (Fig. 92-9*A*). In that case roughen the base of the middle phalanx, and create a transverse trough. Place a 4-0 nonabsorbable suture in the distal end of the plate in a modified Bunnell fashion. Place drill holes at the lateral margins of the trough; direct them distally but also somewhat laterally so that the extensor mechanism will not be injured or trapped by the passing of the pull-out suture. Pass the ends of the suture from the volar plate through the drill holes, and tie them over a protected button. As the suture is tied, flex the proximal interphalangeal joint, and apply gentle traction on the suture so the distal end of the volar plate is pulled snugly into the trough (Fig. 92-*B*).

If there is not enough of the volar plate left to advance or repair, isolate either slip of the superficialis. Detach it proximally under the A2 pulley, but leave it attached distally. Place a drill hole in the neck of the proximal phalanx, and draw the proximal end of the detached superficialis slip into the hole, using a pull-out 4-0 nonabsorbable suture tied over a protected button (Fig. 92-10). Be sure the superficialis slip is taut when the proximal interphalangeal joint is in 10° to 15° of flexion.

Temporarily transfix the joint with a 0.035-inch smooth wire for 3 weeks. Protect the joint with a dorsal-block splint for an additional 4 weeks. There are other techniques of tenodesis of this joint, most technically more complex.[1,3,6,9,11]

Complications. Any of the ligament repairs or reconstructions can lead to some loss of motion and chronic thickening. A flexion deformity is common.

Metacarpophalangeal Joint

Injuries to the ligaments and dislocations of the metacarpophalangeal joints of the fingers are uncommon. Most of these occur with the fingers in some extension when the ligaments are more lax. This provides some margin for protection so that complete ligament rupture is unusual.

Dislocations

Simple dislocations are easily treated by closed reduction. One must be careful not to make a simple dislocation complex. In simple dislocations the volar plate lies over the metacarpal head palmarward. Therefore, the proximal phalanx should merely be pushed distally and palmarly, not hyperextended with traction—a maneuver in which the volar plate can slip dorsally and prevent reduction.

The pathomechanics of a complex dislocation were highlighted by Kaplan.[17] The key element that makes this complex dislocation irreducible is the interposition of the volar plate between the metacarpal head and the base of the proximal phalanx.[16] This occurs most commonly in the index finger. Clinically, the joint is slightly hyperextended—with the phalanx appearing parallel to the metacarpal—with a tendency for the digit to overlap its neighbor (Fig. 92-11). On the palmar surface the skin is puckered or dimpled. Radiographically, the joint space is widened, the joint surfaces are offset, and the sesamoid appears to lie within the joint (Fig. 92-12).

Treatment should include a single attempt at closed reduc-

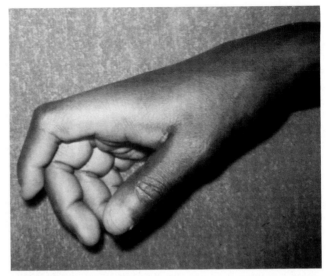

FIGURE 92-11. Complex metacarpophalangeal dislocation with the finger parallel to the metacarpal.

tion under a good anesthetic in the operating room. If this fails—and it usually does—open reduction can proceed promptly.

Technique. The dorsal and palmar approaches each have strong advocates. For the dorsal approach,[14] make a straight dorsal incision over the joint. Incise the extensor and dorsal capsule in the midline. The volar plate is then seen. Split it in the midline with a knife, but do not damage the articular surface of the metacarpal head. Flex the wrist to relax the flexors and reduce the joint. Push the separate halves of the plate over and around the head of the metacarpal if necessary. Repair the capsule, extensor, and skin separately. Splint the hand with the metacarpophalangeal joints flexed for a few days; then begin active motion, preventing hyperextension with a dorsal-block splint.

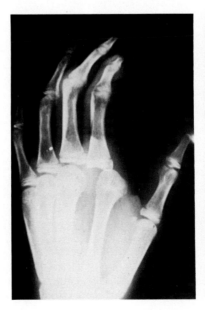
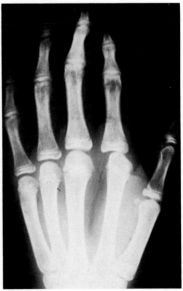

FIGURE 92-12. The phalanx is offset at the metacarpophalangeal joint, lying parallel to the metacarpal in a complex dislocation.

For the palmar approach make an incision that connects the midaxial line with the transverse midpalmar crease. Take great care to avoid injuring the digital artery and nerve (especially the radial), which are pressed against the deep surface of the skin by the metacarpal head. Gently retract the nerves and arteries. Incise the A1 pulley, and retract the flexor tendons and lumbrical. The metacarpal head now dominates the field (Fig. 92-13A). Incise carefully between the sides of the volar plate on the deep transverse metacarpal ligament longitudinally. Insert a sturdy but narrow-angled dental probe or skin hook around the volar plate, and extricate it from between the phalangeal base and the metacarpal head. The joint will snap into the reduced position (Fig. 92-13B). Because the volar plate is still attached to the phalanx, no repair is needed. Close the skin. Immobilize the hand with the metacarpophalangeal joints flexed for a few days, then start active motion. Prevent hyperextension with a dorsal-block splint for 3 to 4 weeks.

Complications.   Injury to the neurovascular bundles occurs in the palmar approach with a deep, forceful skin incision. Redislocation can occur if hyperextension is not prevented.

Collateral Ligament Injuries

Collateral ligament injuries of the metacarpophalangeal joint injuries frequently are missed. To test for collateral ligament stability, the metacarpophalangeal joint must be flexed maximally. The injury seems to occur predominantly in the ulnar three fingers and to the radial side.[15] If there is *not* an associated displaced avulsion fracture, closed treatment with the metacarpophalangeal joints flexed 45° for 3 weeks is advised.

If there is an associated avulsion fracture that is displaced 3 mm or more, open repair should be done.

Technique.   Make a longitudinal incision in the dorsum of the web space on the affected side of the digit. Incise the transverse fibers of the hood, and retract them. Incise the capsule of the joint dorsal to the collateral ligament parallel to its dorsal margin. Dissect the ligament, and mobilize it. If there is an attached avulsion fracture of adequate size attached to the ligament, reduce it and fix it with one or two smooth 0.035-inch Kirschner wires (Fig. 92-14A and B). If the fragment is too small, place a pull-out suture around it. Drill a hole obliquely connecting the cortex on the opposite side of the phalanx to the site of the intended ligament attachment. Pass the pull-out suture through this hole and over a protected button. Repair the transverse fibers of the hood with 5-0 nonabsorbable suture, and close the skin. Immobilize the hand with the metacarpophalangeal joints flexed 45° for 3 weeks.

When chronic these ligament tears often are only minimally symptomatic. If they prove disabling, surgical treatment can be difficult.

Technique for Chronic Injuries.   Make the same approach as described in the preceding section. Tease out and mobilize the ligament carefully to its maximum length. Repair it to the phalanx by the pull-out suture technique. Close as previously described.

Complications.   Loss of motion can result from repairing the ligament tightly with the joint in extension.

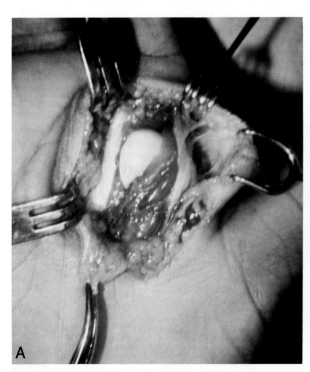 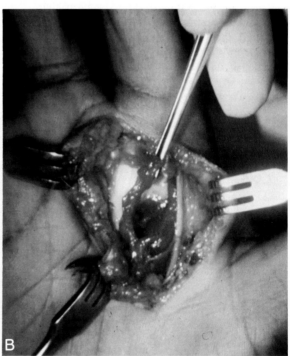

FIGURE 92-13.   (*A*) When the skin is opened prior to reduction, the metacarpal head dominates the field. The flexor tendons lie ulnarly, the lumbrical and digital nerve radially, and the volar plate dorsally, blocking reduction. (*B*) The volar plate (held by the forceps) has been extricated and the joint reduced.

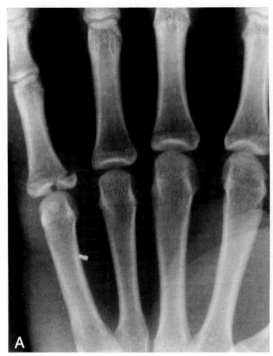
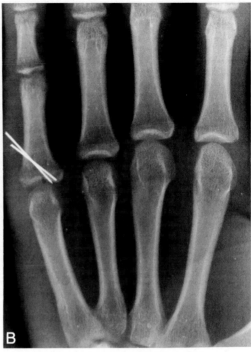

FIGURE 92-14. (*A*) A displaced articular fracture usually is attached to the collateral ligament. (*B*) Kirschner wire fixation of the displaced fracture often must be done by placing the wire in the phalanx first.

Carpometacarpal Joint

Dislocations and ligamentous injuries of the carpometacarpal joints are virtually synonymous and will be considered so for this discussion.

The commonest site for subluxation or dislocation is at the base of the fifth metacarpal.[18] The fifth and fourth metacarpals may dislocate together,[20] or all four may do so. Careful evaluation of AP, lateral, and oblique radiographs reveals the diagnosis.[19] Often an intra-articular fracture is associated with dislocation of the fifth and fourth metacarpals.

For dislocations without fracture closed reduction usually is possible. Immobilization with the wrist extended, the metacarpophalangeal joints flexed, and the interphalangeal joints extended for 3 to 4 weeks can succeed, but frequent evaluation for redislocation is necessary. Closed reduction with percutaneous pinning is preferable. The pins should transfix the metacarpal to the appropriate carpal. Small associated fractures with some articular incongruity are unimportant.[21]

If redislocation occurs, closed reduction fails, or a substantial intra-articular fracture is present and remains significantly displaced after closed reduction, open reduction must be performed.

Open Reduction: Acute Dislocation

Technique.   Make a dorsal longitudinal or oblique incision over the affected joint. Protect the sensory nerve branches and veins. Retract the extensor tendons, and visualize the injured joint. Carefully retract the ruptured ligaments and debride any small loose fragments about the joint. Gently reduce the joint. Align any intra-articular fracture, and transfix it with one or two smooth 0.035-inch Kirschner wires. If no fracture is present, reduce the dislocation and secure it with a 0.035-inch smooth wire placed obliquely from the metacarpal across the joint into the appropriate carpal bone. Ligament repair is not necessary. Close the skin, and splint the hand for 3 to 4 weeks, but allow full finger motion after the first few days. Remove the pins at 6 weeks.

If the dislocation is chronic and symptomatic, an open reduction can still be attempted as previously described. More extensive dissection with excision of scar is necessary to achieve reduction. If symptomatic post-traumatic arthrosis is present (usually with subluxation and not with dislocation), a resection arthroplasty is useful.

Open Reduction: Chronic Dislocation

Technique.   Make the same approach described with open reduction. Incise and reflect the scarred ligaments by subperiosteal dissection. Resect the proximal 1 cm of the base of the metacarpal. Repair the ligaments with 4-0 nonabsorbable suture. Close the skin. Splint the hand for 3 to 4 weeks but permit early finger motion.

Others advocate carpometacarpal arthrodesis instead of arthroplasty.[35] One must be careful to preserve the transverse metacarpal arch by fusing the fourth and fifth metacarpals in some flexion.

Complications.   As noted, redislocation can occur after closed reduction alone or after removing the pins following percutaneous or open placement. Sensory nerve injury is common, so care is imperative. Pinning metacarpals to adjacent metacarpals can lead to a "pancake" hand from flattening of the transverse metacarpal arch.

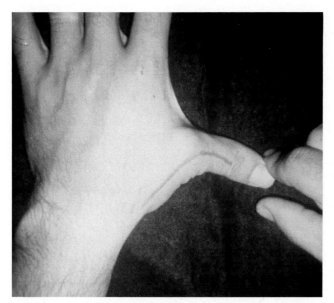

FIGURE 92-15. Complete instability to radial stress of the MP joint of the thumb. (Neviaser, R.J., Wilson, J.N., Lievano, A.: Rupture of the Ulnar Collateral Ligament of the Thumb—Correction by Dynamic Repair. J. Bone Joint Surg. **53-A:**1357–1364, 1971.)

THUMB

The anatomy of the joints of the thumb is sufficiently different from that of the other digits to consider some review. The metacarpophalangeal joint is supported by strong collateral and accessory collateral ligaments as well as a volar plate. The adductor pollicis and abductor pollicis brevis insert into sesamoids in the volar plate, and each tendon has an expansion or aponeurosis into the extensor. The motion at this joint is widely variable. The trapeziometacarpal joint consists of two saddle surfaces in apposition. Although it has a relatively loose capsular support, a key ligament is the palmar trapeziometacarpal ligament.

Metacarpophalangeal Joint

Dislocations

Dislocations of the metacarpophalangeal joint usually are dorsal and amenable to closed treatment. Occasionally, they may prove to be irreducible due to interposition of the volar plate between the base of the proximal phalanx and the head of the metacarpal. When this situation is present, open reduction is needed.

Technique. Make a chevron incision on the radial aspect of the joint, and bring the apex somewhat palmarly. Be careful of the radial digital nerves. Partially release the flexor tendon pulley, and retract the flexor pollicis longus. Incise longitudinally between the radial collateral ligament and the edge of the volar plate. Introduce a stiff-angled probe or a skin hook behind the volar plate, and extricate it from the joint. Reduction will occur promptly and spontaneously. Close the skin. After initial immobilization for comfort for a few days, allow motion with an extensor-block splint.

Ulnar Collateral Ligament Ruptures

Ulnar collateral ligament ruptures of the metacarpophalangeal joint are common injuries that continue to receive much attention. The diagnosis can be made on clinical examination by applying gentle radial stress to the thumb.[23,24] If there is no apparent end point of resistance and angular deformation is more than 15° greater than the uninjured thumb (Fig. 92-15), complete rupture is likely. In questionable cases, stress radiographs with local or nerve block anesthesia can be helpful (Fig. 92-16). These tests should not be done in the presence of a significant articular fracture but, contrary to prevailing opinion, can be of value with a small avulsion fracture. The fracture is not always attached to the ligament (Fig. 92-17), and the position of the fracture fragment does not ensure the location of the ruptured ligament end.

When an acute rupture is present, operative repair provides the greatest security that a stable joint will result. In the major-

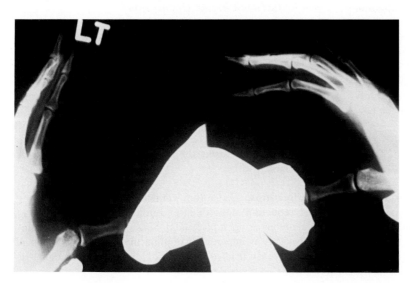

FIGURE 92-16. Comparative stress radiographs showing instability of the left thumb.

ity of cases, the ruptured ligament displaces so that the adductor aponeurosis lies interposed between the ruptured end of the ligament and the proximal phalanx (the Stener lesion).[28] Because this cannot be determined by physical examination, stress or plain radiographs, or arthrography, surgical repair is necessary.

Technique. Make a chevron incision on the ulnar side of the joint. Do not extend either limb across the web lest a contracting scar result. Elevate the flap, being careful to protect the dorsal sensory branch of the radial nerve. The torn ligament may be seen at the proximal edge of the adductor aponeurosis. Divide the aponeurosis at the edge of the extensor, and reflect for later repair. Inspect the joint for loose fragments. Repair any rent in the dorsal capsule. Mobilize the ligament, and place a 4-0 nonabsorbable suture in the distal end in a modified Bunnell fashion. Roughen the base of the proximal phalanx where the ligament is to be attached. Drill a hole obliquely to the opposite cortex. Pass both ends of the suture through the hole, and penetrate the skin. Reduce the joint, and tie the suture over a protected button. Repair the aponeurosis to the extensor. Close the skin. Immobilize in plaster for 3 to 4 weeks, and then have the patient begin exercising. Remove the button after an additional week.

When chronic instability is present, it usually results in weakness of thumb function. If post-traumatic arthritis is present, arthrodese the joint (see Chapter 100). If the joint is not arthritic, the following reconstructive procedure is valuable,[25] although many other techniques using tendon grafts have been reported.[22,27,29]

Technique. Use the same approach as with the acute injury. Protect the digital nerves dorsally and palmarly. Isolate the major tendon of insertion of the adductor pollicis and detach it. Be certain to leave sufficient tendinous tissue to accept a pull-out suture. Create a broad U-shaped flap based on the metacarpal, and mobilize it carefully. Drill a hole in the ulnar midaxial line of the proximal phalanx 10 to 12 mm distal to the joint, and extend it through the opposite cortex. Enlarge the opening on the ulnar side to accept the adductor tendon. Imbricate or advance the flap of scarred collateral ligament to the residual soft tissue at the phalangeal base with the joint reduced, using 4-0 nonabsorbable suture. Place a 4-0 nonabsorbable modified Bunnell suture in the adductor tendon, and pass it through the proximal phalanx to exit percutaneously on the radial side. With the thumb adducted tie the suture over a protected button, making sure the adductor tendon is pulled well into the ulnar hole of the phalanx (Fig. 92-18). Repair the aponeurosis and skin separately. Immobilize in plaster for 4 weeks. Have the patient start exercising, and remove the button and pull-out suture 1 week later.

Complications. A loose ligament repair may leave a lax joint. Motion loss is common. Pain can persist from unappreciated arthritis.

Radial Collateral Ligament Ruptures

The radial collateral ligament of the metacarpophalangeal joint is less commonly injured than its ulnar counterpart. The clinical findings often show the thumb lying in ulnar deviation, a finding confirmed by radiographs (Fig. 92-19). The proximal

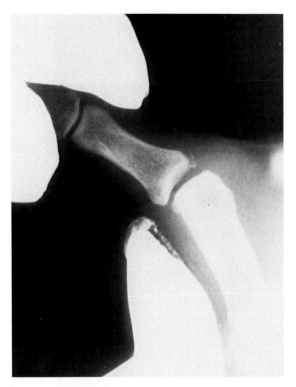

FIGURE 92-17. Stress radiograph in which "avulsion" fracture follows phalanx, suggesting it is not attached to the ligament.

phalanx is deviated ulnarly by the strong pull of the adductor pollicis with no radial collateral ligament to provide stability.

Although anatomically the Stener lesion cannot exist on the radial side, unless the thumb is casted in a reduced position, the ligament will not heal. The adductor pollicis deviating the phalanx keeps the ligament displaced. Therefore, in the acute stage, casting the thumb in a reduced position for 4 weeks should result in stability.

Unfortunately, these injuries usually are recognized in the chronic state. If there is post-traumatic arthritis, an arthrodesis should be done. If the joint is not arthritic, utilize the following reconstruction.[26]

Technique. Make a chevron incision on the radial side of the joint over the metacarpophalangeal joint. Protect the sensory

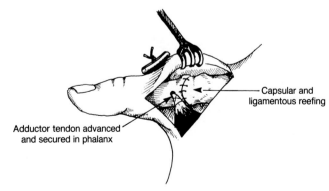

Capsular and
ligamentous reefing

Adductor tendon advanced
and secured in phalanx

FIGURE 92-18. Capsuloligamentous complex is reefed, and tendon of the adductor pollicis is advanced and inserted into a drill hole in the midaxial region of the proximal phalanx.

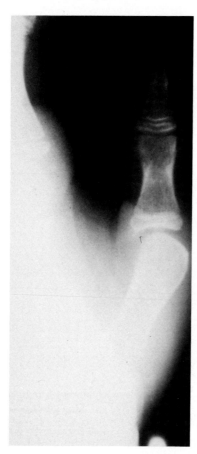

FIGURE 92-19. Radial collateral ligament rupture leaves the phalanx subluxated ulnarly by the strong pull of the adductor pollicis.

nerve. Isolate and detach the tendon of the abductor pollicis brevis with sufficient tendon length to hold a suture. Create a U-shaped flap based proximally of the scarred collateral ligament mass on the radial side. Drill a hole 10 to 12 mm distal to the joint in the radial cortex and through the ulnar cortex. Enlarge the radial hole with a curette. Imbricate or reef the ligament flap with the joint reduced. Pass a 4-0 nonabsorbable suture through the abductor pollicis brevis tendon in a modi-

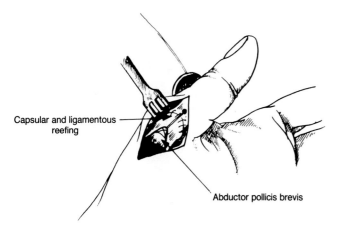

Capsular and ligamentous reefing

Abductor pollicis brevis

FIGURE 92-20. Capsuloligamentous complex is reefed, and tendon of the abductor pollicis brevis is advanced to a drill hole on the radial side of the phalanx in the midaxial plane.

fied Bunnell fashion. Pass both ends of the suture through the drill hole in the proximal phalanx and out through the skin on the ulnar side. Secure this suture over a protected button, making sure the tendon fits snugly in the radial hole (Fig. 92-20). Close the skin. Immobilize the thumb and hand for 3 to 4 weeks. Start the patient on exercises; remove the button and suture 1 week later.

Complications. These are the same as under ulnar collateral ligament tears described earlier.

Volar Plate Ruptures

Hyperextension injuries of the metacarpophalangeal joint are common, even more so than dorsal dislocations. The diagnosis can be made acutely by eliciting tenderness over the volar plate and detecting hyperextensibility of this joint compared to the opposite thumb. Unlike the finger proximal interphalangeal joints, the volar plate detachment occurs proximally from the metacarpal. Acute injuries can be treated with dorsal-block splinting (restricting the last 20° of extension) for 4 weeks.

For patients with chronic hyperextensibility at the metacarpophalangeal joint, a capsulodesis is helpful.[30]

Technique. Make a palmar zig-zag incision, and retract the digital arteries and nerves. Incise the A1 pulley in its proximal portion, and retract the flexor pollicis longus. Incise the interval between the sides of the volar plate and the accessory collateral ligaments. Free the plate proximally, and excise the sesamoids subperiosteally. Using an osteotome or dental chisel, create a transverse trough in the metacarpal neck. Drill a hole through each edge of the trough obliquely through the metacarpal. Test the fit of the proximal edge of the volar plate into the trough; be sure that when the plate is seated, the metacarpophalangeal joint remains at 15° of flexion. If less flexion is evident, trim a tiny bit from the free edge of the volar plate, and recheck the position of the joint. Once this is correct, weave a 4-0 nonabsorbable suture through the free proximal edge of the plate in a modified Bunnell technique. Pass the suture ends through the drill holes and the skin. Tie the suture over a protected button, drawing the volar plate securely into the trough. The metacarpophalangeal joint should show a 15° to 20° flexion deformity. Transfix the joint obliquely with a 0.035-inch smooth Kirschner wire to maintain the position. Suture the accessory collateral ligaments to the edges of the volar plate with 5-0 nonabsorbable suture. Close the skin. Utilize plaster external protection for 4 weeks, but allow interphalangeal joint flexion at 1 week. Remove the plaster and pin at 4 weeks. Allow exercises with an extension-block splint for 2 more weeks, then remove the button, suture, and splint.

Complications. A permanent flexion contracture is common. Recurrent hyperextensibility is the result of a loose capsulodesis or insecure fixation to the phalanx.

Trapeziometacarpal Joint

The most common dislocation or ligament injury at this joint is the Bennett's fracture–dislocation, discussed chapter 95. Trapeziometacarpal dislocation without fracture is far less common but quite difficult to treat. Although it has been thought that the palmar ligament ruptures, Burkhalter[31] explored some acutely dislocated thumbs and found that this was not so. Rather, the metacarpal was rotated (supinated) out of its periosteal sleeve. He noted that when the thumb was pronated maximally, the metacarpal rotated back into the sleeve. If these injuries were treated with percutaneous transarticular pinning and held in plaster for 6 weeks in this position, recurrent dislocations did not occur. Thus, there should be little need to operate in the acute phase of this injury.

For chronic dislocations or for recurrent instability with post-traumatic arthritis, arthroplasty or arthrodesis is preferred. See chapters 100 and 101. If there is no significant arthritic change, ligamentous reconstruction should be undertaken. The most widely accepted technique is the use of the flexor carpi radialis as described by Eaton.[32,34]

Technique. Make an incision along the radial margin of the thumb metacarpal, and curve it palmarward as it approaches the wrist flexor crease, ending over the flexor carpi radialis. Do not injure the sensory nerves. Elevate extraperiosteally the thenar muscle origin from the trapezium and metacarpal, retracting them distally. Incise the roof of the tunnel of the flexor carpi radialis. Using a gouge, create a tunnel in the metacarpal base from dorsally between the extensor pollicis longus and brevis, exiting at the palmar beak of the metacarpal. Do not enter the joint.

Split the flexor carpi radialis longitudinally for 6 cm, leaving the insertion intact. Proximal exposure of the tendon is done through two transverse incisions over the tendon. Pass the tendon through the trough. Reduce the joint, and pin it with a smooth 0.035-inch Kirschner wire, but avoid spearing the tendon slip. Pull the tendon slip taut, and suture it to the dorsal periosteum of the metacarpal. Route it beneath the extensor pollicis brevis and abductor pollicis longus proximally across the joint and back under the remaining intact portion of the flexor carpi radialis. Then turn it back to the palmar periosteum of the metacarpal, and suture it there. Place additional sutures wherever the slip changes direction (Fig. 92-21). Close the wound, and immobilize in plaster for 4 weeks. Remove the Kirschner wire at that time, and splint for 1 more week. Start the patient on exercises, but do not expect maximal return of motion for up to 4 months.

An alternative to using part of the flexor carpi radialis is to use one of the slips of the abductor pollicis longus. The most common insertion for the commonly present second slip is the trapezium.[33] This natural anchor can be used to advantage.
Technique. Make an incision starting at the dorsal ulnar side of the proximal third of the first metacarpal. Start longitudinally, and then curve the incision palmarward over the trapezium, and continue it along the anterior border of the first dorsal compartment. Isolate the slip of the abductor pollicis longus that attaches to the trapezium, and detach it 8 cm proximally. Use a gouge or drill to make a hole in the metacarpal parallel but distal to the trapeziometacarpal joint from dorsal to palmar. Pass the abductor pollicis longus tendon through the hole. Reduce the joint, and tighten the tendon. Loop it back to itself, and suture it to its trapezial insertion. Reinforce the new ''ligament'' by spreading it out and suturing it to the capsule on each side of the tendon wherever it crosses the joint (Fig. 92-22). Pin the joint with a smooth wire if necessary.

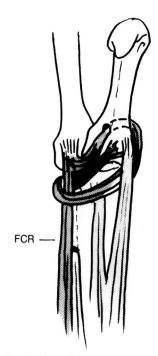

FIGURE 92-21. Stabilization of the trapeziometacarpal joint by one-half of the flexor carpi radialis (*FCR*) (Eaton).

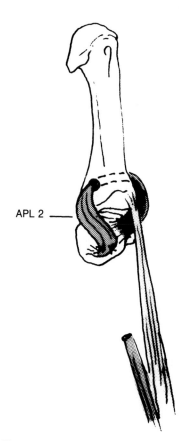

FIGURE 92-22. Using the accessory slip of the abductor pollicis longus (APL) to stabilize the trapeziometacarpal joint.

Immobilize in a thumb spica for 6 weeks. Remove the cast and pin at that time.

Complications. Persistent subluxation can result if the new ligament is not tightened sufficiently with the joint reduced.

REFERENCES

Interphalangeal Joint (Fingers)

1. Adams, J.P.: Correction of Chronic Dorsal Subluxation of the Proximal Interphalangeal Joint by Means of a Criss-Cross Volar Graft. J. Bone Joint Surg. **41-A:**111, 1959.
2. Agee, J.M.: Unstable Fracture Dislocations of the Proximal Interphalangeal Joints of the Fingers: A Preliminary Report of a New Treatment Technique. J. Hand Surg. **3:**386, 1978.
3. Curtis, R.M.: Treatment of Injuries of the Proximal Interphalangeal Joints of the Fingers. In Adams, J.P. (ed.): Current Practice in Orthopaedic Surgery, II. St. Louis, C.V. Mosby, 1964.
4. Eaton, R.G., and Malerich, M.M.: Volar Plate Arthroplasty of the Proximal Interphalangeal Joint: A Review of Ten Years' Experience. J. Hand Surg. **5:**260, 1980.
5. Johnson, F.G., and Greene, M.H.: Another Cause of Irreducible Dislocation of the Proximal Interphalangeal Joint of a Finger. A Case Report. J Bone Joint Surg. **48-A:**542, 1966.
6. Kleinert, H.E., and Kasdan, M.L.: Reconstruction of Chronically Subluxated Proximal Interphalangeal Finger Joint. J. Bone Joint Surg. **47-A:**958, 1965.
7. McElfresh, E.C., Dobyns, J.H., and O'Brien, E.T.: Management of Fracture–Dislocation of the Proximal Interphalangeal Joints by Extension-Block Splinting. J Bone Joint Surg. **54-A:**1705, 1972.
8. Neviaser, R.J., and Wilson, J.N.: Interposition of the Extensor Tendon Resulting in Persistent Subluxation of the Proximal Interphalangeal Joint of the Finger. Clin. Orthop. **83:**118, 1972.
9. Palmer, A.K., and Linscheid, R.L.: Chronic Recurrent Dislocation of the Proximal Interphalangeal Joint of the Finger. J. Hand Surg. **3:**95, 1978.
10. Spinner, M., and Choi, B.Y.: Anterior Dislocation of the Proximal Interphalangeal Joint. A Cause of Rupture of the Central Slip of the Extensor Mechanism. J. Bone Joint Surg. **52-A:**1329, 1970.
11. Swanson, A.B.: Surgery of the Hand in Cerebral Palsy and Muscle Origin Release Procedures. Surg. Clin. North Am. **48:**1129, 1968.
12. Thompson, J.S., and Eaton, R.G.: Volar Dislocation of the Proximal Interphalangeal Joint (Abstract). J. Hand Surg. **2:**232, 1977.
13. Wilson, J.N., and Rowland, S.A.: Fracture–Dislocation of the Proximal Interphalangeal Joint of the Finger. Treatment by Open Reduction and Internal Fixation. J. Bone Joint Surg. **48-A:**493, 1966.

Metacarpophalangeal Joint (Fingers)

14. Becton, J.L., Christian, J.D., Jr., Goodwin, H.N., et al.: A Simplified Technique for Treating the Complex Dislocation of the Index Metacarpophalangeal Joint. J. Bone Joint Surg. **57-A:**698, 1975.
15. Dray, G., Millender, L.H., and Nalebuff, E.A.: Rupture of the Radial Collateral Ligament of a Metacarpophalangeal Joint to One of the Ulnar Three Fingers. J. Hand Surg. **4:**346, 1979.
16. Green, D.P., and Terry, G.C.: Complex Dislocation of the Metacarpophalangeal Joint. Correlative Pathological Anatomy. J. Bone Joint Surg. **55-A:**1480, 1973.

17. Kaplan, E.B.: Dorsal Dislocation of the Metacarpophalangeal Joint of the Index Finger. J. Bone Joint Surg. **39-A:**1081, 1957.

Carpometacarpal Joint (Fingers)

18. Bora, F.W., Jr., and Didizian, N.H.: The Treatment of Injuries to the Carpometacarpal Joint of the Little Finger. J. Bone Joint Surg. **56-A:**1459, 1974.
19. Green, D.P., and Rowland, S.A.: Carpometacarpal Dislocations (Excluding the Thumb). In Rockwood, C.A., and Green, D.P. (eds.): Fractures. Philadelphia, J.B. Lippincott, 1975.
20. Hsu, J.D., and Curtis, R.M.: Carpometacarpal Dislocations on the Ulnar Side of the Hand. J. Bone Joint Surg. **52-A:**927, 1970.
21. Petrie, P.W.R., and Lamb, D.W.: Fracture-Subluxation of Base of Fifth Metacarpal. Hand **6:**82, 1974.

Metacarpophalangeal Joint (Thumb)

22. Alldred, A.J.: Rupture of the Collateral Ligament of the Metacarpophalangeal Joint of the Thumb. J. Bone Joint Surg. **37-B:**443, 1955.
23. Campbell, C.S.: Gamekeeper's Thumb. J. Bone Joint Surg. **37-B:**148, 1955.
24. Coonrad, R.W., and Goldner, J.L.: A Study of the Pathological Findings and Treatment in Soft-Tissue Injury of the Thumb Metacarpophalangeal Joint. J. Bone Joint Surg. **50-A:**439, 1968.
25. Neviaser, R.J., and Adams, J.P.: Complications of Treatment of Injuries to the Hand. In Epps, C.H. (ed.): Complications in Orthopaedic Surgery. Philadelphia, J.B. Lippincott, 1978.
26. Neviaser, R.J., Wilson, J.N., and Lievano, A.: Rupture of the Ulnar Collateral Ligament of the Thumb (Gamekeeper's Thumb). J. Bone Joint Surg. **53-A:**1357, 1971.
27. Smith, R.J.: Post-traumatic Instability of the Metacarpophalangeal Joint. J. Bone Joint Surg. **59-A:**14, 1977.
28. Stener, B.: Displacement of the Ruptured Ulnar Collateral Ligament of the Metacarpophalangeal Joint of the Thumb. J. Bone Joint Surg. **44-B:**869, 1962.
29. Strandell, G.: Total Rupture of the Ulnar Collateral Ligament of the Metacarpophalangeal Joint of the Thumb. Acta Chir. Scand. **118:**72, 1959.
30. Milch, H.: Recurrent Dislocation of Thumb. Capsulorrhaphy. Am. J. Surg. **6:**237, 1929.

Carpometacarpal Joint (Thumb)

31. Burkhalter, W.E.: American Society for Surgery of the Hand Correspondence Newsletter No. 18, 1981.
32. Eaton, R.G., and Littler, J.W.: Ligament Reconstruction for the Painful Thumb Carpometacarpal Joint. J. Bone Joint Surg. **55-A:**1655, 1973.
33. Neviaser, R.J., Wilson, J.N., and Gardner, M.M.: Abductor Pollicis Longus Transfer for Replacement of the First Dorsal Interosseous. J. Hand Surg. **5:**53, 1980.
34. Eaton, R.G., and Dray, G.J.: Dislocations and Ligament Injuries in the Digits. In Green, D.P. (ed.): Operative Hand Surgery. New York, Churchill Livingstone, 1982.
35. Green, D.P.: Dislocations and Ligamentous Injuries in the Hand. In Evarts, C.M. (ed.): Surgery of the Musculoskeletal System. New York, Churchill Livingstone, 1983.
36. Milford, L.: The Hand. In Crenshaw, A.H. (ed.): Campbell's Operative Orthopaedics, 7th ed. St. Louis, C.V. Mosby Co., 1987.

CHAPTER 93

Principles of Stable Internal Fixation in the Hand

GOTTFRIED SEGMÜLLER

There is still no general agreement among hand surgeons as to whether stable internal fixation is a necessary and safe adjunct in the overall treatment of fractures and fracture sequelae of the skeleton of the hand. The anatomy of the hand, the lack of muscle endowments to surround the bones, a minimal layer of subcutaneous tissues, and the tendon system that clings to the skeleton like a glove are thought to be incompatible with the exposure of the fracture site and the use of implants for stable internal fixation.[3,4,24,25]

However, for more than half a century, Kirschner wire stabilization has been an accepted practice and is still considered useful for clearly unstable fractures by many.[5,7,10,11,13–16,22–24] Percutaneous pinning—especially for oblique phalangeal fractures—or Kirschner wire fixation following open reduction[5,11,13] is encouraged. However, the unavoidable plaster cast immobilization for several weeks following surgery increases the risks inherent in any operative procedure. In addition, there are the inevitable shortcomings of nonoperative fracture treatment, such as swelling, bone atrophy, dystrophy, and joint stiffness. Thus, an increasing number of authors have confirmed our finding that the advantages of stable internal fixation outweigh the disadvantages of the operative trauma to the soft tissue in hand surgery.[1,7–9,12,17,19–21,26] However, experience in hand surgery and adherence to the known principles of "atraumatic" operative technique, as well as a sound knowledge of the principles and techniques of stable bone fixation, are mandatory for surgeons utilizing open reduction and internal fixation in hand surgery.

In the last two decades, increasingly refined operative techniques have been developed in rapid succession in the large field of hand surgery. This is especially true for microsurgery, tendon surgery, and nerve surgery. In the field of skeletal reconstruction, bone grafts are now stabilized by rigid internal fixation rather than by Kirschner wires. Today, it is our task to make the experience of refined operative techniques available to peripheral skeletal surgery. The well-known and excellent functional adaptability of the hand to severe and irreversible damage caused by trauma is an insufficient argument against an increased use of reconstructive procedures on the skeleton of the hand. The aim of any responsible further development of peripheral skeletal surgery is to minimize permanent functional loss of the hand.

Today, it is indeed possible to utilize a biomechanically conceived osteosynthesis which effectively neutralizes all muscle forces acting upon the bones in the rehabilitation phase. In this way, bone regains its load-carrying capacity immediately following surgery. As many of these biomechanical principles and techniques are still unknown to many hand surgeons, we consider it necessary to elucidate some of them as they apply to hand surgery.[6–8,12,17,21]

PRIMARY STABILITY BY INTERFRAGMENTARY COMPRESSION

Stability is achieved by increasing friction between two pressure-resistant elements by means of compression. It has been demonstrated conclusively in numerous animal experiments, as well as by clinical experience, that static compression does not have any deleterious effects on living bone.[18] It is, therefore,

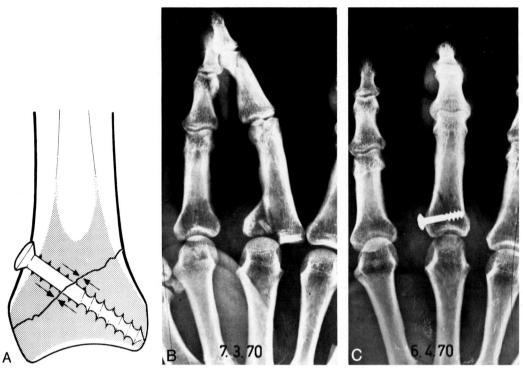

FIGURE 93-1. (*A*) The lag screw principle, using the screw with short thread (cancellous bone screw) is depicted. The section of the screw that carries the thread lies in the distant mobile free fragment; the section without the thread, in the fragment that forms the buttress. (*B* and *C*) The lag screw principle applied to an intra-articular fracture at the base of first phalanx, third digit.

safe to use the mechanical advantages of compression in reconstructive skeletal surgery of the hand in order to obtain the stability necessary to engage in a rehabilitation program immediately following surgery. Four techniques used in hand surgery are described.[21]

Lag Screw Technique

The lag screw technique is used when there is a well-defined fracture plane, either oblique or spiral, without comminution

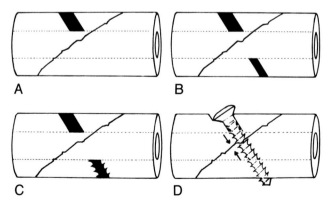

FIGURE 93-2. The lag screw principle using a cortical screw with whole-length thread. (*A*) The gliding hole (wide caliber) is drilled in the near cortex, forming the buttress. (*B*) The far cortex is drilled (using a small caliber for the screw core). (*C*) Cutting the thread in the far cortex only. (*D*) The screw takes hold only in the opposite cortical bone, producing interfragmentary compression.

or bone defects (Fig. 93-1). Almost any small size fragments may be stabilized using small screws (i.e. 1.5 mm, 2.0 mm, and 2.7 mm in diameter) that are adapted to the size of the skeleton of the hand (Fig. 93-2). The only precondition is a fracture plane which, following reduction, offers full resistance to pressure by the compressing metal implant.

Neutralization Plate Technique

The addition of a neutralization plate to the lag screw technique increases the spectrum of the compression principle considerably (Fig. 93-3). Especially in hand surgery, where short bones and, therefore, short oblique fractures are typical, the stability attained by the lag screw alone must often be protected by the neutralization plate. The lever arms in the anatomy of the hand may appear to be short, and muscle action may accordingly be "minimal." However, experience demonstrates that operative technical shortcomings, such as minimal deviation of the direction of a screw, or misjudgment of the type of spiral fracture may critically reduce the stability of fixation, which then will be unable to resist the forces generated, despite the short lever-arm systems in the hand. On the basis of these experiences, we advocate the use of a neutralization plate in cases in which the security of fixation is questionable.

Dynamic Compression Plates

Plates of all sizes for hand surgery may be used as self-compressing plates, since oval holes permit eccentric positioning of the screws, therefore approximating the bone ends when

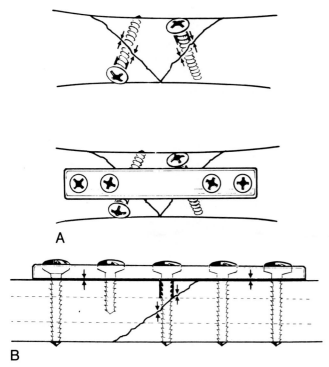

A

B

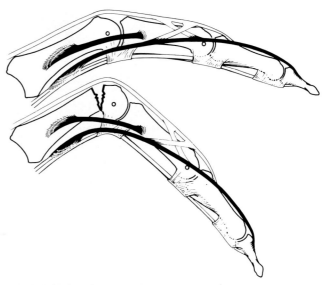

FIGURE 93-4. The anatomic and biomechanical characteristics of the hand. Disruption on the tension side occurs as a result of bending stress through extrinsic and intrinsic tendon systems at the level of the metacarpophalangeal joint.

FIGURE 93-3. Neutralization plate I and II. (*A*) The single screws produce interfragmentary compression of the large fragments. This arrangement cannot withstand the physiologic functional load under all circumstances; therefore, a plate protects the already stabilized fracture zone against muscle actions that occur with use. (*B*) If the fracture plane permits, interfragmentary compression can be achieved with single screws which, at the same time, fix the plate. Accordingly, the central screw is inserted to act as a lag screw with a gliding canal in the first cortex.

driven home. This compression technique is now used whenever a plate is applied on the hand skeleton in the absence of a bone defect.[2,19]

Tension Band Techniques

The anatomic and biomechanical characteristics of the hand favor the use of tension band techniques more than in most anatomic areas of the body (Fig. 93-4). Metacarpals, phalanges, the carporadial segment, and the forearm are stressed mainly by bending, and less by extension, torsion, or axial loading while in use. The main muscle action results in compression on the palmar side and distraction on the extensor side. This bending stress, arising from functional loading, may easily be neutralized and counteracted by restoration of the tensile strength, either by the dorsally placed tension band plate or the tension band wire technique. Not only are bending and distracting forces neutralized, but functional muscle action converts these forces into compression forces that become active within the plane of the fracture.

For successful treatment using these tension band techniques, it is mandatory that torsion and shearing, ever-present biomechanical characteristics of hand function, be taken care of efficiently. Interlocking of the fragments is a prerequisite for the simple tension band wire technique; whenever interlocking of irregular fracture surfaces is missing, rotational displace-

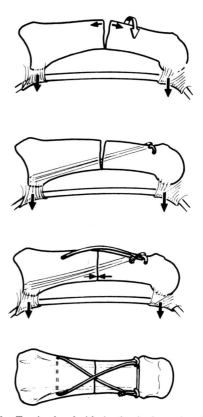

FIGURE 93-5. Tension band with simple wire loop placed dorsally. A superficially placed figure-of-eight wire loop stabilizes the diaphysis against bending. Interfragmentary postoperative compression is increased on the flexor side by the postoperative bending stress arising from functional load. Parallel Kirschner-wires are used for rotational stability.

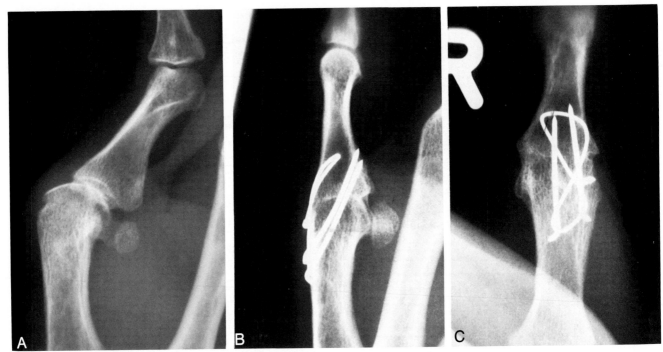

FIGURE 93-6. Tension band technique applied for fusion of the first metacarpophalangeal joint. (*A*) Destruction of the metacarpophalangeal joint following low-grade infection. (*B*) The dorsally placed wire loop is carried through a burr hole distally and around the Kirschner-wires proximally. (*C*) Torsional forces are neutralized by the parallel Kirschner-wires.

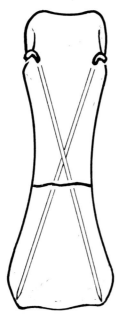

FIGURE 93-7. Crossed Kirschner-wires, applied correctly, are anchored in the proximal and distal metaphysis and cross proximal (or distal) to the fracture level.

ment is abolished by the use of double parallel Kirschner wires (Figs. 93-5 and 93-6). Instead of the wire technique, the tension band plate technique is used whenever neutralization of shearing or torsion is mechanically rather difficult, such as in the case of a small comminution zone, a small gap by loss of bone substance, or when a pressure-resistant bone graft is being used. Again, restoration of tensile strength of the fractured bone and neutralization of torsional forces are the goals to be achieved.

Preconditions for all tension band techniques are:

1. The presence of a bending load with anatomic function
2. Bony buttressing on the compression side (palmar aspect)
3. Adequate neutralization of torsional forces

When these conditions are met, we use tension band techniques as the main internal fixation method based on compression.

PRIMARY STABILITY BY NONCOMPRESSION TECHNIQUES

The goal of stabilization by compression cannot always be realized, and in such cases techniques of internal fixation without compression may prove useful. These must be strictly distinguished from compressive techniques, since the regimens of postoperative rehabilitation will differ.

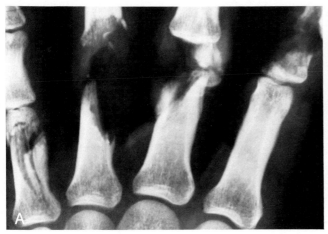

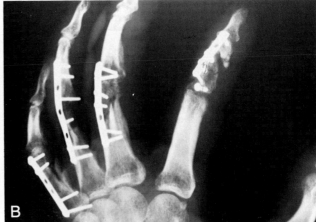

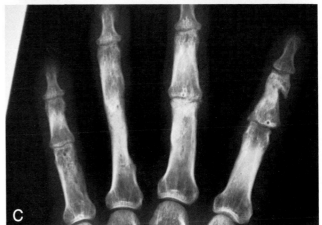

FIGURE 93-8. Bridge plate. (*A–C*) If a bone defect is not filled with a pressure-resistant corticocancellous graft, it should be loosely filled with cancellous bone chips as an alternative. All functionally imposed forces have to be taken up by the metallic implant alone, without any bone partnership. Therefore, the system is exposed to alternating tension, bending, and torsion moments. During the phase of bony consolidation, it can withstand these stresses only if a strong plate is used and when functional aftertreatment is restricted.

Kirschner Wires Crossed

There is no question that the majority of all fractures of the skeleton of the hand lend themselves to well-planned, well-conducted, conservative, and nonoperative treatment. Fixation by Kirschner wires is not at all outdated. Their use is considered the most gentle method of operative stabilization by many authors, and we do not hesitate to encourage their use as long as their application provides enough stability to allow for unrestricted postoperative functional rehabilitation. When applied correctly, anchored in the proximal and distal metaphysis, and not crossing at the fracture level, but rather proximal or distal to it, crossed Kirschner wires may provide adequate fixation of the fragments, especially at the level of the middle phalanx (Fig. 93-7). However, with comminution or even small bone defects, this technique must be abandoned.

Bridge Plate (Strut Plate)

A zone of comminution is bridged by a simple stabilizing plate, without compression. This plate, which is not based on a perfect partnership of reduced bone fragments and metal implants, must resist by itself all functionally generated forces. Therefore, it must be of adequate size and mechanical strength. This difficulty may also be overcome by replacing a shattered bone zone by an autologous, corticocancellous, pressure-resistant bone graft, bridged by the metal plate (Fig. 93-8).

Stability produced by noncompressive techniques, a decision which has to be made by the surgeon at the time of operation, demands a modified postoperative rehabilitation program. Use of removable static splints may be necessary for a varying period of time.

REFERENCES

1. Allgöwer, M.: Cinderella of Surgery—Fractures? Surg. Clin. North Am. **58:**5, 1978.
2. Allgöwer, M., Ehrsam, R., Ganz, R., Matter, P. and Perren, S.M.: Clinical Experience with a New Compression Plate "DCP." Acta Orthop. Scand. [Suppl.] **125,** 1969.
3. Barton, N.J.: Fractures of the Hand. J. Bone Joint Surg. **66-B:**159, 1984.
4. Barton, N.J.: Fractures of the Shafts of the Phalanges of the Hand. Hand **11:**119, 1979.
5. Belsky, M.R., Eaton, R.G., and Lane, L.B.: Closed Reduction and Internal Fixation of Proximal Phalangeal Fractures. J. Hand Surg. **9-A:**725, 1984.
6. Black, D., Mann, R.J., Constine, R., and Daniels, A.U.: Comparison of Internal Fixation Techniques in Metacarpal Fractures. J. Hand Surg. **10-A:**466, 1985.

7. Brown, P.W.: The Management of Phalangeal and Metacarpal Fractures. Surg. Clin. North Am. **53**:1393, 1973.

8. Crawford, G.P.: Screw Fixation for Certain Fractures of the Phalanges and Metacarpals. J. Bone Joint Surg. **58-A**:487, 1976.

9. Foucher, G., Merle, M., and Michon, J.: Traitement "Tout en Temps" des Traumatismes Complexes de la Main avec Mobilisation Précoce. Ann. Chir. **31**:1059, 1977.

10. Fyfe, I.S., and Mason, S.: The Mechanical Stability of Internal Fixation of Fractured Phalanges. Hand **11**:50, 1979.

11. Green, D.P., and Anderson, J.R.: Closed Reduction and Percutaneous Pin Fixation of Fractured Phalanges. J. Bone Joint Surg. **55-A**:1651, 1973.

12. Jabaley, M., and Freeland, A.E.: Rigid Internal Fixation in the Hand: 104 Cases. Plast. Reconstr. Surg. **77**:288, 1986.

13. Joshi, B.B.: Percutaneous Internal Fixation of Fractures of the Proximal Phalanges. Hand **8**:86, 1976.

14. Lister, G.: Intraosseous Wiring of the Digital Skeleton. J. Hand Surg. **3**:427, 1978.

15. Lord, R.E.: Intramedullary Fixation of Metacarpal Fractures. JAMA **164**:1746, 1957.

16. McCue, F.C., Honner, R., Johnson, M.C., Jr., and Gieck, J.H.: Athletic Injuries of the Proximal Interphalangeal Joint Requiring Surgical Treatment. J. Bone Joint Surg. **52-A**:937, 1970.

17. Pannike, A.: Osteosynthese in der Handchirurgie. Berlin, Springer-Verlag, 1972.

18. Perren, S.M., Huggler, A., Russenberger, M., Allgöwer, M., Mathys, R., Schenk, R., Willenegger, H., and Müller, M.E.: The Reaction of Cortical Bone to Compression. Acta Orthop. Scand. [Suppl.] **125**, 1969.

19. Perren, S.M., Russenberger, M., Steinemann, S., Müller, M.E., and Allgöwer, M.: A Dynamic Compression Plate. Acta Orthop. Scand. [Suppl.] **125**, 1969.

20. Segmüller, G.: Operative Stabilisierung am Handskelett. Bern, Verlag Hans Huber, 1973.

21. Segmüller, G.: Surgical Stabilization of the Skeleton of the Hand. Bern, Hans Huber Publishers, (Distributed in the USA by Williams & Wilkins), 1977.

22. Stark, H.H.: Troublesome Fractures and Dislocations of the Hand. American Academy of Orthopedic Surgeons: Instructional Course Lectures, vol. 19. St. Louis, C.V. Mosby Co., 1970, pp. 130–149.

23. Strickland, J.W., et al: Phalangeal Fractures in a Hand Surgery Practice: A Statistical Review and In-depth Study of the Management of Proximal Phalangeal Shaft Fractures. J. Hand Surg. **4**:285, 1979.

24. Strickland, J.W., Steichen, J.B., Kleinman, W.B., and Flynn, N.: Factors Influencing Digital Performance after Phalangeal Fracture. *In* Strickland, J.W., and Steichen, J.B. (ed): Difficult Problems in Hand Surgery. St. Louis, C.V. Mosby, 1982, p. 126.

25. Tubiana, R.: Le Traitement Chirurgical des Fractures Récentes des Métacarpiens et des Phalanges. *In* Traumatismes Ostéo-articulaires de la Main. Paris, Exp. Scientifique Francaise, 1971.

26. Tupper, J.W.: Technique of Bone Fixation and Clinical Experience in Replanted Extremities. Clin. Orthop. **133**:165, 1978.

CHAPTER 94

Indications for Stable Internal Fixation in Hand Injuries

GOTTFRIED SEGMÜLLER

PRIMARY RECONSTRUCTION

Even in severely displaced fractures, adequate stability for bone healing may be achieved by simple closed reduction and external splinting. The intact tendon sleeve, arranged in a circular fashion around the bone, tends to stabilize the skeleton following closed reduction of the fracture. All that is needed is a static splint on which the finger is gently fixed without any pressure. Twelve days of continued immobilization may be followed by 2 weeks of rehabilitation utilizing a removable splint; thereafter, mobilization without a splint may be permitted. Satisfactory stability, however, is not to be expected in the presence of comminuted fractures or in the absence of some interlocking between the fragments that are reduced (Fig. 94-1). In these cases, primary reconstruction, as well as internal fixation,[4–6,8,9,13] is mandatory. In a few cases only external fixation by the use of a external fixator may be indicated.

The following indications for primary reconstruction are discussed in this chapter:

Unstable fractures
Open fractures with or without injuries to tendons and nerves
Multiray and multilevel fractures
Articular fractures
Fractures with substantial bone loss, including defect fractures, articular fractures with bone loss, and comminuted fractures (devitalized bone fragments)

Unstable Fractures

When unstable fractures in the hand are to be stabilized rigidly, the operative techniques used include compression techniques (lag screw, neutralization plate, compression plate, tension band plate, or tension band wiring) (Fig. 94-2) and noncompression techniques (crossed Kirschner wires, strut plate, or bridging plate).[12]

We prefer the dorsal approach to the digit and to the metacarpals, using a dorsal straight incision through the midline of the extrinsic extensor tendon over the proximal phalanx or parallel to the extrinsic tendon dorsal to the metacarpal. In our experience, a lateral paratendinous approach is not necessary to separate the intrinsic from the extrinsic tendons, even when a buttress-type plate or a strut plate is applied. The dorsal approach through the middle of the extrinsic tendon preserves the integrity of the intrinsic system, which is of much greater importance than the extrinsic system, especially at the level of the proximal phalanx, proximal interphalangeal joint, and the proximal end of the middle phalanx. The lateral approach, by definition, includes damage to the intrinsic tendon system.

A postoperative rehabilitation program is instituted to minimize early tenodesis and to encourage function of the extensor tendon apparatus. Considering the extremely close relationship between the gliding structures of the tendons and the underlying bone, no fracture treatment of the hand is conceivable without at least a minimal, but well-planned rehabilitation program. Any surgical approach to the phalanges for internal fixation requires a professional rehabilitation program such as is used following tendon reconstruction in hand surgery.

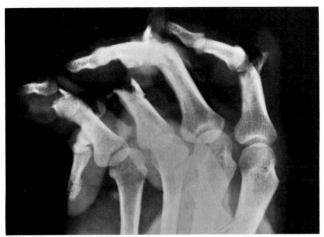

FIGURE 94-1. An unstable, comminuted, open serial fracture that requires primary and stable reconstruction.

Open Fractures With or Without Injuries to Tendons and Nerves

The ratio of soft tissue to bone at the level of the phalanges and metacarpals differs greatly from the same ratio in many other anatomic regions of the body. Moreover, the close contact of a large section of vulnerable peritendinous tissue with the bone surface is the key feature of fracture pathology of the hand.

There is also a characteristic mechanism of injury, as shown by Strickland and colleagues[15] in their retrospective study of the incidence and nature of phalangeal fractures. They found that direct blow and crush injuries accounted for 80% of the total, whereas indirect force was instrumental in only 20% of the fractures. These facts explain why, in their series, 44% of the patients had additional tendon injuries involving flexors

and extensors. It is obvious that the incidence of open fractures of the hand is significantly higher than that of any other site (38% in our series) (Fig. 94-3).

The functional restoration of digits with open fractures, which has been poor in various series, must be analyzed in terms of primary *versus* secondary reconstruction. Primary, global reconstruction of all traumatized structures of the hand yields far better results than does late reconstruction. Delayed or deferred skeletal reconstruction must be limited to exceptional situations; such a decision is mainly organizational in nature. Effective primary care requires emergency surgery performed by a staff of experienced hand surgeons able to deal with a wide variety of bone and associated soft-tissue lesions.

Multiray Fractures and Multilevel Fractures

Even multiple fractures of the hand are not an absolute indication for stable internal fixation in order to regain some function. However, with serial fractures, it is much easier to establish a rehabilitation program in the course of bone healing when the function—i.e., the load transmission—of the skeleton is restored immediately. Moreover, the needs and the duration of this program are modest compared to the rehabilitation program following any nonoperative treatment of multiple fractures in the same hand. It is also accepted that financial considerations, as well as the loss of working capacity, must be evaluated when the treatment of fractures of such complexity is planned. Primarily, however, immediate internal fixation is indicated by the predictability of optimal functional restoration of the hand.

The longitudinal arch of the hand includes the carpal bones, the metacarpals, and the metacarpophalangeal joints, as well as the phalanges, as components of a stable functional chain. Any fracture, especially those occurring at different levels of the

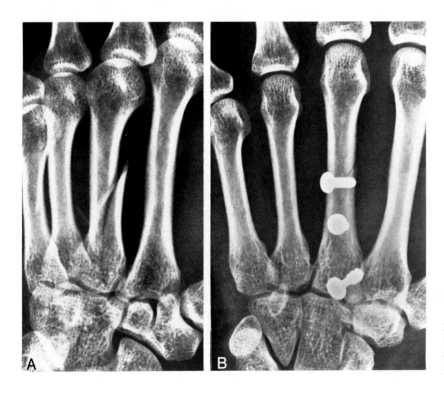

FIGURE 94-2. Unstable spiral fracture of the third metacarpal. (*A* and *B*) Stabilization was achieved by using the lag screw compression technique.

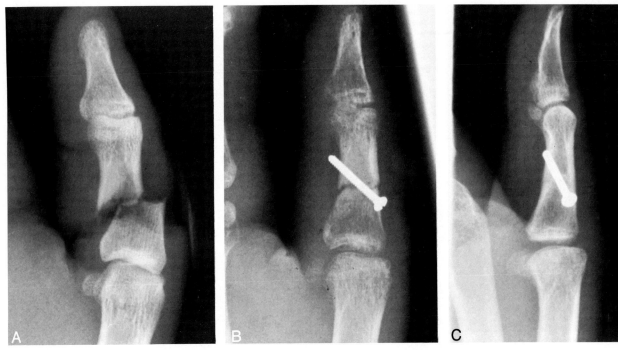

FIGURE 94-3. (*A*) Open fracture of the thumb. (*B*) Severance of bone, extensor tendon, flexor tendon, nerves, and arteries. (*C*) Reconstruction of all structures following simple lag screw stabilization of bone.

system, may cause a break in the slightly winged longitudinal arch. The lever-arm system of the extensor, as well as the flexor tendons, is thrown into disarray. A typical transverse series of fracture dislocation which interrupts the longitudinal arch of all long fingers is the fracture dislocation of the second to fifth metacarpal at their proximal ends—i.e., at the carpometacarpal junction (Fig. 94-4). Often, the ulnar marginal metacarpals, which are more mobile in their carpometacarpal joints, tend to become displaced from articulation, whereas the more stable second and third metacarpals frequently suffer fractures near their base. Open reduction and stabilization of the second to fifth arch is mandatory.

Serial fractures of the metacarpal shafts, usually in the form of long spiral fractures, produce a palmar tilt of the distal fragment, a marked shortening of the metacarpals, and a rotation in the form of supination on the ulnar aspect of the hand; eventually, pronation on the radial aspect of the hand also occurs. With a fracture of the third metacarpal, the very important central pillar of the hand is unstable. Instability, therefore, concerns the transverse as well as the longitudinal metacarpal arch of the hand. We agree with Tubiana that any palmar tilt should be corrected surgically, since muscle balance is otherwise markedly disturbed.[16]

Articular Fractures

Monocondylar or bicondylar fractures of the second phalanx require anatomic reduction in all the fingers, as does an impaction fracture at the base of the second phalanx. Internal or percutaneous pinning is a suitable treatment mode that is associated with a low risk of infection. Internal stable fixation, by contrast, is associated with additional advantages, such as perfect anatomic reduction and permanent stability throughout

the entire phase of bone healing. With internal fixation, the rehabilitation program need not make allowances for the care of percutaneous Kirschner wires, early removal of metal implants, or secondary losening of implants. Rather, its aim is immediate functional recovery, despite the presence of stabilizing implants *in situ*. The same holds true for those fractures that occur at the base of the thumb, such as instable, transverse, extra-articular fractures; the large spectrum of intra-articular fractures (Bennett) (Fig. 94-5); and finally, the Rolando-type fracture.

Stable internal fixation in the management of fractures at the base of the first metacarpal bone incorporates all of the techniques based on compression: single or double lag screws of the cortical type, a tension band plate and tension band wiring, and a neutralization plate.

The "saddle" joint (first carpometacarpal joint), with its convex/concave articular planes at 90° which provide movements in planes of abduction/adduction and flexion/extension, requires extensive exposure in order to visualize all components of the joint. Stabilization must resist the moments of forceful actions, such as opposition, flexion, and rotation. The stabilization of unstable fractures, both extra-articular and intra-articular, at the base of the thumb (Fig. 94-6) may serve as an example for planning of stable internal fixation.

Exposure

The incision must allow for a dorsal, ulnar, and radial approach to the first carpometacarpal joint. Make a large incision starting beside the first metacarpal at its ulnar border and swinging over and parallel to the carpometacarpal joint space to the radial side. This may be prolonged if necessary, to permit an additional palmar approach described by Gedda.[7] This incision

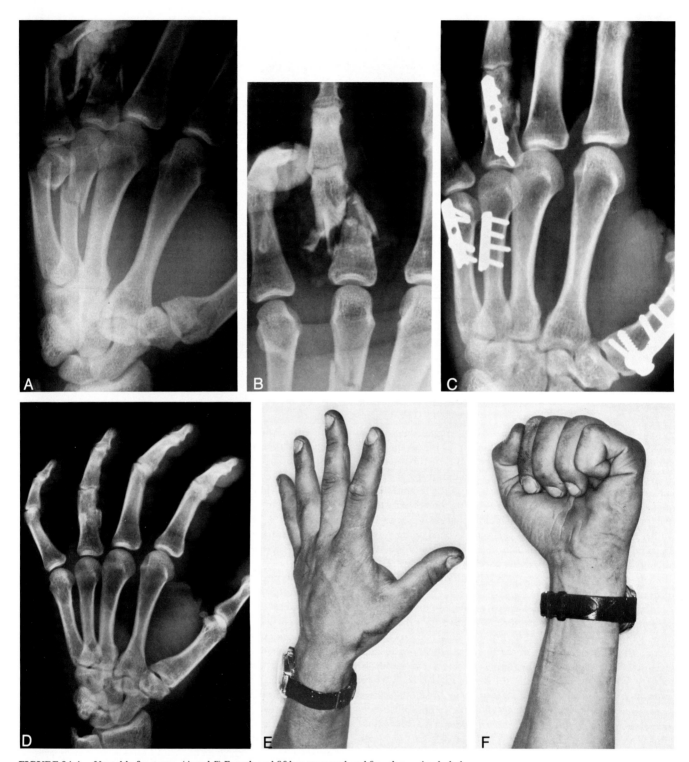

FIGURE 94-4. Unstable fractures. (*A* and *B*) Fourth and fifth metacarpal and fourth proximal phalanx (The fracture of the first metacarpal is stable.) (*C* and *D*) Compression techniques for the first, fourth, and fifth metacarpal and a strut plate (2.0 mm) in the proximal phalanx. The fractures healed within 9 weeks; remodelling of the bone took 6 months. (*E* and *F*) Functional performance following removal of implants.

FIGURE 94-5. Oblique intra-articular fracture. (*A* and *B*) Three-point fixation by lag screws. The position of the screws varies according to the fracture plane.

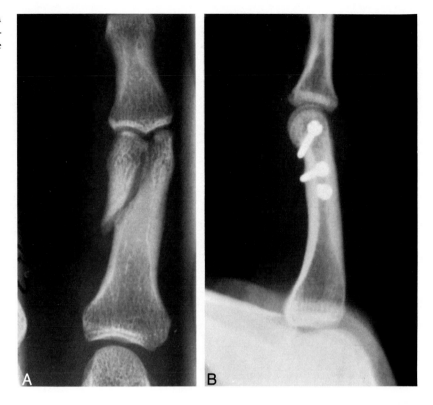

FIGURE 94-6. Unstable extra-articular fracture at the base of the first metacarpal. (*A* and *B*) Stabilization with a 2.7 mm neutralization plate. The first and second proximal screws are crossing the oblique fracture, functioning as lag screws in the plate.

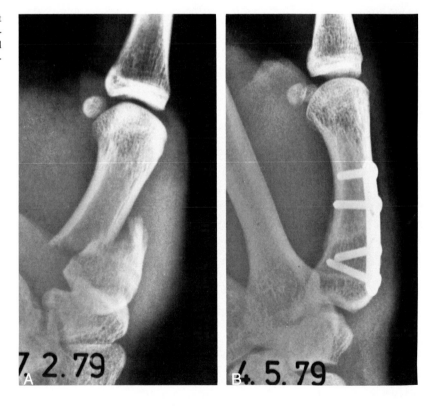

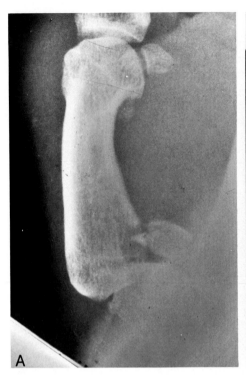
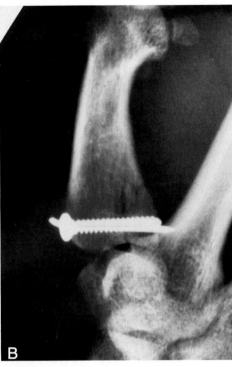

FIGURE 94-7. Bennett's fracture with a small fragment and subluxation. (*A* and *B*) Reconstruction and compression by lag screw, with additional rotational stability afforded by placement of a Kirschner wire.

is necessary in order to visualize the sometimes small fragment starting from the ulnar border and extending all the way down to the articular surface. This exposure is achieved by stripping off the origin of the radial head of the first dorsal interosseous muscle from the base of the first metacarpal. The fragment may thus be reduced perfectly and stabilized by a preliminary Kirschner wire, and then by one, or preferably, two, 2.0-mm cortical lag screws. If reduction is difficult, or if several frag-

ments are present, extend the transverse section of the incision, allowing for a wide exposure of the joint itself. Incise the joint capsule transversely; in even more difficult conditions, sever the abductor pollicis longus rather close to its insertion. Thereafter, the joint space may be enlarged by distraction, thereby facilitating inspection of all the components of the articulation. The articular surface may then be reconstructed precisely. Following reconstruction and preliminary fixation by two Kirschner wires, different combinations of stabilization may be required:

> One lag screw (adequate only for a rather large fragment)
> Two lag screws placed in appropriate angles to the fracture plane
> One lag screw and one Kirschner wire, added to increase rotational stability (Fig. 94-7)
> One lag screw plus tension band wiring in the case of a capsular avulsion fracture on the dorsal aspect
> A Neutralization plate for multifragmented fractures, especially of the Rolando type (Fig. 94-8).

A spectrum of techniques and implants must always be available, especially in treating articular fractures, so that any type or form of joint destruction, in any given case, may be managed properly.

Fractures With Substantial Bone Loss

Since the hand is exposed to machines and tools in labor, and to trauma in sport activities, it is, more than any other anatomic area of the body, subject to open fractures with loss of bone substance and with defects of soft tissue, as well with severance of extensor and flexor tendons in some cases.[15] We have come to the conclusion that these multistructural lesions are amena-

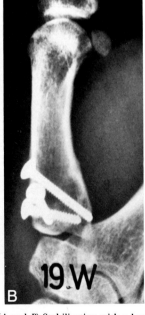

FIGURE 94-8. Rolando's fracture. (*A* and *B*) Stabilization with a lag screw (2.0 mm); the position of each screw is determined according to the various fracture planes.

ble to integrated reconstruction of all injured tissues in one operative session, starting with reconstruction of the skeleton. In this way, emergency surgery of the hand has become a primary, "global" surgical reconstruction of all tissues. Emergency operative sessions, therefore, are time-consuming and are often difficult to fit into a regular operative program.

Emergency surgery facilities in a hospital may not suffice for the demands of this type of primary reconstructive surgery;[5,6,8,9] nonetheless, primary total reconstruction may be expected to give the best functional results.

The technique of bone grafting in hand surgery has changed fundamentally over the last decade (Fig. 94-9). Until recently,

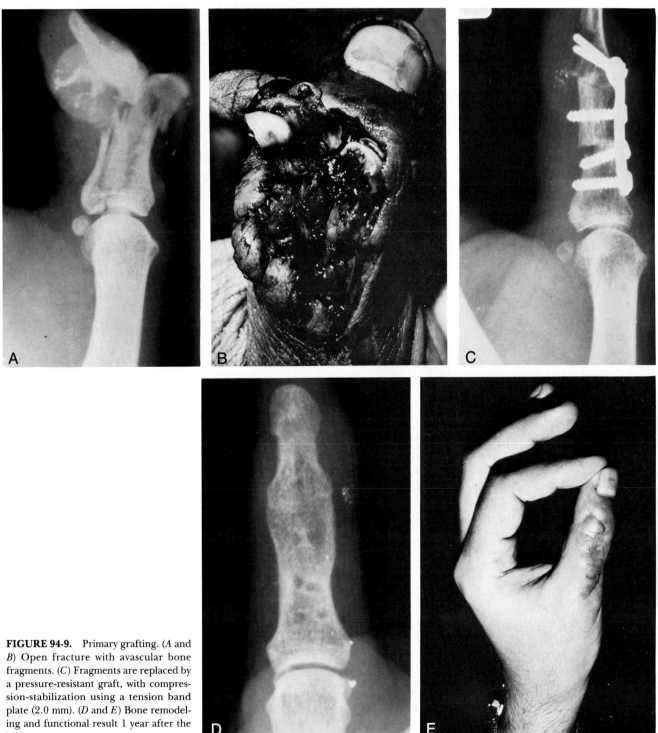

FIGURE 94-9. Primary grafting. (*A* and *B*) Open fracture with avascular bone fragments. (*C*) Fragments are replaced by a pressure-resistant graft, with compression-stabilization using a tension band plate (2.0 mm). (*D* and *E*) Bone remodeling and functional result 1 year after the injury.

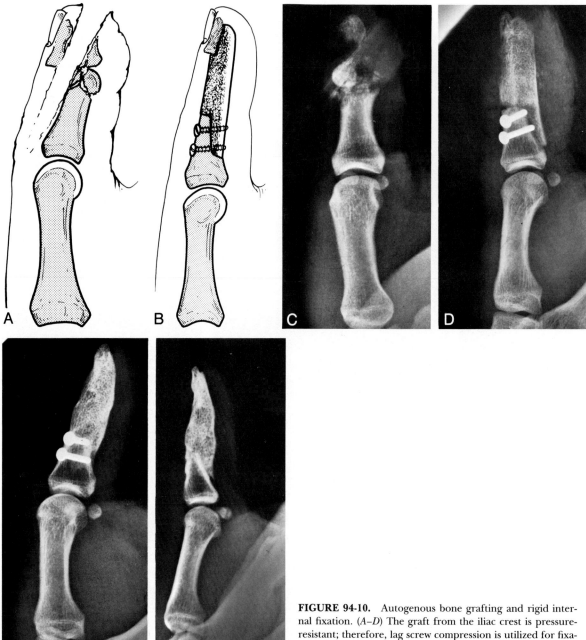

FIGURE 94-10. Autogenous bone grafting and rigid internal fixation. (*A–D*) The graft from the iliac crest is pressure-resistant; therefore, lag screw compression is utilized for fixation. (*E, F*) No resorption occurs, and rapid remodeling of the bone graft takes place.

solid bone grafts that were tightly fitted into a bone defect without stabilization by any other means than Kirschner wire were utilized. Revascularization and remodeling of the graft took several months or years; therefore, additional external immobilization was unavoidable and prolonged.

Numerous experimental studies have shown that cellular elements from the intertrabecular spaces of transplanted autogenous cancellous bone may survive, and that revascularization and remodeling of cancellous bone, used in the form of chips as well as cubes, is quick and safe under adequate biologic and mechanical conditions (Fig. 94-10). Integral to the success of the graft in primary or secondary reconstructive procedures of the hand are the favorable biologic qualities of the graft itself, and of the graft bed. The anatomy of the hand offers an almost unlimited vascular supply by virtue of its abundant vascular distribution and numerous collateral arteries at the level of the wrist, the mid carpus, and the digits. Of utmost biologic importance is the composition of the graft itself, which should always include cancellous bone elements, in addition to compact bone. Osteoid deposition with a dense layer of osteoblasts covering the transplanted trabeculae has been demonstrated within 10 days of surgery in experimental animals. New trabeculae graft themselves in different directions onto the necrotic trabeculae. Finally, necrotic trabeculae serve as scaffolding, supporting the build-up of new structures.[11] The osteolysis of the nonrevitalized trabeculae follows much later, since they remain embedded in a newly formed trabecular bone system.

Besides these important biologic needs, a mechanical prerequisite has been recognized and generally accepted—namely, uncompromised immobilization, which means abolition of even the slightest motion between graft and graft bed. Even "micro-movements" mechanically prevent the undisturbed ingrowth of capillaries from the graft bed. In order to achieve a high rate bone fusion (over 80% of the cases), the following basic principles must be adhered to:

A well-vascularized graft bed with emphasis on the best possible quality of the soft parts involved (including the addition of vascularized flaps if necessary) must be created.

Autogenous corticocancellous grafts of every shape and size, with a varying quantitative ratio of compact and cancellous bone, are taken from the pelvic crest. Allografts, as well as autologous cortical grafts, have limited indications only.

A mechanically quiet environment is achieved when all involved muscular activity at the site of reconstruction is neutralized by compression techniques of internal fixation (and also external fixation).[12,13]

Defect Fractures

If we warn against external plaster fixation lasting longer than 3 weeks, this applies even more so in the presence of defect fractures, which would necessitate additional immobilization. The most suitable treatment is primary bone grafting combined with internal fixation in order to achieve permanent mechanical stabilization of the grafted area (Fig. 94-11). Instead of the firm, wedged-in cortical grafts that were formerly used, we now predominantly rely on corticocancellous grafts. The perfectly fitting carpentry of Bunnell is replaced by internal fixation techniques. A tension band technique is used in combination with a pressure-resistant corticocancellous graft; a bridge or strut plate is acceptable when a defect is filled in with cancellous bone chips only. The stability attained primarily must last through the entire period of revascularization and remodeling.

Articular Fractures With Bone Loss

Disruption of the articular components often hinders reconstruction of the joint with preservation of mobility. Replacement of a destroyed joint in the hand by Silastic spacers or by

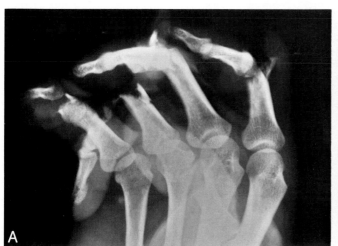 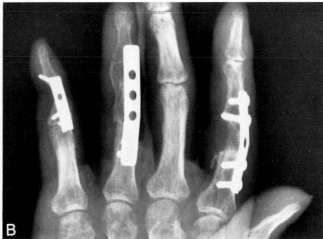

FIGURE 94-11. Serial multistructural lesions of the digits. The second and fourth proximal interphalangeal and fifth distal-interphalangeal joints are sacrificed. (*A* and *B*) Fragments are replaced by autogenous bone grafts, and stabilization is achieved by strong strut plates that bridge the grafted area since no pressure-resistant graft was used.

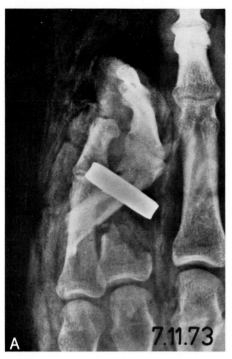

FIGURE 94-12. Compound, comminuted fracture of the first phalanx. (*A* and *B*) Meticulous reduction of fragments is not attempted; rather, replacement of partially avascular fragments by autogenous bone graft is undertaken. Preoperative state and programmed procedure. (*C* and *D*) Stabilization of the fracture and grafting with the use of lag screws and neutralization plate. Remodeling of the phalanx occurred within 9 months.

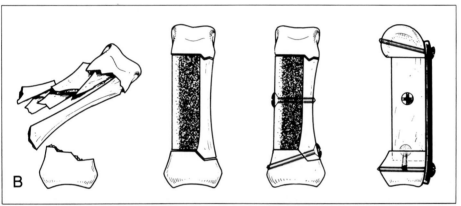

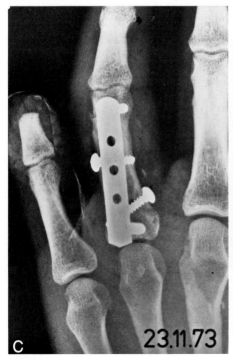

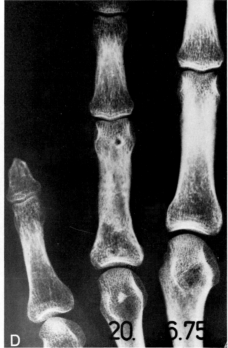

any cemented alloplastic material should not be the first choice in young individuals who are engaged in manual activities, since long-term results are not guaranteed. Painfree stability, achieved by joint fusion, may be a preferable solution in view of the overall function of the hand.

Comminuted Fractures (Devitalized Bone Fragments)

Devitalized or poorly vascularized fragments in a zone of comminution may delay fracture healing, prolong immobilization, and lead to nonunion, stiffness in the hand, and poor functional restoration. In cases involving large zones of comminution, there is less hazard in using primary bone grafts then in performing painstaking open reduction and fixation of the small, partially devitalized fragments. No attempt is made to reduce single fragments. A strut plate is used for stabilization instead of compression (Fig. 94-12). The advantage of this technique lies in the control of length and rotation of a metacarpal or phalanx. Also, some blood supply to loose fragments may be preserved by not attempting a meticulous reduction of these fragments. Finally, wound healing takes place under stable conditions. Revascularization of the grafting material proceeds rapidly, and osseous healing and remodeling is demonstrated on radiography within 3 months. In some severely comminuted fractures, we advocate use of a treatment program similar to that proposed for defect fractures or severe articular fractures. The postoperative care of the patients, however, is modified. Full functional loading is not permitted for a period of 3 weeks, nor is mobilization against resistance. An active rehabilitation program is, nevertheless, instituted immediately upon healing of the soft tissue.

SECONDARY RECONSTRUCTION

Rotational deformities, palmar tilting of distal fragments, and shortening of the metacarpals frequently follow fracture treatment. Disruption of the transverse arch of the hand, as well as the longitudinal arch, may cause an unfavorable cosmetic appearance, as well as impaired action of grasping. With modern techniques of adequate stabilization following correction, the indications for secondary reconstructive procedures have become numerous, and the safety of the procedures has increased considerably. The most common secondary reconstruction procedures are fusion, osteotomy, and treatment of nonunion.

Fusions

Sensibility is the single most important component leading to functional integrity of the hand; this is followed by mobility. So mobility may be sacrificed, rather than tactile gnosis and stability. Painful and limited function of a joint may, therefore, be treated by fusion with great benefit to the patient (Fig. 94-13). The prerequisites, however, include morbidity of only a short duration, no plaster cast fixation during the phase of bone healing, maintenance of optimal flexion and rotation, and a high rate of union.

According to a number of authors, the rate of nonunion following fusion rarely exceeds 5%. The techniques of stable

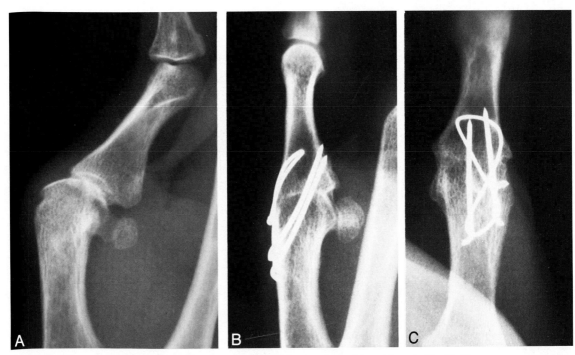

FIGURE 94-13. Fusion of the first metacarpophalangeal in a patient with septic arthritis. (*A–C*) Tension band techniques (wire technique) are now used at the level of the metacarpophalangeal-joints, as well as of the proximal and distal interphalangeal joints.

internal fixation for arthrodesis have been exceptionally successful; as a result, the indications for finger joint fusions have become numerous.

Techniques

Tension Band Technique.   Charnley[1] introduced external fixation to achieve fusion of the knee joint. Similar small devices were described by Stellbrink and Tupper and others.[3,14,17] These require space between the fingers. Tension band techniques are now preferred, since they are adequate biomechanically with the flexor power greatly exceeding that of the extensor tendons. Two Kirschner wires guarantee rotational stability, while the tension band cerclage on the extension side effectively neutralizes all distraction forces caused by bending stress. The tension band wire technique is now being used mainly at the metacarpophalangeal joint of the thumb, at the proximal interphalangeal joints, and also at the level of the carpometacarpal joint of the thumb. The technique may also be adequate in other articulations of the hand.

Tension Band Plate.   A rather large bone graft may be necessary following septic arthritis, bone necrosis, or post-traumatic bone defects. Stabilization of a corticocancellous bone graft may be achieved by a 1.5-mm or 2.0-mm tension band plate (Fig. 94-14). Initial and lasting stability will permit immediate postoperative resumption of active motion, thereby minimizing stiffness of the adjacent joints caused by tenodesis. Osseous consolidation without complication was achieved in 96.7% of patients in a series of 63 cases.[12] By eliminating unnecessary prolonged immobilization, modern techniques of stabilization are of considerable assistance in avoiding trophic disturbances, such as reflex dystrophy.

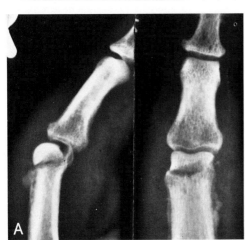
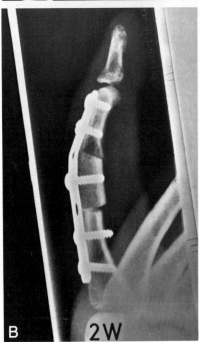
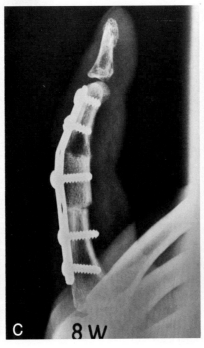
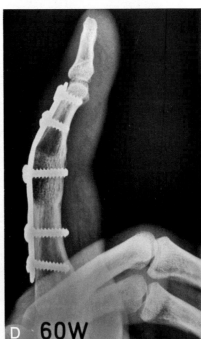

FIGURE 94-14.   Fusion of the proximal interphalangeal joint using a tension band plate. (*A* and *B*) Avascular sequestrum, osteitis, and septic arthritis are treated by extensive debridement, pressure-resistant corticocancellous bone graft, and tension band plate. (*C* and *D*) The graft is perfectly immobilized. Revascularisation occurs within 8 weeks, and remodeling of the graft takes place within 1 year.

Osteotomy

Rotational deformities, as well as abduction and adduction deformities of the phalanges and metacarpals following trauma, are no longer acceptable to the patient. However, correction may depend on the safety and predictability of the operative procedure. There is also a risk of postoperative impairment of function from interference with the gliding mechanism of the tendons following osteotomy and internal fixation (Fig. 94-15). With modern techniques, however, the indications for corrective osteotomy may be extended widely at any level of the skeleton of the hand.

Techniques

Lag Screw Technique. Bunnell (1958) pointed out that, compared with fractures, the time needed for union of a corrective osteotomy is considerably longer, and that nonunion can easily occur. Moreover, secondary displacement may lead to further malposition and additional functional loss. At the level of the condyles of the phalanges, the plane of osteotomy is oblique, and stability by compression is achieved by a single lag screw. Postoperative immobilization is limited to the period of wound healing. Thereafter, full active motion is encouraged. For 6 more weeks, however, a static extension splint is applied only at night, in order to avoid extensor tendon adhesions in the flexion position.

Tension Band Plate. The tension band plate technique is the method of choice. The angles of correction are determined in 2 or 3 planes before operation. The correction of the axes is then controlled intraoperatively by 2 guiding Kirschner wires, placed to visualize the angle of correction. In our experience, it is seldom necessary to apply a bone graft (Fig. 94-16). Even a lack of buttressing on the palmar aspect following open wedge osteotomy is acceptable. The gap, however, is bridged by a strut plate—which must be of adequate size and strength—rather than by a tension band plate. The osteotomy is performed at the level of displacement, if possible, rather than at the metaphysis of the phalanx.

As with fresh fractures, we use the dorsal approach, splitting the extrinsic extensor tendon and displacing it laterally by subperiosteal dissection. The skin is not dissected from the extensor tendon structures. The small plate is placed as a tension band plate dorsally, beneath the extensor tendon, and early active motion is permitted. Function is not significantly impaired if functional postoperative care is instituted.

Treatment of Nonunion

Except in defect fractures, bony consolidation in the hand skeleton is excellent, and non-union is rare. Bone destruction by infection and by inadequate internal fixation are recognized as the main etiological factors in the development of nonunion. Autogenous graft material is used to restore and maintain length, rather than to promote osseous consolidation (Fig. 94-17). Our experience affirms the well-known statement of Pauwels that there is no need to change the biological substrate at the site of nonunion;[10] rather, all active shearing and bending forces must be neutralized adequately by mechanical means. In hand surgery, this is achieved by rigid internal fixation, based on one of the compression techniques.

CONCLUSION

Fractures of the hand skeleton result in as much worker's compensation expenses as do fractures of the long bones.[2,15] Digital

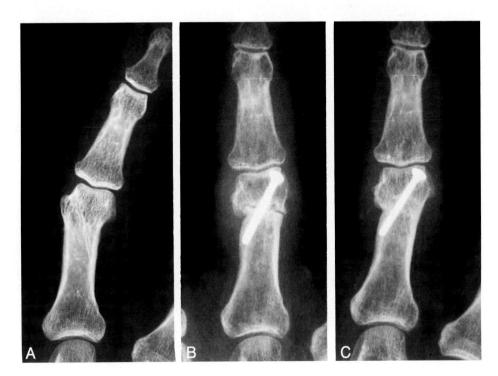

FIGURE 94-15. Osteotomy of the first phalanx. (*A–C*) Lag screw fixation of the oblique, subcapital osteotomy.

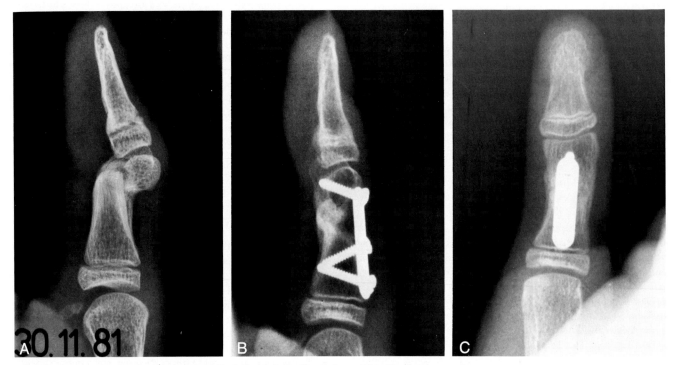

FIGURE 94-16.   Osteotomy of the proximal phalanx of the thumb in a child. (*A–C*) Open wedge osteotomy resulted in full correction of the deformity. No bone graft was needed during growth of the skeleton.

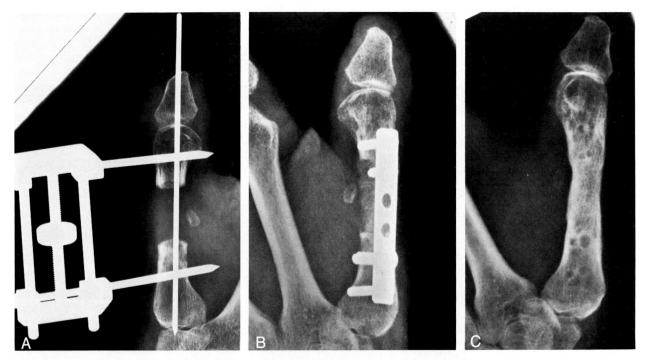

FIGURE 94-17.   Osteotomy of the first metacarpal. (*A–C*) Lengthening procedure (after MATEV), with bridge plate stabilization following autogenous bone grafting.

performance following management of comminuted fractures, as well as of simple fractures of the hand, falls far short of normal functional restoration (Strickland). Today, an increasing number of upper extremity fractures are multistructural lesions, including flexor and extensor tendons, as well as neurovascular structures and the integument. Early reconstruction of the skeletal load-bearing function is now considered to be a prerequisite for further repair of other functionally important soft tissue structures. A full understanding of the principles, techniques, and biomechanics of internal fixation, as applied to hand surgery, is mandatory.

REFERENCES

1. Anderson, R.: Fractures of the Radius and Ulna. A New Anatomical Method of Treatment. J. Bone Joint Surg. **16**:379, 1934.
2. Bunnel, S.: Surgery of the Hand. Philadelphia, J.B. Lippincott, 1956.
3. Charnley, J.C.: Positive Pressure in Arthrodesis of the Knee Joint. J. Bone Joint Surg. **30-B**:478, 1948.
4. Dabezies, E.J., and Schutte, J.P.: Fixation of Metacarpal and Phalangeal Fractures with Miniature Plates and Screws. J. Hand Surg. **11-A**:283, 1986.
5. Foucher, G., Merle, M., and Michon, J.: Traitement "Tout en Temps" des Traumatismes Complexes de la Main avec Mobilisation Précoce. Ann. Chir. **31**:1059, 1977.
6. Foucher, G., Van Genechten, F., Merle, M., and Michon, J.: Single Stage Thumb Reconstruction by a Composite Forearm Island Flap. J. Hand Surg. **9-B**,245, 1984.
7. Gedda, K.O.: Studies on Bennett's fracture. Anatomy, Roentgenology and Therapy. Acta Chir. Scand. (Suppl. 193), 1954.
8. Jupiter, J.: The Management of Multiple Fractures in One Upper Extremity: A Case Report. J. Hand Surg. **11-A**:279, 1986.
9. Meuli, C., Meyer, V., Segmüller, G.: Stabilization of Bone in Replantation Surgery of the Upper Limb. Clin. Orthop. **133**:179, 1978.
10. Pauwels, F.: Grundsätzliches über Indikation und Technik der Umlagerung bei Schenkelhalspseudarthrose. Langenbeck Arch. Klin. Chir. 262, 404, 1949.
11. Segmüller, G.: Spongiosaregeneration in der Milliporekammer. Helv. Chir. Acta **34**:5, 1967.
12. Segmüller, G.: Surgical Stabilization of the Skeleton of the Hand. Bern, Hans Huber Publishers (Distributed in the USA by Williams & Wilkins), 1977.
13. Segmüller, G.: Stabile Osteosynthese und Autologer Knochenspan bei Defekt- und Trümmerfrakturen am Handskelett. Handchir. **13**:209, 1981.
14. Stellbrink, G.: Aeusseres Fixationsgerät für Fingerarthrodesen. Chirurg **40**:422, 1969.
15. Strickland, J.W., Steichen, J.B., Kleinman, W.B., and Flynn, N.: Factors Influencing Digital Performance after Phalangeal Fractures. In Strickland, J.W., Steichen, J.B. (ed): Difficult problems in hand surgery. St. Louis, C.V. Mosby, 1982, p. 126.
16. Tubiana, R.: Le traitement chirurgical des fractures récentes des métacarpiens et des phalanges. In Traumatismes ostéoarticulaires de la main. Exp. Scientifique francaise, 1971.
17. Tupper, J.W.: A Compression Arthrodesis Device for Small Joints of the Hand. Hand **4**:62, 1972.

CHAPTER 95

Fractures of the Metacarpals and Phalanges

JESSE B. JUPITER and
MARK A. SILVER

Fractures involving the tubular bones of the hand are undoubtedly the most common of all skeletal injuries.[8] The skeleton of the hand is inherently related to adjacent joints, overlying gliding tendon units, and deforming muscle forces. Although failure to gain union with phalangeal and metacarpal fractures is unusual,[19] the prevention of angular or rotational deformity, articular stiffness, or tendon adhesion is challenging to even the most experienced surgeon. Charnley recognized this when he stated that "the reputation of a surgeon may stand as much in jeopardy from this injury [phalangeal fracture] as from any fracture of the femur."[5]

The vast majority of phalangeal and metacarpal fractures are amenable to successful nonoperative treatment. Yet a nonanatomic outcome can jeopardize overall hand function, leading at times to a prolonged and major disability.[4] Therefore, it is important to identify the fractures that require operative treatment (Table 95-1), the surgical approaches that minimize soft tissue adhesions, and the postoperative management that best encourages joint mobilization and avoids soft tissue contracture.[3]

CLASSIFICATION

Like fractures of long bones, phalangeal and metacarpal fractures call for specific methods of treatment that depend on the fracture pattern and location. A number of features are employed in classifying phalangeal and metacarpal fractures, including anatomic location, fracture configuration, soft tissue integrity, and inherent stability (Table 95-2). These tubular bones are anatomically divided into base, shaft, neck, and articular heads (Fig. 95-1). In the pediatric patient, the epiphyseal zones are found at the bases of the phalanges and the head and neck of the metacarpals. The thumb metacarpal differs in that the epiphyseal center is found at the base.

FUNCTIONAL ANATOMY

The longitudinal and distal transverse arches of the hand pass through the metacarpals, having a common keystone in the metacarpophalangeal joints. The rigid central pillar of the hand passes through the second and third metacarpals, while the mobile carpometacarpal joints of the thumb, ring, and little rays permit mobility at the borders of the hand. The deep transverse metacarpal ligaments connect the four metacarpals of the hand and provide internal support, particularly for the long and ring metacarpals. The extrinsic flexor tendons exert a flexion and adduction force on the distal metacarpals that is enhanced by the short but powerful intrinsic tendons that pass on the palmar side of the midaxis of the metacarpophalangeal joint.

In contrast to the interconnected metacarpals, the phalanges are isolated skeletal units and are subject to the deforming muscle forces of both the extrinsic flexor and extensor tendons as well as the intrinsic tendons. The proximal parts of the proximal and middle phalanges are subject to strong flexor forces, whereas the more distal shafts and neck tend to go into hyperextension because of the pull of the extensor mechanism.

The thumb plays a unique role in all forms of prehensile

TABLE 95-1. PHALANGEAL AND METACARPAL FRACTURES OFTEN REQUIRING INTERNAL FIXATION

Subcondylar proximal phalanx
Palmar base middle phalanx
T or intercondylar proximal/middle phalanx
Displaced avulsion
Rotated spiral
Comminuted
Severely displaced
Extreme soft-tissue trauma
Bennett's/reverse Bennett's

hand function. This is achieved by virtue of the complex configuration of the carpometacarpal joint as well as the transmission of power through the numerous tendon insertions. When the integrity of the thumb skeleton has been disrupted or deformed secondary to fracture malunion, the balance of these forces is disturbed, leading to deformity.

PRINCIPLES OF TREATMENT

The fracture pattern is determined by three radiographic views—anteroposterior, lateral, and oblique. Rotational and angular alignment is checked by evaluating the relationship of the fingernails to each other in both extension and flexion. It may be necessary, after careful assessment of the neurovascular status, to anesthetize the digit or hand in order to better assess rotational alignment and fracture stability.

When manipulative reduction is required and the fracture proves unstable, internal splintage is required. Kirschner wire fixation, particularly when placed percutaneously, is an excellent method of fixation in single or adjacent metacarpal or phalangeal fractures. This technique demands expertise in wire placement as well as image intensification.[2,12,20]

Open reduction and internal fixation is performed using various methods, including interosseous wire[21] and tension band wire techniques[14] as well as more rigid mini screws and plates.[15,23,25,27,28] These are described in chapters 93 and 94.

The postoperative program is directed toward preserving joint motion as well as minimizing adhesions of the gliding structures, such as the tendons and joints. Under the supervision of a hand therapist, the use of static and dynamic splints, anti-edema measures such as Coban* wraps, and active assisted

* 3M Medical Products Division, St. Paul, MN 55144

range-of-motion exercises has proved an effective means of regaining motion and avoiding joint contracture, even in severe combined skeletal and soft-tissue injuries of the hand.

SURGICAL APPROACHES

Metacarpals

In general, longitudinal incisions are preferable to transverse or serpentine approaches on the dorsum of the hand, because venous and lymphatic trauma is less (Fig. 95-2). Approach the long and ring metacarpals through a longitudinal incision between the bones, using a Y-shaped extension if necessary to provide more proximal or distal exposure. Approach the border metacarpals individually through longitudinal incisions, with curving extensions as needed. Exposure of the distal metacarpal shafts, neck, or head is facilitated by cutting through the juncturae tendinae linking the common extensor tendons. Tag these for later reapproximation with 5-0 nylon suture. Next, incise the junction of the sagittal band and extensor tendon to permit access to the metacarpophalangeal joint. This, too, should be reapproximated with fine nonabsorbable suture.

At the shaft level, incise the periosteum carefully, leaving as much attached as possible and preserving the origins of the interosseous muscles. Gently expose the fracture site and remove the hematoma by irrigation with a small-bore needle and the use of a dental pic.

Surgical approaches to the thumb metacarpal are most often required for intra-articular fractures at the base. The palmar approach described by Gedda and Moberg,[11] starts proximally at the wrist crease and extends distally along the metacarpal shaft (Fig. 95-3). The thenar muscles are elevated subperiosteally off the metacarpal shaft, permitting excellent exposure to the palmar aspect of the carpometacarpal joint. This approach is particularly effective for Bennett fractures with small palmar fragments. The radiodorsal approach is preferred for fractures that extend onto the proximal metacarpal shaft. Make the incision along the radial edge of the metacarpal. Identify and preserve crossing branches of the radial sensory nerve as well as the insertion of the abductor pollicis longus tendon. Elevate the thenar muscles subperiosteally off the shaft, if necessary, to improve exposure of the base.

Phalanges

The proximal and middle phalanges can be approached through either dorsolateral or midaxial incisions (Fig. 95-4).

TABLE 95-2. FUNCTIONAL FRACTURE CLASSIFICATION

Location	Pattern	Skeleton	Soft Tissue	Reaction to Motion
Base	Transverse	Simple	Closed	Stable
Shaft	Oblique	Impacted	Open	Unstable
Neck	Spiral	Comminuted		
Condyle (head)	Avulsion			
Epiphysis				

FIGURE 95-1.   The anatomy of the metacarpal and phalanx.

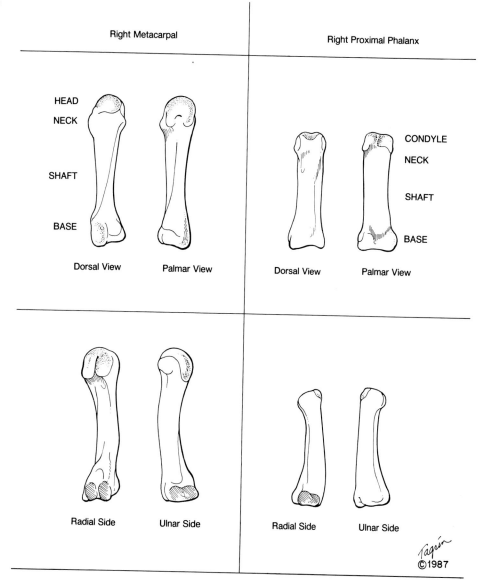

Elevate the dorsal skin flap off the paratenon of the extensor tendon. Preserve the dorsal venous arcade whenever possible. Careful attention to preserving the paratenon and periosteum will help avoid later adhesions between the phalanx and tendon. If more distal exposure of the shaft is necessary, incise the transverse retinacular ligament to allow further mobilization of the extensor mechanism. Mark this interval for later reapproximation.

The proximal interphalangeal joint can be approached straight dorsally between the central extensor tendon and the lateral band or between the lateral band and the collateral ligament. Occasionally, additional exposure can be obtained by osteotomizing the insertion of the central slip onto the base of the middle phalanx and reflecting the tendon proximally. The insertion can later be secured with a tension wire or small screw.

A modified "H" incision is preferred for access to the head of the middle phalanx or distal interphalangeal joint. Exposure of the joint is gained by splitting the extensor tendon longitudinally or in a "Z" fashion.

METACARPAL FRACTURES

Shaft Fractures

Treatment

The treatment of metacarpal shaft fractures has progressed considerably since the 1930s, when virtually all metacarpal fractures were treated by bandaging over roller bandage with little or no attempt to correct displacement. Angulation, shortening, or rotation that cannot be controlled by plaster support requires internal fixation. In addition, fractures associated with soft-tissue crush or open injuries are better managed with internal fixation (Table 95-3).

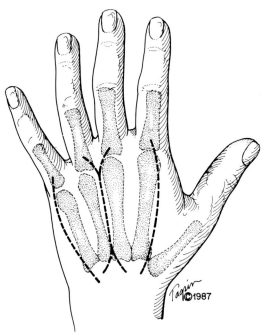

FIGURE 95-2. Dorsal surgical approaches to the metacarpals.

Percutaneous Kirschner wire fixation may be applicable for some transverse shaft fractures.[20] Potential problems are inherent with the placement of the wire through the metacarpophalangeal joint capsule or the extensor tendon mechanism. For multiple transverse fractures or those associated with crushing injuries we prefer dorsally placed tension band plates (Fig. 95-5). Four-hole one-quarter tubular plates using 2.0-mm or 2.7-mm screws are usually used. Some compression can be gained at the fracture line by drilling eccentrically in the farthest holes from the fracture line and placing both screws in simultaneously.[15] If comminution is noted at the fracture line, use a longer plate. In addition, a small amount of cancellous bone graft is readily obtained from the distal radius and should be placed in the zones of comminution.

Spiral and long oblique fractures provide a wide surface amenable to interfragmentary screw fixation (Fig. 95-6). The screws should distribute interfragmentary compression evenly along the entire fracture length. One screw placed perpendicular to the fracture line and one perpendicular to the shaft will assure distribution of compression and offset shear stresses on the implants. With short oblique fractures, a single screw cannot withstand the rotatory, shear, or bending stresses of normal activity. These stresses must be "neutralized" by a plate in order to allow early mobilization (Fig. 95-7).

Postoperative Management

The incisions are closed over a small vacuum drain, wrapped in Dacron batting dressing, and supported in a plaster splint. Active assisted range-of-motion exercises are begun 48 to 72 hours after surgery. Coban wraps around the digits and hand effectively control postoperative swelling. Radiographs should be taken at 1, 3, and 6 weeks after surgery. The patient should be able to start light manual activities at 3 weeks and unrestricted activities by 6 to 8 weeks.

Pitfalls and Complications

The surgeon must be confident that the internal fixation is rigid enough to support the fracture during rehabilitation.

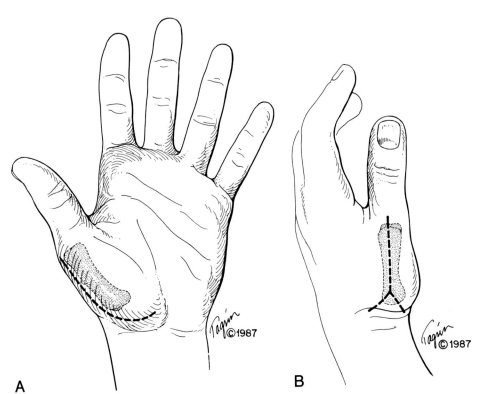

A   B

FIGURE 95-3. Surgical approaches to the thumb metacarpal. (*A*) Palmar. (*B*) Dorsal.

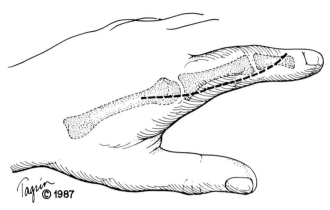

FIGURE 95-4. Surgical approaches to the phalanges.

TABLE 95-3. INDICATIONS FOR INTERNAL FIXATION—METACARPAL SHAFT

Multiple oblique or spiral fractures
Shortened fractures
Open fracture
Displaced border metacarpal (index/little finger)

Leaving the hand immobile until fracture union after an extensive surgical exposure, can result in tendon adhesions or joint contracture. Unforeseen comminution or longitudinal fracture lines may cause the unwary surgeon to place the screws in unsound bone. This can be avoided by studying the fracture pattern once the hematoma has been cleared and before the actual reduction. When a screw is loose because of stripping of the tapped threads, placing a larger screw, redirecting the screw, or using a longer plate can retrieve a stable fixation. Converting to Kirschner wire fixation with tension loops of stainless steel wire is also effective when rigid fixation is inadequate.[14]

Neck Fractures

Fractures of the metacarpal neck are almost always the result of direct impact, with the deformity generally being palmar angulation of the distal fragment; rarely, malrotation may also be present. Excessive flexion of the distal fragment can lead to hyperextension at the metacarpophalangeal joint, interference with grip, and pain over the metacarpal head in the distal palm. While most would agree that more than 10° of palmar angulation is unacceptable in the index and long metacarpals because of their immobile carpometacarpal joints, some controversy surrounds fractures of the metacarpal necks of the ring and little fingers. Several authors have reported acceptable functional results with flexion deformities upwards of 70° in the little finger.[7,16,17] We believe as others[28,30] that reduction should be considered for angulation beyond 30° to 40° in the little and beyond 20° to 30° in the ring finger.

Treatment

Closed reduction of metacarpal neck fractures is readily accomplished by the 90-90 method introduced by Jahss of flexing the proximal interphalangeal joint and using the proximal phalanx to push the metacarpal head into position.[18] Immobilization in this position is not acceptable to hold the reduction in place because of the risk of joint contracture or skin necrosis.

Percutaneous Kirschner wire fixation has proved most effective in stabilizing metacarpal neck fractures, particularly of the little and ring metacarpals. The wires, generally 0.035-inch,

can be introduced transversely, proximal and distal to the fracture, into the adjacent metacarpal; obliquely across the fracture; or longitudinally through the flexed metacarpophalangeal joint. A 14-gauge hypodermic needle placed against the metacarpal functions well as a pin guide. These methods of treatment carry a risk of permanent metacarpophalangeal joint stiffness by virtue of the pins transfixing the extensor mechanism.

We prefer to introduce the Kirschner wires from the base of the metacarpal. Using image intensification, make a small transverse incision over the dorsoulnar aspect of the base of the metacarpal. Create a small window in the metacarpal base. Bend a 0.045-inch Kirschner wire into a gentle arc and hammer it distally up the shaft while holding the fracture reduced in the 90-90 position. The pin should extend into the subchondral bone of the head (Fig. 95-8). Introduce a second pin if motion is felt at the fracture. Cut the pin(s) just beneath the skin and apply an ulnar gutter splint with the metacarpophalangeal joint maintained in flexion. Gentle motion may be initiated 2 weeks after surgery.

Percutaneous pins, placed sagittally from dorsal to palmar and bonded together by methylmethacrylate, have also been advocated as a reliable means of holding the reduction without opening the fracture site.[26] The method, however, carries a risk of the extensor mechanism's being transfixed by the pins or pintract sepsis. This technique is perhaps best reserved for fractures associated with soft-tissue injury or bone loss.

Open reduction and internal fixation should be reserved for grossly displaced fractures, fractures associated with extensive soft-tissue trauma, or fractures seen beyond the time when manipulative reduction can be achieved. Because of the proximity of these fractures to the joint and extensor mechanism, we prefer crossed Kirschner wires looped with a stainless steel wire as a tension band (Fig. 95-9). This technique involves placing two 0.035-inch or 0.028-inch Kirschner wires either crisscrossing the fracture or parallel to the fracture placed dorsal to the midaxis of the bone. A 28-gauge stainless steel wire is placed dorsally over the fracture and just under the points of the wires. Motion may be initiated within 48 to 72 hours after surgery. The Kirschner wires can be removed under local anesthesia in the office.

Pitfalls and Complications

The major difficulty associated with the treatment of metacarpal neck fractures lies in the potential for stiffness of the metacarpophalangeal joint. Open reduction should be avoided if possible; percutaneous techniques are preferable. We generally bury the Kirschner wires just under the skin to avoid pintrack infections.

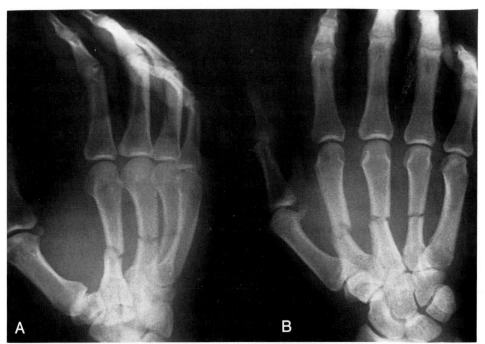

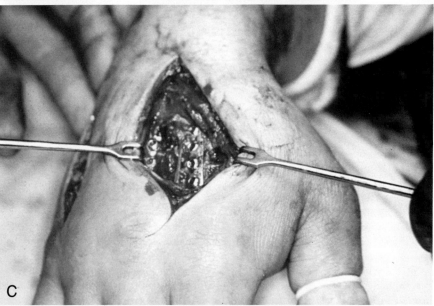

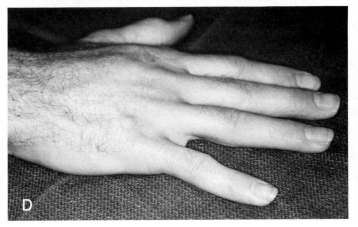

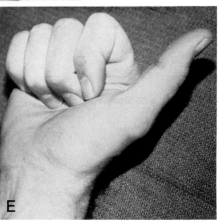

FIGURE 95-5. A 24-year-old laborer had his dominant right hand crushed by a dumpster. There was extensive soft-tissue trauma associated with three metacarpal shaft fractures. (*A, B*) Anteroposterior and oblique views revealed transverse metacarpal shaft fractures. (*C*) Through two longitudinal incisions, one-quarter tubular plates and 2.7-mm screws were applied. (*D, E*) Full flexion and extension were achieved within 6 weeks despite the extensive soft-tissue crush.

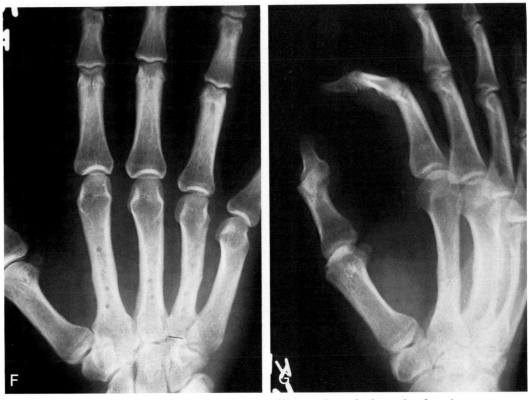

FIGURE 95-5. (*continued*) (*F, G*) Anteroposterior and oblique radiographs 6 months after plate removal.

Head Fractures

Less common injuries, metacarpal head fractures are intraarticular fractures seen most often in young adults as a result of athletic injury.[22] These vary from an osteochondral fracture, to two- or three-part fractures in a sagittal or coronal plane, to grossly comminuted fractures.

Treatment

Treatment planning should include anteroposterior and lateral tomography to determine the operability of the fracture as well as the location of the fragments. For the nondisplaced as well as the very comminuted fractures, splint support and protected motion is preferable.

Open reduction and internal fixation is indicated for the split or three-part fracture. Through a dorsal approach, open the joint capsule longitudinally. Meticulous handling of the small fracture fragments is imperative to avoid further fragmentation or devascularization. Preserve any soft tissue attachments. Provisionally stabilize the fracture with 0.028-inch Kirschner wires, verifying the reduction with anteroposterior, lateral, and oblique radiographs. As a general rule, if the fracture fragment is larger than two to three times the diameter of the screw head, internal fixation with 1.5-mm mini screws is preferred. If secure fixation can be achieved, early mobilization of this joint injury can be started. With smaller fragments, Kirschner wire fixation is recommended. In the setting of impacted fragments, cautious elevation and support with cancel-lous bone graft obtained from the end of the radius can restore the anatomic profile of the metacarpal head.

Postoperative management depends on the stability of the internal fixation. Screw fixation, if rigid, will permit protected motion within 48 to 72 hours after surgery. Kirschner wire fixation should be held in a splint with the metacarpophalangeal joint flexed 70° for 10 to 14 days before motion is started.

Pitfalls and Complications

Inability to fix the fracture fragment securely, increased fragmentation, or excessive soft-tissue stripping can lead to avascular necrosis, loss of reduction, metacarpophalangeal joint stiffness, or post-traumatic arthrosis. Proper preoperative assessment, particularly with tomography, may prevent the surgeon from entering into an unduly difficult reconstruction.

Base Fractures

Fractures at the bases of the metacarpals, particularly the mobile ring and little, require a careful assessment of any intraarticular involvement. These fractures are often the result of crushing injuries and are associated with fracture-dislocations at the carpometacarpal joints. Accurate reduction may offset later post-traumatic arthrosis, particularly in the ulnar metacarpals. In fact the treatment of fractures at the base of the little metacarpal should be approached in a similar manner to fractures of the thumb carpometacarpal joint.

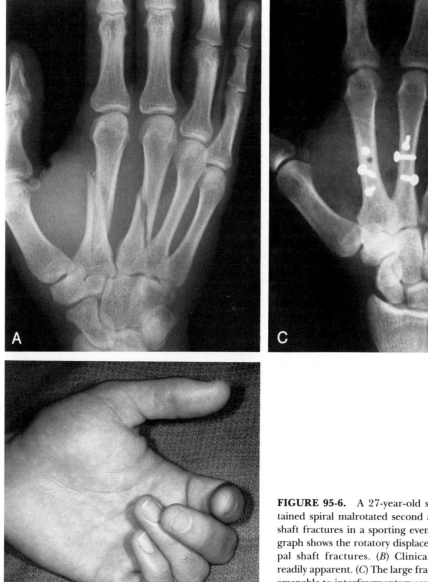

FIGURE 95-6. A 27-year-old surgical resident sustained spiral malrotated second and third metacarpal shaft fractures in a sporting event. (*A*) Oblique radiograph shows the rotatory displacement of the metacarpal shaft fractures. (*B*) Clinically, malrotation was readily apparent. (*C*) The large fracture surfaces proved amenable to interfragmentary screw fixation using 2.7-mm and 2.0-mm screws. Note the arrangement of the screws to offset shear and rotational stresses. The patient made a full functional recovery.

Thumb Metacarpal Fractures

Most thumb metacarpal fractures occur at or near the base. The distinction between intra- and extra-articular fractures is important, particularly in that the thumb metacarpal will tolerate upward of 30° angulation without noticeable deformity or altered function.[13] However, the carpometacarpal joint of the thumb is critical for thumb and hand function, and inadequate treatment can lead to a substantial hand disability. Special radiographic views, including tomography or the Robert anteroposterior view taken with the hand in maximum pronation, are often required to assess the fracture pattern accurately.

Treatment

A number of techniques, all reporting good results, have been advocated for treatment of Bennett's fracture dislocation.[10] The small palmar fragment remains attached to the trapezium and second metacarpal by the stout anterior oblique ligaments, while the shaft of the metacarpal is pulled proximally and radially, allowing the abductor pull to increase the deformity at the base.

Our approach has been directed toward regaining anatomic reduction of the intraarticular fracture. With the aid of image intensification, attempt closed reduction by longitudinal trac-

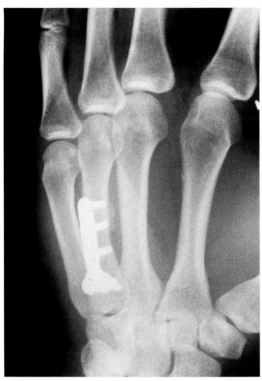

FIGURE 95-7. A 35-year-old laborer sustained a severe crush injury to his left hand. In view of the massive soft tissue trauma, rigid internal fixation was chosen in order to rapidly mobilize the hand. An interfragmentary screw was placed through a small T plate.

tion and compression on the base of the metacarpal. If, indeed, an anatomic reduction can be realized, percutaneous Kirschner wire fixation using 0.045-inch wires will guard against redislocation. The use of a 14 gauge hypodermic needle will facilitate the placement of the Kirschner wires onto the tubular shaft of the metacarpal. Direct one wire into the second metacarpal and a second into the trapezium. Cut the wires off just under the skin, and apply a thumb spica cast for 6 weeks (Fig. 95-10).

If an anatomic reduction cannot be obtained or maintained, open reduction and internal fixation is required. Through the palmar approach of Gedda and Moberg, reduce the fracture and gently hold it with a bone reduction clamp while provisional fixation is made with Kirschner wires. Introduce a 2.0-mm or 2.7-mm cortical screw from a dorsal direction into the fragment, placing the gliding hole in the metacarpal shaft. Use the half-threaded 4.0-mm cancellous screw only as a "bailout" if adequate fixation cannot be achieved, as this type of screw may prove difficult to remove. If small Kirschner wires are used, support the fixation by an additional Kirschner wire between the thumb metacarpal and second metacarpal as well as by a thumb spica cast for 4 to 6 weeks. With stable screw fixation, protected motion may be initiated within 48 to 72 hours after surgery.

Although a Y-shaped intra-articular fracture was described by Rolando, significant comminution is far more common. Preoperative tomography is exceedingly important in determining the operability of these fractures. Often they have been im-

pacted and require support with cancellous bone graft. Place a small "T" or "L" plate on the dorsal surface of the metacarpal to support the reconstruction (Fig. 95-11).

When the comminution is too extensive to allow screw and plate fixation, Kirschner wire fixation, cancellous bone graft, and mini external fixation stabilizing the thumb metacarpal to the index metacarpal can maintain distraction on the joint while healing occurs (Fig. 95-12).

Pitfalls and Complications

Failure to achieve or maintain an anatomic reduction may result early in adduction deformity of the thumb metacarpal, leading to post-traumatic arthrosis. Miniscrew and plate fixation should be employed only by a surgeon experienced in these techniques, since inadequate fixation can lead to collapse of the articular restoration and substantial later disability. When surgically approaching this area, avoid prolonged intraoperative traction on the branches of the radial sensory nerve, which can result in a distressing neuritis.

PHALANGEAL FRACTURES

Shaft Fractures

Phalangeal shaft fractures are common injuries in which the associated complications are significant and the functional disability can be profound. Certainly many are nondisplaced, stable, and readily treated by splintage or buddy straps and others are easily reduced and held by external plaster support. However, because of the intimate relationship of the tendons and joints to the phalangeal shaft, there are certain unstable phalangeal fractures—including displaced, comminuted, spiral, or short oblique (Table 89-1)—that require internal fixation to assure anatomic alignment and restore functional mobility.

Treatment

A large percentage of unstable phalangeal shaft fractures can be successfully treated by percutaneous Kirschner wire fixation (Fig. 95-13). After appropriate anesthesia, apply longitudinal traction through the middle phalanx and flex the metacarpophalangeal joint 60° to 70° with the proximal phalanx flexed approximately 45°.[2] Make angular and rotatory corrections at this juncture. If swelling is not profound, the flare of the head of the proximal phalanx proves to be a reliable landmark—as does the proximal palmar skin crease, which also lies under the flare.[12] The size of the Kirschner wire is determined by the location of the fracture and the size of the bone. Fractures of the base, transverse shaft, and neck are stabilized by one 0.045-inch or two 0.035-inch Kirschner wires placed longitudinally through the metacarpal head, preferably to the side of the extensor tendon and extended distally into the subchondral bone at the condylar levels. The reduction and wire placement are verified by image intensification and confirmed by standard radiographs in three views. Apply either dorsal and palmar

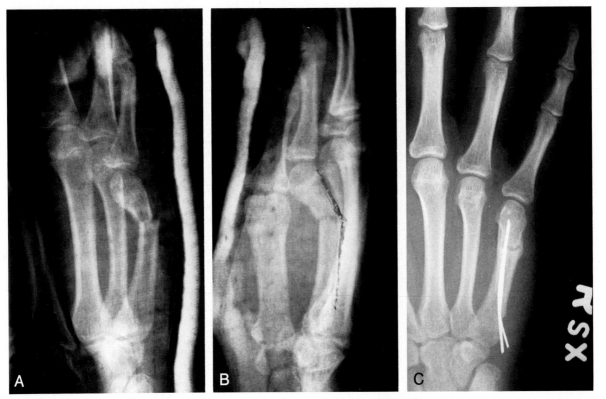

FIGURE 95-8. A 14-year-old student-athlete injured his dominant hand in a football game. (*A*, *B*) An oblique and lateral radiograph shows a displaced neck fracture. The epiphyseal plate was still open. (*C*) Two 0.045-inch Kirschner wires were inserted through a small opening in the base of the metacarpal. The fracture was reduced and held by the 90-90 method while the wires were inserted. Clinical union occurred in 2 weeks, and the wires were removed 1 week later.

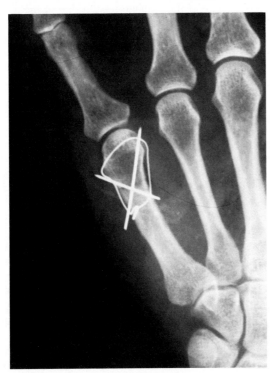

FIGURE 95-9. A 46-year-old woman was thrown from a horse, sustaining multiple injuries. Anteroposterior radiograph shows a fifth metacarpal neck fracture treated by two crossed Kirschner wires and a dorsal stainless steel loop acting as a tension band.

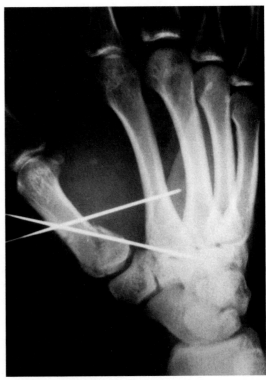

FIGURE 95-10. A displaced Bennett's fracture was treated successfully by a closed reduction and percutaneous Kirschner wire fixation. Image intensification facilitated the pin placement.

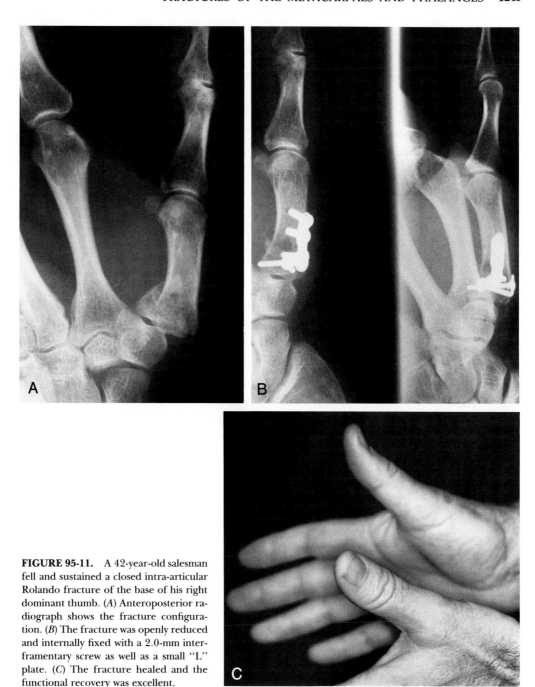

FIGURE 95-11. A 42-year-old salesman fell and sustained a closed intra-articular Rolando fracture of the base of his right dominant thumb. (*A*) Anteroposterior radiograph shows the fracture configuration. (*B*) The fracture was openly reduced and internally fixed with a 2.0-mm interframentary screw as well as a small "L" plate. (*C*) The fracture healed and the functional recovery was excellent.

splints or a plaster cast. Take care that the plaster does not come into contact with the pins, which are left protruding through the skin for ease of removal. The cast is removed at 3 weeks and the pin is removed either then or at 4 weeks, depending on the radiographic appearance. Active assisted range-of-motion exercises should be initiated under the supervision of a therapist.

Spiral or short oblique fracture patterns can be satisfactorily stabilized with parallel Kirschner wires placed across the fracture site. For the index and little fingers, the wires are introduced from the radial and ulnar sides respectively and left protruding through the skin for ease of removal.

Shaft fractures that cannot be well reduced by manipulative reduction, those associated with soft-tissue trauma, and those seen late require open reduction and internal fixation. The shaft can be approached through the interval between the lateral band and common extensor tendon. More distal exposure may require division of the transverse retinacular ligaments, which are marked for later reapproximation. Spiral fractures, for the most part, are amenable to interfragmentary screw fixation using 1.5-mm screws. Directing one screw perpendicular to the phalangeal shaft and a second perpendicular to the fracture line protects the fracture against shear and rotatory stresses. Countersinking the holes keeps the screw heads from

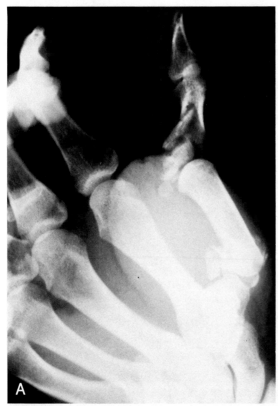

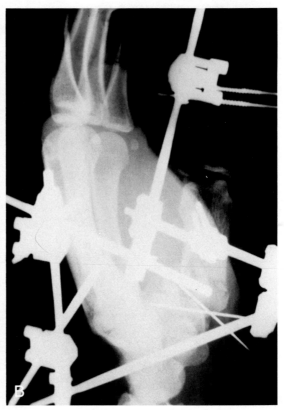

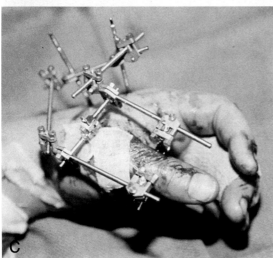

FIGURE 95-12. A 30-year-old tool and die worker had his dominant thumb caught in a lathe, causing extensive skeletal and soft-tissue trauma. (*A*) Anteroposterior radiograph shows a comminuted intra-articular fracture at the base of the metacarpal as well as a severe fracture of the proximal phalanx. (*B*) Following repair of the flexor pollicis longus and the radial digital nerve and artery, an open reduction and internal fixation of the base of the metacarpal was accomplished. The impacted articular fragments were reduced, held with 0.035-inch Kirschner wires and supported by distal radius cancellous bone graft. A mini external fixation unit was placed to prevent settling of the joint reconstruction, maintain the first web space, and maintain reduction of the proximal phalanx fracture. (*C*) Rehabilitation of the hand progressed with the fixator in place.

interfering with the overlying gliding structures. Although plates may prove bulky, if the fracture is a short oblique pattern, the interfragmentary screw will require a "neutralization" plate to protect against shear or rotational forces.

The interosseous wire technique advocated by Lister is most effective for transverse fractures (Fig. 95-14).[21] Its application is straightforward and requires little in the way of instrumentation, and the fixation is less bulky than plates. The disadvantages, however, include the failure to gain a "tension band" effect if the wire loop is placed in the midaxis of the shaft as well as the potential for the oblique Kirschner wire required to "neutralize" rotational forces to interfere with gliding of the

lateral band. A wire loop placed on the dorsal aspect of the shaft in association with transverse or crossed Kirschner wires will effectively function as a tension band.[14]

The technique of interosseous wire fixation starts with the placement of two parallel drill holes with a 0.035-inch Kirschner wire placed just dorsal to the midaxis of the shaft and just proximal and distal to the transverse fracture line. A 20 gauge hypodermic needle passed into the drill holes facilitates the passage of a 26 gauge stainless steel wire through the drill holes with the free ends facing the surgeon. Alternatively, with the hub cut off sharply, the hypodermic needle can also be used to drill the holes.

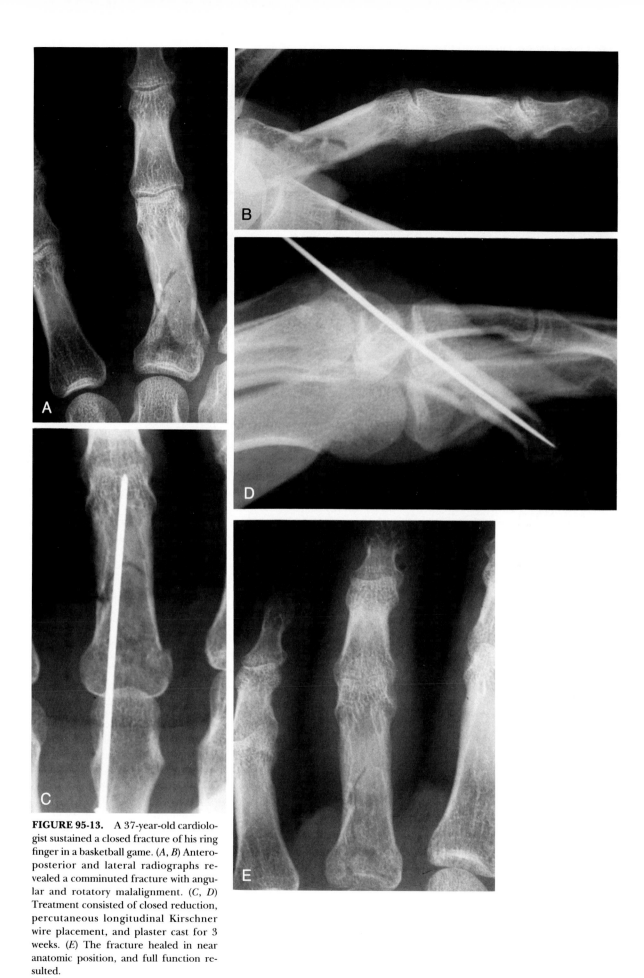

FIGURE 95-13. A 37-year-old cardiologist sustained a closed fracture of his ring finger in a basketball game. (*A, B*) Anteroposterior and lateral radiographs revealed a comminuted fracture with angular and rotatory malalignment. (*C, D*) Treatment consisted of closed reduction, percutaneous longitudinal Kirschner wire placement, and plaster cast for 3 weeks. (*E*) The fracture healed in near anatomic position, and full function resulted.

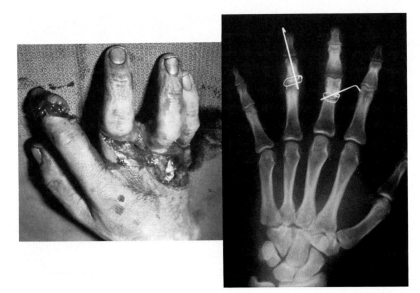

FIGURE 95-14. A 19-year-old right-hand-dominant student caught his right hand in a table saw. Extensive soft-tissue and skeletal disruption resulted. The phalangeal fractures in the long and ring fingers were fixed with an interosseous wire as well as an additional Kirschner wire for rotational control. Revascularization of the involved digits was also required.

At this juncture, pass a 0.035-inch double-ended Kirschner wire obliquely from within the fracture site distally out through the skin. With the fracture held reduced, drive the Kirschner wire into the proximal fragment. Then firmly pull the interosseous wire, twist it manually for three or four turns, and then twist it with a needle holder until the twist is seen to gently bend. Stress the fracture manually to verify the stability of the fixation and cut the twist short and bend it either against the shaft or into a drill hole in the shaft (see Fig. 95-14).

Postoperative Management

Stable internal fixation will permit active motion to be started 48 to 72 hours after surgery. Coban wraps will help reduce digital swelling, and static and dynamic splints will help restore mobility while preventing potential joint contracture. Kirschner wires will usually be removed at 3 to 4 weeks. We prefer to leave interfragmentary screws in place unless they prove bothersome.

Pitfalls and Complications

Following external fixation, excessive soft-tissue stripping, inadequate or loose internal fixation, and prolonged immobilization can result in loss of position or motion. Because of the inherent relationships of the tendons to the phalangeal skeleton, vertically placed screws can risk tendon rupture if left too long.[9]

Articular Fractures

Displaced phalangeal articular fractures, particularly the condylar or bicondylar variants, often require open reduction and internal fixation, as the fragments are small and frequently not only separated but also rotated. Three radiographic views must be obtained to adequately visualize the fracture and degree of displacement.

Treatment

The exposure of the fracture must be sufficient to allow the fracture line and the joint to be visualized, but care must be taken to avoid dissection of the soft-tissue attachments to the condyles. At the proximal interphalangeal joint level, either a dorsal or midaxial incision is recommended, while a modified "H" incision is used over the distal interphalangeal joint. For extremely displaced bicondylar fractures or those with associated impaction of the base of the middle phalanx, we have on occasion obtained added exposure by osteotomizing the insertion of the central slip, which is later replaced and secured with a tension band wire.

Unicondylar fractures are fixed with 1.5-mm lag screws. Small condylar fractures may be held by directing the screw from the opposite cortex, thereby avoiding devascularization of the collateral ligament or fragment by the relatively large screw head.

Bicondylar fractures are often the result of a more severe trauma with a high risk of residual joint stiffness. For this reason we try to obtain fixation rigid enough to permit early postoperative joint mobility. One can securely fix both condyles with a lag screw placed through the mini condylar plate along the side of the shaft. This plate is designed to sit on the side of the shaft, thus avoiding interference with the glide of the extensor mechanism.

Unstable fracture-dislocations of the proximal interphalangeal joints are also difficult fractures to treat and have a high incidence of residual stiffness or joint subluxation. The force couple technique described by Agee has the advantage of maintaining joint reduction while encouraging joint mobility, which not only helps mold a new fibrocartilagenous joint surface on the base of the middle phalanx but also avoids contracture of the soft tissues (Fig. 95-15). Place two parallel 0.045-inch Kirschner wires transversely just distal and proximal to the joint. Drill a 0.062-inch threaded Kirschner wire from dorsal to palmar in the proximal third of the middle phalanx. Bend the distal transverse Kirschner wire 90° on both sides to pass

FIGURE 95-15. A fracture-dislocation of the proximal interphalangeal joint was treated with a closed reduction and application of Agee traction. (*A*) Clinical appearance with traction in place. (*B*) Radiographic appearance, showing reduction. (*C*) Placement technique. (*Left*) Before reduction. (*Right*) After reduction, with rubber band traction assembly in place.

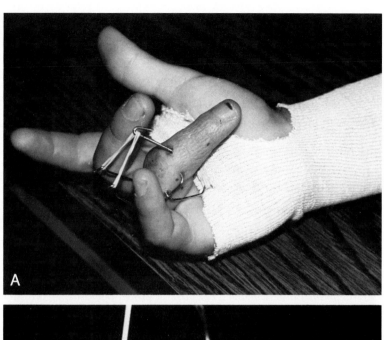

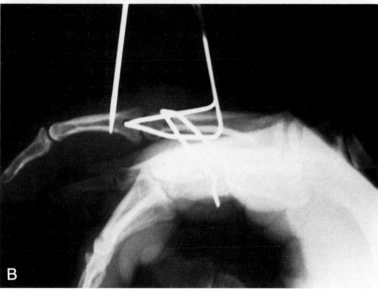

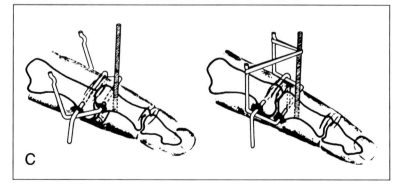

proximally and below the proximal Kirschner wire and bend it again 90° dorsally. Next, bend the proximal transverse wire 90° palmarly on either side of the finger extending palmarward, and connect it beneath the digit by a strap of adhesive tape. Finally, connect the vertical threaded Kirschner wire with the vertical arms of the distal transverse Kirschner wire with a small rubber band, creating a "force couple" that reduces the dislocation. The patient is encouraged to begin active motion, and the device is left in place for a minimum of 4 weeks and preferably for 6 weeks.

Pitfalls and Complications

Their small size, precarious vascular supply, and propensity for associated soft-tissue contracture all make phalangeal articular fractures among the most difficult hand injuries to treat. Excessive exposure and soft-tissue stripping or inadequate skeletal fixation or fragmentation of the condylar fragments will result in loss of joint mobility, arthrosis, or avascular necrosis. Careful preoperative planning is essential for proper operative management.

BIBLIOGRAPHY

1. Agee, J.: Unstable Fracture Dislocations of the Proximal Interphalangeal Joint of the Fingers: A Preliminary Report of a New Treatment Technique. J. Hand Surg., 3:386, 1978.
2. Belsky, M.R., Eaton, R.G., and Lane, L.B.: Closed Reduction and Internal Fixation of Proximal Phalangeal Fractures. J. Hand Surg., 9:725–729, 1984.
3. Belsole, R: Physiologic Fixation of Displaced and Unstable Fractures of the Hand. Orthop. Clin N. Am., 111:393, 1980.
4. Butt, W.D.: Fractures of the Hand, II. Statistical Review. Can. Med. Assoc. J., 86:775, 1962.
5. Charnley, J.: The Closed Treatment of Common Fractures, 3rd ed., p. 150. Edinburgh, Churchill Livingstone, 1974.
6. Crawford, G.P.: Screw Fixation for Certain Fractures of the Phalanges and Metacarpals. J. Bone Joint Surg., 58-A:487–492, 1976.
7. Eichenholz, S.N., and Rizzo, P.C.: Fracture of the Neck of the Fifth Metacarpal Bone—Is Overtreatment Justified. J.A.M.A., 178:425, 1961.
8. Emmett, J.E., and Breck, L.W.: A Review and Analysis of 11,000 Fractures Seen in a Private Practice of Orthopaedic Surgery. J. Bone Joint Surg., 40-A:1169, 1978.
9. Fambrough, R.A., and Green, D.P.: Tendon Rupture as a Complication of Screw Fixation in Fractures in the Hand: A Case Report. J. Bone Joint Surg., 61-A:781, 1979.
10. Gedda, K.O.: Studies on Bennett's Fracture: Anatomy, Roentgenology, and Therapy. Acta Chir. Scand., Suppl. 193, 1954.
11. Gedda, K.O., and Moberg, E.: Open Reduction and Osteosynthesis of the So-Called Bennett's Fracture in the Carpometacarpal Joint of the Thumb. Acta Orthop. Scand., 22:249, 1953.
12. Green, D.P., and Anderson, J.R.: Closed Reduction and Percutaneous Pin Fixation of Fractured Phalanges. J. Bone Joint Surg., 55-A:1651, 1973.
13. Green, D.P., and O'Brien, E.T.: Fractures of the Thumb Metacarpal. Southern Med. J., 65:807, 1972.
14. Gould, W.L., Belsole, R.J., and Skelton, W.H.: Tension-Band Stabilization of Transverse Fractures: An Experimental Analysis. Plast. Reconstr. Surg., 73:111, 1984.
15. Heim, V., and Pfeiffer, K.M.: Small Fragment Set Manual: Technique Recommended by the ASIF Group, 2nd ed. New York, Springer-Verlag, 1982.
16. Horst-Nielson, F.: Subcapital Fractures of the Four Ulnar Metacarpal Bones. Hand, 8:290, 1976.
17. Hunter, J.M., and Cowen, N.J.: Fifth Metacarpal Fractures in a Compensation Clinic Population. J. Bone Joint Surg., 52-A:1159, 1970.
18. Jahss, S.A.: Fractures of the Metacarpals: A New Method of Reduction and Immobilization. J. Bone Joint Surg., 20:178, 1938.
19. Jupiter, J.B., Koniuch, M., and Smith, R.J.: The Management of Delayed Unions and Nonunions of the Tubular Bones in the Hand. J. Hand Surg., 4:457, 1985.
20. Lamb, D.W., Abernethy, P.A., and Raine, P.A.: Unstable Fractures of the Metacarpals: A Method of Treatment by Transverse Wire Fixation to Intact Metacarpals. Hand, 5:43, 1973.
21. Lister, G.: Intraosseous Wiring of the Digital Skeleton. J. Hand Surg., 3:427, 1978.
22. McElfresh, E.C., and Dobyns, J.H.: Intraarticular Metacarpal Head Fractures. J. Hand Surg., 8:383, 1983.
23. Melone, C.P., Jr.: Rigid Fixation of Phalangeal and Metacarpal Fractures. Orth. Clin. N. Am., 17:421, 1986.
24. Rolando, S.: Fracture de la Base Du Premier Metacarpien, et Principalement sur une Variete Non Encore Decrite. Presse Med., 33:303, 1910.
25. Rüedi, T.P., Burri, C., and Pfeiffer, K.M.: Stable Internal Fixation of Fractures of the Hand. J. Trauma, 11:381, 1971.
26. Scott, M.M., and Mulligan, P.J.: Stabilizing Severe Phalangeal Fractures. Hand, 12:44, 1980.
27. Segmüller, G.: Surgical Stabilization of the Skeleton of the Hand. Baltimore, Williams and Wilkins, 1977.
28. Smith, R.J., and Peimer, C.A.: Injuries to the Metacarpal Bones and Joints. Adv. Surg., 2:341, 1977.
29. Steel, W.M.: The A.O. Small Fragment Set in Hand Fractures. Hand, 10:246, 1978.
30. Workman, C.E.: Metacarpal Fracture. Mo. Med., 61:687, 1964.

ANNOTATED BIBLIOGRAPHY

1. Green, D.P., and Rowland, S.A.: Fractures and Dislocations in the Hand. In Rockwood, C.A., and Green, D.P. (eds.): Fractures, 2nd ed. Philadelphia, J.B. Lippincott, 1984. A comprehensive chapter on skeletal trauma in the hand. The authors review the anatomy, pathophysiology, and various treatment approaches to virtually every fracture. A complete bibliography has been compiled.
2. O'Brien, E.T.: Fractures of the Metacarpal and Phalanges. In Green, D.P. (ed.): Operative Hand Surgery, vol 1. New York, Churchill Livingstone, 1982. This chapter leans more to the operative treatment of hand fractures presented in a clear, well-illustrated text by an experienced hand surgeon.
3. Segmüller, G.: Surgical Stabilization of the Skeleton of the Hand. Baltimore, Williams and Wilkins, 1977. Perhaps the landmark book regarding rigid AO internal fixation of the hand skeleton. Dr. Segmüller not only illustrates various applications of plates, screws, and tension band fixations but also presents the biomechanical concepts associated with rigid internal fixation.

CHAPTER 96

Carpal Bone Dislocations and Fractures

MARTIN A. POSNER

Fractures and ligamentous injuries involving the carpal bones comprise a significant percentage of trauma to the upper extremity. Unfortunately, many of these injuries are initially thought to be trivial by the patient, who neglects to seek immediate medical attention. In some cases, the injury is not properly diagnosed, and its seriousness may remain unrecognized until secondary arthritic changes occur. Correct diagnosis and treatment of injuries to the carpus depend on the knowledge of the anatomy and mechanics of one of the most complex joints in the body.

ANATOMY AND KINEMATICS

Our knowledge of the wrist dates back to the mid-16th century, when Vesalius[8] identified and numbered the carpal bones. For several centuries, the precise shape and articulation of each bone was known in detail, but little attention was paid to its ligaments and even less to its movements. In 1833 Sir Charles Bell, in his classic treatise *The Hand: Its Mechanism and Vital Endowments as Evincing Design,* dismissed the wrist with the cursory observation, "In the human hand, bones of the wrist are eight in number and they are so closely connected that they form a sort of ball, which moves on the end of the radius"[2] (Fig. 96-1). It was not until the discovery of x-rays that the study of wrist kinematics began. Bryce, in 1896,[4] noted that the physiologic axis of the wrist was not fixed but shifted as the joint moved from palmar flexion to dorsiflexion. This preliminary work was enlarged by other investigators[25,37,41,42,43] who recognized the complex yet synchronous movements of the carpal bones; movements that impart to the wrist joint both fluidity of motion as well as remarkable strength. Navarro, in work begun in 1919,[33] introduced the concept of the vertical or columnar carpus. Navarro described a central column for flexion and extension, comprising the lunate, capitate, and hamate bones, and two side columns, the medial column for rotation, which included the triquetrum and pisiform, and the lateral or mobile column composed of the scaphoid, trapezium, and trapezoid. Taleisnik, in 1976,[32] modified Navarro's concept: he described the central column comprising the lunate and the entire distal carpal row; the medial or rotational column, the triquetrum; and the lateral or mobile column, the scaphoid. Gilford, in 1943,[11] also contributed to our understanding of wrist kinematics. He described the wrist in terms of a triple-link system with the radius, lunate, and capitate as its central part. The mechanical advantage of a link system is that each joint in the chain (radiolunate and lunate-capitate) moves only half the range of excursion of the entire joint. The disadvantage of this system is the potential instability of the central intercalated mobile segment, which lacks any support and is dependent on the anatomic configurations and ligamentous attachments for stability.[19] The scaphoid is the important bone for carpal stability because, although anatomically within the proximal row of carpal bones, it functionally bridges both carpal rows.

The important ligaments of the wrist are primarily palmar and intracapsular, and detailed studies have shown that there are extrinsic and intrinsic components.[24,32] The important extrinsic ligaments include the radiocapitate, radiotriquetral, and radioscaphoid, all arising palmar on the radial side of the

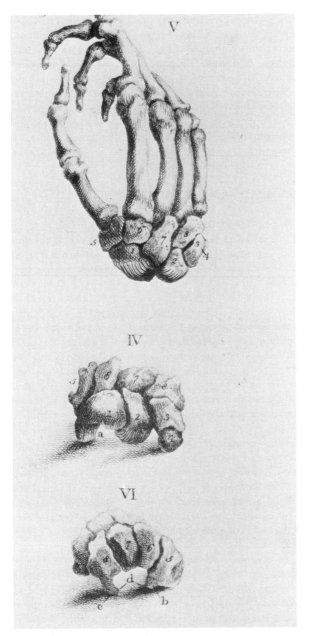

FIGURE 96-1. Anatomic drawings of the wrist in a 19th-century anatomy book by Charles Bell.[2] The carpal bones were commonly referred to by numbers rather than names.

radius. The intrinsic ligaments, or those that arise and insert on the carpal bones, are further subdivided according to length. The longest of these ligaments is the palmar intercarpal deltoid or radiate ligament. Attached to the neck of the capitate, it fans proximally in two limbs to have an inverted "V" configuration as it inserts into the scaphoid and triquetrum. The area between the two limbs is weak and is known as the "space of Poirier." The lunate is within this space, and the absence of intrinsic support between it and the capitate predisposes to midcarpal instability. The dorsal wrist ligaments are far weaker and arranged in thin laminar bands.

DIAGNOSTIC WORKUP

The evaluation of any carpal injury requires a careful physical and radiographic examination. While swelling and loss of mobility are common in most injuries, it is important to determine areas of tenderness. These may be diffuse in severe fractures or dislocations or localized in more subtle injuries. Tenderness localized to a carpal bone or to an intercarpal joint will determine which radiographic views must be obtained and also aid in their interpretation. The neurovascular status of the hand should always be assessed in any wrist injury, particularly the function of the median nerve, which will be compromised in some injuries.

Routine radiographs of the wrist should include three views: anteroposterior, lateral, and oblique (Figs. 96-2 to 96-4). The anteroposterior or supination view may be more informative than the more commonly performed posteroanterior view, particularly with respect to subluxation of the scaphoid. The lateral view with the wrist in neutral position must be a true lateral in order to evaluate any abnormal tilt of the lunate or capitate. Additional radiographic views may be required, depending on the clinical situation, including tomograms or videotape motion studies.[1] Arthrograms may be useful in evaluating injuries to intercarpal ligaments or the triangular fibrocartilage complex.[29] Wrist arthroscopy is an increasingly valuable technique in the evaluation of many ligament injuries.

CARPAL SUBLUXATIONS—DISLOCATIONS

The mechanism of injury of most carpal dislocations is an acute dorsiflexion force to the hand. Combining this force with ulnar deviation and the torque effect of intercarpal supination will result in varying degrees of ligamentous damage.[24] Ligaments that are palmar and radial will be the first to rupture. As the force continues in an ulnar direction, additional ligaments fail in tension. The numerous carpal subluxations and dislocations described in the literature are frequently the result of a similar force to the wrist that varies in intensity and duration. Rotatory subluxation of the scaphoid, dislocation of the lunate, and dorsal intercalated segment instability, although treated here as distinct entities, are varying stages of the same injury. The most commonly encountered carpal subluxations and dislocations are as follows.

Rotatory Subluxation of the Scaphoid

This injury is one of the most common carpal subluxations and occurs with disruption of the ligaments that tether the proximal pole of the scaphoid to the radius. While the intrinsic scaphoid-lunate ligament is torn in all cases, disruption of the radioscaphoid ligament is essential before the bone will rotate. Often the injury is dismissed initially as a "sprain," and months or even years lapse before the correct diagnosis is made. Unfortunately, arthritic changes have often intervened by that time, requiring some type of salvage operation.

Proper treatment at the time of the original injury requires diagnosing a problem whose findings may be far more subtle

FIGURE 96-2. Anteroposterior views of a normal wrist in radial and ulnar deviation. (*A*) In radial deviation the scaphoid is palmar flexed and appears shortened, which can sometimes be misinterpreted as a fracture (*closed arrow*). (*B*) The outline of the scaphoid is more easily visualized in ulnar deviation. These radiographs also demonstrate the relationship of the proximal and distal carpal rows to each other and to the radius and ulna. (*B*) In ulnar deviation there is a sinusoidal curve comprising the radioulna, lunate-triquetral, and capitate-hamate joints (*open arrows*).

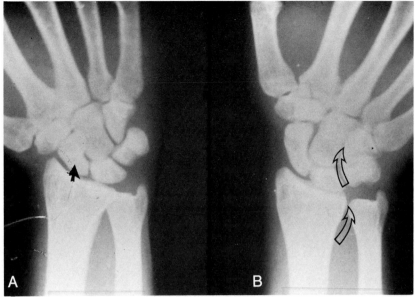

FIGURE 96-3. Lateral radiograph of a normal wrist showing the alignment of the radius, lunate, capitate, and metacarpals. The longitudinal axis of the scaphoid is at an angle of 45° to 60° to the longitudinal axis of the lunate.

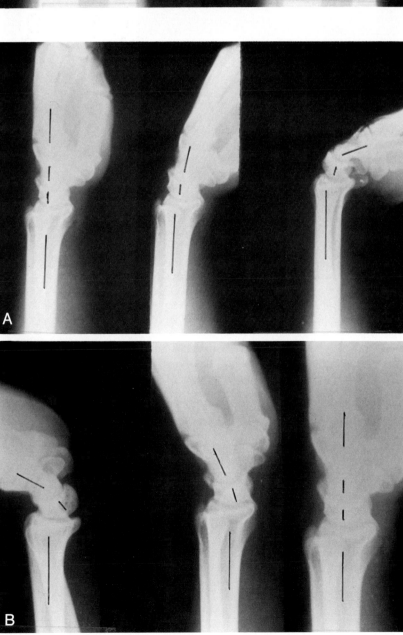

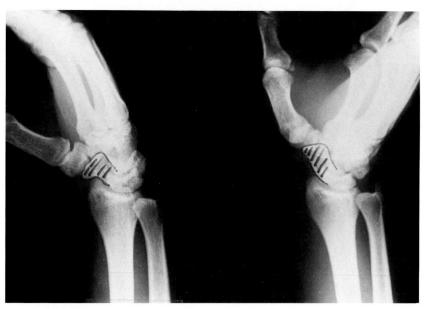

RAD. DEVIATION   ULNAR DEVIATION

FIGURE 96-4. Oblique radiographs of a normal wrist that facilitate visualization of the scaphoid (*shaded*), particularly in ulnar deviation.

than a dislocation. Since the proximal pole of the scaphoid is dorsally tilted, it appears foreshortened on the anteroposterior radiographic view, producing a cortical ring shadow. The lateral radiographic view may show the long axis of the scaphoid to be perpendicular to the long axis of the lunate rather than at the usual angle of 45° to 60°.[23] Any abnormal tilt of the lunate in this view is indicative of a more severe ligamentous injury and will be discussed in the section on carpal instability. The most characteristic radiographic finding is widening of the scaphoid-lunate gap more than 2 mm.[12–14] Best seen with the anteroposterior (supination) view and with the hand in radial deviation, this radiographic finding has been referred to as the "Terry Thomas sign," named after the actor who had a wide space between his two front teeth (Fig. 96-5).[9]

Treatment for rotatory subluxation of the scaphoid requires reduction and prolonged cast immobilization. If reduction cannot be obtained by closed means, surgery is required. The dorsal surgical approach is preferred because it provides excellent visualization of the carpal bones.

Make a transverse incision at the radiocarpal joint with the radial aspect of the incision curved distally for a distance of approximately 2 cm. The ulnar part of the incision can be carried proximally for a similar distance. Elevate skin flaps, taking care to identify and protect the sensory branches of the radial nerve and the dorsal sensory branch of the ulnar nerve. The radial nerve branches are fairly constant in their location as they cross the extensor pollicis longus tendon where it, in turn, crosses both radial wrist extensor tendons. The dorsal sensory branch of the ulnar nerve is more variable in its path and may arise proximal to the ulna head, directly over it or even distal to it.

Divide the extensor retinaculum longitudinally over the fourth compartment. Retract the tendons in the fourth compartment ulnarly, and mobilize the retinaculum radially, dividing the septa between the third and fourth as well as between the second and third compartments. This permits radial re-

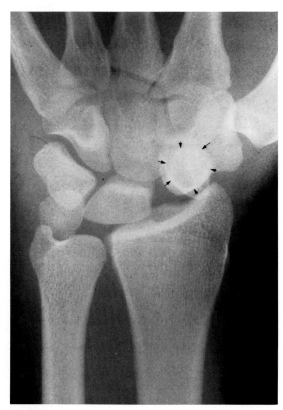

FIGURE 96-5. Radiographic view of a rotatory subluxation of the scaphoid showing the cortical ring shadow (*arrows*) and the wide diastasis between the scaphoid and lunate, commonly referred to as the "Terry Thomas" sign.

traction of the extensor pollicis longus and the extensor carpi radialis longus and brevis tendons. The torn dorsal capsule is readily visualized; if necessary, further divide it transversely in order to permit access to the underlying carpal bones.

Excise any granulation tissue between the scaphoid and lunate. Apply dorsal pressure to the proximal pole of the scaphoid, which will usually reduce the subluxation. Maintain the reduction with at least two nonthreaded Kirschner pins, fixing the scaphoid to the capitate and lunate.[17] Postoperative radiographic confirmation of the reduction is important to determine that the gap between scaphoid and lunate is closed and that there is no midcarpal instability (Fig. 96-6). Leave the pins outside the skin, bending them to facilitate later removal. Following closure of the capsule and dorsal retinaculum, apply a palmar splint, maintaining the wrist in 15° to 20° of palmar flexion. A circular cast can be utilized when the swelling has subsided, usually within 2 weeks. Prolonged immobilization for up to 10 to 12 weeks is recommended.

Although the palmar radioscaphoid ligament is ruptured in all cases and theoretically should be repaired, such a procedure is technically difficult. The ligament is short and relatively inaccessible. In young patients with a severe subluxation and a large scaphoid-lunate gap, however, ligamentous repair should be considered.

In cases where the rotatory subluxation of the scaphoid is chronic, the problems are magnified. Closed reduction should still be attempted, but it is usually unsuccessful, or if obtained it is difficult to maintain, and therefore surgery is necessary to restore articular congruity. Some type of intercarpal stabilization is also required to prevent later carpal instability. Ligamentous reconstructions have been attempted whereby a tendon is passed through drill holes in the carpal bones. These operations are technically demanding, and the results are often poor. Unfortunately, the precise repair or reconstruction of carpal ligaments is not possible at the present time. With significant subluxations the intercarpal arthrodeses remain the most predictable procedures.

Dorsal Perilunate and Palmar Lunate Dislocations

These injuries should be considered together, as the pathomechanics of both are similar. In the perilunate dislocation the entire carpus displaces dorsal to the lunate, which remains in its normal position. A dislocation of this magnitude requires the rupture of many ligaments including the radiocapitate, radioscaphoid, and radiotriquetral. Palmar dislocation of the lunate occurs when the dorsally displaced carpus spontaneously relocates in line with the radius. The radiolunate component of the dorsal radiocarpal ligaments tears, allowing the lunate to be displaced palmarly. The lunate dislocation is therefore the final stage of a perilunate dislocation. Often there is considerable diagnostic overlap between these two types of dislocations. The initial radiograph may fail to show either a pure dorsal perilunate dislocation or a pure palmar lunate dislocation, but, rather, a condition that falls someplace between both extremes.[14]

As with any carpal injury, radiographs are essential in order to determine the precise nature of the injury. The displacement of the capitate dorsal to the lunate in the lateral view is diagnostic of a dorsal perilunate dislocation (Fig. 96-7). The anteroposterior radiographic view is also important because the perilunate dislocation may be transscaphoid, and the fracture fragments of the scaphoid are more obvious in this view. With a pure palmar dislocation of the lunate, the lateral radiographic view will show the "spilled cup" of the lunate as it is tilted palmarly (Fig. 96-8A). The anteroposterior radiographic view is also helpful, because the normal rectangular shape of the lunate becomes triangular (Fig. 96-8B).[16]

The management of both types of dislocations is identical. A closed reduction under appropriate anesthesia, either general or regional block, should be attempted as soon as possible. Local infiltration of anesthesia into the wrist is unsatisfactory, because it does not provide complete muscle relaxation, which is essential if a closed reduction is to be achieved. Apply longitudinal traction to the hand before the reduction, using wire finger traps. The hand is pointed to the ceiling with the elbow flexed to 90°, and countertraction is applied to the upper arm using a 10- to 15-lb weight.

After approximately 10 min, remove the finger traps, and while maintaining longitudinal traction, manipulate the patient's hand. The objective is to restore the midcarpal articulation, which is accomplished by sliding the capitate palmarly over the lunate rather than by simply pushing the lunate back into position.[38] Dorsiflex the patient's wrist with one hand while stabilizing the lunate with the other hand. Gradual palmar flexion of the patient's hand usually permits the capitate to

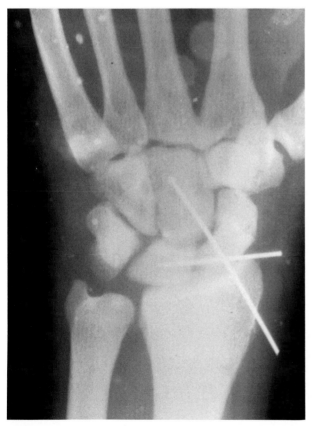

FIGURE 96-6. Postoperative reduction and Kirschner pin fixation of the subluxed scaphoid. Whether to cross the radiocarpal joint with a pin is controversial, and some surgeons would pin only carpals.

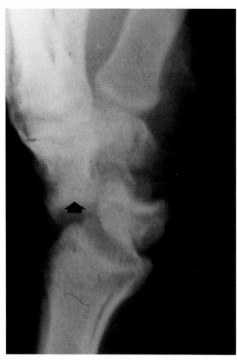

FIGURE 96-7. Lateral radiograph of a perilunate dislocation showing the capitate (*arrow*) displaced dorsal to the lunate, which remains in its normal position.

slide over the concavity in the lunate and snap into place. The reduction is usually stable with the wrist in palmar flexion or even neutral position.

Postreduction radiographs are essential to determine if the carpal bones, primarily the scaphoid, lunate, and capitate, have been restored to their anatomic positions. The lateral radiograph must show that the lunate-capitate midcarpal joint is in alignment and that there is no intercalary segment instability. The anteroposterior radiographic view must show that there is no abnormal separation between scaphoid and lunate. With radiographic confirmation of carpal realignment, initial immobilization is provided utilizing palmar and dorsal plaster splints. After swelling has subsided, usually within 7 to 10 days, a circular cast is applied and maintained for a total of 8 weeks. Prolonged immobilization is preferable to a shorter period of immobilization, even at the risk of causing more wrist stiffness. A stable carpus without intercarpal instability will be more functional than the wrist whose carpus is unstable, even though it may have greater mobility. Pain will usually be greater in the latter situation and will tend to increase as secondary arthritic changes occur.

If anatomic reduction of the carpal bones cannot be achieved by closed measures, open reduction is necessary. Even when reduction can be obtained, it is difficult to maintain by closed means; for this reason, many favor open reduction and internal fixation. There have been varied opinions concerning the operative technique, with some authors favoring a dorsal

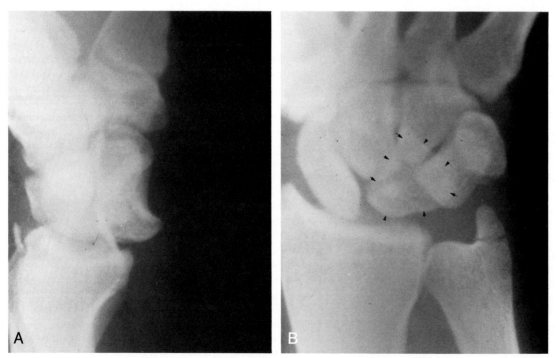

FIGURE 96-8. (*A*) Lateral radiograph of a palmar lunate dislocation showing the "spilled cup" sign. (*B*) The anteroposterior view shows that the dislocated lunate has a triangular shape (*arrows*).

approach, others a palmar approach, and some even a combined dorsal and palmar approach. Generally, a dorsal operative approach is recommended and permits satisfactory visualization, even with a complete palmar dislocation of the lunate. The dorsal approach permits excision of the torn ligaments and granulation issue in the space left by the displaced lunate.

While applying longitudinal traction to the hand, a skid is used to lever the lunate back into position as digital pressure is applied to the bone palmarly. The dorsal approach also facilitates reduction and internal fixation utilizing nonthreaded Kirschner pins of the fracture fragments in a transscaphoid perilunate dislocation. Anatomic reduction of the scaphoid fracture is important to hasten healing. While avascular necrosis of the proximal pole of the scaphoid is common, even when anatomic reduction has been achieved, it does not necessarily result in the fracture failing to heal. Kirschner wires are used to reattach any sizable osteochondral fragments, which are usually from the lunate or capitate, or to reattach a fractured radial styoid. Operative reduction and pin fixation may also be necessary to treat a rotatory subluxation of the scaphoid that occurs following reduction of either type of carpal dislocation. In addition to providing satisfactory visualization of the pathology, the dorsal operative approach avoids damage to the remaining intact palmar ligaments to the lunate, thereby reducing the risk of later avascular necrosis. If, however, a reduction of the dislocated lunate cannot be accomplished through the dorsal approach, a palmar incision is required. The palmar operative approach may also be necessary to decompress the median nerve in the dislocation which causes a carpal tunnel syndrome.

Postoperative immobilization must be more prolonged when the dislocation is transscaphoid, because it must be continued until the fracture heals, which may be as long as 1 year. When healing fails to progress, as demonstrated by serial radiographs and tomograms, bone grafting the fracture site is required. This is discussed in the section dealing with scaphoid fractures.

Dorsiflexion and Palmar Flexion Carpal Instability

As previously noted, the wrist is a complex joint composed of carpal bones arranged in anatomic and functional units. The intercalated proximal carpal row depends on a complex series of ligaments as well as articular congruity for its stability. The scaphoid plays an important role in wrist stability, and its skeletal and ligamentous integrity is responsible for the synchronous movements of the two carpal rows. Its function as a stabilizing force is compromised by ligamentous disruptions or a displaced fracture resulting in collapse of the midcarpal joint. Landsmeer, in 1961,[21] described the deformity as zig-zag in appearance, which will occur whenever a multilink system is axially loaded. Fisk, in 1970,[7] likened the collapse to the bellows of a concertina, and Linscheid et al., in 1972,[23] referred to the problem as intercalated segment instability. Midcarpal instability is the result of more extensive ligamentous damage than occurs with an isolated rotatory subluxation of the scaphoid, although it can also be seen in conjunction with that problem. Generally, the lunate will tilt dorsally, resulting in a dorsal intercalated segment instability pattern. The lateral radiograph shows the lunate dorsiflexed more than 15°, and the scaphoid-lunate angle is greater than 70°. The anteroposterior radiographic view is also abnormal, with the lunate adopting a trapezoidal appearance.

Palmar intercalated segment instability is far less commonly encountered than the dorsiflexed variety. This pattern may be due to rupture or attenuation of the radial carpal ligaments on the ulnar aspect of the wrist, as seen in cases of concomitant injuries to the triangular fibrocartilage complex at the distal radioulnar joint. It may also occur with an incomplete perilunate dislocation or with ulnar displacement of the entire carpus, which may occur in rheumatoid arthritis. Clinically, there is a dorsal depression in the midcarpal joint area. The lateral radiograph shows forward tilting of the lunate with the radiolunate angle greater than 15° and angulation at the lunate-capitate joint. The scaphoid-lunate angle remains normal or may be decreased.

Treatment in either instability pattern requires early recognition of the problem and correction. If reduction by manipulation cannot be achieved by closed means (which is often the situation), operative reduction and pin fixation is required. The wrist is then immobilized for at least 8 weeks. Surgical repair or reconstruction of the torn ligaments has not been satisfactory. Unfortunately, midcarpal instability patterns are often not diagnosed until weeks, months, or even years after the injury. The preferred treatment in many of these chronic cases is a correction of the instability pattern and midcarpal arthrodesis.

Dynamic Instability

While most types of carpal instability are recognized by routine radiographic studies, some may be intermittent or dynamic in nature. These rarer varieties can be subdivided into two groups, primary and secondary. In the primary group instability is the result of loss of intrinsic ligament support to the carpal bones, while in the secondary group the instability is secondary to deformity of the radius or ulna as seen in malunited fractures or following injuries to the distal radioulnar joint. A high index of suspicion is helpful in properly diagnosing these problems because standard radiographs are normal. The patient will usually report "clicking," "clunking," or "snapping" with certain wrist motions. Clinically, there may be an audible and sometimes a palpable snap as the abnormal carpal motion occurs. Tenderness is usually confined to a small area of the carpus. Cineradiography or video motion radiograph studies are necessary to diagnose these problems. Two wrist motions are examined in this radiograph study: (1) palmar and dorsiflexion with the wrist in the lateral position and (2) radial and ulnar deviation with the hand in the anteroposterior position. The forearm must be stabilized during the examination, and the movements are performed slowly, which facilitates interpretation of the radiographs. Rotational motions are not particularly useful and may even obscure the pathology.

Various dynamic instability patterns have been encountered involving the lateral mobile column and the medial rotational column, as well as the central column. These instabilities have included scaphoid-lunate, lunate-triquetral, midcarpal, and even radiocarpal joints.[18,22] The recommended treatment depends on the presence or absence of secondary arthritic changes. If there are no arthritic changes, stabilization of the instability pattern by means of ligamentous reconstruction can be considered. Intercarpal arthrodeses are, however, more predictable procedures and are preferred in the treatment of localized instabilities such as those involving the lunate-triquetral joint.

CARPAL FRACTURES

As with ligamentous injuries to the carpus resulting in subluxation, dislocation, or instability (static or dynamic), fracture of a carpal bone may seriously affect wrist function. The initial evaluation of any wrist injury requires a careful physical examination, localizing areas of tenderness followed by appropriate radiographic studies. Depending on the area of tenderness, special radiographs, aside from the routine anteroposterior, lateral, and oblique views, are necessary. This is often the situation for some of the common carpal fractures that are discussed in the following section.

Scaphoid Fractures

Acute

Fractures of the scaphoid are exceeded in frequency only by fractures involving the distal radius.[34] Occurring most commonly in young adult males following falls on the outstretched palm of the hand, many of these injuries are initially dismissed as a "sprain" by the patient and sometimes even by the physician. The injury should be suspected in any patient with wrist pain and tenderness over the scaphoid, either dorsally within the anatomic snuff box or over the palmar aspect of the bone. Confirmation of a fracture is by radiographic examination; the profile view of the bone on both anteroposterior and oblique

views can be enhanced by placing the wrist in as much ulnar deviation as possible. Occasionally, the initial radiographs may be negative. In such cases the diagnosis of a fracture should still be considered and appropriate immobilization instituted. Repeat radiographs should be taken within 3 weeks, and the injury may then be evident as resorption at the fracture site has occurred.

Scaphoid fractures can be classified in a variety of ways: according to the direction of the fracture line,[30] the degree of stability of the fragments,[5] and the portion of the bone that is fractured. The first method of classification, described by Russe,[30] is based on the relationship of the fracture line to the long axis of the bone and can be subdivided into three types. The horizontal, oblique, or type I, fracture is where the line is horizontal to the wrist but oblique to the long axis of the scaphoid. The transverse, or type II, fracture is where the line is at right angles to the long axis of the scaphoid. Both of these types will usually heal with immobilization. The vertical oblique, or type III, fracture is where the line is vertical to the wrist and oblique to the bone. This type has a high shear component and is relatively unstable and, therefore, healing is problematic (Fig. 96-9).

The method of classification based on anatomic alignment of the fracture is divided into either a stable, undisplaced type or an unstable, displaced type. While the former type will usually heal, the latter type, regardless of the direction of the fracture line, may be associated with carpal instability. A lateral radiograph is critical to determine if there is any abnormal lunate tilt. If present this must be reduced along with the proximal scaphoid fragment.

The third method of classifying scaphoid fractures is according to the portion of the bone injured: proximal, middle, or distal thirds. The majority of fractures involve the middle third and, if there is no displacement or carpal instability, healing should be anticipated in more than 90% of cases. Those fractures in the proximal third have a high incidence of non-

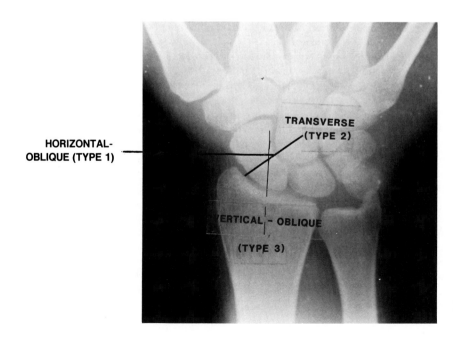

HORIZONTAL-
OBLIQUE (TYPE 1)

TRANSVERSE
(TYPE 2)

VERTICAL - OBLIQUE
(TYPE 3)

FIGURE 96-9. Classification of scaphoid fractures according to Russe.

union and avascular necrosis because of the interruption of the vascular supply, which enters the bone distal to its waist. Fractures in this location may require up to 12 weeks longer to unite than fractures in the middle third. Fractures involving the distal third of the bone are infrequent, but they tend to heal promptly due to the rich blood supply in this area. Occasionally, the distal fracture may be vertical and disrupt the articular surface of the joint, which may require surgery if there is significant joint incongruity. Fractures involving the tuberosity are extra-articular and usually the result of direct trauma. Treatment for these fractures is directed primarily to relieve pain, which can be achieved by use of a palmar splint for several weeks.

The type and duration of immobilization in the treatment of scaphoid fractures are controversial. Recommended treatment is a well-fitted thumb spica plaster or fiberglass cast, immobilizing the wrist in slight palmar flexion, and the thumb, excluding the interphalangeal joint, in opposition.* The elbow joint is included in the cast for the initial 8 weeks of immobilization. Thereafter, a below-elbow thumb spica cast is continued until there is radiographic evidence of complete healing. Unfortunately, many scaphoid fractures are not completely healed when the immobilization is discontinued. Chronic nonunions are often seen in patients who report that their original scaphoid fracture was "healed" after 6 weeks of casting.

Chronic

The scaphoid fracture that remains ununited after several months of immobilization should be differentiated from the fracture that was not recognized until months after the injury. In the former situation union is delayed, but may still occur with continued immobilization, particularly if the fracture is stable and if there is no concomitant midcarpal instability. Radiographs, including trispiral tomograms, are important to determine the potential for the fracture to unite. In the latter situation where the fracture was unrecognized for several months, the likelihood that healing will occur without intervention is poor. While a cast can still be employed as a method of treatment, it should not be continued for as long a period of time as when it is utilized for an acute fracture, before surgery is considered.

Surgery is required for those cases where there is a definite nonunion; that is, when radiographic findings indicate that there is no potential for healing to occur. These findings include sclerotic margins of the fracture fragments, a prominent radiolucency, or a pseudarthrosis. In the absence of classic radiographic signs, yet where there is no evidence of healing as demonstrated on serial radiographs over a period of several months, surgery is still necessary.

The inlay bone graft into the palmar surface of the scaphoid described by Russe[30] remains the most predictable procedure for achieving union. Avascular necrosis of the proximal fragment is not a contraindication to surgery, provided there are no significant secondary arthritic changes. Prolonged postoperative immobilization, however, may be required in such cases.

Make a longitudinal incision over the radial border of the

flexor carpi radialis. Curving the distal portion of the incision radially within the wrist flexion crease for a short distance facilitates the exposure. Retract the tendon ulnarly as the incision is carried down to the joint capsule. Cauterize small branches of the radial artery, which is to the radial side of the exposure, taking care to protect the artery itself. Divide the capsule longitudinally, and if necessary to gain better visualization of the fracture, elevate it off the radius, both radially and ulnarly. Locating the fracture site should not pose any difficulty, since the radial styloid provides an excellent guide. The position of the fracture as it relates to the styloid on the anteroposterior radiographic view can be correlated to what is viewed in the operative field.

Make a long, deep trough across the fracture site into both fragments, curving it slightly to follow the contour of the bone. A power burr facilitates making the trough and eliminates the danger of converting the stable nonunion into one where the proximal fragment becomes unstable. Undercut the entire periphery of the trough with the burr, which aids in stabilizing the graft. Saline irrigation is used throughout the procedure to remove debris and to prevent the bone from overheating. Use the power instrument in your dominant hand and the suction in the other. In this manner, you can control the amount of fluid in the operative area while the assistant supplies the irrigation.

Harvest a bone graft from the ipsilateral ilium. The thick crest itself should not be used, but rather the thin outer cortical table with an adequate amount of cancellous bone. Carefully fashion the graft, using a small bone cutter, to fit snugly within the trough with its cortex on the outside. Gently distract the fracture fragments when inserting the graft. Forceful distraction should be avoided, particularly if the nonunion site is relatively stable. Once the cortical cancellous graft is in place, insert additional cancellous chips to fill any defects.

Internal fixation with nonthreaded Kirschner wires is used only for those cases where there is instability after the graft has been inserted. Carefully repair the capsule and apply an above-elbow thumb spica cast (Fig. 96-10). After 8 weeks, a below-elbow cast is continued until healing has occurred, which should be anticipated in more than 90% of cases. Radial styloidectomy should not be routinely performed as an adjunct of bone grafting. It should be considered only in those rare cases of symptomatic arthritis between the styloid and scaphoid (Fig. 96-11).[34]

In those cases where the proximal fracture fragment involves the proximal pole of the scaphoid and is no longer than one-quarter of the length of the bone, excision is the preferred treatment. Following excision, a coiled tendon or silicone plug can be inserted into the void, although it is usually unnecessary, because there is little likelihood of any subsequent carpal shift. Newer arthroscopic techniques permit removal of small bone fragments, eliminating the need for an arthrotomy.

Lunate Fractures

Fracture of the lunate is, in all likelihood, the result of repeated compressive forces on the bone. It can also occur, but less frequently, from a single severe compression force. While there has been general acceptance of Kienböck's[20] classic description

---

* We recommend including the thumb interphalangeal joint in the cast—eds.

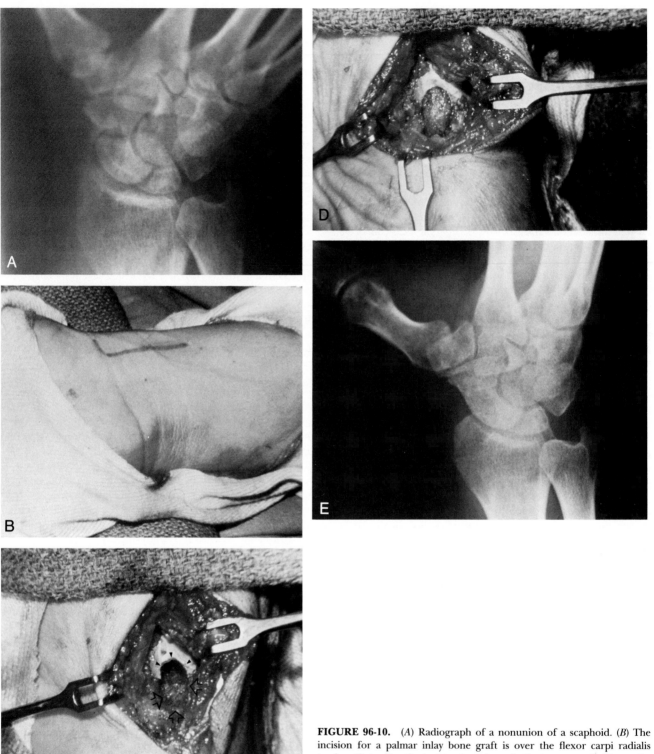

FIGURE 96-10. (*A*) Radiograph of a nonunion of a scaphoid. (*B*) The incision for a palmar inlay bone graft is over the flexor carpi radialis tendon. Extending the incision into the wrist flexion crease facilitates the exposure. (*C*) A deep longitudinal trough is made across the fracture site (arrows) and (*D*) is filled with an autogenous iliac bone graft. (*E*) Radiograph taken 4 months after surgery shows healing of the fracture.

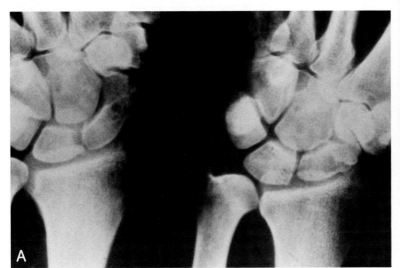
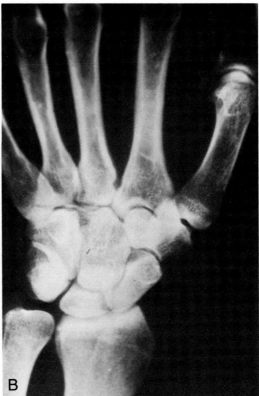

FIGURE 96-11. Impingement exostosis localized to the scaphoid-radial styloid area treated by a styloidectomy.

of lunatomalacea as being the result of avascular necrosis, the precise etiology of these changes, as well as an effective method of treatment, remain unresolved. The diagnosis of this condition is based solely upon radiographs. Usually, the changes are of a chronic nature with fragmentation and collapse of the bone as well as secondary radiocarpal and intercarpal arthritis. Diagnosing the condition at an early stage where there is a brief history of pain and stiffness is difficult, but it should be suspected when there is tenderness confined to the lunate. Trispiral tomograms, particularly in the lateral projection, are often helpful in both diagnosing the problem as well as determining a treatment program (Fig. 96-12). If the bone has not fractured, the objective should be to restore circulation, thereby reducing the likelihood for later carpal collapse. Prolonged immobilization of the wrist for up to 1 year has been successful, although such treatment may be impractical in an adult, working individual. Healing has also been achieved by inserting a bone graft from the adjacent intact triquetrum (Fig. 96-13). Other recommended operations include ulnar lengthening or radial shortening, which are based on the established statistical association of Kienböck's and an ulna minus varient where the distal articular surface of the ulna is proximal to the radius.[10] It remains unclear whether these osteotomies can actually reverse the structural changes in the bone.

Triquetral Fractures

Fractures of the triquetrum are the third most common group of carpal fractures.[3] They can be divided into two types. In the first type there is a chip fracture, usually from the dorsal surface that occurs with injuries forcing the wrist into ulnar deviation and hyperextension. In this position the hamate is pressed against the posterior aspect of the triquetrum and may shear off a fragment. Chip fractures can also occur from a ligament avulsion, as seen in association with other carpal injuries such as a perilunate dislocation or following falls on the palmar flexed wrist. Regardless of mechanism of injury, these chip fractures usually present no long-term problem even if they fail to unite. Initial immobilization for approximately 6 weeks is recommended for symptomatic relief of pain and swelling.

The second type of triquetral fracture, which is less common, involves a fracture through the body of the bone. The fracture is secondary to impingement or a direct blow. Healing with immobilization is usual, and in distinction to fractures of the scaphoid or lunate, avascular necrosis does not occur.

Capitate Fractures

Fractures of the capitate may appear as an isolated injury or in conjunction with other carpal injuries such as a fracture of the scaphoid when the proximal fragment of the capitate is rotated (scaphocapitate syndrome). Usually, the injury follows a fall on the outstretched palm with the wrist forced into dorsiflexion. If the head of the capitate is displaced, operative reduction with internal fixation is required.[14] Nonunions or late, untreated fractures through the neck of the bone do occur and require bone grafting. In those situations where midcarpal arthritis has intervened, a midcarpal arthrodesis is required.

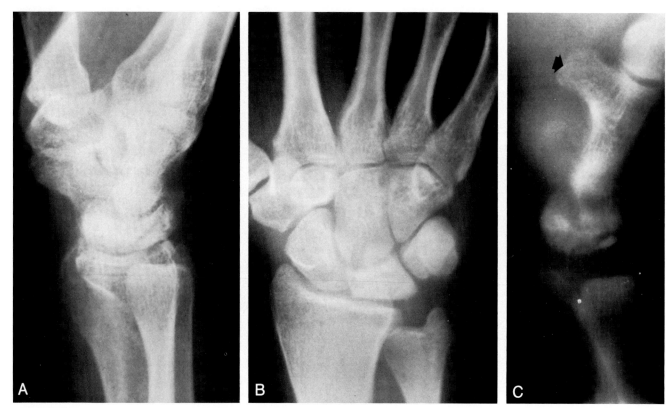

FIGURE 96-12. (*A*) Conventional and (*B* and *C*) trispiral tomograms of Kienböck's disease. The trispiral tomograms clearly show the severity of the problem with fragmentation of the lunate. The lateral view also demonstrates the usefulness of this radiographic technique for visualizing fractures of the hook of the hamate (*arrow*), which is normal in this patient.

Hamate Fractures

Fractures of the hamate involve either the body of the bone or its hook (hamulus). In either fracture a careful radiographic examination including special views and techniques is essential in order to confirm the diagnosis. Fractures of the body of the bone are generally stable and usually heal after 6 to 8 weeks of immobilization.

Fractures to the hook of the hamate may result from direct trauma to the bony prominence, but they are more likely to occur from a sudden or forceful contraction of the attached intrinsic muscles. The fracture should be suspected in baseball players, golfers, and tennis players who report experiencing a painful "snap" in their palm while improperly hitting a ball or even when swinging at and missing the ball.[28,31] Neuropathies of the ulnar nerve, which is in very close proximity to the hook, may be present. Usually, the motor division of the nerve is affected, resulting in weakness of the intrinsic muscles. These fractures are frequently missed, because they cannot be easily seen on routine radiographic views. A fracture of the hook should be suspected in the patient who complains of pain on the ulnar aspect of the wrist or in the hypothenar area of the palm. Tenderness with pressure over the hook or on its ulnar side should be considered as a fracture until proven otherwise. A careful radiographic examination is essential, and in order to be considered complete, the entire hook including its base must be visualized. The anteroposterior radiographic view is not diagnostic, but it may be helpful because an intact hook will usually project a ring or "eye sign".[26] An anteroposterior radiograph without an eye sign should, therefore, arouse suspicion of a fracture. Although carpal tunnel radiographs clearly show the hook in profile, they frequently fail to show its base. This is often the situation in the acute injury where, because of pain, the patient is unable to adequately dorsiflex his or her wrist. Unfortunately, carpal tunnel views that fail to show the entire base of the hook are often interpreted as "negative," and at some later time, many of these cases are discovered to have a fracture.

Trispiral tomography is an excellent radiographic technique to visualize the hamate using both carpal tunnel and lateral views. The advantage of a carpal tunnel tomogram over a conventional carpal tunnel radiograph is that it does not require as much wrist dorsiflexion.[15] This is important in the patient whose wrist pain limits wrist mobility at the time of the examination. Tomography in the lateral projection will clearly define the hook as well as the entire body of the bone. Other diagnostic techniques have also been described in visualizing the bone including computed tomographic (CT) scan and magnetic resonance imaging (MRI).

Although prolonged immobilization can result in healing of the acute hook fracture, excision is the preferred treatment. Make an incision along the radial border of the hypothenar eminence, curving it ulnarly into the wrist flexion crease. Identify the ulnar neurovascular bundle, including the motor and sensory divisions of the nerve. Magnification facilitates identification and protection of these structures. Using subperiosteal

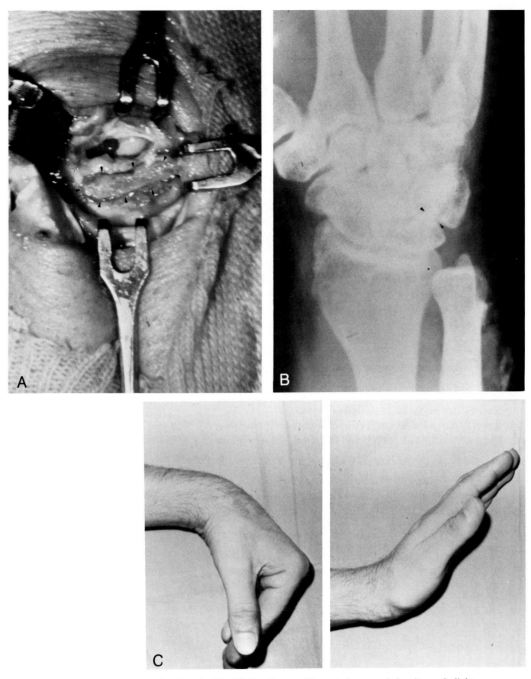

FIGURE 96-13. (A) Radiograph of early Kienböck's disease. There is increased density and slight compression on the radial aspect of the bone but no fragmentation. Circulation was restored by bridging the damaged lunate into the adjacent triquetrum. (B) A trough was made across the lunate-triquetral joint, and an autogenous iliac bone graft was inserted (arrows). After several months the graft consolidated (arrows) and the density of the lunate was restored. (C) Wrist motions were only slightly compromised because the intercarpal fusion was confined to the proximal carpal row and did not cross either the radiocarpal or midcarpal joint.

dissection, detach the intrinsic muscles as well as the transverse carpal ligament. Continue the dissection to the fracture site, and excise the fragment. Take care to avoid any undue retraction on the motor division of the nerve during the procedure. Remove any bony spur at the nonunion site with a rongeur, and close the intrinsic muscles with fine nonabsorbable sutures. A dorsal splint, maintaining the wrist in neutral position or slight flexion for 2 weeks, is used. Return to full activities including racquet sports should be anticipated by 6 weeks.

Pisiform Fractures

The pisiform is actually a sesamoid bone in the flexor carpi ulnaris tendon. The bone glides on the palmar surface of the underlying triquetrum in wrist flexion and extension. A fracture to the pisiform is usually the result of a direct force, as when falling on the palm. It may also occur in those situations where the heel of the hand has been used as a hammer in striking objects. Proper radiographs are essential and must include more than one view. An oblique view may visualize the bone, but fail to show the fracture if it is linear and in the coronal plane. Unless there is severe fragmentation or dislocation of the bone (which may occur with disruption of its ligamentous attachments), initial treatment consists of either a palmar or dorsal splint for several weeks. Chronic problems, including pisotriquetral arthritis, may warrant surgical excision. As with excision of the hook of the hamate bone, excision of the pisiform must be carried out carefully, avoiding injury to the adjacent ulnar neurovascular bundle. The flexor carpi ulnaris is dissected away from the bone without jeopardizing its other distal connections. Once the bone is removed, the periosteum is repaired, thereby reinforcing the insertion of the tendon. A dorsal splint immobilizing the wrist in neutral position or slight flexion is applied and maintained for 2 weeks before gradual return to normal activities is permitted.

REFERENCES

1. Arkless, R.: Cineradiography in Normal and Abnormal Wrists. Am. J. Roentgenol. **96:**837, 1966.
2. Bell, C.: The Hand: Its Mechanism and Vital Endowments as Evincing Design. London, W. Pickering, 1833.
3. Bryan, R.S., and Dobyns, J.H.: Fractures of the Carpal Bones Other than the Lunate and Navicular. Clin. Orthop. **149:**107, 1980.
4. Bryce, T.H.: Certain Points in the Anatomy and Mechanism of the Wrist Joint Reviewed in the Light of a Series of Roentgen Ray Photographs of the Living Hand. J. Anat. Physiol. **31:**59, 1896.
5. Cooney, W.P., Dobyns, J.H., and Linscheid, R.L.: Fractures of the Scaphoid: A Rational Approach to Management. Clin. Orthop. **149:**90, 1980.
6. Gilford, W.W., Bolton, R.H., and Lambrinudi, C.: The Mechanism of the Wrist Joint, With Special Reference to Fractures of the Scaphoid. Guy's Hosp. Red. **92:**52, 1943.
7. Fisk, G.R.: Carpal Instability and the Fractured Scaphoid. Ann. R. Coll. Surg. Engl. **46:**63, 1970.
8. Fisk, G.R.: An Overview of Injuries of the Wrist. Clin. Orthop. **149:**137, 1980.
9. Frankel, V.H.: The Terry-Thomas Sign. Clin. Orthop. **129:**321, 1977.
10. Gelberman, R.H., Bauman, T.D., Menon, J., et al.: The Lunate Bone and Kienböck's Disease. J. Hand Surg. **5:**272, 1980.
11. Gilford, W.W., Bolton, R.H., and Lambrinudi, C.: The Mechanism of the Wrist Joint With Special Reference to Fractures of the Scaphoid. Guy's Hosp. Rep. **92:**52, 1943.
12. Green, D.P.: Carpal Dislocations. *In* Green, D. (ed.): Operative Hand Surgery, vol. 1. New York, Churchill Livingstone, 1982.
13. Green, D.P., and O'Brien, E.T.: Open Reduction of Carpal Dislocations: Indications and Operative Techniques. J. Hand Surg. **3:**250, 1978.
14. Green, D.P., and O'Brien, E.T.: Classification and Management of Carpal Dislocations. Clin. Orthop. **149:**55, 1980.
15. Greenspan, A., Posner, M.A., and Tucker, M.: The Value of Carpal Tunnel Trispiral Tomography in the Diagnosis of Fracture of Hook of the Hamate. Bull. Hosp. Jt. Dis. Orthop. Inst. **45:**74, 1985.
16. Hill, N.A.: Fractures and Dislocations of the Carpus. Orthop. Clin. North Am. **1:**275, 1970.
17. Howard, F.M., and Fahey, T.: Rotatory Subluxation of the Navicular. Clin. Orthop. **104:**134, 1974.
18. Jackson, W.T., and Protas, J.M.: Snapping Scapholunate Subluxation. J. Hand Surg. **6:**590, 1981.
19. Kauer, J.M.G.: Functional Anatomy of the Wrist. Clin. Orthop. **149:**9, 1980.
20. Kienböck, R.: Concerning Traumatic Malacia of the Lunate and the Consequences: Degeneration and Compression Fractures. Peltier, L.F. (trans.). Clin Orthop. **149:**4, 1980.
21. Landsmeer, J.M.: Studies in the Anatomy of Articulation. The Equilibrium of the "Intercalated Bone. Acta Morpho. Neerl. Scand. **3:**287, 1961.
22. Lichtman, D.M., Noble, W.H., and Alexander, C.E.: Dynamic Triquetrolunate Instability. J. Hand Surg. **9:**185, 1984.
23. Linscheid, R.L., Dobyns, J.H., Beabout, J.W., et al.: Traumatic Instability of the Wrist. Diagnosis, Classification and Pathomechanics. J. Bone Joint Surg. **54-A:**1612, 1972.
24. Mayfield, J.K., Johnson, R.P., and Dilcoyne, R.K.: Carpal Dislocations: Pathomechanics and Progressive Perilunal Instability. J. Hand Surg. **5:**226, 1980.
25. McMurtay, R.Y., Toum, Y., Flatt, A.E., et al.: Kinematics of the Wrist. Parts 1 and 2. J. Bone Joint Surg. **60-A:**423, 955, 1978.
26. Norman, A., Nelson, J.M., and Green, S.M.: Fractures of the Hook of the Hamate: Radiographic Signs. Radiology **154:**49, 1985.
27. Posner, M.A.: Injuries to the Hand and Wrist in Athletes. Orthop. Clin. North Am. **8:**593, 1977.
28. Posner, M.A.: Wrist Injuries. *In* Scott, W.N., Nisonson, B., and Nicholas, J.A. (eds.): Principles of Sports Medicine. Baltimore, Williams & Wilkins, 1984.
29. Ranawat, C.S., Harrison, M.O., and Jordan, L.R.: Arthrography of the Wrist Joint. Clin. Orthop. **83:**6, 1972.
30. Russe, O.: Fracture of the Carpal Navicular. Diagnosis, Non-Operative Treatment and Operative Treatment. J. Bone Joint Surg. **42-A:**759, 1960.
31. Stark, H.H., Jobe, F.W., Boyes, J.H., et al.: Fracture of the Hook of the Hamate in Athletes. J. Bone Joint Surg. **59-A:**575, 1977.
32. Taleisnik, J.: The Ligaments of the Wrist. J. Hand Surg. **1:**110, 1976.
33. Taleisnik, J.: Wrist: Anatomy, Function and Injury. Instr. Course Lect. **27:**61, 1978.
34. Taleisnik, J.: Fractures of the Carpal Bones. *In* Green, D. (ed.): Operative Hand Surgery, vol. I. New York, Churchill Livingstone, 1982.
35. Thompson, T.C., Campbell, R.J., Jr., and Arnold, W.D.: Primary and Secondary Dislocation of the Scaphoid Bone. J. Bone Joint Surg. **46-B:**73, 1964.
36. Vaughan-Jackson, O.J.: A Case of Recurrent Subluxation of the Carpal Scaphoid. J. Bone Joint Surg. **38-A:**1198, 1956.
37. Volz, R.G., Lieb, M., and Benjamin, J.: Biomechanics of the Wrist. Clin. Orthop. **149:**112, 1980.
38. Watson-Jones, R.: Carpal Semilunar Dislocations and Other Wrist Dislocations With Associated Nerve Lesions. Proc. R. Soc. Med. **22:**1071, 1929.
39. Weber, E.R.: Biomechanical Implications of Scaphoid Waist Fractures. Clin. Orthop. **149:**83, 1980.
40. Wilson, J.N.: Profiles of the Carpal Canal. J. Bone Joint Surg. **36-A:**127, 1954.
41. Wright, R.D.: A Detailed Study of Movement of the Wrist Joint. J. Anat. **70:**137, 1935.
42. Youm, Y., and Flatt, A.E.: Kinematics of the Wrist, I and II. J. Bone Joint Surg. **60-A:**423, 955, 1978.
43. Youm, Y., and Flatt, A.E.: Kinematics of the Wrist. Clin. Orthop. **149:**21, 1980.

CHAPTER 97

Fractures and Dislocations of the Distal Radioulnar Joint

WILLIAM E. BURKHALTER

ETIOLOGY AND INDICATIONS

Acute fractures of the distal radioulnar joint usually result from extension of a fracture of the distal radius into the joint. In addition to direct injury to the articular surface, ligament injury, either locally at the wrist or at a distance proximally, may bring about instability of the distal radioulnar joint. Often these acute injuries are treated casually because of a feeling that any chronic problem that develops can be easily treated later by resection of the ulnar head (Darrach procedure). However, late reconstructive efforts are not always satisfactory, and early treatment is preferable.

Isolated dislocations of the distal radioulnar joint are unusual. Normally, closed reduction and immobilization in a long arm cast allows return to near normal function. Following reduction, dorsal dislocations should be immobilized in the most stable position (supination) for 4 to 6 weeks (Fig. 97-1). Palmar dislocations are more stable in slight pronation. If residual instability remains, reconstructive procedures become necessary.

Several chronic problems may befall the distal radioulnar joint. First, an untreated palmar or dorsal dislocation may lead to loss of forearm rotation and chronic pain. Gross instability may result from an unhealed triangular fibrocartilage tear with subsequent painful motion and subluxation; this instability may also be encountered following excision of the distal ulna.

Second, articular irregularity of the sigmoid notch of the radius, usually secondary to distal radial fractures, may result in loss of congruity between the radius and ulna distally, thereby mechanically obstructing motion.

Third, the ulna may be relatively long, secondary to shortening of the radius as a result of a radial shaft fracture or arrest of the growth plate either proximally or distally. This leads to impingement and pain on the ulnar side of the wrist.

Last, arthritis of the distal radioulnar joint may follow combined intra-articular radial and ulna fractures, or Colles' fractures, with loss of congruity of the joint surfaces. A combination of instability and arthritis may be seen in diseases such as rheumatoid arthritis, where synovitis causes articular disease and ligamentous disruption.

A great many surgical procedures have been devised to relieve problems of the distal radioulnar joint. These may be subdivided into four main groups: (1) excision of the head of the ulna, (2) ligamentous stabilization, (3) arthroplasty, and (4) shortening of the ulna, with or without arthrodesis of the radioulnar joint.

SURGICAL PROCEDURES

Resection of Ulnar Head (Darrach)

Until recently surgery for any chronic derangement of the distal radioulnar joint has concentrated on excision of the distal ulna as proposed by Darrach.[9,10,11] The indications for the operative procedure were subluxation or dislocations of the distal radioulnar joint as an isolated entity or associated with fractures of the radius. Darrach's operative technique consists of subperiosteal removal of the ulna to clear the distal radioulnar

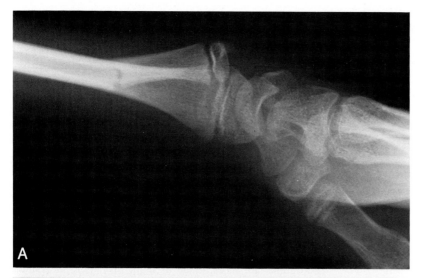

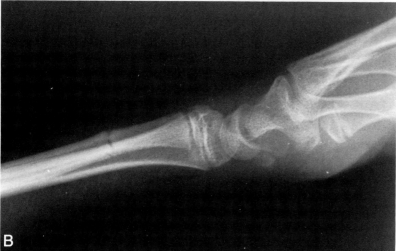

FIGURE 97-1. (*A*) Acute dislocations of the distal radioulnar joint may be accompanied by fracture. (*B*) With dorsal dislocation closed reduction by supination and direct pressure usually result in anatomic restoration of the abnormality.

joint only, leaving the ulnar styloid and its base in place, followed by subperiosteal closure to allow some boney regeneration.

Darrach felt that ulnar regeneration was important in order to improve the strength and function of the wrist postoperatively.[9] Dingman,[13] writing almost 40 years later, felt that the technique of excision or time of postoperative immobilization did not affect the end result. At follow-up in his series, almost all patients with good or excellent results had minimal bone excision initially or considerable boney regeneration after surgery.[13] The strength and stability of these wrists were virtually normal. Kessler and Hecht[28] felt that instability might be a complication of the procedure, but that improved motion and strength were almost always seen in cases in which the etiology was trauma. Although Hartz and Beckenbaugh[23] felt that good results could be obtained by the Darrach procedure for derangement of the distal radioulnar joint secondary to trauma, not all agree. Ekenstam et al.[15] found that in their series only patients with documented arthritis of the distal radioulnar joint benefited from distal ulnar excision in more than 50% of the operated cases. Causes for failure included instability of distal

ulna, continuing pain in the wrist, minimal to no increase in range of motion, and no improvement in grip strength.

As with any excisional arthroplasty, the Darrach procedure usually diminishes pain and increases motion, but usually at the expense of stability of the pseudojoint. This stability or lack of it may be active or passive. Passive instability, which disappears with active use, suggests muscular-stabilizing forces. The stability of the distal radioulnar joint is primarily through the intact triangular fibrocartilagenous complex (TFCC) the pronator quadratus muscle, and a normally placed extensor carpi ulnaris tendon.[8,41] The latter two structures are active stabilizers, while the TFCC acts passively as a ligamentous structure.

The Darrach procedure is probably best indicated for traumatic derangements with secondary arthritis of the distal radioulnar joints. The deranged distal radioulnar joint that is painful and unstable is not improved by distal ulnar excision, which usually makes instability worse. Multiple tendon ruptures of the extensor digitorum communis tendon have also been reported as complications of the Darrach procedure,*[35,44]

* Stein, F.: Personal communication, 1980.

but instability is usually the most distressing complication. Dingman[13] and Kessler[28] have pointed out that instability is usually associated with excessive bone resection. Minimal bone resection and avoiding the procedure in the unstable situation will be rewarded with better results.

Can one stabilize the unstable distal ulna following resection and still allow forearm rotation? Many operations are described to stabilize the ulnar head into the sigmoid notch of the radius utilizing fascia or tendon grafts, although the reported series are small and follow-up inadequate to demonstrate painless forearm rotation. The essential problem with these procedures is that if graft tension is high and immobilization prolonged, then arthritis of the joint with pain and limitation of motion is the likely result.[12] On the other hand if graft tension is low and immobilization short, the instability remains.

Ligamentous Reconstruction

Hui and Linscheid

Since most instabilities of the distal radioulnar joint are dorsal Hui and Linscheid[26] have attempted stabilization of the joint, using a distally based portion of the flexor carpi ulnaris tendon. The authors point out that this is an operative procedure similar to one described in Bunnell's *Surgery of the Hand*. The operative procedure is indicated only for young, vigorous individuals without arthritis of distal radioulnar joint. The procedure as described is not applicable to patients who have already undergone a previous excision of the distal ulna (Fig. 97-2).

The technique of Hui and Linscheid[25] requires two incisions, one palmarly from the pisiform proximally 6 to 8 inches along the flexor carpi ulnaris tendon and another dorsally exposing the dislocated ulnar head. Being careful to protect the dorsal cutaneous branch of the ulnar nerve, drill a hole from proximal to distal, emerging in the area near the base of styloid process of the ulna. Divide a portion of flexor carpi ulnaris tendon proximally and free it distally to its pisiform attachment. Using blunt technique, make an opening in the capsular structures between the pisiform and triquetrum ulnarly. Then pass the tendon slip into the wrist joint and into the osseous hole created in the ulnar head.

Reduce the subluxation of the distal radioulnar joint by supination, and stabilize the two bones with Kirschner wires. Tighten the tendon and suture it back to the pisotriquetral capsule. Shorten the attenuated dorsal radioulnar ligament, and return the extensor carpi ulnaris to its sheath, which is then closed. This "ligament" locks the ulnar carpus to the ulnar head.

Immobilization for 6 weeks with the forearm in supination is followed by protected motion for an additional 6 weeks following removal of the Kirschner wires. The patients universally lose forearm pronation but do not complain of instability.

Tsai and Stillwell Procedure

Tsai and Stillwell[46] use the interosseous membrane and extensor carpi ulnaris as an aid in stabilization after passing the distally based flexor carpi ulnaris tendon through a drill hole in the ulna. The operation of Tsai and Stillwell is applicable to patients with an intact ulnar head as well as those who have undergone ulnar head excision with continuing instability. As in the previous procedure of Hui and Linscheid,[25] a strip of flexor carpi ulnaris with its distal attachment to the pisiform intact is the stabilizing structure (Fig. 97-3).

The technique of Tsai and Stillwell is as follows: Make an incision on the flexor surface of the forearm along the course of the flexor carpi ulnaris tendon. Expose the tendon from muscle-tendon junction to pisiform, and develop a strip from proximal to distal. Release Guyon's canal to avoid ulnar nerve compression with tightening of tendon toward the dorsum. Make an additional incision dorsally, exposing the distal ulna or shaft in the case of previous ulnar head excision. Drill a hole from the medullary canal opening obliquely and proximally, emerging on the dorsal aspect of the ulna. Expose the interosseous membrane close to the ulna distally.

Pass the flexor carpi ulnaris tendon slip, which is still attached to the pisiform, dorsally deep to the ulnar nerve and artery into the medullary end of the ulna and out the dorsal cortical hole. Make parallel incisions in the interosseous membrane perpendicular to the long axis of the forearm, and pass the slip of flexor carpi ulnaris from proximal to distal through these incisions. Supinate the forearm, tighten the tendon slip, and suture it to the interosseous membrane. Loop the remaining extra tendon slip about the extensor carpi ulnaris to maintain this tendon dorsal to the resected ulna.

Postoperative supination is maintained for 6 weeks; then gentle controlled motion is begun with night splint for an additional 2 to 4 weeks. Protection of the new ligament requires approximately 3 months of postoperative support.

In both procedures postoperative immobilization must be in supination; forced pronation must be protected against for several months postoperatively. The extra-articular course of the flexor carpi ulnaris in the latter procedure seems to result in less loss of pronation, but our experiences with the Tsai operative procedure has been only on patients with instability following a Darrach procedure.

Blatt and Ashworth

The palmar capsular transfer of Blatt and Ashworth[3] attempts to reconstruct, as in the operative procedures of Hui and Linscheid[25] and Tsai and Stillwell[46] a new distal palmar to proximal dorsal ligamentous structure.

The technique of the operation Blatt and Ashworth is as follows: Expose the distal ulna dorsoulnarly with the forearm in pronation. Identify and protect the dorsal branch of the ulnar nerve. Expose the resected distal end of the ulna between the fifth and sixth dorsal compartments, and enter the wrist joint by incising the dorsal carpal ligament. Perform a subperiosteal exposure of the distal ulna, and drill one or more holes unicortically from the medullary canal dorsally. Expose the palmar capsule of the wrist, and elevate a rectangular flap of tissue based distally. Suture this flap to the dorsal aspect of the resected ulna. Imbricate the dorsal capsule for additional stability, followed by routine closure.

Fifty of the 62 patients with 69 operative procedures in Blatt and Ashworth's series had rheumatoid arthritis. None of the

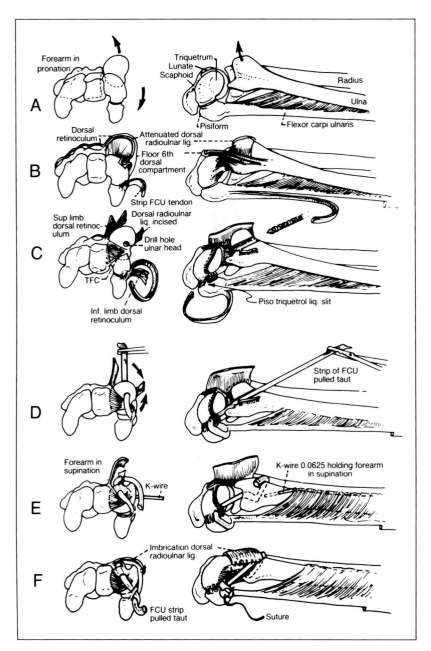

FIGURE 97-2. The technique of ulnotriquetral stabilization is illustrated here as described by Hui and Linscheid. (Hui, F., and Linscheid, R.: Ulno-triquetral Augmentation Tenodesis: A Reconstructive Procedure For Dorsal Subluxation of the Distal Radioulnar Joint. J. Hand Surg. **7:**230, 1982.)

arthritic patients gained or lost wrist range of motion. All patients, regardless of diagnosis, regained full rotation of the forearm, and there were no cases of recurrent dorsal ulnar subluxation or ulnar carpal translation of the hand.

The procedures of Hui and Linscheid,[25] Tsai and Stillwell,[46] and Blatt and Ashworth[3] just described have in common the aim of passively reducing and stabilizing the ulna by creating a new ligament. Several other procedures have been described (Goldner and Hayes,[20] Johnson and Skewsburry,[26] Hill,[24] and Butler*), which are based on a different concept, namely that of using active muscle force to dynamically stabilize the ulna (Figs. 97-4, 97-5). Examination of patients treated by these procedures will be abnormal when the patient's arm is relaxed. These procedures are more applicable to an unstable Darrach

procedure than to a normal but unstable distal radioulnar joint.

The operative procedure according to Goldner and Hayes is as follows. Make a dorsal ulnar incision distal to and proximal to the ulnar-carpal joint. Identify and isolate the dorsocutaneous branch of the ulnar nerve distal to the ulna. If the annular ligament remains, identify it by nonabsorbable sutures; if the annular ligament is not intact, isolate its remnants.

Delicately elevate the periosteum from the distal ulna by sharp dissection. If bone cells remain on the periosteum, it is likely to regenerate a thick, osseous periosteal flap that may impinge on the carpals and cause discomfort later; therefore be meticulous in dissection.

Identify the extensor carpi ulnaris tendon, and retract it on a hernia tape. Identify the extensor digitorum communis tendon to the little finger, and take special care to protect it.

* Butler, B.: Personal communication, 1976.

FIGURE 97-3. The technique of stabilization of the ulna using a sling between flexor–extensor carpi ulnaris according to Tsai and Stilwell (Tsai, T., and Stilwell, J.: Repair of Chronic Subluxations of the Distal Radio Joint Using Flexor Corpi Ulnarus Tendon. J. Hand Surg. **9-B:**289, 1984. Courtesy of British Journal of Hand Surgery.)

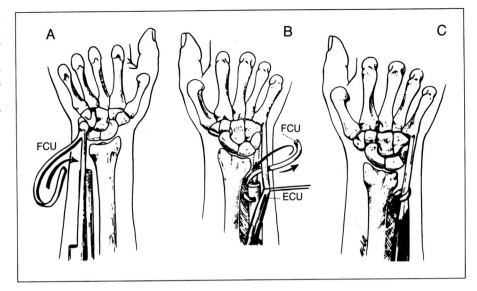

Resect approximately 2 cm of the distal ulna, cutting it just proximal to the point of contact with the radius. Mark the ulna attachment of the pronator quadratus with a suture.

With a rongeur shape the end of the ulna so that the dorsal edge is rounded, and trim the radial aspect so that there is no impingement on tendons to the little finger.

Split the extensor carpi ulnaris from its insertion distally to a point 1 cm proximal to the newly shaped end of the ulna; the split should make a strip on the *ulnar* side of the tendon about one-third the width of the total tendon. It is important to carry it sufficiently proximally so that the remaining tendon is not displaced toward the ulna.

Drill a $7/64$ths (3-mm) hole in the proximal ulna with the forearm held in full supination. Direct the drill hole from dorsal to proximal at a point about 5 mm proximal to the cut end of the ulna. Enlarge the hole with curettes and a $9/64$ths (3.5-mm) drill, using a drill guide and slow speed to avoid breaking the distal cortex. Eliminate bone dust and bone chips by copious irrigation.

Pass the freed segment of the extensor carpi ulnaris through the hole from dorsal to palmar with a needle and 3-0 nonabsorbable suture. Direct the tendon to the ulnar side of the remaining proximal ulna, and suture it back on itself at a point where the tendon entered the bone. This creates a cuff of tendon directly over the end of the ulna, with an extension of bone of about 2 mm. This cuff of tendon stabilizes the remaining extensor carpi ulnaris and tethers it toward the radial side of the ulna; it also acts as a collagen sleeve and collagen base to which the periosteal sleeve proximally and the annular ligament dorsally can be resutured in order to prevent fore and aft or anterior or posterior movement of the proximal ulna.

Wrap the remaining tendon around 180° of the proximal ulna. It is not wrapped around the ulna for 360° because its presence between the ulna and the radius would cause impingement as pronation and supination occur.

Close the periosteum with absorbable suture, and the annular ligament with nonabsorbable white 4-0 suture with a P-3 needle. Perform the closure with the forearm in supination and the elbow flexed; thus the surgeon is sitting to the ulnar aspect of the forearm, and as the closure is being performed, the elbow is flexed with the dorsum of the forearm facing the surgeon.

The forearm is immobilized for 2 weeks, after which gradual pronation, supination, and radial and ulnar deviation are initiated. The wrist is protected for a total of 3 months with a removable splint at night and partial splinting during the daytime. Forceful gripping and extensor stress are not allowed for 6 months. Occasionally, snapping and popping persist for 4 to 6 months, and 1 year must pass before maximum improvment is obtained.

Potential complications of the procedure include (1) neurapraxia of the superficial branch of the ulnar nerve; (2) bone regeneration from an excessively heavy periosteal flap, requiring further periosteal resection and reconstruction of the annular ligament; (3) rupture of the extensor digitorum communis and extensor digiti quinti to the little finger as a result of too vigorous exercise within 3 to 4 weeks after the operation; (4) subluxation of the carpus in patients with severe rheumatoid disease (this was not felt to be due entirely to the ulnar resection, but to the intrinsic disease).

The dynamic stabilization of the distal radioulnar joint by the pronator quadratus has been described by Johnson and Skewsburry.[26] Johnson[27] has described advancing the origin of the quadratus dorsally to stabilize the joint. The Johnson muscle advancement procedure can be performed on patients with an intact ulnar head as well as on those who have already undergone a Darrach procedure.

The Johnson Pronator Advancement

Make an incision over the distal ulnar aspect of the forearm. Identify, but do not open, the tendon sheath of the extensor carpi ulnaris through its entire length. Identify the pronator quadratus muscle distally, and remove its origin from the ulna, working distal to proximal and including as much periosteum as possible with the muscle. Advance the origin 6 to 9 mm dorsally, and suture it to the tendon sheath of the extensor carpi ulnaris with the forearm in full pronation. With Kirschner

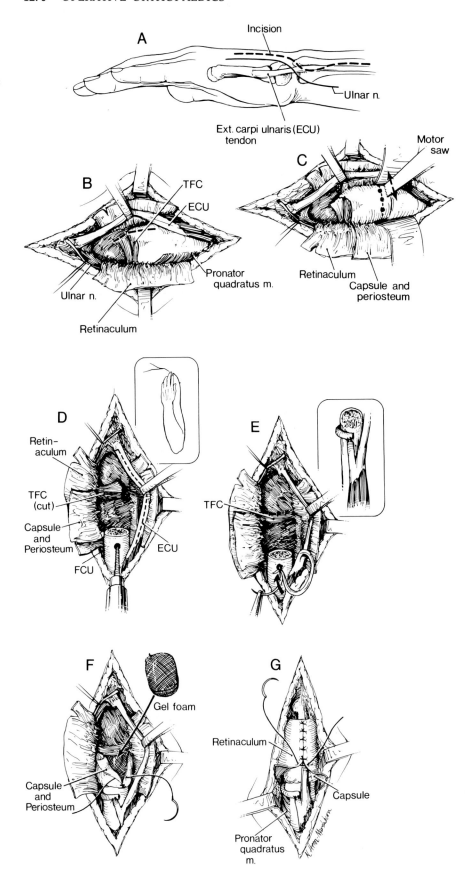

FIGURE 97-4. Technique of operative stabilization of distal ulna using half of extensor carpi ulnaris. (Goldner, L., personal communication, 1987.)

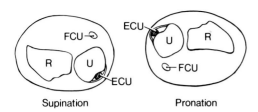

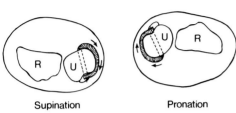

FIGURE 97-5. Diagrammatic illustration of stabilizing effect of transferred extensor carpi ulnaris (*ECU*). *FCU*, flexor carpi ulnaris. (Goldner, L., personal communication, 1987.)

wires transfix the ulna to the radius with the forearm in midposition, and close the wound. The midposition rotation is maintained for 4 weeks, at which time the Kirschner wires are removed and a supervised exercise program begun.

Hemiresection Arthroplasty (Bowers)

Bowers[4,5] has described hemiresection arthroplasty of the distal radioulnar joint accomplished by excising that portion of the distal ulna that articulates with the sigmoid notch of the radius while maintaining the distal ulnar shaft and styloid process. This preserves the triangular fibrocartilage complex, excises the damaged portion of ulnar head, and maintains stability of the distal ulna. The majority of his patients had a diagnosis of rheumatoid arthritis. In those patients with radial shortening secondary to fracture as a cause for arthroplasty, all needed ulnar shortening in addition to the arthroplasty in order to achieve postoperative pain relief. All patients, however, achieved excellent forearm rotation regardless of diagnosis, and instability was not seen after surgery at an average follow-up of 2½ years. (Fig. 97-6)

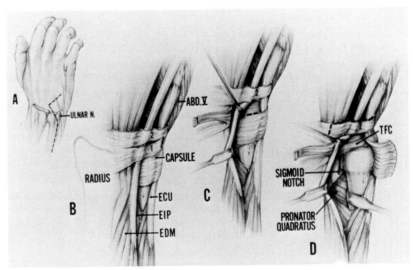

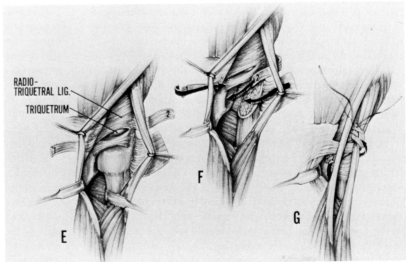

FIGURE 97-6. Surgical exposure of the distal radioulnar joint and technique of Bowers hemiresection arthroplasty is demonstrated. (Courtesy of Elizabeth Roselius.)

The technique of hemiarthroplasty is as follows. With the forearm in full pronation, open the interval between the extensor digiti quinti and extensor carpi ulnaris, exposing the extensor retinaculum and protecting the dorsal cutaneous branch of the ulnar nerve. Two flaps of retinaculum are developed. The more proximal of the two, representing about one-half of the width of the retinaculum, is based radially; the more distal is based ulnarly. Radial retraction of the extensor digiti quinti at this level places the surgeon immediately dorsal to the sigmoid notch of the radius.

Open the capsule close to the radius, allowing enough tissue to remain for later repair. Greater exposure is afforded by extending the longitudinal opening in the dorsal capsule into an "L" configuration ulnarly. The triangular fibrocartilage can easily be visualized throughout its entire extent now. Remove the convexity of the ulnar head with rongeurs, osteotomes, or dental burrs. This resection should preserve the shaft and ulnar-styloid relationship. Suture the ulnarly based dorsal capsular flap over the raw bone of the distal ulna, with the sutures entering the palmar wrist capsule. Rotate the forearm to be certain there is no contact between the radius and ulna.

If inadequate tissue is available to avoid radioulnar contact, place a small "anchovie" of tendon of the palmaris longus into the defect previously occupied by the ulnar head. Suture the distal ulnarly based retinacular flap to the dorsal capsular structure remaining on the sigmoid notch. Pass the proximally based radial flap about the extensor carpi ulnaris and suture it not to itself, but to the distal aspect of the retinaculum of the fourth compartment. Closure is routine and immobilization in neutral forearm rotation is continued for 3 weeks following which mobilization is begun.

Ulnar Ostectomy

There are alternatives to the Darrach procedure, with or without subsequent stabilization operation, for derangements of the distal radioulnar joint. Milch[33] described cuff resection or ulnar shortening for dorsal dislocation of the ulna following a malunited Colles' fracture in one case with good results. More recently Darrow et al.[12] have reported on ulnar shortening for a wide variety of conditions on the ulnar side of the wrist. Although in only 5 of 36 cases was the cause related to a fracture of the distal radius, most patients demonstrated positive ulnar variance. One-half of the patients had signs of instability of the distal radioulnar joint. The authors feel that the shortening decompresses the ulnar side of the carpus, presents a different surface of the distal ulna to the radial sigmoid notch, and tightens the ligament support system on the ulnar side of the wrist. The technique of ulnar shortening as originally described by Milch has been modified because of the availability of rigid internal fixation techniques. (Fig. 97-7)

Make an incision over the distal ulna with subperiosteal exposure of the bone. Adjust a dynamic compression plate (DCP) plate to fit the ulna and insert two distal screws with appropriate technique. Select the site of the shortening ostectomy and make rotational and alignment markings proximal to the ostectomy site. Perform the ostectomy removing an amount of the ulna as determined by preoperative measurements.

Open the wrist joint between the fifth and sixth compartment by incising the dorsal capsule. More extensive exposure of the distal radioulnar and wrist joint can be obtained by stripping the pronator quadratus and interosseous membrane from the distal ulnar fragment. This allows the fragment to be swung outward, exposing the triangular fibrocartilage for possible repair. If required, wedges of bone may be removed from the osteotomy site in order to realign the ulna distally. Reduce the ostectomy and place a compression screw proximally. Observe wrist and forearm motion in order to make certain that there is no mechanical block, impingement, or instability that has not been corrected. Closure is routine following insertion of the remaining screws.

Steindler[42] quoted an article in the German literature by Lauenstein that had another approach to derangements of the distal radioulnar joint following Colles' fractures. The procedure was creation of an ulnar nonunion at the junction of middle and distal third of the ulnar shaft. The damaged distal radioulnar joint underwent arthrodesis (Fig. 97-8). A similar approach was also advocated by Sauve and Kapandji[38,39] and McMurray.[32]

This ulnar nonunion allowed ulnar shortening so that there was no longer ulnar carpal impingement that would limit wrist dorsiflexion and ulnar deviation. In addition the ulnar nonunion added a new distal radioulnar joint, so the patient gained forearm rotation as well. This three-bone forearm operative procedure has been examined by Goncalves, who felt that results were consistently better than those achieved with the Darrach procedure.[21]

In 1966 I saw my first traumatic three-bone forearm. The patient, injured in an explosive incident, lost a significant portion of the middle third of his ulna with muscle and nerve injury. However, he demonstrated no functional deficit except the ulnar nerve problem. Forearm rotation was full and stable, and elbow and wrist motion were normal and stable. No boney reconstruction was conducted.

A few weeks later a patient with long-standing ulnar nonunion with bone loss underwent surgery. At the time of internal fixation, the normal forearm rotation, which existed preoperatively, was lost. A fibrous ankylosis of the distal radioulnar joint had occurred with the patient preferentially rotating through the ulnar nonunion. The bone graft subsequently became infected, and following removal of graft and metal, normal forearm rotation was again present without instability.

Forearm rotation in both of the patients was occurring through the proximal radioulnar joint, which was normal: through the intact interosseous membrane proximally; and distally through the ulnar nonunion. The radial shaft, which is uninjured, and that portion of the ulna distal to the nonunion were moving as a unit. The intact interosseous membrane distally and the normal distal radioulnar joint ligamentous structures stabilized the ulna to the radius. The uninjured radius and the ulnar shaft nonunion create the three-bone forearm radiographically, but functionally the forearm remains a two-bone system. The radius and distal ulnar fragment act as a single unit, while the ulna proximal to the nonunion acts as the other member. These two units are stabilized by the intact interosseous membrane.

Deliberate creation of an ulnar nonunion in the distal one-third of the forearm is yet another alternative to the Darrach procedure for derangement of the distal radioulnar joint. No arthrodesis of the distal radioulnar joint need be per-

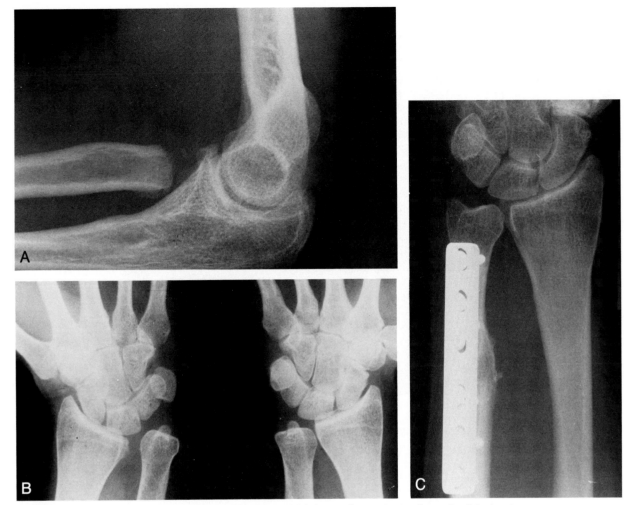

FIGURE 97-7.   Following an axially loaded forearm injury with injury to the proximal radius and radial head excision, instability of the distal radial ulnar joint may occur. This is a so-called Essex-Lopresti injury, and in such a case, ulnar shortening is the procedure of choice to tighten up the ulnar side of the wrist and shorten the ulna. This is the Milch procedure.

formed.[1,22,43] Radial shortening following fracture, premature epiphyseal closure and Colles' type fractures are all examples of conditions that bring about disparity of normal radioulnar length, with or without articular damage to the distal radioulnar joint. The relatively long ulna may result in attritional changes in the TFCC or chondromalacia of the lunate or ulnar head, in addition to limited wrist motion and forearm rotation.

In this group of patients, simply shortening the ulna as advocated by Milch[33] and Darrow et al.[12] should eliminate the length discrepancy, decompress the ulnar side of the carpus and hopefully improve motion. If, however, there has been significant damage to the articular surface of the distal radioulnar joint, painful rotation may not be relieved even though the length disparity is corrected.

Based on our experience with the three-bone forearm, we felt that partial ostectomy of the ulnar shaft would substitute for ulnar shortening or the standard Darrach procedure. Excision of a portion of ulna would reduce the subluxated ulnar head with improved wrist dorsiflexion and ulnar deviation as well as forearm rotation. The amount of ulnar shortening is essentially determined by the patient's anatomy. Ulnar side decompression of the carpus is achieved as in ulnar shortening. Although rotational forces are no longer operative through the distal radioulnar joint, the ulna, through its soft tissue attachment to the distal radius, is able to take some load from the carpus. While this relative unloading of lunate by ulnar ostectomy may expose the lunate to increased forces, we have not seen or heard of any cases of Kienböck's disease occurring in these patients. If inadequate bone is removed at the time of creation of the ulnar nonunion, reconstitution of the ulna may occur. In this situation loss of forearm rotation will result because of the fibrous ankylosis of the distal joint that usually occurs quite rapidly. Reexcision in the area of the ostectomy will once again return forearm rotation to previous levels.

The technique of partial ulnar ostectomy with or without distal radioulnar fusion is as follows. If there is no plan to perform a distal radioulnar arthrodesis, make an incision on the subcutaneous border of the ulna at the junction of the middle and distal thirds of the ulna. Incise the periosteum, expose the bone, and remove approximately 2.5 to 3 cm of the

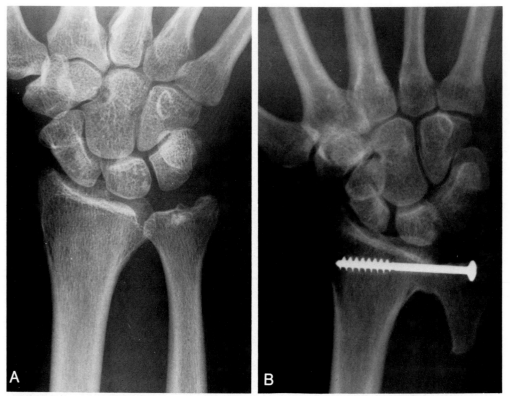

FIGURE 97-8. Derangements of the distal radioulnar joint, as in the case of a 25-year-old man, may be treated by a wide variety of operative procedures. In this case arthrodesis of the distal radioulnar joint coupled with a partial ostectomy of the ulna restored full function.

ulnar shaft. Remove the periosteum, but leave the interosseous membrane intact. Routine closure follows, ranging the forearm to determine whether or not full passive motion is present. After surgery forearm rotation is begun on the day following surgery in a wrist control splint.

If distal fusion is to be added to the partial ostectomy, then make a slightly curved incision paralleling the course of the dorsal cutaneous branch of the ulnar nerve. Expose the ulnar head by dividing the dorsal capsule in the interval between the extensor carpi ulnaris and the extensor digiti quinti. Incise the dorsal capsule close to the sigmoid notch, leaving some tissue for later repair. Extend the incision ulnarly from the longitudinal limb, exposing the ulnar head. If there is minimal or no length discrepency between the radius and ulna, remove the cartilagous surfaces of the distal radioulnar joint with dental burrs to cancellous bone. Expose the shaft of the ulna, and make an additional incision over the head of the ulna medial to the extensor carpi ulnaris. Supinate the forearm, and use Kirschner wires to temporarily hold the ulna to the radius in the sigmoid notch. Insert a lag screw or an overdrilled cortical screw from the ulna into the radius. Following this, remove 2 to 3 cm of ulna proximal to the arthrodesis site. Check forearm and wrist motion, and remove the Kirschner wires. Suture the dorsal capsule back to the sigmoid notch area, and close the wound.

Mobilization of the forearm is begun the day following in a wrist control splint. If the ulna must be shortened, this should be done before the arthrodesis, and the distal ulnar fragment

stabilized with the Kirschner wires before screw insertion. Our results with this operation on 72 procedures have been reviewed. The cases cover the time from 1975 to 1983. On 26 occasions arthrodesis of the distal radioulnar joint was required at the time of ulnar ostectomy, usually for rheumatoid arthritis.[22]

The procedure does require an intact interosseous membrane, and is not indicated in patients with Monteggia or Essex-Lopresti fracture-dislocations.[17,34] The ulnar ostectomy will reduce the length discrepency, but without an intact interosseous membrane between the radius and proximal ulnar fragment, excess instability will result. In cases with length discrepency and an inadequate interosseous membrane proximally, ulnar shortening is the procedure of choice (Fig. 97-9).

Although a major cause of derangement of the distal radioulnar joint is union with deformity of distal radius fracture, what is the fate of the joint with osteotomy of the radius?[19] Talesnick and Watson[49] feel that loss of palmar tilt of the distal radial articulation is likely to result in radiocarpal problems. Shortening and radial deviation are more likely to be associated with difficulties with forearm rotation. If the problem is simple shortening of the radius, then a Darrach procedure or ulnar shortening should relieve the problem. However, radial deviation of the distal fragment will result in weakness of grasp and poor cosmesis. In general, young, more active patients are the ones who require radial osteotomy. Fernandez[17] believes that a Darrach procedure should be performed in addition to the radial osteotomy if there is shortening of more than 12 mm, if

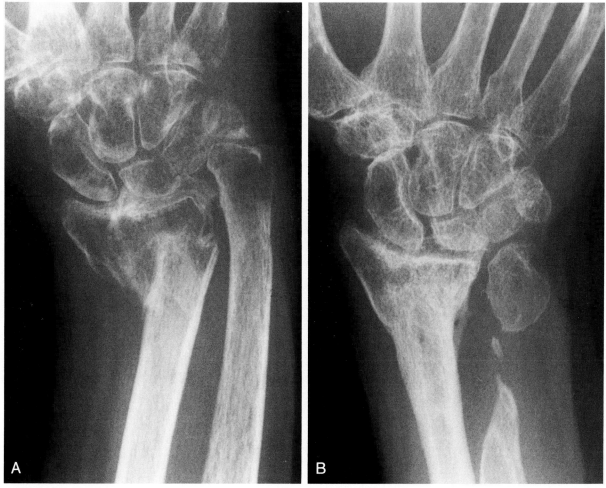

FIGURE 97-9. In patients with malunited fractures, extreme osteoporosis may be seen. In these patients an opening wedge ostectomy may create problems, and a closing wedge ostectomy with ulnar shortening may be an acceptable alternative.

arthritis exists in the distal radioulnar joints, or if there is subluxation of the joint. In addition, he feels preservation of the distal radioulnar joint in this group of patients is important in order to avoid a decrease in grip strength. A Darrach procedure was, however, necessary in 5 of 20 patients undergoing osteotomy.[17]

Although previous osteotomies of the distal radius have been of the opening wedge type, we feel that a closing wedge osteotomy coupled with a partial ulnar ostectomy offers an alternative. This procedure allows correction of the deformity in the sagittal, frontal, and horizontal plane, preserves the distal radioulnar joint, avoids the necessity of bone graft, and allows extremely early motion of wrist and forearm. Distal radioulnar joint fusion is not necessary (see Fig. 97-8).[27]

RADIOULNAR JOINT IN RHEUMATOID ARTHRITIS

What is the place of the Darrach distal ulna excision in rheumatoid arthritis? Since 1943[40] the Darrach procedure has been utilized for the unstable distal radioulnar joint in rheumatoid arthritis with generally excellent results. The great majority of patients note diminished pain and increased forearm rotation.[6,28,34,36] However, there have been concerns about ulnar translation of the carpus on the remaining radius and instability of the remaining distal ulna, or at least our inability to stabilize it after resection.

Swanson[44] has suggested that at the time of excision of the ulnar head, an ulnar silicone prosthesis be added to cover the resected end of the ulna (Fig. 97-10). Ligament stabilization can then be carried out without the concern of bony impingement between radius and ulna. Although the procedure is applicable to other conditions with derangements of the distal radioulnar joint, its major usefulness seems to be in those patients with rheumatoid arthritis. In Swanson's original series[44] with a short follow-up, there were no cases of carpal translation ulnarly with use of the ulnar head prosthesis. Gainor and Schaberg,[19] however, were unable to show that ulnar translation was prevented by the prosthesis. They felt that either spontaneous radiolunate fusion or reactive bone in response to the translation were more important in avoiding the clinical problem of ulnar translation (Fig. 97-11). Boney resorption beneath the

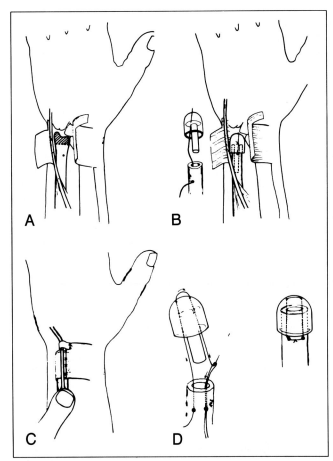

FIGURE 97-10. The technique of ulnar resection and coverage with a silicone cup using Swanson's technique. (Swanson, A.: Implant Arthroplasty for Disabilities of the Distal Radio-Ulnar Joint. Orthop. Clin. North Am. **4**:373, 1973.)

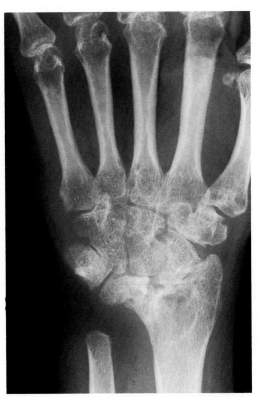

FIGURE 97-11. In the presence of excision of the distal ulna in a rheumatoid arthritic, ulnar translation is a possibility. Protection from ulnar translation is afforded by formation of reactive osteophytes to support the ulnarly translating carpus or spontaneous radial lunate fusion, as in this case.

prosthesis with subsequent instability has been reported. The instability has required removal of the ulnar head prosthesis in a number of patients. These articles suggest no advantage to the use of the prosthesis over a simple Darrach procedure.[20,47]

In spite of this there is a group of rheumatoid arthritic patients that does poorly following simple distal ulnar excision. This group comprises the patients who show early evidence of intercarpal subluxations and ulnar translation of the hand on the distal radius. As pointed out by Gainor and Schaberg,[19] the absence of a bony stabilizer or bony shelf ulnarly on the radius in a wrist that already shows ulnar translation is likely to result in further translation with distal ulnar excision. Black et al.[2] have previously described erosion of the radius in the area of sigmoid notch in rheumatoid patients. They felt that erosion in this area suggested that a distal ulnar excision was contraindicated because of the likelihood of ulnar translation.

In patients without a bony shelf or with erosion of the ulnar aspect of the distal radius, I feel that partial ulnar ostectomy, proximal to a distal radioulnar fusion, should be considered. Maintaining the distal ulna in a reduced position in the sigmoid notch offers ulnar support to the carpus, and the proximal ulnar nonunion adds forearm rotation to the distal stability. This arthrodesis of the distal radioulnar joint more than com-

pensates for the loss of ligament support that occurs in rheumatoid arthritis. This is the same pattern of motion that exists in the traumatic three-bone forearm (Fig. 97-12).

Noting that patients with spontaneous radiolunate fusion do well, Linscheid and Dobyns[30] have suggested yet another alternative to prevent ulnar translation, a surgical radiolunate fusion. They note generally good preservation of the midcarpal joints so that the motion loss is well tolerated.

SELECTION OF OPERATIVE PROCEDURES

At the present time there is feeling among surgeons that normal anatomy should be restored. This is based on failures with some previous reconstructive procedures. Selection of a surgical procedure should be based on as much sound information as possible. In this case joint exploration must determine which of the many alternatives should or could be used.

In the case of ulnar plus variance with a normal or near normal distal radioulnar joint, ulnar shortening is the procedure of choice. Although there may be a problem with union of the osteotomy and prolonged immobilization may increase considerably the rehabilitation problems, a good result should occur. Usually, instability, which may coexist with this condition, will also be improved.

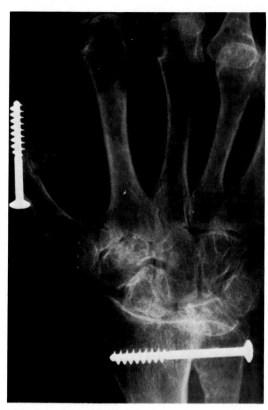

FIGURE 97-12. Partial ostectomy of the ulna with distal radioulnar fusion is a reasonable alternative in the rheumatoid arthritic patient. This offers an ulnar-translating buttress much like the reacting osteophyte and still allows forearm rotation.

With an unstable distal radioulnar joint, which is otherwise normal in a young patient, I would try to create a stabilizing ligament from distal palmar to proximal dorsal. The three procedures described by Hui and Linscheid,[25] Tsai and Stillwell,[46] and Blatt and Ashworth[3] have been mentioned. I would select the procedure of Hui and Linscheid, realizing a pronation loss is to be expected. The palmar capsuloplasty of Blatt and Ashworth seems to have its greatest application in the patient with rheumatoid arthritis, but long-term published results are lacking.

If the distal radial joint is abnormal with cartilage damage or early arthritis, but no real length abnormality, the hemiarthroplasty of Bowers[4] is my suggestion. This is an excellent alternative to the Darrach procedure without the concerns of instability. It can be retrieved with an arthrodesis distally with bone graft and partial ulna ostectomy proximally if it fails for any reason.

In the case of the unstable Darrach procedure, there is probably no 100% successful procedure. The ligament procedure of Tsai and Stillwell,[46] using in some combination the flexor carpi ulnaris and extensor carpi ulnaris sling procedure, is my selection.

In the patients with rheumatoid arthritis, with arthritis and instability of the distal radioulnar joint, with or without tendon ruptures, I avoid the Darrach procedure. While the Bowers[5] procedure seems to have replaced the Darrach in the rheumatoid patients, it is not an easy operation to do; there are many

pitfalls. I prefer an arthrodesis of the distal radioulnar joint and a partial ostectomy of the ulna. The procedure is equally applicable to patients with or without early ulnar carpal translation, and requires no immobilization of wrist or forearm after surgery, unless dictated by other procedures.

Realizing that motion is important, but also realizing that motion without control is a deterrent to normal elbow, wrist, and hand use, arthrodesis must be kept in mind. Stability is more important than motion without control as far as elbow, wrist, and hand functions are concerned. A torn interosseous membrane with a previously resected distal ulna is a case in point, which can be improved by creation of a one-bone forearm with improvement of overall function even though motion is lost.

REFERENCES

1. Ballard, A., and Sulkowsky, J.: Three-Bone Forearm, A Salvage Procedure for the Treatment of Persistent Ulnar Defect. Presented at the annual meeting of the Clinical Orthopaedic Society, Denver, Oct. 1976.
2. Black, M., Boswick, J., and Wiedel, J.: Dislocation of the Wrist in Rheumatoid Arthritis. Clin. Orthop. **124:**184, 1979.
3. Blatt, G., and Ashworth, C.R.: Volar Capsule Transfer for Stabilization Following Resection of the Distal End of the Ulna. Orthop. Trans. **3:**13, 1979.
4. Bowers, W.: Distal Radio-ulnar Joint. *In* Green, D. (ed.): Operative Hand Surgery. New York, Churchill Livingstone, 1982.
5. Bowers, W.: Distal Radio-ulnar Joint Arthroplasty and the Hemiresection Interposition Technique. J. Hand Surg. **10-A:**169, 1985.
6. Clayton, M.: Surgical Treatment at the Wrist in Rheumatoid Arthritis. J. Bone Joint Surg. **47-A:**741, 1965.
7. Cooney, W. Dobyns, J., and Linscheid, R.: Complications of Colles' Fracture. J. Bone Joint Surg. **62-A:**613, 1980.
8. Dameron, T.: Traumatic Dislocation of the Distal Radio-ulna Joint. Clin. Orthop. **83:**55, 1972.
9. Darrach, W.: Forward Dislocation at the Inferior Radio-ulnar Joint With Fracture of the Lower Third of the Radius. Ann. Surg. **56:**801, 1912.
10. Darrach, W.: Anterior Dislocation of the Head of the Ulna. Ann. Surg. **56:**802, 1912.
11. Darrach, W., and Dwight, K.: Derrangements of the Inferior Radioulnar Articulation. Med. Rec. **87:**708, 1915.
12. Darrow, J., Linscheid, R., Dobyns, J., et al.: Distal Ulnar Resession for Disorders of the Distal Radioulnar Joint. J. Hand Surg. **10-A:**482, 1985.
13. Dingman, P.: Resection of the Distal End of the Ulna (Darrach Procedure). J. Bone Joint Surg. **34-A:**803, 1952.
14. Dobyns, J., and Linscheid, R.: Fractures and Dislocations of the wrist. *In* Rockwood, C., and Green, D. (eds.): EDS Fractures. Philadelphia, J.B. Lippincott, 1975.
15. Ekenstam, F., Engkvest, O., and Wadin, K.: Results From Resection of the Distal End of the Ulnar After Fracture of the Lower End of the Radius. Scand. J. Plast. Reconstr. Surg. **16:**177, 1982.
16. Essex-Lopresti, P.: Fractures of the Radial Head With Distal Radio-ulnar Dislocations (2 cases) J. Bone Joint Surg. **33-B:**244, 1951.
17. Fernandez, D.: Correction of Post-traumatic Wrist Deformity in Adult by Osteotomy, Bone Graft and Internal Fixation. J. Bone Joint Surg. **64-A:**1164, 1982.
18. Frykman, G.: Fracture of the Distal Radius Including Sequalae Shoulder-Hand-Finger Syndrome, Disturbances in the Distal Radio-ulnar Joint and Impairment of Nerve Function. Acta. Orthop. Scand. [Suppl.] **108:**27, 1967.

19. Gainor, B.J., and Schaberg, J.: The Rheumatoid Wrist After Resection of the Distal Ulna. J. Hand Surg. **10-A:**837, 1985.

20. Goldner, J.L., and Hayes, M.G.: Stabilization of the Remaining Ulna Using One-half of the Extensor Carpi Ulnarus Tendons After Resection of the Distal Ulna. Orthop. Trans. **3:**330, 1979.

21. Goncalves, D.: Correction of Disorders of the Distal Radio-ulnar Joint by Artificial Pseudoarthrosis of the Ulna. J. Bone Joint Surg. **56-B:**462, 1974.

22. Hales, W., and Burkhalter, W.: The Three-Bone Forearm Procedure in Reconstruction of the Distal Radio-ulnar Joint. Presented at the annual meeting of the ASSH, Las Vegas, Jan. 1985.

23. Hartz, C.R., and Beckenbaugh, R.: Long Term Results of Resections of the Distal Ulnar for Post-traumatic Conditions. J. Trauma **19:**219, 1979.

24. Hill, R.B.: Habitual Dislocation of the Distal End of the Ulna. J. Bone Joint Surg. **21-B:**780, 1939.

25. Hui, F., and Linscheid, R.: Ulno-triquetral Augmentation Tenodesis: A Reconstructive Procedure for Dorsal Subluxation of the Distal Radioulnar Joint. J. Hand Surg. **7:**230, 1982.

26. Johnson, R., and Skewsbury, M.: The Pronator Quadratus in Motion and in Stabilization of the Radius and Ulna at the Distal Radio Ulnar Joint. J. Hand Surg. **1:**205, 1976.

27. Johnson, R.: Muscle Tendon Transfer for Stabilization of the Distal Radioulnar Joint. Presented at the annual meeting of the ASSH, Las Vegas, Jan. 1985.

28. Kessler, I., and Hecht, O.: Present Applications of the Darrach Procedure. Clin. Orthop. **72:**254, 1970.

29. Linscheid, R., and Dobyns, J.: Rheumatoic Arthritis of the Wrist. Orthop. Clin. North Am. **2:**649, 1971.

30. Linscheid, R., and Dobyns, J.: Radio-Lunate Arthrodesis. J. Hand Surg. **10-A:**821, 1985.

31. McDougall, A., and White, J.: Subluxation of the Inferior Radioulnar Joint Complicating Fractures of the Radial Head. J. Bone Joint Surg. **39-B:**278, 1957.

32. McMurray, T.P.: A Practice of Orthopaedic Surgery. Baltimore, Williams & Wilkins, 1949.

33. Milch, H.: Cuff Resection of the Ulna for Malunited Calles Fracture. J. Bone Joint Surg. **23:**311, 1941.

34. Mikic, Z., and Helal, B.: The Value of the Darrach Procedure in the Surgical Treatment of Rheumatoid Arthritis. Clin. Orthop. **127:**175, 1977.

35. Newmeyer, W.L., and Green, D.P.: Rupture of Extensor Tendors Following Resection of the Distal Ulnar. J. Bone Joint Surg. **64-A:**178, 1982.

36. Rana, N., and Taylor, A.: Excisions of the Distal End of the Ulna in Rheumatoid Arthritis. J. Bone Joint Surg. **55-B:**96, 1973.

37. Sarmiento, A., Pratt, G., Berry, N., et al.: Colles' Fracture Functional Bracing in Supination. J. Bone Joint Surg. **57-A:**311, 1975.

38. Sauve, and Kapandji: Constitution dun Ligament Annulaire Pericubital Inferieur. Bull. Mem. Soc. Natl. Chir. **59:**628, 1933.

39. Sauve, and Kapandji: Nouvelle Technique de Traitement Chirurgical de Luxations Recidivantes Isolees de l'Extremite Inferieure du cubitus. J. Chir (Paris) **47:**589, 1936.

40. Smith-Peterson, M., Aufranc, O., and Larson, C.: Useful Surgical Procedures for Rheumatoid Arthritis Involving Joints of the Upper Extremity. Arch. Surg. **46:**764, 1943.

41. Spinner, M., and Kaplan, E.: Extensor Carpi Ulnars Joint Its Relationship to Stability of the Distal Radio-ulna Joint. Clin. Orthop. **68:**124, 1970.

42. Steindler, H.: The Traumatic Deformities and Disabilities of the Upper Extremity. Springfield, Ill., Charles C. Thomas, 1946.

43. Sulkowsky, J.M., Ballard, A., and Burkhalter, W.B.: The Three-Bone Forearm—A Salvage Procedure for Treatment of Ulnar Non-union. Presented at the annual meeting of the AAOS, Las Vegas, Feb. 1977.

44. Swanson, A.: Implant Arthroplasty for Disabilities of the Distal Radio-Ulnar Joint. Orthop. Clin. North Am. **4:**373, 1973.

45. Taleisnik, J., and Watson, K.: Midcarpal Instability Caused by Malunited Fractures of the Distal Radius. J. Hand Surg. **9-A:**350, 1984.

46. Tsai, T., and Stilwell, J.: Repair of Chronic Subluxations of the Distal Radio Joint Using Flexor Corpi Ulnarus Tendon. J. Hand Surg. **9-B:**289, 1984.

47. White, R.: Resection of the Distal Ulna With or Without Implant Arthroplasty in Rheumatoid Arthritis. J. Hand Surg. **11-A:**514, 1986.

CHAPTER 98

Fractures of the Distal Radius

ROBERT M. SZABO

> The nature of this injury once ascertained, it will be a very easy matter to explain the different phenomena attendant on it, and to point out a method of treatment which will prove completely successful.
>
> —Abraham Colles, 1814[8]

Unfortunately, the end result of the treatment of distal radius fractures often leaves much to be desired. The fracture that Abraham Colles described was nonarticular and occurred from a fall on the outstretched hand in a somewhat osteoporotic individual. Presently, all distal radius fractures with dorsal displacement are referred to as "Colles' fractures" regardless of the fracture configuration, degree of comminution, age of the patient, or mechanism of the injury. Because of their frequency, Colles' type fractures are often regarded and treated casually. Controversy and confusion are found throughout the literature as to what is the best way to treat a fracture of the distal radius. The fundamental principle of treatment is the restoration of anatomy with the hopes of producing full painless motion of the wrist. The method selected to achieve this objective can only be determined after careful study of the individual fracture pattern.

ANATOMY

The distal radius is biconcave, triangular in shape, and covered with hyaline cartilage. A smooth anteroposterior ridge divides the articular surface into two facets: a triangular lateral facet, which articulates with the scaphoid, and a quadrilateral medial facet, which articulates with the lunate.[27] The medial surface of the distal radius forms a semicircular notch covered with hyaline cartilage, which articulates with the ulna head. This articulation enables the radius to swing around the ulna. The lateral surface elongates into a prominent styloid process, which gives attachment to the brachioradialis muscle (Fig. 98-1).

The cortical bone in the area of the distal radial metaphysis is quite thin. There is normally an average of 23° of radial angulation in the anteroposterior plane.[34] Average radial length as measured from the tip of the radial styloid to the ulna head is 12 mm, although variance can be considerable[14] (Fig. 98-2).

DEFINITIONS

"Given an eponym one may be sure (1) that the man so honored was not the first to describe the disease, the operation, or the instrument, or (2) that he misunderstood the situation, or (3) that he is generally misquoted, or (4) that (1), (2), and (3) are all simultaneously true."[27]

Colles' Fracture

A Colles' fracture is defined as being a complete fracture within the distal inch of the radius with dorsal displacement of the distal fragment.[2]

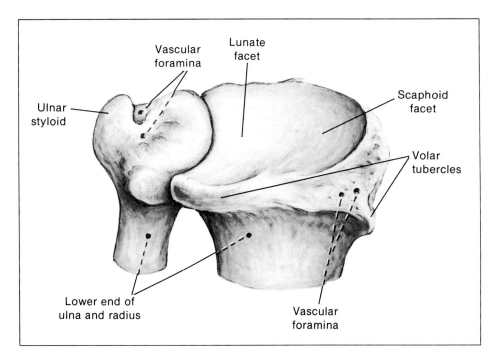

FIGURE 98-1. Anterior distal end of the radius and ulna. (Kaplan, E.B., and Taleisnik, J.: The Wrist. *In:* Spinner, M. (ed.): Kaplan's Functional and Surgical Anatomy of the Hand, 3rd ed.: Philadelphia, J.B. Lippincott, 1984.)

Smith's Fracture

A Smith's fracture is a complete fracture within the distal inch of the radius, however, with palmar and proximal displacement of the distal fragment.

Barton's Fracture

Confusion arises when one tries to define a Barton's fracture. Barton, in his original article,[3] describes a "subluxation of the wrist consequent to a fracture through the articular surface of the carpal extremity of the radius." The controversy in his day was that this injury was frequently not recognized but rather diagnosed and treated as a wrist "sprain." Barton describes the mechanism of injury as a force met by the palm of the hand that drives the carpal bones against the dorsal edge of the articulating surface of the radius creating a dorsal fracture and subluxation of the carpus. He then says, "[rarely a] fracture of similar character occurs on the *palmar* side of the radius from the application of force on the back of the hand."[3] Thus, one may describe a dorsal Barton's fracture or a palmar Barton's fracture rather than inaccurately coin the term a *"reverse" Barton's fracture*. Until the day comes when we drop eponyms from the scientific language, we need at least to agree on what we are describing.

PATHOMECHANICS

The injury produced depends on the position of the wrist, the magnitude and direction of force, and the physical properties of the bone. A fall on the outstretched hand with the wrist in 40° to 90° of dorsiflexion will produce a distal radius fracture with dorsal displacement.[16] The radius probably first fractures in tension on its palmar surface followed by compression on the

dorsal surface, resulting in dorsal comminution. The lunate in particular can exert a compressive force on the distal radius, producing a so-called "die punch" fracture.[41] The ulnar styloid fracture component of the Colles' fracture results from a force transmitted through an intact triangular fibrocartilage complex.

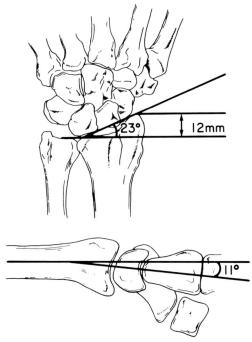

FIGURE 98-2. Measurement of normal average radial angulation, radial length, and palmar angulation. (Szabo, R.M., and Weber, S.C.: Comminuted Intra-Articular Fractures of the Distal Radius. Clin. Orthop. Rel. Res. in press.)

Fractures of the distal radius with palmar displacement are attributed to more than one mechanism of injury. Smith[42] claimed this injury results from a fall on the back of the flexed hand. This mechanism of injury is not always implicated, but rather many of these fractures also result from a fall on the outstretched extended hand. A fall with the forearm in supination followed by pronation around a fixed extended wrist may in fact be the more common mechanism of injury.[12,50]

Radial styloid fractures result from an avulsion (tensile) force generated through the palmar radiocarpal ligaments. Careful evaluation of other ligamentous injuries (i.e., perilunate dislocations with or without spontaneous reduction) should be given to the patient with a radial styloid fracture.

CLASSIFICATIONS

Several classifications exist for distal radius fractures.[16,18,32,50] However, since there is such a great variation in the fracture types, no simple classification can be relied on either to guide optimal treatment or be of prognostic value.

Frykman (Colles')

Frykman[16] introduced in 1967 a comprehensive classification of the Colles' type fractures based on the extent of involvement of the articular surface of the radiocarpal and distal radioulnar joints. Type I is an extra-articular radial fracture; type II, an extra-articular radial fracture with an ulna fracture; type III, an intra-articular fracture of the radiocarpal joint without an ulna fracture; type IV, an intra-articular radial fracture with an ulna fracture; type V, a fracture of the radioulnar joint; type VI, a fracture into the radioulnar joint with an ulnar fracture; type VII, an intra-articular fracture involving both radiocarpal and radioulnar joints; and type VIII, an intra-articular fracture involving both radiocarpal and radioulnar joints with an ulnar fracture.

Thomas (Smith's)

Thomas[50] has further classified Smith fractures: type I, a transverse distal radial fracture with palmar and proximal displacement; type II, a palmar-lip fracture of the distal radius with dislocation of the carpus (a palmar Barton's fracture); type III, an oblique fracture of the distal radius and tilted palmarly.

When evaluating authors' results and recommendations for treatment, the reader is urged to analyze which *types* of fractures are being discussed in any given series.

TREATMENT

General Principles

Treatment begins after careful examination of the patient. Sensibility is monitored in the alert individual with particular attention given to the status of the median nerve. If decreased median nerve function is found in the presence of a swollen wrist, carpal canal pressures are measured and used to distinguish median nerve contusion from an acute compressive neu-

ropathy. The patient with a median nerve contusion may be observed while immediate operative decompression is recommended for the acute carpal tunnel syndrome.[19] Next, the radiographs are analyzed, and the direction of displacement, degree of shortening and comminution, articular involvement, and ipsilateral carpal injuries are determined.

The best results are achieved with anatomic restoration and healing of the fracture; therefore the goal of treatment is to obtain and maintain anatomic position. This goal must be met without compromising nerve function or digital motion.

Most minimally displaced, noncomminuted distal radius fractures are well managed with closed reduction and immobilization in mild flexion (10° to 20°) and ulnar deviation (15°) followed by early mobilization. This group includes Frykman type I and II and Smith type I and III fractures. Immobilization in both pronation[5,31] and supination[14,39,40] have been advocated empirically, but no significance in results has been demonstrated in prospective trials comparing the two.[40,51,52] As the hand is more functional in a neutral or slightly pronated position, this is probably the preferred position for immobilization. Reduction is performed by traction to the hand either manually or with Chinese finger traps and countertraction to the humerus with the elbow flexed. The displacement is reduced gently after disimpaction of the fracture. Initial immobilization is maintained with above-elbow dorsal and palmar plaster slabs in the position previously mentioned.

Sarmiento et al.[39,40] have reported improved early results with cast-bracing for Colles' fractures; however, others have demonstrated no anatomic or functional advantage to this form of treatment.[46] I have used plaster, as it is more readily available and easy to work with. The plaster splints are well molded so that three-point pressure is applied to maintain reduction. The plaster is trimmed just proximal to the proximal palmar wrist crease and around the base of the thumb to allow full finger flexion and thumb opposition. Radiographs are taken after reduction and at frequent intervals over the next few weeks. When swelling decreases, the splints may become loose and need to be replaced. Usually, after 3 to 4 weeks, the elbow is set free and immobilization of the wrist is continued for a total of 6 weeks. Gentle wrist exercises begin, and the patient wears a removable palmar splint for an additional few weeks.

The comminuted displaced distal radius fracture offers a greater treatment challenge. The majority of authors agree that the results of treatment correlate directly with restoration of normal anatomy.[1,2,7,9,15,16,18,20–23,25,28,35,41,48,49] Two general techniques have been advocated to manage these injuries: percutaneous pinning, and traction maintained by transfixing pins either incorporated in plaster or with an external fixation device.

Percutaneous Pinning

Percutaneous pinning has been tried in many ways with a variety of implants.[4,6,11,17,30,37,38,41,43–45] This technique is limited to those fractures in which anatomic reduction can be obtained by traction and where no more than two intra-articular fragments are present.

I prefer a technique similar to that described by Clancy.[6] After fracture reduction is obtained and checked with a C-arm recorder, insert two crossed 0.062 inch smooth Kirschner wires percutaneously with a wire driver. Introduce the first wire at the radial styloid between the first and second dorsal wrist extensor compartments at a 45° angle with the long axis of the radius and 10° dorsally. Engage the Kirschner wire into the ulnar cortex of the proximal radius and go no further. Palpate the radial artery in the anatomic snuff box and avoid it. Introduce the second Kirschner wire between the fourth and fifth dorsal wrist extensor compartments, starting at the ulnar corner of the distal radius, avoiding the semicircular notch. Direct this wire 45° to the long axis of the radius and 30° palmarly, and insert it into the radial cortex of the proximal radius, but go no further. Under fluoroscopy, check the stability of the fracture, quality of reduction, and position of the Kirschner wires (Fig. 98-3).

Cut both Kirschner wires below the skin, or bend the wires and leave them superficial to the skin, and then place the extremity in well-padded, long-arm dorsal and palmar plaster splints. At 4 weeks after surgery, convert this form of immobilization into a below-elbow cast, maintaining the wrist in neutral position. Remove the pins at 6 to 8 weeks, and continue immobilization with a below-elbow cast for an additional 2 weeks.

Sometimes this technique will produce distraction of the fracture fragments, and union will be delayed. We have seen late recurrence of deformity by early mobilization, and therefore, continue protection of the wrist until the fracture is clinically and radiographically healed.

External Fixation

If the articular surface of the radius is comminuted into more than two fragments, I have adopted the use of external fixation.[9,20,21,29,53] While pins and plaster have been the main form of treatment for those fractures that cannot be held reduced by plaster alone,[5,7,10,23,24,26,41,47] external fixation has the advan-

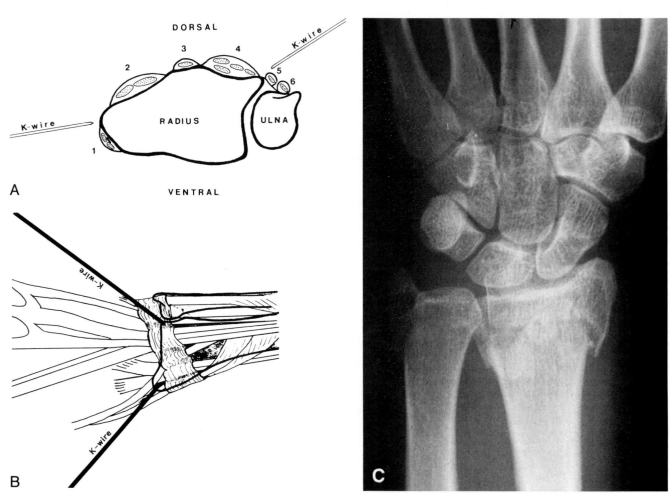

FIGURE 98-3. Technique for percutaneous Kirschner wire fixation of Colles' fractures. (*A*) Schematic cross section of the distal parts of the radius and ulna, demonstrating the extensor canals and the starting points for both Kirschner wires. (*B*) Dorsal view of the wrist, showing correct placement and orientation of both Kirschner wires for insertion into the distal part of the radius while avoiding the extensor tendons. (*C* and *D*) Anteroposterior and lateral radiographs of distal radius fracture suitable for percutaneous pinning. (*E* and *F*) Postoperative radiographs demonstrating anatomic reduction and proper fixation. (*A* and *B* from Clancy, G.J.: Percutaneous Kirschner Wire Fixation of Colles' Fractures. J. Bone Joint Surg. [Am] **66:**1008, 1984.)

tages of being adjustable should fracture displacement occur, and avoids the complications of circumferential plaster. External fixation relies on the principle of "ligamentotaxis," where a distraction force applied to the carpus aligns the fracture fragments via intact ligaments. DePalma[11] has shown in Colles' fracture created in the laboratory that disruption to the carpal ligaments is rare. As some authors have gained experience with open reduction of distal radius fractures, however, injury to these soft tissues has often been noted.[31] Distraction with external fixation will frequently improve length and alignment; however intra-articular displacement may be increased and palmar tilt is often not restored. In selected cases where traction restores length and intra-articular alignment, I use external fixation as the definitive treatment (Fig. 98-4).

When intra-articular fragments do not reduce with traction alone, I prefer to perform open reduction and internal fixation of the main fragments most commonly through a dorsal approach to obtain restoration of the articular surface. The previously applied external fixator then functions as a neutralization device (Fig. 98-5).

Smooth Kirschner wires are used for supplemental fixation, avoiding the extensive dissection and periosteal stripping required to fix the fracture with a plate. External fixation is maintained for 8 to 10 weeks, after which protected range of motion exercises are started. If additional internal fixation has been used, I usually remove the pins a few weeks before removing the external fixation device.

Several commercially available external fixation frames are available, each with small advantages over one another. In general, two threaded 3-mm half pins are inserted distally and proximally in the following manner. Make a longitudinal skin incision over the proximal half of the index metacarpal along its radial aspect. Dissect the subcutaneous tissues bluntly, and retract to avoid the small branches of the radial nerve. Use a 2-mm drill to penetrate the proximal cortex of the index metacarpal at its metaphyseal flare, passing through the fibers of the extensor carpi radialis longus tendon insertion.

Insert the first pin by hand through this hole in the index metacarpal, and go into the base of the long finger metacarpal but not beyond this point. Insert a second pin parallel to the first in a similar fashion with the aid of a guide or the distal portion of the external fixation frame (this technique will vary, depending on which external fixation frame is chosen). The depth of penetration of the second pin should be no further than the ulnar cortex of the index metacarpal.

Make a 3-cm longitudinal skin incision along the midradial aspect of the radius, beginning about 10-cm from the distal wrist crease. Once again dissect the subcutaneous tissues

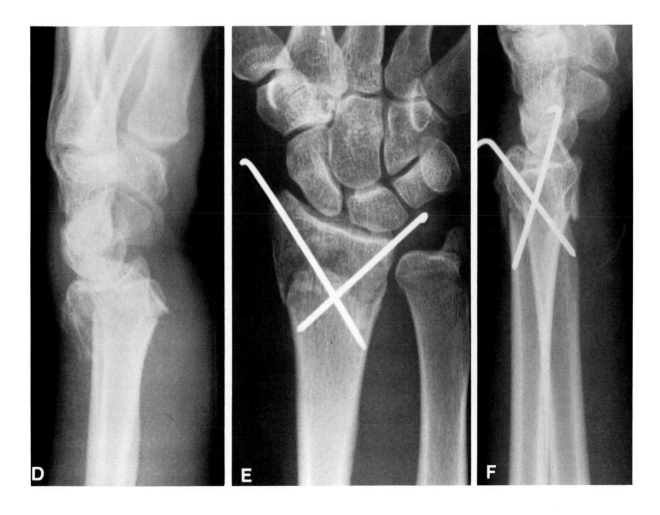

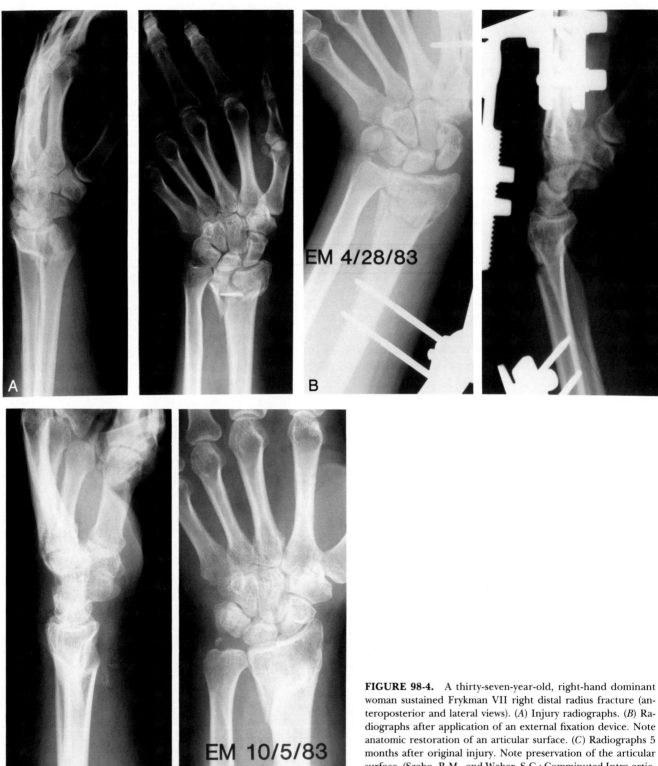

FIGURE 98-4. A thirty-seven-year-old, right-hand dominant woman sustained Frykman VII right distal radius fracture (anteroposterior and lateral views). (*A*) Injury radiographs. (*B*) Radiographs after application of an external fixation device. Note anatomic restoration of an articular surface. (*C*) Radiographs 5 months after original injury. Note preservation of the articular surface. (Szabo, R.M., and Weber, S.C.: Comminuted Intra-articular Fractures of the Distal Radius. Clin. Orthop. Rel. Res. in press.)

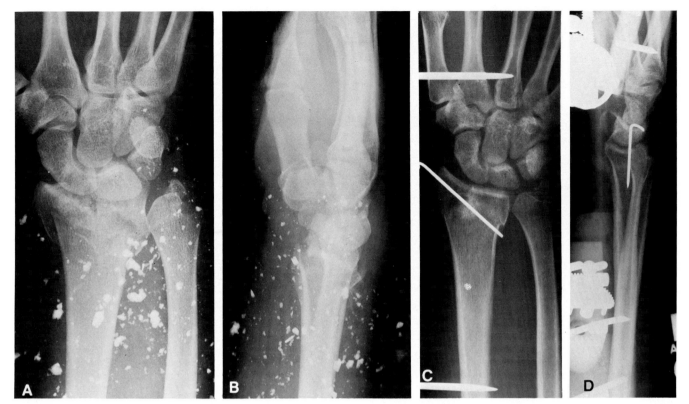

FIGURE 98-5. Comminuted distal radius fracture sustained in car accident with metal particles imbedded in the skin. (*A* and *B*) Preoperative radiographs, anteroposterior and lateral views. (*C* and *D*) Postoperative radiographs, anteroposterior and lateral views, demonstrating application of external fixation with supplemental percutaneous pin fixation. The external fixation device used in this case was a WristJack.

bluntly, and protect the sensory branch of the radial nerve. Retract the abductor pollicis longus and extensor pollicis brevis dorsally. Use a 2-mm drill to penetrate the radial cortex of the radius at the level of the insertion of the pronator teres. Hand drill a 3-mm threaded half pin into this hole, while aiming at the ulnar shaft until it penetrates the ulna cortex of the radius.

Insert a second pin distal and parallel to the first with the aid of a guide or the proximal portion of the external fixation frame. Close skin incisions loosely, and apply sterile dressings to the wounds. Apply the external fixation frame loosely.

Perform fracture reduction with usual techniques, either with an assistant or the use of Chinese finger traps. Tighten the external fixator.

Obtain anteroposterior and lateral radiographs to confirm proper position of the fixation pins, as well as alignment of the fracture. Final adjustments can be made with the fixator. However, if alignment cannot be obtained, open reduction and additional internal fixation should be considered. Further incisions and pin placement will be dictated by the fracture fragments that do not align with distraction alone.

Do not forget the distal radioulnar joint. If the distal radioulnar joint is severely comminuted or the distal ulna is dorsally subluxed, a long-arm plaster splint maintaining the wrist in supination may be needed for additional immobilization.

At the time of this writing, I am evaluating a new external fixation device called the WristJack (developed by Dr. John M. Agee, 77 Scripps Drive, Sacramento, California, 95825). Its mechanics permit independent adjustment of length, fracture alignment in the lateral and anteroposterior plane, and the position of the wrist in the flexion–extension plane. Distraction and flexion have a detrimental effect on the functional position of the hand, creating excess tension forces on the extensor tendons and resulting in a "clawing" of the hand (an intrinsic minus or actually an extrinsic extensor plus position). Clawing of the fingers is associated with hand stiffness. This observation, along with the fact that it is more difficult to rehabilitate the hand when the wrist is in the flexed position, has led to the development of the WristJack, which allows for Colles' fracture fixation with the wrist in the extended position. It is my observation that the WristJack may prove to be a real contribution to those of us who struggle with this fracture. A multicenter study is in progress in order to evaluate its potential.

Internal Fixation

Open reduction and plate fixation is reserved for managing the displaced, intra-articular distal radius fracture with palmar dislocation of the carpus (Smith fracture, type II) (Fig. 98-6). Experience has shown that this fracture seldom is stable. Although acceptable reduction can often be obtained by closed

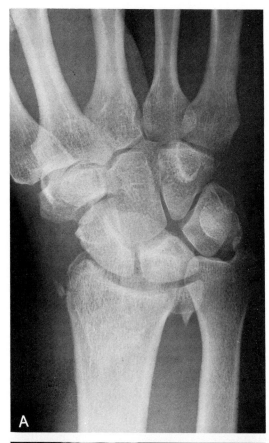

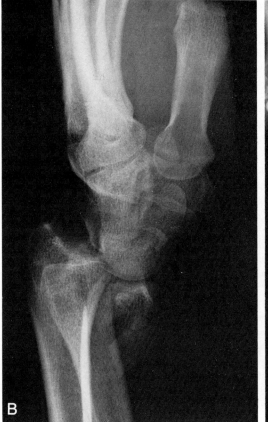

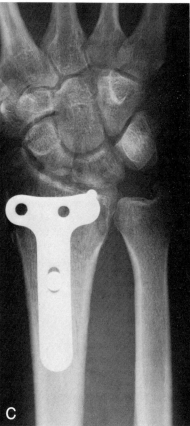

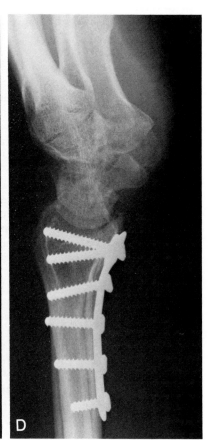

FIGURE 98-6. (*A* and *B*) Comminuted Smith type II distal radius fracture, anteroposterior and lateral preoperative radiographs. (*C* and *D*) Anteroposterior and lateral radiographs demonstrating postoperative reduction and fixation with a palmar T-plate.

means, redisplacement of the fracture is common. There are two surgical approaches to the distal radius that are useful to apply a plate palmarly. They are described here as techniques A and B.

Technique A

Make an anterior incision, starting at the distal wrist crease along the radial border of the flexor carpi radialis tendon and extend it 6 to 8 cm proximally. Identify the flexor carpi radialis tendon and the radial artery. Incise the deep fascia between the flexor carpi radialis and radial artery. Divide the pronator quadratus at its radial insertion. Insert retractors on the ulnar and radial aspects of the radius, and analyze the fracture pattern. Select a small fragment T-plate that will fit the width of the distal radius. Determine the length of the plate with respect to the proximal extension of the fracture so that the final result will provide stable internal fixation. Fix the plate first to the proximal fragment. The fracture is reduced by the buttress effect of the plate. If the distal fragments are large, additional fixation is obtained with cancellous screws through the horizontal holes in the plate. Obtain radiographs to confirm the fracture reduction and the position of the internal fixation device. Reattach the pronator quadratus, and close the tissues in layers.

Technique B

Technique B utilizes a modified carpal tunnel incision. This incision allows extension into the carpal tunnel should release be necessary and avoids the palmar cutaneous branch of the median nerve and radial artery, which are vulnerable in technique A.

Make an incision paralleling the ulnar crease, cross the distal wrist crease in an ulnar direction, and then curve back to the midline. Extend the incision 6 to 8 cm proximally from the distal wrist crease. Split the fascia proximal to the flexor retinaculum medial to the tendon of the palmaris longus. Identify and tag the median nerve. Incise the fascia and, if necessary, the flexor retinaculum (transverse carpal ligament) along the ulnar border of the median nerve. Retract the median nerve, palmaris longus, flexor pollicis longus, and flexor carpi radialis radially, and the flexor digitorium superficialis and flexor digitorium profundus ulnarly. Insert the T-plate and complete the procedure as described in technique A.

After surgery, the extremity is placed in a bulky plaster-reinforced compression dressing until suture removal. Immobilization continues for a total of 5 to 6 weeks in a short-arm cast. The wrist is placed in neutral to 15° of dorsiflexion, not in palmar flexion, particularly if the carpal tunnel is opened.

COMPLICATIONS

Failure to obtain anatomic reduction can result in secondary deformity of the distal radius, midcarpal instability, and arthritis.[28,49] Median nerve damage may occur in the form of acute and late carpal tunnel syndrome, contusion, or stretch. Ulnar nerve damage has also been reported. Radial nerve damage occurs with the placement of external fixation pins percutane-

ously and can be avoided by a skin incision and proper identification of the sensory branch. A painful, stiff hand and reflex sympathetic dystrophy are best prevented by minimizing swelling, starting digital motion immediately, not immobilizing in extreme positions, and avoiding constrictive dressings. The rate of complications related to fixation pins is as high as 60% in some series.[53] Pin loosening is the most common; however metacarpal fractures, pin track infections, and intrinsic muscle tie down have all been experienced. Distal radioulnar joint dissociation and arthritis may require further reconstructive surgery to restore wrist motion (pronation–supination) and eliminate pain. Flexor tendon adhesions and tendon ruptures[54] (particularly extensor pollicis longus ruptures)[13] are also known complications. Although the preceding list is not complete, it represents the majority of those complications that I have encountered.

RECONSTRUCTIVE SURGERY FOLLOWING FRACTURES OF THE DISTAL RADIUS

Reconstructive surgery following fractures of the distal radius including operations directed at correcting the distal radioulnar joint problem, carpal tunnel release, radiocarpal or limited intercarpal arthrodesis, or tendon transfers or reconstructions are described elsewhere in this textbook. Corrective osteotomy of the distal radius is not, however, and is the subject of this discussion.

Radial osteotomy is considered when the dorsal angulation of the distal radius is more than 25° and when there is significant shortening (6 mm) of the radius. This amount of deformity will usually result in a symptomatic patient. Contraindications to osteotomy include advanced degenerative changes in the wrist, significant intra-articular incongruency, fixed carpal malalignment, or a stiff hand. The surgical technique used is that described by Diego L. Fernandez[15] (Fig. 98-7).

Careful preoperative planning includes examination of the radiographs of both the affected and the normal wrist. Particular attention is directed at the ulnar variance in order to restore the normal anatomic relationship to the distal radioulnar joint. The osteotomy must correct the palmar tilt in the sagittal plane, the ulnar tilt in the frontal plane, and rotational deformities in the horizontal plane.

Make a 10-cm dorsoradial incision parallel to the radius beginning 2 cm distal to Lister's tubercle. Expose the radius subperiosteally between the extensor carpiradialis brevis and extensor digitorium comminus tendons. Mark the osteotomy site with an osteotome (about 2.5 cm proximal to the wrist joint).

Insert a 0.045-cm Kirschner wire perpendicular to the radius 4 cm proximal to the osteotomy site. Insert a second 0.045-cm Kirschner wire into the distal radius so that it subtends an angle with the first Kirschner wire that is 5° more than the amount of deformity (see Fig. 98-7).

Make the osteotomy parallel to the joint surface while protecting the soft tissues with subperiosteal retractors. This may be facilitated by placing a fine Kirschner wire along the articular surface of the radius to act as a guide. Open the osteotomy dorsally until the two Kirschner wires are parallel to each other

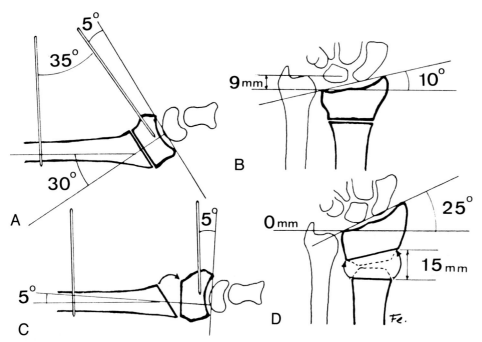

FIGURE 98-7. Preoperative planning of the osteotomy. (*A*) For correction in the sagittal plane, the dorsal tilt (30° in this patient) is measured between the perpendicular to the joint surface and the long axis of the radius on the lateral radiograph. The Kirschner wires are introduced so that they subtend the angle that corresponds to the dorsal tilt plus 5 degrees of volar tilt (30° + 5° = 35° in this patient). (*B*) After opening the osteotomy by the correct amount, the Kirschner wires lie parallel to each other. (*C*) For correction in the frontal plane, shortening (9 mm in this patient) is measured between the head of the ulna and the ulnar corner of the radius on the anteroposterior radiograph. The lines for the measurement are perpendicular to the long axis of the radius. The ulnar tilt is reduced to 10° in this patient. (*D*) In order to restore the ulnar tilt to normal (average, 25°), the osteotomy is opened more on the dorsoradial than on the dorsoulnar side. (Fernandez, D.L.: Correction of Post-Traumatic Wrist Deformity in Adults by Osteotomy, Bone Grafting, and Internal Fixation. J. Bone Joint Surg. **64-A:**1169, 1982.)

(a small Lamina spreader is useful for this maneuver). Open the osteotomy on the radial side to correct radial shortening. Rotate the distal fragment to correct any pronation or supination deformity. Shape a corticocancellous iliac crest graft into a trapezoid to fill the gap created by the osteotomy. Pack the area further with cancellous graft material.

Maintain the reduction with oblique, crossed Kirschner wires and obtain radiograph in both anteroposterior and lateral planes. Obtain rigid fixation by applying a contoured T-plate to the dorsum of the radius; then remove the Kirschner wires (this step is optional; it is acceptable to use only the Kirschner wires for fixation, however postoperative immobilization until union will have to be maintained). Lister's tubercle may be removed for better fit of the plate. Examine the distal radioulnar joint clinically and radiographically. If needed, then perform a Lowenstein or Darrach procedure. (See Chapter 97, on distal radial ulnar joint). Close the tissues in layers, making certain there is good coverage of the plate.

After surgery, immobilize the wrist in a long-arm bulky plaster-reinforced dressing for 2 weeks. At 2 weeks remove the sutures, and begin protective active range of motion exercises. The osteotomy usually is healed in 8 to 12 weeks, at which time unrestricted activity is allowed.

For correction of distal radius fractures with palmar tilt (Smith fractures) a palmar opening wedge osteotomy is performed by an approach identical to that described above for the acute care of Smith type II fractures (technique B).

REFERENCES

1. Anderson, R., and O'Neil, G.: Comminuted Fractures of the Distal End of the Radius. Surg. Gynecol. Obstet. **78:**434, 1944.
2. Bacorn, R.W., and Kurtzke, J.F.: Colles' Fracture. A Study of Two Thousand Cases from the New York State Workmen's Compensation Board. J. Bone Joint Surg. **35-A:**643, 1953.
3. Barton, J.R.: Views and Treatment of an Important Injury to the Wrist. Med. Examiner **1:**365, 1838.
4. Brennwald, J., and Pfeiffer, K.: Radiusfraktur Loco Classico. Ther. Umsch. **37:**743, 1980.
5. Carother, R.G., and Boyd, F.J.: Thumb Traction Technic for Reduction of Colles' Fracture. Arch. Surg. **58:**848, 1949.
6. Clancy, G.J.: Percutaneous Kirschner Wire Fixation of Colles' Fractures. J. Bone Joint Surg. **66-A:**1008, 984.
7. Cole, M.M., and Obletz, B.E.: Comminuted Fractures of the Distal End of the Radius Treated by Skeletal Transfixion in Plaster Cast. J. Bone Joint Surg. **48-A:**931, 1966.
8. Colles, A.: On the Fracture of the Carpal Extremity of the Radius. Edinb. Med. Surg. J. **10:**181, 1814.
9. Cooney, W.P., Linscheid, R.L., and Dobyns, J.H.: External Pin

Fixation for Unstable Colles' Fractures. J. Bone Joint Surg. **61-A:**840, 1979.

10. Dabezies, E.J., Chuinard, R.G., and Kitziger, R.F.: Distraction Pinning for Radial Metaphysis Fractures. Orthopaedics **1:**294, 1978.

11. DePalma, A.F.: Comminuted Fractures of the Distal End of the Radius Treated by Ulnar Pinning. J. Bone Joint Surg. **34-A:**651, 1952.

12. Ellis, J.: Smith's and Barton's Fractures: A Method of Treatment. J. Bone Joint Surg. **47-B:**724, 1965.

13. Engkvist, O., and Lundborg, G.: Rupture of the Extensor Pollicis Longus Tendon After Fracture of the Lower End of the Radius—A Clinical and Microangiographic Study. Hand **2:**76, 1979.

14. Fahey, J.H.: Fractures and Dislocations About the Wrist. Surg. Clin. North Am. **2:**19, 1957.

15. Fernandez, D.L.: Correction of Post-Traumatic Wrist Deformity in Adults by Osteotomy, Bone-Grafting, and Internal Fixation. J. Bone Joint Surg. **64-A:**1164, 1982.

16. Frykman, G.: Fractures of the Distal End of the Radius, Including Sequelae-Shoulder, Hand, Finger Syndrome, Disturbance in the Distal Radioulnar Joint and Impairment of Nerve Function. Acta Orthop. Scand. [Suppl.] **108:**27, 1967.

17. Garner, R.W., and Grimes, D.W.: Percutaneous Pinning of Displaced Fractures of the Distal Radius. Orthop. Rev. **6:**87, 1977.

18. Gartland, J.J., and Werley, C.W.: Evaluation of Healed Colles' Fractures. J. Bone Joint Surg. **33-A:**895, 1951.

19. Gelberman, R.H., Szabo, R.M., and Mortensen, W.W.: Carpal Tunnel Pressures and Wrist Position in Patients with Colles' Fractures. J. Trauma **24:**747, 1984.

20. Gjengedal, E.: Compound Fracture of the Distal End of the Radius Treated with Hoffman's Method of External Fixation. Tidsskr. Nor Laegeforen. **99:**24, 1979.

21. Grana, W.A., and Kopta, J.A.: The Roger Anderson Device in the Treatment of Fractures of the Distal End of the Radius. J. Bone Joint Surg. **61-A:**1234, 1979.

22. Grana, W.A., and Randel, R.L.: Roger Anderson Device for Distal Radius Fractures. AORN J. **28:**1036, 1978.

23. Green, D.P.: Pins and Plaster Treatment of Comminuted Fractures of the Distal End of the Radius. J. Bone Joint Surg. **57-A:**304, 1975.

24. Hammond, G.: Comminuted Colles' Fracture. Am. J. Surg. **54:**617, 1949.

25. Hobart, M.H., and Kraft, G.L.: Malunited Colles' Fracture. Am. J. Surg. **53:**55, 1941.

26. Kain, T., Mandel, R.J., Snedden, H.E., et al.: Comminuted Distal Radius Fractures: Two Methods of Treatment. Clin. Orthop. **128:**369, 1977.

27. Kaplan, E.B., and Taleisnik, J.: The Wrist. *In* Spinner, M. (ed.): Kaplan's Functional and Surgical Anatomy of the Hand, 3rd ed. Philadelphia, J.P. Lippincott.

28. Knirk, J.L., and Jupiter, J.B.: Intra-Articular Fractures of the Distal End of the Radius in Young Adults. J. Bone Joint Surg. **68-A:**647, 1986.

29. Ledoux, R.A., Theibaut, A., and Van der Ghinst, M.: Bipolar Fixation of Fractures of the Distal End of the Radius. Int. Orthop. **3:**89, 1979.

30. Lucas, G.L., and Sachtjen, K.M.: An Analysis of Hand Function in Patients with Colles' Fractures Treated by Rush Rod Fixation. Clin. Orthop. **155:**172, 1981.

31. Mayer, J.H.: Colles' Fracture. Br. J. Surg. **27:**629, 1940.

32. Melone, C.P.: Articular Fractures of the Distal Radius. Orthop Clin. North Am. **15:**217, 1984.

33. Mohanti, R.C., and Kar, N.: Study of Triangular Fibrocartilage of the Wrist Joint in Colles' Fracture. Injury **11:**321, 1979.

34. Morissy, R.T., and Nalebuff, E.A.: Distal Radial Fracture with Tendon Entrapment—A Case Report. Clin. Orthop. **124:**206, 1977.

35. Nigst, H.: Fractures of the Distal Radius in the Adult: Anatomy, Trauma Mechanisms, Fracture Types, and Typical Associated Injuries. Unfallheilkunde **82:**1, 1979.

36. Ravitch, M.: Dupuytren's Invention of the Mikulicz Enterotome with a Note on Eponyms. Perspect. Biol. Med. **22:**170, 1979.

37. Roth, B.: Experience with Percutaneous K-Wire Osteosynthesis in Distal Radius Fractures. Helv. Chir. Acta **44:**35, 1978.

38. Ruiz, G.R.: Percutaneous Pinning of Comminuted Colles' Fractures. Clin. Orthop. **155:**290, 1981.

39. Sarmiento, A., Pratt, G.W., Berry, N.C., et al.: Colles' Fractures—Functional Bracing in Supination. J. Bone Joint Surg. **57-A:**311, 1975.

40. Sarmiento, A., Zagorski, J.B., and Sinclair, W.F.: Functional Bracing of Colles' Fractures—A Prospective Study of Immobilization in Supination Versus Pronation. Clin. Orthop. **146:**175, 1980.

41. Scheck, M.: Long Term Follow-up of Treatment of Comminuted Fractures of the Distal End of the Radius by Transfixation With Kirschner Wires and Cast. J. Bone Joint Surg. **44-A:**337, 1962.

42. Smith, R.W.: A Treatise on Fractures in the Vicinity of Joints and on Certain Forms of Accidental and Congenital Dislocations. Dublin, Hodges and Smith, 1854.

43. Speed, J.S., and Knight, R.A.: The Treatment of Malunited Colles' Fractures. J. Bone Joint Surg. **27-A:**361, 1945.

44. Spira, E., and Weigl, K.: The Comminuted Fracture of the Distal End of the Radius. Reconstr. Surg. Traumatol. **11:**128, 1969.

45. Stein, A.H., and Katz, S.F.: Stabilization of Comminuted Fractures of the Distal Inch of the Radius: Percutaneous Pinning. Clin. Orthop. **108:**174, 1975.

46. Stewart, H.D., Innes, A.R., and Burke, F.D.: Functional Cast-Bracing for Colles' Fractures—A Comparison Between Cast-Bracing and Conventional Plaster Casts. J. Bone Joint Surg. **66-B:**749, 1984.

47. Suman, R.K.: Unstable Fractures of the Distal End of the Radius (Transfixion Pins and a Cast). Injury **15:**206, 1983.

48. Szabo, R.M., and Weber, S.C.: Comminuted Intra-Articular Fractures of the Distal Radius. Clin. Orthop. in press.

49. Taleisnik, J., and Watson, H.K.: Mid Carpal Instability Caused by Fractures of the Distal Radius. J. Hand Surg. **9:**350, 1984.

50. Thomas, F.B.: Reduction of Smith's Fracture. J. Bone Joint Surg. **39-B:**463, 1957.

51. Van der Linden, W., and Ericson, R.: Colles' Fracture. How Should Its Displacement be Measured and How Should It be Immobilized? J. Bone Joint Surg. **63-A:**1285, 1981.

52. Wahlstrom, O.: Treatment of Colles' Fracture. A Prospective Comparison of Three Different Positions of Immobilization. Acta Orthop. Scand. **53:**225, 1982.

53. Weber, S.C., and Szabo, R.M.: The Severely Comminuted Distal Radius Fracture as an Unsolved Problem. J. Hand Surg. **11-A:**157, 1986.

54. Younger, C.P., and DeFiore, J.C.: Rupture of Flexor Tendons to the Fingers after a Colles' Fracture. J. Bone Joint Surg. **59-A:**828, 1977.

CHAPTER 99

Wrist and Intercarpal Arthrodesis

H. KIRK WATSON and
MICHAEL I. VENDER

In the past, treatment of carpal instabilities has entailed many forms of ligament reconstruction,[17,39] but with a few exceptions, these reconstructions have not provided lasting, good results. Degenerative arthritis of the wrist has been treated with proximal row carpectomy[19,38] and total wrist arthrodesis.[6,18,34,35] Proximal row carpectomy results in loss of power and depends on maintenance of the noncongruous radiocapitate articulation. Total wrist arthrodesis results in total loss of motion and is rarely indicated. This chapter emphasizes the role of intercarpal arthrodesis (limited wrist arthrodesis) in the treatment of wrist instabilities and degenerative disorders.

The elimination of pain by joint fusion is a well-known, readily accepted concept.[4,41,58] In the case of certain intercarpal arthrodeses, the benefits of fusion can be obtained with a very acceptable sacrifice of motion. When two or more carpal bones are fused, there is a compensatory increase in motion between the unfused bones. This increased motion probably is achieved by increased stretching of the capsule and is not fully obtained until 9 to 12 months postfusion.

Congenital fusions of most adjacent carpal bones have been described and provide excellent examples of adaptability with good motion and durability.[8,31,40,65] These are asymptomatic and do not undergo late degenerative changes.

INTERCARPAL ARTHRODESIS FOR DEGENERATIVE DISORDERS

Over 90% of cases of degenerative arthritis of the wrist fit into three patterns.[55,58] The most common pattern is termed *SLAC wrist*—scaphoid-lunate advanced collapse. This pattern is caused by abnormal articular alignment between the scaphoid and radius with subsequent degeneration of the radioscaphoid joint.[55] Carpal collapse follows, and the capitate migrates proximally. Shear load in the capitate-lunate articulation eventually leads to destruction. Approximately 55% of cases of naturally occurring degenerative wrist arthritis follow the SLAC pattern.

The second pattern is triscaphe degenerative change, between the trapezium, trapezoid, and distal scaphoid. This pattern comprises 24% of arthritis.[11]

The third pattern is a combination of the first two, SLAC plus triscaphe arthritis. This is seen in 10% of cases.

The remaining cases consist predominantly of degeneration between the distal ulna and lunate and the radiolunate and lunate-triquetral joints.

Congenital, incomplete separation of carpal bones can lead to arthrosis resembling degenerative arthritis. This occurs most commonly at the lunate-triquetral joint and also occurs between the scaphoid and trapezium.[45,65]

Anatomy

The radioscaphoid joint is the site of initial pathology in about 70% of cases of degenerative arthritis of the wrist (cases of SLAC and SLAC plus triscaphe arthritis), while nearly all cases involve the scaphoid in one of its articulations.

The susceptibility of the radioscaphoid joint to degenerative arthritis is based on the shape of the scaphoid's proximal articular surface and the shape of its corresponding articular surface on the distal radius. The scaphoid is oval or elliptical proximally. The radius has two articular fossae: a corresponding elliptical fossa for the scaphoid, which narrows in dorsal-palmar measurement as it approaches the radial styloid, and a more spherical one for the lunate (Fig. 99-1).

In the normal wrist, motion between the radius and scaphoid is allowed only in directions that maintain large articular congruity. In pathologic conditions, such as rotary subluxation and fractures of the scaphoid, the scaphoid is not maintained in its correct alignment and the articular surfaces are no longer congruous. This can be visualized if one compares the proximal articular surface of the scaphoid to a teaspoon that sits in a second teaspoon, representing the scaphoid fossa of the radius (Fig. 99-2). The handle of the scaphoid spoon lies just dorsal and radial to the position of the relaxed thumb. Flexion–extension and all wrist motion occurs with full-spoon contact. If the scaphoid spoon handle is swung in front of the palm, the contact surface of the spoons is changed. The scaphoid spoon comes to lie on the radial edge of the radius spoon. This concentrated load along the contacting edge causes rapid destruction of the radioscaphoid joint, starting radially and progressing proximally to involve the entire radioscaphoid joint.

The joint between the radius and lunate is almost never involved in degenerative arthritis. The spherical shape of the joint ensures cartilage loading in a perpendicular manner, even in cases of large displacement of the lunate (e.g., palmar or dorsal intercalated segment instability). Cartilage can withstand great stress when loaded perpendicularly, while shear stresses may lead to destruction.

Scaphoid-Lunate Advanced Collapse Wrist

SLAC degeneration is most commonly seen following rotary subluxation and nonunion of the scaphoid. It is a predictable sequence of degenerative changes initially involving the radioscaphoid joint[55] (Fig. 99-3). As rotation of the scaphoid and radioscaphoid destruction progress, the capitate migrates proximally and radially on the capitate-lunate articulation. The capitate drives off the radial or dorsoradial portion of the distal lunate articular surface (at times wedging between the scaphoid and lunate), causing a cartilage shear stress with eventual destruction of the capitate-lunate joint. With further carpal collapse, hamate-lunate destruction is seen. This midcarpal phenomenon can occur with a silastic scaphoid in place.

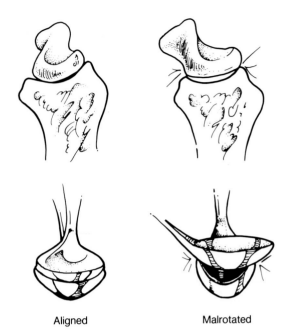

FIGURE 99-2. The proximal scaphoid and the elliptical fossa of the radius can be compared to two spoons. Normally, they are congruous, with even load distribution. With rotary subluxation of the scaphoid, the distal handle moves to a more palmar position with respect to the forearm, and the spoon surfaces malalign. Instead of congruous loading, there is high stress loading at the edges.

Reconstruction of the SLAC wrist is based on the fact that the radiolunate joint is highly resistant to degenerative change even in late, severe cases. The articulation of the lunate with radius is spherical in shape. The lunate can be moved palmarly or dorsally, radially or ulnarly, and the proximal articular surface of the lunate will remain perpendicularly loaded. Even with large displacement of the lunate into palmar intercalated segment instability (PISI) or dorsal intercalated segment instability (DISI), the radiolunate joint will be preserved.

By fusing the capitate-lunate joint, the central column assumes the load bearing (Fig. 99-4). The radiolunate joint takes the load, while the radioscaphoid joint is relatively unstressed. Addition of the hamate and triquetrum to the fusion enhances the healing of the arthrodesis but does not seem to change the eventual range of motion. The principal surgery, however, is the capitate-lunate arthrodesis with a silastic scaphoid prosthesis. In cases in which the silastic scaphoid had been left out, the resting wrist tends toward radial deviation. Following SLAC reconstruction there is often pain at the forced extremes of flexion extension for 2 years. However, the wrist will usually take full-load, and the patient can return to heavy labor without activity pain or postactivity ache.

There is a small number of patients in whom degenerative arthritis between the radius and scaphoid can be handled by a silastic scaphoid implant alone.[48] These are tight-ligamented people, and one must be certain that the capitate-lunate joint has normal ligamentous support, there is no tendency for ulnar shifting of the lunate, and there is no evidence of degenerative change between the capitate and lunate. During surgery, with the scaphoid removed, loading of the wrist should demonstrate that ligamentous support is strong and tight enough to prevent

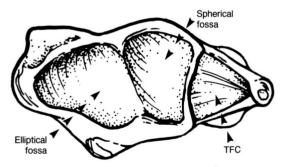

FIGURE 99-1. The end-on view of the distal radius and ulna shows the elliptical fossa for the scaphoid on the radius, and the spheroidal fossa for the lunate on the radius. The triangular fibrocartilage (TFC) contributes to the support of the lunate.

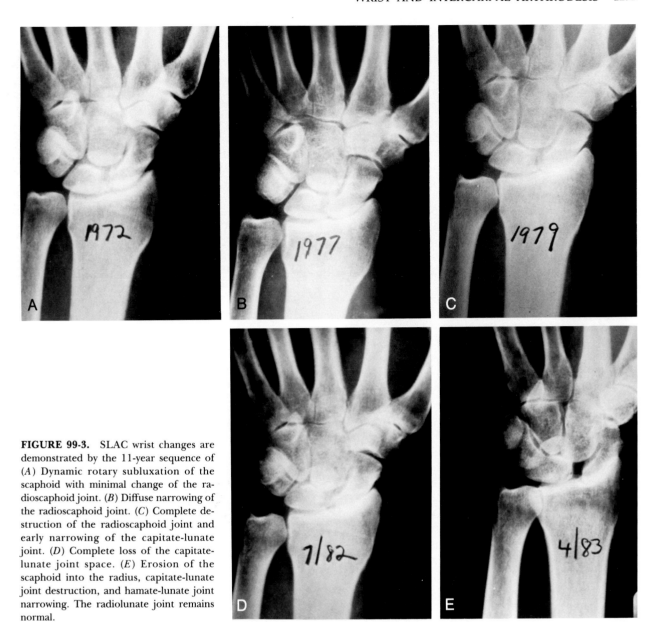

FIGURE 99-3. SLAC wrist changes are demonstrated by the 11-year sequence of (A) Dynamic rotary subluxation of the scaphoid with minimal change of the radioscaphoid joint. (B) Diffuse narrowing of the radioscaphoid joint. (C) Complete destruction of the radioscaphoid joint and early narrowing of the capitate-lunate joint. (D) Complete loss of the capitate-lunate joint space. (E) Erosion of the scaphoid into the radius, capitate-lunate joint destruction, and hamate-lunate joint narrowing. The radiolunate joint remains normal.

the capitate from being driven off the radial side of the lunate. This rare but adequate support should prevent particulate synovitis.

Particulate Synovitis

It is well recognized in the last several years that a destructive process known as particulate synovitis can occur following implantation of silicone material in the bones of the hands and wrist. The pathogenesis appears to be the shedding of finely ground particles of silicone that are picked up by the synovium and have a high propensity for the development of cysts in the bones that share that synovial cavity. We have seen cases of silicone scaphoid replacement with particulate synovitis and cyst formation developing only in the hamate. More typically, however, the particulate synovitis involves all of the bones or most of the bones of the communicating synovium that encompass the silicone replacement. It was our contention for

other reasons that silicone could not be placed in the load column of the wrist without providing a means for load transport through bone. Hence, over the past 15 years, we have never implanted a silicone lunate without also doing a triscaphe limited-wrist arthrodesis. Fortuitously, this seems to prevent particulate synovitis. At least we have not seen a case of particulate synovitis, even long-standing, where a means for load transference through normal bone and cartilage has been provided. Therefore, it is probably valid to state that silicone should not be subjected to significant loading, and silicone should not be subjected to shear force motion. If these rules are followed, silicone can maintain a useful place in our armamentarium.

Triscaphe Degenerative Arthritis

Collapse of the radial column, as in rotary subluxation of the scaphoid, brings the trapezium and trapezoid onto the dorsum of the scaphoid neck, just proximal to the scaphoid's distal

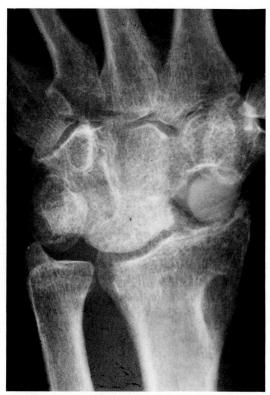

FIGURE 99-4. The radiograph of a SLAC wrist reconstruction demonstrates fusion of the capitate, hamate, triquetrum, and lunate. The scaphoid prosthesis acts as an unloaded spacer. The radiolunate joint is normal.

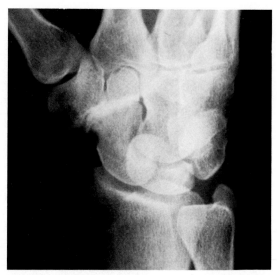

FIGURE 99-5. Sclerosis highlights the degenerative changes in the triscaphe joint.

articular cartilage. Changes in the triscaphe joint are seen when operating for rotary subluxation of the scaphoid (Fig. 99-5). Treatment is by triscaphe arthrodesis (between trapezium, trapezoid, and scaphoid).[7,11,57,59]

Combination of SLAC and Triscaphe Degenerative Arthritis

Combination of these two conditions is usually treated by SLAC reconstruction.[55] The scaphoid replacement of the SLAC reconstruction treats the degenerative triscaphe joint. There are cases in which the triscaphe disease is severe and the changes of the radioscaphoid and capitate-lunate joints are not as severe. Triscaphe arthrodesis alone may suffice in these cases.

Triquetrum-Lunate Arthritis

Symptomatic degenerative change is infrequently noted between the lunate and triquetrum. Congenitally, the lunate and triquetrum commonly fail to completely separate, leaving a coalition proximally, often with inadequate cartilage.[45] This leads to a localized degenerative change, usually in a young patient, and responds nicely to an arthrodesis between the lunate and the triquetrum (Fig. 99-6).

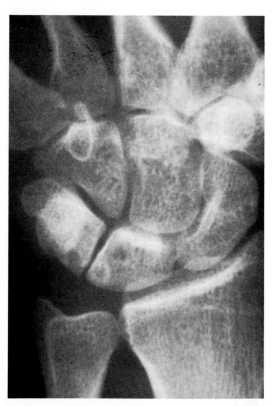

FIGURE 99-6. Congenital incomplete separation of the lunate and triquetrum demonstrates degenerative changes, including cyst formation in the proximal aspect of the joint.

Scaphoid Nonunion

Scaphoid nonunion is a form of rotary subluxation of the scaphoid (see the section entitled "Rotary Subluxation of the Scaphoid" under instability problems), and when untreated progresses to the predictable pattern of SLAC wrist degenerative arthritis[25] (Fig. 99-7). The distal scaphoid fragment is devoid of its proximal tethers and rotates in the same manner as in rotary subluxation of the scaphoid. This causes incongruity in the articulation between the distal scaphoid fragment and the corresponding radial styloid articular surface. The earliest radiographic change is usually a pointing or sharpening of the radial styloid tip. The radiodistal scaphoid fragment joint narrows only to the level of the nonunion, and the shape of the radial styloid articular surface can change from concave to convex. Carpal collapse allows proximal migration of the capitate that drives off the radial or dorsoradial side of the lunate and the proximal scaphoid fragment. Further degeneration occurs between capitate and distal scaphoid fragment, and ultimately the hamate-lunate joint is destroyed.

The radioproximal scaphoid fragment joint is spared because the proximal fragment acts like a lunate. It is a spherical bone in the spherical ulnar portion of the radius' elliptical scaphoid fossa. Even in long-standing cases of nonunion, there is complete preservation of the radioproximal scaphoid fragment articular cartilage.

Wrists without arthritis are treated by fusion of the scaphoid fragments and/or intercarpal arthrodesis (see the section entitled "Scaphoid Nonunion" under instability problems). When early arthritis is limited to the distal aspect of the radioscaphoid joint, as seen by direct visualization, a radial styloidectomy can be performed at the time of scaphoid bone grafting. This eliminates the area of arthritis so the primary problem of the scaphoid nonunion alone can be addressed. Cases not amenable to treatment by the methods discussed are treated by SLAC reconstruction. As discussed under SLAC, excision of the scaphoid and replacement with a silastic prosthesis may be sufficient treatment in a small minority of patients.

Radiocarpal Arthrodesis

There are rare occasions when an isolated destruction of the radioscaphoid joint, or more commonly destruction of the radiolunate or radiolunate and scaphoid joints, is better handled by fusing the lunate or scaphoid or both to the radius. The wrist then functions on the midcarpal joint and will usually produce about 50° to 60° of total motion. It is mandatory that the distal articular surface of the scaphoid and lunate be in normal alignment and configuration with respect to all other carpals.

INTERCARPAL ARTHRODESIS FOR INSTABILITY PROBLEMS

Instability secondary to ligamentous injury is not an all-or-none phenomenon, but varies in degree according to the injury and the load applied.[12,14,23,26–28,33,49–51,62,64] Instability may be static

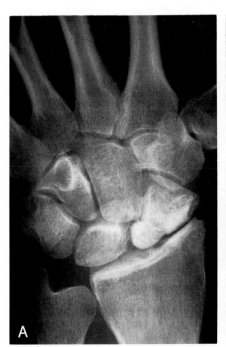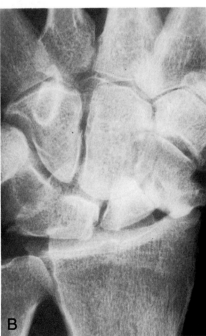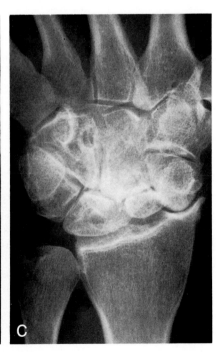

FIGURE 99-7. (*A*) Scaphoid nonunion develops narrowing of the radiodistal scaphoid fragment joint. (*B*) The scaphoid nonunion has developed a large osteophyte on the distal scaphoid fragment. There is destruction of the capitate-proximal scaphoid fragment joint. The radioscaphoid narrowing stops at the site of the nonunion. (*C*) The distal scaphoid fragment has eroded into the radius. Midcarpal joint destruction always follows destruction of the radiodistal scaphoid fragment joint. The radioulnate and radioproximal scaphoid fragment joints remain normal.

or dynamic. If all ligaments supporting a particular bone's position are ruptured, the bone will assume its "neutral anatomy" which is determined only by its shape and position (see "Anatomy" under instability problems). Radiographs demonstrate the instability and show displacement, abnormal radiocarpal and intercarpal angles, and change in the shapes of bones.[15,16,63] Static instability can be demonstrated on resting radiographs, stress radiographs, or cineradiography. Dynamic instability is not demonstrated by radiographic studies, but instead is a clinical diagnosis based on history and physical examination. In dynamic instability partial injury to ligaments can lead to instances when enough stability is present to maintain "normal anatomic" position. However, instability will occur when the wrist is stressed by demanding conditions, such as athletics or manual laboring.

Wrist instabilities result from trauma in which loads applied to either side of the wrist cause ligamentous disruptions and associated fractures. Depending on the patient's anatomy, the exact position of the wrist, and the direction of the stress, various structures will rupture.[29]

Radial side injuries, usually occurring with the wrist in dorsiflexion and the hand in supination, may enter between radius and scaphoid, and radius and lunate, causing rotary subluxation of the scaphoid. This disruption can continue between capitate and lunate and triquetrum, leading to perilunate dislocation. The radial injury could be a scaphoid fracture continuing ulnarward to become a transscaphoid perilunate dislocation. Radial styloid fractures can be part of a fracture-ligamentous injury.[43] Radial side injuries with rotary subluxation of the scaphoid are likely to progress to symptomatic degeneration.

Destructive forces that enter the ulnar side of the wrist are usually the result of pronation–flexion injuries and lead to tears of the ulnar sling mechanism, lunate-triquetrum and hamate-triquetrum instabilities, and injury to the triangular fibrocartilage. Ulnar side injuries, although symptomatic, seldom lead to degenerative arthritis.

Anatomy

Normal anatomy in the wrist is a loaded position, much like a jack-in-the-box, where ligaments serve to restrain carpals from moving in directions determined by the inclination of their articular surfaces. "Neutral anatomy" is the position the bones would assume based solely on shapes and slopes of articular surfaces, that is, with ligament constraints removed. For example, transection of all lunate ligaments releases the lunate to assume its "neutral anatomic position," which is palmar displacement with dorsal tilting, that is, the position of DISI.[20] Instability is a manifestation of the "neutral" versus "normal" anatomy principle.

Rotary Subluxation of the Scaphoid

Rotary subluxation of the scaphoid occurs following rupture of the ligaments that maintain the proximal pole of the scaphoid in its fossa on the radius. These are the radioscaphoid portion of the radioscaphoid lunate ligament, scaphoid-lunate interosseous ligament, and scaphoid attachment of the palmar radioscaphocapitate ligament. The loss of proximal scaphoid tethers

allows the scaphoid to assume a position of palmar flexion (as seen from a lateral view) and rotation.

As noted earlier, a continuation of the force across the wrist between the capitate-lunate and lunate-triquetrum and out through the ulnar sling mechanism will cause a perilunate dislocation. Perilunate dislocations are almost always accompanied by instability.

Static rotary subluxation of the scaphoid is easily diagnosed by the classic findings of a scaphoid-lunate gap; increased scaphoid-lunate angle, with or without dorsal intercalated segment instability; foreshortened scaphoid; and scaphoid ring sign. At times, radiographs will not be positive until stress views are taken.

Dynamic rotary subluxation of the scaphoid is diagnosed by history and physical examination. The most important historical finding is pain with activity, followed by postactivity ache, often lasting 1 to 2 days. Symptoms must be present for a minimum of 6 months before surgery is considered. Physical examination demonstrates loss of palmar flexion and a positive "scaphoid test" (Fig. 99-8). The scaphoid test is performed by placing the examiner's four fingers on the dorsum of the patient's radius and the thumb on the scaphoid tuberosity. The right hand is used to examine the right wrist and vice versa. The wrist is placed in ulnar deviation, which aligns the scaphoid axis with the long axis of the forearm (decreased scaphoid-lunate

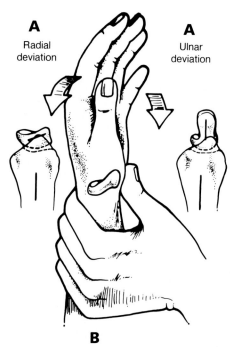

FIGURE 99-8. (*A*) Anteroposterior views of the radius and scaphoid. The scaphoid palmar flexes and its axis lie perpendicular to the long axis of the forearm in radial deviation. The scaphoid dorsiflexes and appears longer. In ulnar deviation the scaphoid assumes an in-line position. (*B*) For testing scaphoid stability the examiner's left fingers are on the patient's dorsal radius, and the examiner's thumb rests on the scaphoid tuberosity. The wrist is placed in ulnar deviation. Thumb pressure on the tuberosity prevents the scaphoid from assuming the more perpendicular position as the examiner's other hand brings the wrist into radial deviation. Pain and hypermobility are present as the proximal scaphoid pole tends to displace dorsally.

angle). As the wrist is brought into radial deviation, pressure is applied and maintained on the scaphoid tuberosity by the examiner's thumb. This prevents the scaphoid from assuming its more palmar flexed position (perpendicular to the forearm), as normally occurs with radial deviation. This provides a stress to rotate the scaphoid and drive the proximal pole dorsally if ligamentous injury will allow this. Pain is the hallmark of a positive test, and the abnormal scaphoid skid can be appreciated. Midcarpal dorsal displacement can also occur. Occasionally, instead of hypermobility, the rotated scaphoid will become almost immobile from long-standing synovitis and secondary capsular fibrosis, and simply applying pressure on the scaphoid tuberosity with radius counter pressure is painful. It is important to first push on the scaphoid tuberosity with counterpressure on the back of the scaphoid to determine if there is local tenderness, which can confuse the examination. The contralateral wrist should always be examined for comparison. The examiner must develop experience in normal wrists to properly evaluate this "test."

Untreated rotary subluxation of the scaphoid leads to degenerative arthritis of the wrist (see Fig. 99-5). The pattern of arthritis seen is quite predictable (see the section entitled "Scapho-Lunate Advance Collapse Wrist" under degenerative disorders, preceding).

Rotary subluxation of the scaphoid has been treated with ligamentous reconstructions,[39] but we feel that ligamentous reconstruction is not a suitable choice for this condition, because even normal ligaments cannot hold the position of the scaphoid if the capitate is not well supported by the lunate (see the section entitled "Kienböck's Disease" under instability problems).

Surgery for rotary subluxation of the scaphoid requires an arthrodesis of the triscaphe joint. This resists the significant moments, tending to maintain the scaphoid in a position perpendicular to the forearm.[54,57,59] The triscaphe arthrodesis has been shown to prevent rotary subluxation and its associated symptoms even in the absence of capitate support from the lunate (see "Kienböck's Disease").[61]

Scaphoid Nonunion

In scaphoid nonunion the distal scaphoid fragment loses its proximal ligamentous tethers, which remain attached to the proximal pole or which may be disrupted in cases of scaphoid nonunion with a scaphoid-lunate gap. Rotary subluxation of the distal scaphoid fragment occurs, either in a static or dynamic manner, causing incongruity and eventual destruction of the joint between the radius and distal scaphoid fragment.

The treatment of choice for nonunion of the scaphoid without arthritis is bone grafting through either palmar or dorsal approaches.[9,10,44,47] Accurate realignment of the two scaphoid fragments is mandatory,[13] as failure to obtain anatomic healing can lead to destruction of the radioscaphoid joint. After failed bone grafting, one form of salvage is to fuse both fragments of the scaphoid to the capitate (with or without refusion of scaphoid fragments). This effectively makes the two scaphoid fragments a single unit with no motion between them. However, this causes some loss of wrist motion. In cases of particularly difficult scaphoid nonunion (e.g., very proximal or distal fractures), bone grafting can be combined with triscaphe arthro-

desis, which will maintain alignment and stability of the distal fragment. This contributes to union and helps prevent symptoms even in cases where the nonunion remains, as much of the symptomatology comes from the instability of the articulation of the radius with the distal scaphoid fragment. Degenerative arthritis should not occur. Midcarpal degenerative joint disease may still be a problem, however. Triscaphe arthrodesis decreases wrist motion compared to primary fusion of the scaphoid fragments alone. In cases of scaphoid nonunion associated with scapholunate gap, a triscaphe arthrodesis should be performed prophylactically, as healing of the nonunion alone would convert the nonunion into a scaphoid-lunate dissociation, which would eventually require a triscaphe arthrodesis.

Scaphoid nonunion should not be treated by an isolated excision of the proximal scaphoid fragment. This removes the ligamentous stabilization of the proximal scaphoid, which may contribute some control of the distal scaphoid fragment through a fibrous nonunion. It also creates a gap that causes an acceleration of carpal collapse and SLAC degeneration. Triscaphe arthrodesis will control the instability of the radiodistal scaphoid fragment and maintain carpal height, thereby preventing proximal migration of the capitate.

Cases of scaphoid nonunion with degenerative change limited to a small area of radioscaphoid joint (i.e., distal nonunions) can be treated with the preceding methods combined with a radial styloidectomy to eliminate the area of radioscaphoid joint involved in arthritis (see "Scaphoid Nonunion" under degenerative disorders). Cases where the styloidectomy would be too large (more proximally located nonunions) or where the degenerative arthritis has progressed beyond the radiodistal fragment joint, are treated by SLAC reconstruction. Seldom, silastic scaphoid replacement alone may be sufficient (see "Scapholunate Advance Collapse Wrist" under degenerative disorders).

Kienböck's Disease

Kienböck's disease with collapse of the lunate allows proximal migration of the capitate, driving the scaphoid into a position of rotary subluxation. Collapsed Kienböck's disease can be thought of as a form of rotary subluxation of the scaphoid, and the major symptoms are secondary to the abnormal scaphoid position and articulation with the radius[61] (Fig. 99-9).

There are many operative and nonoperative methods of treating Kienböck's disease, including simple immobilization, excision of the lunate, excision of the lunate plus dorsal flap arthroplasty,[37] and proximal row carpectomy.[19] More recently emphasis has been placed on the association of ulnar-minus variance with Kienböck's disease, leading to ulnar lengthening[3] and radial shortening[2] as forms of treatment. These would seem to have less value once collapse has occurred because of the secondary scaphoid problem.

Many authors have advocated the use of silastic lunate arthroplasty.[48] Silastic prostheses have no solid core and have little capability to resist compression. They function well with light loads but show progressive compression with heavy loading, leading to overload of surrounding joints (Fig. 99-10), synovitis, and instability. More specifically, compression of the lunate allows proximal migration of the capitate, which forces the scaphoid into abnormal rotation.

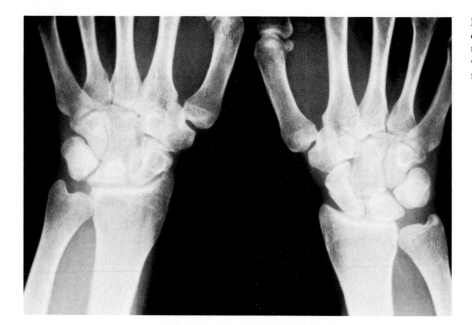

FIGURE 99-9. The radiograph on the left demonstrates proximal migration of the capitate and rotation of the scaphoid in Kienböck's with a collapsed lunate. The radiograph on the right shows the normal wrist for comparison.

Particulate synovitis is probably due to silastic implants that have been placed in a load column. Particles are shed and are picked up by the synovium (Fig. 99-11). Cysts are seen in any bone, even at a distance, associated with particulate synovitis.[36,46,53]

We believe there is no indication for silastic lunate replacement alone. Combining a silastic lunate replacement with a triscaphe arthrodesis provides a pathway for loading through adjacent bone. After triscaphe arthrodesis, load transference is from the capitate to the trapezoid, and more importantly through the capitate-scaphoid articulation. This adequately supports the wrist while unloading the lunate. This should prevent particulate synovitis, as discussed earlier. Taking this a step further, triscaphe arthrodesis is our treatment of choice for Kienböck's disease, without removing the lunate. This is an attempt to preserve the lunate, as it will often revascularize and usually remains asymptomatic even with collapse. If pain or significant restriction of motion persists following arthrodesis,

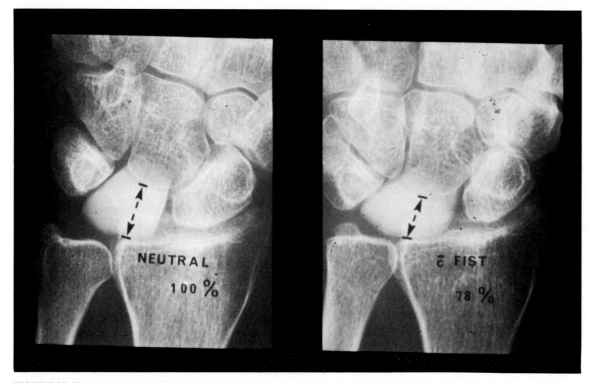

FIGURE 99-10. A silicone prosthesis acts as an adequate spacer when not loaded. The silicone lunate demonstrates significant compression when loaded by simply making a fist. Note the increased scaphoid rotation.

FIGURE 99-11. The radiograph demonstrates particulate synovitis in a patient with a lunate prosthesis for Kienböck's disease. The prosthesis is deformed, and there are cystic changes throughout the carpals.

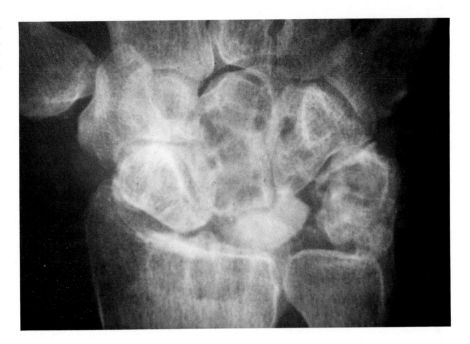

the lunate can easily be replaced with a silastic prosthesis later. Mobilization and rehabilitation would be much quicker after the second procedure, as the arthrodesis has already been achieved.

Dorsal Intercalated Segment Instability

Injury to the palmar radioscaphoid-lunate ligament results in instability of the lunate, allowing it to assume its "neutral anatomic" position of palmar displacement and dorsiflexion. Intercalated collapse of the capitate into palmar flexion and dorsal displacement on the lunate occurs secondarily. Static rotary subluxation of the scaphoid is present and is the cause of symptoms. Triscaphe arthrodesis is the treatment. If arthropathy is present in the radioscaphoid joint, SLAC reconstruction is advised.

Triscaphe arthrodesis, while correcting the rotary subluxation of the scaphoid, does not necessarily correct the DISI deformity itself. However, the arthritis and the symptomatology are from the rotary subluxation of the scaphoid, not the rotated lunate. Even with long-standing severe DISI or VISI (volar intercalated segment instability), degenerative arthritic changes between lunate and radius are almost nonexistent.

Triquetral-Lunate Instability

Injury to the ulnar side of the wrist can lead to instability between the triquetrum and lunate, which must be differentiated from injuries to the ulnar sling mechanism. If instability and tenderness can be localized between the triquetrum and lunate, limited wrist arthrodesis of this joint provides stability and relief of symptoms.[1,21,22,42]

Triquetral-Hamate Instability

The articulation between the hamate and triquetrum allows a large range of motion, with the triquetrum normally moving proximally and distally as well as palmarly and dorsally in relation to the hamate. Before injury occurs in this mobile complex, other more restricting and stabilizing intercarpal ligaments must rupture. Appropriate treatment is usually directed at these more important coexisting instabilities. There is rarely an indication for an isolated hamate-triquetral fusion.[1,22]

Trapezium-Trapezoid-Scaphoid Dissociation

An unusual radial hand dislocation occurs when the injuring load passes between the index and middle metacarpals, between the capitate and trapezoid, and through the trapezoid-scaphoid and trapezium-scaphoid joints. The thumb and index rays, together with the trapezium and trapezoid, dislocate dorsally from the scaphoid. Treatment is with triscaphe arthrodesis.

Capitate-Lunate Instability

Capitate-lunate instability is displacement of the capitate on the lunate, overloading the dorsal ligaments. Ligamentous reconstruction between dorsal capitate and lunate will suffice unless the dorsal capitate-lunate instability is secondary to reversal of the distal radius palmar tilt as in malunion of a Colles' fracture. In this case osteotomy of the distal radius to restore the palmar tilt of the articular surface is the appropriate treatment.[24,52]

WRIST AND RADIOCARPAL ARTHRODESIS

Formal wrist arthrodesis is rarely needed, as the most common, naturally occurring degenerative arthritis of the wrist can be treated with SLAC reconstruction. Radioscaphoid or radiolunate arthrodesis is most commonly utilized after trauma where there is destruction of that portion of the distal radius articular surface.[56] In cases of radius scaphoid fossa destruction, SLAC reconstruction may be a reasonable alternative to radioscaphoid arthrodesis.

For cases of ulnar and/or palmar translocation of the carpus on the distal radius, as seen in rheumatoid arthritis, a fibrous nonunion can be intentionally created between the radius and scaphoid and lunate.[60] This provides strong fibrous stability with good motion.

OPERATIVE PROCEDURES

Triscaphe Arthrodesis

Make a transverse incision on the dorsum of the wrist overlying the triscaphe joint, just distal to the level of the radial styloid tip. Protect dorsal veins and branches of the superficial branch of the radial nerve with a tissue-spreading technique. Open the distal aspect of the extensor retinaculum along the extensor pollicis longus, and approach the triscaphe joint through a transverse capsular incision placed between the extensor carpi radialis longus and brevis tendons (Fig. 99-12). Also make an incision in the capsule over the radioscaphoid to inspect the proximal scaphoid articular surface. Excise about 6 mm of the radial styloid. If radioscaphoid arthritis is found, the procedure of choice should be SLAC reconstruction rather than triscaphe arthrodesis.

With a rongeur remove the articular surfaces of the trapezium, trapezoid, and scaphoid down to cancellous bone. A dental rongeur with a 2 to 3 × 10-mm jaw is an ideal instrument. Harvest bone graft from the distal radius. Place two 0.045-inch Kirschner wires percutaneously through the dorsal trapezoid, and pass them up to the point of entering the scaph-

oid-trapezoid space (Fig. 99-13). Reduce the scaphoid by stabilizing the scaphoid tuberosity with your thumb while holding the wrist in slight radial deviation to prevent overcorrection. Use the scaphoid's articulation with the capitate as a guide to judge reduction. From the dorsal view the scaphoid-capitate joint should be congruous as far proximal as visible. From the lateral view with the wrist neutral, the scaphoid should lie at a 45° angle to the long axis of the radius. There is no need to reduce abnormal rotation of the lunate (see section entitled "Dorsal Intercalated Segment Instability" under instability).

Pack cancellous bone graft into the depths of the fusion site to maintain spacing between the scaphoid and trapezium-trapezoid. Drive the pins across the fusion site and into the scaphoid. An additional control pin from the scaphoid to the capitate may help hold the scaphoid reduction. Densely pack the spaces between the scaphoid, trapezium, and trapezoid with the remainder of the cancellous bone graft, using a dental tamp. Take care to prevent placement of the pins into the radius. Cut the pins off beneath the skin, and close the incision. (Postoperative care is described in a following section.)

The scaphoid should not be overcorrected by placing its long axis in line with the forearm (i.e., decreasing the scaphoid-lunate angle). This will limit the motion obtained after surgery. The average motion following triscaphe arthrodesis, excluding Kienböck's disease, should be 80% of the flexion and extension and 60% of the radial and ulnar deviation in the normal opposite wrist.

Scaphoid-Lunate Advanced Collapse Reconstruction

Make a transverse incision on the dorsum of the wrist at the level of radial styloid tip, protecting dorsal veins and nerves.

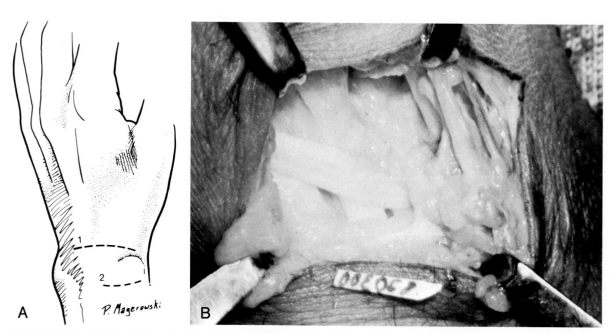

FIGURE 99-12. (*A*) The skin incisions for triscaphe arthrodesis are outlined with the underlying radial styloid for comparison. The proximal incision is over the palpable space between the first and second dorsal compartments. (*B*) The dorsum of a right wrist demonstrates the extensor pollicis longus crossing over the extensor carpi radialis longus and brevis. The triscaphe joint is below where the tendons cross.

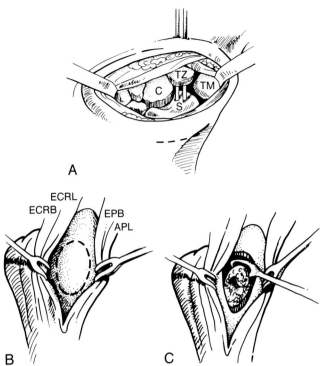

FIGURE 99-13. (*A*) The articular cartilage has been removed from the triscaphe joint. Pins are preset through the dorsal skin into the trapezium. They are driven into the scaphoid after placing the deep bone graft and reducing the scaphoid. The space between the bones should be maintained. *C*, Capitate; *S*, Scaphoid; *TM*, Trapezium; *TZ*, Trapezoid. (*B*) The first and second dorsal compartment tendons are retracted. The constant small periosteal artery is used as a mark for the periosteal incision. An oval cortical window is removed. *APL,* Abductor pollicis longus; *ECRB,* Extensor carpi radialis brevis; *ECRL,* Extensor carpi radialis longus; *EPB,* Extensor pollicis brevis. (*C*) Cancellous bone is removed with a currette. The cortical window is usually replaced.

Identify and retract the extensor pollicis longus, extensor carpi radialis longus and brevis, and extensor digitorum communis and indicis proprius. Make a transverse incision through the capsule at the level of the capitate-lunate joint. Remove the scaphoid, taking care to protect the radial and palmar ligaments. Remove the cartilage from the adjacent surfaces of the capitate, lunate, hamate, and triquetrum, using a dental rongeur. Longitudinal traction is helpful in visualizing the intercarpal joints, especially the capitate-lunate.

Set two pins percutaneously through the capitate. Set one pin from the hamate and one pin from the triquetrum up to the fusion site. Place part of the cancellous graft deep in the fusion site. In cases of the DISI deformity, reduce the capitate on the lunate; this is accomplished by dorsiflexing the hand to match the dorsiflexed lunate while the capitate-lunate joint is distracted by traction. Then drive the pins across to the adjacent bones: capitate to lunate, hamate to lunate, triquetrum to capitate, and triquetrum to lunate. Densely pack the remainder of the bone graft into the fusion site, using a dental tamp. Fill the space remaining from excision of the scaphoid with a silastic scaphoid prosthesis. (Postoperative care is described in a following section.)

The new stemless Dow Corning SLAC scaphoid in the old softer Silastic material is preferable.

Ordinarily, in limited wrist arthrodesis, the space between the joints must be maintained by packing with cancellous bone. In SLAC reconstruction some collapse of the capitate and hamate onto the lunate and triquetrum may be allowed, because no other joints will be affected by the slight degree of collapse. It is mandatory that the capitate be displaced volarly on the volar-center of the lunate. The average motion following SLAC reconstruction should be 65% of flexion and extension and 60% of radial and ulnar deviation in the normal opposite wrist.

Triquetrum-Lunate Arthrodesis

Make an incision on the dorsum of the wrist overlying the triquetrum-lunate joint. Open the extensor retinaculum over the fourth dorsal compartment, and expose the joint between the triquetrum and lunate. With a rongeur remove the adjacent articular surfaces of both bones to cancellous bone, and densely pack the space with cancellous bone harvested from the distal radius. Place two Kirschner wires from the triquetrum to the lunate. Densely pack the remainder of the bone graft into the fusion site, using a dental tamp. Fill the space remaining from excision of the scaphoid with a silastic scaphoid prosthesis. The average motion following triquetrum-lunate arthrodesis should be 85% of flexion and extension and 65% of the radial and ulnar deviation in the normal opposite wrist.

Distal Radius Bone Graft

The distal radius provides a supply of cancellous bone without leaving the operative field and with minimal morbidity.[32]

Make a 3-cm transverse incision approximately 2 cm proximal to the radial styloid, extending from the line of Lister's tubercle dorsally to just palmar to the first dorsal compartment (see Fig. 99-13). Identify the branches of the superficial branch of the radial nerve and dorsal veins, using the spread technique of dissection, and carefully protect them. Make an incision in the interval between the first and second dorsal compartments. This interval is identified by a constant periosteal artery. Elevate the periosteum enough to allow removal of an oval cortical window approximately 2 cm × 1½ cm. Harvest the cancellous bone, and if the cortical window is not used, replace it.

Postoperative Management of Intercarpal Arthrodesis

The postoperative management of triscaphe arthrodesis and SLAC reconstruction are the same. After surgery the patient is placed in a bulky hand dressing and a long-arm posterior plaster splint is applied. One week after surgery the patient is placed in a long-arm finger cast with the thumb included to its tip and the index and middle fingers incorporated in the intrinsic plus position.

Four weeks after surgery the long cast is removed and replaced with a short-arm gauntlet cast. Six to seven weeks after surgery, the cast is removed and radiographs are taken. If healing is adequate the pins are removed in the office using a local anesthetic and the patient is started on hand therapy.

Complications of Intercarpal Arthrodesis

Nonunion is usually between the trapezium-trapezoid complex and the scaphoid. It can be recognized by 8 to 12 weeks on plain radiographs or tomograms, and should be handled aggressively with early regrafting. If insufficient cancellous bone is present in the original distal radius site, the contralateral distal radius can be used. The most probable cause of nonunion is insufficient amount and poor packing of bone graft.

Occasionally, removal of a pin cannot be accomplished in the office, and the patient is returned to the operating room for pin removal.

Progression of degenerative changes subsequent to limited wrist arthrodesis has not been seen up to 10-year follow-ups.

Potential operative complications include injury to branches of the superficial branch of the radial nerve and to the deep branch of the radial artery. The radial artery should be retracted radially from the capsule overlying the triscaphe joint and protected during the procedures.

Wrist Arthrodesis (Senior Author's Preferred Method)

Make a longitudinal incision radially, from the distal index metacarpal distally to the distal 3 inches of the radius proximally. Isolate branches of the superficial radial nerve and veins with the spread technique and protect them. Isolate and retract the extensor pollicis longus and radial wrist extensors. Free the abductor pollicis longus and extensor pollicis brevis from the first dorsal compartment, and retract them palmarly. Elevate the origin of the first interosseous from the index metacarpal. Drill multiple holes to form a groove into the index and middle metacarpals, carpals (trapezoid, capitate, scaphoid, and lunate), and radius. Leave bone palmar and dorsal to the groove. This groove extends from 1 cm into the metacarpals distally to 2 cm into the radius proximally. Gradually widen the groove with larger drills, and connect the drill holes with a dental ronguer. The depth of this groove is just through both metacarpals, through the capitate and lunate, and about the same depth into the radius.

Expose the iliac crest, and obtain a single, large bone graft by taking the outer cortex of the ilium with the cancellous bone attached. Adjust the groove in the wrist to the shape and size of the graft. Cross drill the graft, insert it in place with the wrist in ulnar deviation, and lock it in place by bringing the wrist to neutral radioulnar deviation and neutral flexion. Tamp the graft down, and trim the edges with a rongeur. Pass 0.045-inch Kirschner wires through the metacarpals, graft, and radius (Fig. 99-14), and cut pin ends off beneath the skin.

Postoperative Management

The postoperative bulky dressing and splint are removed approximately 1 week after surgery. A long-arm cast with the thumb, index, and middle fingers included is applied. The cast is removed 4 weeks after surgery. A short-arm gauntlet is applied for 2 (often 4) more weeks. Radiographs are taken out of plaster. If healing is adequate, the pins are removed in the office under local anesthesia.

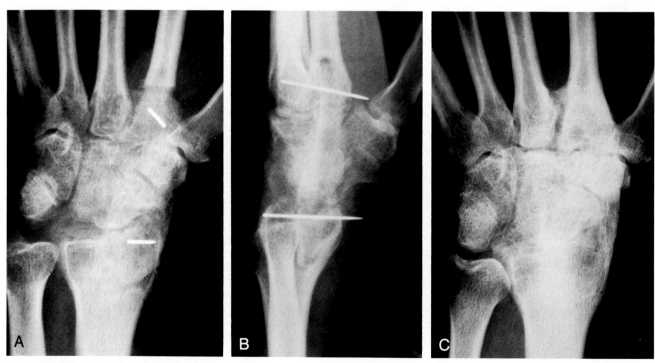

FIGURE 99-14. The (*A*) postoperative anteroposterior and (*B*) lateral radiographs of a wrist arthrodesis demonstrate the graft and groove through the metacarpals, carpals, and radius. (*C*) The anteroposterior radiograph demonstrates the incorporated graft.

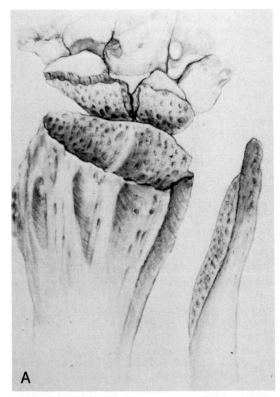

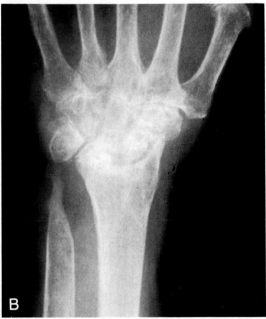

FIGURE 99-15. (*A*) A sketch demonstrates the decortication of the scaphoid, lunate, and radius. Shaping of the distal ulna is demonstrated. (*B*) The radiocarpal fibrous nonunion and matched ulna arthroplasty are demonstrated.

Complications

Avoid injury to branches of the superficial radial nerve and the deep branch of the radial artery. Wound infection is treated with immobilization and antibiotics as needed.

Radiocarpal Fibrous Nonunion in Rheumatoid Arthritis

Make a transverse incision over the radiocarpal joint, curving proximally at the ulnar aspect when distal ulna resection is planned. Identify dorsal veins and nerves by the blunt spread technique and protect them. Open the extensor retinaculum over the first dorsal compartment, and elevate it by cutting the septal attachments, leaving it hinged ulnar to the extensor carpi ulnaris. Perform a synovectomy.

When distal ulna resection is indicated, combine it with a synovectomy of the distal radioulnar joint. Resect the distal ulna in a long, sloping fashion, matching its shape to the radius, but maintaining its length. Resect all the surface opposite the radius from full pronation to supination, leaving the triangular fibrocartilage complex intact.[5]

Reflect the dorsal ligaments and capsule of the wrist radially, and convexly denude the proximal articular surfaces of the scaphoid and lunate to cancellous bone. Create a congruent cancellous concavity in the distal radius, preserving a perimeter of cortical bone. Drive two 0.62-inch Kirschner wires retrograde in a crisscross fashion through the distal radius. After reduction of the radiocarpal joint in a neutral position, drive the pins into the carpus, and cut them off beneath the skin. Lay back the dorsal ligaments, and place the extensor retinaculum across the wrist under the extensor tendons[60] (Fig. 99-15).

Postoperative Management

The postoperative bulky dressing and splint are removed approximately 1 week after surgery. A short-arm thumb spica cast is applied and left in place until 3 weeks after surgery. The pins are removed in the office using local anesthesia. Hand therapy is started with full motion and stress as tolerated, with the intent of producing a nonunion of the radiocarpal joint.

Complications

Delayed healing or wound slough may be seen in patients with rheumatoid arthritis after such extensive surgery. Wound infection is treated with immobilization and antibiotics as needed.

REFERENCES

1. Alexander, C.E., and Lichtman, D.L.: Ulnar Carpal Instabilities. Orthop. Clin. North Am. **15:**307, 1984.
2. Almquist, E.E., and Burns, John F., Jr.: Radial Shortening for the Treatment of Kienbock's Disease—A 5–10 Year Follow-up. J. Hand Surg. **7:**348, 1982.
3. Armistead, R.B., Linscheid, R.L., Dobyns, J.H., et al.: Ulnar Lengthening in the Treatment of Kienbock's Disease. J. Bone Joint Surg. **64-A:**170, 1982.

4. Bertenhaussen, K.: Partial Carpal Arthrodesis as Treatment of Local Degenerative Changes in the Wrist Joints. Acta Orthop. Scand. **52:**629, 1981.

5. Bowers, W.H.: Distal Radioulnar Joint Arthroplasty: The Hemiresection-Interposition Technique. J. Hand Surg. **10-A:**169, 1985.

6. Carroll, R.E., and Dick, H.M.: Arthrodesis of the Wrist for Rheumatoid Wrist: An Evaluation of Sixty Patients and a Description of a Different Surgical Technique. J. Bone Joint Surg. **55-A:**1026, 1973.

7. Carstam, N., Eiken, O., and Andren, L.: Osteoarthritis of the Trapezioscaphoid Joint. Acta Orthop. Scand. **39:**354, 1968.

8. Cockshott, W.P.: Carpal Fusions. Am. J. Roentgenol. **89:**1260, 1963.

9. Cooney, W.P., Dobyns, J.H., and Linscheid, R.L.: Nonunion of the Scaphoid: Analysis of the Results From Bone Grafting. J. Hand Surg. **5:**343, 1980.

10. Cooney, W.P., Linscheid, R.L., and Dobyns, J.H.: Scaphoid Fractures: Problems Associated With Nonunion and Avascular Necrosis. Orthop. Clin. North Am. **15:**381, 1984.

11. Crosby, E.B., Linscheid, R.L., and Dobyns, J.H.: Scapho-trapezial-Trapezoid Arthrosis. J. Hand Surg. **3:**223, 1978.

12. Dobyns, J.H., Linscheid, R.L., Chao, E.Y., et al.: Traumatic Instability of the Wrist. Instr. Course Lect. **24:**182, 1975.

13. Fernandez, D.L.: A Technique for Anterior Wedge-Shaped Grafts for Scaphoid Nonunions With Carpal Instability. J. Hand Surg. **9-A:**733, 1984.

14. Fisk, G.R.: The Wrist. J. Bone Joint Surg. **66-B:**396, 1984.

15. Gilula, L.A.: Carpal Injuries: Analytic Approach and Case Exercises. Am. J. Roentgenol. **133:**503, 1979.

16. Gilula, L.A., Destoute, J.M., Weeks, P.M., et al.: Roentgen Diagnosis of Painful Wrist. Clin. Orthop. **187:**52, 1984.

17. Goldner, J.L.: Editorial. Treatment of Carpal Instability Without Joint Fusion—Current Assessment. J. Hand Surg. **7:**325, 1982.

18. Haddad, R.J., and Riordan, D.C.: Arthrodesis of the Wrist: A Surgical Technique. J. Bone Joint Surg. **49-A:**950, 1967.

19. Inglis, A.E., and Jones, E.C.: Proximal Row Carpectomy for Diseases of the Proximal Row. J. Bone Joint Surg. **59-A:**460, 1977.

20. Kauer, J.M.G.: Functional Anatomy of the Wrist. Clin. Orthop. **149:**9, 1980.

21. Lichtman, D.M., Noble, W.H., and Alexander, C.E.: Dynamic Triquetrolunate Instability. Case Report. J. Hand Surg. **9-A:**185, 1984.

22. Lichtman, D.M., Schneider, J.R., Swafford, A.R., et al.: Ulnar Midcarpal Instability: Clinical and Lab Analysis. J. Hand Surg. **6:**515, 1981.

23. Linscheid, R.L., Dobyns, J.H., Beaubous, J.W., et al.: Traumatic Instability of the Wrist: Diagnosis, Classification, and Pathomechanics. J. Bone Joint Surg. **54-A:**1612, 1972.

24. Louis, D.S., Hankin, F.M., Greene, T.L., et al.: Central Carpal Instability—Capitate Lunate Instability Pattern. Orthopaedics **7:**1693, 1984.

25. Mack, G.R., Bosse, M.J., Gelberman, R.H., et al.: The Natural History of Scaphoid Nonunion. J. Bone Joint Surg. **66-A:**504, 1984.

26. Mayfield, J.K.: Mechanisms of Carpal Injury. Clin. Orthop. **149:**45, 1980.

27. Mayfield, J.K.: Patterns of Injury to Carpal Ligaments. Clin. Orthop. **187:**36, 1984.

28. Mayfield, J.K., Johnson, R.P., and Kilcoyne, R.K.: The Ligaments of the Human Wrist and Their Functional Significance. Anat. Rec. **186:**417, 1976.

29. Mayfield, J.K., Johnson, R.P., and Kilcoyne, R.K.: Carpal Dislocations: Pathomechanics and Progressive Perilunar Instability. J. Hand Surg. **5:**226, 1980.

30. Mazet, R., and Hohl, M.: Radial Styloidectomy and Styloidectomy Plus Bone Graft in the Treatment of Old Ununited Carpal Scaphoid Fractures. Ann. Surg. **152:**296, 1960.

31. McCredie, J.: Congenital Fusion of Bones: Radiology, Embryology, and Pathogenesis. Clin. Radiol. **26:**47, 1975.

32. McGrath, M.H., and Watson, H.K.: Late Results With Local Bone Graft Donor Sites in Hand Surgery. J. Hand Surg. **6:**234, 1981.

33. McMurty, R.Y., Youm, Y., Flatt, A.E., et al.: Kinematics of the Wrist. II. Clinical Applications. J. Bone Joint Surg. **60-A:**955, 1978.

34. Millender, L.H., and Nalebuff, E.A.: Arthrodesis of the Rheumatoid Wrist: An Evaluation of Sixty Patients and a Description of a Different Surgical Technique. J. Bone Joint Surg. **55-A:**1026, 1973.

35. Müller, M.E., and Baudy, W.: Arthrodesis of the Elbow and of the Wrist. *In* Muller, M.E., Allgower, M., Schneider, R., et al.:Manual of Internal Fixation, 2nd ed. New York, Springer-Verlag, 1979.

36. Nagel, D.A., Burton, D.S., and Kaye, R.A.: Silicone Synovitis After Implantation. Orthop. Cap. Com. **8:**1986.

37. Nahigian, S.H., Li, C.S., Richey, D.G., et al.: The Dorsal Flap Arthroplasty in the Treatment of Kienbock's Disease. J. Bone Joint Surg. **52-A:**245, 1970.

38. Neviaser, R.J.: Proximal Row Carpectomy for Posttraumatic Disorders of the Carpus. J. Hand Surg. **8:**301, 1983.

39. Palmer, A.K., Dobyns, J.K., and Linscheid, R.L.: Management of Posttraumatic Instabilities of the Wrist Secondary to Ligamentous Rupture. J. Hand Surg. **3:**507, 1978.

40. O'Rahilly, R.: A Survey of Carpal and Tarsal Anomalies. J. Bone Joint Surg. **35-A:**636, 1953.

41. Peterson, H.A., and Lipscomb, P.R.: Intercarpal Arthrodesis. Arch Surg. **95:**127, 1967.

42. Reagan, D.S., Linscheid, R.L., and Dobyns, J.H.: Lunotriquetral Sprains. J. Hand Surg. **9-A:**502, 1984.

43. Rosenthal, D.I., Schwartz, M., Phillips, W.C., et al.: Fracture of the Radius With Instability of the Wrist. Am. J. Roentgenol. **141:**113, 1983.

44. Russe, O.: Fracture of the Carpal Navicular: Diagnosis, Nonoperative Treatment, and Operative Treatment. J. Bone Joint Surg. **42-A:**759, 1960.

45. Simmons, B.P., and Mckenzie, W.D.: Symptomatic Carpal Coalition. J. Hand Surg. **10-A:**190, 1985.

46. Smith, R.J.: Silicone Synovitis of the Wrist. J. Hand Surg. **10-A:**47, 1985.

47. Sutro, C.J.: Treatment of Nonunion of Carpal Navicular Bone. Surg. **20:**536, 1946.

48. Swanson, A.B.: Silicone Rubber Implants for the Replacement of the Carpal Scaphoid and Lunate Bones. Orthop. Clin. North Am. **1:**299, 1970.

49. Taleisnik, J.: Ligaments of the Wrist. J. Hand Surg. **1:**110, 1976.

50. Taleisnik, J.: Wrist Anatomy, Function and Injury. Instr. Course Lect. **27:**61, 1978.

51. Taleisnik, J.: Posttraumatic Carpal Instability. Clin. Orthop. **149:**73, 1980.

52. Taleisnik, J., and Watson, H.K.: Midcarpal Instability Caused Malunited Fractures of the Distal Radius. J. Hand Surg. **9-A:**350, 1984.

53. Telaranta, T., Solonen, K., Tallroth, K., et al.: Bone Cysts Containing Silicone Particles in Bones Adjacent to Carpal Silastic Implant. Skeletal Radiol. **10:**247, 1983.

54. Watson, H.K.: Limited Wrist Arthrodesis. Clin. Orthop. **149:**126, 1980.

55. Watson, H.K., and Ballet, F.L.: SLAC Wrist: Scapholunate Advanced Collapse Pattern of Degenerative Arthritis. J. Hand Surg. **9-A:**358, 1984.

56. Watson, H.K., Goodman, M.L., and Johnson, T.R.: Limited Wrist Arthrodesis. II. Intercarpal and Radiocarpal Combinations. J. Hand Surg. **6:**223, 1981.

57. Watson, H.K., and Hempton, R.F.: Limited Wrist Arthrodesis. I. Triscaphe Joint. J. Hand Surg. **5:**320, 1980.

58. Watson, H.K., and Ryu, J.: Degenerative Disorders of the Carpus. Orthop. Clin. North Am. **15:**337, 1984.

59. Watson, H.K., Ryu, J., and Akelman, E.: Limited Triscaphoid Intercarpal Arthrodesis for Rotary Subluxation of the Scaphoid. J. Bone Joint Surg. **68-A:**345, 1986.

60. Watson, H.K., Ryu, J., and Burgess, R.C.: Rheumatoid Wrist Reconstruction Utilizing a Fibrous Nonunion and Radiocarpal Arthrodesis. J. Hand Surg. **10-A:**830, 1985.

61. Watson, H.K., Ryu, J., and DiBella, A.: An approach to Kienböck's Disease: Triscaphe Arthrodesis. J. Hand Surg. **10-A:**179, 1985.

62. Weber, E.R.: Concepts Governing Rotational Shift of the Intercalated Segments of the Carpus. Orthop. Clin. North Am. **15:**193, 1984.

63. Yeager, B.A., and Dalinka, M.K.: Radiology of Trauma to the Wrist: Dislocations, Fracture Dislocations, and the Wrist: Dislocations, Fracture Dislocations, and Instability Patterns. Skeletal Radiol. **13:**120, 1985.

64. Youm, Y., McMurty, R.Y., Flatt, A.E., et al.: Kinematics of the Wrist. I. An Experimental Study of Radial-Ulnar Deviation and Flexion-Extension. J. Bone Joint Surg. **60-A:**423, 1978.

65. Zielinski, C.J., and Gunther, S.F.: Congenital Fusion of the Scaphoid and Trapezium. Case Report. J. Hand Surg. **6:**220, 1981.

CHAPTER 100

Small Joint Arthrodesis in the Hand

PAUL R. LIPSCOMB

In the late 19th century, E. Albert of Vienna experimented persistently with the technique of fusion of joints and coined the term *arthrodesis*. He deliberately attempted to produce ankylosis of joints that were unstable.[3]

Arthrodesis of a single small joint (metacarpocarpal, metacarpophalangeal, or interphalangeal) may be indicated for congenital, traumatic, infectious, or degenerative processes that are usually isolated to one or several joints. At other times, as in cases of rheumatoid arthritis or paralytic disorders, significant improvement in hand function may result when arthrodesis of one or more small joints is performed in combination with other reconstructive procedures.

The age, sex, and occupation of the patient and the nature of the traumatic or disease process and its prognosis should affect the decision concerning the best surgical procedure or procedures for each individual.

A number of techniques have been described for arthrodesis of the joints in the hand. These include excision of the joint surfaces, resulting in various configurations that may be approximated and secured by internal fixation with Kirschner pins,[4,14] interosseous wire loops,[23] small screws,[7] compressive apparatuses of various types, and bone grafts. The latter may be removed from the ilium, distal radius, crest of the ulna, metacarpals, or from other sites when excision arthroplasty of other joints is done during the same operative procedure. Some of the various configurations and techniques have been described as end-on mitering,[22] cup and cone,[5] convex–concave,[25] dowel,[20] AO dynamic compression,[2,13,22,27] tension-band,[1,9,11] Herbert bone screw,[7] tenon,[8,14] and figure-eight tension-band wiring[10] methods (Fig. 100-1).

INDICATIONS

Most authors agree that despite enthusiasm for prosthetic replacement, there continues to be an important place in surgery of the hand for small joint fusions. The indications are to correct deformity, relieve pain, and provide stability.[1,15] Fusion may be the best way to correct severe contractures or deformities that result from congenital, traumatic, and paralytic abnormalities and degenerative and rheumatoid arthritis.[3,4,8,15,18,19,22,24,26] Likewise, fusion often is the best way to improve function of fingers with long-standing severe flexion deformities that result from Dupuytrens' contracture or scleroderma (Figs. 100-2–4).[16]

Arthrodesis is the best treatment for traumatic and degenerative arthritis of the metacarpotrapezial joint of the thumb in most patients (usually men) who require firm pinch and grasp with the thumb.[2,5,6,26] Fusion of this joint results in relief of pain, stability of the thumb, and excellent strength.[12,25] Although a minor loss of thumb motion is noted, this is not considered a problem by most patients.

Arthrodesis of the fifth metacarpocarpal joint is occasionally indicated after a traumatic fracture dislocation involving this joint, which normally has more extension than does that of the second, third, and fourth metacarpocarpal joints. For localized severe injuries and in surgical procedures requiring transposition of a digital ray involving the metacarpocarpal joints of the fingers, fusion to the trapezoid, capitate, and hamate bones

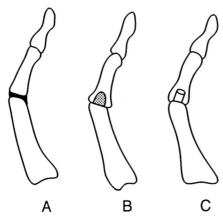

FIGURE 100-1. Configurations used most frequently for arthrodesis of metacarpophalangeal and interphalangeal joints. (*A*) Miter. (*B*) Cup and cone. (*C*) Tenon.

and adjoining metacarpal bases may occasionally be indicated (Fig. 100-5).

Arthrodesis of the metacarpophalangeal joint of the thumb is indicated when it is severely involved by rheumatoid arthritis or advanced degenerative joint disease and by some paralytic disorders (Fig. 100-6).[18,19,22] The most common deformity of the thumb associated with severe rheumatoid arthritis is that of flexion of the metacarpophalangeal joint and hyperextension of the interphalangeal joint. When both of these joints are destroyed and unstable, arthrodesis of both is justified (Fig. 7). In such instances it is desirable that good motion and position be present in the first metacarpotrapezial joint, but unfortunately this may also be severely destroyed. Then, excision of the trapezium and an arthroplasty using an autogenous coiled tendon placed between the properly located base of the first metacarpal and the proximal pole of the scaphoid is the procedure of choice ("anchovy" operation). Occasionally, a severe adduction contracture of the thumb is present, and the contracted thumb web may have to be released by Z-plasty of the skin and section of the adductor tendon before the proximal end of the first metacarpal can be placed in correct alignment with the scaphoid.

In two patients in one series of cases, the indications for compression arthrodesis of finger joints using Kirschner pins and cerclage wire were extended to include the acute stage of septic arthritis when the cartilage was found to have been destroyed.[9] In most similar cases it is preferable to delay formal arthrodesis until the acute stage of infection is under control. It is conceivable that the introduction of Kirschner pins and cerclage wire could, in such instances, cause a superimposed osteomyelitis of the phalanges.

Occasionally, when the interphalangeal joints are normal, or almost so, and the metacarpophalangeal joint of only one or two fingers is severely destroyed and unstable, arthrodesis of the unstable metacarpophalangeal joint may be the procedure of choice. The cup and cone technique may be employed.

Fusion of the metacarpophalangeal joint of the little finger has been recommended as a means of blocking ulnar drift of the other fingers. Unfortunately, with movement in the other metacarpophalangeal joints, the other fingers then underride or override the fused little finger.[15]

Moberg,[21] when attempting to create a thumb flexor grip in patients with quadriplegia, immobilized the interphalangeal joint of the thumb by drilling a large Kirschner wire across the joint and leaving it permanently. Some of the Kirschner wires in the thumb migrated out spontaneously and were replaced with new ones after a few weeks. Surgical arthrodesis was not necessary in any patient. Moberg stated earlier that arthrodesis is contraindicated in digits without sensation.[20] I have occasionally performed arthrodesis of the interphalangeal joint in some quadriplegics and can recall no particular problem with the procedure in these patients.

COMBINATION OF OPERATIONS

Especially for patients who have deformities as a result of rheumatoid arthritis, it is often advantageous to have two surgical teams operating at the same time, thereby achieving a substantial saving in time, morbidity, and money. One surgeon can operate on the hand and wrist while another works on both feet or the knee.

I have long been convinced that for the patient with rheumatoid arthritis needing surgical treatment of the hand and wrist, the final result is usually better when all procedures are done during one operation, thereby requiring one period of postoperative immobilization and rehabilitation (Figs. 8, 9). Of course, one must always operate within the limits of a safe tourniquet time. When the surgical procedure on an upper extremity requires longer than 1½ hours, I prefer to release the tourniquet for 10 to 15 minutes midway in the operation.

ANESTHESIA

When arthrodesis is to be confined to one or two interphalangeal joints, digital blocks with local anesthesia are preferable. Axillary block of the lowermost portion of the brachial plexus or conventional brachial block is efficacious for most surgical procedures involving more than two digits and the metacarpophalangeal and metacarpocarpal joints. When two surgical teams are operating simultaneously, usually for deformities of both upper extremities or of an upper and lower extremity, general anesthesia is almost always preferable and is advisable for children and some apprehensive adult patients.

PREOPERATIVE PLANNING

Interphalangeal Joints

For the interphalangeal joint of the thumb, 15° of flexion is the ideal position for arthrodesis in most patients. For the other digits in males, the distal interphalangeal joints are fused at approximately 25°. However, most women prefer that these joints be fused in only 5° or less of flexion. The fingers function best with the proximal interphalangeal joints arthrodesed in 30° to 40° of flexion. Some believe flexion should be slightly more in the ring finger and most in the little finger. The metacarpophalangeal joint of the thumb is fused in 20° of flexion, and its metacarpotrapezial joint in that position of abduction and rotation that allows best opposition of its tip to the other digits. The remaining metacarpocarpal joints are fused in their accustomed position on the distal carpal bones and to each other.

Interphalangeal and Thumb Metacarpophalangeal Techniques for Arthrodesis

After removal of the hyaline cartilage and most of the subchondral bone, juncture of the ends of the bones to be fused may be either of a mitered, chevron, cup and cone, or similar convex–concave configuration (Fig. 100-1). Autogenous peg grafts may be added. The bone ends may be held together by Kirschner wire pins, stainless steel wire loops, small AO plates and screws, Herbert bone screws that have threads at both ends, or by a tension band and Kirschner wire pins.

I have had most experience with arthrodesis of the interphalangeal joints and the metacarpophalangeal joint of the thumb using the conventional miter technique and that described by Carroll and Hill in 1969,[5] and later dubbed the cup and cone method. Before that time the joint surfaces were excised in an oblique manner (the miter method) and the remaining cancellous surfaces were approximated and held in the desired degree of flexion using crossed Kirschner wires or hypodermic needles that were drilled across the joints to be fused. Tension-band wiring techniques have been reserved for joints with marked destruction and instability and also for those with pseudoarthrosis. For patients with fracture dislocations of one or two severely destroyed interphalangeal joints, primary arthrodesis using a miter configuration is usually the procedure of choice (Fig. 100-2).

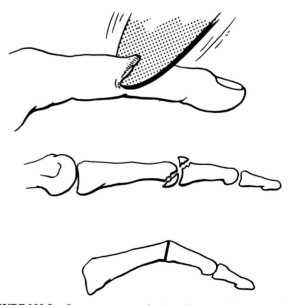

FIGURE 100-2.   Severe trauma to the interphalangeal joints resulting in irreparable damage to hyaline cartilage is best managed by primary or delayed arthrodesis of the joint in the position of function.

SURGICAL TECHNIQUES

Conventional Miter Technique

Approach the proximal interphalangeal joints through a curved incision on the dorsoradial surface. Split the extensor tendon longitudinally, and retract it. Approach the distal interphalangeal joints through an inverted V-, U- or H-shaped incision over the dorsum of the finger. Take care to avoid injury to the nail matrix. Section the collateral ligaments, and resect the capsule. Depending on the joint to be fused, deliver the head of the proximal or middle phalanx into the wound, and excise the condyles at the proper slant, using bone biters or rongeurs. I hesitate to use oscillating saw blades, which often result in bone necrosis because of the heat generated. Next, excise the opposing joint surface at a slant that corresponds with that of the proximal surface so that the correct angle of joint flexion and rotation is produced. Approximate the two cancellous surfaces, and fix them with crossed, smooth Kirschner wires; clip the ends of the wires off beneath the skin. Close and dress the wound, and apply a finger cast joined to a short-arm plaster of Paris cast.

Cup and Cone Method of Carroll and Hill

Expose the proximal and distal interphalangeal joints in the manner described for the miter technique. After the head of the proximal or middle phalanx is dislocated into the wound, trim the cartilage and subchondral bone in such a manner that a dome- or cone-shaped cancellous surface is fashioned. Next, make multiple awl holes in the base of the adjacent middle or distal phalanx at its periphery. Connect the holes, using a small (⅛ inch) osteotome that is directed at a 45° angle toward the center of the bone. Save the cone of bone that is removed by this action. Drill a retrograde smooth Kirschner wire pin through the distal segment, and make a small awl hole at the proper angle in the proximal ball to receive the Kirschner wire. Fit the two phalanges together in the desired angle and rotation. Then drill the wire proximally to transfix the site of arthrodesis, which is impacted during the process. When flexed at the metacarpophalangeal joint, the finger should now point to the base of the tubercle of the carpal scaphoid. Place chips of cancellous bone obtained from the cone that was excised about the site of the arthrodesis, and clip off the Kirschner wire beneath the skin. After the wound is closed and dressed, immobilize the finger in a padded plaster cast that is extended to a short-arm type to ensure against undesirable motion at the site of arthrodesis.

Following the miter or cup and cone technique, the cast is removed at 6 to 8 weeks, and radiographs are obtained. If further immobilization is then deemed appropriate, a finger cast or splint is usually sufficient.

The originators of the cup and cone technique experienced a 5% pseudoarthrosis rate. This rate dropped to 2% when patients with cerebral palsy were excluded.[5]

There are a number of other techniques that encompass the basic configurations of the miter and cup and cone connections, but are modified by the addition of a compression force achieved by placing a lag screw, a Herbert bone screw, an AO plate, or a tension-band wire across the joint surfaces. Others[9,10] advocate compression fixation by placing two

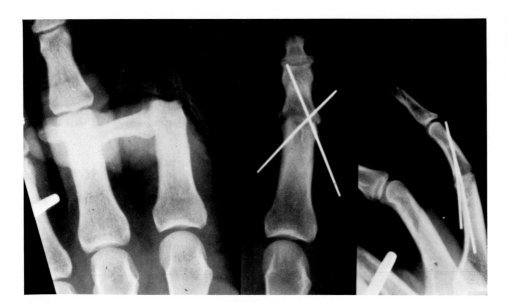

FIGURE 100-3. Severe open fracture dislocation of proximal interphalangeal joint of left index finger treated by cleansing, debridement, and primary arthrodesis with the metaphyses held in position by removable Kirschner wire pins.

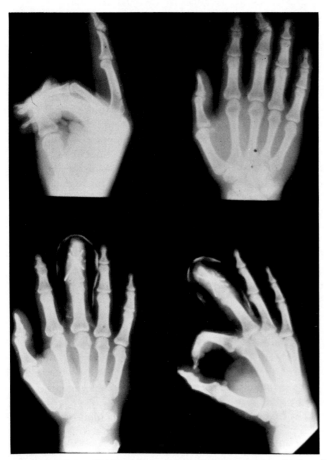

FIGURE 100-4. Old fracture involving distal interphalangeal joint of right long finger with nonunion and poor position of distal phalanx in a young woman. The small bone fragments and articular cartilage were excised, and the prepared bone ends were held in position for fusion in 5° flexion by removable Kirschner wire pins.

Kirschner wires transverse to the longitudinal axis of the bones to be fused and connecting them externally under tension with either modified Charnley clamps, methylmethacrylate cement, or fiberglass or synthetic casting tape. The proponents of compression arthrodesis of the interphalangeal joints and the metacarpophalangeal joint of the thumb generally dispense with the use of external casts and splints after surgery and claim that fusion can be expected in 5½ to 8 weeks rather than in 8 to 12 weeks.[1,2,7,9,10,13,27]

Kovach and associates[11] did a biomechanical analysis of four internal fixation techniques for arthrodesis of proximal interphalangeal joints in cadavers. Articular surfaces of the joints were excised at 30° and the joints were fixed by paired longitudinal 0.065 Kirschner wires compressed with a dorsal figure-eight loop of 26-gauge stainless steel wire. This type of fixation was compared with (1) an oblique Kirschner wire and a tension axis intraosseous wire loop, (2) an oblique Kirschner wire and a neutral axis intraosseous wire loop, and (3) one oblique and one longitudinal Kirschner wire. Of the four techniques studied, the figure-eight tension-band wiring specimens were stronger in anteroposterior bending and torsion but not significantly different in lateral bending stress. There was also significantly less permanent deformation of the fixation with the figure-eight tension-band technique than with the other three techniques evaluated. The authors[11] stressed that this was a preliminary study because of the limited number of techniques evaluated and also because clinical factors such as soft tissue dissection, subcutaneous implant irritation, difficulty of implant insertion, and removal were not addressed.

Thumb Trapeziometacarpal Joint Arthrodesis

Expose the trapeziometacarpal joint by an L-shaped lateral incision that extends from the middle third of the first meta-

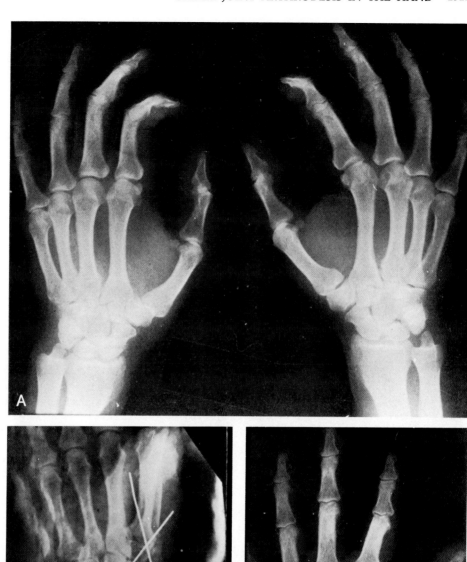

FIGURE 100-5. Radiographs of a 44-year-old man with subluxation and degeneration of trapeziometacarpal joint of left thumb. His occupation required him to remove the bones from 52 hams per hour. (*A*) Both hands and wrists before surgery. Right is normal. (*B*) Method of immobilization after articular surfaces are denuded of cartilage and the site of arthrodesis is fixed with crossed Kirschner wires. A bone graft, removed from the crest of the ulna, is fitted into a slot across the joint. (*C*) The thumb and wrist are immobilized in a short-arm padded plaster of paris cast for approximately 6 to 8 weeks. The distal phalanx of the thumb is left free. Three months after surgery fusion is firm. The bone graft across the fused joint can be visualized. Patient returned to his occupation of deboning hams and reported excellent function, strength, and relief of pain 3 years after surgery.

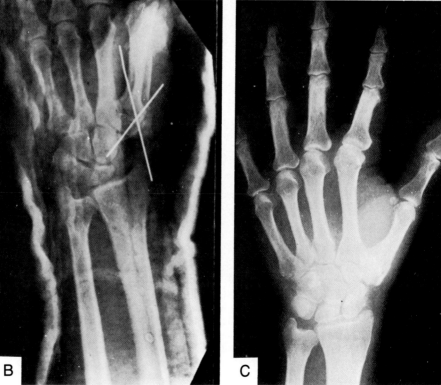

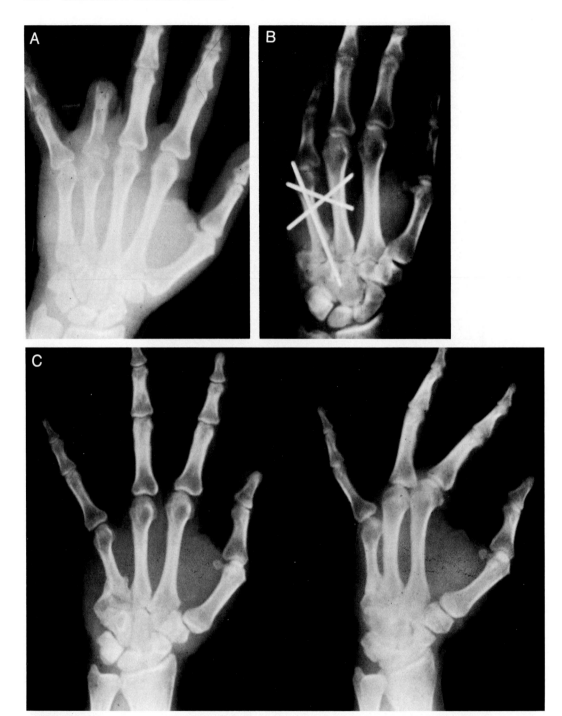

FIGURE 100-6.   (*A*) Recurrence of giant cell tumor, which originally involved left ring finger in its distal half. The base of the proximal phalanx is now involved with evidence of cortical erosion on radial side. (*B*) The remaining fourth digital ray was excised en bloc, and the fifth digital ray was transferred. Its metacarpal was arthrodesed to the capitate and base of the third metacarpal. Fixation was with three Kirschner wire pins. (*C*) Several months later site of arthrodesis was firm, and function and cosmesis were satisfactory. There was no further recurrence of the neoplasm.

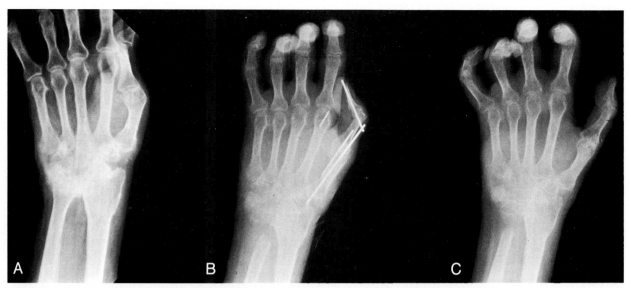

FIGURE 100-7. (A) Due to low-grade rheumatoid arthritis, there is a fixed flexion deformity and marked narrowing of metacarpophalangeal joint and a hyperextension deformity of interphalangeal joint where good space is preserved. There is also deformity of the carpal and distal radioulnar joints. Clinical examination also demonstrated ulnar subluxation of the extensor tendons crossing the metacarpophalangeal joint of index finger. (B) Postoperative radiograph demonstrates fixation of convex–concave arthrodesis of the metacarpophalangeal joint of the thumb and temporary internal fixation with two Kirschner wires. The volar plate of the interphalangeal joint was advanced proximally, and the joint was fixed temporarily in flexion with one Kirschner wire. The extensor tendons were relocated to their normal position over the second metacarpophalangeal joint. After lateral imbrication a short Kirschner wire pin was placed in the metacarpal head to ensure that correct position of the tendons was maintained for several weeks. Note that the distal end of the ulna has been resected. (C) Position of thumb after removal of Kirschner wires. Metacarpophalangeal joint is fused, and interphalangeal joint no longer hyperextends.

carpal to the tip of the radial styloid process, where it is curved ulnarward into the distal wrist crease. With the branches of the superficial radial nerve and the radial artery protected, expose the trapeziometacarpal joint, reflect the capsule, and resect the synovial tissue. Remove articular cartilage from the opposing joint surfaces with an osteotome and small rongeurs. Obtain a graft, 1 cm long and 2 to 3 mm wide, from the shaft of the first metacarpal or from the crest of the upper ulna through a small separate incision. Oppose the roughened base of the first metacarpal to the roughened trapezium, and pack cancellous bone into any interstices. With the metacarpal held in abduction and external rotation, transfix the joint with two 0.045 crossed Kirschner wires, which are then clipped off subcutaneously. The touch pad of the thumb should now face the touch pads of the other digits. Cut a groove with osteotomes across the joint to receive the graft, and impacted the graft into position. After wound closures and dressing, apply a cast to the thumb similar to that used for fractures of the scaphoid until firm union is present.

The Kirschner wires are usually removed 4 to 6 weeks after surgery, but cast immobilization may be required for 8 to 12 weeks. Mobilization of the wrist, thumb, metacarpal and interphalangeal joints usually presents no problem (Fig. 100-6).

COMPLICATIONS AND PITFALLS

Small joint arthrodesis, when performed by most surgeons on carefully selected patients, is fraught with few complications. If the patient has a serious traumatic, infectious, arthritic, or paralytic background, the danger of complications is increased.

Atraumatic technique, which was emphasized by the father of modern hand surgery, Sterling Bunnell,[4] is accompanied by a decreased incidence of complications. Nevertheless, wound infections and loosening of fixative devices will sometimes occur. These are much less serious now than was once the case because of the antibiotics presently available.

If a wound infection does occur, one is tempted to immediately remove the Kirschner pins, wire loops, AO plates, and other fixative devices. Most acute postoperative infections in the hand will respond to opening of the wound, elevation, sterile warm packs, and an antibiotic to which the infecting organism is sensitive. It is well-known that in patients who are on steroid medications, infections are more serious than otherwise.

The incidence of pseudoarthrosis following most procedures for arthrodesis of the small joints is in the neighborhood of 2% to 5%. A fibrous ankylosis that is relatively painless may

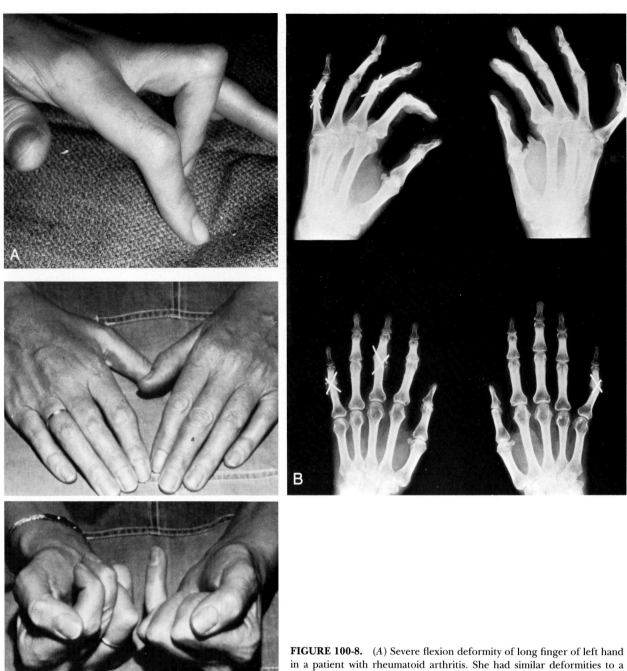

FIGURE 100-8. (*A*) Severe flexion deformity of long finger of left hand in a patient with rheumatoid arthritis. She had similar deformities to a lesser degree in both little fingers. (*B*) Oblique and anterior radiograph views of both hands 5 weeks after arthrodeses. (*C*) Appearance of hands in extended and flexed positions 4 years after operation. Patient had no pain, could again wear gloves, and was pleased with result.

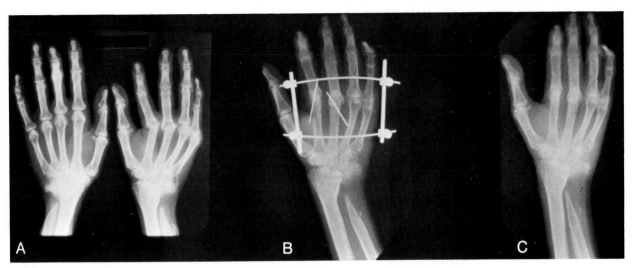

FIGURE 100-9. (*A*) Preoperative radiographs of the hands of a patient with rheumatoid arthritis that had involved primarily the wrists and the metacarpophalangeal joints of her right index and long fingers. She had had previous excision of the distal ends of both ulnas. She desired relief of pain and restoration of strong pinch between the touch pads of the thumb, index, and long fingers. (*B*) Two months after convex–concave compression arthrodeses with Roger Anderson apparatus in position. The transverse Kirschner wires are through the bases of the second and third metacarpals and proximal phalanges. (*C*) Three and a half months after surgery, fusion is firm and patient was pleased with position and function.

be the final result. If considerable pain or a loose and unstable pseudoarthrosis is present, a further attempt to obtain arthrodesis, using rigid fixation and an autogenous bone graft, is warranted for most patients.

REFERENCES

1. Allende, B.T., and Engelm, J.C.: Tension-band Arthrodesis in the Finger Joints. J. Hand Surg. **5:**269, 1980.
2. Braun, R.M., and Rhoades, C.E.: Dynamic Compression for Small Joint Arthrodesis. J. Hand Surg. **10-A:**340, 1985.
3. Bick, E.M.: Source Book of Orthopaedics. Baltimore, Williams & Wilkins, 1936.
4. Bunnell, S.: Surgery of the Hand. Philadelphia, J.B. Lippincott, 1944.
5. Carroll, R.E., and Hill, N.A.: Small Joint Arthrodesis in Hand Reconstruction. J. Bone Joint Surg. **51-A:**1219, 1969.
6. Eaton, R.G.: Replacement of the Trapezium for Arthritis of the Basal Articulations. J. Bone Joint Surg. **61-A:**76, 1979.
7. Faithfull, D.K., and Herbert, T.J.: Small Joint Fusions of the Hand Using the Herbert Bone Screw. J. Hand Surg. **9-B:**167, 1984.
8. Goldner, J.L.: Upper Extremity Surgical Procedures for Patients With Cerebral Palsy. Instr. Course Lect. **28:**37, 1979.
9. Hogh, J., and Jensen, P.O.: Compression Arthrodesis of Finger Joints Using Kirschner Wires and Cerclage. Hand **14:**149, 1982.
10. Khuri, S.M.: Tension Band Arthrodesis in the Hand. J. Hand Surg. **11-A:**41, 1986.
11. Kovach, J.C., Werner, F.W., Palmer, A.K., et al.: Biomechanical Analysis of Internal Fixation Techniques for Proximal Interphalangeal Joint Arthrodesis. J. Hand Surg. **11-A:**562, 1986.
12. Kvarnes, L., and Reikeras, O.: Osteoarthritis of the Carpometacarpal Joint of the Thumb: An Analysis of Operative Procedure. J. Hand Surg. **10-B:**117, 1985.
13. Leonard, M.H.: Compression Arthrodesis of Finger Joints. Clin. Orthop. **145:**193, 1979.
14. Lewis, R.C., Nordyke, M.D., and Tenny, J.R.: The Tenon Method of Small Joint Arthrodesis in the Hand. J. Hand Surg. **11-A:**567, 1986.
15. Lipscomb, P.R.: Surgery of the Arthritic Hand: Sterling Bunnell Memorial Lecture. Mayo Clin. Proc. **40:**132, 1965.
16. Lipscomb, P.R.: Surgery for Rheumatoid Arthritis—Timing and Techniques: Summary. Instructional Course Lecture, The American Academy of Orthopaedic Surgeons. J. Bone Joint Surg. **50-A:**614, 1968.
17. Lipscomb, M.D., Simons, G.W., and Winkelmann, R.K.: Surgery for Sclerodactylia of the Hand: Experience With Six Cases. J. Bone Joint Surg. **51-A:**1112, 1969.
18. Lipscomb, P.R.: Surgery for the Patient With Rheumatoid Arthritis. Tex. Med. **70:**56, 1974.
19. Lipscomb, P.R.: Surgery of the Rheumatoid Hand. *In* Flynn, J.E. (ed): Hand Surgery, 3rd ed. Baltimore, Williams & Wilkins, 1982.
20. Moberg, E.: Arthrodesis of Finger Joints. Surg. Clin. North Am. **40:**465, 1960.
21. Moberg, E.: Surgical Treatment for Absent Single Hand Grip and Elbow Extension in Quadriplegia. J. Bone Joint Surg. **57-A:**196, 1975.
22. Nalebuff, E.A.: Rheumatoid Hand Surgery—Update. J. Hand Surg. **8:**678, 1983.
23. Robertson, D.C.: The Fusion of Interphalangeal Joints. Can. J. Surg. **7:**433, 1964.
24. Szabo, R.M., and Gelberman, R.H.: Operative Treatment of Cerebral Palsy. Hand Clin. **1:**525, 1985.
25. Watson, H.K., and Shaffer, S.R.: Convex–Concave Arthrodesis in Joints of the Hand. Plast. Reconst. Surg. **46:**368, 1970.
26. Weinman, D.T., and Lipscomb, P.R.: Degenerative Arthritis of the Trapeziometacarpal Joint: Arthrodesis or Excision? Mayo Clin. Proc. **42:**267, 1967.
27. Wright, C.S., and McMurtry, R.Y.: AO Arthrodesis in the Hand. J. Hand Surg. **8:**932, 1983.

CHAPTER 101

Arthroplasty of the Hand and Wrist

JOHN J. NIEBAUER

ARTHROPLASTY OF THE WRIST

Principles of Treatment

Arthroplasty using a prosthetic device should be limited to selected cases, specifically, patients with rheumatoid arthritis, bilateral wrist arthritis, or potential bilateral wrist arthritis. Patients with unilateral wrist involvement not caused by rheumatoid arthritis may be more successfully treated with proximal row carpectomy or arthrodesis of the wrist; the latter, certainly, is the procedure of choice in a young person whose wrist will demand heavy use.

Three prosthetic devices—the Meuli, the Swanson, and the Volz—have had adequate clinical trial, and all have some problems. I prefer the Volz prosthesis, since it is durable, causes no excessive tissue reaction, and is relatively simple to insert.[2] My main use of this prosthesis is in the patient with rheumatoid arthritis. The alternatives are arthrodesis and synovectomy. Arthrodesis of both wrists in a badly crippled patient is a poor solution. Synovectomy of both wrists, as described by Straub and Ranawat,[17] may have a primary good result, but with long-term follow-up many of these wrists develop subluxation.

The Volz prosthesis is manufactured in two sections. The distal section, which in the newest model is a single vitallium stem, is made for insertion into the long finger metacarpal, usually through a portion of the capitate. The proximal component is inserted into the intramedullary canal of the radius (Fig. 101-1) and articulates loosely with an ultrahigh-molecular-weight polyethylene-covered section. The prosthesis is available in one metacarpal component size and two radial component sizes (small and standard). Trial components are also available.

The greatest problem associated with the prosthesis in severe wrist deformity is to balance the muscles about the wrist so that the hand goes neither into radial nor ulnar deviation.[12,18] This is particularly difficult to overcome in patients with complete destruction of the carpus and a 30° to 40° fixed ulnar deviation deformity of the hand, since the tendons and other structures on the ulnar side of the wrist are short and the finger extensors slip to the ulnar side of the capitate, which is the axis of the wrist and prosthesis motion. This problem is accentuated when the prosthesis is inserted, since unrelieved tight structures are made functionally shorter. In this situation, it is usually necessary to lengthen the flexor carpi ulnaris and extensor carpi ulnaris tendons and, most often, reconstruct a sling from part of one of the radial wrist extensors to keep the finger extensors located over the center of the axis of flexion and extension of the prosthesis.

Operative Procedure

An axillary block anesthesia is preferred, and a tourniquet is used. It is particularly important in patients with severe rheumatoid arthritis to avoid traumatizing the skin or impairing the veinous drainage any more than necessary. Therefore, after exsanguinating the arm, make a long, longitudinal incision on the dorsum of the wrist. At the level of the dorsal retinaculum, peel the soft tissues away widely from side to side.

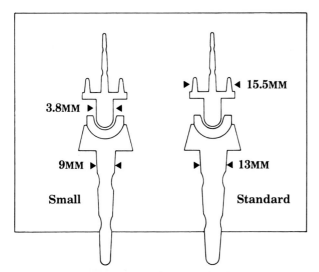

FIGURE 101-1. Volz prosthesis.

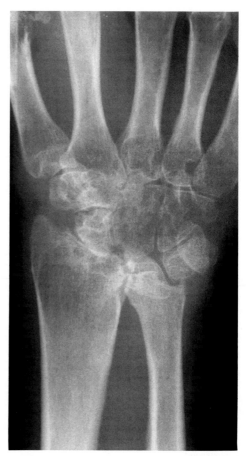

FIGURE 101-2. Rheumatoid arthritis with destruction of wrist.

In the rheumatoid patient the exposure is made by transecting the dorsal carpal ligament along the ulnar side of the sixth dorsal compartment and then reflecting it radialward to its insertion. A synovectomy of the extensor apparatus is then done. The dorsal capsule of the wrist and radioulnar joint is usually infiltrated with pannus, which must be excised. Trim the end of the ulna back to the level of the resected radius. Perform a complete synovectomy of the wrist, removing any bony debris as well. It is usually necessary to excise the greater part of the carpus with a rougeur, leaving the trapezium, to obtain enough room for the prosthesis without unduly resecting the end of the radius.

Then place the wrist in acute flexion and transversely transect the radius with a saw as distally as possible. Take care to preserve the volar capsule of the wrist when removing the bony debris and synovium. Thoroughly curette the intramedullary canal of the radius. Open the proximal end of the long finger metacarpal with an awl and curette it. Determine if the cortex of the bone is intact by turning the curette around in the intramedullary canal. Irrigate the whole area, and insert the trial prosthesis. If, at this time, structures on the ulnar side of the wrist are tight and prevent radial deviation, then lengthen both the flexor carpi ulnaris and the flexor carpi radialis tendons. The capsule must be thoroughly released on the ulnar side of the wrist (Figs. 101-2 and 101-3).

Dry the intramedullary canals of the radius and the long finger metacarpal, and insert soft cement with a syringe. This is facilitated by first inserting a large-bore needle into the canals. Position the distal segment first and then the radial segment. Reduce the prosthesis, and hold it in position until the cement has set. Excess cement is then trimmed away.

Close the wound by bringing the transverse dorsal carpal ligament beneath the extensor tendons and suturing it over the end of the ulna to its original position. If the finger extensors fall to the ulnar side of the longitudinal axis of the prosthesis, then form a loop from one-half of the tendon of the extensor carpi radialis longus or brevis as in Figure 101-4 to create a sling to keep the extensor apparatus of the fingers over the axis of the prosthesis. Then adjust and suture tenotomies, which

have been done in the extensor carpi ulnaris and flexor carpi ulnaris tendons. If the radial wrist extensors have been destroyed, they must be supplemented by transfers or tendon grafts to reproduce their integrity.

Remove the tourniquet and elevate the armboard by dropping the operating table. When the post-tourniquet flush has subsided and the bleeding is controlled, close the wound.

In patients with severe rheumatoid arthritis with multiple tendon ruptures, one must be prepared to replace the ruptured tendons with transfers or grafts. It is essential to the success of the operation that if the radial wrist extensor tendons are destroyed, their function be restored.[7] It is also sometimes necessary to replace the dorsal capsule when no dorsal retinaculum is available. In these cases the patient's opposite lower extremity is prepared so that grafts may be removed from toe extensors or the dorsal fascia of the foot may be used to replace the dorsal wrist capsule.

No drains are used, but the wound is dressed wet with Bunnell's solution* and is kept wet for several days by repeated applications of Bunnell's solution, supported by a short-arm split cast.

In patients with osteoarthritis or post-traumatic arthritis with an intact radioulnar joint, the wrist joint is approached

---

* Bunnell's solution is 0.5% acetic acid and 40% glycerin in sterile water.

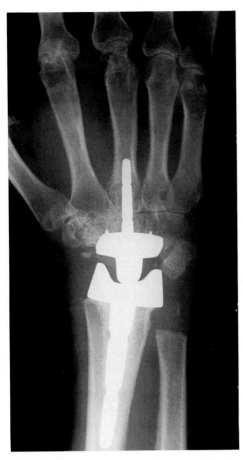

FIGURE 101-3.   Appearance following insertion of Volz prosthesis.

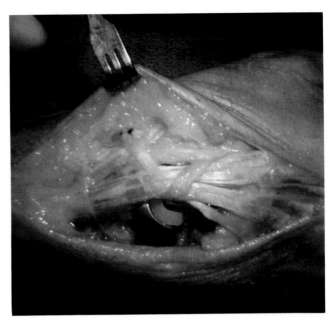

FIGURE 101-4.   Sling about finger extensors constructed from one-half of the extensor carpi radialis longus.

through a longitudinal incision on the ulnar side of the third dorsal compartment. Radially reflect the extensor pollicis longus and tendons radial to it by subperiosteal dissection with the dorsal retinaculum. In a similar manner, turn the periosteum up from the dorsal edge of the radius to the radioulnar joint, which is not opened. Make a cruciate transection of the capsule, and resect the carpus and radius. The procedure is otherwise similar to that used in the patient with rheumatoid arthritis.

Postoperative Care

If no tendon transfers have been done and the wrist is stable, then active exercises should be begun at the end of a week. A dynamic splint is used for another 2 weeks, and a night splint is used for as long as a month following surgery.

If much reconstruction tendon work and tendon transfers have been required, then it is necessary to continue immobilization for a period of 3 weeks and then start the above routine. Active exercises and dynamic splints are most effective.

Pitfalls and Complications

If the cast is changed during the first week, the prosthesis can dislocate during a cast change. However, this can be done if necessary by changing the cast in sequence—first the dorsal

half, then the volar half. If the prosthesis dislocates at this stage, it can usually be simply reduced.[6] Infection is always a worry with any prosthetic device; therefore, during the surgery the patients receive prophylactic antibiotics that are continued until the wound is healed. The hand may go into radial or ulnar deviation if the tendons have not been balanced properly. Gravity alone and the existence of a previous ulnar deviation deformity may cause the hand to go into ulnar deviation. This can be alleviated by the use of a night splint. If the deformity continues to increase, then appropriate tendon transfers should be considered, such as increasing the strength on the radial side of the wrist by the use of the brachial radialis tendon transferred into the extensor carpi radialis longus. A failed prosthesis can be converted to an arthrodesis by the use of an iliac bone graft, although extraction of the prosthesis from the radius may be difficult and can cause a fracture, particularly in osteoporotic patients.

PROSTHETIC REPLACEMENT OF THE METACARPOPHALANGEAL JOINTS

Principles of Treatment

The primary indication for prosthetic replacement of the metacarpophalangeal joints is disabling rheumatoid arthritis in an older patient. It should be realized that rheumatoid arthritis cannot be cured by a prosthetic replacement of a joint and that pannus formation may occur even in the synovial tissue that lines a pseudoarthrosis. Thus, early changes in the metacarpophalangeal joints with intact cartilaginous surfaces should be treated by a lesser procedure such as synovectomy and possibly crossed intrinsic transfers. A hand of a patient with rheumatoid arthritis of long duration that functions well and is painless and stable should probably be left alone. The main indication for a prosthetic replacement is destruction of the metacarpophalangeal joints with palmar subluxation and beginning fixed hyperextension deformity of the proximal interphalangeal joints. If this deformity is allowed to progress, the proximal interphalangeal joints will subluxate dorsally secondary to the deformity at the metacarpophalangeal joints.

Prosthetic replacement of the metacarpophalangeal joints with the prostheses currently available should not be used in post-traumatic arthritic hands where there will be much stress on the prosthetic device, since all devices show a tendency with time to loosen or break.[15] A complete solution to this problem has not been found.

A number of devices are available to the surgeon. The device that I use is a silicone prosthesis that is reinforced with Dacron. The stems are covered with Dacron for bony or fibrous tissue ingrowth. Ties that extend from the hinge blocks are tied into the proximal phalanx and the metacarpal. The tie into the proximal phalanx is then tied into the extensor tendon, which helps keep the extensor tendon centralized over the middle of the joint and aids in extension of the proximal phalanx. The stems become quickly fixed into the intramedullary canals, and this allows for early motion without displacement of the prosthesis. Four sizes are available. This prosthesis has been modified since its introduction (Fig. 101-5).[8,13–15] If the patient has an appreciable degree of ulnar drift, the operation should be combined with crossed intrinsic transfers and should include advancement and reinsertion of the first dorsal interosseous tendon.

It has not been my practice to use this prosthesis, or any variation of it, for the metacarpophalangeal joint of the thumb since arthrodesis of this joint usually is the indicated procedure. A determination of how functional a hand will be after reconstruction should evaluate hand function, that is, the fingers and the thumb functioning as a unit, before embarking on reconstruction of the metacarpophalangeal joints. A good result should permit full extension of the metacarpophalangeal joints, no further subluxation and flexion, and extension of about 40°.

Operative Procedure

Two dorsal surgical approaches may be used: (1) longitudinal incisions over the metacarpophalangeal joints and (2) a transverse incision at the level of the metacarpophalangeal joints. The longitudinal incision over the metacarpophalangeal joints is preferred if crossed intrinsic transfers are planned. Otherwise, the approach provided by the transverse incision is adequate (Fig. 101-6).

For the transverse approach, make the incision from the ulnar side of the little finger metacarpophalangeal joint to the radial side of the index metacarpophalangeal joint. Protect the vascular structures in the valleys between the metacarpal heads. The extensor apparatus is usually found subluxed to the ulnar side of its respective metacarpophalangeal joint. To free-up the extensor apparatus, it is necessary to run the line of dissection along the ulnar side of the extensor apparatus distally onto the proximal phalanx, separating it from the lateral band (Fig. 101-7). If a crossed intrinsic transfer is to be done, transect the lateral band quite distally, near the interphalangeal joint.

Separate the extensor tendon and shroud ligament from the underlying capsule and reflect them to the radial side of the joint. Excise the dorsal capsule, which is usually grossly infiltrated with pannus. Detach the collateral ligaments from the metacarpal heads, and transect the metacarpal heads at about the insertion of the collateral ligaments. This permits extensive exposure of the joint, and a synovectomy of the joint is then done with a rongeur (Figs. 101-7 and 101-8).

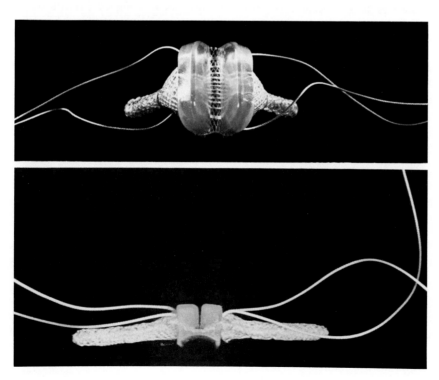

FIGURE 101-5. Reinforced silicone prosthesis with Dacron-covered stems for ingrowth of tissue.

FIGURE 101-6.   Surgical approach to metacarpophalangeal joints.

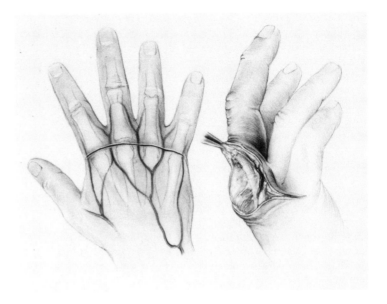

If the phalanges have dislocated palmar to the metacarpals, then they must be freed from the palmar capsule by transecting the attachment of the palmar capsule to the proximal phalanx. Take care to avoid the flexor tendons. This should allow the proximal phalanx to be brought up into the reduced position in relation to the metacarpal. There should be about 1.5 cm between the resected end of the metacarpal and the phalanx to allow easy insertion of the prosthesis.

If the subchondral bone of the proximal phalanges is dense, then it is best drilled by a Hall drill. The intramedullary canals of the proximal phalanges and of the metacarpals are then cleaned out with broaches (Fig. 101-9).

Using the Hall drill and a small drill point, drill holes on the dorsum of the metacarpal and proximal phalanx to accept the ties for the prosthesis (Fig. 101-10). The largest prosthesis that can be used should then be inserted into the metacarpals and

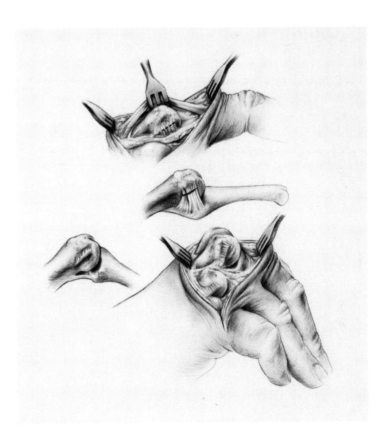

FIGURE 101-7.   Exposure of metacarpophalangeal joint.

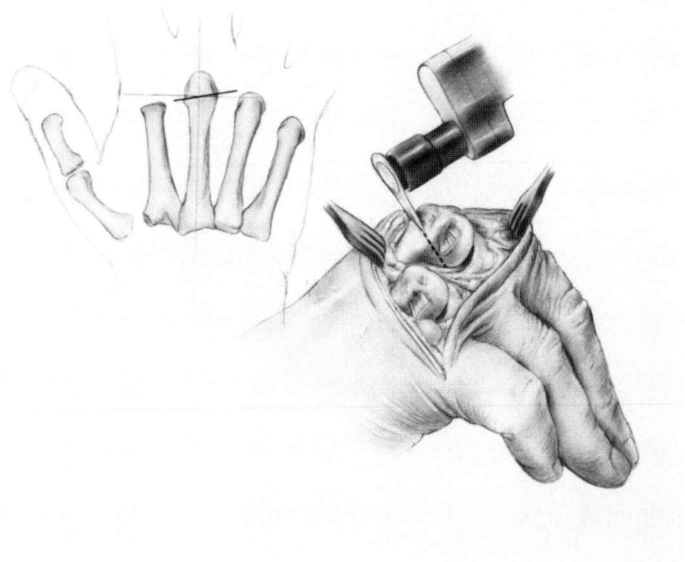

FIGURE 101-8.   Transection of metacarpal heads.

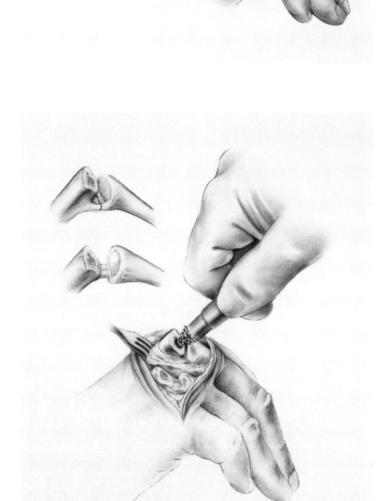

FIGURE 101-9.   Intramedullary canals are cleaned out with a broach to accept the prosthesis.

FIGURE 101-10.   The prosthesis is tied into the metacarpal and base of the proximal phalanx.

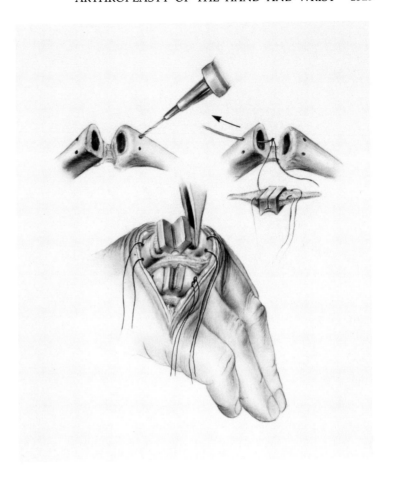

proximal phalanges. Trial prosthesis are used for size determination.

Using a bent crochet hook or a needle, pull the proximal ties up through the holes and put the prosthesis in place. Tie the ties down tightly over the dorsum of the metacarpals. Bring the distal ties through the proximal phalanges and up through the extensor apparatus and tie them into the extensor apparatus, thus keeping the extensor apparatus on the dorsum of the reconstructed joint (Fig. 101-11).

Reflect the extensor tendon over on itself and suture it to the shroud ligament to assist in keeping the tendon centered over the dorsum of the joint. Remove the tourniquet and control bleeding, mainly by removing all constrictions and elevating the arm by dropping the operating table in relation to the armboard.

Close the skin, dress the hand wet with Bunnell's solution, and apply anterior and posterior splints with the metacarpophalangeal joint splinted in extension.

Postoperative Care

If no other reconstructive procedures were necessary, then mobilization exercises can be started in 5 days. With more severe deformities, it is advantageous to use dynamic splints for 3 weeks to hold the metacarpophalangeal joints in extension and to avert forces that may push the fingers into ulnar deviation. By that time the stems will become fairly well fixed in the intramedullary canals. During surgery and for 5 days after surgery the patient is administered antibiotics.

Pitfalls and Complications

Even though a complete synovectomy has been done at the time of surgery, synovial-like tissue, which histologically appears to be pannus, may occur around the prosthesis. This varies tremendously from one person to the next. If the rheumatoid arthritis is unremitting and advancing, then this will be more prominent.

Resorption of bone about the stems of the prostheses may occur, particularly in patients with osteoporosis, leading to loss of stability of the prosthesis. Use and gravity will cause the fingers to go into ulnar drift.

As with other such devices, fracture of the prosthesis may occur. It has been seldom necessary to remove or change the prostheses when they have broken.[8,9]

Particles of silicone that break off from prostheses have been reported in adjacent lymph nodes. Particles from the prostheses can be seen in the tissue surrounding the prostheses, as is noted when all silicone devices are used.

ARTHROPLASTY OF THE CARPOMETACARPAL JOINT OF THE THUMB

Principles of Treatment

By far the most common reason for reconstructing the carpometacarpal joint of the thumb is pain caused by osteoarthritis,

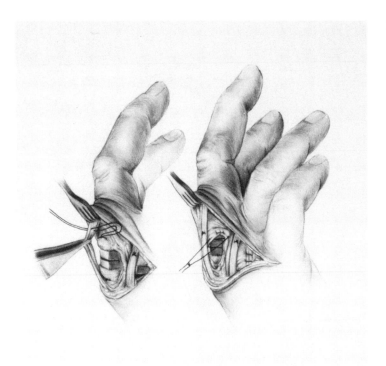

FIGURE 101-11. The distal tie is placed through the extensor tendon.

which is a common disease in postmenopausal women. It is significant that the pain is often most severe early in the disease. Early on, this problem should be treated by conservative measures, since the pain may subside and the patient may be willing to tolerate some deformity rather than undergo a surgical procedure. It should be realized that a number of women wish to have the procedure done because of appearance rather than because of pain or loss of thumb function.

Rheumatoid arthritis, except in juvenile rheumatoid arthritis, usually initially produces a flexion deformity of the metacarpophalangeal joint of the thumb. Thus, the base of the thumb metacarpal is not levered out of the carpometacarpal joint by the adducted thumb ray. In this situation, the deformity is best treated by arthrodesis of the metacarpophalangeal joint in a few degrees of flexion. When there is an adduction contracture of the thumb ray, then the base of the thumb metacarpal must be stabilized with a prosthesis, the adduction contracture released, and the metacarpophalangeal joint arthrodesed. Arthrodesis of the trapezial metacarpal joint is the preferred procedure in a laborer's hand.[3,11]

Excisional arthroplasty, that is, excision of the trapezium, gives a good result if there is not a fixed adduction deformity of the thumb metacarpal. I consider it an excellent operation with few complications and certainly without the worries that attend a prosthetic replacement.[1,4,5,10]

A large number of prosthetic devices are available to the surgeon: Ashworth, Braun, Eaton, Kessler, Linschied (Mayo total joint), Niebauer (Sutter), Steffee, and Swanson. None is faultless.

I prefer a Dacron silicone prosthesis, the stem of which is covered with Dacron mesh to facilitate the ingrowth of bone and fibrous tissue from the surrounding intramedullary canal of the thumb metacarpal. The heavy Dacron tie at the base of

the prosthesis is used to fix the prosthesis to the index metacarpal as described in the following technique (Fig. 101-12). I excise the distal ties for fixation into the thumb metacarpal, since they are unnecessary. The prosthesis comes in several sizes. I prefer the smallest size.

I particularly prefer this prosthesis for use when there is adduction deformity of the thumb metacarpal and a beginning hyperextension deformity of the metacarpophalangeal joint. In this situation, particularly if there are arthritic changes and destruction in the metacarpophalangeal joint, it may be necessary to arthrodese the metacarpophalangeal joint and thoroughly stabilize the base of the thumb ray after first doing a Z-plasty in the thumb web, and, if necessary, releasing the adductor muscle of the thumb. I have not found it necessary to use supplementary ligamentous procedures with the trapezoid prosthesis, particularly when the base of the prosthesis is supported by the proximal half of the trapezium.

Operative Procedure

An axillary block anesthesia is preferred. Exsanguinate the arm and apply a tourniquet. Make a zig-zag incision, centered over the radial side of the carpal metacarpal joint of the thumb (Fig. 101-13). Identify the branches of the superficial branch of the radial nerve in the subcutaneous tissue, and retract them ulnarward.

Expose the metacarpophalangeal joint of the thumb through a longitudinal incision extending from the thumb metacarpal onto the trapezium. With sharp dissection, peel back the capsule on either side of both bones to fully expose the joint. Transect the proximal end of the thumb metacarpal with a saw through the subchondral bone. The line of transection is

FIGURE 101-12. Trapezium prosthesis. The stem is covered with Dacron for tissue ingrowth. The ties at the base of the stem are unnecessary.

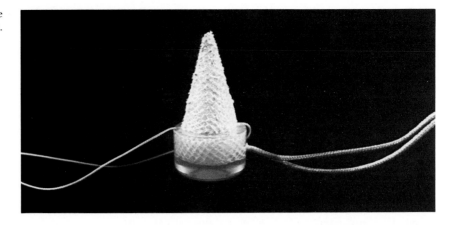

mainly transverse to the thumb metacarpal, but it must also include any osteoarthritic spurs or ossifications on the medial side of this joint, so that the thumb metacarpal can be reduced completely.

I prefer to resect the distal third of the trapezium with an osteotome rather than resect it completely, since this forms a good base on which the prosthesis can rest. The plane of resection is angled slightly proximal to the longitudinal axis of the bone (Fig. 101-14). It is probably not necessary to excise the entire trapezium even in the presence of scaphotrapezial arthritis, since the forces on that joint produced by the thumb ray are greatly diminished by insertion of the prosthesis. However, the surgeon should base his decision on the source of the patient's pain.

Using a Christmas Tree type broach, ream out the intramedullary canal of the thumb to accept the stem of the prosthesis. A trial prosthesis then may be used to determine fit.

Identify the articulate facet on the radial side of the index metacarpal and drive a $^3/_{32}$-inch drill with a transverse hole in the end through it so that it exits on the dorsum of the index metacarpal. Make a 1-cm incision on the dorsum of the metacarpal over the drill point. Pull a doubled No. 32 stainless steel wire back through the drill hole, insert the stem of the prosthesis into the intramedullary canal of the thumb metacarpal, and pull the ties attached to the base of the prosthesis back onto the dorsum of the hand, where they are tied into the periosteum of the metacarpal (see Fig. 101-14).

Place sutures in the capsule, and after all sutures have been carefully laid and the capsule well delineated, close it. At times the closure may be reinforced by a slip from the abductor pollicis longus, although this is usually unnecessary.

Remove the tourniquet, elevate the arm by dropping the operating table, and remove all constrictions about the arm. Control bleeding, close the skin, and apply a thumb spica splint using wet dressings of Bunnell's solution.

Postoperative Care

In approximately 1 week the splint is removed, the sutures are removed, and a new thumb spica cast is applied. Check-up radiographs are taken. Immobilization with the thumb in ab-

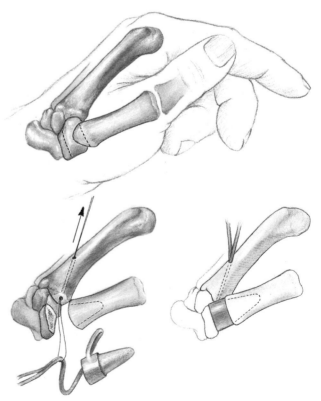

FIGURE 101-14. Insertion of trapezium prosthesis: the ties on the base of the stem of the prosthesis have been deleted.

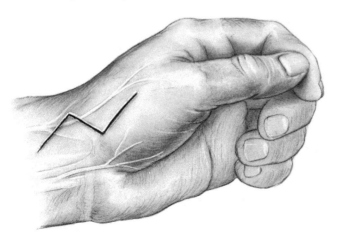

FIGURE 101-13. Incision for insertion of prosthesis.

duction is continued for 6 weeks when the cast is removed, and the patient is placed on exercises.

Pitfalls and Complications

During surgery the patient is placed on prophylactic antibiotics. As when other prostheses are used, if the patients have dental procedures, they should be covered by antibiotics to avoid seeding of bacteria to the prosthetic device. It is important to immobilize the thumb for a period of 6 weeks so that the prosthesis becomes well encapsulated, which will prevent flakes of silicone from being distributed through the wrist and causing a panarthritis.[16] It is more difficult to stabilize a prosthesis if the entire trapezium must be excised, and supplementary stabilization procedures may then be considered necessary, particularly if the patient has had an adduction deformity of the thumb metacarpal. Subluxation of the prosthesis has been one of the reported complications. A failed prosthesis can be easily converted to an excisional arthroplasty, since there is usually heavy, reactive capsular structure about the prosthesis.

REFERENCES

1. Amadio, P.C., Millender, L.H., and Smith, R.J.: Silicone Spacer on Tendon Spaces for Trapezium Resection Arthroplasty: Comparison of Results. J. Hand Surg. **3-A:**237, 1982.
2. Brace, D.W., and Millender, L.H.: Failure of Silicone Rubber Wrist Arthroplasty in Rheumatoid Arthritis. J. Hand Surg. **11-A:**175, 1986.
3. Bunnell, S.: Surgery of the Hand, 3rd ed. Philadelphia, J.B. Lippincott, 1956.
4. Burton, R.I., and Pellegrini, V.D.: Surgical Management of Basal Joint Arthritis of the Thumb: I. Long-Term Results of Silicone Implant Arthroplasty. J. Hand Surg. **11-A:**309, 1986.
5. Burton, R.I., and Pellegrini, V.D.: The Surgical Management of Basal Joint Arthritis of the Thumb: II. Ligament Reconstruction with Tendon Interposition Arthroplasty. J. Hand Surg. **11-A:**324, 1986.
6. Dennis, D.A., Clayton, M.L., Ferlic, D.C., and Patchett, C.E.: Bilateral Traumatic Dislocations of Volz Total Wrist Arthroplasties: A Case Report. J. Hand Surg. **10-A:**503, 1985.
7. Dennis, D.A., Ferlic, D.C., and Clayton, M.L.: Volz Total Wrist Arthroplasty in Rheumatoid Arthritis: A Long-Term Review. J. Hand Surg. **11-A:**483, 1986.
8. Derkash, R.S., Niebauer, J.J., and Lane, C.S.: Long-Term Follow-up of Metacarpal Phalangeal Arthroplasty with Silicone Dacron Prosthesis. J. Hand Surg. **11-A:**553, 1986.
9. Goldner, J.L., Gould, J.S., Urbaniak, J.R., et al.: Metacarpophalangeal Joint Arthroplasty (Niebauer Type): Six and a Half Years' Experience. J. Hand Surg. **2:**200, 1977.
10. Kvarnes, L., and Reikeras, O.: Rheumatoid Arthritis at the Base of the Thumb Treated by Trapezium Resection or Implant Arthroplasty. J. Hand Surg. **10-B:**195, 1985.
11. Kvarnes, L., and Reikeras, O.: Osteoarthritis of the Carpometacarpal Joint of the Thumb: An Analysis of Operative Procedures. J. Hand Surg. **10-B:**117, 1985.
12. Lamberta, F.J., Ferlic, D.C., and Clayton, M.L.: Volz Total Wrist Arthroplasty in Rheumatoid Arthritis: A Preliminary Report. J. Hand Surg. **5-A:**245, 1980.
13. Niebauer, J.J.: Dacron-Silicone Prosthesis for the Metacarpal-phalangeal and Interphalangeal Joints. *In* Cramer, L.M., and Chase, R.A. (eds.): Symposium on the Hand, vol. 3, pp. 96–105. St. Louis, C.V. Mosby, 1971.
14. Niebauer, J.J., and Landry, R.M.: Dacron-Silicone Prosthesis for the Metacarpophalangeal and Interphalangeal Joints. Hand **3:**55, 1971.
15. Niebauer, J.J., Shaw, J.L., and Doren, W.W.: Silicone-Dacron Hinge Prosthesis: Design, Evaluation and Application. Ann. Rheum. Dis. Suppl. **28:**56, 1969.
16. Poppen, N., and Niebauer, J.J.: Tie-in Trapezium Prosthesis: Long-Term Results. J. Hand Surg. **3:**445, 1978.
17. Straub, L.R., and Ranawat, C.S.: The Wrist in Rheumatoid Arthritis. J. Bone Joint Surg. **51-A:**1, 1969.
18. Tolbert, J.R., Blair, W.F., Andrews, J.G., and Crowninshield, R.D.: The Kinetics of Normal and Prosthetic Wrists. J. Biomech. **18:**887, 1985.

CHAPTER 102

Gunshot, Crush, and Frostbite Injuries of the Hand

ROBERT LEE WILSON and
JAMES J. CREIGHTON, JR.

While injuries of the hand are rarely life-threatening, a high degree of disability can result from gunshot wounds, crush injuries, injection injuries, and frostbite. Completely normal hand function is indeed rare after these major injuries. The goal of primary care for a mutilating hand injury is to save all viable tissue that can be utilized to provide basic hand function. Such reconstruction includes a stable wrist, a mobile radial digit with sensation, and a cleft between the remaining fingers.[21] The initial treatment must be based on sound judgment. Attempts to salvage a functionally useless or doomed part will only delay the patient's rehabilitation. Many treatment options are open, including debridement and observation, amputation,[5] replantation, or primary reconstruction.[9,25,43] In order to select the most appropriate form of treatment, the surgeon must understand all the alternatives.

A patient with any of these major injuries is first assessed in the emergency room and subsequently reevaluated in the operating room. After potentially life-threatening injuries have been stabilized, attention is turned to the hand and upper extremity. When examining or treating injuries involving multiple tissues, priorities must be established (Table 102-1). In the emergency room, vascularity may be determined by observing the nailbeds, sticking the fingertip with a pin, or using a Doppler device. With gunshot wounds and crush injuries, the possibility of a compartment syndrome must always be considered. If a digit or part of the hand is avascular, a decision must be made whether to amputate or attempt revascularization. Skin and soft tissues are evaluated, realizing the possible need for grafting or application of a flap. Obvious bony deformities are sought. Radiographs are taken to assess whether fractures or dislocations are present. Sensibility and muscle function are evaluated to determine the possibility of a nerve injury. Lastly, tendon function is tested. Tetanus prophylaxis is given and antibiotic medication is considered. A sterile dressing and temporary splint are applied to the extremity, and the patient is taken to the operating room.

In the operating room undertake a tissue-oriented evaluation and establish priorities of treatment.[72] If the hand or a portion of it is avascular but the tissue distally is not irreversibly destroyed, a decision to revascularize or amputate must be made. Factors to consider include the age and health of the patient, as well as the type and level of the potential amputation.[47,62,71] Although viable skin and subcutaneous tissue must be preserved, skin that is crushed must be debrided. If primary wound closure is not possible, critical sensitive tissues (nerves, tendons, open joints) must be preserved for later coverage. An exposed nerve should be evaluated for continuity and areas of local damage.

Bony stability must be restored, maintaining length and alignment. Perform fasciotomies when indicated. Debride devitalized tissue, repeatedly if necessary, and remove all foreign material. When there is any question of tissue viability or contamination, the wound is left open for 3 to 5 days with frequent reevaluation. To prevent joint contractures, a postoperative dressing is applied, immobilizing the hand in the optimal position. The safe or intrinsic-plus position places the metacarpal phalangeal joints in flexion and the interphalangeal joints in extension.[34] The wrist is rested in 30° to 40° extension. The basic goal in a severely injured hand having an adequate blood supply is to obtain primary wound healing, to prevent infec-

TABLE 102-1. PRIORITIES IN EVALUATION AND TREATMENT FOR THE UPPER EXTREMITY

1. Circulation/Compartment
2. Skin
3. Nerves
4. Bones
5. Joints
6. Tendons

tion,[21] and to provide a satisfactory environment for further reconstructive surgery.

GUNSHOT INJURIES

Principles of Treatment

Gunshot injuries in the hand demonstrate a wide range of complexity from initial management to subsequent reconstructive care. Published series categorize these injuries with respect to bullet velocity[17] and range from the gun.[13] This ballistic information is useful in predicting the magnitude of tissue damage and will guide decisions about therapeutic intervention.

The important ballistic characteristics with respect to long-term prognosis are bullet design, jacket size, and missile velocity. Historically, there have been three theories of wounding from missile injuries: the momentum, power, and kinetic energy theories.[31,12] The *kinetic energy theory* has gained overall acceptance. This wounding theory states that the energy at wounding is directly proportional to the missile mass and the square of its velocity, $E = \frac{1}{2}MV^2$. Thus, an increase in bullet mass increases its energy linearly, whereas an increase in missile velocity increases the energy exponentially. Therefore, velocity has a much greater effect on bullet energy. Pistol bullets, which have an average velocity of 600 to 1200 feet per second, are regarded as low-velocity. In contrast, bullets from military and hunting rifles traveling at greater than 2000 feet per second are classified as high-velocity. Dziemian,[17] DeMuth[13] and others[2,12,16] have compared the wounding characteristics of various bullets. The .38 caliber revolver and the .30 caliber military bullet have similar bullet weights but significantly different velocities. The military bullet, with a velocity four times that of the civilian weapon, has a 16-fold greater missile energy.

Harvey[30] has discussed the pathophysiology of missile wounds with respect to missile velocity. The involved tissue in low-velocity missile wounds is pushed apart by the bullet as it proceeds forward, creating a longitudinal wound tract with a small peripheral zone of crush. Tissue damage from a high-velocity missile is magnified by the *temporary cavity phenomenon*, which is responsible for the explosive appearance of these wounds (Fig. 102-1). Temporary cavitation results from a sudden disruptive force caused by forward missile penetration with concomitant surrounding tissue expansion. The size of the cavity created is related to bullet ballistics (disruptive force) and the elastic characteristics of the involved tissue (retentive force). Experiments demonstrate that specific gravity and elastic tissue content are the most important factors in predicting cavity production.[12] These studies correlate well with the clinical appearance of high-velocity wounds, in which massive tissue destruction of cortical bone is often found in conjunction with an innocuous-looking entrance skin wound. Unlike a low-velocity wound tract, temporary cavitation from high-velocity missiles creates a variable zone of injury, depending on the characteristics of the tissues along the bullet path. Pressure gradients develop as the temporary cavity equilibrates with surrounding tissues. Collapse of the temporary cavity ensues, creating a force that may draw fragments into the wound from surrounding areas.[33] While wound contamination is often alluded to, no well-controlled bacteriologic studies have been reported. Nevertheless, infection should always be considered possible after a high-velocity missile injury. By contrast, contamination is not a significant factor following low-velocity wounds. Heat sterilization of missiles does not occur.[66]

Tetanus prophylaxis should be emphasized.[53] This includes a tetanus toxoid booster for all immunized patients and Hypertet for those not previously immunized. Use of broad-spectrum antibiotics is recommended. Low-velocity wounds do not routinely call for antibiotic use in their management. Indeed, wounds that eventually require antibiotic usage may have had inadequate initial debridement.[33] For high-velocity war wounds to the upper extremity, Burkhalter[7] describes the routine use of intravenous antibiotics until meticulous skin and wound debridement can be performed.

Surgical Treatment

Low-velocity wounds from small caliber missiles often appear quite benign. Recommended management includes initial wound cleansing with skin and subcutaneous debridement only, followed by copious irrigation of the wound tract. Do not perform wide excision of entrance and exit wounds with exploration and surrounding muscle debridement.

Since the low-velocity missile pushes the surrounding soft tissue away from its path, the less-confined structures such as tendons and nerves are often found undamaged within the palm of the hand. However, when an injury occurs in the digits, tendons and nerves may not be spared, owing to the fibrosseous constraint of tendons and envelopment of the neurovascular bundles by Grayson's and Cleland's ligaments. Digital nerve paresthesias should be documented and followed closely with static two-point testing or von Frey evaluation.[46] All low-velocity hand wounds require control of soft-tissue swelling with supportive dressings and joint immobilization in the intrinsic-plus position.

The presence of open fractures associated with low-velocity missiles is not an indication for extensive wound debridement,[29] though the skeletal injury should be stabilized to assist in rehabilitation.[19] External fixators permit wound care and observation while imparting skeletal support. This stabilization may be used as the definitive form of treatment or as a temporizing measure until surrounding soft tissues permit definitive internal fixation or external immobilization. Duncan and Kettlecamp[16] have emphasized the importance of skeletal fixation and noted that bone instability produces the greatest long-term disability following low-velocity bullet injuries. In their review, infection and soft-tissue injuries did not significantly contribute to residual impairment (Fig. 102-2).

FIGURE 102-1. (*A*) This wound and radiograph demonstrate an injury from a low-velocity (0.22 caliber) bullet. (*B*) Wounds from a high-velocity bullet (rifle) demonstrate massive bone and soft tissue injury.

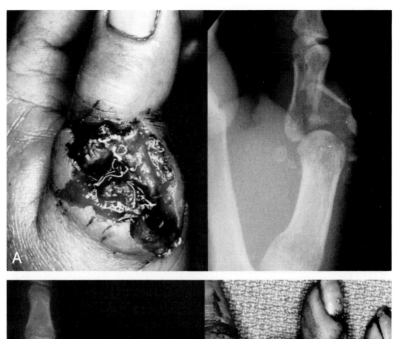

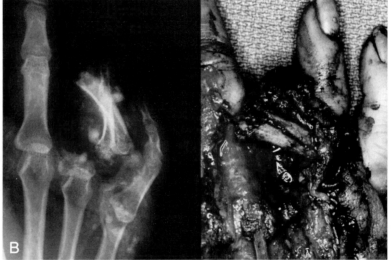

FIGURE 102-2. Skeletal stabilization achieved with Kirschner wire fixation and external fixator.

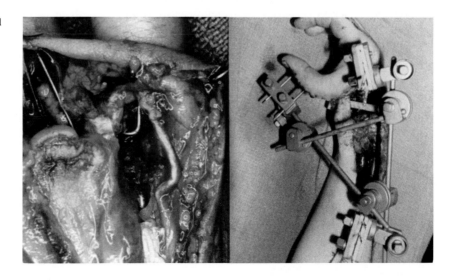

Intra-articular injuries require more aggressive initial surgical debridement, with documentation of articular damage and ligamentous injury. Lead synovitis has been addressed by Watson, who emphasizes the need for early removal of lead missiles from joints.[69] Bullets retained in soft tissues are found to become rapidly encapsulated by fibrous tissue and therefore eliminated from body circulatory fluid.[68] Bullets within joints that do not become surrounded by fibrous tissue, however, are in continual contact with synovial fluid. It has been suggested that joint motion and peripheral friction increase systemic lead absorption, leading to a potentially fatal complication.

Burkhalter[7] reviewed a series of hand injuries that occurred in Vietnam and recommended early surgical debridement and delayed wound closure for high-velocity missile injuries. A second debridement within 36 to 48 hours of the primary operation enables reevaluation of the variable zone of traumatized peripheral soft tissue. Temporary skeletal stabilization may be obtained using Kirschner wire spacers or external fixation devices until definitive reconstructive procedures are performed. If vascular reconstruction is required, stable skeletal fixation must be achieved prior to microvascular reconstruction.

If wound debridement allows for visualization of a transected nerve after a high-velocity bullet injury, accurate documentation of the condition of the injured nerve and its location is important for secondary reconstruction.[36] Primary nerve repair should not be attempted at the time of initial debridement, as primary microneural repair is unlikely to be successful. Instead, tag the nerve ends with a wire suture, which may assist in subsequent location of the nerve when performing a delayed nerve repair or grafting.

Soft-tissue coverage of a hand following high-velocity missile injuries is performed as quickly and safely as possible. This can be achieved by use of a free skin graft, a local rotation flap, distant random or axial pattern flaps or composite primary free flap coverage.

Postoperative Care

Use a supportive dressing with continuous elevation of the arm to control postoperative edema. Plaster reinforcement of the surgical dressing assists in immobilization of the extremity. The fingertips must be visualized for circulatory evaluation at all times. Selection of intravenous antibiotics is determined by the bacteriologic studies obtained at the initial procedure or at the second debridement. Close clinical monitoring of the patient's course is of paramount importance. Indications for reexploration include unexplained temperature rise, foul-smelling dressings, and unexplained pain not controlled by routine analgesics.

The soft-tissue reaction to the injury and any subsequent debridement must be stable before a supervised therapy program is begun. While an attempt to control edema is advisable, maneuvers such as massage, finger wrapping, and fluidotherapy must take into consideration any tendon, ligament, or bone reconstruction that has been performed.

Pitfalls and Complications

The initial treatment and subsequent evaluation of a hand following high-velocity bullet injuries should not overlook the potential for swelling within the intrinsic muscle compartments or in the carpal tunnel region.[6,7] The need for surgical decompression of the interosseous compartments is difficult to determine clinically. However, this decision may be assisted by the use of commercially available compartment pressure monitors.[28,59] Often, the need for decompression is based on the clinical presentation of a massively swollen hand with closed metacarpal fractures and without penetrating palmar lacerations. Decompression of the four dorsal interosseous compartments is simply performed through two longitudinal incisions, allowing release of the dorsal fascia over the adjacent muscles.[55] This intrinsic decompression prevents subsequent myofibrosis and contractures of the interossei, and will facilitate remobilization of the hand. Palmar release of the median and ulnar nerves is recommended when swelling in the palmar carpal region creates a tense palm and measurable loss of sensibility.

SHOTGUN WOUNDS

Principles of Treatment

DeMuth,[13] Paradies[46] and others[15] have outlined the basic ballistic and wounding properties of shotgun wounds, which differ significantly from rifle or pistol wounds. The shotgun is capable of inflicting a large number of projectiles into its target and producing a complex wound. Energy studies demonstrate that, at 40 yards, shotgun projectiles have lost more than half their original energy, regardless of the size of the pellets.

Muzzle constriction (choke) is a ballistic consideration that affects wounding from a shotgun. This narrowing concentrates the shot, thereby delivering a large number of pellets at a greater distance. The velocity of individual shot pellets is not affected significantly by choke or barrel length. Luce and Griffin,[39] in a review of gunshot wounds of the upper extremity, found that ballistic information often had no predictive value for the presence or absence of injury to the vascular or nervous systems. DeMuth and others[13] described shot patterns on the basis of yards from barrel to target. The most significant wounding occurs within 15 yards; at this range most of the shot charge is contained within the wound.

When evaluating and managing a wound that occurs at close range, keep the shot wadding in mind. This substance is often composed of organic material such as cattle hair, burlap, cardboard, or plastic. Always seek this nidus for bacterial colonization when treating short-range shotgun wounds.

With shotgun wounds, other areas of the body are often injured and must be thoroughly evaluated. Deadly complications can occur with injuries to the neck, thoracic, and abdominal regions. Do not underestimate the injuring potential of an isolated pellet, especially with a close-range injury.

Surgical Treatment

Initial wound care of a shotgun injury varies considerably; each wound requires individual treatment and consideration based upon anatomic location. For close-range shotgun wounds, follow the basic principles outlined for high-velocity bullet wounds. This includes early debridement with reexploration and redebridement. The shot wad must always be sought during wound debridement when no exit wound exists.

Massive damage to bone, nerves, and vessels may occur, even in the presence of only a small skin wound. Pay particular attention to any potential vascular injury in the region of the initial trauma. Proximal and distal vascular control must be gained before removal of the wadding in the region of a vessel; this prevents unexpected hemorrhage if the lumen of the damaged vessel was occluded by parts of the wadding. Tissue swelling must be expected after these injuries, and release of closed compartments by fasciotomy should be performed when indicated.[28] The presence of a distal neurologic deficit is not, by itself, an indication for extensive wound exploration.

Pitfalls and Complications

The complication most often reported following shotgun injuries at close range is causalgia. War experience and a variety of case reports demonstrate that a partial nerve injury can lead to a subsequent reflex sympathetic dystrophy.[60] Awareness of this problem allows prompt treatment during the postoperative rehabilitation period. The complexities of shotgun injuries are often compounded by the psychosocial aspects surrounding the incident. The stigmata of this violent episode are often visible and disabling. Appropriate initial treatment and prompt secondary reconstructive procedures give the patient the best chance of returning to the highest functional level of activity.

CRUSH (ROLLER OR WRINGER) INJURIES

Principles of Treatment

True crush injuries of the hand and arm result from compression between motor-driven rollers. These may occur in the work place, as from a printing press or by home laundry machines—the classic "wringer arm."[38,42] The severity and character of the trauma produced by rollers or wringers are determined by a number of factors.[20,56] Clearance between the rollers; the rollers' surface, whether steel or rubber; and the temperature are critical. The speed of the roller determines, in part, the force applied; greater speeds frequently produce skin avulsion. The length of time the extremity is compressed and the technique of extraction are important.

Three forces are involved in roller or wringer injuries.[1] A compression force is created by the large extremity entering the small gap between the rollers. Compression accounts for the edema and tissue contusion. A friction-abrasion force may tear the skin and characteristically will produce a distally based flap. Third, the shearing force will move soft tissues over deeper fixed structures, producing lacerations, avulsions, or subcutaneous hematomas. The degree of injury is proportionate to the size, clearance, duration of entrapment, and the method of extraction.

The depth of injury produced by such compression and shearing forces is not readily evident. Skin that has been completely separated from its blood supply will undergo necrosis.[67] Hemorrhage may separate the subcutaneous tissues from the deep fascia and require drainage. Bleeding beneath the fascial

envelope of the forearm can produce increased pressure (see Chapter 16), muscle ischemia, and Volkmann's contracture. Ischemic contracture can also occur in the hand with involvement of the intrinsic muscles.[77] If the severely crushed, edematous hand is painful on passive intrinsic stretch testing, perform interosseous decompression. Initial evaluation should include radiographs of the extremity up to the point of compression. Fractures occur in 25% of roller injuries.[42] A frequently unrecognized injury in the hand is dislocation of the basal (trapezial-metacarpal) joint of the thumb. This occurs when the transverse arch in the hand has been flattened and compressed (Fig. 102-3).[75]

In the past, the most common crush or roller injury was that produced by the household laundry wringer; these devices have now become rarities. The majority of injuries occur in patients under age 15, and particularly in children between 3 and 5. The most severe injury is usually located at the area most proximally involved.[43] Damage commonly occurs up to the level of the elbow, with more proximal trauma occurring in younger patients. The most frequent injuries are friction burns from abrasion and soft-tissue contusion, sometimes leading to tissue necrosis. Lacerations, joint injuries, and vascular trauma occur much less frequently.[64]

A variety of treatments have been recommended, including compression bandages,[57] enzymes, cold packs, and stellate ganglion blocks. The initial treatment after assessment for serious (i.e., neurocirculatory) injury includes cleansing and suturing any lacerations and reducing any dislocations. Distally based flaps and cyanotic skin margins are not improved with com-

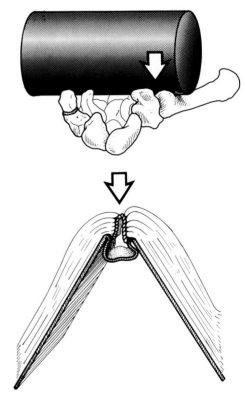

FIGURE 102-3. Roller or crush injuries extending to the level of the wrist can dislocate the basal (trapezial-metacarpal) joint (*A*) similar to breaking the binding of a book (*B*).

pression dressings. These should be avoided; a light, nonconstrictive dressing or open care is preferable. If the patient does not have critical problems or full-thickness skin loss, observation may be on a daily basis. The rare patient with major soft-tissue injury or vascular damage requires prompt treatment. The greatest difficulty is assessing the initial depth of a wringer injury in a child. The most common operative procedure is skin grafting. Antibiotics are limited to those patients who demonstrate obvious contamination.[27]

Surgical Treatment

Management of major crush injuries includes a careful tissue-oriented examination. Circulatory status must be assessed and documented using a Doppler device and arteriograms as needed. Increased forearm compartment pressure requires decompression. With open wounds, debridement and closure, probably on a delayed basis, are required. Skin loss requires resurfacing with grafts, flaps,[44] or a combination of both.[37] A common injury is a palmar laceration with a distally-based skin flap and crush of the thenar and hypothenar muscles.

The significance of nerve injuries following crushing trauma is difficult to evaluate initially. When wounds require debridement, the major nerve trunks should be evaluated if accessible. Neurapraxia is common following a major crush injury. Radiologic evidence of fractures or dislocations testifies to the great force associated with the injury. Fractures require stabilization and immobilization. Tendon injuries are repaired primarily, if possible. Crush injuries involving the dorsum of the hand usually are associated with tendon and joint damage. Injuries that involve both surfaces of the hand often result in amputation of some parts. After initial treatment, apply a supportive dressing with the hand and wrist immobilized in the safe position. Until stable, the wound is reevaluated every 24 to 48 hours.

Postoperative Care

Management immediately after the injury is directed toward the particular problems that have occurred (i.e., skin loss, fracture alignment, etc.). Once the wound has stabilized, a prompt remobilization program is aimed at overcoming the most common problems: chronic edema and stiff joints.[76]

The best way to limit or decrease edema is through elevation and active motion. Further help can be obtained with retrograde massage and a mechanical compression pump. Thermoelastic gloves provide continual compression and warmth. Prevention of joint stiffness and fixed joint contractures is a major problem following a joint injury. All joints are remobilized within the limits of pain tolerance. The aim is to move each joint through as great an arc of motion as possible, at least three times a day, and preferably once an hour. When the patient has less pain, dynamic splinting may be added to the exercise program.

Although splinting the hand in the safe position will prevent the most serious joint contractures (metacarpophalangeal joint extension and proximal interphalangeal joint flexion), this attitude will increase the chance of the patient's developing an intrinsic muscle contracture. Even if the interossei are not compromised initially, persistent dorsal edema will predispose to intrinsic muscle involvement and contracture. An exercise program that stretches the intrinsics can prevent this.

Active motion mobilizes joints that are becoming stiff and restores gliding tendon function. Motion encourages healing and increases wound strength but will only prolong an infection if one is present. Persistent drainage from a wound indicates inadequate debridement, with retained foreign material or necrotic tissue. The best means to prevent stiffness in the hand following serious trauma is protected early motion.

Pitfalls and Complications

Other problems besides chronic edema and joint stiffness can arise after crush injuries. These include scar contractures, muscle-tendon adherence, nerve compression, and chronic pain.[8] Wounds in which there is marked flaying reflect detachment of the skin. The blood supply of these flaps is usually poor and distally based. Tests for circulation (compression, tourniquet, and fluorescein dye) are often unsatisfactory. All obviously nonviable skin should be excised. Borderline tissue flaps should be sutured without tension and observed. At 3 to 5 days after injury, tissue viability should be clarified and the wound should be debrided of all necrotic tissue.

Wounds with skin loss should be closed with skin grafts or composite tissue flaps, depending on their size and location. Initially detached skin may be defatted and used as a full-thickness skin graft if it has not been too severely traumatized.[60] Should there be any question as to the quality of this tissue, a split graft will provide satisfactory wound closure. If future reconstructive surgery will be required (i.e., bone graft or nerve reconstruction), primary flap coverage should be undertaken.

A scar contracture can be produced by the skin graft used for wound closure or by a surgical incision required for fasciotomy. The latter can be prevented by selective application of the principles for incision placement.[38] Skin grafts may be eliminated secondarily by resection, either serially or following tissue expansion. A graft may be replaced by a flap if additional tissue is required, once the contracture is released. This is especially important if the location is one that will receive considerable pressure with future use or that will be subject to tissue breakdown (e.g., palm) or is one where primary closure might not solve the problem (e.g., wrist flexion crease). Occasionally, contractures can be released with a Z-plasty or a local flap.

While a compartment syndrome should always be considered following a severe crush injury, direct muscle injury with necrosis and fibrosis is more common.[27] With open injuries, selective muscle debridement is required. Adherence of injured muscles or tendons is common, but it should result in little loss of motion if the hand is promptly remobilized and joint motion does not become a problem in itself. Tenolysis is an alternative to be considered only when all the other tissues in the extremity are healed and the wound is stable. However, adherence proximal to the muscle-tendinous junction will not respond to a lysis, and should not be attempted when trying to improve distal motion.

External nerve compression can occur following a crush injury at sites where a nerve passes adjacent to traumatized muscle or injured fixed tissues (e.g., ligaments or bone). An intraneural injury is even more likely when an extremity is crushed, however, and a difficulty arises in deciding the basis of the resulting neuropathy. Is this the result of external compression or internal fibrosis of the nerve? The production of paresthesias upon percussion over the nerve trunk is not helpful in making this distinction. Electromyograms and nerve conduction velocity studies may prove more useful.

The development of prolonged pain after major trauma, especially crushing injuries, unfortunately is not rare.[4] Several weeks after the initial trauma the patient should be able to control pain with a non-narcotic medication. Management of pain once it becomes a chronic problem requires the combined efforts of many individuals. When pain can be controlled, using supportive splinting and other therapy modalities (such as the transcutaneous electrical stimulator), the patient will be able to participate in an exercise program. The possibility of the patient developing a reflex sympathetic dystrophy must be recognized from the onset. Successful management of this condition requires early recognition and a rapid response to achieve a satisfactory result.

While the list of complications that can arise after a crush injury is extensive, two pitfalls must be recognized to prevent further difficulties. The major problem after a mutilating injury is failure to recognize the depth and significance of the original injury. When the primary injury is underestimated, any subsequent treatment decisions will probably be faulty. The most critical element after a major crush injury is the correct timing of treatment. The judgment needed to arrive at such decisions correctly arises from knowledge and experience.

INJECTION INJURIES

Principles of Treatment

High-pressure injection injuries of the hand caused by paint or grease occur frequently. While the wound initially may appear innocuous, these injuries are surgical emergencies that require prompt exploration, decompression, and debridement.[41]

Injection guns put out a fine stream of paint or grease under pressures that range from 600 to 4,000 pounds per square inch. The material fired at such velocity through a small nozzle enters the skin and then spreads along fascial planes, tendon sheaths, or neurovascular bundles—the paths of least resistance.[35] Tissue within the hand may be mechanically damaged by pressure and rendered ischemic. The material injected produces an acute chemical inflammation, which may be associated with further soft-tissue and vascular damage.[11]

If the wound is not treated, or if foreign material is not completely removed, chronic inflammation, fibrosis, foreign body granulomas (oleomas), and sinus formation with chronic tissue breakdown may occur. Paint is likely to produce an acute inflammatory response, while grease will give rise to a delayed chemical reaction with fibrosis and stiffness. Injection guns that achieve higher pressures will allow more matter to enter the hand. Results from several studies have shown the greater the volume of material that has been injected, the greater amount of soft-tissue damage that occurs.[26]

Initially, the patient may only complain of burning discomfort at the injection site. Within a short time, however, the finger may become distended, pale, and numb, with throbbing pain. Subsequently, greater pain and mottling of the skin appear. When a considerable volume of material has been injected, enlargement of the finger is prompt. The left hand is involved twice as frequently as the right, and the patients are usually male. Injection sites are commonly the distal segments of the index and middle fingers. The thumb and palm are damaged less frequently.

Grease gun injuries are more frequent than wounds with paint guns.[41] Radiographs of the hand and finger may demonstrate how far the grease or paint has extended. Many greases are radiopaque because of the lead that has been added as a lubricating agent. If plain films are not revealing, xerogradiographs may provide useful information.[10] Patients can develop systemic effects, which include fever, lymphangitis, and an elevated white count. These signs usually appear within 2 days after the injury and may last from 4 to 5 days.

Surgical Treatment

High-pressure injection injuries require immediate surgery. Explore a finger through a modified midlateral incision[56]; a zigzag approach, while providing better exposure, is more likely to result in a skin slough. Continue the incision in a curvilinear fashion and extend it past the wrist into the forearm as needed. Separate incisions may be used if felt to be indicated.

Local anesthestic blocks in the palm are contraindicated, and the extremities should not be wrapped with a pressure bandage before application of the tourniquet.[35] Remove all the abnormal material (grease or paint). Excise any fat or fascia that is involved. Resect tendon sheaths in part if they are involved, taking care to leave essential portions of the fibro-osseous sheath system. A small curette or rongeur may be helpful in removing the material. Nerves and arteries that are functional but have a foreign substance embedded in them should be left intact and not resected.

Despite a meticulous dissection, it is inevitable that some foreign material will remain. Grease solvent and paint remover have been found inefficient and will only cause further tissue damage. Pack wounds open with the intention of performing a secondary exploration and closure at 2 to 3 days, or close them loosely over drains. On occasion, skin grafts may be required to close wounds if critical tissues are exposed. Wound cultures should be performed at the time of all surgeries. While many authors recommend antibiotic coverage for 2 weeks, the use of prophylatic antimicrobial drugs is not clearly indicated unless an active infection is present.[41] Immobilize the hand in the safe position.

Postoperative Care

The wounds should be reevaluated in 2 to 3 days. Once it is determined that all foreign material has been removed and healing has started, consideration should be given to a remobilization program. Do not attempt to close or cover small defects with skin grafts. Instead, mobilize the entire hand, using a whirlpool for further debridement if needed. When not exercising, the patient's hand should be placed at rest in a position so that contractures, particularly flexion contractures at the middle joint, will not occur. Eventual impairment is related to the amount of tissue destroyed by the foreign material. Paint gun injuries inflict greater damage than do grease guns. Injections into the palm, as contrasted to the digits, have a better prognosis.[26]

Pitfalls and Complications

The most frequent complications from injection injuries result from failure to debride the wound sufficiently and from closing the wound too early. While much has been written about the toxicity of both grease and paint, injected paint thinner is the most difficult to detect and completely remove.[63] Injection injuries from paint thinner should never be closed primarily, but carefully reevaluated every 48 hours. Such wounds may require multiple debridements and exploration.

Delay in initiating treatment leading to an adverse result often occurs because the patient or primary care physician is unaware of the significance of an injection injury.[26] While prompt surgery is recommended, this by itself, does not always ensure a good result.[26] Indeed, it is possible to obtain satisfactory results even with delayed surgical treatment, particularly with grease gun injuries.[62]

The question of amputation must always be considered. Retention of a digital tip that has required extensive soft tissue and skin resection is fruitless. Wound healing will be delayed and the patient will be left with an atrophic finger with little function. In one study, the average period of disability after an injection injury was seven months.[26] Owing to this prolonged mobidity, several authors[35,52] recommend early amputation, especially with a paint gun injury. Patients who have undergone early amputation often return to work within 6 to 8 weeks of the injury.

Late complications include skin breakdown, ulceration, and sinus formation with discharge of foreign material. Infection rarely occurs if it is possible to obtain wound healing within 2 weeks of the original injury. Retention of foreign material, necrotic tissue, and chronically open wounds will lead to sepsis.

FROSTBITE

Principles of Treatment

A broad spectrum of injury can occur in the hand following prolonged cold exposure. The diagnosis of frostbite does not represent a finite set of physical conditions. Injury classification and management protocols have been presented, but little information is available that enables a consistent prediction regarding the severity of the injuries. The two factors felt to determine the extent of tissue damage, the severity of the temperature and the duration of exposure, are usually not known. Systemic conditions such as atherosclerosis, smoking, and alcohol intoxication are variables that influence the development of frostbite and its response to treatment. A classification system, based on prognostic factors has been proposed by Mills et al.,[45] grouping the injuries according to superficial frostbite and deep frostbite. Superficial frostbite affects only the skin, as opposed to deep frostbite, where subcutaneous as well as neurovascular structures are involved.

Recent work demonstrates two pathophysiologic processes responsible for cell injury: (1) specific cell injury through crystalization of intra-cellular fluid, and (2) progressive ischemic necrosis arising from hemodynamic changes and increased sympathetic tone.[50,70,71]

Surgical Treatment

Management of the patient with frostbite requires evaluation of all possible tissues. Mills[45] has published a summary of acute frostbite management which emphasizes rapid restoration of core body heat. Caution is advised during this rewarming to monitor for cardiac arrhythmias. The rapid rewarming of the frozen extremity in a 40° to 44°C water bath quickly reverses both cellular and systemic responses. Rewarming is quite painful, requiring axillary or wrist anesthetic nerve blocks, or both, to control the pain. This anesthesia may break the sympathetic pain cycle, which is serving to produce peripheral vasoconstriction.

Many other supplemental treatments have been reported, each addressing the spectrum of disease seen in the frozen extremity. Antibiotics are used, but not routinely. While preservation of skin blisters ensures a germ-free environment, inevitable rupture requires meticulous wound care to prevent secondary infection. Medical lysis of vascular thrombi with heparin, low molecular weight dextran, or vasodilating agents have yielded variable results.[14,18,24,61] Recently, metabolites of arachidonic acid—prostaglandins and thromboxanes—have been postulated as causing progressive vascular changes seen in frozen tissue.[54] If further studies demonstrate that the role of these metabolites is similar to that known to mediate dermal burn ischemia, then the use of antiprostaglandin or antithromboxane agents may decrease the amount of ischemic damage seen in frostbitten hands.

The surgical role in the treatment of ischemic digits following frostbite in the acute stage is controversial. Early surgical intervention is not warranted, with the possible exception of an escharotomy when viable distal tissue is jeopardized. Ischemic digits are allowed to demarcate unless secondarily infected. This separation may require 2 or 3 months. Another approach is advised by Page and Robertson,[47] who feel that preservation of a long segment of a necrotic finger interferes with the rehabilitation of the hand. They recommend early amputation of nonviable tissue at 3 to 4 weeks to allow active remobilization of the remaining digits.

Formal digital amputation is performed, with nerve resection and wound closure to the level of viable tissue. Attempted preservation of digital length with inadequate soft tissue coverage often leads to subsequent stump breakdown and will only prolong the patient's rehabilitation.

Postoperative Care

Throughout the recovery period, the rehabilitation staff must be aware of potential joint contractures. These can be prevented by an early joint mobilization program. Skin desensitization and edema control are initiated as soon as possible, and motion is encouraged in noninvolved joints. Intrinsic contracture from muscle fibrosis secondary to ischemia can severely limit composite flexion of the frostbitten digit and can significantly decrease the grasping ability of the hand. House and Fiedler[32] report that surgical correction of intrinsic deformity has not been necessary in frostbitten hands if properly managed.

Pitfalls and Complications

Early complications following frostbite include wound breakdown, hypersensitivity, and chronic osteomyelitis, which often limit rehabilitation following the initial treatment. For this reason, wound care and levels of amputation are of utmost importance. The neurologic changes seen following frostbite will gradually improve except over gangrenous areas. Cutaneous atrophy and thinning of digital pulp beds can be correlated with sympathetic nervous system injury.

Late complications are seen primarily in young, skeletally immature patients and affect the epiphyseal growth plate. As outlined by Bigelow and Silke,[3] epiphyseal changes are related to both a direct effect of freezing on the epiphyseal cartilage as well as vascular damage to the plate. In young patients, the thumb is infrequently involved. This is felt to be related to the infantile posturing of the thumb, clasped into the palm.

REFERENCES

1. Adams, J.P., and Fowler, F.D.: Observations in Wringer Injuries. J. Bone Joint Surg. **43-A:**1179, 1961.
2. Adams, R.W.: Small Caliber Missile Blast Wounds of the Hand. Am. J. Surg. **82:**219, 1951.
3. Bigelow, D.R., Boniface, S.T., and Ritchie, G.W.: The Effects of Frostbite in Childhood. J. Bone Joint Surg. **45-B:**122, 1963.
4. Brown, H.: Closed Crush Injuries of the Hand and Forearm. Orthop. Clin. N. Am. **2:**253, 1970.
5. Brown, P.W.: Sacrifice of the Unsatisfactory Hand. J. Hand Surg. **4:**417, 1979.
6. Bunnell, S.: The Early Treatment of Hand Injuries. J. Bone Joint Surg. **33-A:**807, 1951.
7. Burkhalter, W., Butler, B., Metz, W., and Omer, G.: Experiences with Delayed Primary Closure of War Wounds of the Hand in Viet Nam. J. Bone Joint Surg. **50-A:**945, 1968.
8. Carter, P.R.: Crush Injury of the Upper Limb. Orthop. Clin. N. Am. **14:**719, 1984.
9. Chase, R.A.: The Damaged Index Digit. A Source of Components to Restore the Crippled Hand. J. Bone Joint Surg. **50-A:**1152, 1968.
10. Crabb, D.J.M.: The Value of Plain Radiographs in Treating Grease Gun Injuries. Hand **13:**39, 1981.
11. Craig, E.V.: A New High-Pressure Injection of the Hand. J. Hand Surg. **9-A:**240, 1984.
12. DeJong, P., Sawyer, P.N., and Wesolowski, S.A.: The Role of Regional Sympathectomy in the Early Management of Cold Injury. Surg. Gynecol. Obstet. **115:**45, 1962.
13. DeMuth, W.E., Jr., and Smith, J.M.: High-Velocity Bullet Wounds of Muscle and Bone: The Basis of Rational Early Treatment. J. Trauma **6:**744, 1966.
14. DeMuth, W.E., Jr.: The Mechanism of Shotgun Wounds. J. Trauma **11:**219, 1971.
15. Drye, J.C., and Schuster, G.: Shotgun Wounds. Am. J. Surg. 438–443, 1953.
16. Duncan, J., and Kettelkamp, D.B.: Low-Velocity Gunshot Wounds of the Hand. Arch. Surg. **109:**395, 1974.
17. Dziemian, A., Mendelson, J.A., and Lindsey, D.: Comparison of the Wounding Characteristics of Some Commonly Encountered Bullets. J. Trauma **1:**341, 1961.
18. Edwards, E., and Leeper, R.W.: Frostbite: An Analysis of Seventy-One Cases. J.A.M.A. **149:**1199, 1952.
19. Elton, R.C., and Bouzard, W.C.: Gunshot and Fragment Wounds of the Metacarpals. South. Med. J. **68:**833, 1975.
20. Entin, M.A.: Roller and Wringer Injuries: Clinical and Experimental Studies. Plast. Reconstr. Surg. **15:**290, 1955.
21. Entin, M.A.: Salvaging the Basic Hand. Surg. Clin. N. Am. **48:**1063, 1968.
22. Fitzgerald, R.H., Jr., et al.: Bacterial Colonization of Mutilating Hand Injuries and Its Treatment. J. Hand Surg. **2:**85, 1977.
23. Flatt, A.E., and House, J.H.: Frostbite of the Hand. J. Iowa Med. Soc. **52:**53, 1962.
24. Flatt, A.E.: Digital Artery Sympathectomy. J. Hand Surg. **5:**550, 1980.
25. Friedland, A.E., Jabaley, M.E., Burkhalter, W.E., and Chaves, A.M.V.: Delayed Primary Bone Grafting in the Hand and Wrist After Traumatic Bone Loss. J. Hand Surg. **9-A:**22, 1984.
26. Gelberman, R.H., Madison, J.L.P., and Jurist, J.M.: High-Pressure Injection Injuries of the Hand. J. Bone Joint Surg. **57-A:**935, 1975.
27. Golden, G.T., Fisher, J.C., and Edgerton, M.T.: "Wringer Arm" Re-evaluated: A Survey of Current Surgical Management of Upper Extremity Compression Injuries. Ann. Surg. **177:**362, 1973.
28. Halpern, A.A., and Mochizuki, R.M.: Compartment Syndrome of the Interosseous Muscles of the Hand. Orthop. Rev. **9:**121, 1980.
29. Hampton, O.: The Indications for Debridement of Gunshot Wounds of the Extremities In Civilian Practice. J. Trauma **4:**368, 1961.
30. Harvey, E.N., Korr, I.M., Oster, G., and McMillen, J.H.: Secondary Damage in Wounding Due to Pressure Changes Accompanying the Passage of High-velocity Missiles. Surgery **21:**218, 1947.
31. Hennessy, M.J., Banks, H.R., Leach, R.B., and Quigley, T.B.: Extremity Gunshot Wound and Gunshot Fracture in Civilian Practice. Clin. Orthop. **114:**296, 1976.
32. House, J.H., and Fidler, M.O.: Frostbite of the Hand. Op. Hand Surg. **47:**1553, 1982.
33. Howland, W.S., and Ritchey, S.J.: Gunshot Fractures in Civilian Practice. J. Bone Joint Surg. **53-A:**47, 1971.
34. James, J.I.P.: Fractures of the Proximal and Middle Phalanges of the Fingers. Acta Orthop. Scand. **32:**401, 1962.
35. Kaufman, H.D.: High-pressure Injection Injuries: The Problems, Pathogenisis and Management. Hand **2:**63, 1969.
36. Keggi, K.J., and Southwick, W.O.: Early Care of Severe Extremity Wounds: A Review of Viet Nam Experience and Its Civilian Applications. Inst. Course Lect. **19:**186, 1970.
37. Kleinman, W.B., and Dustman, J.A.: Preservation of Function Following Complete Degloving Injuries to the Hand: Use of Simultaneous Groin Flap, Random Abdominal Flap and Partial-Thickness Skin Graft. J. Hand Surg. **6:**82, 1981.
38. Littler, J.W.: Hand, Wrist and Forearm Incisions. In Littler, J.W., Cramer, L.M., and Smith, S.W. (eds.): Symposium on Reconstructive Hand Surgery. St. Louis, C.V. Mosby, 1974, pp. 87–97.
39. Luce, E.A., and Griffin, W.O.: Shotgun Injuries of the Upper Extremity. J. Trauma **18:**487, 1978.
40. MacCollum, D.W.: Wringer Arm: A Report of 26 Cases. N. Engl. J. Med. **218:**549, 1938.
41. Mann, R.J.: Paint and Grease-gun Injuries of the Hand. J.A.M.A. **231:**933, 1975.
42. Matev, I.: Wringer Injuries of the Hand. J. Bone Joint Surg. **49-B:**722, 1967.
43. McCullough, J.H., Boswick, J.A., Jr., and Jonas, R.J.: Household Wringer Injuries: A Three-Year Review. J. Trauma **13:**1, 1973.
44. McGregor, I.A.: Flap Reconstruction in Hand Surgery: The Evaluation of Presently Used Methods. J. Hand Surg. **4:**1, 1979.
45. Mills, W.J., Jr.: Frostbite: A Discussion of the Problem and a Review of the Alaskan Experience. Alaska Med. J. **15:**27, 1973.

46. Omer, G.E., Jr.: Injuries to Nerves of the Upper Extremity. J. Bone Joint Surg. **56-A:**1615, 1974.

47. Page, R.E., and Robertson, G.A.: Management of the Frostbitten Hand. Hand **15:**185, 1983.

48. Paradies, L.H., and Gregory, C.F.: The Early Treatment of Close-range Shotgun Wounds to the Extremities. J. Bone Joint Surg. **48:**425, 1966.

49. Pulvertaft, R.G.: Reconstruction of the Mutilated Hand. Scand. J. Reconstr. Surg. **11:**219, 1977.

50. Quintanilla, R., Krusen, F., and Essex, H.: Studies on Frostbite with Special Reference to Treatment and the Effect on Minute Blood Vessels. Am. J. Physiol. **149:**149, 1947.

51. Rakower, S.R., Shahgoli, S., and Wong, S.L.: Doppler Ultrasound and Digital Plethysmography to Determine the Need for Sympathetic Blockade After Frostbite. J. Trauma **18:**713, 1978.

52. Ramos, H., Posch, J.L., and Lie, K.K.: High-Pressure Injection Injuries of the Hand. Plast. Reconstr. Surg. **45:**221, 1970.

53. Robles, N.L., and Walska, B.R.: Current Concepts of Tetanus Prophylaxis. Am. J. Surg. **118:**835, 1969.

54. Robson, M.C., and Heggers, J.P.: Evaluation of Hand Frostbite Blister Fluid as to Pathogenesis. J. Hand Surg. **6:**43–46, 1981.

55. Rowland, S.A.: Fasciotomy. Oper. Hand Surg. **14:**565, 1982.

56. Sangvinetti, M.V.: Reconstructive Surgery of the Roller Injuries of the Hand. J. Hand Surg. **2:**134, 1974.

57. Schulz, I.: Wringer Injury. Surgery **20:**301, 1946.

58. Selke, A.C. Jr.: Destruction of Phalangeal Epiphyses by Frostbite. Radiology, **93:**859, 1969.

59. Sheridan, G.W., and Masten, F.A., III: Fasciotomy in the Treatment of the Acute Compartment Syndrome. J. Bone Joint Surg. **58-A:**112, 1976.

60. Sherman, R.T., and Parrish, R.A.: Management of Shotgun Injuries: A Review of 152 Cases. J. Trauma **3:**76, 1963.

61. Shumaker, H.B., Jr., and Kilman, J.W.: Sympathectomy in the Treatment of Frostbite. Arch. Surg. **89:**575, 1964.

62. Stark, H.H., Wilson, J.N., and Boyes, J.H.: Grease-Gun Injuries of the Hand. J. Bone Joint Surg. **43-A:**485, 1961.

63. Stark, H.H., Ashworth, C.R., and Boyes, J.H.: Paint-Gun Injuries of the Hand. J. Bone Joint Surg. **49-A:**637, 1967.

64. Stone, H.H., Cantwell, D.V., and Fullenwider, J.T.: Wringer Arm Injuries. J. Pediatr. Surg. **2:**375, 1976.

65. Tajima, T.: Treatment of Open Crushing-Type of Industrial Injuries of the Hand and Forearm: Degloving, Open Circumferential, Heat-Press and Nailbed Injuries. J. Trauma **14:**995, 1974.

66. Thoresby, F.P., and Darlow, H.M.: The Mechanisms of Primary Infection of Bullet Wounds. Br. J. Plast. Surg. **54:**359, 1967.

67. Tubiana, R., Stack, H.G., and Hakstian, R.W.: Restoration of Prehension After Severe Mutilations of the Hand. J. Bone Joint Surg. **48-B:**455, 1966.

68. Viegas, S.F., and Calhoun, J.H.: Lead Poisoning from a Gunshot Wound to the Hand. J. Hand Surg. **11-A:**729, 1986.

69. Watson, N., and Songcharden, G.P.: Lead Synovitis in the Hand: A Case Report. J. Hand Surg. **10-B:**423, 1985.

70. Weatherby, R.C.A., White, B., Patton, C., and Sjostrom, B.: The Pathogenesis of Frostbite. J. Surg. Res. **4:**17, 1964.

71. Weatherby, R.C.A., White, B., Patton, C., and Sjostrom, B.: Experimental Studies in Cold Injuries: III—Observation on the Treatment of Frostbite. J. Plast. Reconstr. Surg. **36:**10, 1965.

72. Weeks, P.M., and Wray, R.C.: Management of Acute Hand Injuries. St. Louis, C.V. Mosby, 1978.

73. White, J.C.: Timing of Nerve Suture After a Gunshot Wound. Surg. **48:**946, 1960.

74. Wilson, R.L., and Carter-Wilson, M.S.: Rehabilitation After Amputations in the Hand. Orthop. Clin. N. Am. **14:**851, 1983.

75. Wilson, R.L., and Liechty, B.W.: Complications Following Small Joint Injuries. Hand Clin. **2:**329, 1986.

76. Wilson, R.L., and Reynolds, C.C.: Joint Stiffness. In McFarlane, R.M. (ed.): Unsatisfactory Results in Hand Surgery. Edinburgh, Churchill-Livingstone, 1987.

77. Wolfort, F.G., et al.: Immediate Interossei Decompression Following Crush Injury of the Hand. Arch. Surg. **105:**826, 1973.

78. Ziperman, H.H.: The Management of Soft-Tissue Missile Wounds in War and Peace. J. Trauma **1:**361, 1961.

CHAPTER 103

Principles of Nerve Repair

ROBERT M. SZABO and
MICHAEL MADISON

Acute traumatic damage to a peripheral nerve may occur as a result of traction, contusion, compression, or laceration. The mechanism of injury will determine the nature of the lesion, its management, and its prognosis.

A nerve trunk can be stretched by as much as 15% of its length without injury. Much of this elasticity derives from the geometry of the nerve. "The nerve trunk runs an undulating course in its bed; the funiculi run an undulating course in the epineurium; and the nerve fibers run an undulating course inside the funiculi."[13] The straightening of these undulations provides elasticity in the physiologic range of stretching. As the nerve is stretched beyond this amount, the axons (efferent) and dendrites (afferent), which have little tensile strength, fail before the surrounding connective tissues (epineurium and perineurium), which are stronger. When the tensile strength of the perineurium is exceeded, which occurs at about 20% stretching, the nerve tears in two. In the region between the elastic limit and the mechanical limit, the nerve fibers will be damaged to varying degrees without gross disruption of the nerve trunk. Traction injuries may occur in association with fractures, either at the time of injury or during reduction or fixation, in dislocations and stretch injuries, and in gunshot wounds. Although spontaneous recovery is typical of most of these, complete nerve loss can also occur.

Contusion injuries from a blunt blow to the nerve carry a similar prognosis to traction injuries, with spontaneous functional recovery the norm. Recovery from compression injuries depends on how long the nerve has been compressed and the degree of compression.

A lacerated nerve has no chance of spontaneous recovery, and the discontinuity must be surgically repaired. If the wound is a clean one from a sharp object such as a knife or glass, the damage to the nerve is likely to be local, unlike a crush, traction, or missile wound in which damage may extend a considerable distance proximally and distally. The likelihood of functional recovery following accurate surgical repair depends on which nerve is involved, the level of the injury, the condition of the wound, and most importantly, the age of the patient. Results of nerve repair in children are always better than in adults. More distal injuries have a better prognosis for recovery than proximal ones, and a pure motor or sensory nerve has a better prognosis than a mixed nerve.

Seddon[10,11] proposed a simple classification of nerve injuries based on degree of damage rather than on mechanism of injury. *Neurapraxia* is a minor injury resulting from traction or compression in which ischemia and/or local demyelination interfere with nerve function. Damage to motor function is usually greater than to sensation, and recovery is within hours or days. *Axonotmesis* is a moderate injury in which continuity of axons is disrupted with Wallerian degeneration distal to the lesion. The endoneurial tubes remain intact, however, so that regenerating axons can reestablish their functional connections; and good recovery, usually within a year, is likely. *Neurotmesis* is a severe injury with disruption of both axons and connective tissues of the nerve. Fibrosis, loss of coaptation, and loss of continuity mitigate against spontaneous recovery. Surgical repair is indicated.

Sunderland[12] has classified peripheral nerve lesions into five types, representing increasing degrees of damage (Table

103-1). Millesi has added a second variable, the degree of fibrosis, to Sunderland's classification (see Chapter 111).

NATURAL HISTORY OF NERVE INJURY

Experimentally, a sharp surgical division of a peripheral nerve is the model that has been best studied; traction and crush injuries are less well understood. Within a month following laceration, the distal portion of the nerve, cut off from trophic support of proximal cell bodies, undergoes Wallerian degeneration. This involves disintegration of the axon and myelin sheath, which are absorbed by macrophages and Schwann cells, leaving a tubule along the pathway of the former axon. Proximal to the lesion some retrograde degeneration will occur as well; this is likely to be greater in more proximal lesions.

Within about 96 hours, the cell bodies whose axons or dendrites have been severed will enlarge and their metabolic activity will greatly increase. At the same time, axon sprouting will occur at the proximal stump. Provided that the two severed ends are still congruently opposed, axon sprouts will grow at a rate up to about 1 mm/day down the endoneurial tubules of the degenerating distal axons to eventually reestablish connection with the sensory, motor, and sympathetic end points. Spontaneous recovery from mild axonotmesis may take from 1 to 6 months, with more proximal lesions requiring greater time to heal.

In more severe lesions, several factors mitigate against successful natural recovery. The chief of these is loss of coaptation. Obviously, if the nerve is completely transected, then retraction of the severed ends and motion of the extremity will destroy coaptation and axon sprouts will not grow into the distal endoneurial tubules. Following a noncongruent repair, malaligned axon sprouts either will grow into epineurial tissues and reach a blind end or will grow into inappropriate tubules to establish connections that are nonfunctional. A second obstruction to successful natural repair is the development of fibrosis in the vicinity of the lesion. Fibrosis may distort the nerve architecture, thereby destroying coaptation; it may create a barrier at the lesion that is difficult for the axon sprouts to traverse; and it may tether the nerve to surrounding tissues, impairing its mobility. In general, extensive soft-tissue injuries with a major inflammatory response will lead to a greater degree of fibrosis. In traction, crush, and missile injuries, fibrosis may extend a considerable distance proximally and distally.

The management of peripheral nerve lesions must be designed to enhance the natural pathways of repair. This involves the reestablishment and maintenance of coaptation, avoidance of traction, and excision of excessive fibrosis.

CLINICAL ASSESSMENT OF PERIPHERAL NERVE INJURY

Severence of a peripheral nerve causes acute loss of sensory, motor, and sympathetic functions of that nerve distal to the lesion. Clinically, the acute picture is often confused by associated injuries. Fractures and dislocations; damage to muscles, tendons, or vascular structures; and head injury or altered psychological state can either mask or mimic a peripheral nerve injury. Assessment of peripheral neuropathy should be done as early as possible after stabilization of the patient's other injuries so that proper therapy can be planned.

A number of diagnostic tests have been devised to evaluate the function of a peripheral nerve (Table 103-2); these are well reviewed by Omer.[8] Accuracy and consistency in performing the initial diagnostic tests is critical, since these are the standard by which one will later judge whether the injury is spontaneously recovering, and hence whether surgery is indicated. Sometimes assessment can be made only by surgical exploration, as in young children or head trauma victims.

INDICATIONS FOR SURGERY

When nerve damage is suspected in the context of an open wound, direct inspection of the nerve at the time of irrigation and debridement is indicated. If the wound is clean, the mechanism of injury is a sharp laceration, the patient's condition is stable, and the surgical team and its facilities are available, then an acute primary repair may be undertaken. When this constellation of circumstances is not encountered, a delayed primary repair at 8 to 15 days is performed. When delayed pri-

TABLE 103-1. CLASSIFICATION OF NERVE INJURIES

Injury	Anatomy	Functional Loss	Recovery
First-degree	No disruption of axon; no Wallerian degeneration	Variable, usually more motor than sensory	Spontaneous, in hours to weeks; simultaneous distal and proximal recovery
Second-degree	Disruption of axon with Wallerian degeneration; endoneurial tubules intact	Complete sensory, motor and sympathetic loss	Spontaneous; proximal to distal motor recovery up to 1 year
Third-degree	Disruption of endoneurium, fascicles, and axons; perineurium intact; fibrosis and neuroma common	Complete	Spontaneous; proximal to distal motor recovery slower with some permanent motor and sensory loss likely
Fourth-degree	Extensive disruption with only some connective tissue continuity; fibrosis and neuroma common	Complete	Little spontaneous recovery without surgery
Fifth-degree	Complete disruption	Complete	No recovery without surgery

(After Sunderland, S.: Nerves and Nerve Injuries, 2nd ed. Edinburgh, Churchill Livingstone, 1978.)

TABLE 103-2. TESTS OF PERIPHERAL NERVE FUNCTION

Test	Effect of Neurotmesis	Comment
1. Sudomotor activity	Loss of sweating in affected distribution	Test by starch-iodine, Ninhydrin, or palpation; correlates loosely with sensory loss
2. Wrinkle test	Deinnervated skin immersed in warm water for 30 minutes will not wrinkle	
3. Volitional muscle action	Lost distal to lesion	Palpate the muscle belly rather than simply looking at distal motion. Test all muscles (distal to proximal) to localize lesion. Nerve block of parallel nerves may be useful.
4. Electromyography	Fibrillation action potentials in deinnervated muscle	Seen several weeks after neurotmesis
5. Nerve conduction velocity	Stimulus distal to lesion is not seen proximally, or velocity is reduced in partial lesion.	A true sensory test, unlike nos. 6–8, which are sensibility tests depending on cortical integration
6. Static and moving two-point discrimination	Lost; recovery shows increasing acuity.	May be confused by overlapping receptive fields; difficult to administer consistently
7. Semmes-Weinstein monofilaments	Lost; recovery shows increasing acuity.	Nos. 7 and 8 are threshold tests, best suited to follow nerve status after compression injury when nerve is intact
8. Tuning fork or vibrometer	Lost; recovery shows increasing acuity.	
9. Tinel's sign	In recovery, percussion over regenerating front produces tingling in area of distribution.	Failure to progress distally is indication for surgery.
10. Pick-up test	Lost; with recovery, speed and accuracy improve.	Reflects functionality of the repair (combined sensory, motor, and cortical function)

mary repair is to be done, at the time of acute exploration of the wound the nerve ends may be tagged with wire suture to facilitate later identification. Tagging is not critical, since later surgery is based on identifying normal nerve proximal and distal to the lesion and dissecting toward the injury, rather than on searching for suture tags in a bed of scar. However, the wire is useful for locating nerve ends on radiographs. If the severed ends can be easily approximated, then they may be loosely sutured together to resist retraction during the interval before the delayed repairs.

Early repair is preferable in a clean wound, since extensive nerve retraction has not yet occurred, and therefore less mobilization is required. However, the delay of 1 or 2 weeks after injury may offer some advantages besides allowing the surgical team opportunity to prepare. The post-traumatic edema of the cut ends has time to resolve, and the nerve cell bodies greatly increase their anabolic activity in association with axon sprouting. The extent of proximal and distal damage to the nerve is easier to assess. The location of early axon sprouts can help define a necrotic terminus of the proximal stump.

In a closed injury with a suspected neuropathy, after an acute compartment syndrome is ruled out, quantitative diagnostic tests should be performed (see Table 103-2) to serve as a standard by which the recovery (or lack of recovery) of the deficit may be measured. These tests must be performed in a meticulous and consistent way so that comparisons are valid. Although no single test is infallible, the combined weight of several tests with similar results allows reasonably secure diagnosis. The patient should be reevaluated at intervals of 4 to 6 weeks.

Secondary repair (i.e., more than 2 weeks after injury) is indicated in heavily contaminated wounds, when soft-tissue coverage is poor and requires flaps, when the amount of nerve damage cannot be assessed early (e.g., gunshot wounds, head injuries), or when diagnosis is initially missed. Some motor recovery may be expected following repairs as late as 1 year after injury; partial sensory recovery may result from repairs as late as 2 years after injury. However, success is less likely the longer one delays, since muscle atrophies and endoneurial tubules undergo fibrosis.

ANATOMIC BASIS OF NERVE REPAIR

The anatomic goal of neurorraphy is, simply, to exactly realign the axons so that regenerating axon sprouts will reconnect to their preinjury end points. A number of factors will frustrate the surgeon's attempt to achieve this. Edema in the proximal stump and shrinkage of the distal stump prohibit exact coaptation of formerly congruent ends, as will any distortion caused by less-than-perfect suture technique. A greater problem is segmental loss of even a few millimeters of nerve due to necrosis resulting from the injury. The pioneering studies of Sunderland in mapping the topography of the fasciculi in the peripheral nerves reveal a complex arrangement of branching, anastomosis, and wandering pathways. Consequently, the number, size, arrangement, and neurologic content of the fascicles as seen in cross section will vary along the nerve. With greater segmental loss, the cross-sectional arrangements of the two ends will be increasingly dissimilar and the possibility of excellent coaptation will diminish accordingly.

Sunderland's diagram of the fascicular topography of a segment of the musculocutaneous nerve (Fig. 103-1) has been often reproduced and stands as a graphic display of the impossibility of obtaining perfect coaptation following segmental loss. Jabaley and co-workers[5,16] have found that in several regions of the median and radial nerves the fascicular topography is considerably less variable than in Sunderland's diagram and that precise coaptation of most fascicles is theoretically possible despite segmental loss. Even over a longer distance encompassing various fascicular plexi, a bundle of axons tends to remain in the same quadrant of the nerve.

If segmental loss is minimal, correct rotational alignment can be ensured by aligning epineurial features (vessels) at the two stumps and by sketching the cross-sectional appearance of the two ends and approximating them accordingly. When segmental loss is greater, a sketch of the cross-sectional fascicular arrangment can be compared with published "maps," which may facilitate alignment. Finally, intraoperative electrical stimulation can be used to distinguish predominantly motor from sensory fascicles. With the patient awake and the tourniquet released, stimulation of the distal stump may identify motor fascicles and stimulation of the proximal stump may identify sensory fascicles. Silent fascicles proximally are presumed to be motor, and silent fascicles distally are presumed to be sensory.[4]

A staining technique based on acetylcholinesterase has been shown to help differentiate motor from sensory fascicles within a nerve. Because it requires 24 hours of incubation time, it is not usually suitable for intraoperative use, although it has provided confirmation of mapping of fascicles done by other means. Similar histochemical techniques with shorter development times show promise,[9] but they are not now in general use.

TECHNIQUES OF NEURORRHAPHY

There are three surgical techniques of neurorrhaphy in current use: epineurial repair, fascicular repair, and group fascicular repair. Each technique is appropriate to certain circumstances. Appreciation of microneuroanatomy is essential to understanding the techniques of nerve repair (Fig. 103-2).

Epineurial repair is the standard, classic method of nerve repair carried out by placing several sutures peripherally in the epineurium after aligning the nerve ends according to fascicular pattern and epineurial landmarks. This technique has the advantage of being less technically demanding, less traumatic to the nerve ends, and of placing less suture material in the repair site. Epineurial repair is indicated for small nerves, for nerves with only one or two fascicles, and for primary repair of a clean laceration in a larger nerve.

In fascicular (also called funicular) repair, individual fascicles are dissected free of enveloping epineurium and sutured fascicle to fascicle through the perineurium. In principle, this should lead to a more precise coaptation and hence a greater potential for recovery. In practice, fascicular repair is technically demanding, inevitably causes some trauma to the nerve ends, and leaves suture material within the nerve, which may stimulate a fibrotic response. Nonetheless, in the hands of those skilled in the technique, fascicular repair produces good results, especially in nerves with two to five large fascicles, or in repairs where epineurium constitutes a large part of the cross-sectional area of the nerve.

Group fascicular repair is similar in principle to fascicular repair except that recognizable groups of fascicles are joined instead of individual fascicles. The repair of more than five fascicles or groups is impractical, since it excessively injures the

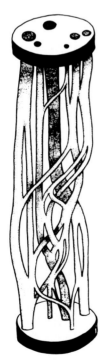

FIGURE 103-1. Fascicular topography of a segment of the musculocutaneous nerve. (Sunderland, S: Nerves and Nerve Injuries, 2nd ed. p. 32. Edinburgh, Churchill-Livingstone, 1978.)

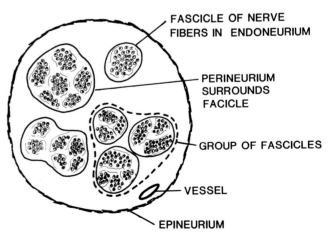

FASCICLE OF NERVE
FIBERS IN ENDONEURIUM

PERINEURIUM
SURROUNDS
FACICLE

GROUP OF FASCICLES

VESSEL

EPINEURIUM

FIGURE 103-2. Cross section of a peripheral nerve indicating principal structures.

nerve end and leaves too much suture material within the wound. Group fascicular repair is the technique employed in nerve grafting.

Epineurial and fascicular repair may be combined, as in repair of a laceration of the median nerve at the wrist where fascicular repair of the motor component may be combined with epineurial repair to approximate sensory elements. The choice of technique depends on the topography of the nerve at the site of the lesion. The superiority of fascicular or group fascicular repair over epineurial repair has not been clearly demonstrated either clinically or experimentally. The immediate environment of wound healing, the condition and age of the patient, and the skill of the surgeon are probably more important than the type of neurorrhaphy.

NERVE GRAFTING

Where segmental loss prohibits end-to-end repair without excessive tension, interfascicular nerve grafting is indicated. This technique has been developed and refined by Millesi,[6,7] whose series shows a high percentage of good to excellent results. The nerve stumps are stepcut and the fascicles debrided of enveloping epineurial tissues. Corresponding fascicles or groups of fascicles are identified by geometry and/or electrodiagnostic tests. Graft segments of a length sufficient to bridge the gap without tension are sutured through the perineurium to connect appropriate fascicles or groups of fascicles in the proximal and distal stumps. Although the regenerating axons must cross two suture lines, it is considered that the prognosis is better for crossing two suture lines without tension than one suture line under tension. Typically the sural nerve is used as the graft; this can yield a usable graft segment up to about 40 cm long. The lateral antebrachial cutaneous nerve may also be used.[14]

Although it is well known that nerve repair under tension has a poor prognosis, what constitutes "excessive" tension (and thus an indication for grafting) is not universally agreed. Wilgis[15] suggests that if an 8-0 suture cannot close the gap, tension is too great. Millesi[6] recommends grafting gaps greater than 2.5 cm with the extremity in a functional position. By mobilizing the nerve proximally and distally and flexing the joints it crosses, gaps of several centimeters may easily be closed. Flexion of the elbow beyond 90° or the wrist beyond 40° to close a gap is contraindicated. The surgeon must judge the potential morbidity of postoperative immobilization of the joints in a flexed position against the morbidity of nerve grafting in light of his own skills and experience.

Surgical Technique

Prep and drape the entire extremity into the operative field, since often it is necessary to mobilize the nerve proximally and distally for considerable distances. Prep and drape one or both lower extremities if nerve grafting is a possibility. Apply a tourniquet to each extremity being draped. Use a generous, extensile incision. In freeing the nerve, work toward the lesion, that is, distally in the proximal portion and proximally in the distal portion. Keep exposed portions of the nerve moist with saline-soaked sponges.

The nerves should be handled very gently using a jeweler's forceps to grasp only the epineurium. Avoid applying any pressure to the fascicles, which may result in further injury. Magnifying loupes are used in the initial identification of the nerve and its dissection. However, when the final preparation of the nerve ends and suturing needs to be done, an operating room microscope will facilitate proper grouping of similar nerve fascicles, aligning of epineural land marks with proper orientation, and more accurate placement of sutures. Microsurgical instruments are used in performing nerve repair and nerve grafting techniques.

Technique for Epineurial and Group Fascicular Repairs

Place a moist wooden tongue depresser beneath the end of the nerve. While an assistant applies gentle traction on the nerve end with a jeweler's forceps, use a Weck blade to sharply cut back the nerve ends until reaching noninjured tissue. Inspect the proximal portion of the cut ends under the microscope to look for bulging axons. Repeat these steps on the opposite nerve end. When both ends have been freshened until normal-looking structures are seen, the repair can begin.

Inspect the epineurium for longitudinal blood vessels as a landmark to orient the nerve. Also, inspect the fascicular pattern of the proximal and distal stumps for orientation. The assistant can take the tension off the nerve by grasping the proximal and distal nerves about 1 cm away from the repair and approximating the nerve ends. If the tension is observed to be great or proximation is not possible, then consider further mobilization of the nerve or grafting.

If performing an epineurial repair, after alignment of the nerve, pass the appropriate suture both proximally and distally in the epineurium only and tie the knot firmly. Pass a second suture 180° opposite to the first suture in a similar fashion. Use the minimal amount of sutures necessary to close the entire epineurium on the anterior side, and repeat this, having turned the nerve around, on the posterior side. A nonabsorbable 9-0 suture (nylon) is used for larger nerves, and a 10-0 nonabsorbable suture is used for smaller nerves (Fig. 103-3).

In a fascicular repair, identify the fascicles proximally and distally by observing the cross-sectional anatomy under the microscope. Coapt the ends of the matching funiculae, placing 10-0 nylon interrupted sutures through the interfascicular epineurium and the perineurium of the individual fascicles. Avoid all tension (Fig. 103-4).

In a grouped fascicular repair, identify groups of fascicles by observing proximal and distal cross-sectional anatomy and join these groups with interrupted 10-0 nylon suture placed in the interfascicular epineurium.

In mixed fascicular and epineural repair line up the major group of fascicles that can be identified and perform a grouped fascicular repair. Then repair the epineurium circumferentially around the entire nerve as described under epineurial repair.

Nerve Grafting

Explore and prepare the nerve stumps as described above. Examine the cross-sectional anatomy and isolate the fascicle

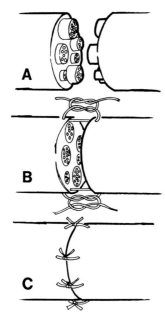

FIGURE 103-3. Epineurial repair.

groups. Measure the distance between the two stumps in the extended position of the elbow joint and the extended position of the wrist joint. Pass a 10-0 nylon stitch between the fascicles of the graft, catching the interfascicular epineurium, and then pass this stitch into the proximal stump of one group of fascicles. Now approximate the distal end of the graft to the stump of the corresponding distal fascicle group in similar fashion.

The usual donor site for providing nerve graft material is the sural nerve. The use of this nerve creates an insignificant sensory loss at the lateral side of the foot below the lateral ankle. Locate the nerve behind the lateral malleolus with a 1-cm longitudinal incision. Tag the nerve with an umbilical tape. A few centimeters proximal to this incision, make a small transverse incision. Pull on the nerve distally with slight tension so that it can be easily palpated in the proximal incision. Two to three more incisions placed proximally at equal intervals are used to harvest the entire segment of sural nerve. Other sources of donor nerve include the lateral and medial antebrachial cutaneous nerves and the terminal articular branches of

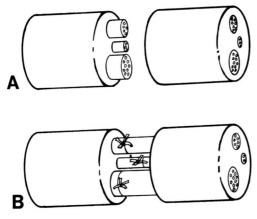

FIGURE 103-4. Fascicular repair.

the posterior interosseous nerve; however, the sural nerve provides the most tissue with the least morbidity.

Finally, it is essential to document in the operative notes exactly where the location of repair is in relation to surface anatomy. Each juncture should be measured and noted so that after surgery one can follow the progression of the Tinel sign. On occasion, particularly when using a long interfascicular graft, progression may cease at the distal nerve juncture. One would know this is happening clinically if the progression of Tinel ceases at the same point it was noted for the distal juncture.

The wounds are closed as usual and drained if appropriate. However, avoid suction drains placed close to a nerve repair or nerve graft since they may disrupt the suture line.

POSTOPERATIVE CARE

The extremity is immobilized in the exact position it is in during the operation for 10 to 14 days. Once wound sutures are removed, the extremity is placed in a plaster cast in a position to relax all suture lines. For example, a median nerve repair in the forearm would require the wrist to be in slight flexion and the elbow placed at 90° of flexion. Continue immobilization for a total of 6 weeks; however, at 4 weeks start to straighten out the joints that have been splinted in a position for the purpose of avoiding tension on the nerve suture line.

REHABILITATION

Preoccupation with the technical intricacies of nerve repair should not cause the surgeon to lose sight of his goal, which is a functional patient. In some cases in which nerve repair is feasible, the patient may nonetheless be better served by other procedures, such as tendon transfers. If an older patient is well adapted to his disability, it may be better not to intervene despite the possibility of improved function.

It is inevitable that following nerve repair some regenerating neurons will make connections to sensory or motor end points different from those to which they were formerly connected. Consequently, although they recover sensory function and transmit signals to the brain, the meaning of these signals is garbled if they are evaluated in the cortex according to preinjury habits of interpretation. The patient must be reeducated to correlate sensory input with external reality. In children, this is readily accomplished. Older patients are less flexible and may in the end ignore sensory information supplied by heterotopically regenerated nerves. In such a case, the anatomically "successful" nerve repair is in vain. An aggressive program of therapy aimed at sensory reeducation may considerably improve the clinical results of nerve repair by training the patient to adapt to the altered arrangement of the peripheral axons.

REFERENCES

1. Cabaud, H.E., Rodkey, W.G., and Nemeth, T.J.: Progressive Ultrastructural Changes After Peripheral Nerve Transection and Repair. J. Hand Surg. **7A:**353, 1982.

2. Dellon, A.L., and Munger, B.L.: Correlation of Histology and Sensibility After Nerve Repair. J. Hand Surg. **8**:871, 1983.

3. Frykman, G.K., Wolf, A., and Coyle, T.: An Algorithm for Management of Peripheral Nerve Injuries. Orthop. Clin. North Am. **12**:239, 1981.

4. Gaul, J.S. Jr.: Electrical Fascicle Identification as an Adjunct to Nerve Repair. Hand Clin. **2**:709, 1986.

5. Jabaley, M.E., Wallace W.H., and Heckler, F.R.: Internal Topography of Major Nerves of the Forearm and Hand. J. Hand Surg. **5**:1, 1980.

6. Millesi, H.: Interfascicular Nerve Grafting. Orthop. Clin. North Am. **12**:287, 1981.

7. Millesi, H., Meissl, G., and Berger, A.: The Interfascicular Nerve Grafting of the Median and Ulnar Nerves. J. Bone Joint Surg. **54A**:727, 1972.

8. Omer, G.E. Jr.: Evaluation of the Extremity With Peripheral Nerve Injury and Timing for Nerve Suture. AAOS Instructional Course Lectures **33**:463, 1984.

9. Riley, D.A., and Lang, D.H.: Carbonic Anhydrase Activity of Human Peripheral Nerves: A Possible Histochemical Aid to Nerve Repair. J. Hand Surg. **9-A**:112, 1984.

10. Seddon, H.J.: Three Types of Nerve Injury. Brain **66**:237, 1943.

11. Seddon, H.J.: Surgical Disorders of the Peripheral Nerves. Edinburgh, Churchill Livingstone, 1972.

12. Sunderland, S.: Nerves and Nerve Injuries, 2nd ed. Edinburgh, Churchill Livingstone, 1978.

13. Sunderland, S.: The Anatomical Basis of Nerve Repair. *In* Jewett, D.L., and McCarroll, H.R. Jr. (eds.): Nerve Repair and Regeneration. St. Louis, C.V. Mosby, 1980.

14. Tank, M.S., Royce C.L. Jr., and Coates, P.W.: The Lateral Antebrachial Cutaneous Nerve as a Highly Suitable Autograft Donor for the Digital Nerve. J. Hand Surg. **8A**:942, 1983.

15. Wilgis, E.F.S.: Nerve Repair and Grafting. *In* Green, D.P. (ed.): Operative Hand Surgery, 2 vol. Edinburgh, Churchill Livingstone, 1982.

16. Williams, H.B., and Jabaley, M.E.: The Importance of Internal Anatomy of the Peripheral Nerves to Nerve Repair in the Forearm and Hand. Hand Clin. **2**:689, 1986.

CHAPTER 104

Compression Neuropathies of the Upper Extremity

JULIO TALEISNIK

Compression neuropathies are mechanical entrapments of nerves in areas that are anatomically vulnerable. The intrinsic response of the nerve is similar, regardless of the location of the injury or the nature of the offending agent. Thus, the sequence of pathologic changes within the median nerve and the resulting clinical progression are the same whether the entrapment is secondary to synovitis within the carpal tunnel or to a bone fragment from a fracture of the distal radius. Likewise, release of the compression will reverse these changes, partially or completely, or if damage to the nerve is irreversible, in chronic entrapment, release will at least stop their progression. All three major nerves of the upper extremity may be injured by compression in locations where they are anatomically most vulnerable: the carpal, radial, cubital, and ulnar tunnels and deep to fibrous bands and tendinous arches of origin at the level of the elbow and forearm. Therefore, the clinical evaluation of an entrapment syndrome, and the determination of the site of compression, are greatly aided by a knowledge of the anatomic distribution of a nerve and its function. Electrodiagnostic studies may help to corroborate this clinical impression, but are not a substitute for a thorough examination.

Some clinical conditions, such as hypothyroidism, diabetes, and alcoholism, increase nerve vulnerability through metabolic and hormonal effects. These may not only favor the onset of nerve entrapments, but may also be the cause of peripheral polyneuritis, thereby interfering with a satisfactory recovery of nerve function. These conditions must be investigated when suspected.

The mechanism whereby surgical decompression works is not entirely understood. The frequently dramatic response to treatment can only be explained by the reversal of a vascular lesion.[2,3] According to this theory the mechanical factor responsible for producing the compression would generate an obstruction to venous return, followed by segmental anoxia, capillary vasodilatation, and edema.[2,16] The nerve edema itself further aggravates the compression and leads to abnormal axonic and cellular exchange.[3,15] Surgical release at this stage is a very rewarding procedure. Prolonged compression results in intraneural fibrosis, following which nerve recovery is less likely to occur after decompression.

GENERAL PRINCIPLES OF TREATMENT

The onset of symptoms of nerve compression may be acute and rapidly progressive or gradual. Indications for surgery include (1) failure of nonsurgical management (splinting, injections of steroids, elastic gloves for carpal tunnel syndrome in pregnancy or hypothyroidism, avoidance of activities); (2) acute, rapidly progressive involvement; (3) severe, chronic syndromes; (4) recurrence; and (5) the presence of motor involvement. The surgical release should be performed under tourniquet control, unless the site of compression is too proximal in the arm. Exsanguination by elevation of the arm alone is preferable to exsanguination by elastic wrapping, because it will allow easier visualization of partially filled, small potential bleeders, which can be tied or coagulated before releasing the tourniquet. This must be done in all cases, but particularly after prolonged aspirin intake or in patients with spontaneous or induced (e.g., by kidney dialysis) coagulopathies, to reduce postoperative bleeding and swelling.

Frequently decompression does not require hospitalization and is performed under regional anesthesia. Local anesthesia is an excellent choice, particularly for the less involved decompressions, such as decompression of the median nerve at the wrist or of the ulnar nerve at the wrist or elbow. A tourniquet may still be used, because it is well tolerated for these brief procedures.

The choice of treatment of the nerve itself depends on its examination under direct vision, the location of the entrapment, and the clinical findings. Severe strangulation from a scarred down or thickened epineurium must be released by an anterior epineurotomy. If a true neuroma in continuity is present, an internal neurolysis is justified. An internal neurolysis may also be required during reoperations for failure of previous decompression or for recurrence. In my experience internal neurolysis is more frequently used for the median nerve at the level of the carpal tunnel, when there is thenar atrophy or palsy with constant loss of sensibility. Because internal neurolysis carries the risk of damage to the interfascicular plexus, it should be limited to the more distal areas of peripheral nerves (i.e., median and ulnar nerves at the wrist), where interfasciculation is minimal.[2] Use a magnification of 3.5× or higher. Gently tease the nerve fascicles apart with sharp-pointed, curved scissors, taking care to preserve small vessels; leave the bed of the nerve undisturbed. In my experience this is a rewarding procedure in young patients when preoperative pain is not excessive and when constant sensory loss is the main presenting complaint. The postoperative dressing should be well padded and comfortable. Protective plaster splinting is used in most cases and is usually removed after 3 to 5 days, unless tendon origins or insertions were divided, in which case protection by immobilization is longer.

COMPRESSION NEUROPATHIES OF THE MEDIAN NERVE

Compression of the median nerve typically occurs within the carpal tunnel or deep to the origin of the pronator teres. A third form of median nerve entrapment is the isolated compression of the anterior interosseous nerve.

Carpal Tunnel Syndrome

Compressive neuropathy of the median nerve within the carpal tunnel may result from the presence of any space-occupying lesion under the transverse carpal ligament. The most frequent cause is a flexor tenosynovitis; other causes are fractures and dislocations of the floor of the canal and tumors. The diagnosis is strongly suggested by the patient's history. Typically, the patient is a postmenopausal female with nocturnal numbness and burning pain along the median nerve distribution and paresthesias, all of which are increased by elevation and repetitive activities. Radiation of symptoms proximal to the wrist is not unusual. On examination sensibility may be reduced throughout the area normally supplied by the median nerve, except for the distribution of the palmar cutaneous branch, which does not enter the carpal canal.[17] Numbness may extend to the ulnar digits in some patients. Sudomotor activity may be diminished. This is easy to detect clinically by sliding a metal object (i.e., a pen), between the patient's fingers, which are held together.

The object will slide much easier on dry skin than on skin with normal perspiration. In more advanced cases there is thenar weakness or atrophy. The Tinel's and Phalen's tests are positive. The examiner may exacerbate numbness by direct digital compression of the median nerve proximal to the transverse creases at the wrist. Radiographs of the wrist, including carpal tunnel views, and nerve conduction studies, complete the diagnostic workup. When doubt persists as to the correct diagnosis, an injection of a small amount of a steroid preparation into the carpal tunnel (*not* into the nerve) will serve as both a therapeutic and a diagnostic aid.

Operative Technique and Postoperative Care

Start the incision at the interthenar level in the midpalm, and continue it proximally to a point where the ulnar margin of the ring finger ray intersects the distal wrist crease (Fig. 104-1). For a simple carpal tunnel release, this exposure will suffice. In many cases the approach is facilitated by extending the incision along the wrist crease in a radial direction to a point just ulnar to the flexor carpi radialis tendon. Expose the transverse carpal ligament, and divide it longitudinally close to its ulnar attachments. Distally, this division should reach the fatty envelope surrounding the vessels of the superficial palmar arch. With the median nerve under direct vision, undermine the skin, and elevate it proximally to visualize the transverse carpal ligament as it blends into the palmar carpal ligament. Complete the division of these two structures. Elevate the entire radial flap of skin, together with its subcutaneous tissue, ligament, and the intact palmar cutaneous branch of the median nerve and its divisions; this exposes the median nerve[17] (Fig. 104-2). Removal of a strip of transverse carpal ligament is not necessary. If additional exposure at the wrist or distal forearm is required (e.g., for a flexor tenosynovectomy, or for the reduction and fixation of a carpal dislocation or radius fracture, or for the additional release of the ulnar nerve at the wrist), prolong the incision proximally, or in a proximal and ulnar direction.

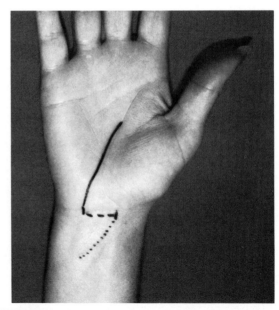

FIGURE 104-1.   Approach to the carpal tunnel. The more proximal third is used when a more extensive exposure is required (see text).

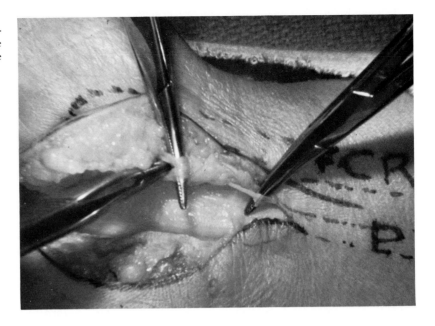

FIGURE 104-2. The radial flap of skin, subcutaneous tissue, and transverse carpal ligament contain the intact palmar cutaneous branch of the median nerve and its branches.

If an anterior neurolysis is needed, first perform a longitudinal epineurotomy on the radial side of the nerve, away from the ulnar entry of the segmental circulation.[2] Gently tease fascicles with sharp-pointed, small, curved scissors, using 3.5× or higher magnification, preserving small intraneural vessels. Leave the dorsal bed of the nerve undisturbed. Release the tourniquet and secure hemostasis. Close only the skin, and apply a well-padded dressing with plaster reinforcement. Encourage immediate full motion of all digits and shoulder. Bulky dressings and splinting are usually removed 3 to 5 days after operation, to permit wrist mobilization. Gradual return to full activities is allowed thereafter.

Pitfalls and Complications

Complications and pitfalls are secondary to misdiagnosis or to technical factors. Conditions associated with peripheral neuropathies must be suspected, recognized when present, and treated before operation or concurrently with the surgical release. For instance hypertrophic synovium should be removed. Upton and McComas[18] proposed a "double crush syndrome" as a hypothesis to explain the failure of distal decompressions in nerves subject to compression in multiple sites. Complications secondary to technical factors include improper placement of the incision (usually too far radially); injury or entrapment of the palmar cutaneous nerve or its branches (Fig. 104-3); and poor exposure, resulting in incomplete division of the transverse carpal ligament, or in injury to the superficial palmar arch. Transverse incisions at the wrist crease for decompression of the carpal tunnel should not be used.

A rare complication is a tendency of the flexor tendons to the little finger to sublux during strong gripping. This is, fortunately, a transient problem. Complications from deficient postoperative management usually result from swelling and edema

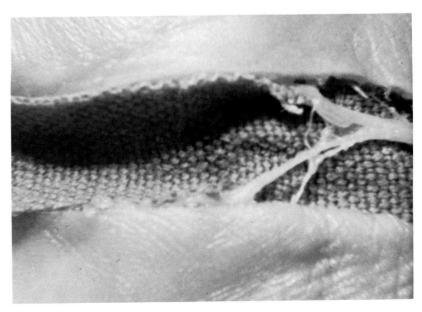

FIGURE 104-3. Palmar cutaneous branch of the median nerve and its divisions crossing an incision placed too far radially.

and poor control of pain, leading to loss of finger or wrist motion (particularly if a synovectomy was performed) and to reflex sympathetic dystrophy. The benefits of a good postoperative dressing, an aggressive motion program, and elevation cannot be emphasized enough.

Pronator Syndrome

The symptoms arising from the compression of the median nerve at this level—numbness in the radial three and one-half digits and thenar weakness—may easily be attributed to a carpal tunnel syndrome. Important in the differential diagnosis are (1) the location of the pain, in the anterior aspect of the proximal forearm; (2) aggravation of pain by resisted pronation; (3) the presence of numbness within the territory of the palmar branch of the median nerve; (4) a positive nerve percussion sign in the forearm rather than at the carpal tunnel; and (5) a negative Phalen's test. Exactly the same pronator syndrome may also result from compression in areas other than that deep to the arch of origin of the pronator teres, namely under the origin of the flexor digitorum superficialis, beneath the lacertus fibrosus, and from a supracondylar process com-

bined with a ligament of Struthers. The latter two conditions should be suspected when symptoms are aggravated by elbow flexion against resistance with forearm supination.[1,2,14] Symptoms arising from a typical pronator entrapment are aggravated by forearm pronation against resistance, preferably checked with the elbow in extension and the wrist palmarflexed to relax the flexor digitorum superficialis.[3,9,13,14] Finally, symptoms that are increased by resisted flexion of the flexor superficialis to the long finger suggest entrapment beneath the superficialis arch of origin.[3,14] Special diagnostic procedures include electrodiagnostic studies and, when a supracondylar syndrome is suspected, radiographs to include the distal humerus in four projections, designed to show a supracondylar process. In 1% of limbs, this anomalous spur is connected to the medial epicondyle by the ligament of Struthers, forming a fibro-osseous tunnel through which the median nerve (exceptionally the ulnar nerve) passes.[14]

Operative Technique and Postoperative Care

When there is evidence of compression under an arcade of Struthers (Fig. 104-4A), the surgical exposure should be cen-

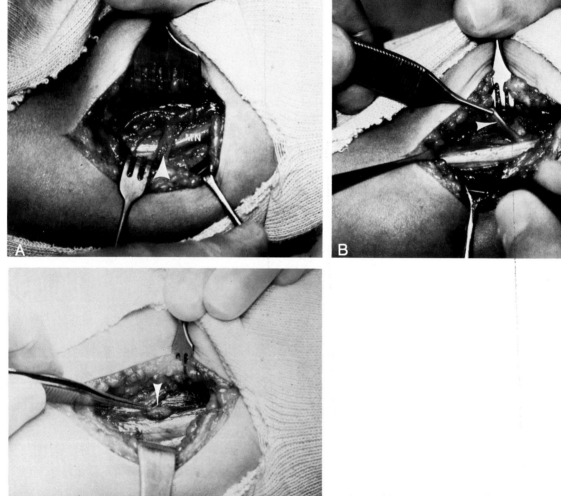

FIGURE 104-4. Entrapment of the median nerve (MN) under a ligament of Struthers. (*A*) Initial appearance. (*B*) The ligament divided and elevated (*arrow*). (*C*) Supracondylar process (*arrow*).

FIGURE 104-5.   Extensive approach for the exposure of the median nerve at the elbow and proximal forearm.

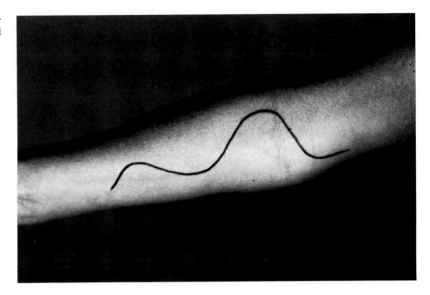

tered at the radiographic projection of the supracondylar process. In these cases I prefer to not only divide the ligament of Struthers (Fig. 104-4*B*), but also to excise the supracondylar process (Fig. 104-4*C*). If a ligament of Struthers is not found, the area of compression must be found by further dissection distally. For these particular cases, and for all others clinically involving areas other than the supracondylar process, decompression of the median nerve for pronator syndrome should include a routine division of the lacertus fibrosus.

Begin the incision along the projection of the medial neurovascular bundle, just 5 cm proximal to the elbow flexure. Continue it in a gentle curve along the elbow flexure, and extend it distally past the superficialis arch (Fig. 104-5). All three possibly offending structures—lacertus, pronator teres, and superficialis arch—are thus exposed. First, identify the median nerve proximal to the lacertus (Fig. 104-6*A*). From this point the goal of the procedure is, simply, to free the nerve of all constricting bands and arches. It is important to follow the nerve as it passes

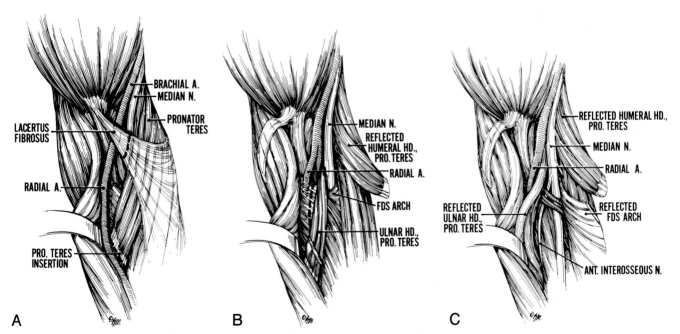

FIGURE 104-6.   (*A*) "The lacertus fibrosus may act as a compressive band across the flexor muscle mass in supination; it should be divided with any exploration of the median nerve." (*B*) "Exposure of the median and anterior interosseous nerves by reflection of the humeral head (superficial head) of the pronator teres also exposes the arch of the superficialis." (*C*) "The radial origin of the superficialis muscle is elevated by subperiosteal dissection to expose the deep volar compartment and the anterior interosseous nerve." (With permission of Eversmann, W.W., Jr.: Entrapment and Compression Neuropathies. *In* Green, D.P.: Operative Hand Surgery. New York, Churchill Livingstone, 1982.)

between the two heads of the pronator teres. Detach the superficial head from its distal conjoined tendon with the deep head, using a step-cut[14] or a long oblique incision designed to allow reattachment of the superficial head with relative lengthening. Reflect the superficial head ulnarly (Fig. 104-6B).

When clinical examination suggests entrapment under the arch of origin of the flexor digitorum superficialis, detach the flexor from its radial insertion, (Fig. 104-6C) or simply divide it along its fibers between its radial and ulnar halves. Reattach the superficial pronator at a point proximal to its original insertion.

After skin closure, apply a well-padded compression dressing and a posterior plaster splint with the elbow flexed at right angles and the forearm in semipronation. Shoulder and finger motion are encouraged immediately after operation. After 3 to 5 days, immobilization is discontinued, and the patient is allowed to resume elbow flexion–extension and forearm rotation.

Pitfalls and Complications

Just as for the carpal tunnel syndrome, misdiagnosis and technical factors are responsible for avoidable complications. The most important is failure to release constriction at one of the four sites of possible entrapment. Accidental damage to branches of the median nerve is avoided by initial exposure and dissection of the nerve along its lateral, branch-free aspect.

Anterior Interosseous Syndrome

Unlike the entrapment syndromes of the entire median nerve, the compression neuropathy of the anterior interosseous nerve results exclusively in loss of motor function, without sensory deficit. The typical finding is weakness or paralysis of the muscles innervated by this nerve: the radial half of the flexor digitorum profundus, the flexor pollicis longus, and the pronator quadratus. The patient complains of a vague aching pain in the anterior forearm. There is frequently a history of a single episode of strong contraction of elbow, wrist, and finger flexors, accompanied by pain and followed shortly thereafter by motor loss. The patient is unable to end-pinch between index and thumb; the lack of long flexors results in a hyperextension attitude of the distal joints of these two digits.[11] Weakness or paralysis of the pronator quadratus may be demonstrated by asking the patient to pronate against resistance, with the elbow flexed to neutralize the stronger pronator teres. The diagnosis is usually confirmed by electromyographic studies. Compression may be caused by one of many structures, including accessory muscles, aberrant vessels, or tendinous bands. Surgical decompression is the treatment of choice, designed to expose the nerve from its origin and to release all structures crossing its path with a potential for causing undue constriction.

Operative Technique and Postoperative Care

Persistence of palsy after a period of 6 to 8 weeks, without electromyographic or clinical evidence of improvement, is an indication for operation.[14] The surgical technique and postoperative management are very similar to those used in the pro-

nator syndrome. The anterior interosseous nerve originates from the median just distal to the proximal border of the pronator teres and should be exposed as it traverses between the two heads of the pronator teres, under the aponeurotic origin of the flexor digitorum superficialis, and deep between the flexor pollicis longus and the radial half of the flexor digitorum superficialis. Just as for exposure in the pronator syndrome, divide the lacertus fibrosus, and if necessary, detach the superficial head of the pronator teres and the origin of the flexor digitorum superficialis (see Fig. 104-6A and B). Rarely does the nerve traverse deep to the entire pronator teres. Distally, end the dissection when the branches to the deep flexors are visualized. Although it is exceptional to completely detach the pronator teres or the origin of the flexor digitorum superficialis, this may be needed to complete visualization of the median and anterior interosseous nerves (see Fig. 104-6C). When anterior subcutaneous transposition of the median nerve is deemed necessary (a very infrequent occurrence in my experience), reattach the origin of the flexor digitorum superficialis deep to the median but superficial to the anterior interosseous nerve. Also, place the pronator beneath the median nerve in these patients. The postoperative management is essentially identical to that following treatment of the pronator syndrome.

Pitfalls and Complications

Pitfalls are similar to those described for the carpal tunnel and pronator teres syndromes. The main problem is an error in diagnosis, particularly in patients with an incomplete syndrome involving either the thumb or the index long flexors, but not both[4] (Fig. 104-7). In these patients the presenting findings may lead to the erroneous diagnosis of tendon rupture and a negative tendon exploration.

COMPRESSION NEUROPATHIES OF THE ULNAR NERVE

The ulnar nerve may be entraped at the elbow (the cubital tunnel syndrome), or at the wrist, within Guyon's canal (the ulnar tunnel syndrome).

Cubital Tunnel Syndrome

The presenting complaint is usually numbness along the ulnar nerve distribution, frequently accompanied by grip weakness, rarely by wasting of the intrinsic musculature. These symptoms are identical to those arising from ulnar entrapment at the wrist. The differential diagnosis is aided by eliciting other symptoms and by a careful examination. Aching or pain referred to the medial aspect of the elbow; tenderness, particularly at the edge of the arch of origin of the flexor carpi ulnaris; a positive percussion test within the cubital tunnel; and reproduction or aggravation of numbness by full elbow flexion are helpful to localize the entrapment to the elbow. Less frequently, the motor changes involve extrinsic muscles, particularly the long flexors to the ring and little fingers, or the flexor carpi ulnaris, in which case a proximal nerve entrapment becomes obvious. Likewise, numbness including the ulnar half of

FIGURE 104-7. Incomplete anterior interosseous nerve syndrome. (*A*) preoperative loss of flexion of the right thumb; (*B*) postoperative result.

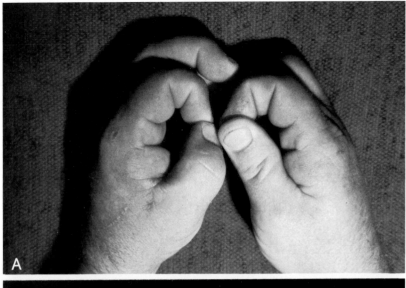

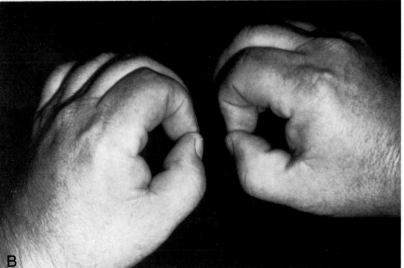

the dorsum of the hand indicates compression proximal to the origin of the dorsal cutaneous branch of the ulnar nerve, and therefore, proximal to the canal of Guyon. Electrodiagnostic studies showing a reduction of conduction velocity greater than 33% are significant.[3]

The causes of compression are many, including trauma, deformity (e.g., cubitus valgus), spurs or bone fragments within the floor of the cubital tunnel (Fig. 104-8), tumors, abnormal muscles, and a nerve that subluxes or dislocates repeatedly over the medial epicondyle.

Choice of Operative Technique

The choice of operative technique is greatly influenced by the etiology of the compression and by other factors, specifically, the patient's age and the presence or absence of systemic conditions such as diabetes or alcoholism. In my practice I have elected to decompress the nerve by division of the arch of origin of the flexor carpi ulnaris[20] when clinical findings (e.g., a localized nerve percussion sign) suggest isolated entrapment of

the nerve beneath the arch, when the nerve presents a constricting groove caused by this arch as visualized during operation (Fig. 104-9), and in nerves that may be vulnerable to manipulation (in older patients or in cases of diabetic or alcoholic neuropathy). Anterior submuscular transposition[6,7] is reserved for neuropathies associated with elbow deformity, abnormalities of the cubital canal, and the subluxing or dislocating ulnar nerve, particularly in the younger population and in the more severe cases with evidence of motor involvement. In my experience the only indication for medial epicondylectomy has been the ulnar neuropathy associated with a nonunion of a fracture of the medial epicondyle.

Operative Technique and Postoperative Care

Decompression. Start the incision equidistant from the olecranon and the medial epicondyle, and extend it 3 to 4 cm proximally and 6 to 8 cm distally to the cubital tunnel. (Although an incision convex anteriorly and palmar to the medial epicondyle is free from subsequent pressure, it may divide

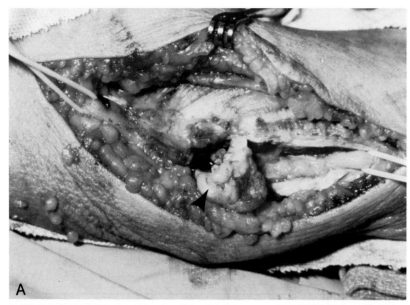

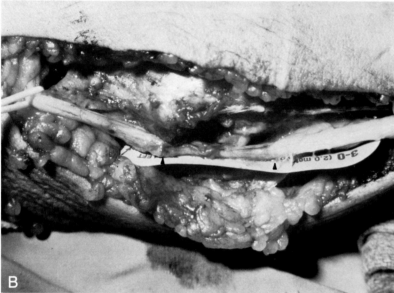

FIGURE 104-8. (*A*) Compression of ulnar nerve at the elbow by large osteochondral body (*arrow*). (*B*) Severe nerve constriction is seen (*between arrows*) after osteochondral fragment is removed.

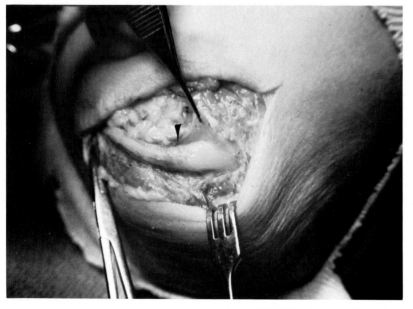

FIGURE 104-9. Well-defined constriction of the ulnar nerve (*arrow*) seen after division of the arch of origin of the flexor carpi ulnaris.

small cutaneous branches and produce annoying postoperative paresthesias. If such an approach is selected, expose and preserve cutaneous branches, and perform the decompression beneath them.) Isolate the ulnar nerve before it enters the cubital canal. Delineate the arch of origin of the flexor carpi ulnaris, elevate it from the nerve, and divide it, keeping the underlying nerve under direct vision and protected. It is prudent to extend this division distally between the two heads of the muscle to allow plenty of room for the nerve.

Release the tourniquet for careful hemostasis. In my experience it is not necessary to suture the split heads of the flexor carpi ulnaris beneath the nerve; closure is limited to the skin. Apply a well-padded dressing. The arm is supported in a sling for a few days. Immediate active flexion–extension of the elbow is encouraged.

Although subluxation of the nerve following decompression is a possibility, I have not encountered this complication in practice. On the contrary, nerves that are tense as bow-strings proximal to the constricting tendinous arch, snapping over the medial epicondyle during elbow flexion–extension, recover a normal excursion after decompression.

Anterior Submuscular Transposition. The exposure needs to be greater than that for decompression alone. Center the incision between olecranon and medial epicondyle, and extend it along the axes of humerus and ulna, therefore avoiding the majority of the cutaneous nerves crossing this area[6] (Fig. 104-10). Expose the deep fascia, and raise the entire lateral skin flap on this plane to expose the flexor-pronator muscle origin. Next, identify the ulnar nerve proximally, and elevate it gently on a moistened wide Penrose drain. Split the two heads of the flexor carpi ulnaris, as is done for decompression alone. As the ulnar nerve is freed, short branches to the joint may need to be divided. Those to the ulnar head of the flexor carpi ulnaris must be preserved; carefully separate them proximally from the main trunk, in order to allow mobilization of the nerve. Next, identify the *lateral* border of the flexor-pronator origin. Further lateral is the median nerve; the purpose of this procedure is to place the ulnar nerve alongside the median.

Using blunt dissection from lateral to medial, elevate the flexor-pronator origin. Once the entire muscle mass is raised, detach it from its origin and turn it distally (Fig. 104-11A). At this stage an aponeurotic structure common to the flexor superficialis arch and the humeral head of the pronator teres may be found; divide it to avoid kinking of the nerve around it[5] (Fig. 104-12). The ulnar nerve can now be transposed next to the median nerve. The following step is most important; palpate the medial intermuscular septum as a tense, sharp band that must be excised. If an arcade of Struthers is present, release it to avoid kinking the nerve (see Fig. 104-11A). Release the tourniquet, and carefully secure hemostasis. Reattach the flexor-pronator origin, using nonabsorbable sutures, and reapproximate both heads of the flexor carpi ulnaris with fine resorbable sutures (see Fig. 104-11B). Close the skin. Apply a well-padded dressing from the hand to the upper arm, with a posterior plaster splint for further support. Plaster immobilization is discontinued at 2 weeks, when active flexion–extension exercises of the elbow are allowed several times daily, while support of the elbow in flexion continues in a sling. As soon as full active motion is restored, usually at 3 to 4 weeks after surgery, free use of the extremity is allowed.

Ulnar Tunnel Syndrome

Entrapment at this level may result in pure motor, sensory, or mixed symptoms. Shea and McClain[10] described three ulnar nerve compression syndromes at and distal to the wrist. In type I the entrapment takes place proximal to or within the canal of Guyon, resulting in mixed motor and sensory deficit. Type II is purely motor, secondary to compression in the canal of Guyon, or at the hook of the hamate, in relation with the origins of the abductor digiti minimi and the flexor digiti minimi, and within the substance of the opponens digiti quinti. Type III is due to pressure on the superficial branch of the ulnar nerve, without associated muscle weakness or atrophy.

A careful evaluation will be extremely helpful in localizing the precise site of compression. Palpation of the deep structures within the hypothenar region may suggest a mass, not

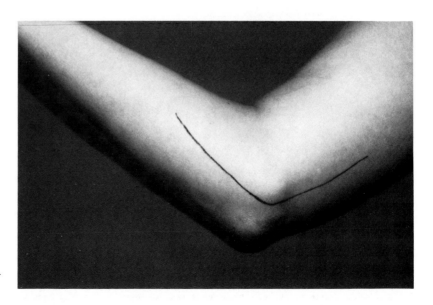

FIGURE 104-10. Approach for anterior transposition of the ulnar nerve.

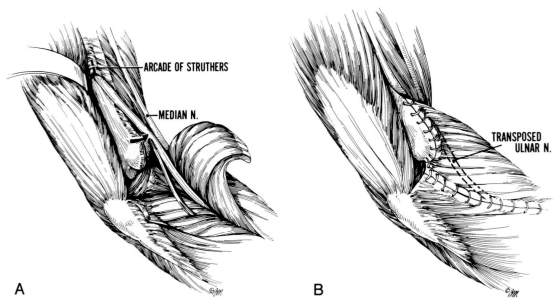

A   **B**

FIGURE 104-11. (*A*) "After submuscular transposition, care must be taken to prevent angulation of the ulnar nerve at the arcade of Struthers. The branches to the flexor carpi ulnaris should be preserved." (*B*) "Completion of the submuscular transposition by repair of the flexor muscles to the medial epicondyle." (With permission of Eversmann, W.W., Jr.: Entrapment and Compression Neuropathies. *In* Green, D.P.: Operative Hand Surgery. New York, Churchill Livingstone, 1982.)

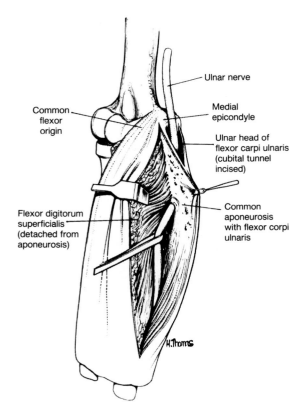

FIGURE 104-12. "Right elbow. The anatomic structures about the medial aspect of the elbow. Note the relation of the ulnar nerve as it enters the cubital tunnel and then exits by perforating the common intermuscular septum between the [flexor digitorum superficials] and [flexor carpi ulnaris] to course distally along the forearm." (With permission of Inserra, S., and Spinner, M.: An anatomic factor significant in transposition of the ulnar nerve. J. Hand Surg. **11-A:**80, 1986.)

infrequently a ganglion within the canal. The Allen's test should be done, because thrombosis or aneurysm of the ulnar artery may be the cause of the neuropathy. Radiographs, including a carpal (ulnar) tunnel view, and electrodiagnostic tests complete the preliminary workup. Additional tests may be done when vascular compromise is suspected. This syndrome may be secondary to space-occupying lesions (ganglions, aneurysms, lipomas) (Fig. 104-13), fractures of the bony walls of the canal of Guyon, anatomic variations of the canal, accessory or aberrant muscles, or repeated blunt trauma to the hypothenar region. Except for this last condition, when cessation of trauma may lead to complete resolution of symptoms, and for the type III neuropathies, the ulnar tunnel syndrome is best treated by surgical means.

Operative Technique and Postoperative Care

Decompression of the canal of Guyon should routinely be accompanied by a release of the carpal tunnel, even in the absence of clinical or electrodiagnostic evidence of median nerve entrapment. This combined procedure does not add to the postoperative morbidity and eliminates a potential cause of later problems. Conversely, I do not explore the ulnar nerve during carpal tunnel releases, *unless* there is preoperative clinical or electrodiagnostic evidence of ulnar nerve involvement at the wrist. Use the extended incision described for the approach to the carpal tunnel (see Fig. 104-1). Once the transverse carpal ligament is released, expose the ulnar neurovascular bundle proximal to the Guyon canal, and follow it distally. Divide the palmar carpal ligament, and expose sensory and motor branches of the nerve. Divide all constricting bands or vascular arches crossing the nerve. When a ganglion is found, it usually originates from the pisotriquetral joint and must be excised in

FIGURE 104-13. Aneurysm of the ulnar artery within the canal of Guyon (ulnar tunnel) producing an ulnar tunnel syndrome.

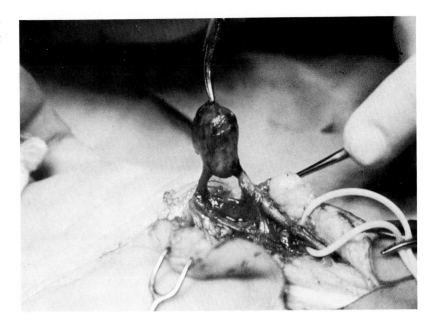

its entirety. The postoperative care is identical to that described for the carpal tunnel release.

Pitfalls and Complications

Pitfalls and complications are similar to those secondary to carpal tunnel syndromes. The only additional pitfall is failure to recognize the existence of a vascular component within this syndrome.

COMPRESSION NEUROPATHIES OF THE RADIAL NERVE

Although the radial nerve can be entrapped as it crosses the lateral intermuscular septum in the arm (most frequently in conjunction with displaced fractures of the humerus), or at the distal forearm and wrist,[19] the two more frequent and typical compressions are the posterior interosseous nerve syndrome and the radial tunnel syndrome.

Posterior Interosseous Nerve Syndrome

After the radial nerve bifurcates, just proximal to the elbow, its posterior interosseous branch passes between the two heads of the supinator muscle under an inverted fibrous arch, the arcade of Frohse, formed by the thickened edge of origin of the superficial head[12] (Fig. 104-14). Entrapment is most common at this level, although it may also occur further distally within the supinator. It may be associated with space-occupying lesions (lipomata, ganglions, synovitis) or with fractures of the neck and dislocations of the head of the radius. Posterior interosseous nerve compression may also be iatrogenic, for instance following internal fixation of fractures of the proximal radius, where the nerve is extremely vulnerable, as it may lie directly on the periosteum at a level opposite the tuberosity of the radius[12] (Fig. 104-15). This syndrome is purely motor. The brachioradialis and extensor carpi radialis longus muscles are

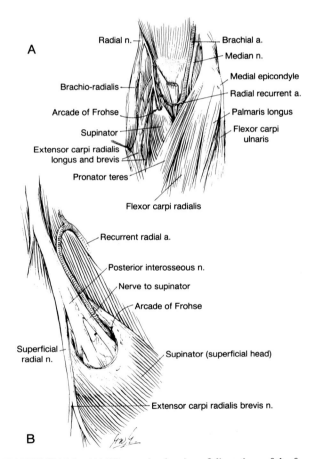

FIGURE 104-14. (A) "Composite drawing of dissections of the forearm at the level of the elbow. (B) Enlarged view of posterior interosseous nerve and its relationship to the supinator muscle. The arcade of Frohse is readily seen. The motor supply to the extensor carpi radialis brevis arises most frequently from the superficial radial nerve." (With permission of Spinner, M.: Injuries to the Major Branches of Peripheral Nerves of the Forearm. Philadelphia, W.B. Saunders, 1972.)

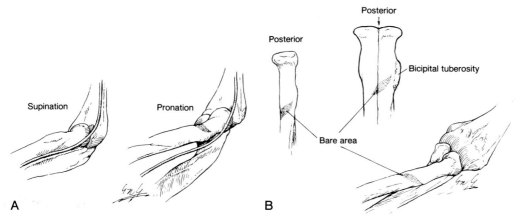

FIGURE 104-15. (*A*) "In supination when the bare area of the proximal radius is present, the posterior interosseous nerve comes to lie against the periosteum of the radius. (*B*) Details of the bare area are noted." (With permission of Spinner, M.: Injuries to the Major Branches of Peripheral Nerves of the Forearm. Philadelphia, W.B. Saunders, 1972.)

never involved, since their innervation is proximal to the arcade of Frohse. Frequently, the extensor carpi radialis brevis is also spared, because its innervation may originate more proximally, or it may appear to arise from the superficial bifurcation of the radial nerve (see Fig. 104-14). The complete syndrome involves loss of extension to all digits and to the extensor carpi ulnaris. The patient can dorsiflex the wrist but with a radial deviation. It is important to remember that middle and distal digital joints may still be extended through their intact intrinsics. Partial syndromes may involve just the extensor digitorum communis, with extension of thumb and index fingers still preserved (Fig. 104-16). Early in the compression syndrome, a less striking clinical picture may be present, with just paresis or paralysis of isolated digits. Patients with rheumatoid arthritis may present an identical attitude of the hand from either a posterior interosseous nerve compression, or from ruptures or dislocations of the extensor digitorum communis tendons. A careful examination should assist the clinician in differentiating these two entities. In suspected cases of nerve compression, electromyographic studies are usually diagnostic.

Operative Technique and Postoperative Care

Persistence, without improvement, of a posterior interosseous nerve palsy for 6 to 8 weeks is an indication for operative intervention. Although a limited incision may be used to expose just the dorsal interosseous nerve (Fig. 104-17), it is preferable to visualize the main trunk of the radial nerve as part of the procedure. Therefore, start the incision 4 to 5 cm proximal to the elbow flexion crease at the interval between the brachioradialis laterally and the brachialis medially. Distally, continue the incision dorsally and laterally to the interval between the extensor carpi radialis brevis (ECRB) laterally and the extensor digitorum communis (EDC) medially (Fig. 104-18). Carry out deeper dissection first at the proximal end of the incision; identify the radial nerve; and tag it with a wide, moist Penrose drain. Next, at the distal end, develop the plane between ECRB and EDC, exposing the oblique fibers of the supinator muscle (Fig. 104-19). Wider exposure is accomplished by partial detachment of the ECRB from the lateral epicondyle. While the plane between ECRB and supinator is safe, that between su-

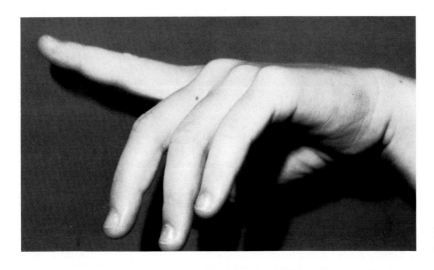

FIGURE 104-16. Incomplete dorsal interosseous nerve syndrome.

FIGURE 104-17. Superficial head of supinator (S) straddling deep branch of radial nerve (held up by Penrose drains).

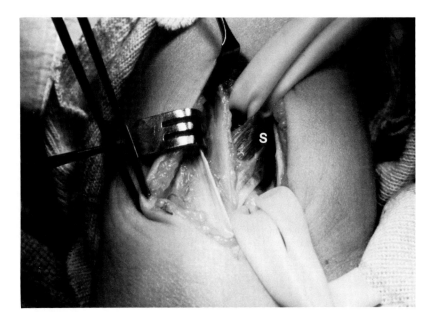

pinator and EDC must be developed only if necessary, and gently, because branches cross this plane from the posterior interosseous nerve to the finger extensors.[12] The distal border of the supinator may now be defined, under which the branches of the interosseous nerve are seen to fan out. Identify and split the proximal arcade of Frohse as the nerve disappears beneath it. With the nerve now properly exposed, divide the superficial head of the supinator (see Fig. 104-17). Also, divide any fibrous bands and vascular arches (the radial recurrent vessels or "leash of Henry"[2]), and remove tumors or other lesions. Loosely reapproximate the origin of the ECRB, and close the superficial fascia and skin. Apply a well-padded compression dressing with a posterior plaster splint for support. Immediate exercises for the shoulder and fingers are encouraged. Since this approach is carried out entirely between anatomic planes, all immobilization may be discontinued after 3 to 5 days.

Pitfalls and Complications

In addition to pitfalls common to other entrapment syndromes, differentiation of the posterior interosseous nerve syndrome from extensor tendon ruptures or dislocations in the patient with rheumatoid arthritis is important. Furthermore, avoid forceful dissection between the supinator muscle and the EDC.

Radial Tunnel Syndrome

Radial tunnel syndrome is painful, without sensory or motor deficit. The radial tunnel starts proximally as the radial nerve lies deeply between brachioradialis and brachialis and extends distally to the distal border of the supinator muscle.[8] Within this tunnel nerve entrapment may occur at one of four levels: under fibrous bands just proximal to the supinator, under the

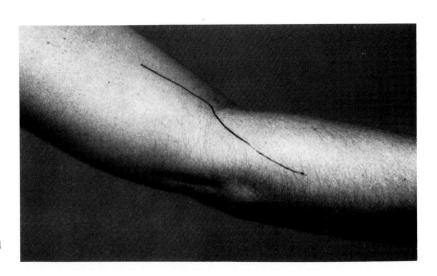

FIGURE 104-18. Approach for the radial nerve and its bifurcation at the elbow and proximal forearm.

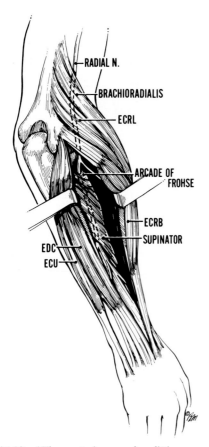

FIGURE 104-19. "The posterior muscle-splitting approach to the radial tunnel and the arcade of Frohse." ECU, extensor carpi ulnaris; ECRB, extensor carpi radialis brevis; ECRL, extensor carpi radialis longus; EDC, extensor digitorum communis. (With permission of Eversmann, W.W., Jr.: Entrapment and Compression Neuropathies. *In* Green, D.P.: Operative Hand Surgery. New York, Churchill Livingstone, 1982.)

radial recurrent vessels, beneath the arcade of Frohse, and under the medial tendinous origin of the extensor carpi radialis brevis.[8] At the onset the clinical presentation resembles an acute tennis elbow, with pain and localized tenderness over the lateral epicondyle, increased by wrist and finger extension against resistance. There may be a temporary response to local

injections of steroids, followed by gradual aggravation and a change in the location and characteristics of the pain. Radiation proximally and distally, weakness of grip, limitation of full elbow extension, and maximum tenderness anteriorly, along the projection of the radial nerve, suggest a radial tunnel syndrome. Paresthesias in the distribution of the superficial radial branch imply a more proximal entrapment, at a point where both divisions of the main trunk are simultaneously vulnerable, such as beneath the fibrous bands proximal to the arcade of Frohse. Maneuvers that actively or passively tense up offending structures are helpful. Symptoms that are increased by active forearm supination against resistance with the elbow flexed at 90° to neutralize the brachioradialis ("long supinator") and biceps, or by passive pronation, point to the arcade of Frohse and the supinator. The addition of passive flexion of the wrist, or its active extension, suggest entrapment by the ECRB tendon. Aggravation of pain by resisted extension of the long finger with the elbow fully extended[8] is also suggestive, although not pathognomonic, of the presence of a radial tunnel syndrome. Electrodiagnostic tests are usually not helpful. The patient's response to very localized injections of a local anesthetic may also assist in differentiating a radial tunnel syndrome from a tennis elbow.

Operative Technique and Postoperative Care

The muscle-splitting approach described by Roles and Maudsley[8] is simple and sufficient. Make an incision approximately 6 cm long, starting at the elbow crease and projected longitudinally over the radial head (Fig. 104-20). Expose the brachioradialis, and split its fibers by blunt dissection. Immediately beneath is the superficial radial nerve, under a fascial layer of variable thickness. Further retraction in a lateral direction will show the edge of the extensor carpi radialis longus. Retract this as well to expose the deep branch of the radial nerve and the oblique fibers of the supinator (Fig. 104-21A). Divide the more proximal fascial bands. Ligate and sever the radial recurrent vessels. Delineate both margins of the superficial head of the supinator, and divide the muscle. Fully expose the posterior interosseous nerve (Fig. 104-21B). The contribution of the extensor carpi radialis brevis to this syndrome may now be evaluated by passively pronating the forearm, while simultaneously palmar flexing the wrist. Palpate the aponeurotic edge of the ECRB, and visualize it in relation to the nerve. If it is believed

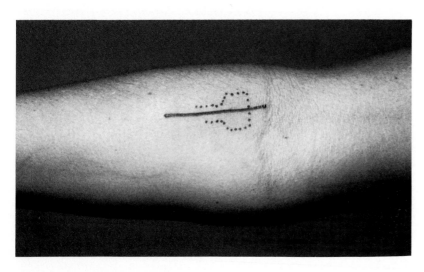

FIGURE 104-20. Limited approach to the radial tunnel.

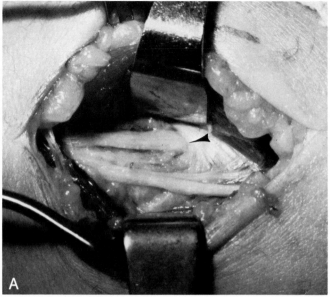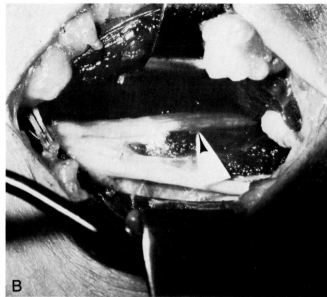

FIGURE 104-21. Superficial and deep branches of the radial nerve. (*A*) The deep branch is seen as it passes under the arcade of Frohse (*arrow*). (*B*) Compression of the deep branch seen (*arrow*) after superficial head of supinator is divided.

to be a contributory factor, release it. Loosely approximate the deep fascia, and close the skin. Apply a well-padded compression dressing from above the elbow to beyond the wrist, with the forearm and wrist in neutral. Immediate finger and shoulder motion are encouraged. After 3 to 5 days, all immobilization is discontinued.

Pitfalls and Complications

The only problem I have encountered is a transient, and distressing, partial paresis of the finger extensors. When operative findings prove the presence of constriction, the long-term results are rewarding.

REFERENCES

1. Barnard, L.B., and McCoy, S.M.: The Supracondyloid Process of the Humerus. J. Bone Joint Surg. **28:**845, 1946.
2. Eversmann, W.W., Jr.: Entrapment and Compression Neuropathies. *In* Green, D.P. (ed.): Operative Hand Surgery. New York, Churchill Livingstone, 1982.
3. Eversmann, W.W., Jr., and Ritsick, J.A.: Intraoperative Changes in Motor Nerve Conduction Latency in Carpal Tunnel Syndrome. J. Hand Surg. **3:**77, 1978.
4. Hill, N.A., Howard, F.M., and Huffern, B.R.: The Incomplete Anterior Interosseous Syndrome. J. Hand Surg. **10-A:**4, 1985.
5. Inserra, S., and Spinner, M.: An Anatomic Factor Significant in Transposition of the Ulnar Nerve. J. Hand Surg. **11-A:**80, 1986.
6. Learmonth, J.R.: A Technique for Transplanting the Ulnar Nerve. Surg. Gynecol. Obstet. **75:**792, 1942.
7. Leffert, R.D.: Anterior Submuscular Transposition of the Ulnar Nerve by the Learmonth Technique. J. Hand Surg. **7:**147, 1982.
8. Roles, N.C., and Maudsley, R.H.: Radial Tunnel Syndrome. Resistant Tennis Elbow as Nerve Entrapment. J. Bone Joint Surg. **54-B:**499, 1972.
9. Seyffarth, H.: Primary Myoses in the M. Pronator Teres as Cause of Lesion of the N. Medianus (the Pronator Syndrome). Acta. Psychiatr. Neurol. **74**(suppl.):251, 1951.
10. Shea, J.D., and McClain, E.J.: Ulnar-Nerve Compression Syndromes at and Below the Wrist. J. Bone Joint. Surg. **51-A:**1095, 1969.
11. Spinner, M.: The Functional Attitude of the Hand Afflicted With an Anterior Interosseous Nerve Paralysis. Bull. Hosp. Joint Dis., **30:**21, 1969.
12. Spinner, M.: Injuries to the Major Branches of Peripheral Nerves of the Forearm. Philadelphia, W.B. Saunders, 1972.
13. Spinner, M.: Injuries to the Major Branches of Peripheral Nerves of the Forearm, 2nd ed. Philadelphia, W.B. Saunders, 1978.
14. Spinner, M.: Management of Nerve Compression Lesions of the Upper Extremity. *In* Omer, G.E., and Spinner, M. (eds.): Management of Peripheral Nerve Problems. Philadelphia, W.B. Saunders, 1980.
15. Sunderland, S.: Nerves and Nerve Injuries. Baltimore, Williams & Wilkins, 1968.
16. Sunderland, S.: The Nerve Lesion in the Carpal Tunnel Syndrome. J. Neurol. Neurosurg. Psychiatry **39:**615, 1976.
17. Taleisnik, J.: The Palmar Cutaneous Branch of the Median Nerve and the Approach to the Carpal Tunnel. An Anatomical Study. J. Bone Joint Surg. **55-A:**1212, 1973.
18. Upton, A.R.M., and McComas, A.J.: The Double Crush in Nerve Entrapment Syndromes. Lancet **1:**359, 1973.
19. Wartenberg, R.: Cheiralgia Paraesthetica (Isolierte Neuritis des Ramus Superficialis Nervi Radialis). Z. Gesamte Neurol. Psychiatr. **141:**145, 1932.
20. Wilson, D.H., and Krout, R.: Surgery of Ulnar Neuropathy at the Elbow: 16 Cases Treated by Decompression Without Transposition. Technical Note. J. Neurosurg. **38:**780, 1973.

CHAPTER 105

Neuromas

ALAN E. FREELAND and
MICHAEL E. JABALEY

Classification
Diagnosis
Prevention and Treatment
  Neurorrhaphy and Nerve Grafting
  Decompression
  Simple Excisional Neurectomy
  Centrocentral Coaptation
  Transposition
Postoperative Care
Pitfalls and Complications

After a nerve is partially or completely divided, the regenerating axons of the proximal segment seek to reenter their original endoneurial tubes and reestablish contact with their respective end organs. Repair of the Schwann's cell–endoneurial barrier optimizes this process. If axons escape to the outside at the repair site, if repair is not performed, or if amputation is the interrupting process, the regenerating axons of the proximal segment of the injured nerve form a nodule in the substance of the nerve or at the terminal end of its transected proximal segment (a neuroma).

Grossly, the nodule is rubbery to firm in consistency, well-circumscribed, white, and may adhere by scar to adjacent skin, muscle, fascia, tendon, periosteum, or bone.[38] Histologically, there is a disorganized admixture of axons, frequently in whorl-type patterns surrounded by Schwann's cells, fibroblasts, a variable amount of collagen, macrophages, and capillaries.[14] Myofibroblasts have been consistently identified by electron-microscopy in painful neuromas. These cells may serve as histologic markers of a symptomatic neuroma, but their pathophysiologic role, if any, in its symptomatology has not yet been determined.[17]

Only neuromas containing sensory nerve fibers can be symptomatic. The digital nerves of the hand, the palmar and ulnar cutaneous nerves, and the dorsal sensory branches of the radial and ulnar nerves are pure sensory nerves, which are particularly vulnerable to painful neuroma formation. Upon division 20% to 30% of the neuromas formed by these nerves will become symptomatic.[21] Furthermore, common digital nerves in ray amputations seem more inclined to be painful than those of digital amputations.

CLASSIFICATION

Neuromas have been classified by Sunderland.[33] The three major categories are (1) neuromas-in-continuity; (2) neuromas in completely severed, unrepaired nerves; and (3) amputation stump neuromas. Neuromas-in-continuity include those with the perineurium intact, those with partial nerve division, and those that form following nerve repair or grafting.

DIAGNOSIS

Patients who form symptomatic neuromas will have a central focus of burning or sharp, aching pain at the site of the nerve injury. The pain may radiate peripherally in the sensory distribution of the injured nerve or proximally in the distribution of the nerve trunk. A dysesthetic "trigger area" is also found in the same site and may radiate peripherally in the distribution of the injured nerve on percussion. This is equivalent to a nonadvancing Tinel's sign and may be called a "neuroma sign." Relief of these signs and symptoms with an injection of local anesthetic will confirm the diagnosis.[38] The addition of triamcinolone acetate to the injection produces a collagenase effect and may soften adjacent scar enough to be curative in some cases.[24,25,31] Up to 10 mg of triamcinolone acetate (a 10-mg/ml concentration is diluted 1:1 with 1% lidocaine) is used and may be repeated three times at 1- to 3-week intervals. Patients should be warned of depigmentation of the skin and atrophy of the subcutaneous fat that may accompany triamcinolone injection.

PREVENTION AND TREATMENT

If medicine is an inexact science, then the cause, prevention, and treatment of neuromas epitomize areas of incomplete knowledge within our profession. Proximity to skin, bony prominences, the working surface (palm) of the hand, traction and compression by scar, and local trauma, either individually or in composite, have been advanced as physical reasons for neuroma pain. Personality, pain tolerance, sympathetic imbalance, and secondary gain may also play a role in the production of symptoms and extent of recovery. Any or all these factors may be operative at various times. An awareness of them makes diagnosis easier.

It should be strongly emphasized that careful identification of transected nerve ends and their repair or removal away from the injury site at the time of primary wound treatment is an extremely effective preventive measure. Nevertheless, some patients will still develop painful neuromata. The signs are identifiable early, and prompt treatment is considerably more effective than later measures. The evolution of symptoms and clinical course makes the result of delayed treatment considerably less predictable.

Symptomatic neuromas alone can impair hand function and be disabling, but a diathesis similar to that seen in the patient who develops reflex sympathetic dystrophy is common and occurs more frequently than one would expect by chance alone in patients developing symptomatic neuromas of the hand. Indeed, symptomatic neuromas of the hand may be complicated by reflex sympathetic dystrophy, which will be refractory to treatment until the noxious stimuli to the nociceptors is eliminated. This impairment and consequent disability are worsened by the complication of reflex sympathetic dystrophy.[23]

Recently, neuroma formation has been linked to the neurohormonal influences of sensory end organs, particularly those of the skin.[8,9,26–28,30,32,36] Transposition of a severed nerve end to a protected environment away from skin, bony prominences, and the working surface of the hand, as well as the avoidance of tension on the nerve may provide the best physical protection of the severed proximal nerve end, and thus prevent, improve, or eliminate symptoms. In addition transposition may remove the nerve ending from local neurohormonal influences at the site of injury.

Operative intervention for symptomatic neuromas is indicated on confirmation of the diagnosis by injection of local anesthesia and when physical measures such as desensitization and injection with triamcinolone acetate fail to provide relief.

Neurorrhaphy and Nerve Grafting

As noted earlier prevention is the best treatment for neuromas. Take care when operating in the vicinity of the sensory nerves of the hand, particularly in ganglion excisions, the decompression of DeQuervain's stenosing tenosynovitis of the first dorsal compartment, carpal tunnel decompression, and in tendon repair and reconstruction.[37] Identify and repair post-traumatic and iatrogenic lacerations of these nerves for optimal recovery.

Secondarily identified lacerations may require nerve grafting if direct suture cannot be performed. In either instance the preferred treatment for prevention of painful neuromas is to restore the continuity of the nerve.

Decompression

When a neuroma-in-continuity forms with the perineurium intact due to repetitive or cumulative trauma in entities such as bowler's thumb, jeweler's thumb, surgeon's thumb, or similar injuries, and does not respond to nonoperative measures, decompression of the nerve should be considered.[5,13,15,19,29,34] In such cases a neurolysis is done, and the perineural sleeve of scar is removed. In some instances the nerve may be translocated intact deep to muscles such as the adductor of the thumb.[1]

Simple Excisional Neurectomy

Following digital amputation it has been recommended traditionally that each digital nerve end be identified, mobilized, placed under gentle tension, then sharply divided and allowed to retract 6 to 10 mm into healthy tissue proximal to the amputation stump (Fig. 105-1). Although this prevents painful symptomatic neuromas in some instances, it is not completely reliable or uniformly successful. Crushing, coagulation, freezing, chemical injections, nerve ligation, and capping in the local area of nerve division have all been recommended, and their record is no better.

If a symptomatic neuroma forms and does not respond satisfactorily to triamcinolone acetate injection, desensitization, transcutaneous electrical nerve stimulation, or other nonoperative measures, surgery may be indicated. Neuroma resection has set a benchmark by which other methods may be gauged[35] (Fig. 105-2). Nevertheless, there is a high incidence of recurrent symptomatic neuroma following efforts at neuroma resection, and this type of treatment has not been quite as satisfactory as methods of transposition and of centrocentral coaptation, which are described later.

For simple excisional neurectomy to be successful in the treatment of amputation neuromas, a stump revision must be performed when a bony prominence is present in order to

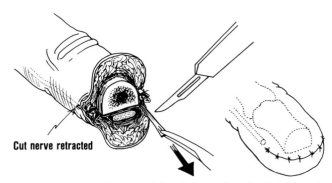

Cut nerve retracted

FIGURE 105-1. At the time of digital amputation, the digital arteries are identified and ligated. The digital nerve is placed under a gentle tension and cut proximally so that following transection it will lie 6 to 10 mm proximal to the amputation stump, away from bony prominences and scar so that it is protected from repetitive trauma.

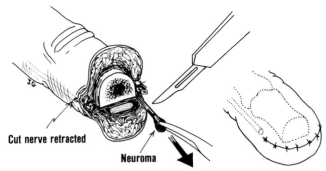

Cut nerve retracted

Neuroma

FIGURE 105-2. To perform simple excisional neurectomy, the nerve is dissected free from its surrounding scar. The adjacent digital artery is identified, and the neuroma is dissected away from it to prevent injury. When the nerve is freely mobile, enough gentle traction is placed on the nerve so that 1 or 2 cm of its terminal portion can be resected. The proximal nerve stump is then allowed to retract into uninjured soft tissue.

eliminate this as a source of potential trauma to the nerve end. Nevertheless, the course following simple excisional neurectomy is all too often one of initial improvement followed by recurrence of symptomatology as the anatomic neuroma reforms in its new position. A second simple excisional neurectomy may occasionally be helpful after the failed initial procedure, but subsequent procedures after a second such operation seem to offer diminishing returns. Neither silicone capping nor funicular excision with epineural ligation improves the results of simple excisional neurectomy.

It is becoming apparent that nerves, much like tendons, are capable of gliding a variable distance in the tissue that surrounds them. To the extent that this gliding is diminished by scar adhesion, traction on the nerve may occur and may sometimes produce symptoms. We now attempt to restore this gliding by early motion following neuroma surgery.[37]

Centrocentral Coaptation

Centrocentral coaptation is the joining of two like-size diameter nerves or fascicles to either end of an autologous nerve or fascicle transplant, artificially created by sharply dividing and then resuturing one of the nerves or fascicles 5 to 10 mm from its cut end[8,9,26] (Fig. 105-3). Perform the junctures between the central nerve or fascicle and the transplant so that the physiologic regeneration of the central axons will course past both the suture lines and join by interdigitating at the midportion of the transplant (Fig. 105-4). If more than one centrocentral fascicular anastomosis is done at the same area, offset the suture lines stepwise to minimize the chances of axonal compression by interfascicular connective tissue proliferation.

Axonal regeneration appears to cease after an overlap of 2 to 5 mm within the midportion of the transplant when the increased intraneural pressure created by this juncture mechanically reduces its axoplasmic flow, thus, centrally inhibiting the neural protein synthesis.[22] Similarly, this mechanism minimizes the size of the intraneural neuroma within the transplant. Why a similar neuroma size reduction does not occur with fasciculectomy and epineurial suture or with silicone capping is uncertain.

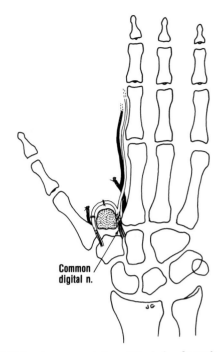

Common digital n.

FIGURE 105-3. A ray amputation of the index finger has been performed. The digital arteries are ligated. The common digital nerves have been joined by centrocentral coaptation. *It is important* to appreciate that this is not a simple joining of the ends, but that a deliberate transection and suture has been performed, creating a degenerate section between the two suture lines.

Another theory explaining the inhibition of symptomatic neuroma formation by centrocentral union is that macromolecular proteins in the distal nerve stump and sensory receptors in and adjacent to the skin as well as in the flaps of the amputation stump (called target-derived neurotrophic factors) stimulate axonal regeneration locally at the site of injury and centrally at the nerve cell body by retrograde axoplasmic transport. They

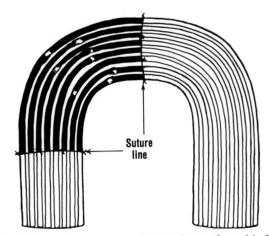

Suture line

FIGURE 105-4. The centrocentral coaptation performed in Figure 105-3 is transposed and shows that the axons have coursed past the suture lines and are joined by interdigitating at the midportion of the transplant. Here the axons recognize each other as "nontarget structures." Therefore, the neuroma formed is small and nonsensitive. There must be no tension at the suture lines.

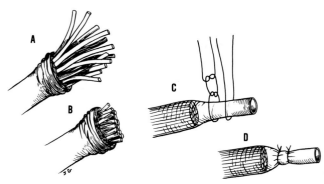

FIGURE 105-5. Although funicular excision with epineural ligation is not in itself a satisfactory method of preventing or treating symptomatic neuromas, it may be a mechanism by which the funicular ends may be protected from trauma at the time of nerve transposition. (*A*) The epineurium is mobilized proximally, exposing the funicular ends. (*B*) The funicular ends are cut proximally. (*C* and *D*) The epineurium is then restored over the funicular ends and doubly ligated with care not to traumatize the funicular ends during ligation.

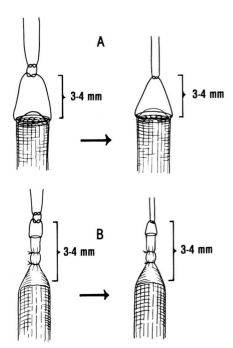

FIGURE 105-6. Technique of nerve transposition in either (*A*) a freshly cut nerve end or (*B*) a nerve prepared by funicular excision with epineural ligation. A knot is tied 3 to 4 mm distal to the freshly cut nerve end or the neuroma, creating a small obstruction. This prevents the nerve end of neuroma from abutting directly into soft tissues, muscle, or bone when it is transposed.

may also guide the regenerating axons to their target end organs when nerve repair or grafting is performed. In the case of an unsatisfied proximal nerve end, these neurotrophic factors may contribute to neuroma formation and, perhaps, to its symptoms.[8,9,26–28,30,32,36]

Centrocentral coaptation may insulate the central nerve or fascicle stumps from neurotrophic influences and confine the regenerating axons to a nontarget environment, thereby allowing the regenerative process to cease. This procedure is excellent for those cases of hand narrowing performed by ray resection with or without digital transposition for digits with fulminant infection, osteomyelitis, destructive joint sepsis, malignant tumor, or in cases of traumatic amputation where the residual portion of the digit is useless or impairs function in the rest of the hand.

Although centrocentral coaptation can be performed and could conceivably be useful as a secondary procedure after neuroma formation, it seems that primary treatment of the severed digital nerves at the time of ray resection is preferable. Its use in secondary cases where other means have failed is uncertain at this time, and its efficacy remains to be proven. When performed the centrocentral anastomosis should be protected by good full-thickness cover and should be placed as far from the skin suture lines as possible.

Transposition

Although cut nerve ends or symptomatic neuromata with poor full-thickness skin coverage can be protected by local or distant flap coverage,[3] it is far more simple and practical to transpose the nerve to a protected environment. Such an area with better blood supply, less scar, and less tension seems to have a salutory effect on a painful neuroma. Transposition has the additional benefits of physically removing the nerve end from areas of direct trauma, such as the working surface of the hand; bony prominences (especially amputated bone ends); severely scarred areas; and local neurohormonal influences. At the present time there are three types of translocation procedures

for cut nerve ends: subcutaneous,[12,16] intraosseous,[2,7,11,20] and intramuscular.[4,17,18]

In order to protect the nerve end or the neuroma from direct trauma in the area to which it is transposed, place a resorbable suture through the epineurium without violating the nerve or through the capsule without violating the neuroma (Figs. 105-5 and 105-6). Tie a knot 3 to 4 mm distal to the freshly cut nerve end or the neuroma; the knot separates the nerve end or neuroma from direct contact to the structures to which it is transposed. Following transposition of any type, inspect the nerve trunk to be sure it is under no tension.

In diffusely dysesthetic digital amputation stumps with one palpable, sensitive digital neuroma and one nonpalpable, insensitive neuroma, consideration should be given to translocating both. If this is not done, the remaining digital neuroma often becomes significantly more painful even though the translocated neuroma becomes asymptomatic.

Dorsal Subcutaneous Transposition

Dissect the neuroma and its fibrous capsule-in-continuity with its nerve proximally, and mobilize it so that it can be translocated without tension. Select a dorsal, scar-free site away from bony prominences and local pressure or trauma. The area selected should place the neuroma dorsal to muscle, thus placing the muscle between the neuroma and the working surface of the hand. The web space is preferred for neuromas of the digital stumps and the area between the metacarpals for those involving the common digital nerves of the palm[12,16] (Fig. 105-7).

Intraosseous Transposition

Intraosseous transposition of the cut proximal end of a sensory nerve or of a neuroma with or without sensory neuroma resection gives results at least comparable to those of dorsal subcutaneous transposition.[2,7,11,20] Either of two techniques for intraosseous transposition may be used (Fig. 105-8). An obstructing knot prevents compression of the cut proximal nerve end or neuroma against intramedullary bone. The epineurium may also be sutured to the periosteum or to the bone at the site of its entry into the intramedullary canal. In either technique there should be no tension on the nerve at any point, and the angle the transposed nerve makes as it enters and courses through the bone should not be too acute. If one elects to transpose a transected nerve into bone, it is important to avoid tension on the proximal stump at any position in the arc of motion of adjacent joints.

Intramuscular Transposition

Although this procedure has long been advocated, there now is evidence in both laboratory animals and humans that neuroma formation is minimized by placing the transected proximal end of a nerve directly into muscle substance.[4,17,18] The operative technique is similar to that of dorsal subcutaneous transposition. While the procedure of neuroma excision and implantation of the transected nerve end into the brachioradialis has

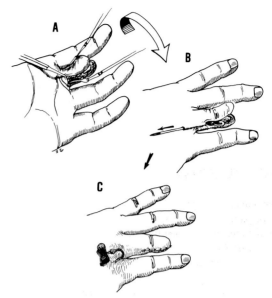

FIGURE 105-7. (*A*) Symptomatic digital neuromas are dissected free following careful ligation of the digital arteries. Sutures are attached to the neuromas with care to involve only capsular and not neural structures. (*B*) The sutures are then attached to a needle, and after tunneling subcutaneously, the needle is brought out in the dorsal web space. (*C*) The nerve is checked to be sure it is neither kinked nor under tension. It is then tied either subcutaneously or over a dental roll to secure its position.

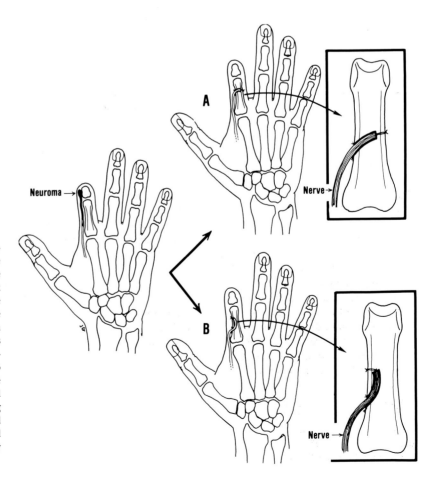

FIGURE 105-8. Technique of intraosseous implantation. The neuroma and nerve proximal to it are dissected free of scar and surrounding tissue. A hole large enough to accommodate the nerve without constriction is drilled into the distal diaphysis of the phalanx. Excising the neuroma does not influence results but does allow a smaller hole to be drilled in the bone to accommodate the nerve. (*A*) The nerve is secured to the opposite cortex. (*B*) The nerve is secured to adjacent cortex. An alternative method is to secure the epineurium to periosteum with a single small suture on either side and leave the nerve end free within the bone. In this illustration both suturing techniques are shown in combination. Two small holes may be drilled with a Kirschner wire or a small drill to accommodate the suture ends so that they may be tied directly to the cortex.

been a successful method of treating symptomatic neuromas of the superficial radial nerve, similar procedures placing digital nerves into the intrinsic muscles of the hand have been most discouraging.[18] Perhaps muscle contracture, a relatively large excursion in relation to muscle size, pressure, traction on the nerve during hand use, or some combination of these, is at fault. Therefore, this procedure is not recommended. Intramuscular transposition with the neuroma intact gives similarly poor results.

POSTOPERATIVE CARE

After skin closure, provide a supportive and protective dressing is until pain at the operative site is minimal. Ordinarily, in the case of a successful operation, this takes 3 to 6 weeks. Remove the sutures 7 to 10 days after surgery. Thereafter, the patient removes the protective dressing or splint three to four times a day for therapy. This includes modalities of motion, scar softening, and physical-desensitizing measures. Warm-water soaks, massage, and active range of motion exercises are routinely used. The Jobst pump* or an Isotoner glove† may be used to diminish swelling. The Isotoner glove is worn at night. Vibration may be soothing and also may be desensitizing to the scar area. Other physical measures to soften and desensitize the scar are used. Silicone elastomer‡ maintained in place with Coban§ may be worn at night. Paraffin wax baths deliver deep heat and may be soothing; in addition when carefully combined with massage, they may help to stretch and soften the scar. These measures are continued until the patient's pain is well within tolerance or resolved. Once the pain is within the patient's tolerance, the program may be converted from an outpatient program to a home program. A positive, supportive attitude by the therapist and the physician as well as a program directed at functional recovery, desensitization of the stump and scar, and early return to manual activities including work and recreation play a very important role in patient recovery.[6,10,23,39]

PITFALLS AND COMPLICATIONS

The principles of prevention of a symptomatic neuroma in cases of nerve division include repair by direct suture in freshly lacerated lesions and by nerve grafting, either primarily or secondarily, in those cases with nerve loss or where direct suture cannot be accomplished without tension. In elective amputations centrocentral anastomosis is the preferred method for managing the digital nerves in ray resection, while dorsal subcutaneous or intraosseous transposition is preferred for partial amputations of the digits. For traumatic amputations the condition of the wound at the time of surgery may dictate whether the transected nerves are managed initially by simple excision or by a nerve-manipulating procedure. If the wound is contaminated or if further dissection would jeopardize tissue viability,

* Jobst Institute, Inc., Box 653, Toledo, OH 43694

† Aris Isotoner, Inc., 417 Fifth Avenue, New York, NY 10016

‡ Smith & Nephew Rolyan, Inc., N93 W14475 Whittaker Way, Menomonee Falls, WI 53051

§ Medical Products Division/3M, St. Paul, MN 55101

the transected nerve ends should be managed by simple excision; either centrocentral anastomosis or transposition of the neuroma may be deferred and done either as a delayed primary procedure when wound conditions permit or secondarily should a symptomatic neuroma develop. Naturally, prevention of a symptomatic neuroma is preferrable to its treatment.

The principles of treatment of a symptomatic neuroma include nerve grafting for symptomatic neuromas when there is a distal nerve available, the procedures described under the section on decompression for neuromas that form in continuity with the perineurium intact due to repetitive or cumulative trauma, and either dorsal subcutaneous or intraosseous transposition for symptomatic neuromas when no suitable distal nerve is present. When digital amputations are revised to ray amputations, centrocentral coaptation is an excellent method of managing the transected digital nerves. Simple excision, although setting the standard for comparison, does not provide as good a result as has been demonstrated by the previously described procedures for established symptomatic neuromata.

The principles of nerve transposition in instances of symptomatic neuroma include physically removing the free nerve end from areas of scarring, bony prominences, and the working surface of the hand. Such translocation may also remove a freshly cut nerve end from local neurohormonal influences arising from denervated cutaneous sensory end organs. The free nerve end must be under no tension and should lie in well-vascularized tissue. There must be no kinking of translocated nerves. When nerve transposition fails, the possibility of excessive nerve tension, pullout or kinking should be considered. A single additional surgical procedure to investigate these causes and to redo or relocate the nerve should be considered.

As in translocation in centrocentral anastomosis, tension on the suture lines or kinking in the nerve substance may lead to failure, and should be meticulously avoided. In case of failure a single additional surgical procedure to investigate the cause and redo the anastomosis or relocate the nerve ends should be considered.

Although neuroma formation elsewhere in the body is suppressed by intramuscular transposition of the proximally transected nerve, this method has proved ineffective in control of neuroma pain in the hand, apparently because of muscle contracture, a relatively large excursion in relation to muscle size, pressure, traction, or some combination of these.

Success of intervention for a symptomatic neuroma correlates with the time from its formation. Chronic pain syndromes and the establishment of central pain are time related and involve psychosocial and economic factors. The longer a patient suffers with an untreated painful neuroma, the less likely any modality is to have much affect. For this reason treatment should be completed expeditiously and an attempt made to return the patient to work, even if only light duty, as soon as possible.

It seems that one reoperation after a failure of initial surgical treatment of a painful neuroma may be successful and is indicated. If this does not solve the problem, further operative intervention is likely to produce sharply diminished returns. Although further surgery is sometimes indicated, one should also begin to consider alternative approaches. For example the patient might be referred to a chronic pain clinic as an alternative to further surgical treatment. Although this method is no panacea, some otherwise recalcitrant patients have been relieved.

REFERENCES

1. Belsky, M.R., and Millender, L.H.: Bowler's Thumb in a Baseball Player: A Case Report. Orthopaedics 3:122, 1980.
2. Boldrey, E.: Amputation Neuroma in Nerves Implanted in Bone. Ann. Surg. 118:1052, 1943.
3. Brown, H., and Flynn, J.E.: Abdominal Pedicle Flap for Hand Neuromas and Entrapped Nerves. J. Bone Joint Surg. 55-A:575, 1973.
4. Dellon, A.L., Mackinnon, S.E., and Pestronk, A.: Implantation of Sensory Nerve Into Muscle: Preliminary Clinical and Experimental Observations on Neuroma Formation. Ann. Plast. Surg. 12:30, 1984.
5. Dobyns, J.H., O'Brien, E.T., and Linscheid, R.L.: Bowler's Thumb: Diagnosis and Treatment. J. Bone Joint. Surg. 54-A:751, 1972.
6. Fisher, G.T., and Boswick, J.A., Jr.: Neuroma Formation Following Digital Amputations. J. Trauma 23:136, 1983.
7. Goldstein, S.A., and Sturim, H.S.: Intraosseous Nerve Transposition for Treatment of Painful Neuromas. J. Hand Surg. 10-A:270, 1985.
8. Gonzalez-Darder, J., Barbera, J., Abellan, M.J., et al.: Centro-Central Anastomosis in the Prevention and Treatment of Painful Terminal Neuroma. J. Neurosurg. 63:754, 1985.
9. Gorkisch, K., Boese-Landgraf, J., and Vaubel, E.: Treatment and Prevention of Amputation Neuromas in Hand Surgery. Plast. Reconstruct. Surg. 73:293, 1984.
10. Grant, G.: Methods of Treatment of Neuromata of the Hand. J. Bone Joint Surg. 33-A:841, 1951.
11. Hemmy, D.C.: Intramedullary Nerve Implantation in Amputation and Other Traumatic Neuromas. J. Neurosurg. 54:842, 1981.
12. Herndon, J.H., Eaton, R.G., and Littler, J.W.: Management of Painful Neuromas in the Hand. J. Bone Joint Surg. 58-A:369, 1976.
13. Howell, A.E., and Leach, R.E.: Bowler's Thumb. J. Bone Joint Surg. 52-A:379, 1970.
14. Huber, C.G., and Lewis, D.: Amputation Neuromas. Arch. Surg. 1:85, 1920.
15. Kisner, W.H.: Thumb Neuroma: A Hazard of Ten Pin Bowling. Br. J. Plast. Surg. 29:225, 1976.
16. Laborde, K.J., Kalisman, M., and Tsai, T.M.: Results of Surgical Treatment of Painful Neuromas of the Hand. J. Hand Surg. 7:190, 1982.
17. Mackinnon, S.E., Dellon, A.L., Hudson, A.R., et al.: Alteration of Neuroma Formation by Manipulation of Its Microenvironment. Plast. Reconstruct. Surg. 76:345, 1985.
18. Dellon, A.L., and MacKinnon, S.E.: Treatment of the Painful Neuroma by Neuroma Resection and Muscle Implantation. Plast. Reconstruct. Surg. 77:427, 1986.
19. Marmor, L.: Bowler's Thumb. J. Trauma 6:282, 1966.
20. Mass, D.P., Ciano, M.C., Tortosa, R., et al.: Treatment of Painful Hand Neuromas by Their Transfer Into Bone. 20 Cases. Plast. Reconstruct. Surg. 74:182, 1984.
21. Nelson, A.W.: The Painful Neuroma: The Regenerating Axon Versus the Epineural Sheath. J. Surg. Res. 23:215, 1977.
22. Ochs, S., and Hollingsworth, D.: Dependence of Fast Axoplasmic Transport in Nerve on Oxidative Metabolism. J. Neurochem. 18:107, 1971.
23. Omer, G.E.: Symposium on Pain: Evaluation and Treatment of the Painful Upper Extremity. J. Hand Surg. 9-B:20, 1984.
24. Pataky, P.E., Graham, W.P., III, and Munger, B.L.: Terminal Neuromas Treated With Triamcinolone Acetonide. J. Surg. Res. 14:36, 1973.
25. Robbins, T.H.: The Response of Tender Neuromas and Scars to Triamcinolone Injections. Br. J. Plast. Surg. 30:68, 1977.
26. Samii, M.: Centrocentral Anastomosis of Peripheral Nerves: A Neurosurgical Treatment of Amputation Neuromas. In Siegfried, J., and Zimmerman, M. (eds.): Phantom and Stump Pain. New York, Springer-Verlag, 1981.
27. Seckel, B.R.: Discussion of Treatment and Prevention of Amputation Neuromas in Hand Surgery. Plast. Reconstruct. Surg. 73:297, 1984.
28. Seckel, B.R., Upton, J., Jones, H.R., et al.: Rapid Regeneration of the Chronically Damaged Facial Nerve Following Ipsilateral Free Gracilis Transfer. Plast. Reconstruct. Surg. 71:845, 1983.
29. Siegel, J.M.: Bowling-Thumb Neuroma. JAMA 192:263, 1965.
30. Slack, J.R., Hopkins, W.G., and Pockett, S.: Evidence for a Motor Nerve Growth Factor. Muscle Nerve 6:243, 1983.
31. Smith, J., and Gomez, N.: Local Injection Therapy of Neuromata of the Hand With Triamcinolone Acetonide. A Preliminary Study of Twenty-Two Patients (Method of Treatment, Results). J. Bone Joint Surg. 52-A:71, 1970.
32. Stoeckel, J., and Thoenen, H.: Retrograde Axonal Transport of Nerve Growth Factor: Specificity and Biological Importance. Brain Res. 85:337, 1975.
33. Sunderland, S.: Nerves and Nerve Injuries, 2nd ed. New York, Churchill Livingstone, 1978.
34. Thirupathi, R., and Forman, D.: The Jeweller's Thumb: An Occupational Neuroma. Orthopaedics 6:438, 1983.
35. Tupper, J.W., and Booth, D.M.: Treatment of Painful Neuromas of Sensory Nerves in the Hand: A Comparison of Traditional and Newer Methods. J. Hand Surg. 1:144, 1976.
36. Varon, S., and Adler, R.: Trophic and Specifying Factors Directed to Neuronal Cells. Adv. Cell Neurobiol. 2:115, 1981.
37. Wilgis, E.F.S.: The Significance of Longitudinal Excursion in Peripheral Nerves. Hand Clinics 2:761, 1986.
38. Williams, H.B.: The Painful Stump Neuroma and Its Treatment. Clin. Plast. Surg. 11:79, 1984.
39. Wilson, R.L., and Carter-Wilson, M.S.: Rehabilitation After Amputations in the Hand. Orthop. Clin. North Am. 14:851, 1983.

BIBLIOGRAPHY

Brown, P.W.: Complications Following Amputations of Parts of the Hand. In Boswick, J.A., Jr. (ed.): Complications in Hand Surgery. Philadelphia W.B. Saunders, 1986.

Eaton, R.G.: Painful Neuromas. In Omer, C.E., and Spinner, M. (eds.): Management of Peripheral Nerve Problems. Philadelphia, W.B. Saunders, 1980.

Herndon, J.H.: Neuromas. In Green, D.P. (ed.): Operative Hand Surgery. Churchill Livingstone, New York, 1982.

Omer, G.E.: Problems of Primary and Secondary Nerve Repair and Grafts. In Sandzen, S.C., Jr. (ed.): Current Management of Complications in Orthopaedics: The Hand and Wrist. Baltimore, Williams & Wilkins, 1985.

Omer, G.E., Jr.: The Painful Neuroma. In Strickland, J.W., and Steichen, J.B. (eds.): Difficult Problems in Hand Surgery. St. Louis, C.V. Mosby, 1982.

CHAPTER 106

General Principles for Restoration of Muscle Balance Following Paralysis in Forearm and Hand

PAUL W. BRAND

EVALUATION OF PATIENT: WORK AND ATTITUDES

A surgeon can move muscles around and attach tendons to new insertions. Therapists can help the patient to understand new patterns of control of the hand. Only the patient, however, can heal the wound and then make the hand work. In this process one of the most important variables is the attitude of the patient and his or her willingness to accept the disciplines of recovery.

The very best results occur when the patient is self-employed, has no one to blame but him- or herself for the injury, and has everything to gain by a speedy return to work. The poorest results occur when a patient blames someone else for the injury and is angry and resentful. This is compounded when the patient is convinced of obtaining a larger financial reward if he or she has residual disability. The outlook is still worse if the patient already has a poor self-image, has been a failure, and now views the injury as a lasting excuse for continued dependency.

No plan for reconstructive surgery should be finalized until the patient's own attitudes and personality have been evaluated and until he or she has been brought fully into the picture. Before outlining any program the surgeon must encourage patients to talk and present their own ideas about the future. It is important to know how the patient has been influenced by others—family, employer, and above all by the attorney. If the patient has been fortunate enough to be seen by the surgeon before talking to a lawyer, it may be possible for the surgeon to recommend a legal advisor who works for a fee rather than for a proportion of the take and who understands the harm that is done to the process of recovery by delays in the financial settlement and by any hint that it might be financially beneficial to the patient to maximize the disability.

When a patient is already angry, it is worthwhile to spend time or get help for the patient to come to terms with these emotions, so that the process of rehabilitation may start with a single-minded and uncomplicated determination to do well.

One must also determine the patient's own attitude about the worth of any complex procedure. An operation that would be obviously indicated for a young manual worker may be inappropriate for a retired person who can manage what he needs to do with the ranges of useful motion that remain.

In planning tendon transfers there is often a choice between a very simple procedure, using synergistic transfers, and one that is more complex, requiring the retraining of nonsynergists. Here age must be taken into account. Children and young people can easily bring back into their consciousness the mechanisms of control of any muscle in the upper limb and can reprogram their nervous system to make it fit a different pattern. This may be almost impossible for some elderly people of even the highest intelligence. The wheels of their mind have created ruts that have deepened over years of efficient use. The ruts remain even when new pathways are established, and it is not good use of mental concentration to have to direct it constantly away from useful activity to the watching and avoiding of old ruts and mental pathways. For such people synergistic muscles should be used, and only one movement restored at a time.

1369

QUANTITATIVE EVALUATION OF MUSCLES

Every muscle has two major variables that identify its potential as compared with other muscles. The first is its capability for creating tension and the second is the distance, or excursion, through which its tension may be sustained.

No one who is unable to work out the mechanical effect of his or her actions should plan to move muscles or tendons around. I do not suggest that a mathematical equation needs to be worked out in each case. However, the surgeon and therapist need to use simple, round figures that will help them to know whether any given tendon transfer will provide enough but not too much tension to restore balance and whether a given muscle will be capable of providing the range of motion needed by the joints.

I will not at this time enter into a detailed account, available elsewhere,[1,2] of the way in which muscles may be evaluated, but will simply display a list (Table 106-1) and a composite graph (Fig. 106-1) of all the muscles of the forearm and hand. Figure 106-1 shows the tension capability on the vertical scale and the potential range of excursion on the horizontal scale. Both of these scales are relative. The numbers for tension represent each muscle as a percentage of the combined tensions of all muscles below the elbow. The excursions are the average of the fiber lengths of each muscle in a medium-sized forearm or hand, measured while all muscles are in their position of physiologic rest.

Most muscles whose tendons cross only one joint actually use only one-half to two-thirds of the excursions that are calculated from the fiber lengths. Those muscles whose tendons cross several joints more often utilize their whole potential excursion, but even these manage to work within the central half to two-thirds of their potential most of the time, by means of extending one of the joints while flexing others.

No surgeon should ever assume that a given nerve injury must result in the classic pattern of muscle loss for that injury. There are a host of variations in patterns of innervation and of injury and disease, so that the only reliable way to evaluate patterns of paralysis is to have a hands-on clinical test of every movement while the examiner's fingers feel for the tightening of the tendons. At surgery it is good if some clinical testing can be repeated while the tendons are exposed, if the patient is awake, or at least that a needle electrode may be used to stimulate the muscles that are about to be used, to confirm their vitality, strength, and potential for excursion.

Changes in Muscle Strength After Transfer

It has been commonly taught that muscles can be expected to lose one grade of strength after transfer. This rule is based on the Medical Research Council (MRC) system of grading of muscle tension, which was developed in Britain during World War II and has been widely used ever since. The grades are 0 to 5, where 5 is normal and 1 is a twitch without movement of a joint. Three of the grades refer to the ability of a muscle to oppose gravity (unable to move against gravity, able to move against gravity, able to move against gravity and resistance).

Because the effect of gravity on muscle is highly variable, depending on what limb segment has to be moved, and because movement against gravity is a very small part of the work of muscles in the upper limb, the MRC scale gives a much wider spread at the lower end of the scale. For this and other reasons, Yahr and Beebe[3] suggested that it would be more reasonable to use a simple percentage scale where 100% is normal. Some may prefer to record 0 to 10, where 10 is 100%. I have an impression that grade 1 on the MRC scale is about 5%; 2 is perhaps 10%; 3 might be 25%; 4, 60 to 70%; and 5, 100%.

Thus the old "rule" (MRC scale) that said a muscle would lose 1 grade of strength on transfer was never a real numeric statement but was more of a general warning not to expect as much tension out of a muscle after it has been transferred as it had before.

The point to make here is that the basic concept of "loss of strength" is wrong. A muscle has the same nerve supply, the same blood supply, and the same number of sarcomeres after it has been rerouted as it had before.

There is a change in the *effectiveness* of a muscle after transfer; this change is not due to loss of active muscle tension but to the increased passive drag on the muscle caused by the effect of the elastic properties of passive soft tissue. All the soft tissue in and around a muscle has to be lengthened with the muscle as it moves and exerts an elastic restraint. In the normal situation of a muscle, the length–tension curve of this tissue is low (Fig. 106-2) and becomes steep only toward extremes of movement. When a muscle is moved to another part of the limb, it becomes surrounded by scar tissue that binds it to the tissues along the new pathway. Scar tissue has a short, steep length–tension curve and may severely limit the excursion of a muscle after transfer. If great care is taken to pass the tendon through yielding fatty tissue only, without using a large wound of access, then the postoperative scar will bind the tendon only to tissues that can be easily moved and stretched and have a low length–tension curve. If an open wound of access cuts through fascia or retinaculum, or if bone is scratched or periosteum is cut, then scar may bind the tendon directly to an immovable structure, and the postoperative range of excursion will be very short indeed. In either case the actual tension produced by the muscle will be the same as it was before. The change is that the tension will be useful only for a short distance on either side of the position in which the muscle and tendon rested while the wound was healing. When wider excursion is attempted, the energy of the muscle will be used up in stretching or attempting to stretch scar tissue.

The lesson to be learned from this is that whenever possible no fascia or other immobile tissue should be cut or wounded in the same wound as a transferred tendon. This is why it is wise to use only a small wound proximally where the muscle or tendon is to change direction and only a small wound distally where the tendon is to be attached. The tendon should be tunneled between the two incisions with no open wound. First detach the tendon from its original site of insertion; then, after any necessary freeing up, pull it out through the proximal incision. Then pass tendon-tunneling forceps from the incision of proposed insertion to the proximal incision. Open the jaws to receive the tendon end, and withdraw the forceps distally with the tendon following.

TABLE 106-1. NORMAL MEAN FIBER LENGTHS, MASS FRACTIONS, AND TENSION FRACTIONS FOR ADULTS*

Mean Resting Fiber Length (cm)		Mass Fraction (%)		Tension Fraction (%)	
BR	16.1	BR	7.7	Supinator	7.1
ECRL	9.3	ECRL	6.5	FCU	6.7
FDS (ring finger)	7.3	FCU	5.6	PT	5.5
FDS (index finger)	7.2	PT	5.6	ECU	4.5
FDS (little finger)	7.0	ECRB	5.1	ECRB	4.2
FDS (middle finger)	7.0	FDS (middle finger)	4.7	FCR	4.1
FDP (ring finger)	6.8	FDP (middle finger)	4.4	ECRL	3.5
FDP (index finger)	6.6	FCR	4.2	FDP (middle finger)	3.4
FDP (middle finger)	6.6	FDP (ring finger)	4.1	FDS (middle finger)	3.4
Lumbrical (middle finger)	6.6	ECU	4.0	First DI	3.2
FDP (little finger)	6.2	Supinator	3.8	APL	3.1
ECRB	6.1	EDP (index finger)	3.5	AP	3.0
EDC (middle finger)	6.0	FDP (little finger)	3.4	FDP (ring finger)	3.0
Lumbrical (ring finger)	6.0	FPL	3.2	PQ	3.0
EDC (little finger)	5.9	FDS (ring finger)	3.0	FDP (little finger)	2.8
EDQ	5.9	FDS (index finger)	2.9	FDP (index finger)	2.7
FPL	5.9	APL	2.8	FPL	2.7
EDC (ring finger)	5.8	EDC (middle finger)	2.2	Second DI	2.5
EPL	5.7	AP	2.1	BR	2.4
EDC (index finger)	5.5	EDC (ring finger)	2.0	Third DI	2.0
EIP	5.5	PQ	1.8	FDS (index finger)	2.0
Lumbrical (index finger)	5.5	EPL	1.5	FDS (ring finger)	2.0
FCR	5.2	First DI	1.4	ODQ	2.0
PT	5.1	FDS (little finger)	1.3	EDC (middle finger)	1.9
PL	5.0	EDQ	1.2	OP	1.9
Lumbrical (little finger)	4.9	PL	1.2	Fourth DI	1.7
APL	4.6	ADQ	1.1	EDC (ring finger)	1.7
ECU	4.5	EDC (index finger)	1.1	ADQ	1.4
EPB	4.3	EIP	1.1	EPL	1.3
FCU	4.2	EDC (little finger)	1.0	FPB	1.3
ADQ	4.0	OP	0.9	First PI	1.3
APB	3.7	FPB	0.9	Second PI	1.2
AP	3.6	APB	0.9	PL	1.2
FPB	3.6	Second DI	0.7	APB	1.1
FDQ	3.4	EPB	0.7	EDC (index finger)	1.0
PQ	3.0	Third DI	0.6	EDQ	1.0
Supinator	2.7	ODQ	0.6	EIP	1.0
First DI	2.5	Fourth DI	0.5	Third PI	1.0
OP	2.4	First PI	0.4	EDC (little finger)	0.9
Second PI	1.7	Second PI	0.4	FDS (little finger)	0.9
Third DI	1.5	FDQ	0.3	EPB	0.8
Fourth DI	1.5	Third PI	0.3	FDQ	0.4
ODQ	1.5	Lumbrical (index finger)	0.2	Lumbrical (index finger)	0.2
First PI	1.5	Lumbrical (middle finger)	0.2	Lumbrical (middle finger)	0.2
Third PI	1.5	Lumbrical (ring finger)	0.1	Lumbrical (ring finger)	0.1
Second DI	1.4	Lumbrical (little finger)	0.1	Lumbrical (little finger)	0.1

Abbreviations: ADQ, abductor digiti quinti; AP, adductor pollicis; APB, abductor pollicis brevis; APL, abductor pollicis longus; BR, brachioradialis; DI, dorsal interosseous; ECRB, extensor carpi radialis brevis; ECRL, extensor carpi radialis longus; ECU, extensor carpi ulnaris; EDC, extensor digitorum communis; EDCI, extensor digitorum communis index; EDCL, extensor digitorum communis little; EDCM, extensor digitorum communis middle; EDCR, extensor digitorum communis ring; EDQ, extensor digiti quinti; EIP, extensor indicis proprius; EPB, extensor pollicis brevis; EPL, extensor pollicis longus; FCR, flexor carpi radialis; FCU, flexor carpi ulnaris; FDP, flexor digitorum profundus; FDQ, flexor digiti quinti; FDS, flexor digitorum superficialis; FDSM, flexor digitorum superficialis middle; FPB, flexor pollicis brevis; FPL, flexor pollicis longus; ODQ, opponens digiti quinti; OP, opponens pollicis; PI, palmar interosseous; PL, palmaris longus; PQ, pronator quadratus; PT, pronator teres; R, ring; S, supinator.

* From Brand, P.W.: J. HAND SURG. **6:** 209–219, 1981.

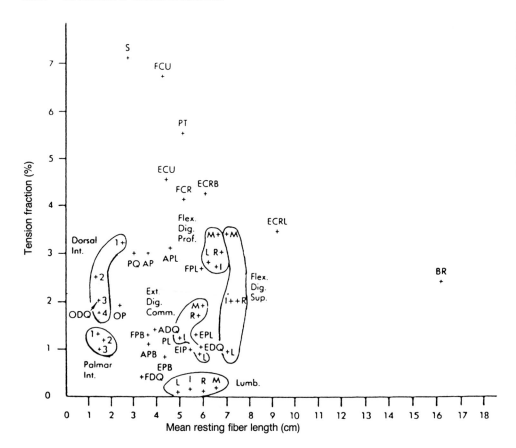

FIGURE 106-1.   Using values from Table 106-1, this diagram shows the relationship between fiber length and tension-producing capability. Some muscle groups are circled for clarity. (From data in Brand, P.W., Beach, R.B., and Thompson, D.E.: Relative Tension and Potential Excursion of Muscles in the Forearm and Hand. J. Hand Surg. **6:**209, 1981.) (See Table 106-1 for key to abbreviations.)

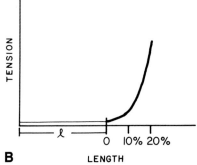

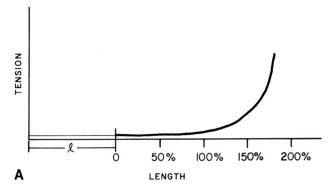

The disciplines that make for success include the following: (1) the tendon-tunneling forceps should have a smooth, rounded nose, widening to a viper head, quite close to the nose, and then narrowing back to a straight shaft as far as the handles. This ensures that any resistance that is felt during passage will be at or near the advancing end (Fig. 106-3). It should be possible to open the jaws of the tunneling forceps without increasing the width of the tunnel. (2) The surgeon must know the anatomy of the pathway, having passed forceps of the same pattern along the chosen path previously, at least in a fresh cadaver arm, so the feel of the structures is familiar. (3) The forceps must never be forced through if resistance is felt. It must be withdrawn a little and probed until yielding tissue is found. (4) If a tendon or graft is to be passed through the carpal tunnel (often a good path), the nose of the tunneler

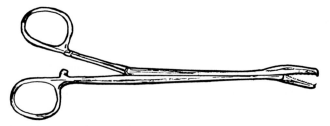

FIGURE 106-2.   (*A*) Normal paratendonous material. Resting length "1". Requires almost no tension to lengthen up to 100%, then gradual increase until elastic limit, in this case at about 160%. (*B*) Scar tissue replacing paratendon. Resting length "1." Requires tension to lengthen from the start. Elastic limit between 10% and 20%. Note: If the scar is short, the percentage of lengthening must also be short.

FIGURE 106-3.   Tendon tunneler. The essentials of a tendon tunneler are (1) it must have a smooth blunt nose; (2) its thickest point should be just behind the nose (the "viper" head); (3) it should be possible to open the jaws and the handles without stretching or tearing the tissues of the tunnel. (From Brand, P.W.: *In* Rob, C., and Smith, R. (eds.): Operative Surgery, 3rd ed. Stoneham, Mass., Butterworth Publishers, 1977.)

must be deep to all tendons and sheaths. The feel of the floor of the tunnel is hard and irregular and quite unmistakable; it is quite safe for the tunneler to press on the floor. If the passage of the tunneler pulls the fingers into flexion, it means that the tunneler is in among the tendons. It must be pulled back and rerouted more deeply on the floor. I have never known adhesions to be a problem in this uninjured skeletal plane; this plane also is well clear of the median nerve.

Changes in Excursion of Muscle After Transfer

Surgeons often wonder what happens if they transfer a muscle that has short fibers to replace a muscle that had long fibers. Assuming that the new muscle will have a shorter excursion, will it eventually develop longer fibers to match the requirement of its new task?

The answer is that it will not. If the patient exercises well and uses the muscle effectively, the result will be gradual lengthening of the paratendinous soft tissues to maximize available excursion. However, the number of sarcomeres in series in each fiber will remain the same. The only way to lengthen a muscle fiber is to keep it on the stretch, at rest. The only way to do this without shortening the fibers on the opposite side of the limb is to operate and attach the tendon at a higher relative tension. Muscle fibers respond to constant tension by adding sarcomeres in series until normal resting tension is reestablished.

There is a danger in attaching transferred muscles at high tension, because the muscle may respond by involuntary contractions that cause avulsion at the suture line.

The best way to handle the problem is to make the attachment of a transferred tendon at a tension just above normal resting tension (for a wrist-moving muscle this might be about 1 cm of distal pulling of tendon from its relaxed position), and then place the limb in the postoperative cast in a posture to relax that tension until the wound has healed, in 3 to 4 weeks. When the posture is allowed to return to normal, the transferred muscle will tend to give electromyography discharges and will obtrude into consciousness for 1 or 2 weeks until new sarcomeres have grown and relaxed the tension. This whole process brings the new muscle enough into consciousness to be of some assistance in the process of reeducation.

EVALUATION OF MECHANICAL BALANCE AT EACH JOINT

The calculation that is needed here involves moment or torque at a joint. This is the product of the tension of the muscle and the lever arm or moment arm at the joint. A weak muscle may produce a high torque at a joint if it crosses the joint far enough from its axis to have a long lever. However, in so doing it will use up a lot of excursion and thus may be able to produce only a limited range of motion of the joint. A stronger muscle may produce the same torque by crossing the joint nearer to the axis and requiring less excursion, allowing a wider range of joint motion.

If one knows the leverage, or moment arm of a tendon at each joint that it crosses, then the excursion needed at that joint may be calculated by multiplying the moment arm in

centimeters by the number of degrees of required motion of the joint measured in radians (1 radian = 57.3 degrees, Fig. 106-4). This also may be checked at surgery when a tendon is transferred. The joint is moved through some multiple of 60° (approximately 1 radian), checked by a geometric triangle (Fig. 106-5), while the resulting motion of the tendon is measured on a millimeter scale. For example, after performing a tendon transfer for intrinsic muscle function at the metacarpophalangeal joint of the middle finger, the surgeon may hold the proximal part of the tendon, pulling it gently, while he flexes the metacarpophalangeal joint through 90° (about 1.5 radians). If the tendon moves 15 mm, that proves that it is lying 10 mm in front of the axis of the metacarpophalangeal joint. By doing this the surgeon is able to make sure that the tendon is positioned correctly. If, with the same metacarpophalangeal angular motion, the tendon moves only, say, 8 mm, the surgeon knows that he or she has inadvertently passed the tendon *behind* the metacarpal ligament rather than in front of it, and the tendon will be a weak metacarpophalangeal flexor unless it is rerouted. (See Fig. 106-6, where flexor tendon is moving at a digital joint.)

Figure 106-7 shows a cross section of the wrist, based on mechanics rather than anatomy. It shows the relationship of each tendon to the axes of flexion–extension and of radioulnar deviation of the wrist. The number of dots marking each tendon indicates the tension fraction of the muscle. Thus, it is possible to calculate the torque available for each movement by multiplying the available tension by the measured distance from the relevant axis. While planning tendon transfers it may be good to sketch a diagram like Figures 106-7 and 106-8 to demonstrate the new balance that will be achieved after paralysis and then after tendon transfers.

If one muscle is used to provide tension to two different tendon insertions, the surgeon must make sure that the excursion required of each tendon is the same for the same range of motion. Otherwise, the tendon with the bigger moment arm will begin to move more, and then, because it is linked to a tendon that moves less, the faster-moving tendon will fall slack and exert no tension. Note, for example, that in radial palsy, a pronator teres attached to both extensor carpi radialis longus (ECRL) and extensor carpi radialis brevis (ECRB) will actually be effective for extension only on ECRL insertion, which is the least effective extensor. The pronator should be attached only to the ECRB, or to a better balanced pair of insertions.

EVALUATION OF CHANGES IN PASSIVE STRUCTURES FOLLOWING PARALYSIS

One of the remarkable features of the hand is that tissues in very close proximity to each other exhibit sharply contrasting responses to imposed mechanical stress. Tendons, tendon sheaths, and ligaments respond to repetitive tensile stress by a steep elastic curve of resistance before 10% of elongation has occurred. Paratenon and areolar tissue between tendons respond to repetitive tensile stress by allowing more than 100% lengthening with minimal elastic resistance. Skin occupies an intermediate position, and muscle allows about 100% of passive lengthening from its fully relaxed position. The last 50% of muscle lengthening requires significant tension, the energy of

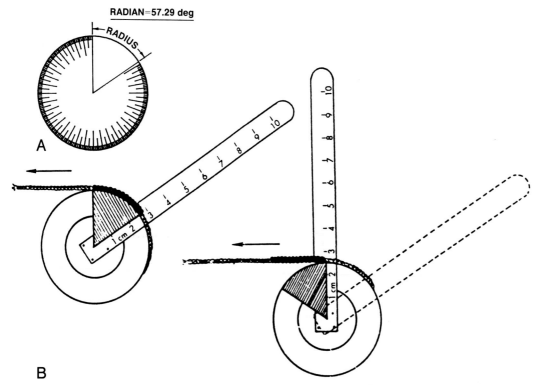

FIGURE 106-4. (*A*) A radian. The length of a radius, measured on the circumference, is joined to the center by two radii. (*B*) Way in which the lengthwise movement of a tendon may be used to measure the moment arm of a joint. If the joint moves 57.29°, the length of rope that runs off the pulley must be equal to its moment arm at the joint (i.e., radius of pulley). (Brand, P.W.: Clinical Mechanics of the Hand. St. Louis, C.V. Mosby, 1985.)

which is stored and used to supplement the active contraction of the stretched muscle.

In contrast to all these highly variable responses to *repetitive* stress, all of the preceding tissues have a rather constant response to long-term changes in their *resting tension.*

If, for any reason, muscle, fascia, or skin is held in a slightly stretched position for several days at a time, the tissue begins to undergo structural change to adapt to the new length and to restore the resting tension that was characteristic of the tissue before the change. A muscle fiber when kept on the stretch begins to add sarcomeres to increase its resting length, thus reducing tension. Collagen bands become progressively absorbed and are replaced by new collagen that is no longer under tension. Skin cells in the germinal layer show many mitotic figures and finally settle down having experienced a true growth, and thereby a reduction of the slight tension that had been imposed upon it.

Conversely, if any of these tissues are allowed to rest in a position where they are totally slack and loose, the tissue elements will begin to be absorbed and reoriented in a shortened position. Muscle fibers will show loss of sarcomeres until normal physiologic resting tension is restored in the new posture.

The normal physiology of muscle–joint interaction is largely dependent on the harmony between active muscle contraction and the viscoelastic changes in the passive soft tissues. For example a stretched muscle uses elastic recoil to provide most of the force when it begins to contract, and conversely most of the active contractile force of a muscle, as it nears its limit of shortening, is used up in stretching out its opposing muscles and is thus not available for its primary function of moving the joints. Similarly, the elastic stretching and recoil of skin and connective tissue participates in all joint motion, and the feedback of its sensory nerves provides the best monitor of joint position and proprioception.

One of the first effects of paralysis is to unbalance the hand. This results in a collapse of various joints toward the posture in which the unparalyzed muscles are shortened and in which the soft tissues on the "paralyzed" side are stretched to the point at

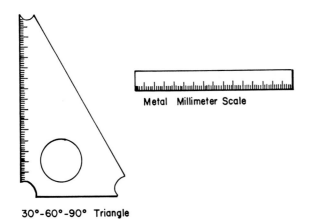

FIGURE 106-5. A 30°–60°–90° triangle. The corners are cut off to allow the triangle to be tucked into web spaces where the actual joint axis is deep in tissue. (Brand, P.W.: Clinical Mechanics of the Hand. St. Louis, C.V. Mosby, 1985.)

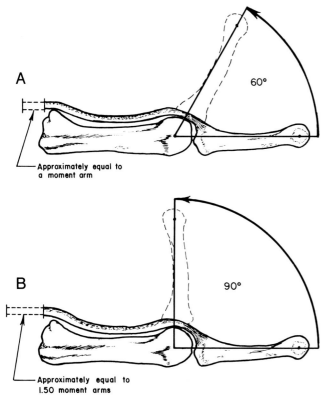

FIGURE 106-6. (*A*) For 60° of joint movement, tendon movement is approximately equal to a moment arm. (*B*) For 90° of joint movement, tendon moves a distance approximately equal to 1.50 moment arms. (Brand, P.W.: Clinical Mechanics of the Hand. C.V. Mosby, St. Louis, 1985.)

which their elastic tension equals the diminished tonus of the shortened unparalyzed muscles.

This new position of equilibrium is unstable. The unparalyzed muscles rest at a tension below their normal resting tension and will begin the process of losing sarcomeres to restore tension in the shortened position. The stretched skin and other soft tissues will begin to be lengthened by growth to get rid of their unnatural state of tension.

These initial compensations result in further destabilization of the equilibrium until some joints reach a point beyond which they cannot move. This whole process is seen in ulnar palsy, where there may be minimal clawing soon after injury but severe deformity after several months. It is also seen in radial palsy if the wrist is not supported at night as well as day and in the thumb in median palsy, in which the dorsal tissues of the thumb web become progressively narrower, and the ligaments at the base of the thumb change their length and density, so that after 1 or 2 years it may become almost impossible to fully oppose the thumb even after effective tendon transfers.

Muscle balance has been emphasized here because it is often neglected. A recognition of its importance will result in a greater insistence on maintaining a normal functional position of the hand *at rest* as well as during activity until muscle balance is restored. It should also stimulate the surgeon to operate earlier to restore muscle balance.

EVALUATION OF TRICK MOVEMENTS DEVELOPED AFTER PARALYSIS

"Trick" movements are the various attempts by an active person to get things done in spite of the limitations of paralysis. It

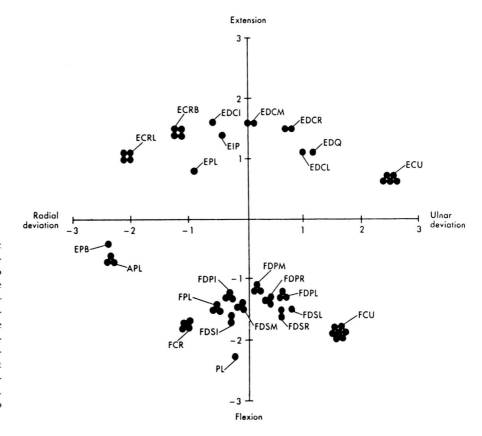

FIGURE 106-7. This is not an anatomic diagram; it is a simplified mechanical statement of the capability of each muscle to affect the wrist joint. The positions of the tendons in relation to the axes of flexion–extension and of radioulnar deviation represents their moment arms at the wrist. The number of dots in each cluster is an indication of the tension capability of that muscle–tendon unit rounded off to the nearest whole number. (Brand, P.W.: Clinical Mechanics of the Hand. St. Louis, C.V. Mosby, 1985.) (See Table 106-1 for key to abbreviations.)

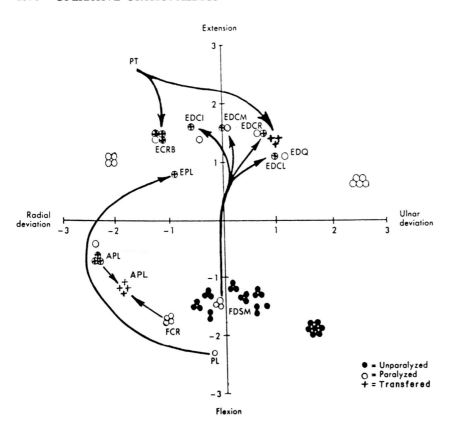

FIGURE 106-8. My preferred pattern of transfer for radial palsy. Note: When normal muscle ● is transferred to site of paralyzed muscle ○, the symbol ⊕ indicates activation of paralyzed tendon, while original tendon becomes ○. (Brand, P.W.: Clinical Mechanics of the Hand. St. Louis, C.V. Mosby, 1985.) (See Table 106-1 for key to abbreviations.)

is the good patient who finds a way around his or her disability and it is only a foolish surgeon or therapist who decries these efforts unless there is a serious reason for preventing their use.

A trick movement is a way of using the hand that would never be used if the hand were normal. When the normal way to hold an object or to perform an action is no longer possible, some people react passively and wait for the doctor to do something. Others are determined to move ahead and find a way to do the job with whatever resources remain in the hand. The good things about such unorthodox patterns of movement are that the *will* to work is maintained. When someone succeeds in accomplishing an objective, they gain confidence and maintain personal pride. These are assets beyond price. Also, the quality of muscles and skin and joint motion are maintained in better condition than when the limb is passive in a splint.

There are two bad things about trick movements. These are (1) when tissues become stretched or contracted as a result and (2) when the trick becomes dominant so that it persists after tendons have been transferred.

Tissue changes have already been mentioned, and examples have been given from paralysis of each of the three main nerve paralyses. Of the trick movements that may be troublesome as a habit after tendon transfer, one of the worst is the lateral squeeze pinch that is developed by almost every patient who has a low ulnar median palsy (Figs. 106-9, 106-10). These people have no easy way to use their thumbs except by simultaneous contraction of the extensor pollicis longus (EPL) and flexor pollicis longus (FPL). Each of these muscles, while opposing each other at the interphalangeal and metacarpophalangeal joints have a common vector for adduction at the carpometacarpal joint of the thumb. To make this work the two muscles have to contract together. The FPL overcomes the

EPL at the two distal joints where its moment arms are greater, while the EPL keeps the carpometacarpal joint in extension for which it has a better leverage than the FPL has for flexion. The resulting ugly pinch is strong and becomes frequently used. The late deformities are flexion contracture of the interphalangeal joint and shortening of the dorsal skin and fascia of the web. Even when these are correctable by surgery, the *habit* pattern of using the EPL for pinch tends to persist. It is most difficult to get rid of when it has been used for many months or years and in older patients. The reason that this abnormal pinch is so bad is that it is directly opposite to the new pattern that the surgeon will use to restore normal pinch. The newly transferred abductor-opponens transfer may be hard to reeducate, while the EPL is easy to use by force of habit. The EPL also has a better moment arm to pull into supination than the new transfer has for pronation. The patient's instinctive tendency to contract the EPL on attempted pinch is the cause of many failures of opponens transfers.

To prevent the development of this habit pattern, the thumb may be splinted forward, or held out by a C-splint. However, if a tendon transfer is to be delayed many months, it is not likely that a patient will agree to remain restrained. If the pattern is already firmly established at the time surgery is planned, one should think about the advisability of *using* the habit, rather than fighting it, by transferring the EPL around the wrist, or through the distal forearm to be attached to the stump of its own tendon to serve as an abductor-extensor of the thumb. Then the attempt to use the trick movement will serve to enhance the true opponens action. This transfer leaves the thumb with inadequate thumb supination, and therefore should be used only in older patients or when there is likelihood of failure of regular transfers.

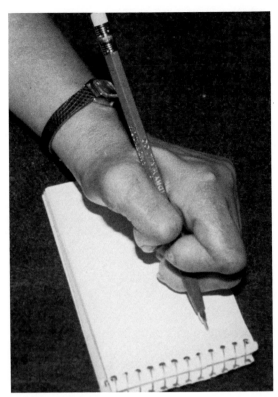

FIGURE 106-9. The lateral squeeze pinch, which is used by patients who have low median and ulnar paralysis of the thumb. The thumb squeezes with all joints in flexion except the carpometacarpal joint, which is in extension and supination. (Brand, P.W.: Clinical Mechanics of the Hand. St. Louis, C.V. Mosby, 1985.)

TIMING OF TENDON TRANSFERS

There is no doubt that the best time for a muscle balance operation in any case of irreparable nerve loss is as soon as possible after wounds have healed and there is tissue homeostasis. This allows no time for harmful secondary stretching or contractures or for the development of trick movements or habit patterns.

For this purpose tissue homeostasis may be judged by a return of normal skin mobility, joint mobility, hand volume, and skin temperature. I suggest the use of a simple skin thermometer for comparing the affected side with the normal side. A hand volumeter is also a useful instrument for monitoring the resolution of any inflammatory state in the tissues of the hand. The patient should see and note the progress of the graph of these records, which will also be used after surgery to mark progress in recovery from the operation and the mobilizing of joints and tendons. The patient will learn to associate raised temperatures with inflammation and will note how his or her hand volume increases when hanging the hand down and how it decreases after a period of elevation and moderate exercise.

If tendon transfers are done while there is still tissue inflammation as marked by lack of free skin mobility, elevated local temperature, and hand volume, then the postoperative inflammation is likely to be more severe and the adhesions around transferred tendons more difficult to resolve.

It is also necessary for the patient to have time before surgery to learn about and understand the implications of the operation and to identify the muscle and tendon to be transferred, so that there may be no loss of time in the critical period after the postoperative cast is removed.

The whole problem of timing is much more difficult when the nerve has been repaired and is in process of recovery. Far too many surgeons assume that they have to wait until they are absolutely certain that no recovery is possible before they decide to operate for restoration of muscle balance. They are afraid of some recovery occurring after they have done a tendon transfer and being told that their operation was unnecessary and possibly harmful.

As so frequently occurs today, the plan of treatment is dominated more by the fear of lawsuits than by the good of the patient. The right approach to this problem is first to make a realistic estimate of the probability of good recovery of the involved muscles. This is done with the recognition of the fact that muscle recovery is good when the nerve repair is accurate and without tension and is in the same limb segment as the affected muscle. The likelihood of good recovery is fair when the nerve injury and repair is in the limb segment proximal to the muscle, and it is poor when the injury is two segments proximal. An ulnar nerve division above the elbow, for example, will almost never result in good recovery of the intrinsic muscles in the hand. A median nerve above the elbow has a slightly better likelihood of recovery, but the secondary stiffness and contracture that results from the necessary 1- to 2-year wait to make sure is more harmful than any disability that might result from an early transfer that is followed 1 or 2 years later by recovery of the thenar muscles. If an operation is to be done early, in a case where later recovery is possible, it is wise to select a tendon for transfer that will not leave a significant defect by its loss from the donor site. For example in a high median palsy, while the thumb is still fully mobile passively, it is quite appropriate to use the extensor indicus proprius around the ulnar border of the wrist to restore abduction to the thumb. This muscle might be inadequate if it had to oppose contracted tissues and a negative habit pattern 1 or 2 years later. In the same way a palmaris longus, extended by free grafts through the carpal tunnel, is just fine for a new case of intrinsic palsy of the fingers, before the support of the volar plates and other tissues is lost by being stretched and before the interphalangeal joints become stiff in flexion.

The whole situation must be fully explained to the patient, and the pros and cons recorded in writing, so that the patient may know and choose between the possible harm of operating early and the more probable harm of waiting until much later.

REFERENCES

1. Brand, P.W.: Clinical Mechanics of the Hand. St. Louis, C.V. Mosby, 1985.
2. Brand, P.W., Beach, R.B., and Thompson, D.E.: Relative Tension and Potential Excursion of Muscles in the Forearm and Hand. J. Hand Surg. 6:209, 1981.
3. Yahr, M.D., and Beebe, G.W.: Recovery of Motor Function. *In* Woodhall, B., and Beebe, G.W. (eds.): Peripheral Nerve Regeneration: A Follow-Up Study of 3,656 World War II Injuries (V.A. Medical Monograph). Washington, D.C., U.S. Government Printing Office, 1956.

CHAPTER 107

Radial Nerve Palsy

LARRY K. CHIDGEY and
ROBERT M. SZABO

Radial nerve palsy most frequently results from penetrating injuries about the lower arm and the upper forearm and from fractures of the middle to distal third of the humerus. An alteration in the ability to grasp and release constitutes the major functional impairment.

Riordan[28] has separated grasp into three phases. Phase 1 constitutes opening the hand widely and requires the long extensors of the fingers and the thumb and abduction of the first metacarpal, as well as intrinsic muscle action. Phase 2 involves surrounding the object and requires combined long flexors and intrinsic action. Phase 3 is gripping the object between the fingers and the palm, or between the fingers and the thumb, and requires strong action of the long flexors. Phase 3 also requires stabilization of the wrist by the wrist extensors; otherwise the strong pull of the finger flexors would pull the wrist into flexion, causing a loss in power grip strength. Opening the hand for release requires the long extensors and the intrinsic muscles to perform as in Phase 1 of grasp. In high radial nerve palsy, grasp Phases 1 and 3 and the ability to release are severely impaired. In posterior interosseous nerve palsy, at least one of the radial wrist extensors is intact for wrist stability during Phase 3 of grasp. Therefore, only grasp Phase 1 and release are affected. Reconstruction for radial nerve palsy is directed at rebalancing the grasp-release mechanism necessary for normal hand function.

ANATOMY

The radial nerve (Fig. 107-1) originates from the posterior cord of the brachial plexus. Contributing nerve fibers can be traced from the fifth, sixth, seventh, and eighth cervical roots, with the largest contribution usually from the seventh. The nerve enters the upper arm posteriorly, accompanying the profunda brachii artery between the long and medial heads of the triceps. The radial nerve does not travel in the spiral groove of the humerus, but lies on the upper part of the medial triceps, separated from the underlying bone by a layer of muscle averaging 3.4 mm in thickness.[40] The nerve is in direct contact with the humerus only in the distal arm, where it pierces the lateral intermuscular septum.

Innervation to the triceps is variable. Linell[20] suggested four branches to the triceps: a branch to the long head arising about 7.1 cm below the tip of the acromion, a branch to the medial head arising about 9.5 cm below the acromial tip, the nerve to the lateral head arising about 10.1 cm, and another larger branch to the medial head about 11.2 cm below the acromial tip. Sunderland[36] found more variability, with 5 to 10 branches typically found. Because the branches to the triceps arise high in the arm, paralysis of the triceps from a fracture of the humerus is unlikely.

The radial nerve pierces the lateral intermuscular septum about 10 cm proximal to the lateral epicondyle and enters the anterior arm between the brachialis and the brachioradialis. The motor branches to the brachioradialis, and the extensor carpi radialis longus are given off in this area above the elbow. A branch is often extended to the brachialis, as well, but the predominant innervation of this later muscle is the musculocutaneous nerve.[29] The radial nerve divides into a superficial and deep branch at about the level of the lateral epicondyle. The

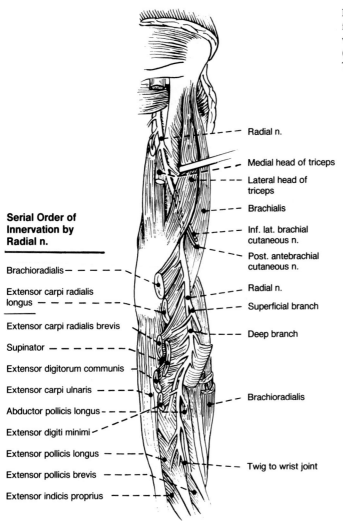

FIGURE 107-1. The radial nerve as it courses through the arm and forearm. The serial order of innervation to the forearm muscles is quite variable but in general follows a proximal-to-distal pattern as outlined. (Modified from Hollinshead, W.H.: Anatomy for Surgeons, Volume 3, The Back and Limbs, 3rd ed. New York, Harper & Row, 1982.)

Labels in figure:

Radial n.
Medial head of triceps
Lateral head of triceps
Brachialis
Inf. lat. brachial cutaneous n.
Post. antebrachial cutaneous n.
Radial n.
Superficial branch
Deep branch
Brachioradialis
Twig to wrist joint

Serial Order of Innervation by Radial n.

Brachioradialis
Extensor carpi radialis longus
Extensor carpi radialis brevis
Supinator
Extensor digitorum communis
Extensor carpi ulnaris
Abductor pollicis longus
Extensor digiti minimi
Extensor pollicis longus
Extensor pollicis brevis
Extensor indicis proprius

level of bifurcation varies from 4.5 cm above the lateral epicondyle to 4 cm below, with division at or below the epicondyle more common.[20] At about this same level, the radial nerve gives a branch to the extensor carpi radialis brevis. Salsbury[29] found this branch to arise from the superficial branch of the radial nerve in 56% of cases, from the deep branch in 36%, and from the angle formed by the two in 8%. With the exception of the frequent branch to the extensor carpi radialis brevis, the superficial branch of the radial nerve is purely sensory. After the bifurcation of the superficial and deep branches, the superficial branch continues distally and dorsally under the cover of the brachioradialis. It emerges from under this muscle at the junction of the middle and distal thirds of the forearm to continue subcutaneously along the dorsoradial aspect of the forearm to supply a variable area of skin on the lateral part of the dorsum of the wrist and hand.

The deep branch of the radial nerve is often referred to as the posterior interosseous nerve. It is purely motor with the exception of several sensory branches to the wrist joint at its most terminal extent. The posterior interosseous nerve passes from the proximal anterior forearm to the posterior forearm through the supinator muscle which it innervates. The proximal margin of the supinator forms a fibrous arch, referred to as

the arcade of Frohse, through which the nerve passes. The posterior interosseous nerve exits the supinator approximately 8 cm below the elbow joint and it immediately divides into multiple branches. Spinner[34] has observed that the branches seem to be arranged into two major groups. The first group supplies the superficial layer of extensor muscles (the extensor digitorum communis, the extensor digiti minimi, and the extensor carpi ulnaris); the second group supplies the deep layer (the abductor pollicis longus, the extensor pollicis longus and brevis, and the extensor indicis proprius). The serial order of innervation is quite variable, but in general follows a proximal to distal pattern (Fig. 107-1).

PRINCIPLES OF TREATMENT

Tendon transfers for radial nerve palsy have been considered relatively predictable and reproducible. Some authors[2,7] have therefore advocated early definitive tendon transfers to the exclusion of neurolysis or neurorrhaphy in the face of a high radial nerve lesion or a segmental nerve defect. We feel this approach denies the patient a potentially superior result. Civilian nerve injuries resulting in neurapraxia or axonotomesis have a high recovery rate.[1] If recovery is delayed, then neurolysis has been found extremely valuable. Functional return following neurolysis in neurapraxia or axonotomesis can be excellent. The myelin sheaths are still intact, or at least properly aligned, allowing selective reinnervation of the muscles by the same regenerating axons as before injury. This restores independent control of the individual muscles, a characteristic which is never achieved with primary nerve repair, nerve graft, or tendon transfers.

After neurotomesis, return of at least some muscle function after primary radial nerve repair or nerve grafting can be expected in 77% of patients.[22] Even if the return in muscle function is small, when combined with definitive tendon transfers, the result is often superior to that achieved by tendon transfers alone. Therefore, initial emphasis should be placed on the nerve injury.

Initial treatment of radial nerve palsy depends on the nature and severity of the inciting injury. In general, closed injuries such as crush injuries, low velocity gunshot wounds, and closed fractures result in neurapraxia or axonotomesis, and should be treated initially with observation. In open injuries, such as open fractures and lacerations, the nerve should be explored during the initial irrigation and debridement of the wound.

The reported incidence of high radial nerve palsy associated with humeral shaft fractures has ranged from 2% to 15%.[8,12–14,17–19,21,24,26,31,33] Several factors have been related to prognosis in these patients. Partial paralysis indicates continuity of the nerve and is a good prognostic sign. Functional recovery can be expected. Kaiser et al.[19] feel that patients suffering a comminuted, middle third fracture of the humerus with immediate onset radial nerve palsy have the poorest prognosis for nerve recovery. The poor prognosis is felt to be related to the high energy involved in this fracture. They suggest early exploration of nerves with this fracture pattern. Holstein and Lewis[14] have suggested that a spiral oblique fracture of the distal humerus places the radial nerve at particular risk for entrapment in the fracture site. They feel early exploration is indicated if this fracture pattern is associated with a radial nerve palsy. In contrast, Pollock et al.,[26] who had a 92% spontaneous recovery rate irrespective of the fracture pattern, recommend initial observation in all closed humerus fractures with

associated radial nerve palsy. If nerve function shows no signs of improvement in 3 to 4 months, then exploration of the nerve with neurolysis or neurorrhaphy is performed.

Our experience also suggests spontaneous recovery in the majority of fractures. In all closed fractures of the humerus associated with a radial nerve palsy we treat the nerve injury expectantly if the fracture can be reduced closed. Most patients can be expected to recover in 1 to 4 months. In 3 to 4 weeks, if recovery has not already begun, the extent of the nerve damage is assessed by electromyography. If no neurologic recovery is observed in 3 to 4 months, we explore the nerve with neurolysis or neurorrhaphy as needed. If reduction is blocked by any soft tissue interposition, especially if the fracture is of the distal spiral oblique type, we explore the nerve and reduce and internally fix the fracture. If manipulation results in an acute radial nerve palsy of immediate onset, then early exploration should be considered. Radial nerve palsies that are delayed in onset, even after manipulation, may be observed.

Segmental defects are repaired with interfascicular grafts. Functional nerve return can be expected in up to 77% of patients.[22] We have observed muscle function return even after grafting defects up to 15 cm. As a general rule, nerve regeneration is reported to progress at a rate of 1 mm per day.[32] Lesions above the elbow may progress at a slower rate. We have occasionally been surprised to find, after having given up on the nerve repair, that some muscle function is beginning to return.

The importance of maintaining supple joints free of deformity with the use of splints and physical therapy while awaiting nerve recovery, and prior to considering any tendon transfers, cannot be overemphasized. Splinting must be individualized. A simple palmer cock-up splint may increase the grip strength 3 to 5 times.[9] Most patients are well served by such a splint. A patient requiring greater excursion of the fingers may prefer a dynamic splint with an extension assist for both the wrist and metacarpophalangeal joints[25,37,38] (Fig. 107-2).

SURGICAL TECHNIQUES

To consider the operative treatment of a patient with radial nerve palsy, the surgeon should be familiar with the funda-

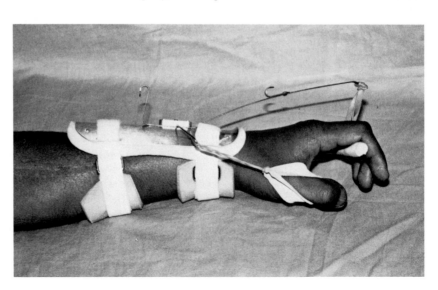

FIGURE 107-2. A dynamic splint with an extension assist for the wrist metacarpophalangeal joints of the fingers and abduction/extension assist for the thumb.

mental principles of tendon transfers and biomechanics (see Chapter 106). In selecting radial nerve transfers, approach each patient individually, with attention to age, occupation, and recreational goals. Familiarize yourself with the limitations and usefulness of the different available transfers (Table 107-1). The transfers discussed here assume an isolated radial nerve palsy.

In planning incisions for tendon transfers, consider the resulting effects on tendon gliding from the inevitable adhesions that will form. Avoid longitudinal incisions along the path of the transfer that tend to form adhesions through their entire length between the transferred tendon and the overlying fascia and skin. Incisions passing directly over tendon junctures are especially troublesome, and may inhibit the transferred tendon from gliding. Make small transverse incisions to mobilize muscle-tendon units if the unit is freely dissectable from its surrounding structures. If the muscle to be transferred requires significant dissection, avoid incisions that will run in a direct line with the proposed path of the transfer. The skin is fairly mobile in the forearm, and adequate exposure can often be obtained by simple retraction without extensive skin incisions.

Little controversy exists in choosing the motor to restore wrist extension. Transfer the insertion of the pronator teres to the extensor carpi radialis brevis at its musculotendinous junction. Avoid the dual insertion of the pronator teres to the extensor carpi radialis brevis and extensor carpi radialis longus.[3,4,9] Brand[6] clearly describes the biomechanical reasons why such dual insertion should be avoided. Consider both radial wrist extensors as ropes attached to two different-sized pulleys on the same shaft (Fig. 107-3). If each rope is wrapped around its respective pulley and pulled separately, more rope will unwrap from the larger pulley, which has a larger moment arm. If the two ropes are tied together and tension placed on the knot, the rope around the larger pulley (larger moment arm) will become loose because a longer length of rope is pulled off the larger pulley than the smaller one. The rope to the smaller pulley remains tight, and is therefore the only one effective in turning the shaft. The extensor carpi radialis longus has a smaller moment arm for wrist extension than the extensor

carpi radialis brevis. With insertion of the pronator teres into both radial wrist extensors, as the pronator teres begins to contract, the extensor carpi radialis brevis with its larger moment arm for wrist extension will become slack, and the extensor carpi radialis longus will be the only effective wrist extensor. Wrist extension will be weaker than if the pronator teres had only been transferred to the extensor carpi radialis brevis. The extensor carpi radialis longus has a larger moment arm for radial deviation of the wrist than for wrist extension; therefore with a dual insertion of the pronator teres, attempted wrist extension will result in significant radial deviation.

Flexor Carpi Ulnaris ("Standard") Transfer

In older patients and in those who are difficult to rehabilitate or have less need for independent digital control, use what has come to be known as the "standard" or flexor carpi ulnaris transfer.[15,16,28,30] Transfer the pronator teres to the extensor carpi radialis brevis; the flexor carpi ulnaris around the ulnar side of the forearm to the extensor digitorum communis; and the palmaris longus to the rerouted extensor pollicis longus. One disadvantage of this set of transfers is the inadequate excursion of the flexor carpi ulnaris to accommodate both wrist and finger extension; therefore, the patient is unable to fully extend both the wrist and the fingers at the same time. Brand[6] has also pointed out the dominance of radial forces after this transfer. We have not found this a significant problem in the carefully selected patient. The flexor carpi ulnaris transfer for finger extension has been the most reproducible of the transfers for finger extension. If the palmaris longus is not present, use the flexor digitorum superficialis to the ring finger, which is divided between the A1 and A2 pulleys.

Technique. The incisions for the flexor carpi ulnaris transfer are shown in Figure 107-4. Under tourniquet control, expose the pronator teres insertion through a 7-cm longitudinal mid-axial incision (*Incision 1*) over the middle third of the radius, while the forearm is held in neutral rotation. Identify the insertion of the pronator teres by developing the interval be-

TABLE 107-1. TRANSFERS FOR RADIAL NERVE PALSY

	Transfer	Advantage	Disadvantages
"Standard" transfer	PT → ECRB FCU → EDC PL → rerouted EPL	Requires little retraining Predictable	Unable to extend fingers & wrist simultaneously Dominance of radial forces across the wrist
FCR transfer	PT → ECRB FCR → EDC PL → rerouted EPL	Maintains FCU as an ulnar wrist flexor—important in heavy laborer	Unable to fully extend fingers & wrist simultaneously
Modified Boyes transfer	PT → ECRB FDS III → EDC FDS IV → EIP & EPL FCR → APL & EPB	Able to extend wrist and fingers simultaneously; independent control of index & thumb from other fingers for pinch	Potential flexion or extension deformities of the donor finger PIP joints Transfer not synergistic with potential for difficult rehabilitation. Potential for adhesions at interosseous membrane

ECRB = Extensor carpi radialis brevis; PT = Pronator teres; EDC = Extensor digitorum communis; FCU = Flexor carpi ulnaris; PL = Palmaris longus; EPL = Extensor pollicis longus; FCR = Flexor carpi radialis; APL = Abductor pollicis longus; EPB = Extensor pollicis brevis; EIP = Extensor indicis proprius; FDS III = Flexor digitorum superficialis to the long finger; FDS IV = Flexor digitorum superficialis to the ring finger.

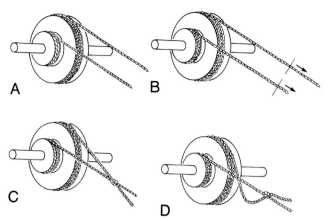

A   B

C   D

FIGURE 107-3. (*A*) Two ropes attached to two different-sized pulleys on the same shaft. (*B*) If each rope is pulled separately, more rope will unwrap from the larger pulley. (*C*) If the two ropes are tied together and tension placed on the knot (*D*), the rope around the larger pulley will become loose because a longer length of rope is pulled off the larger pulley than the smaller one. The rope to the smaller pulley remains tight and is the only one effective in turning the shaft. (Brand, P.W.: Clinical Mechanics of the Hand, St. Louis, C.V. Mosby, 1985.)

tween the brachioradialis and the extensor carpi radialis longus, taking care to protect the sensory branch of the radial nerve. Even in the presence of radial nerve palsy, trauma to the sensory branch may produce a painful neuroma. The insertion of the pronator teres is predominantly muscular, with very little tendinous component. To gain sufficient tendinous length, elevate the pronator teres off the radius with a 3-cm strip of periosteum (Fig. 107-5). In adults, the periosteum is thin and this strip is usually small, so handle it with care (Fig. 107-6). Bring the pronator teres out proximally from underneath the brachioradialis, and pass it superficially over the brachioradialis and extensor carpi radialis longus to the extensor carpi radialis brevis. By simply pronating the forearm the extensor carpi radialis brevis is easily exposed. The periosteal strip of the pronator teres will later be woven through the extensor carpi radialis brevis tendon just distal to the musculotendinous junction, but mobilize all the muscle-tendon units prior to completing any junctures.

To expose the flexor carpi ulnaris (Fig. 107-7*A*), make a longitudinal incision (*Incision 2*) along the palmer ulnar forearm directly overlying the flexor carpi ulnaris muscle belly. Distally, start the incision at the proximal wrist crease just proximal to the pisiform. Continue the incision proximally to the junction of the middle and proximal thirds of the forearm. After placing a tag suture in the flexor carpi ulnaris tendon, detach it from its insertion on the pisiform. Use the tag suture to provide traction on the tendon and to mobilize the flexor carpi ulnaris from its underlying extensive origin from the ulna and its overlying origin from the fascia. Stop this mobilization 5 cm distal to the flexor carpi ulnaris origin to avoid damaging its innervation from the ulnar nerve. Expose the extensor digitorum communis tendons through a 3-cm oblique incision (*Incision 4*) in the distal forearm, going in a proximal-radial to distal-ulnar direction. Tunnel a tendon passer subcutaneously from the ulnar margin of Incision 4 to the proximal extent of Incision 2. With this tendon passer, bring the flexor carpi ul-

naris subcutaneously around the ulnar side of the forearm to lie along the ulnar aspect of the extensor digitorum communis. If the bulk of the distal muscle belly of the flexor carpi ulnaris in its new position seems excessive, then it may be brought out of its tunnel and trimmed from its tendon.

If a palmaris longus is present, it is transferred to the rerouted extensor pollicis longus (Fig. 107-7*B*). Expose the palmaris longus distal insertion into the palmar fascia through a 1-cm transverse incision (*Incision 3*) at the proximal wrist crease. Expose the proximal tendon and muscle belly of the palmaris longus through the proximal portion of Incision 2. Divide the palmaris longus tendon distally, and deliver it into the proximal portion of Incision 2. Make a 2-cm transverse incision (*Incision 5*) over the radial aspect of the wrist just distal to the radial styloid, and expose the extensor pollicis longus tendon in the dorsal extent of this incision. Identify and divide the extensor pollicis longus tendon proximal to the dorsal retinaculum (*Incision 4*) and deliver this tendon from its dorsal compartment into Incision 5. Tunnel a tendon passer subcutaneously from Incision 5 to the proximal extent of Incision 2, and deliver the palmaris longus tendon across the palmar aspect of the forearm into Incision 5 to meet the rerouted extensor pollicis longus. At this time, deflate the tourniquet and achieve hemostasis; close Incisions 2 and 3.

The junction between the pronator teres and the extensor carpi radialis brevis is made last, because the tenodesis effect caused by flexing and extending the wrist is used to make sure the tension of the finger and thumb transfers are appropriate and result in synchronous motion. The juncture of the periosteal strip of the pronator teres to the extensor carpi radialis brevis may be tenuous and intolerant of the repeated wrist manipulations involved with setting the tension of the finger and thumb transfers.

For the flexor carpi ulnaris to extensor digitorum communis transfer we prefer an end-to-side juncture rather than an end-to-end juncture. Some patients have demonstrated improved motor return even a few years after injury. Dividing the extensor digitorum communis tendons for an end-to-end juncture deprives the patient of a potentially superior result, should any motor function return after the transfers have been completed.

Pass the flexor carpi ulnaris tendon through a slit in each of the extensor digitorum communis tendons in a proximal-ulnar to distal-radial direction at a 45° angle (Fig. 107-7*A*). Determine the site where the flexor carpi ulnaris is passed through the extensor digitorum communis tendons by fully flexing the wrist and fingers to make sure the juncture is proximal enough to remain unrestricted by the dorsal retinaculum. Suture each extensor digitorum communis tendon individually to the flexor carpi ulnaris with 4-0 nonabsorbable braided Dacron. The tension under which the transfers are sutured is critical. Set the tension by placing the metacarpophalangeal joints and the wrist joint in full extension; then suture the flexor carpi ulnaris tendon under slight tension.

For the palmaris longus to extensor pollicis longus transfer, place the thumb interphalangeal and metacarpophalangeal joints in full extension and the carpometacarpal joint in full radial abduction. Weave the palmaris longus tendon three times through the extensor pollicis longus tendon and suture it with 4-0 nonabsorbable braided dacron, as described by Pulvertaft[27] (Fig. 107-7*C*). Pull the palmaris longus tendon distally

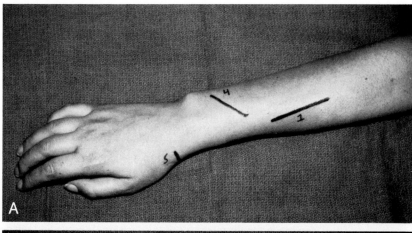

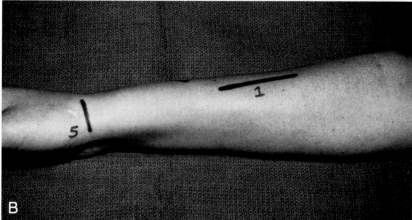

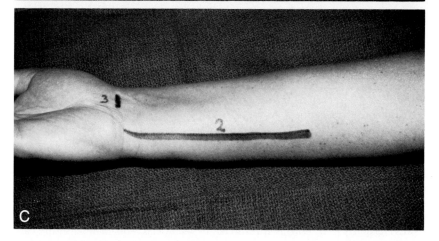

under mild tension while completing this juncture. Move the wrist, fingers, and thumb through a full range of motion to ensure that motion is synchronous and no restrictions are caused by the junctures.

Next, set the tension for the wrist transfer by placing the wrist joint in maximum extension. Pull the pronator teres, under slight tension, to the extensor carpi radialis brevis tendon just distal to the musculocutaneous junction. Weave the pronator teres through the extensor carpi radialis brevis tendon and suture it in place (see Fig. 107-5). Assess the tension of

all the transfers once again by rotating the wrist through a range of motion. With the fingers fully extended with flexion of the wrist, and with the fingers flexed into the palm with extension of the wrist, a synchronous tenodesis effect should be present. In older patients, or in patients who may be difficult to reeducate, suture the musculotendinous units under moderate tension to provide an extra component of sensory feedback through the stretch reflex.[5] Close the remainder of the wounds while maintaining the wrist and fingers in maximum extension and the thumb in maximum extension and radial abduction.

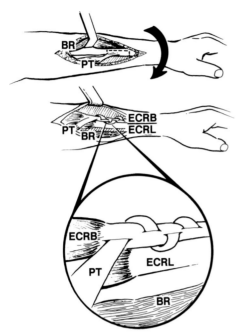

FIGURE 107-5.   Pronator teres (PT) to extensor carpi radialis brevis (ECRB) transfer. The pronator teres is elevated off its radius insertion with a 3-cm strip of periosteum and then passed superficial to the brachioradialis (BR) and the extensor carpi radialis longus (ECRL).

Apply dressings and splints, as described under postoperative care.

If the palmaris longus is not present, use the flexor digitorum superficialis tendon to the ring finger to the rerouted extensor pollicis longus for thumb extension and abduction. Make a 1-cm transverse incision in the distal palm over the fourth metacarpophalangeal joint and divide the flexor digitorum superficialis tendon between the A1 and A2 pulleys. Deliver the tendon into the midforearm through Incision 2 and

tunnel it subcutaneously into Incision 5 to meet the rerouted extensor pollicis longus. The juncture and tension are identical to those described for the palmaris longus transfer.

Flexor Carpi Radialis Transfer

Patients who wish to return to heavy labor may have difficulty, should the flexor carpi ulnaris be sacrificed for transfer. The flexor carpi ulnaris is a strong ulnar deviator and an important wrist stabilizer, and it is necessary for such activities as hammering. In these patients, select the flexor carpi radialis to provide finger extension.[5,35,39] The flexor carpi radialis also has a greater excursion than the flexor carpi ulnaris.[6] This allows more extension of the fingers with wrist extension.

Technique.   For wrist extension, use the pronator teres to extensor carpi radialis brevis exposed through a 7-cm longitudinal midaxial incision (*Incision 1*) (Fig. 107-8) along the middle third of the forearm, as previously described. Expose the insertion of the flexor carpi radialis and palmaris longus through a 1-cm transverse incision (*Incision 2*) at the proximal wrist crease, extending from the radial side of the flexor carpi radialis tendon to the radial side of the palmaris longus. Take care not to damage the palmar cutaneous branch of the median nerve with this incision. Expose the proximal muscle bellies of the flexor carpi radialis and palmaris longus through a 3-cm transverse palmar incision (*Incision 3*) at the level of the junction of the proximal and middle thirds of the forearm. Divide the tendons of the flexor carpi radialis and palmaris longus distally, free both of these muscle-tendon units of their fascial attachments by blunt dissection, and deliver both into Incision 3 (Fig. 107-9A). Expose the extensor digitorum communis tendons through a 3-cm oblique incision (*Incision 4*) in the distal forearm, moving in a proximal-ulnar to distal-radial direction. Into this incision, tunnel the flexor carpi radialis subcutaneously around the radial side of the forearm superficial to the

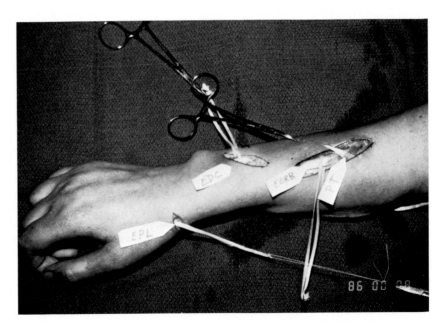

FIGURE 107-6.   In adults, the strip of periosteum elevated off of the radius with the pronator teres (PT) is thin and should be handled with care.

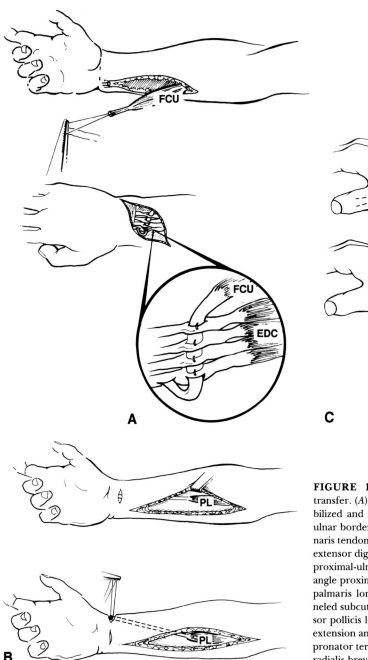

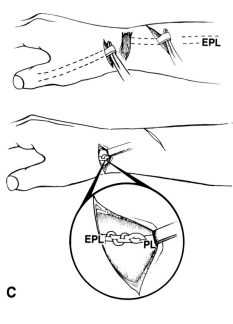

FIGURE 107-7. The flexor carpi ulnaris transfer. (*A*) The flexor carpi ulnaris (FCU) is mobilized and tunneled subcutaneously around the ulnar border of the forearm. The flexor carpi ulnaris tendon is passed through a slit in each of the extensor digitorum communis (EDC) tendons in a proximal-ulnar to distal-radial direction at a 45° angle proximal to the dorsal retinaculum. (*B*) The palmaris longus (PL) is mobilized (*C*) and tunneled subcutaneously to meet the rerouted extensor pollicis longus (EPL), providing simultaneous extension and radial abduction to the thumb. The pronator teres is transferred to the extensor carpi radialis brevis for wrist extension.

brachioradialis, extensor carpi radialis longus, and brevis. Make a 2-cm transverse incision (*Incision 5*) over the radial aspect of the wrist just distal to the radial styloid, and expose the extensor pollicis longus tendon in the dorsal extent of this incision. Return to Incision 4, and identify and divide the extensor pollicis longus tendon at its musculotendinous junction. Deliver the extensor pollicis longus from its dorsal compartment into Incision 5. Tunnel the palmaris longus subcutaneously from Incision 3 to meet the rerouted extensor pollicis longus tendon in Incision 5. Deflate the tourniquet, achieve hemostasis, and close Incisions 2 and 3.

The junction between the pronator teres and the extensor carpi radialis brevis is made last (see earlier section on "Standard" transfer).

Pass the flexor carpi radialis tendon through a slit in each of the extensor digitorum communis tendons in a proximal-radial to distal-ulnar direction at a 45° angle (Fig. 107-9*B*). Determine the site at which the flexor carpi radialis is passed through the extensor digitorum communis tendons by fully flexing the wrist and fingers to make sure the juncture is proximal enough to be unrestricted by the dorsal retinaculum. Suture each extensor digitorum communis tendon individually to the flexor

FIGURE 107-8. Incisions for the flexor carpi radialis transfer.

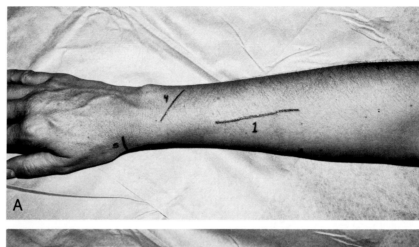

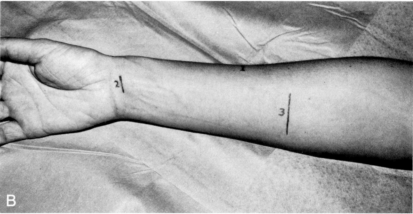

carpi radialis with 4-0 nonabsorbable braided dacron. Set the tension in the flexor carpi radialis to extensor digitorum communis transfer by placing the metacarpophalangeal joints and the wrist joint in full extension. Suture the flexor carpi radialis tendon under slight tension.

For the palmaris longus to extensor pollicis longus and pronator teres to extensor carpi radialis brevis transfers, do exactly as described earlier under standard transfer. Close the remaining wounds while maintaining the wrist and fingers in maximum extension and the thumb in maximum extension and radial abduction. Apply dressings and splints, as described under postoperative care.

If the palmaris longus is not present, use the flexor digitorum superficialis tendon to the ring finger to the rerouted extensor pollicis longus for thumb extension and abduction (see description under standard transfer).

Modified Boyes Transfer

For young patients who may require a greater range of motion in the fingers independent of wrist motion and who are cooperative rehabilitation candidates, use a modification of the transfer described by Boyes.[4,10] The flexor digitorum superficialis of the middle and ring fingers are passed through windows in the interosseous membrane to act as finger extensors. The flexor digitorum superficialis tendon of the middle finger is sutured to the extensor digitorum communis of all four

fingers, while the flexor digitorum superficialis tendon of the ring finger is sutured to the extensor indicis proprius and the extensor pollicis longus. This provides independent control of the index finger and thumb from the other fingers for the pinch function. The flexor carpi radialis is brought around the radial side of the forearm to the abductor pollicis longus to provide thumb abduction. Boyes describes insertion of the pronator teres into both the extensor carpi radialis longus and extensor carpi radialis brevis for wrist extension. We insert the pronator teres only into the extensor carpi radialis brevis for the reasons described earlier. In young patients, retraining the out-of-phase flexor digitorum superficialis to act as a finger extensor has not been a major problem.

Technique. Under tourniquet control, expose the pronator teres insertion through a 7-cm longitudinal midaxial incision (*Incision 1*) (Fig. 107-10) over the middle third of the radius while the forearm is held in neutral rotation. Isolate and mobilize the pronator teres with a 3-cm strip of periosteum, as previously described. Make a 2-cm transverse incision (*Incision 2*) in the distal palm over the third and fourth metacarpophalangeal joints, and identify the flexor digitorum superficialis tendons of the middle and ring fingers between the A1 and A2 pulleys (Fig. 107-11A). Identify the proximal flexor digitorum superficialis muscle-tendon units through a 3-cm transverse palmar incision (*Incision 3*) at the junction between the mid and distal forearm. Divide the flexor digitorum superficialis ten-

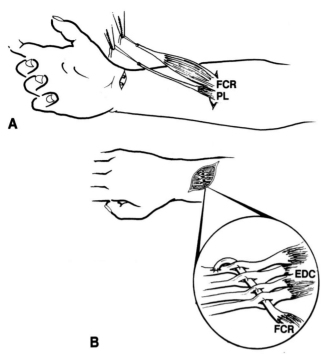

FIGURE 107-9. The flexor carpi radialis transfer. (*A*) The flexor carpi radialis (FCR) and the palmaris longus (PL) are mobilized through the same forearm incision. (*B*) The flexor carpi radialis is tunneled around the radial border of the forearm and passed through a slit in each of the extensor digitorum communis (EDC) tendons to provide finger extension. The palmaris longus is transferred to the rerouted extensor pollicis longus for thumb abduction and extension while the pronator teres is transferred to the extensor carpi radialis brevis for wrist extension.

dons between the A1 and A2 pulleys and deliver the tendons into Incision 3. At a level just proximal to the pronator quadratus through Incision 3, excise two 1-cm by 2-cm openings from the interosseous membrane, one on each side of the anterior interosseous artery, taking care to protect this and the posterior interosseous artery on the dorsal side of the membrane. Expose the extensor digitorum communis, extensor indicis proprius, and extensor pollicis longus tendons through a 3-cm transverse incision (*Incision 4*) just proximal to the wrist. Pass the divided flexor digitorum superficialis tendons through the interosseous membrane, with the superficialis tendon of the long finger passing radially between the profundus tendons, and the flexor pollicis longus tendon and the superficialis tendon of the ring finger passing to the ulnar side of the profundus tendons. Through a 2-cm transverse incision (*Incision 5*) at the base of the thumb, divide the flexor carpi radialis tendon just proximal to the flexor retinaculum. Through this same incision, expose the abductor pollicis longus and the extensor pollicis brevis in the first compartment. Deflate the tourniquet and achieve hemostasis. Close Incisions 2 and 3.

Retract the extensor digitorum communis tendons ulnarly, and weave the ring finger superficialis tendon first through the extensor pollicis longus, and then through the extensor indicis proprius tendon, while maintaining the index metacarpophalangeal, thumb, and wrist in extension and pulling the superfi-

cialis tendon distally under moderate tension (Fig. 107-11*B*). The juncture should be made proximal enough to the extensor retinaculum to avoid impingement when the wrist and fingers are flexed simultaneously. When bringing the superficialis through the interosseous membrane, pull the tendon distal enough to present the muscle belly into the interosseous window to prevent adhesions. Pass the superficialis of the long finger through a slit in each of the extensor digitorum communis tendons, in a proximal-radial to distal-ulnar direction at a 45° angle (Fig. 107-11*C*). Suture each extensor digitorum communis tendon individually, as the superficialis tendon is brought under moderate tension distally, and the finger metacarpophalangeal joints and wrist joint are held in extension. Weave the flexor carpi radialis through the abductor pollicis longus and extensor pollicis brevis, with the thumb in full radial abduction and the flexor carpi radialis under mild tension (Fig. 107-11*D*). Rotate the thumb through a range of motion to ensure that there is no impingement of this later juncture with the first dorsal compartment tunnel. Finally, complete the pronator teres to extensor carpi radialis brevis juncture, as previously described. Close the remainder of the incisions, and apply dressings and splints, as described under postoperative care.

POSTERIOR INTEROSSEOUS NERVE PALSY

In isolated posterior interosseous nerve palsy, the brachioradialis, extensor carpi radialis longus, and, in most cases, the extensor carpi radialis brevis innervations are intact. Therefore, a wrist extensor need not be replaced in these patients. Since all of the radial wrist extensors are intact, a significant amount of radial deviation may occur with wrist extension. In this group of patients use the flexor carpi radialis for finger extension. The palmaris longus or flexor digitorum superficialis of the ring finger may be transferred to the rerouted extensor pollicis longus to restore thumb extension and abduction. For patients requiring a greater range of fingers motion, use the flexor digitorum superficialis of the middle and ring fingers, passed through windows in the interosseous membrane, to act as finger and thumb extensors, and the flexor carpi radialis to provide thumb abduction. Sacrificing the ulnar deviating force of the flexor carpi ulnaris will exaggerate radial deviation caused by the radial wrist extensors. Therefore, we do not use the flexor carpi ulnaris to obtain finger extension in posterior interosseous nerve palsy.

"EARLY" TENDON TRANSFERS

While awaiting nerve recovery, transfer of the pronator teres to the extensor carpi radialis brevis as an "internal splint" has been suggested by Burkhalter.[9] This transfer allows the patient to remain brace-free. If neurologic return does not occur, nothing has been lost and the remainder of the definitive transfers can be completed. This transfer is useful in selected cases. Patients with a poor prognosis for relatively early nerve

FIGURE 107-10. Incisions for the flexor digitorum superficialis (modified Boyes) transfer.

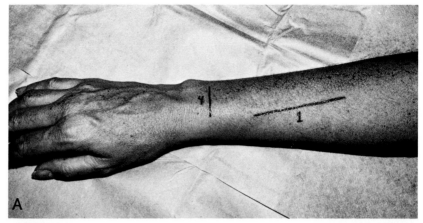

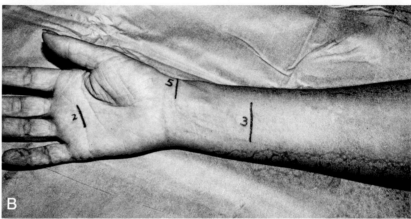

recovery, owing to a high radial nerve laceration; a large defect requiring a long graft; and a nerve graft, or nerve repair performed in a less than optimal tissue bed; are all considered candidates. Some patients will not tolerate bracing, either because of noncompliance or job-related conditions. We also consider early pronator teres to extensor carpi radialis brevis transfer in these patients. As with any tendon transfer, early transfers cannot be considered until a full or near-full passive range of motion has been achieved and "tissue equilibrium," as described by Steindler,[3] is present.

POSTOPERATIVE CARE

Immediate postoperative care is similar in each of the transfers. After the incisions have been closed, apply a bulky plaster-reinforced compression dressing that maintains the elbow at 90° of flexion, the forearm in neutral, the wrist at 45° of dorsiflexion, the metacarpophalangeal, the proximal interphalangeal, and distal interphalangeal joints of the fingers at 0° and the thumb at maximal extension and abduction. No immobilization of the fingers or thumb is required for the isolated pronator teres to extensor carpi radialis brevis "early" transfer. Remove the dressing 10 days postoperatively for suture removal. Apply a long-arm cast, maintaining forearm, wrist, and fingers in the same position. This cast is worn for approximately 3 more weeks and then changed to a removable short-arm splint, maintaining the wrist in 45° of dorsiflexion, metacarpophalangeal joints in 20° of flexion, and the proximal and distal interphalangeal joints are left free. Supervised physical therapy is started at this time. The splint is discontinued 2 to 3 weeks later, unless an extensor lag at the metacarpophalangeal joints or the wrist is present, in which case nighttime splinting is continued until this has resolved.

COMPLICATIONS

Use of the flexor digitorum superficialis may result in either a flexion contracture or a hyperextension deformity at the proximal interphalangeal joint. Littler[23] has suggested that these deformities can be eliminated, at least to the point where no functional impairment is present, by dividing the flexor digitorum superficialis tendon proximally between the A1 and A2 pulleys instead of at its insertion.

The importance of synergistic transfers becomes a question when the flexor digitorum superficialis (a finger flexor) is transferred to the extensor digitorum communis or the extensor pollicis longus (finger extensors). Many authors[6,10] feel the flexor digitorum superficialis is an easy muscle to retrain, and in young patients this seems to be true. We avoid this transfer in older patients who may have difficulty with reeducation.

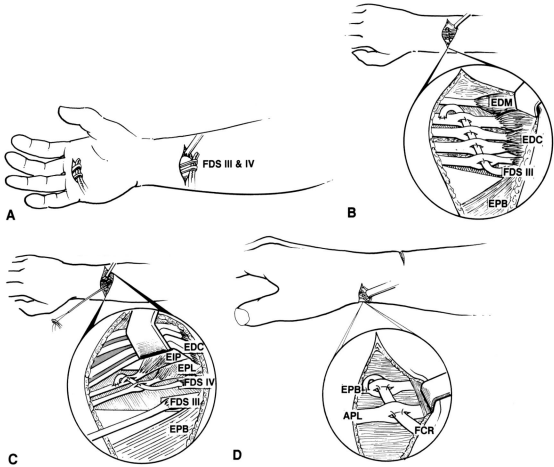

FIGURE 107-11. The flexor digitorum superficialis (modified Boyes) transfer. (*A*) The flexor digitorum superficialis tendons to the long and ring fingers (FDS III & IV) are divided distally between the A1 and A2 pulley and delivered into the mid forearm. (*B*) The two flexor digitorum superficialis tendons are passed through windows in the interosseous membrane to the dorsal forearm. The flexor digitorum superficialis to the ring finger is transferred to the extensor pollicis longus (EPL) and extensor indicis proprius (EIP) to provide index and thumb extension independent of finger extension. (*C*) The flexor digitorum superficialis to the long finger is passed through a slit in each of the extensor digitorum communis (EDC) tendons in a radial to ulnar direction to provide finger extension. The extensor digiti minimi (EDM) is not included in this transfer if the extensor digitorum communis tendon to the little finger is present. (*D*) The flexor carpi radialis (FCR) is transferred to the abductor pollicis longus (APL) and extensor pollicis breves (EPB) to provide thumb abduction. The juncture is made distal to the dorsal retinaculum. The pronator teres to extensor carpi radialis brevis transfer provides wrist extension.

REFERENCES

1. Bateman, J.E.: Trauma to Nerves in Limbs. Philadelphia, W.B. Saunders, 1982, p. 167.
2. Bevin, A.G.: Early Tendon Transfer for Radial Nerve Transsection. Hand 8:134–136, 1976.
3. Boyes, J.H.: Tendon Transfers in the Hand. In Medicine in Japan in 1959. Proceedings of the 15th General Assembly of the Japan Medical Congress 5:958–969, 1959.
4. Boyes, J.H.: Tendon Transfers for Radial Nerve Palsy. Bull. Hosp. Joint Dis. 21:97–105, 1960.
5. Brand, P.W.: Tendon Transfers in the Forearm. In Flynn, J.E. (ed.): Hand Surgery, 2nd ed. Baltimore, Williams and Wilkins, 1975.
6. Brand, P.W.: Clinical Mechanics of the Hand. St. Louis, C.V. Mosby, 1985.
7. Brown, P.W.: The Time Factor in Surgery of Upper-Extremity Peripheral Nerve Injury. Clin. Orthop. 68:14–21, 1970.
8. Bryer, B.F.: Management of Humeral Shaft Fractures. Arch. Surg. 81:914–928, 1960.
9. Burkhalter, W.E.: Early Tendon Transfer in Upper Extremity Peripheral Nerve Injury. Clin. Orthop. 104:68–79, 1974.
10. Chuinard, R.G., Boyes, J.H., Stark, H.H., and Ashworth, C.R.: Tendon Transfers for Radial Nerve Palsy: Use of Superficialis Tendons for Digital Extension. J. Hand Surg. 3:560–570, 1978.
11. Frohse, F., and Frankel, M.: Die Muskeln des Menschlichen Armes. Vol. 2. In von Bardeleben, K. (ed.): Handbuch der Anatomie des Menschen. Jena, Fischer, 1908.
12. Garcia, A., and Maeck, B.H.: Radial Nerve Injuries in Fractures of the Shaft of the Humerus. Am. J. Surg. 99:625–627, 1960.
13. Goldner, J.L., and Kelley, J.M.: Radial Nerve Injuries. South. Med. J. 51:873–883, 1958.

14. Holstein, A., and Lewis, G.B.: Fractures of the Humerus with Radial-Nerve Paralysis. J. Bone Joint Surg. **45-A:**1382–1388, 1963.

15. Jones, R.: On Suture of Nerves, and Alternative Methods of Treatment by Transplantation of Tendon. Br. Med. J. **1:**641–643, 1916.

16. Jones, R.: Tendon Transplantation in Cases of Musculospiral Injuries not Amenable to Suture. Am. J. Surg. **35:**333–335, 1921.

17. Kettelkamp, D.B., and Alexander, H.: Clinical Review of Radial Nerve Injury. J. Trauma **7:**424–432, 1967.

18. Klenerman, L.: Fractures of the Shaft of the Humerus. J. Bone Joint Surg. **48-B:**105–111, 1966.

19. Kaiser, T.E., Franklin, H.S., and Kelly, P.J.: Radial Nerve Palsy Associated with Humeral Shaft Fractures. Orthopedics **4:**1245–1251, 1981.

20. Linell, E.A.: The Distribution of Nerves in the Upper Limb, with Reference to Variabilities and their Clinical Significance. J. Anat. **55:**79, 1921.

21. Mast, J.W., Spiegel, P.G., Harvey, J.P., and Harrison, C.: A Retrospective Study of 240 Adult Fractures. Clin. Orthop. **112:**254–262, 1975.

22. Millesi, H., Messil, G., and Berger, A.: Further Experience with Interfascicular Grafting of the Median, Ulnar, and Radial Nerves. J. Bone Joint Surg. **58-A:**209–218, 1976.

23. North, E.R., and Littler, J.W.: Transferring the Flexor Superficialis Tendon: Technical Considerations in the Prevention of Proximal Interphalangeal Joint Disability. J. Hand Surg. **5:**498–501, 1980.

24. Packer, J.W., Foster, R.R., Garcia, A., and Grantham, S.A.: The Humeral Fracture with Radial Nerve Palsy: Is Exploration Warranted? Clin. Orthop. **88:**34–38, 1972.

25. Penner, D.A.: Dorsal Splint for Radial Palsy. Am. J. Occup. Ther. **26:**46–47, 1972.

26. Pollock, F.H., Drake, D., Bovill, E.G., Day, L., and Trafton, P.G.: Treatment of Radial Neuropathy Associated with Fractures of the Humerus. J. Bone Joint Surg. **63-A:**239–243, 1981.

27. Pulvertaft, R.G.: Tendon Grafts for Flexor Tendon Injuries in the Fingers and Thumb. A Study of Technique and Results. J. Bone Joint Surg. **38-B:**175–194, 1956.

28. Riordan, D.C.: Tendon Transfers in Hand Surgery. J. Hand Surg. **8:**748–753, 1983.

29. Salsbury, C.R.: The Nerve to the Extensor Carpi Radialis Brevis. Br. J. Surg. **26:**95, 1938.

30. Scuderi, C.: Tendon Transplants for Irreparable Radial Nerve Paralysis. Surg. Gynecol. Obstet. **88:**643–651, 1949.

31. Seddon, H.J.: The Practical Value of Peripheral Nerve Repair. Proc. R. Soc. Med. **42:**427–436, 1949.

32. Seddon, H.J.: Surgical Disorders of the Peripheral Nerves, 2nd ed. Edinburgh, Churchill-Livingstone, 1975, p. 31.

33. Shaw, J.L., and Sakellarides, H.: Radial-Nerve Paralysis Associated with Fractures of the Humerus. A Review of Forty-Five Cases. J. Bone Joint Surg. **49-A:**899–902, 1967.

34. Spinner, M.: The Radial Nerve. In Injuries to the Major Branches of Peripheral Nerves of the Forearm. Philadelphia, W.B. Saunders, 1972.

35. Starr, C.L.: Army Experience with Tendon Transference. J. Bone Joint Surg. **4:**3–21, 1922.

36. Sunderland, S.: Metrical and Non-Metrical Features of the Muscular Branches of the Radial Nerve. J. Comp. Neurol. **85:**93, 1946.

37. Thomas, F.B.: A Splint for Radial (Musculospiral) Nerve Palsy. J. Bone Joint Surg. **26:**602–605, 1944.

38. Thomas, F.B.: An Improved Splint for Radial (Musculospiral) Nerve Paralysis. J. Bone Joint Surg. **33-B:**272–273, 1951.

39. Tsuge, K., and Adachi, N.: Tendon Transfer for Extensor Palsy of Forearm. Hiroshima J. Med. Sci. **18:**219–232, 1969.

40. Whitson, R.O.: Relation of the Radial Nerve to the Shaft of the Humerus. J. Bone Joint Surg. **36-A:**85, 1954.

CHAPTER 108

Median Nerve Palsy

STEVEN M. GREEN

In spite of advances in understanding and treating nerve injuries, surgical reconstruction for paralysis of median innervated muscles remains a common procedure. This chapter discusses the functional anatomy of the intrinsic muscles and the techniques of opposition transfer, as well as the methods available to restore function in cases of extrinsic median palsy. Median nerve palsy is most often the result of lacerations or compression syndromes. It is also seen in cases of peripheral neuropathy, such as diabetes, traction injuries to the brachial plexus, and infections such as polio and leprosy.

INTRINSIC MEDIAN PALSY

The strongest and most important of the median intrinsic muscles is the abductor pollicis brevis, whose function is to move the thumb away from the palm of the hand (palmar abduction) and rotate (pronate) it towards the pulp of the fingers.[10] Pronation is the main function of the opponens pollicis muscle, although it also assists in palmar abduction. The primary function of the flexor pollicis brevis is metacarpophalangeal joint flexion. It also assists in palmar abduction and pronation.[8]

The term "opposition" describes the position of the thumb when its pulp is directly opposite that of one of the fingers, with the nails parallel.[7] Opposition is a combined motion of thumb metacarpal palmar abduction and pronation, with flexion of the thumb metacarpal, metacarpophalangeal joint, and interphalangeal joint. The converse of opposition is reposition.

The median innervated intrinsics of the thumb characteristically include the abductor pollicis brevis, the opponens pollicis, and the superficial head of the flexor pollicis brevis. There are, however, variations in the innervation of these muscles that may present a confusing clinical picture.[19] Because the innervation of these muscles is so variable, the functional consequence of median neuropathy ranges from mild to severe.[11]

Although tendon transfers to restore opposition are commonplace today, it was not until 1918 that Steindler[22] suggested rerouting the flexor pollicis longus in order to restore thumb mobility. Bunnell,[4] in his classic article of 1938, outlined the basic principles of opposition reconstruction and emphasized that surgery must be individualized to meet the patient's needs, since "each hand is a problem in itself."

Candidates for tendon transfer surgery must have adequate sensibility. The thumb joints should be stable, and the skin and joints must be supple; if not, they must be corrected by therapy or surgery. Occasionally, a Silastic tendon prosthesis is used to preform an adequate subcutaneous pathway for eventual tendon transfer. The function of the extrinsic flexor and extensor tendons must also be evaluated before tendon transplantation is considered.

In restoring thumb opposition, one must consider the excursion and force of the tendon transfer as well as the direction of its pull and the axis of insertion into the thumb (see Chapter 106). Although it may not be possible to fully replace the function of several weakened intrinsic muscles with one tendon transfer, the motor tendon to be utilized in the replacement should match as closely as possible the normal force and excursion of the paralyzed muscles. The force generated by a muscle is proportional to its cross-sectional area, which is 6.0 cm^2 for the usual median innervated intrinsics.[6] The long finger superficialis (cross section: 5.8 cm^2) and the extensor carpi ulnaris (6.2 cm^2) most closely match the thenar forces. Although the ring finger superficialis (3.2 cm^2), the extensor indices proprius (1.7 cm^2), the palmaris longus (1.8 cm^2), and the abductor digiti quinti (2.1 cm^2) are frequently used for tendon transfers, their potential forces are significantly less. Excursion, or the change in length between full relaxation and contraction, depends on mean fiber length, which averages 3.5 cm for the thenar muscles.[6] This figure is surpassed by all the commonly used transfers.

In selecting a tendon for transfer, the surgeon must not substitute one imbalance for another. Choosing a strong motor may improve thumb function, for example, but if a finger flexor is used, the improvement occurs at the expense of grip power.

To produce the motion of opposition, the transfer must pull from the direction of the pisiform, thereby paralleling the fibers of the abductor pollicis brevis, the most important muscle in opposition. Transfers that use a pulley distal to the pisiform encourage metacarpal flexion at the expense of palmar abduction. The reverse is true for transfers that pull more proximal and radial to the pisiform.[7]

Unless there exists a supple subcutaneous bed through which the transfer is to be passed, the motor will not be able to transmit its force of contraction. Therefore, skin resurfacing may be required before a tendon transfer is performed. Although free skin grafts can be used in some areas, flaps are frequently necessary to provide adequate subcutaneous tissue to allow tendon excursion. Alternatively, a Silastic tendon prosthesis can be used to help preform an adequate pathway for eventual tendon transfer.

The most predictable insertion is made into the tendon of the abductor pollicis brevis.[13] Insertions into the ulnar base of the proximal phalanx do not produce greater rotation during opposition, and such insertions may slip about the metacarpophalangeal joint, causing unwanted extension or flexion of the proximal phalanx. Insertions into the extensor mechanism[18] or the metacarpophalangeal joint capsule[1] increase thumb extension and stability, but are only recommended for patients with combined nerve palsies.

SPECIFIC TENDON TRANSFERS

Flexor Digitorum Superficialis

The most popular transfer for restoration of opposition utilizes a superficialis as the motor. This choice was first popularized by Krukenberg,[5] Bunnell,[4] Royle,[20] and Thompson.[24]

Via an oblique or transverse distal palmar incision, incise the proximal flexor tendon sheath and retract the round profundus. Deep to the profundus, the flat superficialis tendon is seen; after passively flexing the digit, cross-clamp and transsect this tendon (Fig. 108-1). If the superficialis is incised more distally, past the chiasm of Campfer, it will be difficult to withdraw the superficialis, as it will become trapped about the lumbrical origin of the profundus. In addition, some patients develop proximal interphalangeal joint hyperextension after distal excision of the superficialis.

Make a second incision in the distal forearm, beginning at the midline 2 cm proximal to the wrist, and curving towards the pisiform. Through this incision, expose the superficialis and withdraw it with a moist gauze sponge. Dissect the distal flexor carpi ulnaris tendon from the ulnar nerve and artery, and protect the artery with a moist tongue depressor passed beneath the tendon. Starting from its insertion, make a 2-cm longitudinal midline split in the flexor carpi ulnaris tendon with a Number 11 scalpel. Then transect the radial portion at the proximal extent of the split, creating a 2-cm tendon stump attached to the pisiform. Pass the superficialis tendon dorsal to the intact flexor carpi ulnaris tendon, so that it emerges on its ulnar side (Fig. 108-2).

Make a third incision on the dorsal-radial aspect of the thumb metacarpophalangeal joint, and pass a large curved clamp superficial to the abductor pollicis brevis tendon and then subcutaneously across the palm, to emerge at the distal forearm incision at the pisiform. Place the end of the superficialis into the clamp and withdraw it toward the thumb. Then loop the cut portion of the flexor carpi ulnaris about the transfer and suture it to itself with 4-0 nonabsorbable suture.

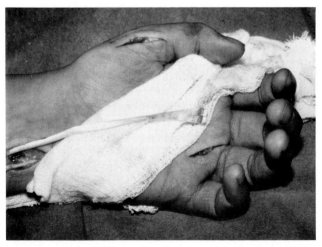

FIGURE 108-1. The three incisions required for an opposition transfer using the ring finger superficialis.

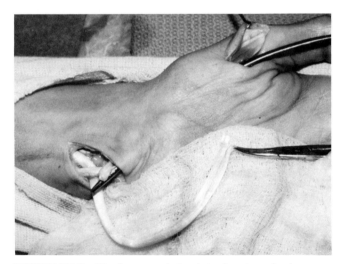

FIGURE 108-2. The flexor carpi ulnaris tendon stump has been created, the superficialis passed beneath the intact portion of the wrist flexor, and a subcutaneous pathway produced with the tendon passer.

The loop should be just large enough to permit excursion of the superficialis tendon without friction (Fig. 108-3). Combining the tendon loop with passage of the tendon transfer under the flexor carpi ulnaris is the most satisfactory method of preventing proximal and radial migration of the tendon transfer.

Finally, pass the superficialis tendon through a perforation in the intrinsic tendon. Use a ruler to measure the passive excursion of the superficialis with the wrist at neutral and the thumb held in opposition to the ring finger. An interweaving suture is then accomplished with the wrist and thumb in this position and with enough tension on the end of the superficialis to generate half of its passive potential (Fig. 108-4). Upon completion of the tendon suture, the thumb should remain in opposition to the middle finger. If not, adjust the tension and place additional tacking sutures between the intrinsic tendon and the superficialis (Figs. 108-5 to 108-7).

Extensor Indicis Proprius

Another useful transfer involves the extensor indicis proprius (EIP).[25] This tendon has excellent excursion, and its use does not weaken grip strength as does the superficialis transfer. However, the EIP is not as forceful (cross section: 1.7 cm^2),[6] and it is an antagonist to the thenar muscles, which makes retraining difficult in some cases.

This tendon lies to the ulnar side of the index communis. Expose it at the metacarpophalangeal joint, and incise it together with a thin longitudinal strip of the extensor hood. Then close the hood with 4-0 or 5-0 nonabsorbable suture to prevent a lag of active extension.

Expose the indicis tendon and withdraw it through a transverse dorsal incision just proximal to the extensor retinaculum. Then make a longitudinal 2-cm incision midaxially over the distal ulna, and with a large clamp pass the EIP subcutaneously into this exposure. Continue the rest of the operation as for the superficialis transfer, except that the ulnar border of the forearm rather than the flexor carpi is used to form the pulley.

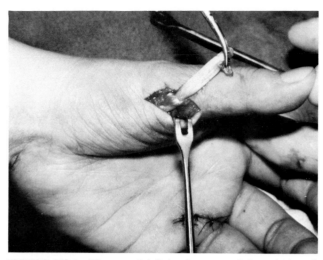

FIGURE 108-4. The superficialis has been passed through the substance of the thenar intrinsic tendon.

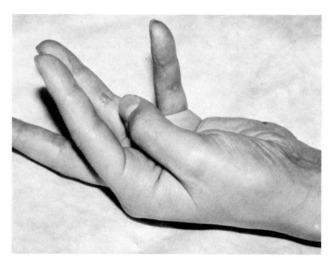

FIGURE 108-5. Lack of active opposition as a result of median nerve palsy.

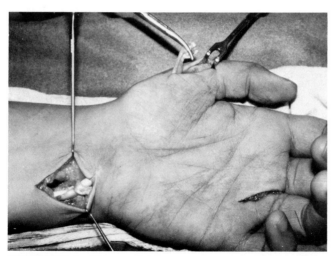

FIGURE 108-3. The superficialis has been transferred and the tendon loop formed.

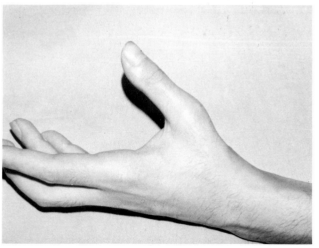

FIGURE 108-6. Same patient as in Figure 108-5 after superficialis transfer (palmar abduction).

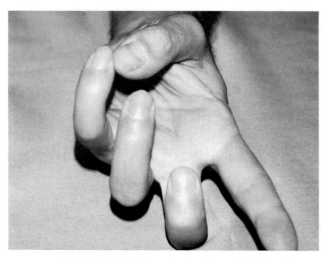

FIGURE 108-7. Same patient (opposition).

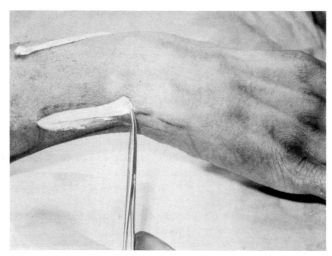

FIGURE 108-9. The insertion of the extensor carpi ulnaris has been transsected.

Extensor Digiti Quinti

Although rarely indicated in patients with isolated median palsy, good results can be obtained by transfer of the extensor digiti quinti (EDQ).[21,23] After exposing this tendon over the dorsal small finger metacarpophalangeal joint and ascertaining the presence of a communis slip from the ring finger, transect the EDQ and bring it out through an additional incision over the distal ulna (Fig. 108-8). Complete the procedure as for the extensor indices proprius transfer.

Extensor Carpi Ulnaris

As an alternative, the extensor carpi ulnaris can provide a forceful transfer.[17] It lacks the excursion of the superficialis group, however, and must be prolonged with a tendon graft.

Expose the wrist extensor through a distal ulnar incision, and transect it as far distally as possible (Fig. 108-9). The extensor pollicis brevis tendon is wholly employed to lengthen the extensor carpi ulnaris; identify its insertion and musculo-

tendinous junction through two separate incisions (Fig. 108-10). After dividing this tendon at its musculotendinous junction, bring it out at the thumb metacarpophalangeal joint, pass it subcutaneously across the palm, and suture it into the extensor carpi ulnaris (Figs. 108-11 and 108-12). Occasionally, the extensor pollicis brevis is hypoplastic, and then a free palmaris graft can be used to prolong the extensor carpi ulnaris.

Although good results can be obtained, the insufficient extensor carpi ulnaris excursion and the less-than-optimal insertion of the extensor pollicis brevis make this tendon transfer a secondary choice, as full opposition is rarely achieved.

Palmaris Longus

In patients with moderate thenar weakness, especially as a consequence of chronic carpal tunnel syndrome, the palmaris longus can be utilized as a transfer.[5,15] Expose the palmaris tendon through a palmar incision and dissect it distally along with a strip of palmar fascia (Fig. 108-13). Expose the abductor pollicis brevis tendon on the radial side of the thumb, and pass

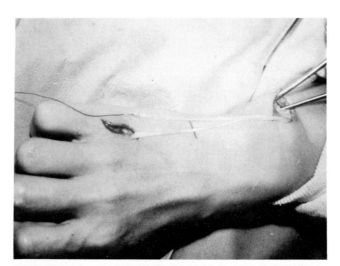

FIGURE 108-8. The EDQ has been divided and a clamp has been used to form a subcutaneous passage between the distal forearm and the thenar eminence.

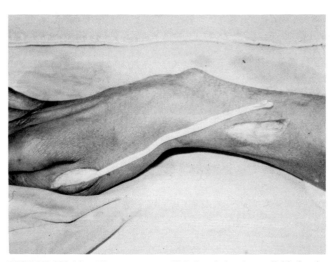

FIGURE 108-10. The extensor pollicis brevis has been divided at its musculotendinous junction and its insertion exposed.

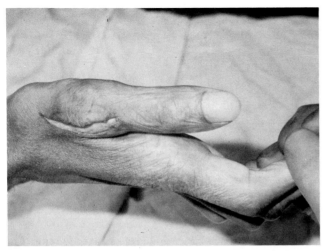

FIGURE 108-11. The transposed extensor pollicis brevis, without traction.

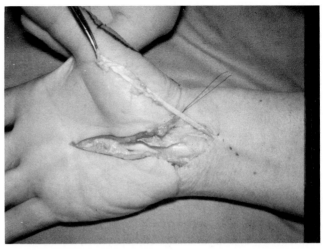

FIGURE 108-13. The palmeris longus has been exposed and prolonged with a strip of palmar fascia.

the prolonged tendon subcutaneously into the intrinsic tendon. This transfer gives fair to good palmar abduction but poor pronation, since no pulley has been constructed near the pisiform, and the line of pull consequently derives from the midline.

Abductor Digiti Quinti

Although technically difficult, transfer of the abductor digiti quinti (ADQ)[14,16] is especially indicated in cases of congenital thenar hypoplasia or when injuries to the forearm prevent transfer of a flexor or extensor. Expose the ADQ along its entire length via a curved hypothenar incision, which continues along the ulnar midaxial border of the small finger. Identify the ADQ muscle, the ulnar artery and nerve, and the neurovascular pedicle to the muscle (Fig. 108-14). Divide the tendon insertion and, with great care for the neurovascular pedicle, divide the attachments to the pisiform and the flexor carpi ulnaris. Then make a second incision about the radial aspect of the thumb, and create a generous subcutaneous channel between the thenar and hypothenar incisions (Fig. 108-15). Turn

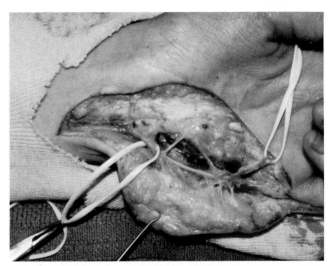

FIGURE 108-14. The ADQ muscle has been exposed and the ulnar nerve and artery carefully dissected and retracted with vessel loops.

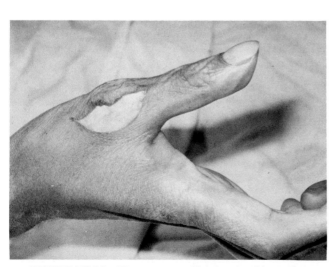

FIGURE 108-12. The extensor pollicis brevis, with traction.

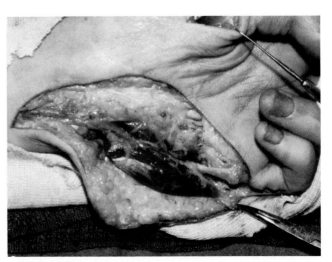

FIGURE 108-15. The origin and insertion of the ADQ have been divided and the conjoined thenar intrinsic tendon exposed.

the ADQ, like the page of a book, towards the thumb, pass it into the tunnel, and suture it into the abductor pollicis brevis tendon. The distinct advantage of this operation is that the ADQ is a synergist, making retraining facile; in addition, the procedure restores the thenar bulk (Fig. 108-16). The operation will be ineffective, however, if the neurovascular pedicle has been damaged or if a constricting subcutaneous tunnel restricts excursion.

POSTOPERATIVE CARE

Postoperative care and rehabilitation for all these transfers are similar. The thumb is immobilized in complete palmar abduction, with the wrist in a neutral position for 4 weeks. During the second postoperative month, a removable orthosis is employed to protect the transfer. This splint is progressively removed in order to encourage active mobility, asking the patient successively to touch the tips of each finger with the thumb, to adduct the thumb to the palm, and, finally, to bring the thumb into radial abduction. Resistive exercises are begun after the second postoperative month, with full use permitted 3 months after surgery. Occasionally, patients are not able to activate the transfer, especially if a digital extensor has been used. In such cases, biofeedback is added to the postoperative rehabilitative program.

Recovery of mobility after an opposition transfer is best determined by measuring the degrees of active palmar abduction and rotation of the thumb. Grip and pinch strength recordings should also be taken and compared with the preoperative measurements, as well as those of the unaffected hand.

COMPLICATIONS

Unsatisfactory results after an opposition transfer are generally a consequence of poor preoperative planning. The patient must be cooperative, and display good sensibility and supple skin and joints. In addition, the effect of the transfer must not further unbalance the extremity. Occasionally, the use of a

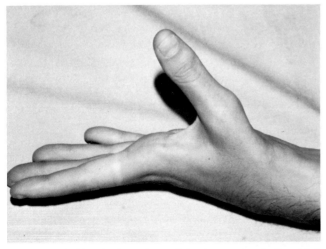

FIGURE 108-16. Active palmar abduction regained after ADQ transfer.

superficialis will result in alteration of the mobility of the proximal interphalangeal joint. If the tendon is cut very near its insertion into the middle of the phalanx in a patient with a lax volar plate, a hyperextension of the proximal interphalangeal joint can ensue. The contrary deformity (i.e., a flexion contracture) can occur if the remaining stumps of the transsected superficialis adhere to the volar aspect of the proximal phalanx and the volar plate. This can be avoided by encouraging early mobility of the donor digit. Inadequate active motion after an opposition transfer can also be a consequence of disruption of the tendon suture, adherence in the palm, or use of a motor with inadequate excursion.

EXTRINSIC MEDIAN NERVE PALSY

In addition to intrinsic thenar weakness, patients with high median nerve injuries demonstrate paralysis of the flexor pollicis longus (FPL), the flexor digitorum superficialis (FDS), the median innervated portion of the flexor digitorum profundus (usually index and middle fingers), and the pronator teres and pronator quadratus. Injury to the anterior interossous portion of the median nerve results in weakness of the FPL, FDP (median portion), and the pronator quadratus.

The most reliable operation for weakness of the FPL is fusion of the thumb interphalangeal joint in 20° of flexion. In patients who need active flexion, a tendon transfer can be carried out. If the superficialis is functioning, one of its tendons can be exposed through a midvolar forearm incision transsected and interwoven into the FPL. The tension of the transfer is correct if, with the wrist at neutral, the interphalangeal joint of the thumb rests in 30° of flexion.

In higher median nerve injuries that also cause denervation of the superficialis, the brachioradialis can be transferred to the FPL through a radiovolar incision. In patients in whom active distal interphalangeal joint (DIP) motion is lost because of paralysis of the profundi, DIP joint fusions can be used if the FDS are intact. If not, then tendon transfers are required. If only the index FDP is weak, it can be sutured into its neighboring profundi. In patients who lack activity of both index and middle profundi, suturing these tendons into the ulnar innervated profundi can likewise be accomplished. This will increase mobility of these digits, but not grip strength, which may be a problem if the superficialis muscles are also weak. For this situation, where added power is a priority, the extensor carpi radialis brevis can be passed through a generous window in the interosseous membrane and interwoven into the paralyzed profundi. Unfortunately, a wrist extensor has significantly less excursion than the profundi and, as a result, full digital mobility cannot be expected. The tension of such a transfer must therefore be adjusted according to the patient's functional needs. A reasonable balance of digital flexion and extension can be achieved if, at the end of the transfer, full digital extension is possible with the wrist in mild flexion.

REFERENCES

1. Brand, P.W.: Tendon Grafting Illustrated by a New Operation for Intrinsic Paralysis of the Fingers. J. Bone Joint Surg. **34-B:**444, 1961.

2. Brand, P.W.: The Hand in Leprosy. In Pulvertaft, R.G. (ed.): Clinical Surgery. Washington, Butterworth 1966.

3. Brand, P.W., Beach, M.A., and Thompson, D.E.: Relative Tension and Potential Excursion of Muscles in the Forearm and Hand. J. Hand Surg. **6:**209, 1981.

4. Bunnell, S.: Opposition of the Thumb. J. Bone Joint Surg. **20:**269, 1938.

5. Camitz, H.: Uber die Behandlung Oppositionslahmung. Acta Chir. Scand. **65:**77, 1929.

6. Cooney, P.W., Linscheid, R.L., and Kai-Nan, A.N.: Opposition of the Thumb: An Anatomic and Bio-mechanical Study of Tendon Transfers. J. Hand Surg. **9A:**777, 1984.

7. Curtis, R.M.: Opposition of the Thumb. Orthop. Clin. N. Am. **5:**305, 1974.

8. Duchenne, G.B.A.: Physiology of Motion (Trans. E.B. Kaplan). Philadelphia, W.B. Saunders, 1959.

9. Huber, E.: Hilfsoperation bei Medianaulahmung. Dtsch. Z. Chir. **162:**271, 1921.

10. Kaplan, E.B.: Functional and Surgical Anatomy of the Hand, 2nd ed. Philadelphia, J.B. Lippincott, 1961.

11. Kirklin, J.W., and Thomas, C.G.: Opponens Transplant: An Analysis of the Methods Employed and Results Obtained in Twenty Five Cases. Surg. Gynecol. Obstet. **86:**213, 1948.

12. Krukenberg, H.: Lieber Ersatz des M. Oppens Pollicis. Z. Ortho. Chir. **42:**178, 1921.

13. Littler, J.W.: Tendon Transfers and Arthrodesis in Combined Median and Ulnar Nerve Paralysis. J. Bone Joint Surg. **31-A:**225, 1949.

14. Littler, J.W., and Cooley, S.G.S.: Opposition of the Thumb and its Restoration by Abductor Digiti Quinti Transfer. J. Bone Joint Surg. **45-A:**1389, 1963.

15. Ney, K.W.: A Tendon Transplant for Intrinsic Hand Muscle Paralysis. Surg. Gynecol. Obstet. **33:**342, 1921.

16. Nicolaysen, J.: Transplantation Des M. Abductor Dig V bei Fehlender Oppositions—Fahigkeit des Daumens. Dtsch. Z. Chir. **168:**133, 1922.

17. Phalen, G.S., and Miller, R.C.: The Transfer of Wrist Extensor Muscles to Restore or Reinforce Flexion Power of the Fingers and Opposition of the Thumb. J. Bone Joint Surg. **29:**993, 1947.

18. Riordan, D.: Tendon Transfers for Nerve Paralysis of the Hand and Wrist. In Adams, J.P. (ed.): Current Practice of Orthopaedic Surgery. St. Louis, C.V. Mosby, 1964.

19. Rowntree, T.: Anomalous Innervation of the Hand Muscles. J. Bone Joint Surg. **31-B:**505, 1949.

20. Royle, N.D.: An Operation for Paralysis of the Intrinsic Muscles of the Thumb. J. A. M. A. **111:**612, 1938.

21. Schneider, L.: Opponensplasty using the Extensor Digiti Minimi. J. Bone Joint Surg. **51-A:**1297, 1969.

22. Steindler, A.: Orthopaedic Operations of the Hand. J. A. M. A. **71:**1288, 1918.

23. Taylor, R.: Reconstruction of the Hand, A New Technique in Tenoplasty. Surg. Gynecol. Obstet. **32:**237, 1921.

24. Thompson, T.C.: A Modified Operation for Opponens Paralysis. J. Bone Joint Surg. **24:**632, 1942.

25. Zancolli, E.A.: Structural and Dynamic Bases of Hand Surgery, 2nd ed. Philadelphia, J.B. Lippincott, 1979.

CHAPTER 109

Ulnar Nerve Paralysis

PAUL W. BRAND

The following motor functions may be affected by damage to the ulnar nerve: flexion and ulnar deviation of the wrist; flexion of the ring and little fingers; independent flexion at the metacarpophalangeal joints of all fingers; interphalangeal extension of all fingers; abduction-adduction of all fingers; adduction-flexion of the carpometacarpal joint; and flexion of the metacarpophalangeal joint of the thumb.

FLEXION AND ULNAR DEVIATION OF THE WRIST

The flexor carpi ulnaris is the strongest muscle in the forearm and an important element in many physical actions, such as swinging an axe, hammer, or club, cutting with a knife, and pounding on the desk. When it is paralyzed, the result is a general sense of weakness in a variety of actions, but there is no total loss of any action, nor is there a specific deformity. For this reason most surgeons do nothing, specifically no tendon transfers, to balance the wrist. For a manual worker in an occupation such as carpentry, who might feel disabled by an ulnar-flexor quadrant weakness, it might be practical to transfer flexor carpi radialis to flexor carpi ulnaris, since the radial-flexor quadrant is unaffected in ulnar palsy.

FLEXION OF THE RING AND LITTLE FINGERS

Flexion of the ring and little fingers is severely weakened in high ulnar palsy, with loss of flexor profundus to both fingers, especially since the surviving median-supplied flexor superficialis to the little finger is less than one-third of the strength of the profundus. In the ring finger, the flexor digititorum superficialis is two-thirds the strength of the profundus, so that two-fifths the flexor strength of the ring finger survives. However, the finger flexor weakness is partially masked by the fact that the paralyzed ulnar-supplied profundus moves with the median-supplied profundus to the middle finger. This cross finger support is variable and only partial, because the actual muscle fibers are not shared but linked by connective tissue, which allows some independence.

Since some extrinsic flexor power remains in the ulnar two fingers, no *deformity* is caused by paralysis of the long flexors. Because deformity is observed more often than functional weakness, substitution is rarely offered for the paralyzed long flexors. If the weakness seems gross, the ring and little finger profundus tendons may be sutured side-to-side to the profundus of the middle finger, so that they move fully together. This does not really add strength; it just shares weakness more evenly. If one adds together the tension fractions (see Chapter 106, Figs. 106-1 and 106-2) of all the muscles that normally combine to flex the little and ring fingers, including the intrinsic muscles, the total is 14.6. Of these, only 2.9, or about one-fifth, survive in high ulnar palsy. The deformity of claw hand can be corrected by replacement of the intrinsic muscles by transfers, with a strength that often amounts to a tension fraction of between 1.0 and 3.0 shared between four fingers. This still leaves a gross weakness of ulnar side grip, only about

25% of normal strength. Yet most forearm muscles remain unparalyzed, and the forearm and hand retain at least 70% of their total tension capability.

A weak ulnar side grip results in a gross disability for all actions that use the width of the hand for controlling radial-ulnar torque. One of the most common actions of the hand is the use of a hammer (Figs. 109-1 to 109-3).

This and all hand movements that require a twist or turn, either in a pronation-supination direction or in the radial-ulnar deviation, require that the object (or the instrument) be held by the hand in such a way as to transmit a torque, by means of a *couple* (Fig. 109-2). The handle of a hammer is moved by a couple when one force pulls upward and a simultaneous force pushes downward, with a distance between them, along the handle.

The hammer head is forced down while the end of the handle may move up, or the whole hammer may move, with F_1 moving more than F_2. As with all forms of torque, the length of the lever arm is just as important as the amount of force (Fig. 109-3). In the case of a couple, twice as much total force is needed for the same torque if the two components are moved 50% closer together. In a medium-sized hand, the width of an effective grip is about 10 cm. In the same hand, if only the index and middle fingers are strong, the *effective* width of the hand is reduced to about 5 cm. Even though such a hand may retain 50% of its power to grip an object, it will have only 25% of its power to *turn* or twist or swing an object. The patient has difficulty describing the weakness, saying only, "I feel that my hand is weak." The dynamometer is not a measure of the dexterity strength of a hand, but only of squeeze power. Most manual tasks demand multidirectional torque, which requires a broad hand with strength at each of its borders.

A further problem associated with paralysis of the finger flexors is the reversal of the metacarpal arch, usually considered to be caused by paralysis of the intrinsic muscles. However, the best muscles to control the arch are those that cross the fifth carpometacarpal joint—the hypothenar muscles and

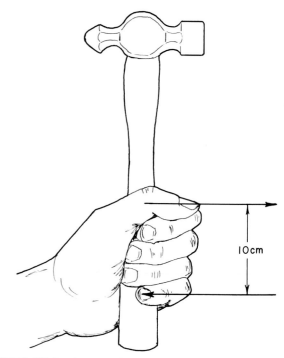

FIGURE 109-2. A normal hand may be about 10 cm wide where it holds a hammer. In the force stroke the thumb web *pushes* while the little and ring finger *pull*. In retracting the hammer, the hypothenar mass pushes, and the index and middle fingers pull.

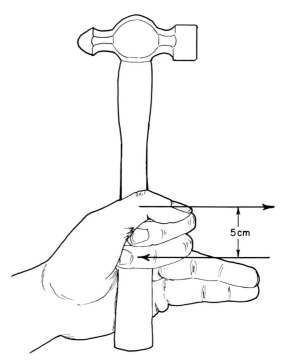

FIGURE 109-3. In high ulnar palsy, the little and ring fingers may be so weak that only the middle finger is able to pull firmly enough to complete the couple. This is only half as wide as in a normal hand. The hammer is unstable and weak. For many tasks involving torque it is better to have strong index and little fingers, even if the middle fingers are weak.

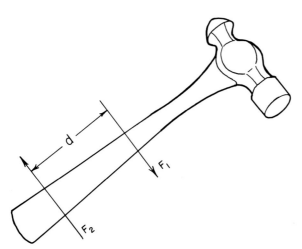

FIGURE 109-1. To strike with a hammer, since there is no fixed axis, it is necessary to produce a force couple. Two forces move in opposite directions. They produce a torque on the hammer proportional to the magnitude of the forces multiplied by the perpendicular distance between them.

the long flexors to the ring and little fingers. Brandsma[3] has noted that ulnar palsy patients who retain ulnar-supplied profundus rarely have severe arch reversal.

Recognition of the importance of the loss of profundus in the ulnar-paralyzed hand should suggest rethinking the patterns of correction. An obvious method to increase ulnar side grip strength is to use the extensor carpi radialis longus to reactivate the flexor profundus tendons to the ring and little fingers. The fiber length of the extensor carpi radialis longus is long enough to allow a good range of finger flexion with a little synergistic relaxation of the wrist. The extensor carpi radialis longus is also strong enough to compensate for the ulnar profundus loss, and helps to rebalance the wrist, which is relatively overpowered on the dorsal radial side in high ulnar palsy.

INDEPENDENT FLEXION AT THE METACARPOPHALANGEAL JOINTS OF ALL FINGERS

The most significant functional loss in ulnar palsy is independent flexion at the metacarpophalangeal joints. It is important because it (1) is the basis for the deformity of claw hand, because uncontrolled extension of the metacarpophalangeal joints results in failure to extend interphalangeal joints; and (2) changes the sequence of flexion of the fingers, making it impossible to flex the proximal segment ahead of the distal segments. Therefore, when the hand closes on an object, the force of grasp is transmitted only through the finger tips rather than through the whole palmar surface of the fingers. This results in high localized tip pressure, leading to inhibition of the use of strength (in sensitive fingers) or in pressure sores and injuries to finger tips (in insensitive fingers) (Figs. 109-4 and 109-5).

Ulnar palsy results in metacarpophalangeal flexion weakness in *all* fingers, not just in the ring and little fingers. Clawing may occur earliest and most obviously in the ulnar side fingers, because the index and middle fingers usually have median-supplied lumbricales. However, the lumbricales can exert only about one-tenth the tension of the combined interossei. The lumbricales may delay the onset of clawing or make it less severe; however, when the end of the finger is pushed backwards, as when pinching against the thumb, the metacarpophalangeal joint retreats into extension and the proximal interphalangeal joints hyperflex. This mechanism is similar to Froment's sign in the thumb. It can be tested in a patient who has no clawing of the index and middle fingers by asking the patient to hold the intrinsic-plus position (metacarpophalangeal joint flexed and interphalangeal joints extended) while the examiner pushes backwards with a finger against the middle of the front of the proximal segment of the patient's finger. If this test causes the finger to "buckle" into proximal interphalangeal flexion, weakness of the intrinsic muscles is indicated, as is a need to rebalance the finger to compensate for present weakness and to prevent clawing later.

INTERPHALANGEAL EXTENSION OF ALL FINGERS

In the normal hand, the intrinsic muscles extend, or help to extend, the interphalangeal joints by three mechanisms. (1)

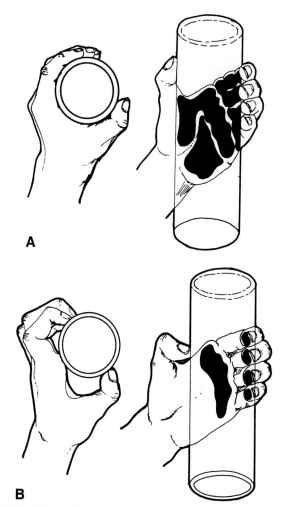

FIGURE 109-4. (*A*) Normal hand grasping a cylinder. The area of skin contact is marked in black. (*B*) Claw hand grasping a cylinder. The area of contact is limited to the fingertips and the metacarpal heads. (Brand, P.W.: Clinical Mechanics of the Hand. St. Louis, C.V. Mosby, 1985.)

Direct action of the lumbricales and those interosseus muscles that insert into the lateral band, all create direct extension of the proximal interphalangeal and distal interphalangeal joints. This mechanism is effective even in radial nerve palsy, which inactivates the long extensors. (2) By holding the metacarpophalangeal joint flexed, without flexing the interphalangeal joints, the long extensors can be prevented from extending the metacarpophalangeal joints and so can be effective on the interphalangeal joints. (3) The unique action of the lumbricales pulls the profundus tendons distally while pulling the lateral bands proximally to facilitate interphalangeal extension with metacarpophalangeal flexion. This action, the weakest of the three, cannot be reproduced by tendon transfer, so we shall consider the other two mechanisms.

By bringing the tendon of any muscle across the palmar side of the intermetacarpal ligament and attaching it to the lateral band, both extension mechanisms are accomplished. Such a transfer flexes the metacarpophalangeal joints and extends the interphalangeal joints, so it corrects both elements of the claw

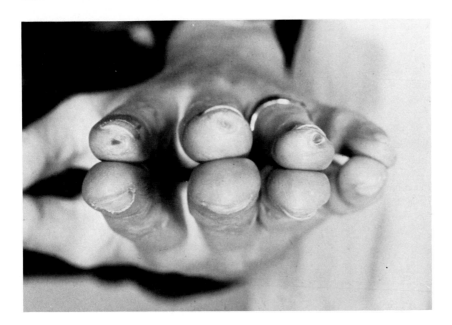

FIGURE 109-5. This patient had loss of sensation from Hansen's disease. The little ulcers and scars are in the most characteristic position for a patient with functional clawing. The high stress occurs just in front of the fingernail at the end of the phalanx. (Brand, P.W.: Clinical Mechanics of the Hand. St. Louis, C.V. Mosby, 1985.)

hand deformity (Fig. 109-6). We have found this pattern most successful. In the normal hand, however, only part of the force of the intrinsic muscles is transferred into the lateral bands. The greater part moves directly into bone and flexes only the metacarpophalangeal joint. This provides freedom for the fingers to flex at the metacarpophalangeal joint with or without interphalangeal extension. Following tendon transfer into the lateral band, with no intrinsic transfer into the proximal phalanx, the total force of the transfer for metacarpophalangeal flexion must also provide tension for interphalangeal extension. In hypermobile fingers, this constant pull on the lateral bands may result in a degree of progressive hyperextension of the interphalangeal joints that can become a true swan-neck deformity. This is common when the flexor superficialis tendon is removed and used for transfer to the lateral band.[1] The proximal interphalangeal joint is thus deprived of a prime flexor, which becomes an uncontrolled extensor.

Because of this complication, the attachment of the transfer for intrinsic replacement to the lateral band should be performed only in fingers that are stable or that have some degree of extension limitation of the proximal interphalangeal joints caused by stiffness, or at least have no range of passive hyper-

extension. In all hypermobile fingers, and especially in those deprived of their flexor superficiales, it is better to attach the tendon transfer to the flexor tendon sheath, as suggested by Brooks[4] and Zancolli.[10,11] In such cases, extension of the interphalangeal joints is accomplished by the long extensors, though at a higher total cost of energy (because the intrinsic metacarpophalangeal flexors must overcome the metacarpophalangeal extension moment from the extrinsic extensors).

ADDUCTION-ABDUCTION OF ALL FINGERS

Adduction-abduction of all fingers is a function of the intrinsic muscles supplied by the ulnar nerve. The median-supplied lumbricales are near enough to the midline of the metacarpophalangeal joints that they have a very small active abduction capability.

Fingers should not be provided with an effective abductor (away from the midline of the hand) unless there is an effective adductor to restore the side-by-side position of all fingers. Most tasks can be accomplished by side-by-side fingers, as long as they have independent flexion and extension. Fingers that can abduct but not adduct are an embarrassment. A spread hand looks strange, and the projecting fingers become caught on the edges of pockets or bags and are subject to injury in the work place.

To control both adduction and abduction, eight separate tendons are needed, one to each side of each finger. Most surgeons find this too many to employ and patient reeducation too difficult. All insertions for the motor replacement of the intrinsics should be on the side of the finger that pulls towards the interface between the index and middle fingers. Thus, the middle, ring, and little fingers will be moved toward the radius and the index finger moved toward the ulna. In addition, a replacement for the first dorsal interosseus may be added to the radial side of the index finger, if deemed necessary (Fig. 109-7).

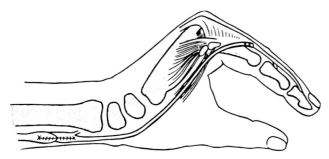

FIGURE 109-6. Tendon transfer to correct intrinsic minus hand. The transferred tendon or graft passes in front of the transverse intermetacarpal ligament and into the lateral band. (Milford, L.: The Hand, 2nd ed. St. Louis, C.V. Mosby, 1982.)

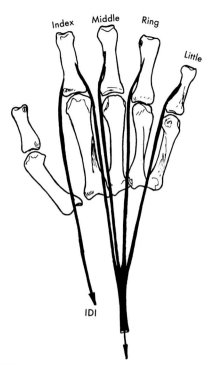

FIGURE 109-7. For correction of ulnar paralysis, a single motor may be used for the radial side of the middle, ring, and little fingers and the ulnar side of the index finger. A separate motor may be used for the radial side of the index finger if necessary. (Brand, P.W.: Clinical Mechanics of the Hand. St. Louis, C.V. Mosby, 1985.)

There are two reasons for adding an index finger abductor. The first is to spread the fingers, as for a piano player or typist. This does not need a strong muscle, and even the extensor indicis proprius, properly rerouted, might be adequate. The second is to stabilize the index finger against the thrust of the thumb in pinch. A normal pinch is not "square," pulp to pulp. There is at least a 30° angle between the thumb nail and the finger nail, so the transverse vector of the thumb force that pushes the finger across the palm is maybe half as great as the vector that pushes the finger backwards (Fig. 109-8A). It would seem, therefore, necessary to have an index finger abductor about half as strong as the flexors. The first dorsal interosseus, at a tension fraction of 3.2 is about right. However, the index finger has no true adduction-abduction axis, but moves around a variable cone.[2] There is also a link between abduction and rotation. Thus, a replacement for first dorsal interosseus will twist the finger while it abducts, so that it faces more across the palm than before, providing a pinch that is less square. The more the first dorsal interosseus pulls, the more it increases the angle between the line of thrust of the thumb and that of the index finger (Fig. 109-8B). This makes the pinch more unstable, requiring support by a force vector that opposes the resultant of the two major flexion forces of the thumb and index finger. In effect, the first dorsal interosseus increases the need for other stabilizing intrinsic muscles.

The converse of this is that if no replacement is made for first dorsal interosseus, but one is provided for the first palmar interosseus on the ulnar side of the finger, the result will be to twist the finger into external rotation and diminish the angle by

which the index finger meets the thumb. The result of an "ulnar-side only" attachment of an intrinsic replacement to the index finger is that the thumb and index finger meet in a true square pinch, with finger and thumb nails parallel and with thumb flexors opposing finger flexors squarely, so that no lateral stabilization is necessary (Fig. 109-8C).

For these reasons routine replacement for first dorsal interosseus is not advised, except as a device for spreading the fingers apart. For the purposes of pinch, the first palmar interosseus (which we call the "opponens indicis") is all that is needed.

If the patient will use a key pinch, rather than a tip or pulp pinch, then there is more reason for a first dorsal interosseus replacement, since it directly supports the side of the index finger against the thumb. However, even in a key pinch this is not necessary if the patient usually pinches against all four fingers together (Fig. 109-8D).

In most cases of paralysis of the intrinsic muscles of the hand, therefore, it is best to use one muscle only as a replacement for the intrinsics to all four fingers, and to extend it by four strands of tendon or tendon graft to be attached to the lateral band on the radial side of the middle, ring, and little fingers, and to the ulnar side lateral band of the index finger.

Choice of Motor for Intrinsic Transfers

The total tension capability of all the intrinsic muscles to the fingers is greater than the total of the flexor profundus. Thus, a powerful muscle for each finger is required to replace the lost tension. In the normal hand, the total intrinsic tension to any finger is divided between multiple insertions, and it would lead to gross imbalance to apply that total tension to any one insertion on only one side of a finger. Most surgeons use much less tension, and use only one muscle, such as a single superficialis tendon, split into four strands in the proximal palm, and taken to the lateral band of each finger. The extensor carpi radialis longus (tension fraction 3.5) may be used, with a free graft split into four insertions, or else two weaker muscles, such as extensor indicis proprius and extensor digiti quinti, with two insertions each.[6]

Following the experience of Fritschi,[7] I have sometimes used the palmaris longus (average tension fraction 1.2) with grafts to all four fingers, and found that it does correct the deformity in cases that are operated on early, before bad habit patterns have developed and before the palmar plate has become grossly stretched. The advantage of using the palmaris is that the operation may be done immediately after any ulnar nerve injury in the arm or upper forearm with the confidence that nothing has been lost, even if the intrinsic muscles recover later. This is an important advantage. It prevents any deformity, and still leaves the option of adding a stronger muscle a year or two later, if the intrinsic muscles have not recovered and if the patient needs more grasp strength.

Zancolli[10] popularized a technique for moving the flexor superficialis tendons from their insertion on the middle phalanx to be attached to the flexor sheath in front of the metacarpophalangeal joint. By doing this ("lasso") operation, the proximal interphalangeal joint is deprived of its prime flexor, but leaves the muscle as a flexor of the metacarpophalangeal joint. This is similar to the old Stiles operation,[9] except that the

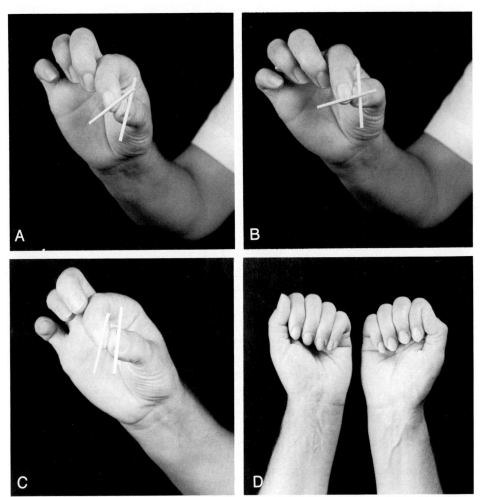

FIGURE 109-8. (*A*) Normal pinch angle of about 30° between markers on thumb nail and finger nail. Pinch is stable by action of intrinsic muscles. (*B*) With index finger abducted, the angle between thumb and finger nails is greater, making an unstable pinch. (*C*) Desireable pinch in ulnar palsy patient. An ulnar-side intrinsic transfer to the index finger acts like a first palmar interosseus and circumducts the index metacarpophalangeal joint, so as to oppose the thumb pulp. This results in a true square pinch that needs no other intrinsic muscle support. (*D*) Key pinch does not demand much intrinsic muscle support of the index finger, providing it is supported by all the fingers flexed together.

insertion is central rather than to the lateral band. It is also rather simple, but it may create long-term problems, because the proximal interphalangeal joint is deprived of a flexor except by contraction of the profundus, which is more effective at the distal interphalangeal joint than at the proximal interphalangeal joint[2] when working against resistance. The same problem results in interphalangeal hyperflexion of the thumb in "Froment's sign" of ulnar palsy. In the fingers the deformity develops slowly, but finally a hyperflexed distal interphalangeal joint and a hyperextended proximal interphalangeal joint give rise to a swan-neck deformity. The lasso operation should be reserved for the late correction of clawed fingers that are somewhat stiff in proximal interphalangeal joint flexion, and therefore unlikely to become straight or hyperextended.

If a lasso operation has been performed, or a Stiles-Bunnell with transfer of the superficialis tendon, and the distal interphalangeal joints begin to show signs of hyperflexion and inability to extend fully, early intervention is best, by performing a profundus tenodesis in the middle segment with the distal interphalangeal joint just short of full extension. This transfers profundus power from distal interphalangeal joints to proximal interphalangeal joints, and provides a more satisfactory hand (Fig. 109-9).

Strength

Various muscles have been used with success for the correction of claw hand. It is easy to misunderstand the exact usefulness of each. Since surgeons and patients are most concerned about *deformity,* procedures such as the Stiles-Bunnell[9] or the lasso of Zancolli[10] are preferred, because these are "strong" correctors of deformity. They are not really strong, however, in that they add *nothing* to the strength of the fingers. They take strength away from proximal interphalangeal flexion and move it proximally to the metacarpophalangeal joint. Even a weak tendon transfer such as palmaris from the wrist area is stronger, be-

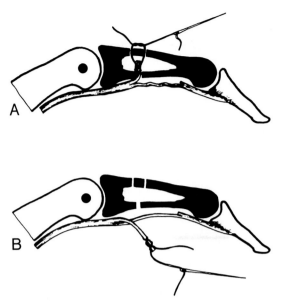

FIGURE 109-9. Profundus tenodesis in the middle segment. (*A*) The profundus tendon is split, and half divided distally. The proximal end of the middle phalanx has a 2-mm drill hole in anterior cortex and 2 × 1 mm holes in dorsal cortex. (*B*) The cut end of the profundus slip is drawn into bone, leaving half profundus in continuity.

cause it *adds* something to the fingers from an area that is unaffected by paralysis. From the point of view of real strength, the Fowler operation[6] using the extensor indicis proprius and extensor digiti quinti (tension fractions 1 + 1 = 2), is better still, and the transfer of extensor carpi radialis longus or extensor carpi radialis brevis (tension 3.5 or 4.2) may be the best of all. Whereas in the immediate postoperative phase both surgeon and patient appreciate quick correction of deformity, it is in the long term that the patient realizes the extent of the weakness and how a "strong correction" sometimes results in "overcorrection" and still does not provide a strong hand.

The Pathway of Transferred Tendons

An advantage of the Bunnell,[5] Fowler,[6] and lasso[10] operations is that the tendons are all long enough for direct transfer, without grafts. If a single superficialis tendon is to be used for four fingers (modified Stiles-Bunnell[5]), the tendon should be withdrawn in the proximal palm, just distal to the carpal ligament roof, so that each tendon strand can be passed to its own finger without having to cross a palmar septum.

In a Fowler's or modified Fowler's operation, the tendons of extensor indicis proprius or extensor digiti quinti must be withdrawn and split back to the carpal area. Then, pick up each strand, using a tunneler that has been passed from the base of each finger, in front of the transverse metacarpal ligament, through the intermetacarpal space, and on to the dorsal incision *without* penetrating the dorsal fascia that overlies the extensor tendons. Pass the tendon strands to the index and middle fingers through the second space, and the two strands to the ring and little fingers through the third space. The strand to the little finger crosses the neck of the fourth metacarpal on the palmar side on its way to the fifth proximal phalanx. Al-

though this route to the little finger sounds complex, and there may be concern that adhesions will occur as the tendon hugs the metacarpal bone, it is not difficult if a curved blunt-nosed tunneler is passed empty from the little finger and angled across until the bone of the fourth metacarpal neck is felt. Slip the tunneler between the bone and the flexor tendons and immediately turn it dorsally, through the intermetacarpal space, and then proximally to the rerouting incision over the carpometacarpal area, where a tendon strand is grasped and pulled through to the finger.

This pathway is less likely to allow two deformities—reversal of the metacarpal arch and continued abduction of the little finger—than the more usual route, which passes through the fourth intermetacarpal space. If adhesions form in this modification of Fowler's operation, they occur at the point of perforation of the interosseus fascia, not to the bone.

When a forearm muscle is used (either the palmaris or the extensor carpi radialis longus), it is anastomosed with a four-tailed tendon graft and then tunneled through the carpal tunnel to the fingers. Divide the extensor carpi radialis longus near its insertion and pull it out proximally, about midforearm. Make a transverse incision in the anterior distal forearm about 5 cm proximal to the wrist crease and centered over the palmaris. Pass a blunt-nosed tunneler into this incision and direct it beneath the tendons of palmaris, flexor carpi radialis, and brachioradialis to appear in the proximal incision over the extensor carpi radialis longus. Grasp the tendon end and pull it through to the distal incision, where it is anastomosed to a four-tailed graft, either of plantaris tendon folded in two and each limb split in two, or a 12-mm wide strip of fascia lata, taken from the lateral thigh and split into four in its distal two-thirds.

Make a rerouting incision in the proximal palm, just distal to the carpal tunnel, and bluntly pass a curved tunneler through a split in the palmar fascia to the bony-ligamentous floor of the carpal tunnel, deep to all tendons and sheaths. Then direct the tunneler toward the distal forearm incision, between the flexor carpi ulnaris and the flexor tendons to the fingers, until it appears in the wound. Grasp the ends of all four tendon strands with the tunneler and pull them into the palm. From here tunnel each strand separately to each finger, and attach it to the lateral band (see Fig. 109-6), or else to the flexor sheath in front of the metacarpophalangeal joint, as suggested by Brooks.[4]

If the extensor carpi radialis brevis is to be used as a motor, divide it at its insertion and withdraw it 10 cm up the forearm, pulling a black thread behind it to identify its sheath. Remove the distal one to 2 cm and attach a four-tailed graft. Grasp the four graft tails with tunneling forceps and pull them back through the sheath, following the thread marker. From there, tunnel each graft through an interosseus space to its own finger. Grafts to the index and middle finger pass through the second space, and grafts to the ring and little finger pass through the third space.

Suture all grafts into position with the wrist flexed (for tendons that pass through the carpal tunnel) or extended (for the extensor carpi radialis brevis and the dorsal route). The metacarpophalangeal joints are flexed and the interphalangeal joints extended (see Fig. 109-6). In this position tendon tension should be minimal or even zero. In the postoperative cast the wrist may be straight and the fingers in full metacarpophalangeal flexion and interphalangeal extension.

ADDUCTION AND FLEXION OF THE CARPOMETACARPAL JOINT AND FLEXION OF THE METACARPOPHALANGEAL JOINT OF THE THUMB

There is a great deal of variation in the pattern of innervation of the short flexor and adductor muscles of the thumb. Sometimes the median nerve supplies enough of the short flexor muscles so that ulnar palsy does not leave much deficit. In other cases, the flexor pollicis longus is the only thumb flexor that survives ulnar palsy. In such cases any attempt at firm pinch results in flexion of the interphalangeal joint and extension of the metacarpophalangeal joint. This functional test may be used to determine the need for tendon transfer. If the patient can pinch strongly without interphalangeal flexion, there is probably no need for a transfer.

If a transfer is needed, the best tendon to use is the flexor superficialis of the middle finger. Divide it in the middle of the proximal segment of the finger and withdraw it in the palm through an incision parallel to and just to the ulnar side of the thenar crease, just distal to the midpalm. Split the palmar fascia—do not cut it—and leave a significant strand to the radial side of the split. By means of an incision on the dorsiradial aspect of the middle segment of the thumb, expose the edge of the dorsal expansion. Insert tendon tunneling forceps halfway between the metacarpophalangeal and interphalangeal joints and direct them subcutaneously to the palmar incision. It is essential that the nose of the forceps appear in the palmar incision *superficial* to the palmar fascia. Thus when the tendon is pulled into the thumb, the radial strand of palmar fascia serves as a pulley, preventing the tendon from losing its angle of approach to the thumb (Fig. 109-10).

The tendon transfer may be attached to the extensor pollicis longus tendon, while the interphalangeal joint is fully extended. Alternatively, half the tendon transfer may be attached to the extensor pollicis longus and the other half closer to the metacarpophalangeal joint, to the tendon of attachment of the abductor pollicis brevis. This double insertion (or yoke) serves as a check to prevent excessive metacarpophalangeal flexion.

The hand is immobilized with the interphalangeal joint extended, the metacarpophalangeal joint flexed, and the thumb in a pinching position. The middle (or donor) finger should be splinted in interphalangeal extension to discourage proximal attachment of the stump of the superficialis tendon.

POSTOPERATIVE CARE

In the postoperative reeducation phase of all these operations, early exercises should involve only one of the two joints in each digit. Apply cylinder plaster casts to the interphalangeal joints (finger and thumb) in the corrected position, while the metacarpophalangeal joints are encouraged to move.

After a few days, the interphalangeal joints are allowed to be free, while the metacarpophalangeal joints are prevented from extending by a knuckle-bender splint. Only when reeducation is proceeding well should both metacarpophalangeal and interphalangeal joints be released at the same time. Even then, if there is a tendency to metacarpophalangeal hyperextension or

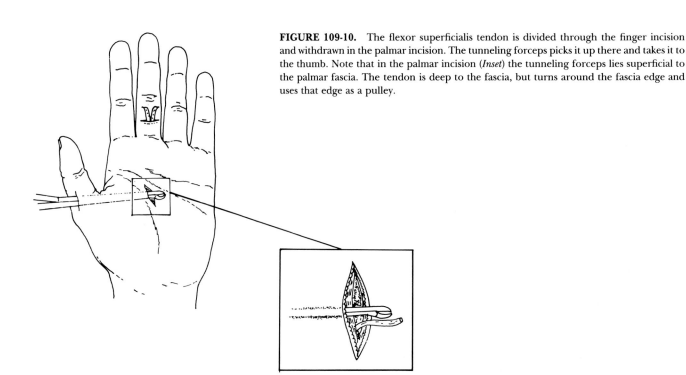

FIGURE 109-10. The flexor superficialis tendon is divided through the finger incision and withdrawn in the palmar incision. The tunneling forceps picks it up there and takes it to the thumb. Note that in the palmar incision (*Inset*) the tunneling forceps lies superficial to the palmar fascia. The tendon is deep to the fascia, but turns around the fascia edge and uses that edge as a pulley.

clawing, the alternating restrictions should be reimposed. In the thumb, the metacarpophalangeal joint is difficult to immobilize, and interphalangeal extension may be continued longer if needed.

REFERENCES

1. Brand, P.W.: Reconstruction of the Hand in Leprosy. Ann. R. Coll. Surg. Eng. **2:**350–361, 1952.
2. Brand, P.W.: Mechanics of Individual Muscles at Individual Joints. In Brand, P.W. (ed.): Clinical Mechanics of the Hand. St. Louis, C.V. Mosby, 1985.
3. Brandsma, J.W.: Personal Communication.
4. Brooks, A., and Jones, D.: A New Intrinsic Tendon Transfer. Presented at the American Society for Surgery of the Hand Annual Meeting, San Francisco, 1975.
5. Bunnell, S.: Surgery of the Intrinsic Muscles of the Hand Other Than Those Producing Opposition of the Thumb. J. Bone Joint Surg. **24:**1–31, 1942.
6. Riordan, D.C.: Tendon Transplantations in Median-nerve and Ulnar-nerve Paralysis. J. Bone Joint Surg. **35-A:**312, 1953.
7. Fritschi, E.P.: Reconstrictive Surgery in Leprosy. Bristol, John Wright & Sons, 1971.
8. Fritschi, E.P.: Surgical Reconstruction and Rehabilitation in Leprosy. New Delhi, The Leprosy Mission, 1984.
9. Stiles, H.J., and Forrester-Brown, M.F.: Treatment of Injuries of the Spinal Peripheral Nerves. London, H. Frowde and Hodder & Stoughton, 1922, p. 166.
10. Zancolli, E.A.: Correccion de la Garra Digital por Paralisis Intrinseca. La Operacion del "Lazo." Acta Orthop. Latino Americana, **1:**65–72, 1974.
11. Zancolli, E.: Structural and Dynamic Bases of Hand Surgery, 2nd ed. Philadelphia, J.B. Lippincott Co., 1979.

CHAPTER 110

Combined Nerve Palsy in the Upper Extremity

JACK W. TUPPER

In instances of direct trauma, early nerve continuity should be obtained by repair or grafting if feasible. Motor nerves have a shorter distance to grow to reach an end point than do sensory nerves, and any return of function will make reconstruction easier. If injury is accompanied by vascular damage, this should be repaired, even if collaterals seem sufficient to keep the fingers pink and warm. Too often high palsies are accompanied by Volkmann's ischemic contracture in muscles that have not been specifically denervated. When there is direct muscle loss, a free neurovascular muscle transfer (gracilis, etc.) may be considered for mass flexor or extensor purposes.[4,7]

Combined palsies have a much greater sensory loss, not only in the skin, but also in deeper proprioceptive fibers, so that joint position sense may be lost. Loss of sudomotor function makes fingers dry and creates difficulty in grasping. Tendon transfers serve best when there is useful sensory feedback.

Combined palsies also suffer a greater muscle-tendon loss, and fewer motor units are available for transfer. There is less choice in regard to muscle fiber length, and cross section and phasic activity, though in the upper extremity, muscles are capable of phasic change after transfer.[5]

The results of rehabilitation depend as much on the patient's natural coordination, adaptability, and motivation as on reconstructive efforts by the surgeon. Probable surgical results should be weighed against those obtainable with a flexor hinge splint,[8] powered either with a single wrist motor or, if necessary, with a cable to the opposite shoulder, as with an amputation prosthesis. A flexor hinge splint can be applied to a flaccid hand without need for amputation, and in some cases it is an alternative that should be considered (Fig. 110-1).

SENSIBILITIES

Proprioception cannot be surgically reestablished but may develop to some extent in the sensation of stretch felt in a transferred muscle.

Tactile sensibility may be obtained to a limited degree for median loss by transfer of skin, either from the radial or ulnar distribution.[9] Local transfer from the radial distribution does not usually cause a problem, but it will not give epicritic sensation. Dorsal radial skin may be rotated after transmetacarpal amputation of the index finger in the manner of Omer[9] to obtain some degree of sensibility between the base of the thumb and index finger for pinch purposes.

An island pedicle from the ulnar aspect of the ring to the thumb may be rewarding, allowing a good thumb-to-little finger pinch, but it is somewhat unpredictable. If this is carried out, the skin should be incised over the whole course of the transfer. A blind passage under a skin bridge may tether the pedicle on a fascial band and contribute to either immediate vascular problems or late sensory loss.

Also occasionally useful, where there is a proximal sensory nerve distal enough for functional purposes, is a free microvascular sensory flap from the toe, although these usually do not function well in high lesions requiring a nerve graft.

MOTOR BALANCE

The only true spare muscles in the upper extremity are the palmaris longus, extensor indicis proprius, and extensor digiti

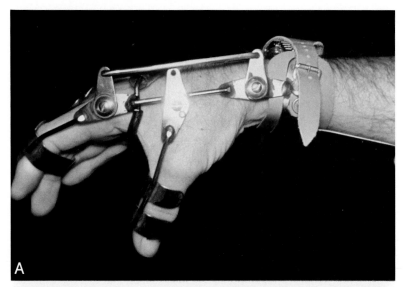

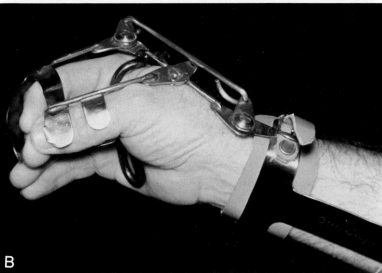

FIGURE 110-1. Flexor hinge splint used to assist hand function when finger and thumb flexors and extensors are paralyzed. This device depends upon the pressure of active wrist flexion and extension. (*A*) Wrist flexion drives the fingers and thumb into extension, allowing "release." (*B*) Wrist extension drives the fingers, and thumb into flexion, allowing "grasp" or "pinch."

minimi, and perhaps the brachioradialis. Other useful structures are the metacarpophalangeal palmar capsules. At times, tenodeses are valuable, and both capsulodeses and tenodeses are more predictable when placed into bone.

TENODESIS AND CAPSULODESIS

Tenodesis

Complete a flexion tenodesis of the distal interphalangeal joints by inserting the profundus tendon into the neck of the middle phalanx through a window in the anterior cortex, just proximal to the articular surface. Then, through a longitudinal dorsal incision, sever the extensor tendon. The joint is pinned for 6 weeks. This type of tenodesis usually remains at about the angle placed.

"Zancolli" Type of Flexion Capsulodesis

Use a distally placed pedicle.[2] The excision and advancement include not only the palmar plate *per se,* but also the intervening

transmetacarpal ligament and the adjoining assessory collateral ligaments. Set the proximal end of the fibrous portion of the palmar plate into metacarpal bone in a manner similar to the tenodeses (Fig. 110-2). Joints are pinned in flexion for about 6 weeks. The pin enters from the metacarpal side of the joint, where it may miss penetrating an extensor tendon.

APPROACH TO COMBINED PALSIES

Low Median–Low Ulnar Palsy

Findings in low median–low ulnar palsy include the following:

1. Dry, insensate tactile skin in all digits
2. Soft (early) or atrophied (late) intrinsics
3. Poor pinch, positive Froment's sign
4. Variable amount of clawing, depending on natural amount of hyperextensibility of the metacarpophalangeal joints
5. Awkward fine motor function

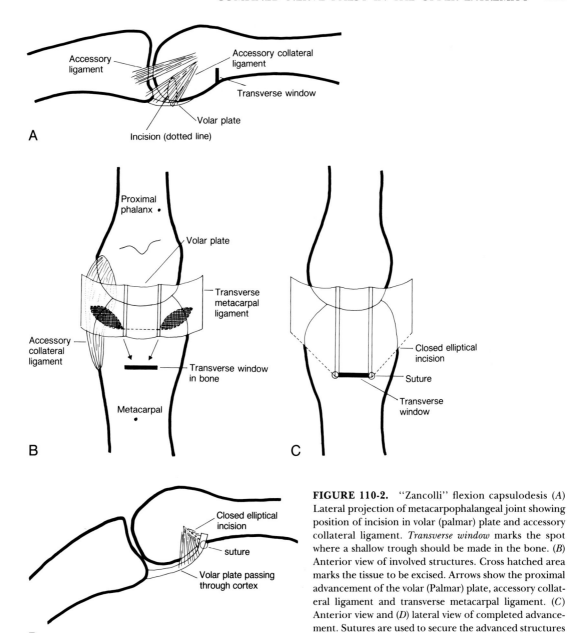

FIGURE 110-2. ''Zancolli'' flexion capsulodesis (*A*) Lateral projection of metacarpophalangeal joint showing position of incision in volar (palmar) plate and accessory collateral ligament. *Transverse window* marks the spot where a shallow trough should be made in the bone. (*B*) Anterior view of involved structures. Cross hatched area marks the tissue to be excised. Arrows show the proximal advancement of the volar (Palmar) plate, accessory collateral ligament and transverse metacarpal ligament. (*C*) Anterior view and (*D*) lateral view of completed advancement. Sutures are used to secure the advanced structures into bone.

Functions needed and the structures available are noted in Table 110-1.

A transmetacarpal amputation of the index finger may be carried out, leaving a fairly large piece of dorsal radially innervated skin for the thumb web. The dorsal skin from the thumb may also be rotated to the more palmar surface of the thumb, to oppose the new web skin. If the patient refuses to have the index finger amputated, some improvement may be obtained by rotation flaps from the dorsum of the proximal phalanx of the index and the entire dorsum of the thumb. If there has been tactile skin damage, a free neurovascular toe skin flap may be considered.

TABLE 110-1.   TENDON TRANSFERS FOR LOW MEDIAN–LOW ULNAR PALSIES

Function Needed	Structures Available
1. Tactile sensation	1. Radially innervated skin, free neurovascular toe skin flap
2. Flexion stability of the metacarpophalangeal joints	2. Extensor carpus radialis longus, extensor carpi radialis brevis, extensor carpi ulnaris, all superficiales, extensor interphalangeals, adductor palmaris longus, all profundi, extensor palmaris brevis, EPB, B.R., MP volar plate
3. Thumb opposition	
4. Thumb adduction	

TABLE 110-2. TENDON TRANSFERS FOR HIGH MEDIAN–HIGH ULNAR PALSIES

Function Needed	Structures Available
1. Tactile sensation	1. Radially innervated skin
2. Stability of the metacarpophalangeal joints	2. Extensor carpi radialis longus, extensor carpi radialis brevis, extensor indicis proprius, extensor digiti minimus, brachioradialis, biceps, palmar plates
3. Finger flexion	
4. Thumb flexion	
5. Thumb opposition	
6. Wrist flexion	
7. Pronation	

An opponensplasty may be performed using the extensor indicis proprius around the ulnar side of the wrist and into the thumb abductor brevis insertion. There is usually just enough length on the tendon to accomplish this. It provides a somewhat weak opponens action, but in the presence of complete tactile sensory loss, it may well be sufficient. If a stronger opponensplasty is required, either the extensor carpi ulnaris or extensor carpi radialis brevis can be passed around the ulnar side of the wrist, prolonged with a graft, and inserted in similar fashion. Before any tendon is used for one purpose, it is important to be certain that that tendon is not better used for some other purpose.

For adductorplasty, the superficialis of the ring may be transferred across the palm, beneath the flexors, to the adductor insertion in the manner of Littler.[3]

Stabilization of the metacarpophalangeal joints can be accomplished by a combination of tendon grafting and capsuloplasties. Flexion capsuloplasties of the Zancolli type alone may be sufficient, but the middle superficialis may be split, with one part placed in the adjacent lateral bands of the middle and ring fingers, followed by a flexion capsuloplasty to the index and little fingers. The partially\active control of the deficit helps to prevent any stretching of the passive capsuloplasties.

High Median–High Ulnar Palsies

In high median–high ulnar palsies, the following features will be missing:

1. All tactile sensation
2. All intrinsics
3. Both wrist flexors
4. All finger and thumb flexors
5. Both pronators

Possibilities for repair are noted in Table 110-2.

A flexor hinge splint[8] should be considered prior to tendon transfer since it is able to function on one wrist extensor and may give an indication of how additional transfers and tenodeses will function.

Use of radially innervated skin can be considered, as in low median–low ulnar palsy. (Free neurovascular transfer of toe skin is not likely to provide any improvement in a high lesion, particularly in adults). The metacarpophalangeal is stabilized by multiple palmar flexion capsuloplasties. The brachioradialis is transferred into the superficialis, along with completion of flexion tenodeses of the distal joints for finger flexion. The

thumb may be included as the same motor. Also to be considered is transfer of the extensor carpi radialis longus, plus a tendon graft, through the carpal tunnel into the flexor brevis insertion in the proximal phalanx of the thumb. Flexion tenodesis of the distal joint of the thumb can be performed to stabilize the joint at 0° to 20° of flexion. The extensor indicis proprius is passed ulnarward around the wrist for an opponensplasty. The extensor digiti minimi, is employed with a tendon graft between the second and third metacarpals dorsopalmarly for an adductorplasty. The extensor carpi ulnaris is transferred into the flexor carpi ulnaris for wrist flexion. The biceps could later be transferred to the radius opposite the biceps tubercle for pronation, if this should be necessary, but this should not be done initially.

With recent improvements in microsurgical technique, in cases of sharp radial nerve severances many of the terminal motor nerves, after branching under the supinator, can and should be repaired early, if feasible.

High Median–High Radial Palsies

In high median–high radial palsies, the following features will be missing:

1. Median tactile sensation
2. All wrist extensors
3. Flexor carpi radialis
4. Thumb extension
5. Thumb flexion—extrinsic and intrinsic
6. Thumb opposition
7. All finger extensors
8. All superficiales
9. Profundus—index and middle
10. Pronators
11. Brachioradialis

TABLE 110-3. TENDON TRANSFERS FOR HIGH MEDIAN–HIGH RADIAL PALSIES

Function Needed	Structures Available
1. Median sensation	1. Ulnar sensation
2. Wrist extension	2. Flexor carpi ulnaris
3. Finger extension	3. Profundus, ring and little
4. Thumb extension	4. Hypothenar muscles
5. Thumb flexion	5. Biceps
6. Index and middle flexion	

TABLE 110-4.   TENDON TRANSFERS IN HIGH ULNAR–HIGH RADIAL PALSIES

Function Needed	Structures Available
1. Wrist extension	1. All superficiales
2. Thumb extension	2. Index and middle profundus
3. ? Thumb adduction	3. Flexor pollicis longus
4. Finger extension	4. Flexor carpi radialis
5. Flexion stability of the metacarpophalangeal joints of the ring and little fingers	5. Palmaris longus
6. Profundus flexion of the ring and little fingers	6. Pronator teres

Possibilities for tendon transfer are noted in Table 110-3.

In the case of high median–high radial palsy, the biceps is kept in its ordinary place for its supinatory function, although under some conditions it might be transferred, as in a Steindler procedure for finger flexion, if more power is needed. Sensation is, again, a major problem in this combination.

Among the procedures to consider is an island pedicle transfer of the ulnar ring to thumb for thumb to little finger pinch. It may be possible to use a spring-loaded flexor-driven (flexor carpi ulnaris) hinge splint or flexor carpi ulnaris to extensor carpi radialis brevis transfer. A wrist extensor or flexor can power a flexor hinge splint[8] and the use of this splint alone may provide sufficient help. Use of a hinge splint may also indicate whether a subsequent extensor tenodesis of the thumb and fingers and a flexor tenodesis of the thumb will be of value. The index and middle profundus tendons can be tapped into the functioning ring and little finger profundus for finger flexion. A Huber transfer of the hypothenar muscles may be carried out as an opponensplasty if sensation can be given to the thumb.[6]

High Ulnar–High Radial Palsies

In high ulnar–high radial palsies, the following features will be missing:

1. Ulnar sensation
2. Ulnar intrinsics
3. Flexor carpi ulnaris
4. Ring and little finger profundus
5. Flexion stability of the metacarpophalangeal joints of the ring and little fingers
6. All wrist extensors
7. All finger extensors
8. Thumb extensors
9. Supinator
10. Brachioradialis

Possibilities for tendon transfer are noted in Table 110-4.

Among the transfers to be considered in high ulnar–high radial palsies are: pronator teres into extensor carpi radialis brevis,[1] middle finger superficialis into the extensor digitorum communis, palmaris longus to extensor pollicis longus, flexion capsuloplasty to stabilize the metacarpophalangeal joints, and tapping the ring and little finger profundus into the profundus of the middle finger. Later, if it proves necessary, the ring finger superficialis tendon can be passed under the flexors to the adductor insertion, but often such a procedure is not required.

REFERENCES

1. Brand, P.W.: Clinical Mechanics of the Hand. St. Louis, C.V. Mosby, 1985.
2. Brown, P.W.: Zancolli Capsulorrhaphy for Ulnar Claw Hand. J. Bone Joint Surg. **52-A:**868–877, 1970.
3. Hamlin, C., and Littler, J.W.: Restoration of Power Pinch. J. Hand Surg. **5:**396–401, 1980.
4. Ikuta, Y., Kubo, T., and Tsuge, K.: Free Muscle Transplantation by Microsurgical Technique to Treat Severe Volkmann's Contracture. Plast. Reconst. Surg. **58:**407–411, 1976.
5. Leffert, R.D., and Meister, M.: Patterns of Neuromuscular Activity Following Tendon Transfer in the Upper Limb: A Preliminary Study. J. Hand Surg. **1:**181–189, 1976.
6. Littler, J.W., Stephen, G.E., and Cooley, M.D.: Opposition of the Thumb and its Restoration by Abductor Digiti Quinti Transfer. J. Bone Joint Surg. **45-A:**1389–1396, 1963.
7. Mantkelow, R.T., and McKee, N.: Free Muscle Transplantation to Provide Active Finger Flexion. J. Hand Surg. **3:**416–426, 1978.
8. Nickel, V., Petty, J., and Garrett, A.: Development of Useful Function in the Severely Paralyzed Hand. J. Bone Joint Surg. **45-A:**933–952, 1963.
9. Omer, G., et al.: Neurovascular Cutaneous Island Pedicles for Deficient Median Nerve Sensibility. J. Bone Joint Surg. **52-A:**1181–1192, 1970.

CHAPTER 111

Brachial Plexus Injuries

H. MILLESI

TYPES OF LESIONS

The typical patient with a brachial plexus injury is a young male who has been involved in a motorcycle accident (Table 111-1). Other traffic accidents or sport accidents are less frequently the cause of a brachial plexus injury, and the resultant lesions are generally less severe. Open injuries to the brachial plexus may result from stabbing, but these lesions are rather rare. Gunshot wounds usually lead to only partial lesions.

A common mechanism of injury is compression trauma to the shoulder with fixation of the brachial plexus between the clavicle and the first rib. In such cases the patient's head continues to move away from the shoulder and a traction lesion results. The position of the arm at the time of injury influences which roots are most exposed to traction. The plexus may be compressed. If the humerus is fractured, the plexus is exposed to uncontrolled traction.

Open Injury

In case of an open injury with clean transection of parts of the brachial plexus, primary repair is indicated. A blunt injury has to be treated according to the rules of peripheral nerve surgery; in such instances the brachial plexus should be repaired in a second stage.

Closed Injury

In the case of a fracture of the clavicle, compression of the brachial plexus by the fragments of the clavicle is possible. Repositioning and osteosynthesis are indicated if there is an ipsilateral plexus injury. A fracture of the transverse processes of the cervical vertebrae may also cause external compression of parts of the brachial plexus. Operative decompression is indicated.

With comcomitant rupture of the subclavian artery and subclavian vein, a huge hematoma forms which compresses the brachial plexus. Vascular surgery to repair the artery or the vein is indicated as an emergency procedure. The question arises whether immediate repair of the brachial plexus should be performed. Usually these patients have suffered severe trauma and severe loss of blood. Because a surgeon with experience in brachial plexus surgery might not be available, vascular repair should be performed, with the vascular surgeon using an incision which will allow for later brachial plexus repair. No attempt should be made to identify the individual parts of the brachial plexus, other than what is necessary for the vascular repair, because this will increase the fibrosis and make the secondary operation more difficult.

Most patients with brachial plexus lesions have suffered a closed injury and do not show the above-mentioned complications. However, they may have suffered craniocerebral trauma or futher injuries to the extremities which obviously would require more immediate attention than a closed brachial plexus injury. Although there is no indication for emergency surgery for a brachial plexus injury, the question has been raised as to whether early exploration is indicated.[3,4] An advantage to early surgery is that the lack of fibrous tissue makes exploration easier. On the other hand, the extent of the damage is much more difficult to assess because the damaged parts have not yet developed the inevitable fibrosis. Thus it is more difficult to

TABLE 111-1. CAUSES OF BRACHIAL PLEXUS INJURIES

	Number of Cases
Motorcycle accidents	176
Car accidents	26
Other traffic accidents	22
Other accidents	19
Gun shots	3
Cuts	1
Total	247

identify those lesions which may have a chance for spontaneous recovery.

DIAGNOSIS

The lesions differ according to the location of injury, the lateral extension, and the degree of damage.

Location of Injury

Supraganglionic Lesions

In the case of an avulsion of the nerve roots, the lesion is between the spinal ganglion and the medulla (supraganglionic). There is no proximal stump and no neuroma formation. The characteristics of these lesions are summarized in Table 111-2.

If the avulsed root can be extracted from the intervertebral canal and situated outside, then the avulsion is recognized easily during surgical exploration. If, after a root avulsion, the spinal nerve remains within the intervertebral canal, the situation is not as clear. If such a spinal nerve is transected, part of the cross section may show fibrosis and degeneration but with the sensory fibers still intact. The measurement of evoked potentials can establish whether conduction to the central nervous system is possible.

Infraganglionic Lesions

With rupture, the spinal nerve is interrupted and the roots remain intact (infraganglionic lesion). There is a proximal stump with neuroma formation. The characteristics of such lesions are summarized in Table 111-3.

Trunk Lesions

At the trunk level a lesion may be proximal or distal. The long thoracic nerve, which exits the individual spinal nerves at the very proximal level, remains intact in these cases. The suprascapular nerve is usually involved. The pectoral nerves may or may not be damaged according to the level of injury (Table 111-4).

Spinal Cord Lesions

In a spinal cord lesion the long thoracic nerve, the suprascapular nerve, and the pectoral nerves are intact (Table 111-5). A

TABLE 111-2. CHARACTERISTICS OF SUPRAGANGLIONIC BRACHIAL PLEXUS INJURY WITH AVULSION OF ROOTS

Anatomic Pathology	Sequelae	Clinical Findings
No proximal stump	*No neuroma*	No sign of Tinel's sign
Dural and arachnoid lesion with avulsed roots	Meningocele	Myelographic leak
		Roots not visible on CT
Dorsal rami interrupted	Denervation of dorsal neck muscles	Changes in EMG of these muscles
Nerve fibers to skin in continuity with their neurons in the spinal ganglion	No Wallerian degeneration of sensory nerve fibers	Nerve conduction positive in spite of loss of sensation

TABLE 111-3. CHARACTERISTICS OF RUPTURE OF SPINAL NERVE WITH ROOTS INTACT

Anatomic Pathology	Sequelae	Clinical Findings
Spinal nerve interrupted; proximal stump in continuity with the respective neurons	Formation of a neuroma	Tinel's sign positive
No lesion of dura and arachnoid	No meningocele	Myelography negative
Roots in continuity		Roots visible on CT and myelography
Dorsal rami of spinal nerve in continuity	Deep dorsal neck muscles intact	EMG normal
Nerve fibers to skin not in continuity with their neurons in the spinal ganglion	Sensory nerve fibers undergo Wallerian degeneration	Nerve conduction abnormal

TABLE 111-4. CHARACTERISTICS OF TRUNK LESIONS IN BRACHIAL PLEXUS INJURIES

Lesion	Function
Long thoracic nerve intact	Serratus anterior muscle functioning
Anterolateral pectoral nerve intact	Pectoralis major muscle partially innervated
Suprascapular nerve involved	Supraspinatus and infraspinatus muscles paralyzed
Upper trunk lesion	Paralysis of shoulder muscles Paralysis of biceps brachii
Middle trunk lesion	Paralysis of muscles innervated by radial nerve
Lower trunk lesion	Paralysis of ulnar-innervated and most median-innervated muscles

TABLE 111-5. CHARACTERISTICS OF SPINAL CORD LESIONS IN BRACHIAL PLEXUS INJURIES

Lesion	Function
Long thoracic nerve intact	Serratus anterior muscle functioning
Pectoral nerves intact	Pectoral muscles functioning
Suprascapular nerve intact	Supraspinatus and infraspinatus muscles functioning
Posterior cord lesion	Paralysis of muscles innervated by axillary and radial nerves Paralysis of latissimus dorsi, teres major, teres minor, and subscapularis muscles
Lateral cord lesion	Paralysis of biceps and pronator teres; partial paralysis of forearm muscles innervated by median-nerve
Medial cord lesion	Paralysis of forearm muscles innervated by ulnar nerve intrinsic muscles of the hand; partial paralysis of forearm muscles innervated by median nerve

cord lesion may be suspected if the Tinel–Hoffmann sign is located in the infraclavicular fossa.

Combined Lesions

Brachial plexus injuries often involve more than one specific lesion. For example, a single spinal nerve may have both a supraganglionic lesion and an infraganglionic lesion. Neighboring nerve roots may have suffered an avulsion and a rupture, respectively. A frequent occurrence is the combination of a trunk lesion with a spinal cord lesion.

Such combinations lead to difficulties in diagnosis. Both false-positive and false-negative results occur with myelography and computed tomography.

Lateral Extension

A complete brachial plexus lesion involves all five roots (C5, C6, C7, C8, and T1). The brachial plexus may receive a major additional source from C4 or T2. In the case of a prefixation, the brachial plexus consists of the roots C4, C5, C6, C7, and C8; in the case of a postfixation it includes the roots of C6, C7, C8, T1, and T2 (Table 111-6).

The partial brachial plexus lesions can be divided into two types. In type 1 lesions, all roots are involved but to different degrees. Initially there might be a complete brachial plexus lesion with partial recovery. Recovered muscles have to be regarded as weaker than normal muscles, which may be important if palliative surgery is considered.

In type 2 lesions, some roots are damaged while others are completely intact. In this case palliative surgery can be performed without too much difficulty.

The following specific lesions are differentiated according to the lateral extension of the injury:

Upper brachial plexus lesion (C5, C6)
Extended upper brachial plexus lesion (C5, C6, C7)
C7 lesion
Lower brachial plexus lesion (C8, T1)
Peripheral lesion involving the suprascapular, the axillary, and the musculocutaneous nerves which simulates an upper brachial plexus lesion

Degree of Damage

The extent of damage caused by a brachial plexus injury has been classified by Sunderland[24] into five degrees:

First degree—conduction block without morphologic changes. This can be recognized by electrophysiologic examination. If after several days the conductivity of motor nerve fibers distal to the lesion remains intact in spite of a paralysis, a first-degree lesion can be assumed. Complete spontaneous recovery is possible.

Second degree—loss of continuity of axons with other structures intact. This lesion cannot be recognized as easily as a first-degree lesion. Complete spontaneous recovery is still possible. In these cases there is no indication for surgery. However, the occurrence of external compression and the development of fibrosis may influence the spontaneous recovery in a negative way. The amount of fibrosis was not considered in Sunderland's original scheme, but may be classified as follows[17,17a]:

TABLE 111-6. INVOLVEMENT OF INDIVIDUAL NERVE ROOTS IN 83 PATIENTS WITH COMPLETE BRACHIAL PLEXUS PALSIES*

	C4	C5	C6	C7	C8	T1	Total
Avulsion	1	22	39	68	53	43	226
Interruption	5	58	41	10	6	9	129
Lesion in continuity	0	3	3	5	24	29	64
Total							419

* Brachial plexus configurations: *normal* (C5–T1), 77 patients; 385 affected nerve roots; *prefixation of C4* (C4–T1), 2 patients, 10 affected nerve roots; *strong contribution of C4* (C4–T1), 4 patients, 24 affected nerve roots.

TABLE 111-7.   COMBINED EVALUATION SYSTEM FOR EXTENT OF BRACHIAL PLEXUS INJURIES

Degree	Continuity*	Fibrosis*	Prognosis	Surgical Procedure
I	Conduction block	None	Spontaneous recovery	None
I A	Conduction block	Fibrosis of epifascicular epineurium	No spontaneous recovery	Epifascicular epineurotomy
I B	Conduction block	Fibrosis of interfascicular epineurium	No spontaneous recovery	Epifascicular epineurectomy; interfascicular epineurectomy (for partial lesion)
II	Axons interrupted	None	Spontaneous recovery	None
II A	Axons interrupted	Fibrosis of epifascicular epineurium	No spontaneous recovery	Epifascicular epineurotomy
II B	Axons interrupted	Fibrosis of interfascicular epineurium	No spontaneous recovery	Epifascicular epineurectomy Interfascicular epineurectomy (for partial lesion)
III†	Axons interrupted; endoneural structures damaged; perineurium intact	None	Partial spontaneous recovery	None
III A	Axons interrupted; endoneural structures damaged; perineurium intact	Fibrosis of epifascicular epineurium	No spontaneous recovery	Epifascicular epineurotomy
III B	Axons interrupted; endoneural structures damaged; perineurium intact	Fibrosis of interfascicular epineurium	No spontaneous recovery	Epifascicular epineurectomy Interfasicular epineurectomy (for partial lesion)
III C	Axons interrupted; endoneural structures damaged; perineurium intact	Fibrosis of endoneurium	No spontaneous recovery	Resection plus nerve grafting
IV N	Fascicular structures interrupted; continuity preserved by fibrotic connective tissue with ingrowing neuroma	Continuity preserved by fibrotic connective tissue with ingrowing neuroma†‡	No useful spontaneous recovery	Resection plus nerve grafting
IV S	Fascicular structures interrupted	Continuity preserved by fibrotic tissue only (no conduction possible)	No spontaneous recovery	Resection plus nerve grafting
V	Complete loss of continuity		No spontaneous recovery	Nerve grafting Nerve transfer

* Continuity rating from Sunderlend, S.: A Classification of Peripheral Nerve Injuries Producing Loss of Function. Brain **74:** 491, 1951; Fibrosis rating from Millesi, H.: Eingriffe an peripheren Nerven. In Gschnitzer, F., Kern, E., and Schweiberer L., (eds): Chirurgische Operationslehre, Urban & Schwarzenberg, München, Wien, Baltimore, 1986, p. 1–88.

† Extremely rare because with this amount of damage fibrosis will almost always develop.

‡ A few nerve fibers may reach the distal stump and produce some conduction along the damaged segment.

Type A fibrosis—the epifascicular epineurium has become fibrotic and the whole nerve is compressed like a tight stocking

Type B fibrosis—the interfascicular epineurium has also become fibrotic

Type C fibrosis—the content of the fascicles of the endoneurium has become completely fibrotic

Note: If type A or type B fibrosis is combined with a first- or second-degree lesion, spontaneous recovery will be impeded and neurolysis is indicated.

Third degree—loss of continuity of axons and endoneural structures with intact perineurium. Type A or B fibrosis is possible; the content of the fascicles may have become completely fibrotic (type C) if the lesion is very severe or if a long time has elapsed since the injury. With type A or B fibrosis, neurolysis is indicated. With type C fibrosis, neurolysis cannot effect regeneration, and resection with replacement of the involved fascicles by nerve grafts is indicated.

Fourth degree—continuity is preserved only by connective tissue. This connective tissue can be completely fibrotic, in which case there is no chance for nerve fibers to grow beyond the lesion. In other cases a neuroma may grow into the connective tissue that still unites the two stumps; in such instances some nerve fibers may reach the distal stump, and, therefore, some conduction may be elicited during intraoperative stimulation. However, there is no chance for a functional recovery. In all fourth-degree lesions resection and repair by nerve grafts are indicated.

Fifth degree—complete loss of continuity

Different degrees of involvement are possible in combined lesions. The differentiation between these different degrees is made during intraoperative dissection with or without nerve stimulation (Table 111-7).

INDICATIONS FOR SURGERY AND EXPECTED RESULTS

In a simple first- or second-degree brachial plexus lesion there are good chances for spontaneous recovery and no surgery is indicated. However, in a first- or second-degree lesion with epifascicular fibrosis (type I A or II A), there are usually initial signs of recovery with subsequent failure to improve or even some deterioration. Exploration is indicated, and after neurolysis a complete return of function is possible. The same is true for first- or second-degree lesions with interfascicular fibrosis (type I B or II B).

In a third-degree lesion there is some chance of spontaneous recovery, but this takes longer and the recovery will always be less than complete. Pure third-degree lesions without fibrosis are rare; usually there is a type A or B fibrosis. This can be converted into a pure third-degree lesion, by internal neurolysis, after which recovery may occur. However, if the endoneural space has become completely fibrotic (type III C), there is no chance of spontaneous recovery. In such cases the fascicles should be resected and the continuity repaired by nerve grafts.

In a type IV N lesion with neuroma formation, some nerve fibers may get into the distal stump. Usually regeneration takes a long time and the muscles may have already reached an atrophic and fibrotic stage before this can occur. Therefore, spontaneous recovery cannot be expected in these lesions and surgical repair is indicated. This is also the case for a complete fibrosis with a fourth-degree lesion (type IV S) without neuroma formation.

Likewise, if there is a loss of continuity (grade V), there is no chance for spontaneous recovery.

In patients with complete loss of continuity or type III C, IV N, and IV S lesions, continuity must be restored. Because of the complexity of the structure of the brachial plexus and the long distance between the site of the lesion and the target organs, only partial recovery can be expected. Except in infants, the return of intrinsic hand function has not been observed.

The main goal of surgery is the return of active elbow flexion. If this occurs, the result can be regarded as satisfactory. In addition, some control of the shoulder joint, with the correction of subluxation, and the return of some protective sensation can be expected. If some forearm muscles become active, the result can be regarded as good. It is the experience of surgeons involved with brachial plexus surgery that the development of pain syndromes is less frequent in patients treated operatively than in those who are not treated. In some instances pain is relieved by surgery.

TECHNIQUES FOR EXPLORATION

Ventral Approach through a Zig-Zag Incision

Position the patient supine with the affected arm abducted and the head turned to the contralateral side. Prepare and drape the ipsilateral side of the neck, the shoulder, the upper arm, the forearm, and the ipsilateral side of the thorax. Place a cushion under the dorsal side of the ipsilateral thorax, to lift the thorax.

There are two incisions (Fig. 111-1). The main incision follows the clavicle. In the distal third of the clavicle, the incision turns toward the axilla, traverses the pectoralis major muscle, turns laterally for a short length along the free border of the pectoralis major muscle, then toward the inner side of the humerus; it turns again to proceed along the midline of the medial aspect of the upper arm. The second incision begins behind the sternocleidomastoid muscle at the level of the angle of the mandible. It briefly follows the dorsal border of the

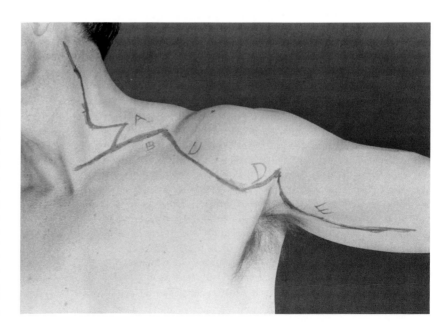

FIGURE 111-1. A patient with a brachial plexus lesion is prepared for surgery. The contour of the clavicle, the supraclavicular groove, the infraclavicular groove, the free border of the pectoralis major muscle, and the axillary groove, as well as the contour of the humeral head, are clearly visible. The line of the main incision follows the clavicle, traverses the pectoralis major muscle, follows the free border of the pectoralis major muscle to the medial side of the upper arm, and proceeds along the midline of the medial side of the upper arm. An additional incision follows the posterior border of the sternocleidomastoid muscle, traverses the supraclavicular fossa in zig-zag-fashion, and meets the main incision in its medial third. By this incision the flaps *a, b, c, d,* and *e* are outlined.

sternocleidomastoid muscle, then traverses the supraclavicular fossa to meet the main incision in its medial third. This is done to avoid an acute angle between the two incisions, which might cause problems for the skin. At the level where this incision traverses the supraclavicular fossa, it is zig-zag–shaped. It is not always necessary to use the whole length of this incision.

Raise skin flaps as follows: between the two incisions and above the supraclavicular fossa (see Fig. 111-1, flap A); on the medial side of the main incision above the infraclavicular fossa (flap B); on the lateral side of the main incision (flap C); at the level of the ventral axillary fold (flap D); and at the upper arm (flap E).

After lifting flap A, expose, ligate, and resect the external jugular vein in order to gain easy access to the supraclavicular fossa. The dissection penetrates the loose connective tissue of the supraclavicular fossa and reaches the scalenus anterior muscle. Identify the phrenic nerve. By following the phrenic nerve, the root of spinal nerve C4 is exposed, and sometimes also that of C5, because the phrenic nerve may have some fibers from this root. Continue in this way until the level of C5 is reached, even in the presence of an avulsion of this root or if the entire area has become fibrotic. If the C5 and C6 spinal nerves are intact, exposure is very easy between the scalenus anterior and the scalenus medius muscle. By further dissection define and isolate the transverse colli and superficial cervical arteries and veins and the omohyoid muscle. Further exploration leads to the middle trunk and the C7 spinal nerve. Before further dissection beneath the clavicle, expose the infraclavicular fossa. This is done by raising flap B and defining the sulcus between the pectoralis major and the deltoid muscle. In this groove the cephalic vein is met. For better exposure of the infraclavicular fossa, detach the clavicular origin of the pectoralis major muscle. After transection of the deltopectoral fascia, the lateral cord is encountered. Dorsal to the lateral cord is the posterior cord, and medially the subclavian artery. By dissection between the subclavian artery and the lateral cord, expose the medial cord. In these areas there are branches from the lateral and the medial cords to the pectoralis major muscle which should be spared.

If this area is scarred and fibrotic, explore the lateral part of the brachial plexus in the axillary groove lateral to the minor pectoralis muscle. Separate the pectoralis major muscle and the deltoid muscle, taking care to preserve the cephalic vein. Isolate and lift the pectoralis minor muscle. Lateral to this muscle, the most superficial structure encountered is the lateral cord. If this cord is followed laterally, the division into the lateral origin of the median nerve and the musculocutaneous nerve is exposed.

Dorsal to the lateral cord is the posterior cord, which can be followed to its division into the axillary nerve and the radial nerve. On the caudal aspect of this cord, the thoracodorsal nerve and one or two subscapular nerves originate. Medial to the lateral cord is the axillary artery, and further medially is the medial origin of the median nerve. If this is followed in a central direction, the medial cord is encountered, with its division into the medial origin of the median nerve and the ulnar nerve. In this area the medial brachial cutaneous and the medial antebrachial cutaneous nerve leave the medial cord. Further medially is found the axillary vein.

If this area is scarred and dissection turns out to be difficult,

the brachial plexus should be explored from a more lateral level. The principle is always to try to explore the plexus from normal tissue. Lift flaps D and E (see Fig. 111-1) and incise the fascia on the medial aspect of the upper arm. The basilic vein and the medial antebrachial cutaneous nerve are met first; after lifting them, the median nerve is reached. Identify the brachial artery, the ulnar nerve, and the radial nerve and continue the dissection into the axillary groove from below until the musculocutaneous and axillary nerves are met. By isolating and lifting the pectoralis major muscle, the site of operation at the caudal aspect and at the cranial aspect of the axillary groove are united. It is never necessary to transect the pectoralis major muscle. Continue the dissection in the direction of the infraclavicular fossa until the area lateral and medial to the pectoralis minor muscle is exposed and all the structures are isolated at both levels.

The next step is to unite the supraclavicular and infraclavicular fossae by lifting the clavicle. Incise the fascia above the clavicle. Isolate the clavicle from the connective tissue surrounding it on its cranial side and from the subclavian muscle on its caudal side. Identify and protect the suprascapular vessels which run underneath the clavicle. By lifting the clavicle and its neighboring structures, a communication is achieved between the supraclavicular and the infraclavicular fossae. By pulling the clavicle cranially or caudally, the entire brachial plexus is accessible from above or from below, respectively. By following the upper and middle trunk, isolate their divisions until the cords already exposed are reached. By lifting the clavicle cranially and following the medial cord, the inferior trunk can be isolated from the subclavian artery and followed along the medial aspect of the first rib to its division into the C8 and T1 spinal nerves.

The brachial plexus is now exposed in its full length and access is available through several different "windows":

1. The supraclavicular fossa cranial to the omohyoid muscle
2. The space between the omohyoid muscle and the clavicle
3. The space between the clavicle and the subclavian muscle
4. The space between the subclavian muscle and the pectoralis major muscle proximal to the pectoralis minor muscle
5. The space between the pectoralis major and deltoid muscles distal to the pectoralis minor muscle
6. The axillary groove and the medial aspect of the arm

The main point is that by using this type of exposure, no structure traversing the brachial plexus has to be transected.

Exposure of the brachial plexus can be facilitated by an oblique osteotomy of the clavicle, using preformed drill holes for an osteosynthesis with plate and screws. The osteotomy alone does not help very much if the other structures, such as the subclavian muscle, are not transected as well. In this case there is no intact soft tissue available for covering the brachial plexus.

Exposure of the Cervical Plexus and the Accessory Nerve

Using the same incision described for exploration of the supraclavicular fossa, proceed cranially along the dorsal aspect of the sternocleidomastoid muscle. A cluster of nerves (punctum nervosum) is exposed with the transversus colli, the greater auricular and the lesser occipital nerves emerging behind the sternocleidomastoid. Dissection following these nerves and the phrenic nerve leads to C4 and C3. The supraclavicular nerves also can be followed to their origins from C4. By further dissection motor branches can be defined by electric stimulation to the sternocleidomastoid muscle, the trapezius muscle, the levator scapulae muscle, and the rhomboid muscles.

At the level of the scalenus medius muscle, the dorsal scapular nerve emerges and, more caudally, the long thoracic nerve. Slightly lateral and deep to the punctum nervosum a group of lymph nodes is encountered. Deeper to these structures one finds the accessory nerve, emerging from a layer underneath the sternocleidomastoid muscle. The accessory nerve becomes more superficial and gives off one branch to the muscle before it enters the muscle.

Exploration and Transfer of Intercostal Nerves

There are several methods available for exploration and transfer of the intercostal nerves. The nerves can be isolated in full length to the level of the parasternal area, specifically the costal arch, and transferred in order to be coapted directly to the distal stump. To facilitate exploration, resection of a rib is recommended. The disadvantage of this technique is the vast exposure required. An advantage is that coaptation is needed only on one side.

It has been suggested that the intercostal nerves may be dissected more dorsally with the patient in a prone position. The intercostal nerve is then brought above the pleura to the ventral side. After turning the patient on his back, the coaptation to the distal stumps of the brachial plexus is performed.[10]

I prefer to transfer the intercostal nerves followed by interposition of a nerve graft. Expose the intercostal nerves by a longitudinal incision in the midaxillary line between the latissimus and the pectoralis major muscles. Split the serratus anterior muscle along each rib. Incise the periosteum of each rib and lift the periosteum from the rib all around. By lifting the exposed rib, direct access to the intercostal nerve underneath the rib is gained. Isolate the nerve for about 5 cm to 6 cm, transect it, and coapt a nerve graft to the proximal stump. Place the nerve grafts underneath a skin bridge in the direction of the axillary groove on the medial aspect of the arm; this coapts then with the peripheral nerve stumps.

Morelli and Raimondi[18] suggested transection of the intercostal nerves more dorsally at the level of the paravertebral line, in order to have more motor fibers in the nerve trunk. Nerve grafts are then used to achieve an indirect coaptation with peripheral stumps of the brachial plexus.

TECHNIQUES FOR SURGICAL REPAIR

Neurolysis

External neurolysis isolates the nerve trunks from adhesions to the surrounding tissues. An epifascicular epineurotomy (single or multiple) is indicated to decompress the nerve trunk with type A fibrosis.

If there is a moderate degree of interfascicular fibrosis (type B), epineurotomy will not be sufficient. An epifascicular epineurectomy (dissecting the epifascicular tissue) is indicated. With a more extensive degree of interfascicular fibrosis (type C), the interfascicular tissue has to be partially excised in order to achieve decompression (interfascicular epineurectomy).

Neurorrhaphy

A neurorrhaphy with end-to-end coaptation of nerve stumps is only rarely possible with brachial plexus lesions. It follows the usual techniques and is most appropriate in cases of clean transection (e.g., stab injuries).

Nerve Grafting

Restoration of continuity by free nerve grafting is performed using the sural nerve, the medial antebrachial cutaneous nerve, and, occasionally, the superficial branch of the radial nerve. The use of cutaneous nerve segments for nerve grafting has the great advantage that well-defined points of the proximal stump can be coapted to well-defined points of the distal stump. The grafts are placed individually in order to increase the spontaneous revascularization and to avoid central fibrosis. The grafts are long enough to avoid longitudinal tension, and very few stitches are necessary to approximate the graft to the proximal and distal stumps. In recent years the use of fibrin glues has been recommended to shorten the operation time considerably.[20] If the grafts are long enough and the coaptations are absolutely tensionless, only a few approximation stitches between the stumps and the grafts are necessary. In this case, the gain of time by using tissue glue is minimal.

In the case of a root avulsion at C8 and T1, the ulnar nerve is available for use as a nerve graft. Bonney and Birch[4] transplanted the ulnar nerve as a free vascularized nerve graft based on the ulnar artery. Breidenbach and Terzis[6,7] have demonstrated that a free microvascular transfer is possible using the ulnar collateral artery inferiorly as the nutritive vessel without sacrificing the ulnar artery.

If there is a long superior collateral ulnar artery, the ulnar nerve can be transferred as an island flap without interrupting the blood supply. If the blood supply is not interrupted by a complication, this type of nerve graft offers the advantage that it is not dependent on the vascularity of the recipient bed. To achieve connections of well-defined spots from the proximal and the distal stumps is more difficult. Initial expectations that the qualitative result of regeneration would be significantly improved by this method have not been fulfilled. The majority of authors agree that the first signs of recovery might occur somewhat earlier but the final result will be the same as with free nerve grafting with spontaneous revascularization.[1,2,5,15-17]*

The ulnar nerve can also be used as a free graft after the epifascicular epineurium has been removed and the nerve trunk has been split into minor units by interfascicular dissection.[17]

---

* Personal communication, Allieu, 1984.

Nerve Transfer

By transferring the proximal stump of a normal nerve to the distal stump of a denervated nerve, the damaged nerve can be regenerated and some functional recovery achieved. Of course, the patient has to learn to use the impulses of the transferred nerve for a different function, which requires a certain plasticity. Intercostal nerves,[22] the accessory nerve,[12,13] and motor branches of the cervical plexus[8,9] have been used for this purpose.

Muscle and Tendon Transfer

Techniques for muscle and tendon transfers are discussed elsewhere in the book, but should be mentioned here because in some cases neurotization is performed with the intention to transfer the treated muscle for another function. This applies especially to the triceps muscle, which regenerates extremely well and which we have in certain cases neurotized in order to transfer the regenerated muscle to the biceps tendon for elbow flexion. Transferred nerves are also sometimes the nerve fiber donor for a free graft muscle.

SELECTION OF TECHNIQUES ACCORDING TO LESION

In lesions in which continuity is present, the different steps of intraneural neurolysis are performed in order to define the degree of damage. If it becomes clear that the fascicular structure remained intact and that decompression has been achieved, the surgery is ended. If not, the next step has to be carried out until the surgeon is convinced that the damage is of a degree making spontaneous recovery impossible. In this case the damaged part is resected and continuity is restored by nerve grafting.

If continuity has been lost, the proximal and distal stumps are prepared by resection or by interfascicular dissection until normal tissue is available. A special problem is presented by root lesions if an avulsion of the roots cannot be proven or excluded because the spinal nerve is still in the intervertebral canal. In this case the continuity or discontinuity central to the spinal nerve can be investigated.

A restoration of continuity of all structures by nerve grafts is aimed for in level III and IV lesions, especially if the defects are short enough to be bridged by using the available donor nerves. If the lesion is at the level of the spinal nerves (level II), a restoration of continuity of all structures is usually not possible and the decision has to be made as to which parts are to be repaired. Lesions of C8 and T1 have poor prognoses and, therefore, restoration of continuity of these spinal nerves has the lowest priority. The highest priority is attributed to the restoration of elbow flexion. If possible, C6 is united with distal structures which lead to that part of the lateral cord which forms the musculocutaneous nerve. The next most important function is the control of the shoulder joint; thus, it is advisable to attempt to neurotize the suprascapular nerve with fibers coming from C5 or even C4. Nerve fibers of the dorsal aspects of C5, C6, and C7 are united with the posterior cord to provide nerve fibers to the axillary and radial nerves.

In case of root avulsion (level I), an individual plan has to be made for each particular case. If the avulsion involves C8 and T1, the ulnar nerve can be used as a nerve graft. No attempt is made to neurotize the lower cord because attempts to do so have not yielded satisfactory results.[19]

If C6 is not available, C5 can be used for the musculocutaneous nerve and the accessory nerve connected with the suprascapular nerve. If C7 is avulsed, the accessory nerve may be the donor for neurotization of the radial nerve.

If C5 and C6 are avulsed, the accessory nerve may neurotize the suprascapular and the axillary nerve and intercostal nerves may be used for the musculocutaneous. The musculocutaneous nerve also can be neurotized successfully by the accessory nerve.[14] A similar approach is selected in case of an avulsion of C5, C6, and C7.

If all roots are avulsed, the accessory and motor branches of the cervical plexus are used to neurotize the axillary and the suprascapular nerve (Fig. 111-2). The second, third, and fourth intercostal nerves can be connected with the median nerve in order to provide motor and sensory fibers to this territory. Also, the supraclavicular nerves can be the source for sensory fibers to the median nerve. The fifth through eighth intercostal nerves can be used to neurotize the musculocutaneous nerve.

POSTOPERATIVE CARE

After wound closure, immobilization is achieved in the position the patient was in during the operation by a plaster cast which includes the head, the trunk, and the arm. This cast is maintained for 10 days. After this time, passive and active mobilization is initiated for as wide a range of motion as is possible. Electrotherapy of the denervated muscles, using exponential current, is performed. Splinting should avoid extension of muscles, especially of the biceps. There is still some questions as to whether or not the shoulder joint should be immobilized in abduction to maintain the full range of motion. According to my experience, return of active motion in the shoulder joint is always limited and it is, therefore, not necessary to maintain a wide range of passive motion. The use of a custom-made orthosis is recommended.

PALLIATIVE SURGERY

In instances of partial type 2 lesions with intact muscles, procedures to replace lost elbow flexion can be performed. These procedures include transfer of the lateral segment of the pectoralis major muscle,[11] transfer of the latissimus dorsi muscle,[25] and transfer of the common forearm flexor muscles from the medial epicondyle of the humerus to the shaft of the humerus.[23]

In a partial type I lesion, a careful evaluation of the available muscle force is necessary.

To improve the functional result in a regenerating biceps, a shortening of the biceps tendon sometimes helps. The biceps tendon can also be transferred 1 cm or 2 cm distally, in order to provide a better moment arm and better flexion power by sacrificing the supination.

Quite often a simultaneous innervation of the biceps and triceps occurs, and very often the triceps is the stronger muscle. In this case the triceps is mobilized and its tendon trans-

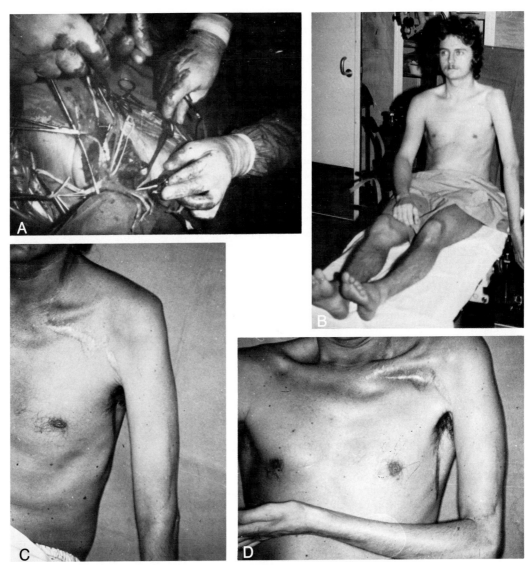

FIGURE 111-2.   A 24-year-old patient suffered severe trauma to the left shoulder in a motor cycle accident. (*A*) The subclavian artery was ruptured and all five roots of the brachial plexus were avulsed. This photograh was taken during vascular repair. (*B*) Five months later the patient is ready for a brachial plexus exploration. All five roots were avulsed (C5, C6, C7, C8, and T1). There was a strong contribution from C4, which was ruptured. This stump was connected by two 15-cm sural nerve grafts with the distal stump of the radial nerve. The dorsal scapular nerve was connected to the distal stump of the axillary nerve. The intercostal nerves III, IV, and V were connected with three sural nerve grafts (6 cm, 8 cm, and 10 cm in length) with the distal stump of the median nerve. The intercostal nerves VI, VII and VIII were united with the distal stump of the musculocutaneous nerve by three nerve grafts (11 cm, 12 cm, and 13 cm in length.): Satisfactory recovery of the biceps and triceps muscles occurred. Because these muscles are innervated simultaneously, if the patient intends to flex the elbow joint, simultaneous contraction of the triceps prevents the flexion. (*C, D*) Strong elbow flexion is possible after transfer of the triceps muscle around the lateral side of the humerus to the biceps tendon. The atypical scar in the pectoralis region resulted from the vascular surgery. It was released by a Z-plasty. In the median nerve area the patient feels light touch, which he localizes to the thoracic wall.

ferred to the palmar aspect and united with the biceps tendon so that both muscles act as flexors. Sometimes the triceps has successfully replaced a nonfunctioning biceps, and in some cases we have initially restored the function of the triceps by nerve transfer, planning a later muscle transfer.

Control of the shoulder joint can be achieved by transferring the horizontal part of the trapezius muscle, including the bony insertion and the acromion, to the humerus, as described by Saha.[21] The active gain of abduction is limited, but usually subluxation can be avoided and some control achieved. An arthrodesis of the shoulder joint is indicated only if the serratus anterior muscle and the other shoulder muscles provide good active motion of the scapula. External rotation of the shoulder can be restored by transferring the pectoralis major or the pectoralis minor to a new insertion. In a supination deformity with lack of pronation, the biceps tendon can be transferred so that its supinating power is abolished. If the flexor carpi ulnaris is available, this muscle can be used to replace the pronator teres.

If elbow flexion has returned but the wrist and finger flexors are still paralyzed, arthrodesis of the wrist joint, using a plate between the radius and the third metacarpal bone, helps to stabilize the hand. The patient can then use the forearm and the stable wrist joint as a supporting limb. If one or two forearm muscles have returned, it is possible to restore a simple gripping function (i.e., key grip) by multiple arthrodeses and tendon transfers.

In old brachial plexus lesions without a chance of regeneration of the ipsilateral muscles, elbow flexion can be achieved by a free muscle transfer, using the gracilis muscle and providing nerve supply by intercostal nerves.

COMPLICATIONS AND PITFALLS

After brachial plexus lesions a hematoma may develop, which has to be drained surgically in order not to impair the result.

Complications with wound healing at the skin level are extremely rare.

After osteotomy and osteosynthesis of the clavicle, bone healing may be complicated.

If long nerve grafts have been used, one has to consider the possibility of a block at the distal side of the coaptation. This can be recognized if the Tinel sign advances along the graft but does not cross over to the distal stump. In this case reexploration is indicated.

Although there is a tendency to form keloidal scars at the level of the neck and the clavicle after brachial plexus surgery, it is rarely necessary to perform a scar correction.

The main pitfall of brachial plexus injury repair is failure of the expected regeneration. This happens quite often without explanation. At present satisfactory results can be expected in about 70% of the cases, leaving as many as 30% of patients with less than satisfactory recoveries.

REFERENCES

1. Alnot, J.Y., Oberlin, C., and Bellaicke, H.: Vascularized Ulnar Nerve Transfer in Total Palsy of the Brachial Plexus. Presented at the Joint Meeting of the Groupe pour l'Avancement de la Microchirurgie and the Deutschsprachige Arbeitsgemeinschaft fur Mikrochirurgie der peripheren Nerven und Gefässe, Strasbourg, May 2–4, 1984.
2. Anderl, H., and Hussel, H.: Erfahrungen mit vaskularisierten Nerventransplantaten. Presented at the Meeting of the DAM f. Mikrochirurgie der peripheren Nerven und Gefässe, Bern, Dec. 5–6, 1986.
3. Bonney, G.: The Case for Early Surgery. Presented at the Symposium on Brachial Plexus Injuries at the St. Mary's Hospital, London, Jan. 24–26, 1983.
4. Bonney, G., and Birch, R.: Surgical Aspects. Presented at the Symposium on Brachial Plexus Injuries by the British Society for Surgery of the Hand, Barbicane Centre, London, Nov. 5–6, 1982.
5. Bonney, G., Birch, R., Jamieson, A.M., and Eames, R.A.: Experience with Vascularized Nerve Grafts. Clin. Plast. Surg. **11:**137, 1984.
6. Breidenbach, W., and Terzis, J.K.: The Anatomy of Free Vascularized Nerve Grafts. Clin. Plast. Surg. **11:**65, 1984.
7. Breidenbach, W., and Terzis, J.K.: The Blood Supply of Vascularized Nerve Grafts. J. Reconstr. Microsurg. **3:**43, 1986.
8. Brunelli, G.: Neurotization of Avulsed Roots of the Brachial Plexus by Means of Anterior Nerves of the Cervical Plexus. Int. J. Microsurg. **2:**55, 1980.
9. Brunelli, G., and Monini, L.: Neurotization of Avulsed Roots of Brachial Plexus by Means of Anterior Nerves of Cervical Plexus. Clin. Plast. Surg. **11:**148, 1984.
10. Celli, L., Mingione, A., and Landi, A.: Nuove Acquisizioni di Tecnica Chirurgica Nelle Lesioni dle Plesso Brachiale: Indicazioni alla Neurolisi, Autoinneste e Trapianti Nervosi. Atti LIX Congresso della Societá Italiana di Ortopedia et Traumatologia, Cagliari, September 29–October 3, 1974.
11. Clark, J.P.M.: Reconstruction of Biceps Brachii by Pectoral Muscle Transplantation. Brit. J. Surg. **34:**180, 1946.
12. Kotani, P.T., Matsuda, H., and Suzuki, T.: Trial Surgical Procedures of Nerve Transfer to Avulsion Injuries of Plexus Brachialis (abstract). Proceedings of 12th Meeting of Societé Internationale Chirurgie Ortopedique et Traumatique (SICOT), Tel Aviv, Israel, October 9–13, 1972, p. 520.
13. Kotani, P.T., Toyoshima, Y., Matsuda, H., Suzuki, T., Ishizaki, Y., Ivani, H., Yamano, H., Inoue, H., Moriguchi, T., Ri, S., and Asada, K.: The Postoperative Results of Nerve Transfer for the Brachial Plexus Injury in Root Avulsion. Proceedings of the 14th Annual Meeting of the Japanese Society for Surgery of the Hand, Osaka, 1971. p. 34
14. Merle, M.: Neurotization of Brachial Plexus Lesions with the Spinal Accessory Nerve—Functional Results. Presented at 2nd Annual Meeting of the American Society for Reconstructive Microsurgery, New Orleans, Louisiana, Feb. 13–15, 1986.
15. Merle, M.: Vascularization Nerve Grafts. Presented at 9th Meeting of the International Microsurgical Society, Brescia, July 27–August 1, 1986.
16. Merle, M., Lebreton, E., Bour, C., Mancaud, M., and Marin Braun, F.: Free Vascularized Nerve Transfer in Brachial Plexus Injuries. Presented at the Joint Meeting of the Groupe pour l'Avancement de la Microchirurgie and the Deutschsprachige Arbeitsgemeinschaft fur Mikrochirurgie d. peripheren Nerven und Gefässe, Strasbourg, May 2–4, 1984.
17. Millesi, H.: Das Problem der Defektbehebung peripherer Nerven. Presented at 9th Meeting of Deutschsprachige Arbeitsgemeinschaft für Mikrochirurgie der peripheren Nerven und Gefässe, Bern, December 5–6, 1986.
17a. Millesi, H.: Eingriffe an peripheren Nerven. In Gschnitzer, F, Kern, E, and Schweiberer, L (eds): Chirurgische Operationslehre, pp 1–88. München-Wien-Baltimore, Urban & Schwarzenberg, 1986.
18. Morelli, E., and Raimondi, P.L.: La Neurotizzazione con Nervi Intercostali. (in press)
19. Narakas, A.O.: Thoughts on Neurotization of Nerve Transfers in Irreparable Nerve Lesions. Clin. Plast. Surg. **11:**153, 1984.
20. Narakas, A.: Brachial Plexus Injury. Presented at 3rd Congress of International Federation of Societies for Surgery of the Hand, Tokyo, November 3–8, 1986.
21. Saha, A.K.: Surgery of the Paralyzed and Flail Shoulder. Acta Orthop. Scand. (Suppl.) **97:**1, 1967.
22. Seddon, H.: Nerve Grafting. J. Bone Joint Surg. **45-B:**447, 1963.
23. Steindler, A.: Reconstruction Work on Hand and Forearm. N.Y. Med. J. **108:**117, 1918.
24. Sunderland, S.: A Classification of Peripheral Nerve Injuries Producing Loss of Function. Brain **74:**491, 1951.
25. Zancolli, E., and Mitre, H.: Latissimus Dorsi Transfer to Restore Elbow Flexion: An Appraisal of Eight Cases. J. Bone Joint Surg., **55-A:**1265, 1973.

CHAPTER 112

Surgery of the Thoracic Outlet

ROBERT D. LEFFERT

Thoracic outlet syndrome is a complex of signs and symptoms that results from compression of the neurovascular structures as they pass out of the chest and neck, through the costoclavicular interval and down into the axilla. Although attention was first focused on the interscalene area, subsequent experience has demonstrated that the dynamic anatomy of the entire region must be understood to treat the disorders that arise there. The changes in the alignment of the shoulder girdle with normal development, age, and disease complicate the problem considerably, but also provide a means of understanding the production of signs and symptoms.[23] Specifically, exaggeration of the normal caudad descent of the shoulder girdle produced by poor posture or local injury can cause compression of the lower trunk of the brachial plexus, as well as the subclavian artery and vein. If there are congenital anatomic abnormalities, such as cervical ribs, long transverse processes, or congenital bands, the effect can be considerably worsened. Although the incidence of cervical ribs in the general population is approximately 0.75%, eight types of congenital fibrous bands have been described that can cause neurovascular compression within the thoracic outlet.[21]

Orthopaedic problems such as malunions and nonunions of the clavicle can also lead to thoracic outlet compression. Disorders of the shoulder joint, such as instability, can be associated with numbness and tingling within the limb. These are manifestations of secondary thoracic outlet syndrome, which will be further discussed.[12]

The patients are often women, by a ratio of approximately five-to-one, and the disorder is seen most commonly between puberty and the fourth decade of life.

DIAGNOSIS OF THORACIC OUTLET SYNDROME

The diagnosis of thoracic outlet syndrome is primarily clinical. Although there are some helpful laboratory examinations, diagnosis is usually made on the basis of a careful history and physical examination.

The symptoms of thoracic outlet syndrome may be quite variable, depending on which structures are being compressed. The vast majority of patients have symptoms of pain and parasthesias that radiate from the neck, upper chest, or shoulder region down the medial aspect of the arm and into the little and ring fingers. Symptoms are often nocturnal, and elevation of the arm appears to aggravate them. Complaints such as inability to hold a hair dryer or to work with the arms above the head are common. These symptoms are caused by compression of the lower trunk of the brachial plexus.

The signs are usually subtle and may be confined to weakness of the ulnar-innervated intrinsic muscles, unless there is more severe compression. There may be panintrinsic weakness and loss of power of the long flexors of the little and ring fingers. When other parts of the brachial plexus are involved, it is much more difficult to make the diagnosis, particularly in terms of differential diagnosis.

Patients with thoracic outlet syndrome rarely may present with signs and symptoms of acute arterial insufficiency or gangrene in the hand. These patients usually have acute occlusion of the subclavian or axillary arteries and often have aneurysms caused by compression of significant cervical ribs.[9] This complication is more often found in older patients with long histories of often undiagnosed symptoms.

Venous compression can cause swelling of the hand and upper limb, which initially will be intermittent, making it difficult to document until such time as it becomes sufficiently established to be seen by the examining physician. Color change due to intermittent venous compression in the absence of thrombosis will produce cyanosis as well as swelling in the limb. Occasionally a patient will present with acute venous thrombosis, so-called Paget-Schroeder syndrome.

Although unilateral Raynaud's phenomenon has been associated with thoracic outlet syndrome, it has often been attributed to selective compression of the sympathetic innervation of the limb within the lower trunk of the brachial plexus. More likely, this phenomenon represents episodes of embolization from an aneurysm located within the subclavian or axillary arteries. In a patient with unilateral Raynaud's phenomenon, the etiology is not caused by collagen disease.

Patients with thoracic outlet syndrome may demonstrate either neck or chest pain as a major component of their problem. When on the left side, it may mimic angina or a myocardial infarction.

Physical examination is most important, not only to achieve positive diagnosis, but also to eliminate other conditions that may be confused with thoracic outlet syndrome. The cervical spine should be carefully evaluated, even though, characteristically, cervical radiculopathy is unusual in the C8 to T1 distribution. Nevertheless, when the symptoms are difficult to interpret, the cervical spine must be ruled out as a site of disease. There may be tenderness over the brachial plexus in the supraclavicular fossa, but this nonspecific finding may accompany either thoracic outlet compression or cervical radiculopathy.

Of the various provocative maneuvers used to elicit thoracic outlet compression, the overhead exercise test and Wright's maneuver are the most consistently positive. The first test is performed by having the patient, in the "hands-up" position, rapidly flex and extend the fingers. In susceptible individuals, this will produce cramping on the affected side within 30 seconds. In addition, placing the arm in the abducted and laterally rotated position will not only obliterate the pulse at the wrist, but also reproduce the symptoms. Lowering the arm to the side restores the pulses and alleviates the symptoms. The mere obliteration of a pulse with any of the provocative positions is not diagnostic of thoracic outlet syndrome, since a large percentage of young women can obliterate a pulse in some position of the arm. The reproduction of the symptoms is crucial. Sometimes they can be enhanced by neck rotation or by deep inspiration. The costoclavicular maneuver or military brace position will reproduce symptoms in patients whose costoclavicular interval has been narrowed, particularly if there has been a clavicle fracture. The classical "Adson maneuver" is performed by having the patient, with the arm dependent, rotate and hyperextend the neck and inspire. This has been the least positive maneuver.

The shoulder girdle must be carefully examined, including tests for instability of the glenohumeral joint. In addition, the finding of an increased venous pattern on the side of the lesion is presumptive evidence of venous hypertension and probable compression or thrombosis.

Manual muscle testing must include the intrinsic muscles of the hand. There may be just-perceptible atrophy of the hypothenar muscles and weakness of adduction of the little finger to the ring finger as the only motor deficit. Rarely, all of the intrinsics will be atrophic. Since the cutaneous distribution of the first thoracic nerve is the medial aspect of the forearm, this differentiates it from the distribution of the ulnar nerve.

Radiographs are essential in evaluation of thoracic outlet syndrome. It is most important to assess the lower cervical spine for the presence of adventitious ribs or long transverse processes at C7. Hypoplastic first ribs may also be seen, and sometimes there is confusion between a cervical rib and a hypoplastic rib, unless one is sure of the vertebral level. This involves being able to count from the atlas caudally to establish that one is, in fact, dealing with a cervical rib. The disc spaces, as well as the intervertebral foramina should be scanned and abnormalities noted. In the lateral view of patients with droopy shoulders, one may be able to clearly define the second dorsal vertebra. These patients may resemble those with thoracic outlet syndrome but have no peripheral signs or symptoms in the limbs.[22]

It is important to examine radiographically the apices of both lungs, with apical lordotic views if necessary, to rule out tumors that can mimic thoracic outlet syndrome. A radiograph of the ipsilateral shoulder should be obtained in those patients who have local findings such as instability of the glenohumeral joint.

Where there is significant concern about possible cervical radiculopathy, myelography may be indicated.

Noninvasive vascular studies have been advocated as a reliable diagnostic test for thoracic outlet syndrome. Because pulses can be positionally obliterated in many normal people, the studies must be interpreted with caution. In cases of intrinsic vascular disease, however, noninvasive studies can be extremely useful.

Arteriography and venography have very limited application to the diagnosis of thoracic outlet syndrome. Since the occlusion of arterial outflow with the position of the arm is common in asymptomatic individuals, an arteriogram adds little unless there is serious consideration of an aneurysm in the subclavian artery or intrinsic vascular disease. Patients with complete cervical ribs may have a significant incidence of aneurysms.[9] Therefore, in such patients, it is prudent to obtain arteriographic studies if the thoracic outlet will be explored through the axilla. Venography is useful in demonstrating thrombosis of the axillary or subclavian vein.

Although it has been claimed that measurement of the velocity of conduction of the ulnar nerve through the thoracic outlet could be used to make a diagnosis of thoracic outlet syndrome,[24,25] the experience of many workers[26] has failed to substantiate this claim. Nevertheless, reports from electrodiagnostic laboratories often indicate no evidence of thoracic outlet syndrome. Such reports should be disregarded, since the test is not of value in this situation. Where it is very useful, however, is in differential diagnosis, since conditions such as ulnar neuropathy at the elbow and carpal tunnel syndrome are readily identified by means of nerve conduction velocity determinations. The electromyographic examination is usually not markedly abnormal in patients with thoracic outlet syndrome unless there has been sufficient compression to have caused denervation. In such cases, it is often possible clinically to detect atrophy and weakness of the ulnar-innervated interosseous and hypothenar muscles. Other patients, however, show fibrillation potentials at rest in these muscles that appear clinically normal.

Because nerve conduction velocity determination is not a reliable means of assessing the proximal parts of the brachial plexus, and particularly those that lie within the thoracic outlet,[26] the use of somatosensory evoked potentials and F responses have received attention as a means of obtaining further objective evidence of neural dysfunction in order to make a diagnosis of thoracic outlet syndrome.[7] Their place has not yet been firmly established, and the diagnosis remains clinical.

The differential diagnosis of thoracic outlet syndrome is listed in Table 112-1.

The question of double crush syndrome and thoracic outlet syndrome is controversial. Carroll and Hurst[4] have written that the coexistence of thoracic outlet syndrome and carpal tunnel syndrome is rare if it exists at all. Nevertheless, patients are observed with well-demonstrated signs of both entities who require treatment. Ulnar neuropathy may coexist with thoracic outlet syndrome.[11] Patients may have hard-to-define combinations of signs and symptoms that appear to be the result of more than thoracic outlet syndrome, and in these cases, one must look for additional lesions to explain the entire picture. Failure to do so will result in failure of treatment.

CONSERVATIVE THERAPY

The general condition of patients with thoracic outlet syndrome varies enormously and, in many cases the symptoms have been present for months or years. Not uncommonly, such patients have been told that their symptoms are of emotional origin, or they have been subjected to unsuccessful conservative or operative treatment. Such patients require objective yet sympathetic evaluation, which may sometimes include psychologic consultation. Some of these patients are clinically depressed, and this has a very deleterious effect on posture, which aggravates the anatomic problem. If such is the case, the surgeon may, according to training and inclination, either treat with antidepressants, or refer for therapy. It is not rare to see patients whose thoracic outlet problems can be lessened by such measures, even though some may ultimately require surgery.

Because the general level of fitness in these patients is often poor, it is worthwhile to inquire about their level of physical activity. Often it is quite limited. Sometimes patients are afraid to exercise for fear of worsening the condition or they have

TABLE 112-1. DIFFERENTIAL DIAGNOSIS OF THORACIC OUTLET SYNDROME

1. Cervical radiculopathy
2. Carpal tunnel syndrome
3. Ulnar neuropathy
4. Brachial plexitis
5. Superior sulcus tumors
6. Coronary artery disease
7. Droopy shoulder syndrome

been so advised by their physicians. If patients have no other serious medical problems, an effort ought be made to mobilize them with whole body exercises. Probably the easiest generalized exercise for such patients is walking, since it does not usually cause much discomfort, although in some patients it may do so.

The problem of obesity can be extremely difficult to manage, since patients do not like to be told that they are overweight. Yet, excess soft tissue can place additional strain on the shoulders, particularly in women who have large breasts, which can aggravate thoracic outlet syndrome. In cases of gigantomastia, reduction mammoplasty as a first step in the treatment of very debilitating thoracic outlet syndrome may be successful. Kay[10] has reported on neurologic deficits with large breasts. The mechanism of thoracic outlet compression makes it likely that this is the locus of the problem. If weight reduction does not produce the desired alleviation of compression, the patient who does reduce will be easier and safer to operate on, especially through the axilla.

The most important part of the conservative management of thoracic outlet syndrome involves correction of those postural abnormalities that can be identified as contributing to the compression, and shoulder girdle strengthening exercises when it is determined that weakened muscles are a significant factor. Unfortunately, when one refers patients with thoracic outlet syndrome to a physical therapy department, it should be made clear to the therapist the genesis of the problem and the necessity of applying appropriate therapy. Very often, stretching and traction are used, which will actually worsen the symptoms. The patient must undergo a thorough analysis by a knowledgeable therapist and then an individual therapy program should be prescribed and monitored to avoid provocative maneuvers.[16]

Patients with significant shoulder girdle disorder may not tolerate the conservative program. Particularly in cases where there is anterior glenohumeral instability, the exercises will often prove provocative because they will tend to reproduce the subluxation. Such patients may be identified from the group of "dead arm syndromes."[12] In all likelihood, many patients with the diagnosis of dead arm syndrome owing to glenohumeral instability are really examples of thoracic outlet syndrome. If this is not recognized, the patients will continue to be symptomatic even if after shoulder repair. An interesting series of patients in whom these two entities co-existed was studied by Leffert and Gumley.[12]

In cases where an activity of daily living or employment seems to be related to symptoms of thoracic outlet syndrome, such activities should be modified, if possible. Overhead activities, carrying heavy loads, or the use of backpacks can be quite provocative to patients with compression within the thoracic outlet.

Conservative measures should be employed with periodic review of the progress or lack thereof, so that the condition does not drag on interminably. This is particularly important in patients whose cases are complicated by litigation, insurance, or workers' compensation. The clinician must attempt to be objective in interpretation of the symptoms, so patients are not unfairly deprived of the benefits of treatment. In addition to periodic reviews, there should be an ultimate time limit beyond which conservative therapy should be viewed as having failed if there is no positive response. One must then decide whether to advise surgery or acceptance of the status quo with hopes that the condition may improve with time.

OPERATIVE TREATMENT

Indications for Surgery

The failure of a carefully supervised program of postural re-education and muscle strengthening conservative treatment measures is the most general indication for surgery.

Patients with significant neurologic deficit, usually of the intrinsic muscles of the hand, but sometimes in the long flexors as well, almost never respond to conservative therapy. If they are subjected to surgery, however, they should know preoperatively that postoperative improvement in the power of the long flexors may actually increase the muscle imbalance in the fingers and cause clawing or make it worse. Such patients should be advised that they may require secondary hand reconstruction for the muscle imbalance if it occurs. For those who have significant sensory loss, the outlook is guarded and somewhat unpredictable.

Patients with impending or established gangrene in the hand are candidates for immediate surgery. Fortunately, they are rare and are usually not seen primarily by the orthopaedic surgeon, but more likely by vascular surgical services.

Probably the most problematic indication for surgery of the thoracic outlet is intractable pain. Only the patient can feel and describe the pain; the surgeon must be able to interpret these complaints appropriately. Constraints of daily routine, vocational or avocational adjustments, sleep disturbance, and history of analgesic usage are all important avenues of inquiry necessary to formulate a decision for surgery.

Because patients with thoracic outlet syndrome often have very complicated medical records, it is important to review the differential diagnosis very carefully before proceeding. The surgeon should discuss with the patient and family the mechanics and objectives of surgery. It is mandatory that all possible complications be explained in detail so that the patient can give an informed consent. If the surgeon senses that a second opinion would be useful, it is essential that the surgeon rendering this opinion have sufficient surgical experience in the area to provide a valid opinion.

If an obese patient has made little attempt to lose weight despite specific instructions, that can be viewed as an indication of poor cooperation. Such patients are told that their surgery is elective and will not be done until they demonstrate genuine evidence of being willing or able to participate in their rehabilitation.

All patients are informed that they will require four units of blood prepared for the operating room. For those who desire autologous blood, donation will have to be sufficiently in advance so that it can be processed and frozen. Because this blood must be thawed prior to surgery, the blood bank should be informed that the patient is going to require the blood on an emergency basis, or not at all. The processing must, therefore, have been completed by the time the surgery begins.

If desired, a vascular or general thoracic surgeon may participate in the procedure. Although the vast majority of cases

are completed without need for such assistance, it is valuable to ensure that such help is available if needed on an emergency basis. For patients who have particular problems such as reoperative surgeries in which complications can be anticipated, consultants may be invited to participate at the beginning of the case. In addition, the operating team should be experienced and adequate in number. Surgery by the axillary route requires three assistants.

Finally, proper instruments must be available and verified as being in working order prior to the skin incision. Vascular and thoracic surgical instrument packs are present in the room should they be needed.

Anesthesia for surgery of the thoracic outlet requires that the patient be completely relaxed if the transaxillary route is used. The newer, short-acting muscle relaxants are particularly well suited to this situation. It is helpful to discuss the time frame for the surgery with the anesthetist prior to commencing surgery so that muscular relaxation may be reversed by the time the incision is closed, thus allowing extubation without delay.

The Surgical Procedures

There is no universal agreement as to which surgical procedure is best for the treatment of thoracic outlet syndrome. Although, historically, scalenotomy was the first procedure to gain favor,[1,2] its anatomic rationale was that the pathologic degeneration resided entirely between the scalene muscles. Release of the anterior scalene should have permanently cured the condition. Unfortunately, the incidence of recurrence following scalenotomy was sufficiently high that other procedures were required.[5] Many workers have considered the first rib to be the common denominator of compression and have concentrated their efforts on means of eliminating it, as well as adventitious ribs or congenital bands that might be encountered in the course of exploration.[6] Roos[19] reported his experience with the transaxillary first rib resection. This has probably been the most often performed operative procedure and as the mainstay of the surgical approach to the problem, will be described in detail. However, a variety of anatomic approaches may be employed for exploration of the thoracic outlet and removal of the first rib. They are listed in Table 112-2.

Claviculectomy may occasionally be required because of malunited or ununited fractures of the clavicle with significant reduction in the costoclavicular interval due to fracture angulation or hypertrophic subclavicular callus. Considerable effort ought to be expended toward retention of the bone if it does not materially increase the risks of the operative procedure. The enthusiasm for claviculectomy for uncomplicated thoracic

TABLE 112-2. ANATOMICAL APPROACHES TO THE THORACIC OUTLET AND FIRST RIB

1. Supraclavicular
2. Transclavicular
3. Subclavicular
4. Axillary
5. Posterior
6. Interpectoral
7. Combined

outlet compression[13] has been very limited, and it is not recommended.

The use of scalenectomy in the treatment of the thoracic outlet syndrome depends on the state of local anatomy. Although it is desirable to avoid reattachment of the scalenes to the bed of the first rib after if it has been resected, I do not routinely resect a portion of the anterior and middle scalenes because of the possibility of injury to branches of the brachial plexus that may actually pass through the muscles. For patients in whom there has been a recurrence caused by scarring within the scalene muscles themselves, one must make a decision whether or not to excise the scarred muscle, with full knowledge of the anatomic variations of the brachial plexus and the possibility that the nerves may be injured. The nerve to the serratus anterior is particularly vulnerable, since it may not always be located lateral to the middle scalene. It may pierce the muscle or even present as two branches which must be gently retracted and preserved.

The Transaxillary Approach[17–20]

The patient, under general endotracheal anesthesia, is placed on the operating table in the lateral decubitus position with the head tilted up. The surgeon faces the patient's back. Position a high standing stool obliquely at the head of the table near the surgeon so that a sterilely gowned assistant may maintain the arm abducted during the procedure. This assistant is able to lower the arm or change its position as required, lest a brachial plexus injury occur from excessive traction, such as might occur if the arm were suspended from the ceiling. Two other scrubbed assistants are necessary, one on either side of the table, to retract the latissimus dorsi and pectoralis major muscles during the course of the procedure. The draping permits movement of the arm as well as access to the upper hemithorax, axilla, shoulder area, and neck.

Make the skin incision transversely between the pectoralis major and latissimus dorsi muscles over the third interspace, just below the axillary hairline. Take care in the female not to prolong the incision onto the breast, since this can cause a hypertrophic scar. Spread self-retaining retractors horizontally in the wound to dissect the fat and render the tissues temporarily ischemic. This eliminates the ligation of superficial vessels. Incise the fascia longitudinally just posterior to the midline, to avoid the intercostobrachial nerve, and then spread it bluntly with the fingers. Carry dissection down through the subcutaneous tissues to the level of the ribcage. Retract the latissimus and pectoralis muscles.

It is imperative that the operator use a headlight or lighted retractors, since overhead lights will not provide sufficient illumination to perform the surgery safely. Dissection is done bluntly with the fingers, by touch, until the surface of the first rib can be palpated. The assistant elevates the arm obliquely to open the outlet. Two vascular structures are usually encountered at this stage of the procedure, each a branch of the subclavian artery and vein, respectively. They should be ligated under direct vision with nonabsorbable sutures or malleable clips. I tend not to use clips because of the possibility of dislodging them during the course of the procedure. These small vessels should not be cauterized because control would be difficult if they were to bleed.

Attention is then turned to identification of the important structures in the field (Fig. 112-1). The anterior scalene muscle attaches to the scalene tubercle, which is located on the inner border of the first rib rather than on its cephalic surface, although occasionally it may extend over to it. Blunt dissection with a small wad of gauze or "palm" will delineate the muscle from the adjacent subclavian artery and vein. Deaver retractors, each held by an assistant on either side of the table, retract the muscles. The most anterior structure in the wound will be the subclavius muscle and its insertion to the superior surface of the first rib. Just behind and adjacent to it is the subclavian vein. The surface of the first rib anterior to the middle scalene muscle may be cleared of its soft tissues by means of a blunt periosteal elevator (Fig. 112-2) and dissecting sponges.

At this stage of the procedure, visualization is limited by the middle scalene, which can be elevated off the first rib with the elevator. It is tempting to divide this muscle sharply at its insertion, but the possibility of injury to branches of the brachial plexus, particularly the nerve to the serratus anterior, make this inadvisable. As the muscle is elevated, it can also be partially retracted by means of the Deaver retractor. Using a rasp (see Fig. 112-2) with a cutting edge that conforms to the outer curvature of the first rib, separate the soft tissues from the bone. Sometimes the first digitation of the serratus anterior muscle may overlap the insertion of the middle scalene on the first rib, and this must be bluntly separated with care. By alternating the rasp, the periosteal elevator and gauze sponges, it is possible to clear the surface of the rib of its muscle attachments. The undersurface should be similarly cleared, although it is not desirable to perform the entire dissection subperiosteally because of the possibility of regrowth of the rib, particularly in young patients. The periosteum must be disrupted, and removed, if possible. This may result in a tear in the adjacent pleura, causing a pneumothorax. During this maneuver, it is advisable to ask the anesthetist to control respirations so that the lung is retracted from the pleura in exhalation. About 30 sec of apnea are usually required. Following this, controlled

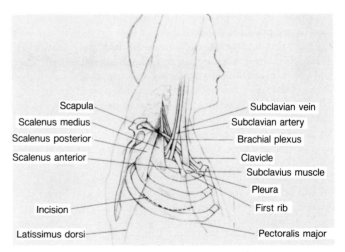

FIGURE 112-1. The anatomy of the right thoracic outlet from the axillary view with the upper extremity and shoulder elevated. (Roos, D.B.: Experience with First Rib Resection for Thoracic Outlet Syndrome. Ann. Surg. **173**:429–442, 1971.)

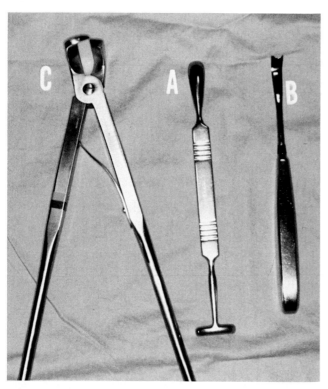

FIGURE 112-2.   Instruments for transaxillary first rib resection. (*A*) Periosteal elevator. (*B*) Rasp for first rib. (*C*) Roos rib cutter.

respiration may be resumed, and the integrity of the pleura may be tested by flooding the wound with normal saline. If the pleura has been breached, there will be air bubbles with respiration, or the fluid will simply funnel down into the pleural cavity. If there is a pneumothorax, one has the option of either draining it by means of a soft rubber catheter at wound closure or inserting a chest tube. Usually a 26 chest tube can be inserted below the incision and into the rent in the pleura without difficulty. It is then connected to underwater seal and suction. A pneumothorax does not significantly prejudice the remainder of the operative procedure, and the tube can be placed just prior to closure.

Turn attention then to the superior surface of the first rib so that the anterior scalene may be defined and detached. The phrenic nerve is not at risk during this maneuver, since it is located at least 2 cm cephalad to the tubercle. Using gentle, blunt dissection, tease the subclavian artery and vein away from the anterior scalene. Since the pleura may rise posteriorly and be adherent to the posterior surface of the muscle, it is helpful to use a long, right-angle clamp to dissect behind the muscle and to shield each vessel in turn as, alternately, half of the muscle is cut sharply at its insertion to the bone. Obviously, all of this is done very carefully under direct vision. When the muscle has been cut, it retracts.

Next, address the tendon of the subclavius muscle. Make an incision at the insertion onto the bone, which covers the superior surface of the rib. The subclavian vein must constantly be kept under direct vision because it is immediately subjacent to the tendon and at significant risk. Once the plane of dissection has been established, however, it is possible to use the perios-

teal elevator and direct it away from the vein as the tendon is elevated from the rib. Failure to accomplish this part of the procedure properly will cause the line of section of the rib to lie at the level of the subclavian vein, where a sharp edge of bone will adhere to it.

Having detached all of the important soft tissue from the first rib, thoroughly explore the outlet for the presence of fibrous bands that are radiographically invisible but which may be quite significant in causing compression of the neurovascular structures. At no time during the dissection should the neurovascular structures themselves be retracted with any considerable tension because of the very real possibility of injury. By positioning the arm appropriately, it is possible to lift the structures off the surface of the rib so that a retractor should not be necessary.

In addition to fibrous bands of various types,[21] other important variations in the local anatomy can be observed. For example, the anterior scalene may actually be overlapped in its insertion by the middle scalene. There may be additional vascular branches, or the presence of a cervical rib. A complete cervical rib may actually attach to the manubrium, but a lesser one may reach to the scalene tubercle. This will make dissection considerably more difficult, but a supraclavicular counterincision should not be required to remove the rib. The rib may have to be removed piecemeal with rongeurs rather than being resectable by means of two neat cuts using rib cutters. This, of course, adds to the time necessary for the procedure, as well as its difficulty. Once the anatomy is clear, a decision is made as to which instruments will be used to remove the rib.

In the ideal case, a rib cutter can be placed posterior to the lower trunk of the brachial plexus, almost to the level of the transverse process, and the rib can be cut at that level. If a straight rib cutter is used, however, the resulting osteotomy will be oblique, leaving a very sharp point on the posterior portion of rib. This is most undesirable. For that reason, most operators have use the rib cutter designed by Roos (see Fig. 112-2), which produces a transverse cut, owing to the inclination of its cutting surfaces. When used on the left side, introduce the rib cutter with its point facing upward, hooking it beneath the rib and closing the jaws before it can be slid posteriorly. For a rib on the right side, the point will face caudad, where it could tear the pleura. In either case, the jaws should be almost closed and under direct vision, so that they can be slid beneath the neurovascular structures and posterior to them. During this period, the anesthetist should maintain apnea in expiration. After verifying that nothing has been caught in the jaws of the rib cutter, firmly close the blades and cut the rib. Then gently slide the instrument forward and open it in the reverse manner in which it was inserted.

Grasp the rib with a Kocher forceps and visualize the anterior attachment to cartilage. Using a standard rib cutter with its blades pointed away from the subclavian vein, divide the rib and gently remove it from the wound. A subtotal resection is completed with at least 2 cm of space behind the lower trunk of the brachial plexus, which means that in most patients, there will be 2 cm or less of posterior rib fragment, measuring from the transverse process. Anteriorly, the line of resection should be medial to the subclavian vein.

At this point in the procedure, retest the integrity of the pleura. There should be complete hemostasis. Digitally explore the outlet and place the patient's arm in all positions to assess whether there is any compression of the neurovascular structures. Usually there is not, although if the second rib is very prominent, it could cause compression. This can be relieved by removal of its middle third.

If there is a pneumothorax, insert a chest tube at this point and then prepare for closure. Antibiotics are given if there has been a pleural leak, but not in an otherwise uncomplicated case.

The arm, which has been intermittently raised and lowered by the assistant, is now returned to the side. No drains are used nor should they be needed. Complete a subcutaneous closure, followed by a subcuticular closure using nonabsorbable suture, which is removed at 2 weeks postoperatively. Apply a small dressing and place the arm in a sling.

Anterior Approaches to the Thoracic Outlet

Anterior approaches to the structures within the thoracic outlet have been advised for resection of cervical ribs, scalenotomy,[1] and resection of the first thoracic rib.[14,15] They provide adequate exposure but allow only limited visualization for subtotal resection of the first rib (Fig. 112-3).

The supraclavicular approach was advocated by Adson[1,2,3] for scalenotomy and resection of cervical ribs. It has the advantage of allowing relatively easy access to the anterior scalene muscle and the vessels.

Make a 7- to 9-cm incision 1 to 2 cm above and parallel to the clavicle, extending from the midpoint of the clavicular attachment of the sternomastoid muscle to the anterior edge of the trapezius. Identify the platysma muscle for later, careful reapproximation. The external jugular vein must usually be ligated. For ease of exposure, carefully divide approximately 50% of the sternomastoid anteriorly, just above its insertion; 1

to 2 cm of trapezius may have to be similarly cut. Divide the omohyoid muscle at its midpoint. The suprascapular and transverse cervical vessels run horizontally and must usually be ligated. Identify the phrenic nerve on the surface of the anterior scalene muscle as it proceeds distally. Carefully retract and preserve it. Detach the anterior scalene muscle and allow it to retract. If scalenectomy is done, carefully inspect the muscle to determine whether any of the branches of the brachial plexus pass through it. In order to detach the muscle safely, carefully dissect the subclavian artery away from it, and the pleura posteriorly. Mobilize the subclavian artery in its extra-adventitial plane and retract it medially, while retracting the brachial plexus laterally. If a cervical rib is present, remove it from its periosteal envelope and resect it. Remove as much of the periosteum as possible. Elevate the middle scalene off the first rib, which then is removed. Using this approach, access to the posterior portion of the first rib is limited, for which reason I do not favor it.

The transclavicular approach should be reserved for postoperative recurrences of thoracic outlet compression in which adherence of the subclavian artery or vein to the anterior edge of the resected rib are strongly suspected.

The subclavicular approach[8] employs a 7-cm skin incision made over the cartilage of the first rib, midway between the clavicle and second rib. Split the pectoralis major in the line of its fibers, exposing the cartilage of the first rib. Open the periosteum of the anterior portion of the first rib with a scissors, and carry out further blunt dissection with a finger or gauze. After the costochondral junction is divided, remove the cartilage with a rongeur. The rib may then be grasped and levered, either caudally or cephalad, for stripping of the anterior and middle scalene muscles. A rasp may be used to further denude the rib, which may then be cut posteriorly with Sauerbruch rib shears.

The significant disadvantages of this exposure are that if any abnormalities of the first rib, including abnormal width or a cervical rib, are encountered, they are difficult to manage because of limited access. The presence of anomalous bands cannot be easily verified or dealt with, and the vessels must be constantly retracted and are at risk in an extremely confined space. Other than for access to the anterior portion of the first rib, this is not a useful incision.

Posterior Approach

The posterior approach is identical with that used for thoracoplasty.[5] Although it is considered a technique that does not involve any disability or disfigurement, it is an extensive approach that traverses the trapezius muscle, as well as the levator scapulae and rhomboids. For this reason, I believe it should be used infrequently, particularly in patients who already have weakness of these muscles and sagging shoulders, as well as those who must do heavy labor following convalescence.

However, the posterior approach is extremely useful for decompression of the thoracic outlet in patients who are extremely muscular or obese and in whom the axillary approach would be technically difficult. Furthermore, it is the preferred approach for reoperations in which a retained posterior segment of rib has become adherent to the brachial plexus and is causing symptoms.

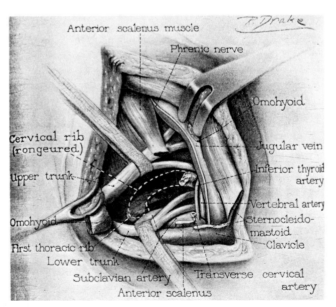

FIGURE 112-3. Anterior approach to the cervical rib. (Adson, A.W.: Cervical Ribs: Symptoms, Differential Diagnosis and Indications for Section of the Insertion of the Scalenus Anticus Muscle. J. Internat. Coll. Surg. **16**:546–559, 1951.)

The patient is placed in the lateral decubitus position, with the affected side up. The arm is prepped and draped free and the entire hemithorax posteriorly is draped past the midline, including the neck to the hairline.

Make a long incision, extending from the superior angle of the scapula, 2 cm medial to its vertebral border, for the length of the bone. An incision too close to the scapula will encounter the anastomotic scapular vessels, causing annoying bleeding. Section the trapezius, levator scapulae, and both rhomboids, taking care to avoid the spinal accessory nerve and dorsal scapular nerve. Introduce a scapular retractor beneath the scapula, which can then be retracted anteriorly and laterally (Fig. 112-4).

Identify the first rib from the level of its transverse process; the rib is not horizontal in most patients, and the second rib may partially obscure its visualization. The posterior scalene may blend with the middle scalene and is attached to the outer surface of the second rib. It is easily detached; then identify and carefully section the middle scalene, which inserts onto the superior surface of the first rib. Anterior to it, the lower trunk of the brachial plexus lies in contact with the rib, with the subclavian artery immediately anterior to it, restrained by the insertion of the anterior scalene to the scalene tubercle. The first digitation of the serratus anterior originates from the outer aspect of the first rib and can be freed with a rasp. The subclavian vein is, of course, anterior to the anterior scalene and must be carefully protected.

Remove the first rib. If a cervical rib is present, it can be easily removed through the same incision. However, it is not possible to deal with a subclavian aneurysm through this approach. Although the rib is resected subperiosteally to protect the adjacent structures, as much of the periosteum as possible should be subsequently removed or displaced to prevent regeneration of the bone.

If a pneumothorax has been produced, insert a chest tube.

Perform closure in layers, taking care to approximate anatomically the very important suspensory muscles of the scapula, including the levator scapulae, rhomboids, and trapezius. The patient is placed in a sling for 3 weeks postoperatively and then shoulder girdle strengthening exercises are begun.

POSTOPERATIVE CARE AND REHABILITATION

In uncomplicated exploration and decompression of the thoracic outlet by the axillary route, there is minimal blood loss and physiologic disturbance. Although there may be moderate postoperative pain, within a day most patients are sufficiently comfortable to move about without the support of a sling for the arm.

If a pleural tear has occurred intraoperatively, then a chest tube is used for 24 hours.

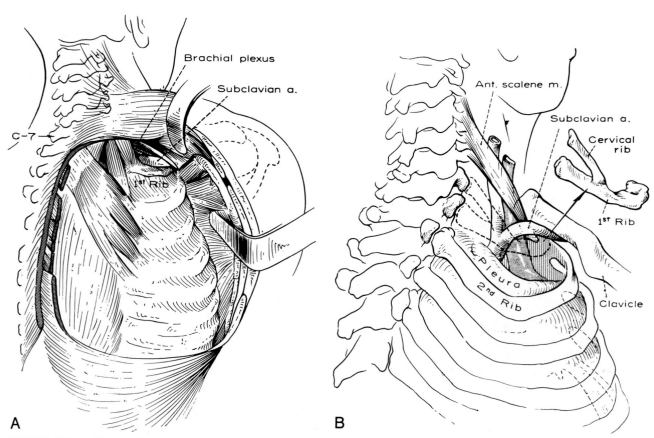

A **B**

FIGURE 112-4. *(A)* Posterior approach for resection of the first thoracic rib. *(B)* A cervical rib has been removed with the first thoracic rib. (Clagett, O.T.: Presidential Address: Research and Prosearch. J. Thorac. Cardiovasc. Surg. **44**:153–166, 1962.)

Most patients are discharged from the hospital on the third or fourth postoperative day.

Within 48 hours of surgery, the dressing may be reduced to a single layer of gauze or removed altogether. Patients are instructed that they may shower as long as the wound is kept dry, and underarm deodorants and powders are prohibited until the sutures are removed.

Patients are advised that they may be active at home, but they are cautioned against heavy lifting or any strenuous activities for 4 weeks after surgery. Then they are advised to resume their preoperative exercise program, if there is significant postural abnormality or weakness of the scapular muscles.

COMPLICATIONS AND PITFALLS

Inadequate Resection

Inadequate resection of the first rib usually results from operator inexperience or timidity. Failure to resect the subclavius tendon anteriorly will produce a line of section of the first rib at the level of the subclavian vein that will then adhere and cause symptoms of venous compression. Because the vein is a thin-walled and easily-torn structure, reoperation is hazardous. It is best performed, if necessary, by the transclavicular route.

Failure to resect sufficient rib posteriorly to clear the lower trunk of the brachial plexus by 2 cm is most common with an anterior approach, but may also occur with a transaxillary procedure. In most cases less than 2 cm of rib should remain from the level of the transverse process, but it is not necessary to disarticulate the rib. If recurrence is thought due to adherence of the lower trunk of the plexus to the rib remnant, this problem is best approached through a posterior, high thoracoplasty approach. The hazards of this procedure stem from the difficulty of separating the periosteum and scar from the nervous structures, which must be carefully defined and lysed while the rib remnant is removed. Preliminary resection of the second rib is an aid to the dissection, which then proceeds to the bed of the first rib with a wider and clearer field.

Pneumothorax

Because an intact periosteal sleeve can result in regeneration of a resected rib, particularly in a young patient, it is advantageous to remove or displace as much of the periosteum as possible. The close adherence of the pleura, however, makes rents in this filmy structure common during the course of the dissection. Since the pleura cannot be directly repaired, either a rubber catheter may be used to drain the pleural cavity during closure and then withdrawn, or a chest tube may be placed through a separate stab wound and connected to underwater suction for 24 hours. Then, after a radiograph confirms the absence of a pneumothorax, the tube may be removed.

Intercostobrachial Neuralgia

The intercostobrachial nerve passes from the chest into the subcutaneous tissues of the arm and innervates the posterior brachium in many patients, down to the level of the olecranon. Since it is located at the midpoint of the axillary incision made over the third interspace, it is liable to injury, either by lacera-tion or traction. If the fascial incision is made perpendicular to the skin incision and somewhat posterior to the midline, injury is less likely. Nevertheless, in many cases, there is some transient numbness along the posterior aspect of the arm, which gradually fades with time. If the nerve is cut, however, the patient may experience very annoying dysesthesia, which can be permanent. Prevention is the best means of dealing with the problem. If there is a neuroma, local nerve blocks may be of some value.

Brachial Plexus Injury

This is the most serious non–life-threatening complication of thoracic outlet surgery. Occasional patients are seen with varying degrees of neural dysfunction in excess of what was present preoperatively. The patient who has increased postoperative loss of intrinsic function in the hand and numbness of the little and ring fingers may have sustained either a direct laceration of the lower trunk or a traction injury. In the first situation, repair is impossible and no improvement is expected. In the second, there is usually little spontaneous recovery. This complication can be avoided by gentle handling of the nerves with minimal or no direct retraction.

The patient who awakens from surgery with numbness of the entire arm and significant motor weakness not present preoperatively has sustained a traction injury to the brachial plexus, which usually results from excessive pull on the arm during the surgery. This complication can result in permanent neurologic loss and pain, and can largely be avoided by carefully monitoring the amount of intraoperative traction. During the procedure, arm traction must be periodically lessened so that a constant pull is not maintained.

Long Thoracic Nerve Injury

Local injury to the nerve on the chest wall or as it comes around or through the middle scalene can result in permanent winging of the scapula owing to paralysis of the serratus anterior. The nerve should be sought and, if identified, carefully protected. Sometimes, separate branches to the digitations of the serratus anterior are seen, in which case these must be preserved. This complication weakens the ability to lift the arm in front of the plane of the body.

Vascular Injury

The subclavian artery and vein are clearly at risk in any procedure within the thoracic outlet. The surgeon must have available appropriate technical ability or surgical assistance for all eventualities. As stated, appropriate instruments must be present in the room, as should four units of blood before the surgery is begun, and the sterile field should be draped to allow additional procedures, including thoracotomy, if necessary.

REFERENCES

1. Adson, A.W., and Caffey, J.R.: Cervical Rib. A Method of Anterior Approach for Relief of Symptoms by Division of the Scalenus Anterior. Ann. Surg. **85**:839, 1927.

2. Adson, A.W.: Surgical Treatment for Symptoms Produced by Cervical Ribs and the Scalenus Anticus Muscle. Surg. Gynecol. Obstet. **85**:687–700, 1947.

3. Adson, A.W.: Cervical Ribs: Symptoms, Differential Diagnosis and Indications for Section of the Insertion of the Scalenus Anticus Muscle. J. Internat. Coll. Surg. **16**:546–559, 1951.

4. Carroll, R.E., and Hurst, L.C.: The Relationship of Thoracic Outlet Syndrome and Carpal Tunnel Syndrome. Clin. Orthop. Rel. Res. **164**:149, 1982.

5. Clagett, O.T.: Presidential Address: Research and Prosearch. J. Thorac. Cardiovasc. Surg. **44**:153–166, 1962.

6. Falconer, M.A., and Li, F.W.P.: Resection of the First Rib in Costoclavicular Compression of the Brachial Plexus. Lancet **1**:59, 1962.

7. Glover, J.L., Worth, R.M., and Bendick, P.J.: Evoked Responses in the Diagnosis of Thoracic Outlet Syndrome. Surgery **89**:86–93, 1981.

8. Hamlin, H., and Pecora, D.: Subclavicular Segmental Resection of First Rib for Correction of Subjacent Neurovascular Compression. Am. J. Surg. **117**:757, 1969.

9. Judy, K.L., and Heymann, R.L.: Vascular Complications of Thoracic Outlet Syndrome. Am. J. Surg. **123**:521–531, 1972.

10. Kay, B.L.: Neurological Changes with Excessively Large Breasts. South. Med. J. **65**:177, 1972.

11. Leffert, R.D.: Anterior Transposition of the Ulnar Nerves by the Learmonth Technique. J. Hand Surg. **7**:147–155, 1982.

12. Leffert, R.D., and Gumley, G.: Dead Arm Syndrome and Thoracic Outlet Syndrome. Orthop. Trans. J. Bone Joint Surg. **9**:44, 1985.

13. Lord, J.W.: Thoracic Outlet Syndromes: Current Management. Ann. Surg. **173**:700, 1971.

14. Nelson, R.M., and Jenson, C.B.: Anterior Approach for Excision of the First Rib. Ann. Thorac. Surg. **9**:1, 1970.

15. Peet, R.M., Hendricksen, J.D., Guderson, T.P., and Martin, G.M.: Thoracic Outlet Syndrome: Evaluation of a Therapeutic Exercise Program. Proc. Mayo Clin. **31**:281, 1956.

16. Rob, C.G., and Standeven, A.: Arterial Occlusion Complicating Thoracic Outlet Syndrome. Br. Med. J. **2**:709, 1958.

17. Roos, D.B.: Transaxillary Approach to the First Rib to Relieve Thoracic Outlet Syndrome. Ann. Surg. **163**:354, 1966.

18. Roos, D.B., and Owens, J.C.: Thoracic Outlet Syndrome. Arch. Surg. **93**:71–4, 1966.

19. Roos, D.B.: Experience with First Rib Resection for Thoracic Outlet Syndrome. Ann. Surg. **173**:429–442, 1971.

20. Roos, D.B.: Congenital Anomalies Associated with Thoracic Outlet Syndrome. Anatomy, Symptoms, Diagnosis and Treatment. Am. J. Surg. **132**:771–8, 1976.

21. Swift, T.R., and Nichols, F.T.: The Droopy Shoulder Syndrome. Neurology **34**:212–215, 1984.

22. Telford, E.D., and Stopford, J.S.B.: The Vascular Complications of Cervical Rib. Br. J. Surg. **18**:557, 1931.

23. Todd, T.W.: The Descent of the Shoulder after Birth. Anatomischer Anzeiger Centralblatt fur die Gesamte Wissenschaftlichje Anatomie **14**:41, 1912.

24. Urschel, H.C., Paulson, D.L., and MacNamara, J.J.: Thoracic Outlet Syndrome. Ann. Thoracic. Surg. **6**:1, 1968.

25. Urschel, H.C., and Rossuk, M.: Management of Thoracic Outlet Syndrome. N. Engl. J. Med. **286**:1140, 1972.

26. Wilbourn, A.J., Lederman, R.J.: Evidence for Conduction Delay in Thoracic-Outlet Syndrome is Challenged. N. Engl. J. Med. **310**:1052–1053, 1984.

CHAPTER 113

Surgical Treatment of the Upper Extremity in Cerebral Palsy

F. WILLIAM BORA, JR.,
and GARY A. MILLER

Cerebral palsy is a nonprogressive perinatal disorder characterized by cognitive, sensory, and motor problems. Some 300,000 children in the United States are affected.[2] The disease is classified on the basis of the observed motor deficit. Spasticity (paraplegia, hemiplegia, and monoplegia) involves abnormal tone. Spastic hemiplegia accounts for about one-third of cerebral palsy cases.[20] Motion disorders include extrapyramidal (athetosis, dystonia) and atonic forms of cerebral palsy in which variations in tone are markedly affected by position and activity. Spasticity and motion disorders may occur together. Spastic patients have the best prognosis for improvement from surgery and orthotics. When a strong element of motion disturbance is present, the results of surgery are often unpredictable,[4,22] and a conservative attitude toward surgical reconstruction is appropriate for these patients.

EVALUATION

Many factors must be considered in planning upper extremity management. These include the patient's cognitive capacity, sensibility, motor disorders, emotional status, and social orientation. If the child denies the limb, it is unlikely he will ever use it despite the improvement gained through surgical reconstruction.[3,22]

Diagnosis

The diagnosis is difficult in the newborn, as the full picture of motor disturbance may not emerge for several years. Factors to be monitored are developmental milestones and disturbances in tone and symmetry, which may appear late in children with cerebral palsy. By 6 months, the Moro, grasp, and tonic neck reflexes should have disappeared, but they may persist in cerebral palsy. Limited spontaneous movement in the neonate should suggest the diagnosis. Increased resistance or lack of resistance to passive motion of the upper limb should also cause concern, particularly if asymmetrical. Affected infants are slow to develop balance and tend to show persistence of perinatal tone reflexes.

Handedness develops normally at about 18 to 24 months. Cerebral-palsied infants may develop hand preference early.[8] This is the result of poor function in the nondominant limb.

By 1 year the normal child has developed pinch. Hand placement by shoulder and elbow control develops at this time. Selective muscle control develops more slowly in the cerebral-palsied child. Thumb opposition develops only in mild cases. Hand placement may be limited by contracture and motion disturbances. As the child grows, sensory and cognitive defects appear and help establish the diagnosis.

Cognition

Cognition includes the processes which indicate intelligence: perception, abstract thinking, and communication. Learning problems are significant in many patients with cerebral palsy, and at least 50% are mentally retarded.[2] A specific intelligence level has not been established as a prerequisite for operative treatment of the upper extremity. In general, only those patients with educable (50–70 I.Q.) or higher cognitive ability can expect functional results from upper extremity surgery.[8] Some surgeons[4,7] maintain that surgery should not be considered in patients whose I.Q. is below 70, as such patients often do poorly. However, Samilson[21] has noted that standard tests of intelligence may be misleading due to the patient's significant motor impairment. The I.Q. should be considered in planning treatment, but should not be the sole determining factor.[2]

Sensibility

Surgical success depends greatly upon sensibility. Tachjdian has reported sensory defects in about 50% of patients with average intelligence.[26] Sensation mediated by thalamic activity, such as light touch and temperature, is usually normal in the patient with spastic hemiparesis. The sensory defects most often affect the cortical functions of stereognosis, position sense, and two-point discrimination.[18] The deficits are due to parietal lobe lesions.

Sensory examination is very difficult in children under age 3 or 4. Some information is gained by observing the child's play. Stereognosis is assessed by having the child close his eyes and raise his hands over his head[6] while identifying and describing the characteristics of objects placed in each hand. If appropriate, two-point discrimination and proprioception are determined. Hoffer[8] considers sensibility to be normal when 5 of 5 objects are identified correctly, graphesthesia is accurate, or two-point discrimination is less than 5 mm. Sensibility is mildly impaired when only 3 of 5 objects are identified, or two-point discrimination is 5 to 10 mm. Moderate to severe impairment applies to hands with greater limitations.

Patients with abnormal sensibility do not gain much from surgery. Prehension requires good proprioception and stereognosis, and may not be an appropriate goal for the hand with poor sensibility. Green[7] has shown that the results of surgery correlate with stereognosis. The patient who exhibits poor stereognosis may exclude the abnormal extremity from use. Such children often have a distorted body image. These patients generally do not benefit from reconstructive surgery.

Motor Examination

The child is examined on several occasions and in different settings to evaluate ability to grasp and release, reach for and transfer objects. The child is observed at play, at specific tasks, while performing activities of daily living, and after periods of stretching.[22] Functional tasks include dressing, toileting, feeding, and side pinch. The activity must be assessed in different settings and at varied table levels because the position of the shoulder and trunk may greatly affect hand function.[22] Hoffer[8] emphasizes the importance of hand placement in planning treatment. The patient is requested to touch the head and then the opposite knee. Performance of this exercise within 5 sec demonstrates good function and, according to Hoffer, is a favorable prognostic sign.

If the patient is able to cooperate, voluntary muscle testing is performed and the individual muscles graded. The observer must judge whether a deficit in muscle function is due to paresis or to overactivity of antagonist muscles. Observe the pa-

tient's use of the more normal hand to position and open the fingers of the other hand for grasp. Joint contractures, spasticity of muscle-tendon units, and increased tone are determined by passive testing. Contracture of the flexor digitorum superficialis, for example, may explain the patient's need to flex the wrist before release.[4] Excess finger flexor tone can be distinguished from wrist flexor tone by testing wrist extension with the fingers passively flexed.

Nerve blocks may aid in distinguishing tone from contracture. For example, it may be difficult to assess the strength of wrist and finger extensors with the wrist held in flexion. Blocking the median and ulnar nerves at the elbow will identify joint contractures, permit evaluation of extensors, and determine if deformity is secondary to increased tone or fixed muscle-tendon contractures.[8] Measurement of the range of motion before and after nerve block determines the need for release of soft tissue and contracture.

The best motors for tendon transfer are those strong muscles under good voluntary control that are phasic with the activity for which transfer is planned.[2] Goldner[4] believes repeated observation of the patient's hand in grasp and release permits determination of phasic activity. Hoffer[9] and others have advocated dynamic electromyography for this purpose. Hoffer[8] contends that a muscle will not change in phasic activity following transfer. Muscles in phase for specific activities will be functional. Muscles active only in release and not grasp, for example, will be effective if transferred to finger extensors. Those muscles active only during grasp are good transfers for wrist extension. Muscles which fire continuously are not candidates for transfer according to Hoffer.[8] Other authors[21] have observed such muscles becoming phasic after transfer. This issue is not yet resolved, and the role of dynamic electromyography remains controversial. Although acknowledging its potential, we do not rely on this technique in planning treatment.

Overall Assessment

It is essential to assess cognitive, sensory, motor, and psychosocial elements in planning management. The overall severity of involvement must be recognized. Green and Banks[7] have devised a grading system for evaluating patients, and this has been modified by Samilson and Morris.[21] An excellent grade denotes the following: good function in activities of daily living, effective grasp and release, excellent control, wrist extension of 45° or more, full active finger extension, and active supination of 50° or more. A grade of good is given to hands used as helpers in activities of daily living, have effective grasp and release with good control, have wrist extension of 15° to 45°, and can actively extend the fingers with the wrist extended. A fair grade denotes hands used as helpers but not effective in dressing, moderate grasp, and release with fair control. A poor grade refers to hands used only as paper weight, with poor or absent grasp and release, poor control, and no finger extension unless the wrist is in maximum flexion.

It is very important to assess the patient's and the family's motivation. Surgery is of value only when the patient and parents are committed to attaining realistic goals. The surgeon should make clear to the parents that a normal extremity will not be the outcome, but that worthwhile improvements in function and cosmesis may result.[22]

Aims of Treatment

Patients may have deficits in function, cosmesis, and hygiene. The spastic hemiparetic patient with reasonable intelligence, good sensibility, motivation, and appropriate parental support should have a good functional extremity as a goal. Planned procedures in such patients have predictable results.[3] Retarded patients with poor sensibility should undergo procedures directed toward improvement of hygiene and prevention of skin maceration.[18] Improvement of cosmesis and hygiene are goals for patients with reasonable intelligence but other limiting factors. Diminished sensibility and voluntary control are not contraindications to surgical treatment, although the expectations are less in such patients.[4]

Age and Timing of Surgery

The patterns of deformity may change during the first several years of life. While the patient's age is only one of the factors to be evaluated before an operation, surgery generally should not be performed before the motor pattern becomes established. In order to prevent deformity and rejection of the extremity, however, surgery should not be overly delayed.

During the first few years, most patients are managed by resting or night splints to preserve thumb abduction, wrist and digital extension, and forearm supination. By age 4 the pattern of persistent deformity becomes evident, and children may become candidates for operative treatment. The optimal time for tendon transfers is between ages 5 and 12 years.[2]

SURGICAL TREATMENT

The most common deformities of the upper extremity appear in Table 113-1. Treatment of the proximal part of the extremity should be carried out before that of the hand. In general, begin with capsulotomies, tenotomies, and tendon lengthenings to correct deformities, proceed to tendon transfers, and conclude with arthrodesis of joints where necessary.

Shoulder

Adduction–Internal Rotation

Adduction–internal rotation is the most common shoulder deformity. It results from spasticity and contracture of the subscapularis and pectoralis major. Internal rotation contracture limits the positioning of the upper extremity and may be managed by passive stretching exercises. For the resistant deformity, subscapularis and pectoralis major lengthening or release is recommended. If the deformity persists, humeral osteotomy may be necessary.

Subscapularis/Pectoralis Major Lengthening Procedure.[4] We prefer a deltopectoral approach, although the procedure may be performed through an axillary incision. Make a longitudinal incision from the coracoid to the border of the pectoralis major insertion (Fig. 113-1A). Identify the deltopectoral groove and develop the interval between the deltoid and pectoralis major (Fig. 113-1B). Protect the cephalic vein.

TABLE 113-1. COMMON DEFORMITIES OF THE UPPER EXTREMITY

	Deformity	Procedure
Shoulder	Adduction–internal rotation	Subscapularis lengthening
		Rotational humeral osteotomy
	Abduction–external rotation	Deltoid recession
		Teres major / Infraspinatus lengthening
Elbow	Flexion	Flexor release
Forearm	Pronation	Flexor-pronator release
Wrist	Flexion	Flexor-pronator release
	Inadequate extension	Transfer FCU → ECRB
		Arthrodesis
Hand	Digital flexion	Z-Lengthening
	Inadequate metacarpophalangeal extension	Transfer FCU → EDC
	Swan-neck	Superficialis tenodesis
		PIP capsulorrhaphy
	Thumb-in-palm	Adductor pollicis myotomy
		Transfer BR → APL
		MCP capsulodesis
		MCP arthrodesis
		Web Z-plasty

Lengthen the subscapularis, bordered inferiorly by the anterior humeral circumflex veins, medially to the glenohumeral joint (Fig. 113-1C). For persistent deformity, release the subscapularis at its insertion into the humerus. If the tendon of the pectoralis major is tight, lengthen it by a stepcut incision. Postoperatively, immobilize the limb in 25° to 30° of abduction and 20° of external rotation for 4 to 6 weeks. Begin active assisted exercises to retain shoulder range of motion at 2 weeks.

More resistant deformities may require an external rotational osteotomy of the proximal humerus. The osteotomy is performed via an anterior approach and is held with crossed pins or with plate fixation.

Abduction–External Rotation

Abduction–external rotation is not commonly encountered.[4,8] Surgical release may be indicated, performed through a "strap" incision, permitting access to the deltoid and the spine of the scapula. Detach the fibers of the anterior two-thirds of the deltoid from their insertion into the humerus and recess the deltoid muscle. Do not disturb the insertion of the scapular portion of the deltoid. Perform a Z-lengthening of the tendons of teres major and infraspinatus. Immobilize the shoulder in a Velpeau bandage (reinforced with plaster) for 2 weeks. Begin active assisted and passive shoulder exercises, while maintaining the limb in a protective Velpeau dressing between exercise periods.

Elbow

Flexion Deformity

Elbow flexion deformity is common, but it is often mild and can be managed by passive stretching exercises. Occasionally, flex-

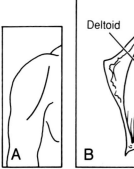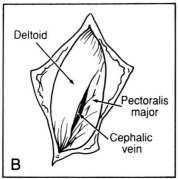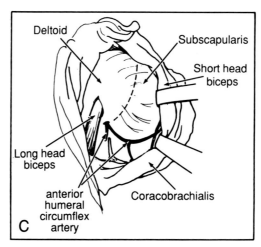

FIGURE 113-1. (*A*) Incision for subscapularis-pectoralis major lengthening. (*B*) Interval between deltoid and pectoralis major. (*C*) Lengthening of subscapularis. Care is taken to avoid the anterior humeral circumflex vessels.

ion contracture becomes sufficiently severe to compromise hygiene, limit reach, interfere with crutch use, and present functional limitations. Flexion deformity caused by contracture or spasticity is treated by biceps tendon lengthening, brachialis tenotomy, recession of the origins of the wrist flexors (excluding flexor digitorum profundus and superficialis), and, if necessary, anterior elbow joint capsulotomy. Preoperative musculocutaneous nerve block may be useful in distinguishing increased tone from contracture.[8] The surgeon must resist the temptation to release flexor muscle origins at the elbow to correct an ipsilateral flexed wrist, flexed fingers, or thumb-in-palm deformity, as this tends to weaken the muscle excessively. Elbow flexion recovers postoperatively provided biceps and brachialis were functioning before the procedure.

Surgical Technique. Make an S-shaped incision in the antecubitum (Fig. 113-2*A*). Excise the lacertus fibrosus. Identify the medial antebrachial cutaneous nerve, and mark it with a Penrose drain (Fig. 113-2*B*). Release the origin of the flexor carpi ulnaris from the medial epicondyle and from its attachment to the proximal ulna. Identify and protect the median nerve and brachial vessels (Fig. 113-2*C*). Release the pronator teres and flexor carpi radialis if there is wrist contracture. Perform a Z-lengthening of the biceps tendon at the musculotendinous junction[17] (Fig. 113-2*D*). The extent of lengthening depends on the angle of contracture and the degree of spasticity; 3 or 4 cm of lengthening are usually appropriate.[4] Identify and protect the radial nerve. Then identify the brachialis aponeurosis and divide its insertion into the ulna, and passively extend the elbow. If the deformity is resistant, incise the anterior elbow joint capsule. Capsulectomy is not required. It may be necessary to release the origin of brachioradialis at the lateral condyle of the humerus. Some authors[4] suggest transferring the ulnar nerve anteriorly to avoid nerve hypermobility postoperatively. If the nerve is under tension in the extended position, it should be transferred anteriorly.

Complete correction of flexion deformity should not be a goal; correction of the major component of the fixed deformity is usually sufficient. At the close of the procedure, release the tourniquet and obtain hemostasis. Introduce a Penrose drain, which is removed at 24 hours. Immobilize the limb in a posterior splint in maximum, unforced extension. This is changed to a plaster cast at the first dressing change. Active elbow flexion is started at 3 weeks postoperatively. Keep the limb in anteroposterior plaster or plastic splints at all other times to preserve extension. This is continued for the first 6 weeks. Night splints are used for an additional 10 weeks.

Forearm

Pronation

Fixed contractures of the forearm in pronation and of the wrist in flexion are common in cerebral palsy. The inability to extend the wrist and supinate the forearm compromises digital motion, power pinch, and grip. Prolonged pronation contracture may produce radial head dislocation.[18] Release of the flexor-pronator origin can provide considerable lengthening and improve appearance and function of an extremity with fixed deformities. In passively correctable deformities that assume a flexed position during grasp, transfer of flexor carpi ulnaris to extensor carpi radialis brevis is recommended. The surgical technique is described in the next section on wrist flexion deformity.

Wrist

Flexion Deformity

Flexion deformities of the wrist and fingers are common in cerebral palsy and interfere with grasp and release. Flexor-pronator release is recommended if both the wrist and fingers are flexed, but if the deformity is limited largely to the fingers, a Z-lengthening tenotomy in the mid to distal forearm is the procedure of choice.

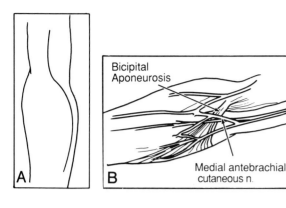

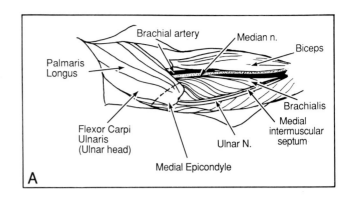

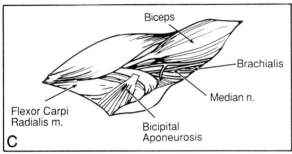

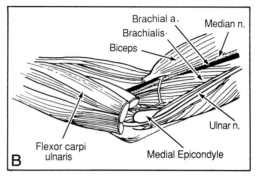

FIGURE 113-3. (*A*) The ulnar nerve is identified and the median intermuscular septum divided. (*B*) The flexor-pronator origins are elevated from the ulna and advanced distally.

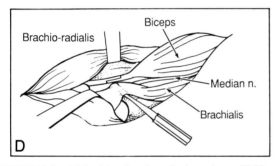

FIGURE 113-2. (*A*) Incision for elbow flexion release. (*B*) The medial antebrachial cutaneous nerve must be protected. (*C*) The bicipital aponeurosis is divided. The median nerve and brachial vessels are identified. (*D*) Z-lengthening of the biceps tendon is performed at the musculotendinous junction. The brachialis insertion is raised from the ulna.

Surgical Technique. Start the incision 5 cm proximal to the medial epicondyle and continue it distally across the antecubitum in a zigzag fashion to the midportion of the proximal forearm. Take care not to damage the medial antebrachial cutaneous nerve in the distal part of the incision and the medial brachial cutaneous nerve posterior to the medial part of the epicondyle. Identify the ulnar nerve and dissect it from its groove (Fig. 113-3*A*). Divide the medial intermuscular septum. Protect the ulnar nerve branches to the flexor carpi ulnaris and the two ulnar heads of the flexor digitorum profundus. Retract the ulnar nerve by vessel loops.

Incise the lacertus fibrosus fascia. Identify and gently retract the median nerve and brachial artery. Take care to preserve the motor branches of the median nerve to the flexor-pronator muscles. This is an exacting dissection and must be performed with patience. Starting distally, elevate the flexor carpi ulnaris and flexor digitorum profundus origins from the

ulna and the interosseous membrane (Fig. 113-3*B*). Continue this dissection proximally along the ulna as far as the ulnar groove. The flexor digitorum superficialis usually must be released from the radius and interosseous membrane. Separate the flexor-pronator muscle mass from the underlying anterior capsule of the elbow, divide it at its origin on the medial part of the epicondyle, and advance it distally about 4 cm. The flexor-pronator muscle mass may be sutured to the underlying tissue at the desired reattachment point. If pronation deformity of the forearm is not a problem, bring the pronator teres origin over the periosteum of the ulna at the proper tension so that pronation of the forearm is not compromised. If a flexion contracture of the elbow persists, release the brachialis. Deflate the tourniquet and obtain hemostasis. Place drains in the forearm and the antecubitum; these should be removed at the first dressing change. By the close of the procedure the wrist should dorsiflex 45° to 60° with the fingers in maximum extension. Use plaster splints to hold the forearm in supination, the wrist in 30° of extension, the metacarpophalangeal joints in 25° of flexion, and the elbow flexed 45° to 90°. At the first dressing change, replace the splint with a cast, which is worn for 3 weeks. Active assisted motion is started after cast removal. Custom-molded anterior-posterior splints that maintain the wrist in extension are worn between treatments for 6 weeks, and then at night for an additional 6 months.

Inadequate Extension

Function in patients with wrist flexion contractures may be improved by Z-lengthening of the wrist flexors: flexor carpi ulnaris, flexor carpi radialis, and palmaris longus. This procedure works best if the patient has active wrist extensor power. Wrist flexor lengthening is not needed if the wrist can be voluntarily extended to at least 10° past neutral, and if the wrist can be actively flexed and assists in finger extension.[5] The procedure is similar to that for lengthening of the digital flexors (see below). The flexor carpi radialis is the first tendon lengthened.[5]

Wrist arthrodesis is indicated only when there is no potential for active finger flexion and extension.[18] Fusion lessens severe flexion deformities and is particularly helpful for athetoid patients.[4] Arthrodesis is performed only after testing hand function in a cast, with the wrist in the position chosen for the procedure. It is contraindicated if the patient depends upon wrist flexion for release or wrist extension for grasp, or if other planned tendon transfers might be compromised by the arthrodesis. The fusion includes the radiocarpal, midcarpal, and carpometacarpal joints. The epiphyses and the distal radioulnar joint are preserved.

When grasp is compromised by inadequate wrist extension from weak extensors, but finger extension can be performed actively with the wrist passively extended, transfer of flexor carpi ulnaris is recommended.[7] The tendon of flexor carpi ulnaris is passed subcutaneously around the ulnar border of the forearm and is transferred to the tendon of extensor carpi radialis brevis (ECRB). The transfer eliminates a deforming force pulling the hand into ulnar deviation and flexion. The procedure has been widely used for many years with good results.[5,14,18,19,22,25] Several prerequisites exist for this transfer. First, there must be satisfactory passive forearm supination and wrist and finger extension. Second, any fixed deformity should be corrected by successive stretching casts and exercises. Finally, there must be adequate digital motor control.

Surgical Technique.[7,18,22,25] Make a 3 cm longitudinal incision radial to the insertion of the flexor carpi ulnaris. Make a second 6 cm longitudinal incision along the palmar-ulnar aspect of the forearm. The two incisions extend over the muscle belly of the flexor carpi ulnaris from the wrist flexor crease to the junction of the middle and proximal thirds of the forearm. Expose the flexor carpi ulnaris, isolate the ulnar nerve, and tag it with a vessel loop posterior to the tendon (Fig. 113-4A). Split the muscle sheath of flexor carpi ulnaris and transect the tendon just proximal to its insertion on the pisiform. Strip the muscle fibers of flexor carpi ulnaris extraperiosteally from the ulna. Free the muscle proximally, without disturbing its nerve supply from the ulnar nerve. Continue the dissection throughout the length of the wound, allowing mobilization of the muscle sufficient to permit its passage in a straight line from its origin to the dorsum of the wrist.

Make a third longitudinal incision over the wrist in line with the long metacarpal, beginning at the distal end of the radius and extending for 5 cm proximally. Incise the extensor retinaculum over the second compartment and identify the extensor carpi radialis brevis. By blunt dissection prepare a tunnel extending from the proximal flexor carpi ulnaris incision to the dorsal radial incision. Construction of this tunnel is facilitated by use of a tendon passer.

Pass the flexor carpi ulnaris tendon around the ulna through the subcutaneous tunnel (Fig. 114-4B). Make a slit in the tendon of extensor carpi radialis brevis with a number 11 blade. Place the wrist in 40° of extension and the forearm in supination; then pass the tendon of flexor carpi ulnaris through the slit in the extensor carpi radialis brevis. The intratendinous suture is by 3-0 nonresorbable suture. Secure the attachment of flexor carpi ulnaris to extensor carpi radialis brevis with additional interrupted sutures. Tension must be sufficient to maintain the wrist in 20° of extension, but should permit passive flexion to 15°. Close the wound and apply a long arm cast with the forearm in supination and the wrist in 20° of extension.

The cast is worn for 4 weeks; then active exercises for ulnar deviation and wrist extension are begun. A bivalved cast or a plastic splint is worn between exercise periods for 2 to 3 months. This program is discontinued when the wrist can be maintained actively in extension. A night brace is worn throughout this time and for an additional 4 months or until there is no tendency toward recurrence.

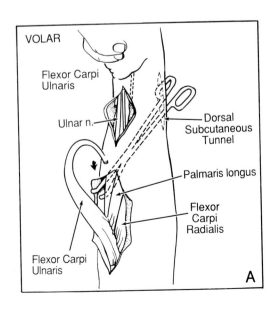

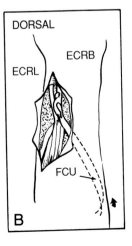

FIGURE 113-4. (*A*) The flexor carpi ulnaris is exposed, released distally, and freed proximally. (*B*) The flexor carpi ulnaris (*FCU*) tendon is passed around the ulna through the subcutaneous tunnel and transferred to extensor carpi radialis brevis (*ECRB*).

Hand

Digital Flexion Deformity

Proximal interphalangeal flexion deformity may be caused by spasticity and myostatic contracture of the flexor digitorum superficialis and flexor digitorum profundus muscles or by paresis of the extensor digitorum communis. Flexion deformity is increased on wrist extension and diminished on wrist flexion. Serial plaster casts with progressive wrist extension may lessen flexion deformity of the digits. If conservative treatment is not effective, surgical lengthening of the spastic or contracted finger flexors is indicated.[5] Lengthening should *not* be performed if the wrist can be voluntarily brought to neutral without excessive digital flexion or if the wrist flexors are weak. With this deformity, lengthening is preferable to flexor-pronator release. The amount of tendon lengthening required may be assessed preoperatively by holding the wrist in maximum extension, placing the metacarpophalangeal joints of the fingers in extension, and then observing the resulting posture of the fingers. Correction should change this finger position to a more functional position for the activities of daily living.

Surgical Technique.[5,25]   Expose the flexor tendons through a midline incision on the palmar surface of the distal forearm (Fig. 113-5*A*). Divide the deep fascia. Identify and protect the ulnar nerve and artery on the radial side of the flexor carpi ulnaris tendon. Isolate the radial artery on the radial side of flexor carpi radialis. Lengthen the flexor digitorum superficialis tendons by stepcut incisions at the musculotendinous junction (Fig. 113-5*B*). Goldner[5] suggests bisecting the tendon for a distance twice that of the proposed lengthening (Fig. 113-5*C*). Divide one slip of the tendon and suture it halfway from the cut end to the intact tendon, after passively extending the fingers. Then, cut the remaining portion of the tendon distally, without disturbing the underlying muscle tissue. This results in a controlled lengthening. With the wrist extended

50°, the proximal interphalangeal joints should be flexed 45°. Repair the incisions with 4-0 resorbable suture.

Release of flexor digitorum profundus at the same operation is not recommended, because grasp is weakened if both extrinsic digital flexors are lengthened. It is best to see how the patient adjusts to lengthening of the superficialis tendons before considering surgery of the flexor digitorum profundus.

Expose the muscle tendon units of the flexor digitorum profundus by retracting the flexor carpi radialis and flexor digitorum superficialis and protecting and retracting the median nerve. Lengthen the flexor digitorum profundus in a manner similar to that used for the flexor digitorum superficialis, but at a different level. Lengthen the flexor pollicis longus if the thumb is held in a flexed position and interferes with pinch and grip.

Patients with wrist flexion contractures may require flexor carpi radialis and flexor carpi ulnaris lengthening. Lengthening is not required if the fingers can be flexed easily while maintaining the wrist in active extension. If the procedure proves necessary, the flexor carpi radialis is the first tendon to be lengthened. Lengthen the tendon of the flexor carpi ulnaris, only if lengthening of the flexor carpi radialis provides insufficient correction. It is essential to lower the tourniquet and achieve meticulous hemostasis at the end of the procedure. Do not close the deep fascia; apply long arm anteroposterior splints to the fingertips, including the thumb, with the elbow at 90°, the forearm supinated, the wrist in 40° extension, and the fingers and thumb in neutral.

Physical therapy for patients undergoing flexor tendon lengthening includes active exercises at 4 weeks after surgery. Bivalved plastic splints are worn between exercise periods. Night splinting continues for 6 months.

Inadequate Metacarpophalangeal Extension

If digital extension is unsatisfactory, a motor should be transferred to the extensor digitorum communis. The procedure is

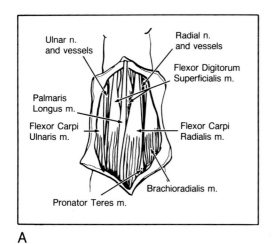
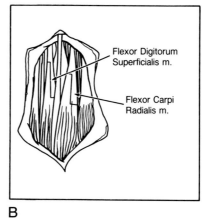
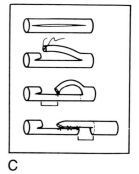

A   B   C

FIGURE 113-5.   (*A*) Exposure of flexor tendons. (*B*) Lengthening of flexor tendons by stepcut incisions. (*C*) Goldner suggests bisecting the tendon for a distance twice that of the proposed lengthening. One slip of the tendon is divided and sutured halfway from the cut end to the intact tendon. The remaining portion is then cut distally.

indicated when there is no significant contracture and a muscle is available for transfer that is synchronous with finger extension.[8] The flexor carpi ulnaris, brachioradialis, and extensor carpi radialis brevis have been recommended for the transfer.[5,16,22,25] We prefer transfer of flexor carpi ulnaris into the extensor digitorum communis because the muscles are synchronous and the transfer produces a tenodesis effect.

Surgical Technique.[22,25] The exposure is similar to that described for the flexor carpi ulnaris to wrist extensor transfer. Make a longitudinal incision that extends along the ulnar-palmar aspect of the forearm, from the palmar wrist crease to the junction of the proximal and middle thirds of the forearm. Expose the flexor carpi ulnaris and identify and protect the ulnar artery and nerve. Divide the flexor carpi ulnaris tendon at its insertion into the pisiform and free it proximally, while carefully preserving the proximal innervation of the tendon. Make a second longitudinal incision over the fourth dorsal compartment. Divide the extensor retinaculum and expose the extensor digitorum communis. Pass the tendon of flexor carpi ulnaris through a subcutaneous tunnel to the dorsal incision. Hold the wrist and metacarpophalangeal joints in neutral. Split the flexor carpi ulnaris tendon into two segments and suture these into each of the tendons of extensor digitorum communis. Adjust the tension so that each finger's metacarpophalangeal joint hyperextends slightly when the wrist is flexed. Apply a long arm cast with the wrist in 30° of extension and the metacarpophalangeal joints in neutral. This position is maintained for 4 weeks, at which point active exercises are started. A splint limiting finger and wrist flexion is worn for 2 months, followed by a night splint for 6 months.

Swan-Neck Deformity

Swan-neck deformity is characterized by hyperextension of the proximal interphalangeal with flexion at the distal interphalangeal joints (Fig. 113-6A). In cerebral palsy, it usually results from muscle imbalance caused by the spastic intrinsics exerting excessive pull on the extensor mechanism. Contraction of the tight or spastic intrinsics results in proximal interphalangeal hyperextension. The tenodesis effect of the extensor digitorum communis while the wrist is flexed also contributes to the deformity. The palmar plate stretches, and the lateral bands sublux dorsally, increasing the hyperextension of the proximal interphalangeal joint. The deformity impairs grasp and pinch. Treatment consists of superficialis tenodesis with or without capsulorrhaphy of the proximal interphalangeal joint, as described by Swanson.[24]

Surgical Technique.[2,5,24,25] Make a midlateral incision from the midportion of the middle phalanx to the base of the proximal phalanx. For the index finger, the incision should be on the ulnar side, and for the little finger on the radial side. Incise the retinacular ligament longitudinally. Gently retract the neurovascular bundle on the side of the incision to the other side. A modified Bruner incision from the middle of the middle phalanx to the proximal palmar crease of the finger also provides good exposure for the procedure. Make an incision in the

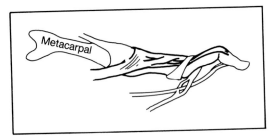

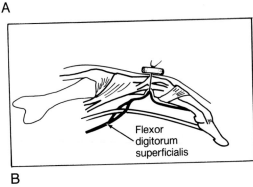

FIGURE 113-6. (A) Swan-neck deformity. (B) The superficialis tendon is drawn into the cavity by passing the suture through the dorsal cortex and tying it over a button.

flexor sheath between the A2 and A4 pulleys; identify each flexor tendon by a vessel loop and retract it.

Expose the palmar aspect of the proximal phalanx by subperiosteal dissection, and drill two small holes, 1 cm apart, in the palmar cortex of the proximal phalanx in a palmar-to-dorsal direction (Fig. 113-6B). Connect the two holes on the palmar aspect using a curette. Roughen the bone for attachment of the tendon. Draw the superficialis tendon into the medullary cavity by a nonresorbable 4-0 suture. Then pass the suture through the palmar cortex defect and out a hole in the dorsal cortex, to the dorsal aspect of the finger, and secure it over a button. Anchor the tendon to the bone with the proximal interphalangeal joint in 30° of flexion. Drill a 0.045-inch Kirschner wire across the joint from the proximal portion of the middle phalanx through the neck of the distal end of the proximal phalanx. Close the flexor sheath with fine resorbable suture. Repair the retinacular ligament and suture the skin. Capsulorrhaphy is required in some cases. Incise the capsule at right angles to the finger. With the joint in 30° of flexion, place 4-0 nonresorbable sutures in the distal end of the proximal flap and the proximal end of the distal flap.

Thumb-in-Palm Deformity

Thumb-in-palm deformity is extremely disabling, as it prevents lateral pinch and grasp. The deformity may be due to adductor spasticity or to spasticity and contracture of flexor pollicis longus. Stretching the metacarpophalangeal joint capsule may produce instability of the joint. Secondary thenar space narrowing may develop. If severe, this can eventually lead to subluxation of the carpometacarpal joint.[25]

Many procedures have been proposed for correction. These

include: metacarpophalangeal and interphalangeal arthrodesis, web space release, tendon transfer, tendon lengthening, and metacarpophalangeal capsulodesis.[2,10,12,13,15,23] For planning correction, the classification scheme of Sakellarides and Mital[18] is helpful.

Type I deformity results from paresis of extensor pollicis longus, with or without instability of the metacarpophalangeal joint. Procedures which have been suggested to correct this include tendon transfer of brachioradialis into abductor pollicis longus and extensor pollicis brevis, and rerouting of extensor pollicis longus.[10,16] We recommend the brachioradialis transfer. Stabilization of the metacarpophalangeal joint by capsulodesis or arthrodesis is indicated if the joint is unstable.[1] Gelberman[2] suggests arthrodesis if the metacarpophalangeal joint shows hyperextension deformity greater than 20°. If performed in a child, the procedure should not interfere with growth of the thumb.[2] Arthrodesis is reserved for cases in which soft-tissue procedures prove unsatisfactory.

Type II deformity is caused by spasticity or contracture of the adductor pollicis. Adductor pollicis contracture is treated by release of the transverse and oblique heads of the muscle. Myotomy is prefered to tenotomy, because it avoids hyperextension of the metacarpophalangeal joint while permitting release of the first metacarpal. Neurectomy of the motor branch to the adductor is performed simultaneously, if severe spasticity is present. Should first dorsal interosseous contribute to the deformity, it is released from the first or second metacarpal, or both.

In Type III deformity, there is paresis of the abductor pollicis longus. Tendon transfer of brachioradialis to the abductor pollicis longus is suggested. Full passive abduction of the first metacarpal and passive thumb extension are prerequisites for tendon transfer.

Type IV deformity is caused by overactivity of flexor pollicis longus. Z-lengthening of the flexor palmaris longus in the distal forearm is required to overcome flexion deformity. Alternatively, some authors[23] suggest the subcutaneous transfer of the flexor palmaris longus to the radial side of the proximal phalanx of the thumb, with tenodesis or arthrodesis of the interphalangeal joint.

Of course, many patients demonstrate more than one type of deformity, and treatment must be individualized accordingly.[23] Deformities of long duration are more likely to demonstrate web space contracture. Z-plasty of the skin of the thumb web and division of the fascia may be necessary. Children's skin, however, has sufficient elasticity to avoid the need for Z-plasty.[5]

Surgical Technique for Capsulodesis of the Metacarpophalangeal Joint.[2]
Make a palmar zigzag incision over the metacarpophalangeal joint. Retract the neurovascular bundles. Incise the A1 pulley and mobilize and retract the flexor palmaris longus. Incise the palmar plate, leaving its distal attachment intact. Release insertions of intrinsics onto the plate. Introduce a 4-0 double-armed wire suture with pullout wire in Bunnell fashion into the palmar plate. Prepare a small groove on the neck of the metacarpal to accommodate the plate. Drill two holes to the dorsum of the metacarpal. Drill a 0.045-inch Kirschner wire through the proximal phalanx, so that it may later be brought across the joint in retrograde fashion. Holding

the joint in 30° of flexion, pass the suture through the apertures and tie it over a button on the dorsum of the thumb. Pass the Kirschner wire across the metacarpophalangeal joint. Hold the thumb in abduction in a plaster cast. Remove the pullout wire at 6 weeks and the Kirschner wire at 8 weeks.

Surgical Technique for Arthrodesis of the Metacarpophalangeal Joint.
Make a radial midlateral incision. Incise the collateral ligament and capsule along the metacarpal head, and dislocate the joint. Carefully remove the articular cartilage from the metacarpal head using a small Rongeur. Remove the articular surface of the proximal phalanx, without disrupting the physes. Drill two 0.045-inch Kirschner wires through the subchondral bone of the proximal phalanx so that they may be passed retrograde across the metacarpophalangeal joint. Hold the joint in 10° of flexion and 10° of lateral rotation and pass the wires. Repair the capsule and collateral ligament with 4-0 resorbable suture. A thumb spica cast is worn for 4 weeks or until firm union.

Surgical Technique for Adductor Myotomy.[22,25]
Make an incision in the thenar flexion crease, from the second metacarpal neck to just proximal to the wrist flexion crease (Fig. 113-7A). If deepening of the web is indicated, use a standard or four-quadrant Z-plasty incision. Make a transverse incision in the web, from the ulnar border of the proximal flexion crease of the thumb to the radial border of the proximal transverse palmar crease; then make two oblique cuts at a 60° angle. After the skin flaps are raised, incise the palmar fascia. Retract the flexor tendons to the index finger radially and those to the long finger ulnarly. Identify and retract the common digital nerve ulnarly. Incise the fascia over the adductor pollicis and first dorsal interosseous (Fig. 113-7B). Retract the first dorsal interosseous radially. Identify the tendon of adductor pollicis. The transverse head of adductor pollicis arises from the distal two-thirds of the long finger metacarpal. The oblique head originates from the capitate and from the bases of the index and

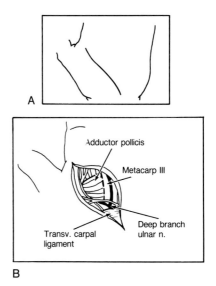

FIGURE 113-7. (A) Skin incision. (B) The first dorsal interosseous is retracted radially and the adductor pollicis identified.

long metacarpals. Release the adductor from its origin; if necessary, release the flexor pollicis brevis, opponens pollicis, and abductor pollicis brevis muscles by elevating their origins from the transverse carpal ligament. Preserve the deep branch of the ulnar nerve and perforating branches of the radial artery. It is rarely necessary to perform neurectomy of the innervation of the adductor pollicis. However, extreme spasticity may require careful dissection and neurectomy of the deep palmar branch of the ulnar nerve, which is the motor branch to the adductor. Release the tourniquet and obtain hemostasis. A cast holds the thumb metacarpal in maximal palmar abduction, the metacarpophalangeal joint in neutral, and the interphalangeal joint in slight flexion. Apply a plastic splint at 4 weeks to maintain the position of abduction and opposition. Active and passive exercises are begun at 4 weeks to rehabilitate thumb function. The cast should be worn for a total of 6 weeks if simultaneous tendon transfers have been performed. Night splints are worn for 6 months to prevent recurrence of the deformity.

Tendon Transfer Brachioradialis to Abductor Pollicis Longus.[22,25] Make a radial longitudinal incision, extending from the radial styloid process to a point 3 cm distal to the lateral epicondyle. Free the insertion of brachioradialis from the radial styloid (Fig. 113-8A). Protect the branches of the superficial radial nerve. The nerve travels along the forearm deep to brachioradialis and can be found adjacent to the radial artery in the proximal forearm. In the distal forearm, the superficial radial nerve emerges from beneath the brachioradialis and penetrates the deep fascia. Dissect the tendon and muscle of brachioradialis free from the antecubital fascia and adjacent muscles to which they are adherent. The muscle must be mobilized proximally as far as possible to gain maximal excursion.

Transect the abductor pollicis longus at its musculotendinous junction proximal to the dorsal retinaculum. Hold the first metacarpal in abduction, weave the distal cut end of abductor pollicis longus through brachioradialis, and suture it with 3-0 nonresorbable suture (Fig. 113-8B). Tension should

allow the first metacarpal to be adducted passively to within 2 cm of the palm, with the wrist in neutral. Tip pinch between the thumb and index must be preserved, and it is necessary to check this after performing the transfer. Persistent extreme flexion of the metacarpophalangeal may be corrected by transferring the proximal end of abductor pollicis longus to the extensor pollicis brevis tendon. Release the tourniquet and obtain hemostasis. Apply an above-elbow cast, with the wrist in neutral, the thumb in neutral, and the first metacarpal in maximal abduction. The cast is removed at 4 weeks, and a short arm plastic thumb spica splint is worn to maintain the thumb in maximal abduction. Active exercises are started at 4 weeks to restore thumb function. Night splints are worn for an additional 6 months.

REFERENCES

1. Filler, B.C., Stark, H.H., and Boyes, J.H.: Capsulodesis of the Metacarpophalangeal Joint of the Thumb in Children with Cerebral Palsy. J. Bone Joint Surg. **58-A:**667–670, 1976.
2. Gelberman, R.: Cerebral Palsy. In Bora, F.W. (ed.): The Pediatric Upper Extremity: Diagnosis and Treatment. Philadelphia, W.B. Saunders, 1986, pp. 323–338.
3. Goldner, J.L.: Outline of Operative Procedures for Reconstruction of the Upper Extremity in Cerebral Palsy. In Keats, S. (ed.): Operative Orthopedics in Cerebral Palsy. Springfield, Ill., Charles C Thomas, 1971, pp. 50–99.
4. Goldner, J.L.: Upper Extremity Surgical Procedures for Patients with Cerebral Palsy. AAOS Instructional Course Lectures, Vol. 28. St. Louis, C.V. Mosby, 1979, pp. 37–66.
5. Goldner, J.L.: Surgical Treatment for Cerebral Palsy. In Evarts, C.M. (ed.): Surgery of the Musculoskeletal System. New York, Churchill Livingstone, 1983.
6. Goldner, J.L., and Ferlic, D.C.: Sensory Status of the Hand as Related to Reconstructive Surgery of the Upper Extremity in Cerebral Palsy. Clin. Orthop. Rel. Res. **46:**87–92, 1966.
7. Green, W.T., and Banks, H.H.: Flexor Carpi Ulnaris Transplant and Its Use in Cerebral Palsy. J. Bone Joint Surg. **44-A:**1343–1352, 1962.
8. Hoffer, M.: Cerebral Palsy. In Green, D.P. (ed.): Operative Hand Surgery. New York, Churchill Livingstone, 1982, pp. 185–194.
9. Hoffer, M., Perry, J., and Melkonian, G.J.: Dynamic Electromyography and Decision Making for Surgery in the Upper Extremity of Patients with Cerebral Palsy. J. Hand Surg. **4:**424–431, 1979.
10. House, J.H., Gwathmey, F.W., and Fuller, M.O.: A Dynamic Approach to the Thumb-In-Palm Deformity in Cerebral Palsy. J. Bone Joint Surg. **63-A:**216–225, 1981.
11. Inglis, A.E., and Cooper, W.: Release of the Flexor Pronator Origin for Flexion Deformities of the Hand and Wrist in Spastic Paralysis: A Study of Eighteen Cases. J. Bone Joint Surg. **48-A:**847–857, 1966.
12. Inglis, A.E., Cooper, W., and Bruton, W.: Surgical Correction of Thumb Deformities in Spastic Paralysis. J. Bone Joint Surg. **52-A:**253–268, 1970.
13. Keats, S.: Surgical Treatment of the Hand in Cerebral Palsy: Correction of Thumb-In-Palm and Other Deformities. J. Bone Joint Surg. **47-A:**274–284, 1965.
14. Keats, S.: Operative Orthopaedics in Cerebral Palsy. Springfield, Ill., Charles C Thomas, 1970.
15. Matev, I.B.: Surgical Treatment of Flexion-Adduction Contracture of the Thumb in Cerebral Palsy. Acta Orthop. Scand. **41:**439–445, 1970.
16. McCue, F.C., Honner, R., and Chapman, W.C.: Transfer of the

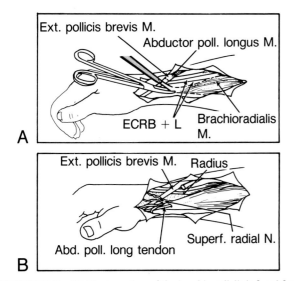

FIGURE 113-8. (*A*) The insertion of the brachioradialis is freed from the radial styloid. (*B*) The distal cut end of adductor pollicis longus is woven through the brachioradialis.

Brachioradialis for Hands Deformed by Cerebral Palsy. J. Bone Joint Surg. **52-A:**1171–1180, 1970.

17. Mital, M.A.: Lengthening of the Elbow Flexors in Cerebral Palsy. J. Bone Joint Surg. **61-A:**515–522, 1979.

18. Mital, M.A., and Sakellarides, H.T.: Surgery of the Upper Extremity in the Retarded Individual with Spastic Cerebral Palsy. Orthop Clin. N. Amer. **12:**127–141, 1981.

19. Omer, G.E., and Capen, D.A.: Proximal Row Carpectomy With Muscle Transfers for Spastic Paralysis. J. Hand Surg. **1:**197–204, 1976.

20. O'Reilly, D.E., and Walentynowicz, J.E.: Etiology Factors in Cerebral Palsy. Dev. Med. Child. Neurol. **23:**633–642, 1981.

21. Samilson, R.L., and Morris, J.M.: Surgical Improvement of the Cerebral Palsied Upper Limb: Electromyographic Studies and Results of 128 Operations. J. Bone Joint Surg. **46-A:**1203–1216, 1964.

22. Smith, R.J.: Surgery of the Hand in Cerebral Palsy In Pulvertaft, G. (ed.): Operative Surgery: The Hand. London, Butterworths, 1977, pp. 215–230.

23. Smith, R.J.: Flexor Pollicis Longus Abductor Plasty for Spastic Thumb-In-Palm Deformity. J. Hand Surg. **7:**327–334, 1982.

24. Swanson, A.B.: Surgery of the Hand in Cerebral Palsy and Swan-Neck Deformity. J. Bone Joint Surg. **42-A:**951–964, 1960.

25. Tachdijian, M.O.: Pediatric Orthopedics, Vol. 2. Philadelphia, W.B. Saunders, 1972, pp. 830–857.

26. Tachdijian, M.O., and Minear, W.L.: Sensory Disturbances in the Hands of Children with Cerebral Palsy. J. Bone Joint Surg. **40-A:**85, 1958.

CHAPTER 114

Surgical Treatment of the Upper Extremity After Stroke

ROBERT L. WATERS and
MARY ANN E. KEENAN

The average life expectancy for individuals surviving the first month following a cerebrovascular accident is greater than 6 years. Consequently, in selected patients surgical procedures that improve limb function may play an important role in improving the quality of life and level of independence.

Stroke is most commonly the result of infarction in the region of the cerebral cortex supplied by the middle cerebral artery or one of its branches. An ascending frontal branch supplies the motor cortex anteriorly, and an ascending parietal branch supplies the sensory cortex posteriorly.

Patients with relatively intact motor control and sensation, but with restricted extension at the wrist, fingers, or thumb as a result of mild flexor spasticity, are candidates for hand surgery to improve function. Those with bilateral hemiplegia caused by multiple strokes have a poor rehabilitation prognosis and are not good candidates for functional surgery. An exception to this general principle is the patient with bilateral hemiplegia due to brain stem infarction but who has intact cognition.

It is essential to understand thoroughly the complex symptomatology of the hemiplegic patient. Good surgical results depend upon careful patient selection. An occupational therapist can assist in performing detailed patient assessment and also in the postoperative rehabilitation program.

EVALUATION

The patient's ability to cooperate with the assessment of upper extremity function provides an appraisal of cognition and communication. To distinguish between an impairment of communication or cognition and a physical deficit, all tests are first performed on the normal side. Communication with the patient should be conducted at a level that produces the most accurate responses. For example, some patients cannot understand spoken communications but will respond to written communication or gestures. Other patients will respond to simple phrases but not to complex sentences. The speech therapist can determine the optimum method of communication.

Cognition is one of the most important factors in determining upper extremity function. It determines the ability of the patient to profit from surgery. The patient must be capable of following simple verbal commands or pantomimed instructions, and must also have sufficient memory to retain what is taught. If problem-solving ability, memory, organization, and attention span are severely impaired, the patient may not function well enough to learn one- or two-handed skills. Most stroke patients without bilateral cortical involvement have sufficient cognition to learn routine independent self-care activities.

Motor Recovery

Recognition of the characteristic patterns of motor impairment allows the surgeon to select those patients who may benefit from surgery. Motor recovery in the paralyzed upper extremity typically follows a consistent pattern, with the greatest amount of spontaneous recovery occurring in the first 6 weeks following stroke. Return of motor function depends primarily on the extent of the lesion and the amount of collateral circulation. Recovery can be arrested at any of the following stages.

The pattern of motor recovery proceeds from proximal to distal in the extremity. In the completely paralyzed extremity, voluntary movement returns first as flexion of the shoulder. Further recovery appears in succession as flexion of the elbow, wrist, and fingers and then as supination of the forearm. Flexor spasticity is greatest at this stage. Any voluntary movement of the affected extremity results in simultaneous flexion of all joints. If there is no further recovery, contractures commonly occur unless the joints are passively extended as part of a daily exercise program.

In general, by the time flexor synergy includes the wrist and fingers extensor motion is also present at the shoulder and elbow. At this stage of recovery there is normally a delay of several seconds between the command to execute a movement and the time that muscle contraction or relaxation occurs.

Selective motion, which is the ability to move a single joint independently of others without involving the entire flexor or extensor synergy pattern, usually returns first at the shoulder and elbow. With the development of selective extension, there is marked improvement in the speed and precision of flexor motor control and a reduction in flexor spasticity.

Simultaneous flexion and extension of all fingers precedes the ability to selectively flex and extend one finger at a time. Independent finger control generally occurs first in the index and middle fingers. Thumb opposition, initially, is to the side of the index finger providing lateral pinch. Full opposition returns later.

Most hemiplegic patients will not use the affected hand, even as an assist, unless they can selectively extend the fingers or thumb without eliciting a simultaneous mass extensor synergy. Without some selective control, it is easier and more practical to use the opposite extremity, even if this entails a change in hand dominance. When it has been determined that neurologic recovery has ceased at a point where some selective extension of the fingers or thumb is present but remains incomplete owing to mild flexor spasticity, surgery to improve function may be indicated in the patient with adequate sensation and cognition.

Sensory Impairment

Functional use of the hand is dependent on sensory awareness as well as motor control. The patient with normal motor function but without sensory perception may use the affected hand on request, relying on visual feedback, but will not routinely use it, even as an assist. Hemiplegic patients prefer to use the uninvolved extremity alone rather than grope with a hand that lacks sensation.

Even slight sensory deficits limit the use of the affected extremity to assist in performing functional tasks because the patient will have persistent problems performing fine manipulative tasks.

When the cerebral infarct involves the entire sensory cortex, the patient will respond to the basic modalities of touch, temperature, and pain once these are perceived subcortically. Depending on the extent of the lesion, the patient may be unable to discriminate higher aspects of sensation such as shape, size, texture, point localization, and proprioception. If the infarct extends posteriorly to the parietal lobe, the patient will have additional perceptual problems involving motion of the limb in space and awareness of the limb itself.

Stroke patients may demonstrate a variety of sensory-integration problems: distorted perception of sensory input, interpretation of that input, and integration of the input with the available motor control to perform purposeful tasks. These deficits are manifested by lack of kinesthetic awareness of body parts, the relation of these parts to each other, and their position in space. Inability to organize and sequence motor acts, and denial or neglect of the affected extremities are other higher sensory deficits.

Kinesthetic awareness may be evaluated by positioning the involved arm in space while the subject looks toward the intact extremity. The patient is then instructed to duplicate the same posture on the uninvolved side. Patients who spontaneously use their involved hand as an assist without visual feedback are able to duplicate the posture of the involved extremity within a few degrees at the shoulder, elbow, forearm, wrist, and metacarpophalangeal joints.

Perceptual deficits are best evaluated by observation of the patient's attempts to perform functional or purposeful tasks. Some screening tests of visual perception, such as foreground-background discrimination, rotation of forms in space, and eye-hand coordination, are useful paper-and-pencil tools that are performed by the therapist to identify likely areas of functional problems. Observation of motor tasks that require sequential planning and execution of individual motions should be included in the sensory-integration evaluation.

Ataxia is frequently present with severe sensory loss, even when the eyes are used for visual feedback. Assessment of speed and precision during motor acts and the patient's ability to cross the midline or change direction should also be evaluated. Sensory integrative deficits greatly influence the patient's rehabilitation because they interfere with the motor performance of the normal limb as well.

Object identification is difficult to use as a test in stroke patients, because their motor deficits result in a decreased ability to handle objects adequately to determine texture and shape.

The most important test of sensory function is careful observation to determine if there is spontaneous purposeful use of the hand. The two-point discrimination test is easily performed and quantitated, and it correlates closely with the patient's overall sensory status. Most patients will use the hand as an assist if motor function is intact, and two-point discrimination is less than 5 mm. Significant functional use is not observed when proprioception is absent, and two-point discrimination is greater than 10 mm at the fingertips or palm.

Vision

Evaluation of vision identifies problems of visual perception and the effects of these aberrations on functional ability. Visual acuity should be tested as well as visual fields.

Homonymous hemianopsia frequently occurs following a cerebrovascular accident, leaving the patient unable to see objects placed on the affected side. This impedes function, because the patient is unable to see half of what is in front of the eyes. Most patients learn to compensate by turning the head, so that homonymous hemianopsia is not a surgical contraindication. Even when homonymous hemianopsia is not present, the patient may experience vertical distortions or visual inattention in the contralateral visual field.

Spasticity

Reaction of the muscles of the hemiparetic upper extremity to quick (phasic) stretch determines the extent of spasticity. The response may be graded as no abnormal response (none), a palpable response that does not block continued passive motion (minimal), a response that blocks passive motion but can be overcome by slow, steady tension (moderate), or a response that produces block to further passive motion that cannot be overcome (severe). The exaggerated flexor response to stretch represents a failure of normal cortical inhibition. When that response is present, there is also a failure of the normal relaxation action of the flexors during extensor movements (reciprocal inhibition), which directly and indirectly interferes with the strength, speed, and range of extension. Clinically, the amount of flexor spasticity is inversely proportional to the amount of extensor control. Repetitive voluntary flexion and extension increases the amount of spasticity.

The precision and speed required for normal hand function makes the least degree of spasticity conspicuous. Even minimal spasticity is associated with loss of fine motor control. If spasticity is moderate or severe, contractures of the elbow, wrist, and fingers will occur if the patient is not placed on a preventive therapy program of daily passive range-of-motion exercises. Functional use of the hand is not possible when moderate spasticity is present in the fingers or thumb. Some patients with moderate flexor spasticity may manually open the hand with their intact extremity and then grasp objects to perform activities that can only be performed two-handed.

The influence of body position on the posture and tone of the hemiplegic upper extremity should be considered. The tonic labyrinthine reflex arises from end organs in the inner ear and is activated when the head is in the upright position. This reflex increases the excitability of the stretch reflex. Thus, flexor spasticity is greater when the patient is sitting or standing than when supine. Therefore, patients should always be examined in the sitting position.

Range of Motion

Range of motion (ROM) is evaluated by the muscle response to slow stretch. The joint is slowly extended over a period of several minutes. This is to avoid the velocity-sensitive components of the muscle spindle that are responsible for causing the monosynaptic phasic stretch reflex. Even when the extremity is extended slowly, some tonic activity may persist. Differentiation between what is presumed to be myostatic contracture and persistent muscle activity can be determined only after anesthetic block of the peripheral nerves or examination of the patient under anesthesia.

TECHNIQUES TO DECREASE SPASTICITY TEMPORARILY

The neurologic recovery phase following a stroke extends for at least 6 months. Definitive surgical procedures are avoided during this time. When no further improvement in spasticity is anticipated, surgical procedures that permanently alter muscle tone and function, such as neurectomies, tendon lengthenings, and transfers, are considered.

Often the spasticity is severe and prevents adequate joint range of motion or maintenance of acceptable limb position, despite the most conscientious and aggressive treatment attempts. Even when joint motion can be maintained by knowledgeable therapists, it may require excessive force, which is painful for the patient, potentially harmful to limbs, and very time consuming. Lesser degrees of spasticity can also impede function or require the use of positioning devices that interfere with the use of an extremity.

Drugs have been used to treat spasticity. Most cause unwanted drowsiness or decrease voluntary muscle strength, and drugs can seriously hamper recovery. Other serious side effects, such as hepatotoxicity, can also occur. None of these medications have proven reliable in the treatment of spasticity in the stroke patient.

The orthopaedic treatment of spasticity focuses on decreasing muscle tone using peripheral procedures to modify the response of the peripheral nervous system or muscle-tendon units. The goals of orthopaedic treatment are to maintain joint range of motion and to improve function during the recovery phase. Maintenance of joint motion preserves muscle fiber length and prevents fixed myostatic contractures from forming.

A combination of peripheral nerve blocks and casting or splinting techniques is commonly used to give temporary relief of spasticity. Lidocaine blocks are useful in temporarily eliminating muscle tone, allowing assessment of an extremity or ranging of a joint. Such blocks are also very helpful when performed prior to cast application, since relieving the spasticity allows for easier limb positioning. Correction of contractual deformities can be obtained by serial cast application at weekly intervals. Serial casting is most successful when a contracture has been present for less than 6 months.

Repeated lidocaine blocks are not practical when severe spasticity prevents daily range-of-motion therapy. In this situation a longer acting agent, such as phenol, is used to block nerve function. Phenol denatures the protein in a peripheral nerve, causing axonal degeneration. The axons then regenerate, because the continuity of the nerve sheath has not been disrupted. This process requires approximately 6 months. The average duration of a phenol block is therefore 6 months. The action of phenol is nonspecific, contrary to original theories, and affects all nerve fibers alike.

Phenol blocks are used only during the period of neurologic recovery to decrease spasticity. It is hoped that by the time the nerve has regenerated, the patient will have recovered control of the effected muscles. If excessive spasticity remains when neurologic recovery has plateaued, then definitive surgery is planned.

Several techniques are available for phenol blocks. The choice of technique depends on the anatomic accessibility of the nerve and the composition of the nerve. The direct injection of a peripheral nerve provides the most complete and longest lasting block. When a peripheral nerve has a large sensory component, direct injection is not recommended, since loss of sensation is undesirable and many patients will, in addition, develop painful hyperesthesia. In some cases it is necessary to dissect free the individual motor branches of a nerve to a muscle and inject each separately. Another approach is to localize the motor points of muscles using an insulated needle and nerve stimulator. Motor point injections do not result in complete relief of spasticity but can be helpful in reducing tone. The duration of effect of motor point blocks is approximately 2 months.

Common Upper Extremity Blocks

Musculocutaneous Nerve Block

When spasticity of the biceps and brachialis muscles interferes with elbow extension, a phenol block of the musculocutaneous nerve provides temporary relief. The block can be performed percutaneously at the bedside or surgically through a small incision on the upper arm (see Fig. 114-8). If the patient is undergoing another surgical procedure, or if heterotopic ossification is present at the elbow, it is preferable to expose the musculocutaneous nerve for direct injection. When performing a surgical block, expose the nerve through an incision on the medial aspect of the arm, beginning at the lower border of the pectoralis major tendon. The nerve is located between the short head of the biceps and the brachialis muscle. Use a nerve stimulator to confirm the identity of the nerve. Protect the surrounding tissues using a moistened gauze sponge, and then inject the nerve with 5% phenol in glycerine. Glycerine is used to provide continued slow release of the phenol. Stimulate the nerve again to confirm that no further conduction is occurring. It is advisable to wear eye goggles during the injection, since the viscosity of the glycerine solution may cause the needle to become disconnected from the syringe and spray the phenol solution.

Perform percutaneous injection of the musculocutaneous nerve using a teflon-coated, insulated needle and a nerve stimulator. Introduce the needle from the medial aspect of the arm and pass it between the lower edge of the short head of the biceps and the brachialis. In a spastic patient this interval is easily identified. Move the needle about while applying stimulation until the point of maximal response is noted. At this location, inject 3 ml of an aqueous solution of 5% phenol. An aqueous solution is used for percutaneous injections to provide better diffusion of the phenol. If any elbow contracture remains following the block, serial casting or drop out casts are used to correct the deformity.

Motor Point Blocks

Spastic forearm flexor muscles causing wrist and finger flexion deformities can be treated by phenol blocks of the motor points. Because of the large sensory component of the median and ulnar nerves at the elbow level, injection of the nerve proper is undesirable. (Also, surgical dissection of the motor branches of these nerves would be extensive.) For these reasons, an attempt is made to localize the point of entry of the motor branches into the muscles, using electrical stimulation on the surface of the forearm. Mark the points of maximal response on the skin. Next, insert a needle coated with teflon for insulation at these points and increase stimulation to further define the motor points of the muscles. When the motor point has been localized, inject 3 ml of a 5% aqueous solution of phenol at each site. No more than five points should be injected in a forearm in one day, to avoid excessive swelling,

inflammation and the risk of compartment syndrome. The onset of the effect of the motor point injections occurs over the ensuing 24 hours and lasts approximately 2 months. The blocks can be supplemented with functional electrical stimulation of the wrist and finger extensor muscles and by casting or splinting techniques.

Ulnar Motor Nerve Block

Spasticity involving the intrinsic muscles of the hand is common but may be masked by extrinsic spasticity. An adducted thumb or swan-neck positioning of the fingers may indicate underlying intrinsic spasticity. Permanent deformity can be avoided by performing a phenol block of the motor branch of the ulnar nerve in Guyon's canal. This block must be made surgically because of the close proximity of the sensory branch of the nerve (see Fig. 114-7). Make an incision on the palmar surface of the hand radial to the pisiform bone and extended distally for 1 inch. The ulnar nerve is easily exposed, as it is branching in the hand. Identify the motor branch, using a nerve stimulator. Protect the surrounding tissues with a moistened gauze sponge and inject the motor branch with 5% phenol in glycerine. The duration of the block is approximately 6 months.

Recurrent Median Nerve Block

When an adduction deformity of the thumb is secondary to spasticity of the median innervated muscles of the thenar eminence, a phenol block of the recurrent motor branch of the median nerve is performed. The block can be performed percutaneously, using a teflon coated needle and nerve stimulator, or as a surgical procedure. When a concurrent ulnar nerve block is needed, the recurrent median nerve is surgically exposed.

The recurrent motor branch of the median nerve enters the thenar mass at the junction of Kaplan's cardinal line and a line drawn along the radial border of the long finger. Kaplan's line is drawn parallel to the proximal palmar crease, beginning at the apex of the first web space. Localize the nerve using a nerve stimulator during the percutaneous injection, as described earlier; then inject 3 ml of 5% aqueous phenol. When a surgical block is performed, a 5% phenol solution in glycerine is used. Casting or splinting may be needed following the block if a contracture is present.

PROCEDURES TO IMPROVE HAND FUNCTION

The selection of hemiplegic patients who will predictably benefit from surgery should follow these general guidelines:

1. It is at least 9 months since the onset of the stroke, and the patient has good cognition, motivation, and willingness to participate in a program including postoperative hand therapy.
2. There is some selective extension of the fingers or thumb.
3. The patient uses the hand spontaneously to perform some functional activities, even as an assist.

4. Proprioception is intact, and two-point discrimination is less than 10 mm, preferably 5 mm at the palm or fingers.

5. The patient has no fixed joint contractures.

Surgery is performed to improve extension at the wrist, thumb, or fingers (or all three) when hand opening is restricted by mild flexor spasticity or myostatic contracture. Preoperatively, local anesthetic block of the median or ulnar nerves differentiates spasticity from contracture. If the restriction is due to spasticity, improved extension occurs following the block, demonstrating that the patient will benefit from surgery.

Thumb

For some patients with voluntary key pinch between the thumb and the side of the index finger, there may be restricted extension owing to adductor pollicis or flexor pollicis longus spasticity. A quick abduction stretch applied to the thumb may elicit a hyperactive adduction response, indicating spasticity of the adductor pollicis. Limited function caused by adductor pollicis spasticity is determined by anesthetic block of the ulnar nerve at the wrist. If improved abduction and extension occurs, release of the adductor and first dorsal interosseous muscle is indicated. This is performed through a dorsal longitudinal incision on the ulnar border of the thumb, extending from the base of the metacarpal to the middle of the proximal phalanx. Release the origin of the first dorsal interosseous muscle from the thumb metacarpal. Detach the insertion of the adductor pollicis from the base of the proximal phalanx. After wound closure, the thumb is immobilized in abduction and extension in a spica cast for 3 weeks. The cast is then removed and active exercises started. A night splint is worn for an additional 3 weeks.

In longstanding deformities, the skin of the web space may be contracted. The web space is lengthened and deepened by performing Z-plasty at the time release of the adductor pollicis and first dorsal interosseous is performed (Fig. 114-1). Place the central limb of the Z along the line of the contracture in the web space. Make the other two limbs of the Z equal in length to the central line and at an angle of 75° to the central line. Handle the flaps carefully to avoid necrosis of the corners. Apply a pressure dressing, along with an abduction splint. The splint should be worn continuously for 3 weeks and as a night positioning device for an additional 3 weeks, to prevent recurrence of the deformity.

If the interphalangeal joint is excessively flexed during pinch, the patient will benefit by interphalangeal stabilization in the neutral position. The benefit of stabilization can be proven preoperatively by externally stabilizing the interphalangeal joint in extension by taping a dorsal splint to the proximal and distal phalanges. Since placing the interphalangeal joint in extension tightens the flexor pollicis longus, this may limit extension at the metacarpalphalangeal or carpal-metacarpal joints, limiting thumb opening. The tension of the flexor pollicis longus should be assessed preoperatively in the dynamic state. If excessive tension is present, it will be necessary to lengthen the tendon of the flexor pollicis longus. Expose the flexor pollicis longus at its myotendinous junction through a small incision on the palmar aspect of the forearm, at the location of the middle and distal thirds of the arm. After identifying

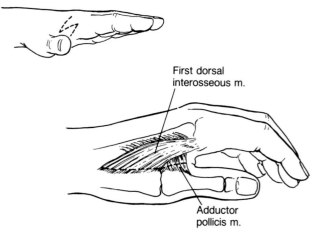

FIGURE 114-1. Z-plasty of thumb web space to release contracted skin in a longstanding adduction deformity. Release of the adductor pollicis tendon and first dorsal interosseous muscle to correct an adduction deformity of the thumb.

the flexor pollicis longus, make an oblique cut in the tendon overlying the muscle belly, leaving the muscle fibers intact. Then, gently extend the thumb, allowing the tendon to slide distally 1 cm. The thumb is immobilized in a splint or cast continuously for 3 weeks after surgery, before a therapy program is begun. A night splint is worn for another 3 weeks, to prevent inadvertent stretching of the tendon.

Stabilization of the interphalangeal joint may be achieved by insertion of a Moberg screw across the joint (Fig. 114-2). Immediate stability is achieved, and postoperative immobilization is not required. For patients with a normal life expectancy (those with hemiplegia due to head trauma, cerebral palsy, etc.), fusion of the interphalangeal joint is performed using the Moberg screw for fixation. Fusion is also performed in patients with fixed flexion deformity to position the interphalangeal joint in neutral and to prevent tension on the digital neurovas-

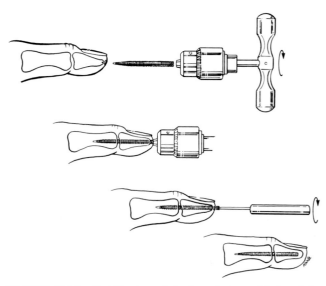

FIGURE 114-2. Stabilization of the interphalangeal joint of the thumb using a Moberg screw.

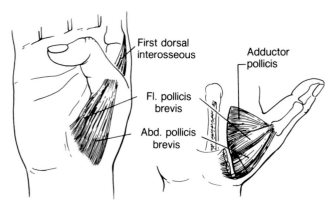

FIGURE 114-3. Proximal release of the thenar muscles, done to correct a flexion and adduction deformity of the thumb, caused by spasticity in all thenar muscles.

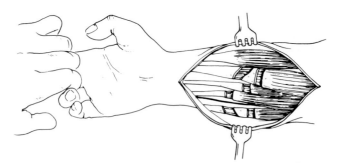

FIGURE 114-4. Fractional lengthening of the individual spastic flexor superficialis and profundus tendons done to improve hand opening.

cular bundles. Make a transverse incision on the dorsum of the thumb overlying the joint. Divide the extensor pollicis longus tendon in line with the incision. Then expose the joint and remove the articular cartilage and subchondral bone from the proximal and distal phalanges, to provide stable surfaces of cancellous bone. Removing this bone and cartilage shortens the thumb and relieves tension on the digital neurovascular structures when a longstanding deformity has resulted in soft tissue contracture. Insert the Moberg screw through the distal tip of the thumb and pass it across the interphalangeal joint in the medullary canal of the phalanges. Approximate the skin and tendon, using interrupted horizontal mattress sutures. When stable fixation has been obtained, no external support is needed while healing occurs.

Occasionally, patients exhibit some selective thumb motion and a potentially useful pinch, which is limited by inadequate thumb opening (extension and abduction) secondary to spasticity of all the thenar intrinsic muscles innervated by the median and ulnar nerve. This condition is more commonly seen in patients whose hemiplegia is due to head trauma and who have mild decorticate or decerebrate rigidity in the upper limb. A preoperative lidocaine block of the median and ulnar nerves enables differentiation of the relative contribution of the thenar intrinsic muscles innervated by both nerves. If all intrinsic muscles restrict thumb opening, proximal release is performed, allowing the thenar muscles to slide distally (Fig. 114-3). Make a curved incision, following the thenar crease on the palm. Release the flexor pollicis brevis, abductor pollicis brevis, and opponens muscles at their origins, and allow them to slide distally. Identify and protect the recurrent motor branch of the median nerve. Retract the long finger flexor tendons, and release the origin of the adductor pollicis from the third metacarpal. Strip the origin of the first dorsal interosseous muscle from the second metacarpal, if needed. After careful wound closure, immobilize the thumb in abduction and extension, using a spica cast for 3 weeks. A night splint is generally worn for an additional 3 weeks.

Fingers

Active finger extension, restricted by mild spasticity or contracture, may be improved by flexor tendon lengthening. Sur-

gical release of the flexor pronator origin has been advocated in the past as a method of treating spastic wrist and finger flexion deformities. This procedure requires extensive dissection, and a supination deformity often results. Lengthening of the individual flexor tendons has proved more reliable.

The control and strength of the finger extensors can be evaluated prior to surgery using lidocaine blocks of the median and ulnar nerves at the elbow to temporarily eliminate the action of the finger flexors. The block also demonstrates the amount of myostatic contracture present in the finger flexors.

Myostatic contracture shortens the active range of muscle excursion. Lengthening of spastic flexor tendons results in partial loss of voluntary flexor strength and contractile range. Because of these factors, overlengthening of the flexor tendons resulting in a loss of flexion range and strength is the most common surgical error. The amount of tendon lengthening is determined preoperatively, and is only half the length necessary (usually 1 to 1.5 cm) to extend the finger from the point of restriction of the voluntary extension to full extension. The temptation to further lengthening should be resisted, since loss of grip strength significantly reduces hand function.

Passive extension of the fingers often reveals that only the superficial tendons appear to restrict motion. However, lengthening of the superficialis tendons alone often uncovers restrictive spasticity in the profundi. Accordingly, both tendons are lengthened an equal amount.

Either fractional lengthening or multiple Z-plasties of the individual tendons are performed (Fig. 114-4). The surgery is performed under tourniquet control, through a curved incision on the palmar surface of the forearm. Identify the wrist, thumb, and deep and superficial finger flexors, protecting neurovascular structures. Divide the palmaris longus tendon. Transect the flexor carpi radialis and flexor carpi ulnaris tendons for Z lengthening, if a wrist flexion deformity is present. Lengthen the flexor digitorum superficialis and flexor digitorum profundus tendons by incising the flexor tendon obliquely at the musculotendinous junction, and then passively extend the digits, allowing the tendons to slide distally. The hand is splinted in the corrected position for 3 weeks after surgery. A vigorous hand rehabilitation program after removal of the splint is essential. Therapy is scheduled for 1 to 2 hours a day, 5 days a week for a minimum of 2 weeks. The program includes functional electrical stimulation of the wrist and finger extensors, and gentle passive range of motion to the wrist and finger flexors. Treatment progresses to include active exercises and activities that maximize wrist and finger-extension response and full grasp of the hand.

Fixed contracture of the proximal interphalangeal joints may be present in longstanding deformities. If so, surgical release is done at the time of flexor tendon lengthening. After a dorsal longitudinal incision is made, retract the skin laterally on either side of the proximal interphalangeal joints to expose the collateral ligaments, palmar plate, and flexor sheath, which are contracted. Release the proximal attachments of the collateral ligaments and palmar plate, and excise the flexor sheath. If the skin on the palmar surface now restricts extension, perform Z-plasty. The proximal interphalangeal joint is transfixed with a Kirschner wire at 25° of flexion for 3 weeks to prevent subluxation.

For patients with severe contractures and in whom insufficient correction is obtained following soft tissue release, proximal interphalangeal fusion obtains bone shortening and prevents excessive tension on the digital nerves and arteries.

Wrist

Inadequate wrist extension may be present, despite satisfactory finger extension. Before a decision is made to lengthen the wrist flexor tendons, however, whether or not the patient will be able to extend the fingers after the wrist flexor tendons are lengthened must be determined. If the finger flexors are shortened because of spasticity or myostatic contracture, finger extension may be lost if only the wrist flexion deformity is corrected. Preoperative evaluation, with the wrist held manually in the corrected position, will determine if satisfactory finger extension occurs. If it does, then wrist flexor tendon lengthening may be safely performed.

If surgery is deemed necessary, it should first be determined which wrist flexor tendons are to be lengthened. Manual palpation usually reveals that the flexor carpi ulnaris is active during attempted hand opening. The contribution of the flexor carpi ulnaris can be determined by anesthetic block of the ulnar nerve at the elbow. If satisfactory wrist extension occurs, then only this tendon is lengthened. If the wrist remains flexed, then the flexor carpi radialis is lengthened also, and the palmaris longus is sectioned.

It is not advisable to transfer the wrist flexors to the wrist extensors in hemiplegic patients. The degree of spasticity, active range of contraction, and the pattern of activity in the individual tendons vary in each patient. No guidelines have been established for the proper amount of tension to secure a transferred tendon. If it is secured too tightly, wrist hyperextension occurs. Fortunately, tendon transfer is seldom necessary. Most patients with selective finger extension will have sufficient wrist extensor strength if the wrist flexors are lengthened.

Wrist flexor lengthening involves Z-plasty lengthening within the tenosynovial sheath of each tendon (Fig. 114-5). Expose the wrist flexor tendons through a curved incision on the distal third of the palmar aspect of the forearm. Divide the palmaris longus tendon. Make a longitudinal cut in the tendon of approximately 3 to 4 cm. Then make hemisection cuts on both the proximal and distal ends of the longitudinal cut at 180° to each other. Place the wrist in 20° of extension and

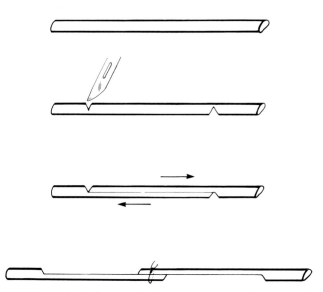

FIGURE 114-5. Z-plasty of the flexor tendons is performed within the tenosynovial sheath. A single suture prevents excessive lengthening.

repair the overlapping ends of the cut tendons with nonabsorbable suture. The wrist is immobilized in 20° of extension for 6 weeks.

SURGERY IN THE NONFUNCTIONAL UPPER EXTREMITY

Surgery in the nonfunctional upper extremity is indicated to correct flexion deformities of the hand, elbow, or shoulder that cause pain, or prevent adequate hygiene, or to improve cosmesis.

Hand

The temptation to release all finger and wrist flexors should be resisted; the wrist may become hyperextended and dislocated dorsally if extensor tone is unmasked after surgery.

When severe wrist and finger flexion deformities are both present, the superficialis-to-profundus transfer is an excellent method of achieving the flexor tendon lengthening necessary to obtain correction.[4] This procedure maintains a restriction to wrist hyperextension if extensor tone is unmasked postoperatively. Expose and identify the superficialis and profundus tendons through an incision on the palmar aspect of the forearm. Then suture the superficialis tendons together distally, using a nonabsorbable suture material. Suture the profundus tendons together proximally in an identical manner. This insures uniform tension on the individual tendons for improved postoperative cosmesis. Divide all of the superficialis tendons distally and transect the profundus tendons proximally. Suture the proximal end of the superficialis en masse to the distal end of the profundus (Fig. 114-6). Allow sufficient lengthening so that the wrist and fingers can be extended to a neutral position without tension. Lengthen the wrist flexors and flexor pollicis longus through the same incision. Unless finger flexion defor-

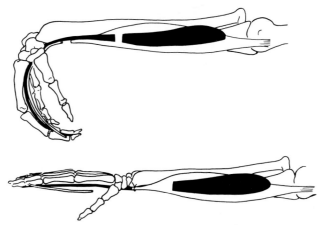

FIGURE 114-6. Superficialis-to-profundus transfer to correct a severe flexion deformity in a nonfunctional hand.

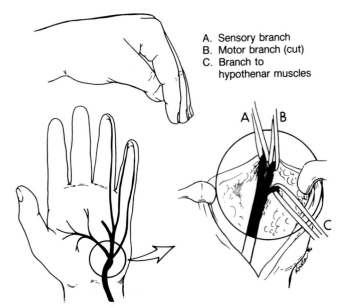

A. Sensory branch
B. Motor branch (cut)
C. Branch to hypothenar muscles

FIGURE 114-7. An intrinsic-plus deformity uncovered following a superficialis-to-profundus transfer.

mities are longstanding and the skin is contracted on the palmar surface, correct fixed contracture of the finger joints, using gentle passive manipulation. Passive manipulation should not be performed in the functional hand, since it results in greater postoperative edema and stiffness than after surgical release.

When excessive finger flexion is present without wrist flexion, sufficient flexor tendon lengthening can be obtained by fractional tendon lengthening. As in the case of the functional hand, usually only the superficialis tendons appear tight on passive stretch of the fingers; however, the profundus tendons should be lengthened as well. Lengthening of the superficialis alone will unmask spasticity in the profundus tendons, preventing satisfactory correction.

When finger flexion deformity is present, the intrinsic muscles are commonly spastic. If surgical attention is directed only to the flexor tendons, the fingers will assume an intrinsic-plus posture after surgery (Fig. 114-7). Evidence of intrinsic spasticity is sought preoperatively by examination of the thumb. If the adductor pollicis is spastic, the intrinsic muscles of the fingers also may be presumed to be spastic. Neurectomy of the motor branch of the ulnar nerve performed at the time of flexor tendon lengthening improves the cosmetic appearance of the fingers and relieves adductor spasticity of the thumb, as well. Expose the ulnar nerve in Guyon's canal through an incision on the palmar aspect of the hypothenar eminence (Fig. 114-7). Identify the motor branch of the nerve, using a nerve stimulator. Then excise a segment of the nerve. Conspicuous intrinsic atrophy is not a problem and is obscured by the slight edema and subcutaneous fat, which is present in most nonfunctional hands, if the patient is well nourished.

Because some patients lack extensor tone, the wrist may remain in a flexed position, because of gravity, after flexor tendon lengthening if the forearm postures in a pronated position. A wrist splint may be prescribed or extensor tenodesis performed at a second operation. Expose the extensor carpi radialis brevis, extensor carpi radialis longus, and extensor carpi ulnaris tendons through a dorsal incision on the forearm. Divide the proximal portion of each tendon, leaving half of the tendon attached to the muscle. Also leave intact the distal insertion of the tendons. Split the detached portion of the tendon longitudinally to the level of the distal radius. Using a

¼-inch drill, make two holes in the cortex of the distal radius. Carefully create a tunnel connecting the two holes, using a small curette. Then, pass the free proximal ends of the three extensor tendons through the bony tunnel in the distal radius. Determine the correct tension by holding the free ends of the extensor tendons, while the arm is held aloft with the wrist unsupported. The wrist should remain in 20° of extension without support. Then sew the extensor tendons to themselves, using nonabsorbable suture. The wrist is splinted in 20° of extension for 8 weeks postoperatively.

Elbow

When an elbow flexion contracture is present, lengthening of the biceps tendon alone will not significantly improve elbow flexion deformity, and attention must be directed to the brachialis muscle, as well. Myostatic contracture is differentiated from spasticity by anesthetic block of the musculocutaneous nerve, axillary nerve block, or by examining the patient under anesthesia. If there is less than 90° of fixed deformity, a musculocutaneous neurectomy is performed. Residual deformity is corrected after surgery by dropout or serial casts.

Even when minimal or no fixed myostatic or joint contracture is present, spasticity may cause the elbow to assume a flexed posture that interferes with function. Among hemiplegics, it is common for the elbow to assume a flexed posture while walking, and it may bounce up and down as a result of clonus. The patient may purposely walk slowly to decrease clonus. Musculocutaneous neurectomy will improve cosmesis and eliminate clonus. Following musculocutaneous neurectomy, the loss of elbow flexion strength is not important, because most stroke patients with excessive elbow flexion have nonfunctional hands. Because the brachioradialis is innervated by the radial nerve, which is left intact, some elbow flexion will persist following surgery, if this muscle was active preoperatively. The loss of musculocutaneous sensation is not bother-

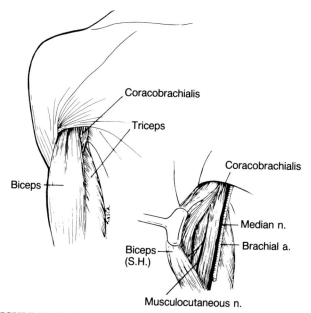

FIGURE 114-8. Exposure of the musculocutaneous nerve in the interval between the short head of the biceps and coracobrachialis muscles.

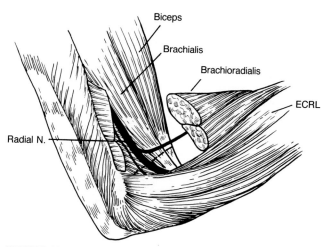

FIGURE 114-9. Release of the brachioradialis, biceps, and brachialis muscles to correct an elbow flexion contracture in a nonfunctional upper extremity.

some. In the patient without volitional brachioradialis control or spasticity, this procedure should not be performed, because musculocutaneous neurectomy will leave a completely flail elbow.

Make a longitudinal incision, extending distally from the tendon of the pectoralis major in the interval between the short head of the biceps and the coracobrachialis. This incision can be extended proximally or distally, if further exploration to locate the nerve is required. Excise a 1-cm segment of the nerve (Fig. 114-8).

When deformity is longstanding and considerable myostatic contracture has occurred, an elbow flexor release is performed. Using a lateral incision, release the origin of the brachioradialis, providing access to the biceps tendon, which is lengthened or tenotomized, and the brachialis, which is myotomized (Fig. 114-9). Some 30° to 40° of correction are usually

obtained, and further elbow extension is blocked by the contracture of the neurovascular structures and skin. Excessive tension on the neurovascular elements is unnecessary and may lead to vascular compromise. It is not usually necessary to release the anterior capsule. Further correction is easily obtained postoperatively by a program of serial casting. Because the skin incision is placed on the side, serial casting does not exert tension on the wound, in contrast to surgical approaches, where the skin incision is placed anteriorly. Because this procedure is usually performed on nonfunctional limbs, full extension is not necessary, and surgery in combination with postoperative serial casting will provide adequate correction.

Shoulder

As with the elbow, passive range-of-motion exercises begun immediately after a stroke prevent severe contractures, which usually occur only in the neglected patient. Once a common deformity, shoulder contracture is now rare.

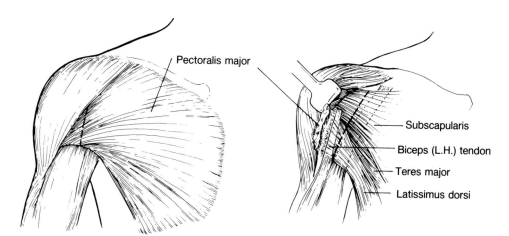

FIGURE 114-10. Release of the pectoralis major, subscapularis, teres major, and latissimus dorsi muscles to relieve an adduction and internal rotation contracture of the shoulder.

Surgical release is indicated when spastic contractures cause severe pain or prevent axillary hygiene.

Four muscles are responsible for adduction and internal rotation contractures of the shoulder: pectoralis major, subscapularis, latissimus dorsi, and teres minor. To determine which muscles contribute to the deformity, abduct the arm and rotate it externally. All but the subscapularis are clinically palpable. If, with the arm at the side, the humerus resists external rotation, the subscapularis may be presumed to be spastic as well.

Surgery is performed through an incision over the insertion of the pectoralis major tendon (Fig. 114-10); release the pectoralis major and subscapularis, and also the teres major and latissimus dorsi, if the latter muscles were tight preoperatively.

REFERENCES

1. Bloch, R., and Bayer, N.: Prognosis in Stroke. Clin. Orthop. **131**:10–14, 1978.
2. Bowman, B.R., Baker, L.L., and Waters, R.L.: Positional Feedback and Electrical Stimulation: An Automated Treatment for the Hemiplegic Wrist. Arch. Phys. Med. Rehabil. **60**:497–501, 1979.
3. Braun, R.M., Mooney, V., and Nickel, V.L.: Flexor-Origin Release for the Pronation-Flexion Deformity of the Forearm and Hand in the Stroke Patient. J. Bone Joint Surg. **52-A**:907–920, 1970.
4. Braun, R.M., Vise, G.T., and Roper, B.: Preliminary Experience with Superficialis to Profundus Tendon Transfer in the Hemiparetic Upper Extremity. J. Bone Joint Surg. **56-A**:446–472, 1974.
5. Garland, D.E., and Waters, R.L.: Orthopedic Evaluation in Hemiplegic Stroke. Orthop. Clin. N. Amer. **9**:291–304, 1978.
6. Garland, D.E., Capen, D., and Waters, R.L.: Surgical Morbidity in Patients with Neurologic Dysfunction. Clin. Orthop. **145**:189–192, 1979.
7. Garland, D.E., Thompson, R., and Waters, R.L.: Musculocutaneous Neurectomy for Spastic Elbow Flexion in Nonfunctional Upper Extremities in Adults. J. Bone Joint Surg. **62-A**:108–112, 1980.
8. Gresham, G.E., Fitzpatrick, T.E., Wold, P.A., et al.: Residual Disability in Survivors of Stroke—the Framingham Study. N. Engl. J. Med. **293**:954–956, 1975.
9. Inglis, A.E., and Cooper, W.: Release of the Flexor-Pronator Origin for Flexion Deformities of the Hand and Wrist in Spastic Paralysis: A Study of Eighteen Cases. J. Bone Joint Surg. **48-A**:847–857, 1966.
10. Jordan, C., and Waters, R.L.: Stroke. In Nickel, V.L. (ed.): Orthopedic Rehabilitation, New York, Churchill Livingstone, 1982, pp. 277–292.
11. McCullough, N.S.: Orthopedic Evaluation and Treatment of the Stroke Patient. American Academy of Orthopaedic Surgeons Instructional Course Lectures. St. Louis, C.V. Mosby, 1975, pp. 21, 24, 45.
12. Page, C.M.: An Operation for the Relief of Flexion Contraction of the Forearm. J. Bone Joint Surg. **5**:233–234, 1923.
13. Perry, J., and Waters, R.L.: Orthopedic Evaluation and Treatment of the Stroke Patient. American Academy of Orthopaedic Surgeons Instructional Course Lectures. St. Louis, C.V. Mosby, 1975, p. 40.
14. Waters, R.L.: Upper Extremity Surgery in Stroke Patients. Clin. Orthop. **131**:30–37, 1978.
15. Waters, R.L.: Surgery of the Hemiplegic Hand. In Fredericks, S., and Brody, G. (eds.): The Neurologic Aspects of Plastic Surgery. St. Louis, C.V. Mosby, 1978, pp. 123–128.
16. White, W.F.: Flexor Muscle Slide in Spastic Hand. J. Bone Joint Surg. **54-B**:453–459, 1972.

CHAPTER 115

Surgical Treatment for Tetraplegia: Upper Limb

ALVIN A. FREEHAFER,
P. HUNTER PECKHAM,
and MICHAEL W. KEITH

Goals of Surgery
Contractures and Abnormalities
  Shoulder Stiffness
  Elbow Extension Contracture
  Elbow Flexion and Supination Contractures
  Wrist Flexion Contracture
  Finger Flexing Deformities
  Finger Clawing
  Finger Extension Deformities
  Olecranon Bursitis
  Heterotopic Bone
Functional Neuromuscular Stimulation
Tendon Transfers
  Restoration of Elbow Extension
  Restoration of Wrist Extension
  Opponens Transfers
  Restoration of Finger Flexion
  Restoration of Finger Flexion and Opposition
Restoration of Thumb Flexion and Adduction
  Transfer of One Motor for Finger Flexion and Opposition
  Suture of Index Flexor
  Tenodeses
Results

Injury to the cervical spinal cord is devastating to the patient, who abruptly acquires a multisystem disease that requires multi- and interdisciplinary care. The intense desire which the tetraplegic has for the return of normal hand function is amplified by his loss of the ability to walk. It is clear today that many tetraplegics benefit from surgical restoration. In the past, resistance to surgical intervention in the upper limbs of tetraplegics predominated, and while this attitude persists to some degree, our experience and that of others[1-4,6,7,9,11-15,17-23,27,31,32] clearly shows the benefits of surgery, and should lead the way to an increasing effort in surgical reconstruction. There are several hundred thousand tetraplegics in the United States who could benefit from restoration of function to their upper limbs.

GOALS OF SURGERY

The goals of surgery in the tetraplegic are to correct abnormalities and deformities in the upper limbs if they exist, and to restore or replace lost function when possible. The selection of these patients is very important. During the first year following the spinal injury all attempts are directed to saving life and preserving remaining function. This allows the comprehensive programs necessary for rehabilitation to be put into place. All persons with tetraplegia should be prepared for discharge from the hospital and entry into society as happy productive citizens. Surgery of the upper limbs should be done when the patient becomes rehabilitated and capable of coping with the existing condition, controlling most daily living activities to the optimum level commensurate with the neurologic deficit, and preventing undesirable contractures and disorders in the upper limbs. We find that it is best to wait 1 year after the spinal cord injury. This period is usually necessary for the patient to be adequately rehabilitated and for the neurologic situation to become stable. Mass reflex spasms are often detrimental, and should be under control if surgery is to be helpful.

CONTRACTURES AND ABNORMALITIES

Contractures in the tetraplegic have not been common in our experience, because we have provided the proper comprehensive care in our spinal cord injury center. They do occur, however, often because of laxity in care by staff or patient.

Shoulder Stiffness

Shoulder stiffness is common but can be overcome, usually by proper positioning and passive and active exercises. Abduction contracture in a shoulder can present a "chicken wing" appearance, probably due to poor posture while at bed rest, excessive scarring from intramuscular injections into the deltoid, and absence of any adductors. This can be corrected by releasing the insertion of the deltoid and reattaching it in a more relaxed position.

Elbow Extension Contracture

Elbow extension contracture occurs infrequently and is usually caused by placing the elbow in the fully extended position and

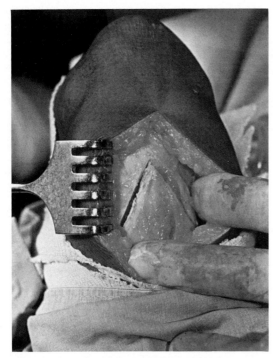

FIGURE 115-1.   A longitudinal incision over the posterior distal arm exposes the triceps tendon where a V cut is made with the apex just 2 to 4 cm proximal to the olecranon process.

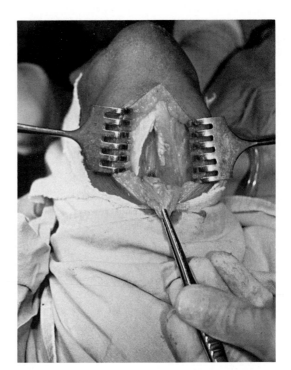

FIGURE 115-2.   The flap is raised, and gentle passive flexion is applied to the elbow.

neglecting range-of-motion exercises. The patients with this problem in our experience had weak elbow flexors and were high tetraplegics.

A longitudinal midposterior and distal arm incision exposes the triceps tendon, where a V cut allows lengthening of the tendon and flexion of the elbow, with a V-Y closure of the tendon. Complete correction at the time of surgery is unwise, and instead should be accomplished with serial casts before and after surgery, using very gentle and passive corrective forces. A long arm cast excluding the wrist and hand is used (Figs. 115-1 to 115-3).

Elbow Flexion and Supination Contractures

Elbow flexion and supination contractures occur together, especially in the neglected patient who spends a lot of time in bed with the elbows flexed and supinated. These are also persons who have good to normal elbow flexion and supination without triceps function; the condition may be considered a contracture of the biceps brachii muscle. Passive extension of the elbow is greatest with the forearm supinated and less with it pronated.

Correction is by serial plaster casts applied with gentle extension of the elbow with the forearm pronated. The long arm cast excludes the wrist and hand. If correction is accomplished, no surgery is done, but when further correction is needed tenotomy of the biceps brachii tendon through a 2-cm longitudinal antecubital incision in the distal arm is performed. Serial casts are continued until the elbow is fully extended and pronated. Casts are changed every 3 days, and a period of 2 or 3

weeks is usually required.[5] More extensive elbow flexion deformities can occur. When more than biceps brachii contracture occurs, more extensive surgery may be required.[30]

Wrist Flexion Contracture

Wrist flexion contractures occur occasionally in patients with spastic, paralyzed wrist flexors. Tenotomies of wrist flexors through small longitudinal incisions, together with plaster casts or splints, are usually helpful. A stiff wrist interferes with function, and is never helpful to the tetraplegic.

Finger Flexion Deformities

Finger flexion deformities sometimes occur, and may be corrected by tendon lengthenings, along with plaster casts and plastic splints. Moderate tightness of finger flexors is useful to the tetraplegic because it improves grasp. The automatic grasp of the hand after tenodesis is extremely valuable to the tetraplegic with a weak hand. Fingers that are closed into the palm are the only ones that need to be corrected. This is done through longitudinal palmar incision ulnar to the midline in the lower forearm; the tendons that are tight are lengthened by Z-plasty.

A C6 (Group III) tetraplegic with no active muscle function of the hand (Fig. 115-4) is independent at a wheelchair level and has the ability to open and close his fingers and thumb. Finger and thumb flexors are a little tight and spastic. By shaking his wrist, he can move the thumb to provide key pinch or palmar pinch. It would be a mistake to alter this particular

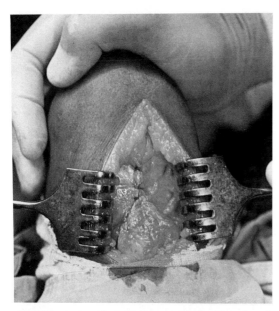

FIGURE 115-3. The V-Y closure with the elbow flexed.

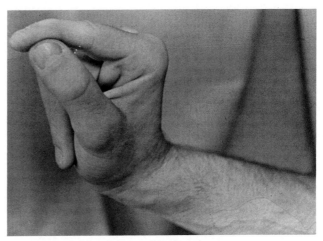

FIGURE 115-4. By shaking the wrist this C6 tetraplegic can move his thumb to get palmar pinch with the index finger.

balance. The tight flexors of the digits work to his advantage. He opens his fingers by gravity flexion of the wrist or by passively extending his fingers; a stiff wrist would totally end this person's ability to function independently.

When should tenotomies be done as opposed to lengthenings? Many surgeons abhor the concept of tenotomy,[4,5] but our experience has been favorable. As long as tendons are outside of tendon sheaths, the tenotomized tendon always heals and does not lead to weakness. If a surgeon has doubts, then tendon lengthening might be more appealing.

Finger Clawing

Severe finger clawing is not common, but when it does occur intrinsic tendon transfer or tenodeses might be indicated.

Finger Extension Deformities

Finger extension deformities occur, and with good occupational therapy some improvement is likely. Tendon transfer to the flexor digitorum profundus is helpful and is discussed later.

Olecranon Bursitis

Olecranon bursitis is very common in tetraplegics because of frequent pressure from leaning on the elbows. This is not a surgical problem, but the bursa should be treated with aspiration if it is large. Elbow pads are the treatment of choice, and almost always lead to healing (Fig. 115-5). Progression to an infected bursitis that needs incision and drainage is devastating. This is sometimes an incurable condition in the tetraplegic. The upper limbs are used for almost every activity, since these two limbs usually are the only ones under some voluntary control. It is impossible to immobilize the elbows unless a plaster cast is applied following the incision and drainage. The use of adequate debridement, open drainage with packing in a plaster

cast, and secondary closure with adequate antibiotics coverage is recommended. Because this condition is so disabling for the tetraplegic, it should be scrupulously avoided by proper care given when the patient is admitted to a spinal cord injury center.

Heterotopic Bone

Heterotopic bone is seen across any joint in the body below the neurologic level of deficit. The most common location in the upper limb is the elbow. Roentgenograms and clinical examination show bone usually coming from the posterior humerus, olecranon fossa, olecranon across the ulnar nerve, and cubital tunnel, often obliterating the groove and covering the nerve. Excision when the bone is mature usually restores good range of motion.

To excise heterotopic bone from the elbow, make a posterior incision, exposing the posterior humerus and olecranon. Identify the ulnar nerve in the arm where it is normal, and follow it to the ulnar groove or the heterotopic bone. Carefully remove pieces of the bone with a rongeur, being careful not to

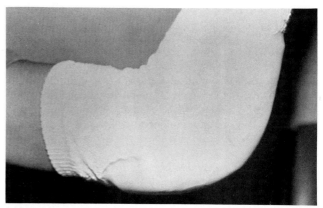

FIGURE 115-5. An elbow pad must be worn at all times except at bathtime in order for the bursitis to disappear. It need not be worn after the bursitis disappears.

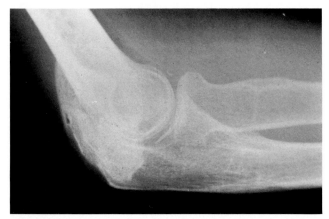

FIGURE 115-6.   Lateral roentgenogram of the elbow shows heterotopic bone.

damage the ulnar nerve. When the bone is removed, elbow motion usually is restored. Then transport the ulnar nerve anteriorly. Apply a bulky dressing and allow early motion (Figs. 115-6 and 115-7).

When heterotopic bone is located elsewhere, the situation must be individualized. We have encountered heterotopic bone in the shoulder and hand, but removal was not necessary.

FUNCTIONAL NEUROMUSCULAR STIMULATION

Surgical approaches in the hand in spinal cord injury may soon be augmented by the use of functional neuromuscular stimulation (FNS). FNS uses low levels of electrical current to elicit contraction in paralyzed muscles, the strength of which is regulated by the applied electrical stimulus. This technique is effective in restoring function in the C5 and C6 tetraplegic who previously has not been considered a candidate for tendon transfer surgery because of the high level of the lesion.[26]

Recently surgery was performed on two such subjects involved in the FNS program, who were not candidates for our usual surgical restoration techniques. The purpose of the surgery was to reduce the number of required motors (in this case electrically stimulated muscles), provide more uniformity in movement of the fingers, and eliminate movement at one joint. The procedures performed were:

1. Arthrodesis of the thumb interphalangeal joint
2. Tenodesis of the flexor digitorum profundus II-V
3. Tenodesis of the extensor digitorum communis II-V
4. Lasso procedure (Zancolli) of the flexor digitorum superficialis II-V (one subject) or tenodesis of FDS II-IV (one subject)

At this early stage of review of these patients' progress, it appears that our goals have been achieved. Surgical enhancement of the hand can also be accomplished by transferring a muscle with an upper motor neuron lesion and utilizing FNS. This provides a large number of possible motors that have previously been considered unavailable for transfer. Recently a transfer of extensor carpi ulnaris to extensor digitorum com-

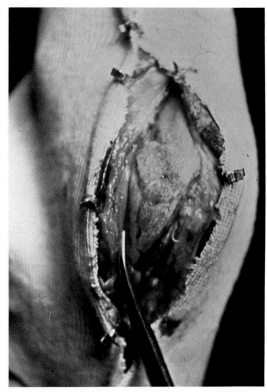

FIGURE 115-7.   Exposure of the heterotopic bone. The hemostat is pointing to the ulnar nerve at the level of the humerus. The heterotopic bone is attached to the humerus below and extends over the olecranon process and medially over the ulnar nerve in the cubital tunnel.

munis for finger extension was performed in one subject. Implanted devices, controlled by radiofrequency have also been utilized. They are surgically placed on the chest with leads and electrodes tunnelled subcutaneously to muscles of the forearm and hand.

The use of functional neuromuscular stimulation to supply additional motor function in such cases of more extensive paralysis is becoming an important adjunct in restoration of hand control in the tetraplegic subject.

TENDON TRANSFERS

Tendon transfers very effectively replace lost upper limb function in the tetraplegic; the goals of this surgery are to provide wrist extension, elbow extension, finger grasp, and thumb pinch. Only when the neurologic situation is stable, at least 1 year has elapsed since the time of spinal injury, and the patient has undergone a program of rehabilitation, should a patient be considered for tendon surgery. Spasticity, autonomic dysreflexia, pain, and psychologic adjustment must be under control if a good result is to be expected.[8,16]

Most patients can be grouped into categories which are frequently seen and based on which treatment can be planned (Table 115-1). There are always some paralytics who are incomplete or who do not fit into any category. The types of surgery done are listed in Table 115-2; not included are the tenotomy and tendon lengthening previously described, which

TABLE 115-1. CLASSIFICATION BY MUSCLE FUNCTION, OBJECTIVES, AND SURGICAL RECOMMENDATIONS

Group	Approximate Level of Lesion	Muscle Function Available	Objective of Transfer	Surgery Performed
Ia	C4	Shoulder shrug only		
Ib	C5	Shoulder control, elbow flexion	Elbow extension	Posterior deltoid transfer
II	C5 with C6 sparing	Above, plus brachioradialis ECRL, ECRB, all weak	Elbow extension	Posterior deltoid transfer
			Wrist extension	Brachioradialis transfer
III	C6	Above are good or normal	Elbow extension	Posterior deltoid transfer
			Finger flexion	Tendon transfer to finger flexors
			Thumb pinch	Adductor or opponens transfer, or tenodesis of flexor pollicis longis
IV	C7	Above + triceps, pronator teres, Flexor carpis radialis, weak finger flexors and extensors	Finger flexion	Transfer to finger flexors
			Thumb pinch	Opponens transfer
V	C8	Paralysis of hand intrinsics	Thumb pinch	Opponens transfer
VI		Incomplete paralysis not fitting the above		

were done in order to remove or adjust paralyzed, spastic, or deforming muscles that were felt to interfere with an optimum result. The muscles used for transfer are listed in Table 115-3. The brachioradialis is used most frequently because it is usually present and is expendable without functional loss to the patient.

Restoration of Elbow Extension

The deltoid muscle has a distinct posterior lobe, which can be separated and transferred to provide another useful function without disturbing shoulder abduction. The posterior portion

TABLE 115-2. OPERATIONS PERFORMED

Intrinsic Transfers
Tenodeses
   Flexor digitorum profundus and flexor
      pollicis longus
   Flexor digitorum profundus
   Extensor digitorum communis
   Flexor pollicis longus
   Extensor pollicis brevis
   Extensor pollicis longus
   Abductor pollicis longus
Opponens transfer alone
   Good voluntary finger grasp
   Automatic or no grasp
Opponens transfer and finger flexor transfer
Opponens transfer and suture index flexor
   digitorum profundus to others
Brachioradialis transfer to flexor pollicis
   longus
Posterior deltoid transfer
Brachioradialis transfer for wrist extension
Extensor carpi ulnaris transfer to finger
   extensors
Extensor carpi ulnaris transfer to extensor
   carpi radialis brevis
Opponensplasty and finger flexor transfers
   using one motor

of the deltoid can be transferred with tendon graft to the triceps to provide elbow extension. We use a modification of the procedure described by Moberg.[23]

Make an incision about 10 to 13 cm in the upper arm posteriorly over the posterior border of the deltoid muscle, and carry it distally to the insertion of the muscle. Because the triceps is paralyzed, atrophied, and flattened in this area, the bulging deltoid muscle is accentuated and can be palpated easily. Expose the deltoid, free the posterior border, and locate and separate the interval between the posterior portion and the rest of the deltoid. Be careful when freeing proximally, so that damage to the axillary nerve is avoided. This dissection should be blunt and one need not come closer than 4 or 5 cm to the nerve.

Make three longitudinal incisions in the foot and leg to expose the tibialis anterior tendon. The upper half of the tendon is covered with muscle, which can be cleared away leaving a long stout tendon for a graft between the freed posterior deltoid and the distal end of the triceps tendon (Figs. 115-8 to 115-11). In patients who walk, use fascia lata for the graft.

Suture the transfer with the arm at the side of the torso, the elbow at 90°, and with the posterior deltoid at the same length it was before it was cut from its insertion. Full flexion and extension of the elbow are done passively and with electrical stimulation, which gives the surgeon a better picture of the muscle function. Do not infiltrate the muscle with local anesthesia.

Immobilize the elbow in 20° of extension in plaster from upper arm to the wrist for 4 weeks, with the hand and wrist left

TABLE 115-3. MUSCLES USED FOR TRANSFER

Brachioradialis
Pronator teres
Flexor carpi radialis
Palmaris longus
Extensor carpi radialis longus
Posterior deltoid
Extensor carpi ulnaris
Flexor carpi ulnaris

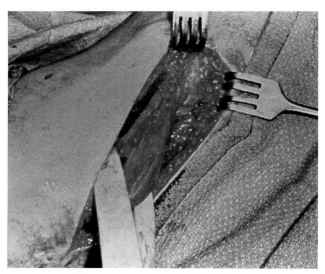

FIGURE 115-8. The posterior lobe of the deltoid is separated.

mobile. After the elbow is removed from plaster, a plastic splint is made for the anterior portion of the elbow to protect it from forced flexion in the first 2 to 3 weeks after the cast is removed. Allow active exercises as soon as the plaster is removed. Stressful activities such as wheelchair pushups and transfers are not allowed for about 3 months following surgery.

Whenever the brachioradialis is used as a transfer, the posterior deltoid transfer should act as an antagonist, which will strengthen the brachioradialis. This procedure can be done either before or after the brachioradialis transfer.

Restoration of Wrist Extension

When wrist extension is poor, the brachioradialis may be transferred to the extensor carpi radialis brevis. The three wrist extensors have different moment arms about the wrist, so only one extensor should be used. The extensor carpi radialis brevis provides the most direct and neutral wrist extension of the three.

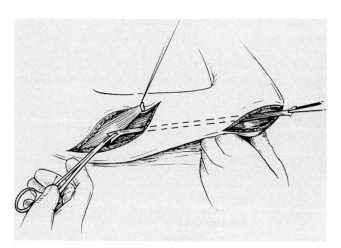

FIGURE 115-9. The tibialis anterior tendon graft, spanning the gap between the deltoid and the triceps tendons just proximal to the olecranon process.

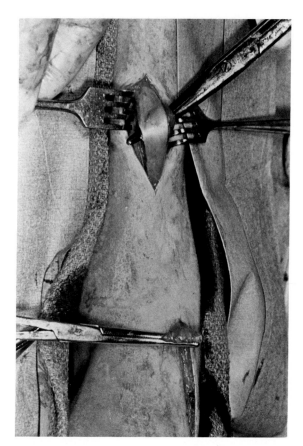

FIGURE 115-10. At the lower part of the figure, the tibialis anterior insertion has been detached and it is being pulled out into the second incision on the lower leg.

Prior to surgery, the brachioradialis is tested with the forearm in pronation with forceful elbow flexion. The examiner must feel the consistency or tightness of the muscle or pluck it, and this must be compared with the normal. The surgeon makes a guess as to the degree of difference. In transferring the brachioradialis for wrist extension, it often fails to do the job if wrist extension is totally absent preoperatively. The presence of active elbow extension enhances by antagonism the force of transferred brachioradialis.[1,6,22,23] Therefore, the posterior deltoid transfer for elbow extension is indicated when elbow extension is absent, either before or after the brachioradialis is transferred.

If contraction of the two radial wrist extensors can lift 10 kg, the long wrist extensor can be used for transfer. Moberg recommends testing under local anesthesia and if the extensor carpi radialis brevis can pull 5 kg the extensor carpi radialis longus can be used for transfer. We use a belt-buckle strain gauge during surgery to decide this if the clinical examination is equivocal.

Make a lateral incision of about 8 to 10 cm in the middle of the forearm. This exposes the brachioradialis; dorsally one can see next to it the extensor carpi radialis longus and the extensor carpi radialis brevis. Identify the lateral cutaneous nerve of the forearm, superficial to the brachioradialis; be careful with it and also protect the sensory branch of the radial nerve, which is deep to the brachioradialis and often intimately attached to its

FIGURE 115-11. The third incision is near the middle and upper one-third of the leg. The muscle is stripped away from the tendon.

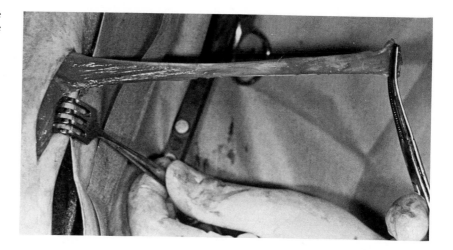

under surface. Distally it emerges from the brachioradialis and becomes superficial. Free the brachioradialis of all surrounding tissues up to the elbow with blunt and sharp dissection. This allows much better excursion of the muscle tendon unit. The tension of the sutured transfer should be such that at elbow flexion of 90°, the forearm neutral in pronation and supination, and the wrist extended about 20°, the end of the brachioradialis tendon should be at the level where it was originally cut. Passive motion and electrical stimulation of wrist extension and flexion give a clear picture of how the completed transfer works (Figs. 115-12 and 115-13).

Opponens Transfers

Opponens transfers are performed to provide pinch strength for the thumb against the fingers. We have found them to reliably provide key pinch, and to provide palmar pinch, as well, in over half of the cases. We most frequently use a varia-

tion of the T. Campbell Thompson modification of the Royle.[10,28,29] The flexor digitorum superficialis is moved to the abductor pollicis brevis, using the distal end of the flexor retinaculum as the pulley. The brachioradialis, pronator teres, or the extensor carpi radialis longus is used to motor the ring flexor digitorum superficialis in the forearm. The extensor carpi radialis longus is used only when it is certain that the extensor carpi radialis brevis is strong enough to maintain strong active wrist extension. The flexor carpi radialis should not be used because the patient then loses strong active wrist flexion.

Make a transverse incision at the base of the ring finger. Cut the superficial flexor at that level and pull it out into a longitudinal palmar incision. Make a longitudinal incision over the ulnar side of the thumb metacarpophalangeal joint and locate the tendon of the abductor pollicis brevis. Bring the ring flexor digitorum superficialis subcutaneously across the thenar eminence and suture it into the abductor pollicis brevis tendon.

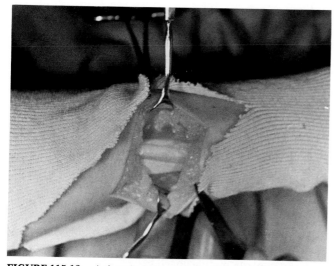

FIGURE 115-12. A short incision on the lateral aspect of the forearm with the wrist to the right shows (from top to bottom) the extensor carpi radialis brevis, the extensor carpi radialis longus, and the brachioradialis.

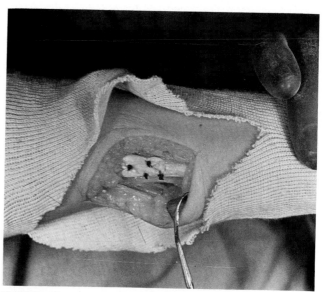

FIGURE 115-13. The brachioradialis is sutured to the extensor carpi radialis brevis.

Make a longitudinal incision in the palmar aspect of the lower forearm, slightly ulnar to the midline; this exposes the ring flexor digitorum superficialis. Make a lateral forearm incision to expose either the brachioradialis, extensor carpi radialis longus, or pronator teres. Suture the muscle for transfer into the ring flexor digitorum superficialis. The tension should be adjusted so that with the elbow at 90°, the thumb touching the index finger, and the wrist neutral, the end of the muscle to be transposed is at a length equal to its position at the point of severance. Moving the wrist in flexion and extension, one should see good pinch as wrist extension begins and opening with wrist flexion. Electrical stimulation is a part of the procedure and is described elsewhere.[6,8,25]

The brachioradialis has good excursion but is firmly bound down, so it must be freed from its surrounding tissues almost to the elbow. The extensor carpi radialis longus also has good excursion, but freeing it is not as important. The pronator teres is a good muscle for transfer, but it is short, and so it sometimes has to be sutured to muscle and to the beginning of the tendons. The pronator teres can be lengthened as much as 2 to 3 cm by including that much periosteum at its distal end.

Restoration of Finger Flexion

Transfers to the flexor digitorum profundus are performed to provide grasp and a firm surface to oppose lateral or palmar thumb pinch. The brachioradialis is preferred, because, in our electrical studies at the time of surgery[8,25] a better length-tension curve and excursion was demonstrated.

Restoration of Finger Flexion and Opposition

The combination of finger flexion and opposition is the procedure most frequently performed. It requires two motors. The same incisions are used, and two tunnels are made subcutaneously. One muscle is attached to the ring superficial flexor, which has been transferred to the abductor pollicis brevis, and the other muscle is woven through the deep finger flexor tendons. The index flexor digitorum profundus is always separated from the others and may be missed if one is not careful.[6] These transfers are useful in C6 and C7 (Group III and Group IV) tetraplegics.

Restoration of Thumb Flexion and Adduction

The brachioradialis is transferred to the flexor pollicis longus to provide thumb flexion and adduction. The thumb interphalangeal joint is fused or pinned.[6,31] When elbow extension is present, it serves as an antagonist and strengthens the force of contraction of the brachioradialis when it is used for transfer.[1,6,22,23]

Transfer of One Motor for Finger Flexion and Opposition

Transfer of one motor for both finger flexion and opposition is done when only one motor is available, and provides surprising

improvement in function. The same incisions are used that were described earlier for restoration of finger flexion and opposition. The brachioradialis is sutured into the ring flexor digitorum superficialis and then into the flexor digitorum profundus.

Suture of Index Flexor

Finger flexor power sometimes is present but weak, with resultant inability to close the index finger, even though the other fingers do fully close. This tendon is always separate from the others and it is easily sutured to the other flexors, which are bound together and work as a unit. The technique described by Omer[6,9,24] for median nerve paralysis may be performed in place of a complete transfer to all of the deep finger flexors.

Tenodeses

Tenodeses are performed in the absence of an active motoring muscle.[6] The tenodeses of the flexor pollicis longus described by Moberg provided key pinch, but the results were not as good as when voluntary motor function could be provided.

The use of extensor tendons for tenodeses may be helpful to move the thumb and fingers out of the palm. Usually wrist flexion automatically opens the thumb and fingers, while wrist extension closes the thumb and fingers. Patients must learn this, because most of the transfers are designed to close the thumb and fingers. There are not enough muscles to provide a balanced hand, and movement of the wrist must not be lost.

We do not perform extensor tenodeses routinely because most patients can learn wrist motion to help finger opening and closing. Tenodeses are done when the preoperative evaluation reveals that wrist motion does not allow automatic opening of the fingers. The extensor digitorum communis, abductor pollicis longus, extensor pollicis longus, and extensor pollicis brevis have all been sutured to the extensor retinaculum in various combinations and at various times. The examiner can usually tell preoperatively which one or combinations need to be tenodesed. Extensor tenodeses can be performed later if digit opening becomes a problem. A short longitudinal incision exposes the extensor retinaculum, and the tendon or tendons are simply attached to it with nylon sutures, so that in wrist flexion the thumb and fingers are open and in wrist extension the digits are able to close.

RESULTS

Grading results in tetraplegics is different from other conditions. Writing, bladder and bowel care, dressing, bathing, grooming, feeding, driving, lifting objects, communication, sex, buttoning, and turning dials are but a few activities which improve after surgery. The comparison of what is achieved with that which existed before surgery in each individual is the way to evaluate results. The patients we observed following tendon surgery almost always functioned better recreationally, educationally, vocationally, and socially.

In our experience, muscle transfers provide better results than tenodeses. When motors for transfer are not available, tenodeses for digit closure are valuable. Tenodeses of the thumb and finger extensors may be used to open the digits when wrist flexion fails to do so, though this should not be done routinely. Patients have to learn to use wrist motion to aid finger opening and closing because the number of motors needed to balance the hand is rarely available.

The tetraplegic functions quite differently from those not paralyzed. The upper limbs serve as "legs" and take considerable weight bearing and stress. This must always be kept in mind when planning reconstructive surgery. Any procedure must be able to stand up to tremendous forces, just as would be expected when doing lower limb surgery. Postoperatively, the tetraplegic must be restricted and given additional assistance for 2 to 3 months, or else tendon transfers will come apart.

We now believe that tendon transfers and tenodeses should be considered for all tetraplegics after 1 year following injury, provided they have undergone an effective rehabilitation program and their neurologic examination is stable. When elbow extension, wrist extension, finger grasp, and thumb pinch are useless, marked improvement in function can usually be achieved with tendon surgery.

REFERENCES

1. Bryan, R.S.: The Moberg Deltoid-Triceps Replacement and Key Pinch Operations in Quadriplegia. Preliminary Experiences. Hand 9:207, 1977.

2. Colyer, R.A., and Kappelman, B.: Flexor Pollicis Longus Tenodesis in Tetraplegia at the Sixth Cervical Level. J. Bone Joint Surg. 63-A:376, 1981.

3. DeBenedetti, M.: Restoration of Elbow Extension Power in the Tetraplegic Patient using the Moberg Technique. J. Hand Surg. 4:86, 1979.

4. Freehafer, A.A.: Care of the Hand in Cervical Spinal Cord Injuries. Paraplegia 7:118, 1969.

5. Freehafer, A.A.: Flexion and Supination Deformities of the Elbow in Tetraplegics. Paraplegia 15:221, 1978.

6. Freehafer, A.A., Kelly C.M., and Peckham, P.H.: Tendon Transfer Surgery for Restoration of Upper Limb Function following Cervical Spinal Cord Injury. J. Hand Surg. 9-A:887, 1984.

7. Freehafer, A.A., and Mast, W.A.: Transfer of the Brachioradialis to Improve Wrist Extension in High Spinal Cord Injury. J. Bone Joint Surg. 49-A:648, 1967.

8. Freehafer, A.A., Peckham P.H., and Keith, M.: Determination of Muscle-Tendon Unit Properties during Tendon Transfer. J. Hand Surg. 4:331, 1979.

9. Freehafer, A.A., Von Haam E., and Allen, V.: Tendon Transfers to Improve Grasp after Injuries of the Cervical Spinal Cord. J. Bone Joint Surg. 56-A:951, 1974.

10. Henderson E.D.: Transfer of Wrist Extensors and Brachioradialis to Restore Opposition of the Thumb. J. Bone Joint Surg. 44-A:513, 1962.

11. Hentz, V.R., and Keoshian, L.A.: Changing Perspectives in Surgical Hand Rehabilitation in Quadriplegia Patients. Plast. Reconstr. Surg. 64:509, 1979.

12. Hentz, V.R., Brown M., and Keoshian, L.A.: Upper Limb Reconstruction in Quadriplegia: Functional Assessment and Proposed Treatment Modifications. J. Hand Surg. 8:119, 1983.

13. Hiensche, D.L., and Waters, R.L.: Interphalangeal Fixation of the Thumb in Moberg's Key Grip Procedure. J. Hand Surg. 9-A:30, 1985.

14. House, J.H., Gwathmey, F.W., and Lundsguard, D.K.: Restoration of Strong Grasp and Lateral Pinch in Tetraplegia due to Spinal Cord Injury. J. Hand Surg. 1:152, 1976.

15. House, J.H., and Shannon, M.A.: Restoration of Strong Grasp and Lateral Pinch in Tetraplegia: A Comparison of Two Methods of Thumb Control in Each Patient. J. Hand Surg. 9-A:22, 1985.

16. Jane, M.J., Freehafer, A.A., Hazel, C., Lindan, R., and Joiner, E.: Autonomic Dysreflexia; A Cause of Morbidity and Mortality in Orthopaedic Patients with Spinal Cord Injury. Clin. Orthop. 169:151, 1982.

17. Lamb, D.W., and Landry, R.: The Hand in Quadriplegia. Hand 3:31, 1971.

18. Lamb, D.W., and Landry, R.: The Hand in Quadriplegia. Paraplegia 9:204, 1972.

19. Lamb, D., and Chan, K.M.: Surgical Reconstruction of the Upper Limb in Traumatic Tetraplegia. J. Bone Joint Surg. 65-B:291, 1983.

20. Maury, M.M., Guillaumat M., and Francois, N.: Our Experience of Upper Limb Transfers in Cases of Tetraplegia. Paraplegia 11:245, 1977.

21. McDowell, C.L., Moberg, E.A., and Graham-Smith, A.: International Conference on Surgical Rehabilitation of the Upper Limb in Tetraplegia. J. Hand Surg. 4:387, 1979.

22. Moberg, E.: The Upper Limb in Tetraplegia. Stuttgart, Georg Thieme Publishers, 1978.

23. Moberg, E.: Surgical Treatment for Absent Single-Hand Grip and Elbow Extension in Quadriplegia. J. Bone Joint Surg. 57-A:196, 1975.

24. Omer, G.E., Jr.: Evaluation and Reconstruction of the Forearm and Hand after Acute Traumatic Peripheral Nerve Injuries. J. Bone Joint Surg. 50-A:1454, 1968.

25. Peckham, P.H., Freehafer, A.A., and Keith, M.W.: The Influence of Muscle Properties in Tendon Transfers. In Brand, P.W. (ed.): Clinical Mechanics of the Hand. St. Louis, C.V. Mosby, 1985, pp. 310–324.

26. Peckham, P.H., Marsolais, E.B., and Mortimer, J.T.: Restoration of Key Grip and Release in the C6 Quadriplegic through Functional Electrical Stimulation. J. Hand. Surg. 5:464, 1980.

27. Raczka, R., Braun, R., and Waters, R.L.: Posterior Deltoid-to-Triceps Transfer in Quadriplegia. Clin. Orthop. 187:163, 1984.

28. Royle, N.E.: An Operation for Paralysis of the Intrinsic Muscles of the Thumb. J.A.M.A. 111:612, 1938.

29. Thompson, T.C.: Modified Operation for Opponens Paralysis. J. Bone Joint Surg. 24:632, 1942.

30. Urbaniak, J.R., Hansen, P.E., Beissinger, S.F., and Aitken, M.S.: Correction of Post-Traumatic Flexion Contracture of the Elbow by Anterior Capsulotomy. J. Bone Joint Surg. 67-A:1160, 1985.

31. Waters, R., Moore, K.R., Graboff, S.R., and Paris, K.: Brachioradialis to Flexor Pollicis Longus Tendon Transfer for Active Lateral Pinch in the Tetraplegic. J. Hand Surg. 9-A:385, 1985.

32. Zancolli, E.A.: Surgery for the Quadriplegic Hand with Active Strong Wrist Extension Preserved. A Study of 97 Cases. Clin. Orthop. 112:101, 1975.

CHAPTER 116

Congenital Hand Deformities

LOUI BAYNE

SYNDACTYLY

Syndactyly (web fingers) represents a developmental failure of separation of the fingers. Syndactyly is usually classified as complete or incomplete, and simple or complex. If the interconnections between the digits extend to the distal end of the digits, the syndactyly is *complete;* if not, it is *incomplete. Simple* syndactyly refers to the abnormal intradigital connections formed by skin, fibrous tissue, or ligaments; *complex* syndactyly refers to abnormal bony intradigital connections. Complex syndactyly is frequently complicated by connections of musculotendinous and neurovascular units. Frequently, complex syndactyly includes three or more digits with interposed incomplete structures. This type of deformity is sometimes referred to as *complicated complex* syndactyly.[15]

Indications for Surgery

The primary reason for surgical intervention is to improve the cosmetic appearance of the hand and to restore its functional capacity. Any deviation from normal appearance is offensive to the individual. Slight webbing, where the web space is advanced distally by more than 1 cm, produces an abnormal appearance and limits the spread of the fingers. It is also difficult to seat a ring properly on a webbed finger. In simple complete and complex syndactyly, the functional loss is even greater. When a complex syndactyly involves two or more digits, careful evaluation of the conjoined digits is necessary to determine if separate functional units can be reconstructed. Quite often essential structures will be absent or shared, and only one functional unit can be salvaged.

Timing of surgical reconstruction is an important factor. Most parents want the deformity corrected as soon as possible. Early intervention should be based on two factors. First, soft-tissue contractures and bony deformity produced by unequal growth of the conjoined fingers should be prevented. Second, separation should be completed before independent finger use is established. With the recent advances in microsurgical techniques, separation of digits can be accomplished at a much earlier age. A good general rule is to separate the thumb and little finger from the adjacent digits before the age of 1 year so that grasp is not impeded. The index finger should be released from the long finger by the second year, and the ring finger should be released before 3 years of age. When multiple digits are involved, the standard principle of never operating on both sides of the digit at one procedure should be followed.

Principles of Treatment

The abnormal anatomy of simple and complex syndactyly vary significantly, and should be considered separately. Simple syndactyly, whether complete or incomplete, involves two digits that are joined by soft tissue. There are three primary concerns in reconstruction of these units:

1. An adequate web space has to be constructed that will have the same depth as the adjacent fingers, will allow at least 30° of abduction of the digits, and will have a sloping contour and tetrahedral shape similar to the adjacent web spaces.

2. The finger flaps should be designed in a zig-zag manner to prevent constriction of the fingers.

3. The fingernail and nail folds should be reconstructed as near to normal as possible. Skin grafts are often necessary because there is never enough skin to completely cover the finger without risking vascular compromise.

Surgical Technique

There are numerous techniques for correction of syndactyly, ranging from simply cutting the web space with scissors to elaborate zig-zag flap formations. For those with a special interest in this topic, a very complete history of the surgical release of syndactyly has been provided by Kelikian.[27] Regardless of the method used, the reconstruction should be planned well in advance.

Simple Syndactyly

My preferred method for surgical release of simple syndactyly is to use a long dorsal flap to create the web space (Fig. 116-1A). The web must be deepened to the proper length to correspond to the adjacent fingers. The length of the flap should be two-thirds the length of the proximal phalanx. Draw the dorsal flap on the dorsal surface of the web space, starting at the midpoint of the metacarpal heads and slanting inward and distally to the midpoint of the proximal phalanx. The end of the flap should be about one-third the width of the base. Draw zig-zag flaps on the dorsal and palmar surface of the conjoined fingers so that they will interdigitate when the fingers are separated (see Fig. 116-1A and B). It is necessary to draw out all flaps and be sure that they will cover the proper spaces before cutting the flaps. This is usually done before the tourniquet is inflated.

Next, elevate the flaps. Start with the dorsal flaps, cutting the points of the flaps and then gradually making them thicker as you progress to the base. This will preserve the small vessels and prevent the necessity of removing the fatty tissue from the flap later. After the dorsal and palmar flaps have been dissected, turn the hand to the dorsal surface and identify and protect the neurovascular structures at the web. Then remove the central fatty tissue and hypertrophied central septum, taking care to preserve the neurovascular structures.

Suture the web flaps first, then the finger flaps. There will then be two areas of skin deficiency on the dorsal inner aspect of each of the adjacent fingers which will require skin grafting (see Fig. 116-1C). I use a full-thickness free-hand graft taken from the groin. The graft is elliptical in shape and the donor site can be closed primarily. Release the tourniquet before application of the dressing to check the vascularity of the flaps and digit. If the color is poor, the points of the various zig-zag flaps can be released to decrease the tension, and circulation will usually return. These defects generally will granulate satisfactorily.

Complex Syndactyly

The treatment of complex syndactyly requires a considerable amount of ingenuity and skill by the hand surgeon (Fig. 116-2). When considering reconstruction of these hands, the correction of the syndactyly is actually a relatively minor consideration. The many bizarre skeletal deformities that are covered by the syndactyly represent the biggest problem. It will be best to discuss these deformities by starting with the least problematic and progressing to the most complicated.

Several principles should be kept in mind in planning surgical correction of any complex syndactyly.

1. Separate the functional digits as early as possible to prevent deformity secondary to adjacent abnormal parts.
2. Separate border digits as early as possible to establish opposable digits for prehension.
3. Realign the skeletal elements on the longitudinal axis to establish a proper growth pattern.
4. Eliminate all parts that will interfere with the normal growth and function of the digits.

Fusions of Nails and Distal Phalanges. The fusion of nails and distal phalanges is an integral part of a complex syndactyly (see Fig. 116-2C and D). The distal phalanges should be divided, especially when they involve unequal fingers. Adequate skin will not be available to cover the defect when the digits are separated, and skin grafting will be necessary. To establish a better contour to the distal phalanx, it may be necessary to take a wedge-shaped graft from the side of the first toe of each foot. These should be full-thickness skin grafts which also incorporate some subcutaneous fat, which will provide a better contour to the distal segment and lateral fold. When a single nail is present it should be divided and each portion reduced in size to be comparable to the adjacent nails. The tuft skin can be re-

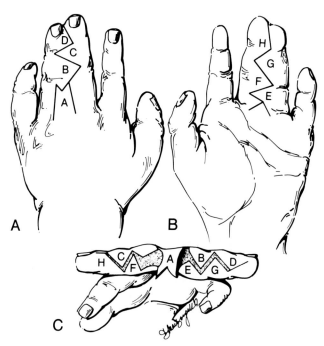

FIGURE 116-1. Incisions outlined on the dorsal (A) and volar (B) surfaces for the syndactylized digits. The dorsal flap has its base at the metacarpal heads and extends distally for two-thirds the length of the proximal segment. (C) The finger flaps are made in a zig-zag manner so as to interdigitate with the volar flaps.

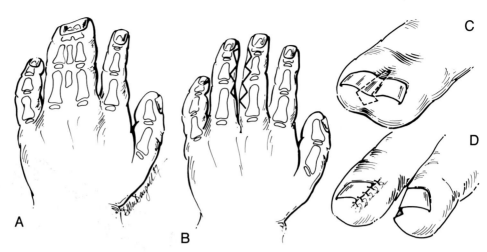

FIGURE 116-2. (*A*) Complex syndactyly showing two digits joined together with remnants of an ill-formed digit. The distal phalanges are fused together and there is a broad common nail. (*B*) The two complete digits are separated and the nonfunctional intervening structure is excised. (*C*) The distal phalanges and nails are trimmed to fit the separated digits. (*D*) By narrowing the nail and debulking the distal tuft, closure can be accomplished.

duced in thickness and the excess skin can be used for the lateral fold of the nail.

Syndactyly with Polydactyly. Frequently you will see syndactyly of two well-formed fingers with a polydactylous element interposed between the digits (see Fig. 116-2*A*). In such cases it is best to remove the extra structures and use the surrounding skin to cover the two adjacent "normal" digits.

Syndactyly with Bizarre Elements. Occasionally in a syndactyly of two or more digits, the skeletal elements of at least one digit will be placed in a transverse axis. It is best in these cases to select the most functional digit, realign its skeletal parts, and eliminate the nonfunctional parts. In these cases it is better to end up with a three-finger hand that is functional than to preserve a functionless digit.

Syndactyly Associated with Acrosyndactyly. In acrosyndactyly, the fingertips are fused together in a cluster formation and the digits are separated by sinuses extending from the dorsal to the palmar skin. It is as if the fingers had been formed previously and then fused together on the ends. Frequently some digits will be deficient and no terminal phalanx will be present. The fingers should be separated early, at 6 months to 1 year of age, especially when multiple digits are involved. Separation should follow the schedule for multiple syndactyly already discussed. The index and little fingers are separated first, followed in 6 months by separation of the long and ring fingers. Locating and maintaining the sinuses will aid in the separation of these fingers. Skin grafting is frequently necessary because of the paucity of skin.

Complications

The most common complication resulting from surgical treatment of syndactyly is the loss of the web correction. This can be the result of infection, maceration of the tissue, loss of skin grafts, or faulty web construction. Infection can be monitored early by temperature elevation, presence of unusual pain, or a bad odor coming from the dressing. Infection should be treated promptly by proper antibiotics. The fingers should be kept separated, and local application of topical antibiotics is frequently useful. Skin grafts can be reapplied when infection is cleared.

Maceration of the skin can occur in large bulky dressings in hot climates. It is best to change the dressing early and frequently. Maceration will cause loss of skin grafts, separation of sutures, and infection. When the skin grafts are lost, frequently the fingers will fuse back together; thus it is necessary to keep the fingers well separated at all times. Special splints can be devised to hold the fingers apart and still allow sufficient air to keep the web dry.

Vascular complications are rare and should always be guarded against. As mentioned, circulation should be checked before the dressing goes on. If there is any question of viability of the digits or flap, the flap should be released until adequate circulation returns. Circulation should be checked frequently after the dressing is applied, and any signs of ischemia should be investigated immediately. Postoperative observation for several days is recommended. The parents should be instructed as to what problems to watch for and told to keep the dressing dry.

Scar formation on the digits can occur when there is a deficiency of skin and tight closure. With growth of the child this deformity can only become worse. It is best to correct any skin contracture by Z-plasty or skin grafting as early as possible.

DUPLICATE THUMBS

Duplication of the thumb is a relatively common anomaly of the upper extremity. The etiology is unknown, but several patterns of inheritance can occur.[42] Sporadic occurrence is the most common.

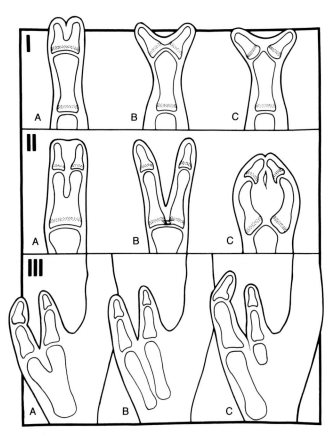

FIGURE 116-3. Classification for thumb duplication. *Type I:* Duplication of distal phalanx. *(A)* Incomplete. *(B)* Complete with base joined by cartilage only. *(C)* Complete. *Type II:* Duplication at the proximal phalangeal level. *(A)* Incomplete. *(B)* Complete with base joined by cartilage. *(C)* Complete. *Type III:* Duplication at metacarpal level. *(A)* Incomplete. *(B)* Complete. *(C)* Mixed.

There is a wide spectrum of degree of thumb duplication. Figure 116-3 illustrates a classification based on the segment of the thumb where the duplication occurs and the extent of duplication (i.e., complete or incomplete).

Principles of Treatment

The basic goal in reconstruction of the thumb is to give the patient a single thumb that is cosmetically pleasing and as near normal in function as possible. It is essential for the surgeon to explain to the parents what they can expect from the surgery. The duplicate thumb is an abnormal thumb and will not appear the same as the opposite thumb. It will be smaller, thinner, and may be limited in function.

Because the thumb plays such an essential role in the function of the hand, the timing of the surgical correction is an important consideration. Delay is necessary in some cases where there is a need to determine which of the two thumbs is most functional. Other factors such as size, progression of deformity, and nail development need to be considered when deciding which thumb is to be salvaged. In some instances it may be necessary to transfer or salvage certain portions of the

ablated part in order to reconstruct a more functional and better-appearing thumb. This correction may be delayed until the child is 1½ to 2 years of age.

Reconstruction of the duplicated thumb requires a basic knowledge of the abnormal anatomy present and the skill to restore the anatomic relationships of the remaining structures. It is necessary to align the growth plates perpendicular to the long axis of the digit. This will ensure that the correction will be maintained as growth continues.

Surgical Techniques

The surgical treatment selected depends on the level of duplication and the degree of involvement (see Fig. 116-3).

Type I Deformities

In type IB and IC deformities in Figure 116-3, where there is a complete duplication of the distal phalanx, it is best to salvage the most functional and cosmetically pleasing part and scavenge the other. In most instances the ulnar part is salvaged.

Make the skin incision in a zig-zag manner so that no longitudinal incisions will cross the flexion crease of the joints. Sufficient skin should be present from the ablated part to reconstruct the lateral surface of the remaining part.

The abnormal anatomic structures that will be present are as follows (Fig. 116-4):

1. The flexor and extensor tendons will be bifurcated.
2. The head of the proximal phalanx will be enlarged to accommodate the two phalanges or the broad conjoined base. There will usually be two separate facets that are congruent with the articular surface of the respective phalanges.
3. Each distal phalanx will have a single collateral ligament.

To reconstruct the distal joint, begin by excising one of the distal phalanges and save the slip of the extensor tendon and as much of its lateral capsule and collateral ligament as possible. Cut off the bifurcated slip of the flexor tendon smoothly to prevent entrapment by the flexor pulley. Use the salvaged collateral ligament and capsule to reconstruct the lateral joint of the remaining part. If the distal phalanx is displaced laterally, it will tighten the remaining collateral ligament and displace the distal phalanx from its congruent articular groove. Both of these factors will impede motion of the distal joint. A wedge resection of the head of the proximal phalanx will sufficiently narrow the head so that capsular and collateral ligament reconstruction can be accomplished without disrupting the normal articular arc of the remaining phalanx (see Fig. 116-4).

Correction of the angulation of the distal phalanx is usually necessary in types IB and IC deformities (see Fig. 116-3). This is accomplished with a closing wedge osteotomy, which will align the physis perpendicular to the long axis of the thumb. Protect the joint reconstruction and osteotomy by an intermedullary Kirschner wire placed from the tip of the distal phalanx to the base of the proximal phalanx.

Occasionally in type IA deformities (see Fig. 116-3), it will

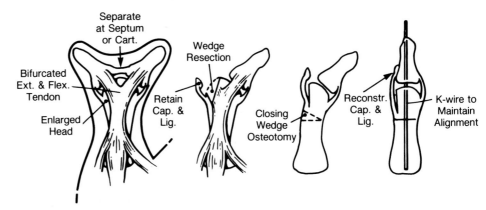

FIGURE 116-4.   Abnormal anatomy and reconstruction techniques for type I thumb duplication.

be necessary to augment the lateral nail fold with a portion of skin salvaged from the lateral surface of the ablated part.

Type II Deformities

Duplications that occur at the proximal phalangeal level will present an additional abnormal anatomy (Fig. 116-5). Reconstruction of type II deformities is much more complicated. It involves the correction of a double angulatory deformity and the salvaging and reconstruction of the intrinsic muscles of the thumb.

The metacarpophalangeal joint is reconstructed in much the same way as the distal joint in type I deformities (see Fig. 116-4). The proximal phalanx is osteotomized to correct the distal joint alignment, and the metacarpal is osteotomized to correct the metacarpophalangeal joint alignment.

The extensor and flexor tendons, because of their more proximal bifurcation and broad septal connections, are subluxated across the distal joint, thus necessitating centralization. Flexor pulley reconstruction at the mid–proximal phalangeal level may be necessary.

The thenar muscles are detached from the radial ablated part and reattached to the proximal phalangeal base and extensor mechanism of the remaining proximal phalanx.

Type III Deformities

Duplications at the metacarpal level vary greatly in degree of deficiency and duplication. When the duplication is an incomplete type IIIA (see Fig. 116-3), the reconstructive procedures are carried out as for a complete duplication, except that the carpometacarpal joint does not need to be reconstructed.

In complete type IIIB duplications (see Fig. 116-3), it is necessary to reattach the radial intrinsic muscles, reconstruct the carpometacarpal joint, and, frequently, to widen the thumb–index web space.

In mixed-quality type IIIC duplications (see Fig. 116-3), the best-appearing thumb has a proximally deficient metacarpal. This thumb will have flexor and extensor function, but is unstable proximally. The more complete radial thumb is thin, angulated, and less functional. Reconstruction requires removal of the radial thumb at the middle portion of the metacarpal and

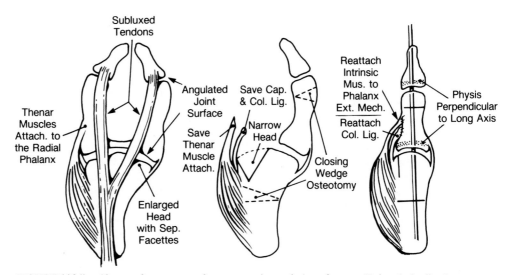

FIGURE 116-5.   Abnormal anatomy and reconstruction technique for type II thumb duplication.

transposition of the ulnar thumb to the radial metacarpal. The extensor pollicis brevis, abductor pollicis brevis, and adductor pollicis are transferred to the transposed part.

Postoperative Care

In all cases the reconstructed thumb is immobilized for 3 weeks, which will allow proper healing of the osteotomy and the reconstructed joints. At this point the immobilization is removed and active mobilization exercises are begun. Further intermittent immobilization is usually not necessary in small children.

Complications

The most frequent complications are recurrent angulation, hypermobility of the joints, and restricted motion of the reconstructed joints.

Recurrent angulation is usually due to failure to align the physis perpendicular to the long axis of the thumb. Thus, as growth proceeds angulation will occur, and will progress unless the angulation is corrected by closing wedge osteotomy. Failure to realign the flexor and extensor tendons across the joint will also produce progressive angulation.

Hypermobility of the reconstructed joint is usually due to poor collateral ligament or capsular reconstruction.

Stiff joints are usually the result of prolonged immobilization or very tight ligament reconstruction.

Loss of abduction is usually related to failure to properly reattach the intrinsic muscles or failure to reconstruct an adequate thumb–index web space.

ABSENT RADIUS

Absence of the radius is a congenital deformity caused by longitudinal failure of formation of parts in the radial or preaxial border of the upper extremity. The radius may be totally or partially absent; total absence is most common.

The etiology of this defect is not completely understood. Heredity has been listed in early reports as the predominant factor.[20] Genetic causes have been recognized due to dominant autosomal genes.[19] Environmental factors have been implicated as causative agents, in particular, prenatal use of thalidomide. In most recent reports, radial dysplasia frequently has been found to occur sporadically.[28]

The deformity is not common, occurring at the rate of 1 in 100,000 live births.[18] The characteristic clinical picture with either partial or complete absence of the radius is a patient with a short forearm which is slightly bowed to the radial side, with a prominent knob distally, representing the end of the ulna. The hand is radially deviated. The thumb may or may not be present. The fingers, particularly the radial digits, are defective to some degree, displaying limited motion and contracture of the middle joints. The greater the radial deficiency, the less support there is for the hand. The greater the radial deviation of the hand, the less effective are the forearm muscles.[37] The function of the hand is affected by the degree of finger deficiency and the loss of wrist support.

Principles of Treatment

Patients with partial or complete absence of the radius with inadequate support of the hand are candidates for surgical reconstruction. The primary consideration in reconstruction is to provide support for the hand. This requires extensive release of soft-tissue contractures and placement of the hand on the end of the ulna. The hand must then be balanced on the end of the ulna by tendon transfers and capsular reefing. The ideal age for reconstruction is from 6 months to 3 years of age.

Many methods of surgical correction for radial deficiencies have been described in the literature.[1,11,13,14,26] The treatment recommended by most authors today is to centralize the hand over the end of the ulna, performing an osteotomy of the ulna when necessary.[3,4,30,37]

Surgical Technique

In most cases, two surgical incisions are used (Fig. 116-6). A transverse wedge incision is made over the end of the ulna to excise the redundant skin and fibrofatty tissue. A Z-plasty incision may also be necessary on the radial surface of the distal forearm and wrist to give extra length to the tight skin on the radial side and to make the wrist flexors more accessible.

Develop the ulnar incision first and expose the distal ulna, being careful not to damage the epiphyseal blood supply. Identify and retract the extensor carpi ulnaris, flexor carpi ulnaris, and dorsal sensory branch of the ulnar nerve. Develop a capsular flap, including the ulnar collateral ligament, with its base distally. This will expose the end of the ulna. Develop the interval between the ulna and carpus along the radial border of the ulna. Release the capsule from its carpal attachment. If preoperative stretching has corrected the radial contracture, attempt to place the lunate over the end of the ulna. If this cannot be done easily, use the radial Z-plasty incision.

Elevate the Z-plasty flaps, and identify and protect the large superficial branch of the median nerve and the radial vascular structures. Divide the flexor carpi radialis, brachioradialis, radial capsule, and other nonessential contracted soft tissues (see Fig. 116-6). Re-expose the distal end of the ulna through the ulnar incision. Flatten the end of the ulna by shaving the cartilage, being careful not to expose the epiphyseal bone. Next, place a Kirschner wire in the center of the distal end of the ulna and drill it from distal to proximal, up the shaft of the ulna, to exit at the olecranon. Then remove the wire, thus providing a pilot track for the final Kirschner-wire fixation.

If the ulna is bowed more than 30°, perform an osteotomy at the apex of the bow. Then place a second Kirschner wire in the middle of the lunate and drill it from proximal to distal through the base of the third metacarpal and out through the knuckle. Withdraw the Kirschner wire distally until only 1 cm is left protruding through the lunate. Then lever the hand over the end of the ulna and place the extruding Kirschner wire in the pilot hole in the end of the ulna. Reduce the hand and drill the Kirschner wire proximally, then withdraw it proximally until the distal end is free of the metacarpal head. The Kirschner wire will also stabilize the ulnar osteotomy, if this needs to be performed (see Fig. 116-6).

If the reduction is still difficult, a resection of up to 3 cm of the shaft of the ulna can be done. It is important that the

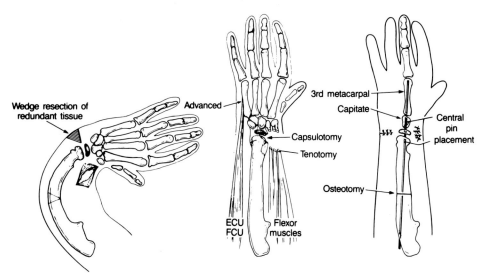

FIGURE 116-6.   Technique for centralization of the hand on the end of the ulna. Two incisions are usually necessary. The radial flexors of the wrist are divided. The extensor carpi ulnaris (*ECU*) and flexor carpi ulnaris (*FCU*) are advanced distally to balance the hand. A Kirschner wire may be used to immobilize the reduction and osteotomy of the ulna.

reduction be easy, because too much tension on the reduction can produce recurrence of the deformity due to soft-tissue tightness. Too much tension on the distal ulnar epiphysis will result in premature closure, loss of growth to the distal ulna, and often recurrent angulation caused by unequal epiphyseal pressure.

Next, rotate the hand to the neutral position between supination and pronation. Balance the hand on the end of the ulna by advancing the extensor carpi ulnaris distally and transferring the flexor carpi ulnaris as far distally as possible and dorsally to the extensor carpi ulnaris. This will reinforce ulnar deviation. Advance the distally based ulnocarpal capsule proximally and suture it to the ulnar periosteum. Before closure, release the tourniquet and evaluate the circulation. Close the incisions in the routine manner. Apply a bulky dressing and reinforce it with long-arm plaster splints.

Postoperative Care

At 2 weeks the dressing is changed, the sutures are removed, and a long-arm plaster cast is applied. Mobilization of the fingers is encouraged at this time. Occasionally in older children the finger flexors are tight and a dynamic outrigger may be used during this period. The cast and the Kirschner wire are removed at 6 to 8 weeks and a short-arm plastic splint is made so that the fingers will be free. The parents are directed to remove the splint several times during the day and mobilize the wrist over the next 3 months. Following this period the splint may be removed during the day and reapplied at night. Intermittent splinting is encouraged for 2 years. The patient should be followed until skeletal maturity.

Complications

There have been no serious complications reported in the literature. In my experience involving 75 surgical cases, there have

been several superficial wound and pintrack infections which have responded to local cleansing and antibiotics. Treatment has not been interrupted.

One vascular complication occurred in a severely contracted deformity where there was a marked webbing of the skin. After centralization and pinning, the hand failed to pink up when the tourniquet was released. The pin had to be removed and the reduction released before the circulation returned. The deformity was treated by casting and splinting, but the final result was poor.

No neurologic complications have occurred in my experience. Recurrence of the deformity has been a frequent complication, primarily caused by surgical failure and progressive bowing of the ulna. Surgical failure was most often caused by inadequate soft-tissue release, which produced recurrence of the deformity and increased tension on the distal ulnar epiphysis.

ABSENT ULNA

Absence of the ulna is only one of the many congenital anomalies that may occur along the ulnar or postaxial border of the upper extremity. Malformations in this deficiency vary more widely than in radial longitudinal deficiencies.[25] Clinically the deformity is characterized by ectrodactyly in various degrees, ulnar deviation of the hand, forearm shortening and bowing, defective elbow motion, and hypoplasia of the proximal part of the upper extremity.

The etiology of this deformity is not well understood. Roberts[39] reported the deficiency in three consecutive generations. There have been no known chromosomal abnormalities reported.[32] The deficiency may occur as part of other recognized syndromes and thus may be inherited in a Mendelian pattern.[43] However, in most reported cases the occurrence has been sporadic, and no teratogenic factor has been found.

Ulnar deficiencies are rare, with reported rates varying from one for every 3.6 radial deficiencies[4] to one for every ten radial deficiencies.[9,33] Ulnar deficiencies have been associated primarily with musculoskeletal defects, such as clubfoot, spina bifida, mandibular defects, fibular defects, femoral agenesis, and absent patella.[33]

Abnormal Anatomy

In congenital ulnar deficiency the abnormalities of the hand contribute greatly to the loss of function. Hand defects are present, to some extent, in all types of ulnar aplasia. Anomalies of the digits vary greatly. Usually some degree of absence occurs along the ulnar border of the hand, but the radial border can be affected as well. Frequently the thumb and several digits are missing. The remaining fingers may be webbed. Absence of the metacarpals and carpal bones corresponds to the absent digits.

Forearm anomalies can be classified as four types.[2,29,33,38] In type I, hypoplasia of the ulna, the distal and proximal epiphyses are present but the growth is suppressed. This produces a short ulna with mild ulnar deviation of the hand and very little functional loss. Treatment is rarely necessary.

In type II deformities only part of the ulna is present, most frequently the proximal portion (Fig. 116-7). This proximal segment provides some stability for elbow motion. The distal

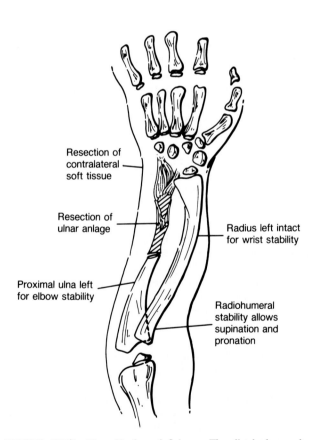

FIGURE 116-7. Type II ulnar deficiency. The distal ulnar anlage attaches to the distal radius and carpal bones and acts as a tethering force on the ulnar side of the forearm.

Labels in figure:
- Resection of contralateral soft tissue
- Resection of ulnar anlage
- Proximal ulna left for elbow stability
- Radius left intact for wrist stability
- Radiohumeral stability allows supination and pronation

anlage is present, but consists of fibrocartilage without longitudinal growth potential.[9] This will, in effect, tether the growing radius, thus producing radial bowing. The radial head may articulate with the capitellum, or, owing to the tethering effect of the ulna–ulnar anlage complex, may become laterally and posteriorly dislocated. If dislocation is pronounced, it will interfere with elbow and forearm motion.

In type III deformities, which are very rare, the ulna is totally absent. The radius is usually straight. The elbow is unstable and the radial head may be dislocated.

In type IV deformities the radius is fused to the humerus. Frequently a fused remnant of the ulna will be seen protruding from the humerus. The ulnar anlage will be present, and will be attached to the distal radius and carpus, causing bowing of the radius and ulnar deviation of the hand.

Principles of Treatment

Treatment of these deformities must be based on evaluation of each case for functional capacity and appearance. Treatment should be predicated on the potential to increase functional capacity, not simply on improving cosmesis.

Indications for Surgery

In type II and IV deformities an anlage is usually present and, if detected early, should be excised, to prevent shortening and bowing of the radius, ulnar deviation of the hand, and subsequent radial head dislocation. Riordan[38] recommends resection of the anlage before 6 months of age.

In older patients with type IV deformities, the anlage should be resected to relieve the tethering force on the hand and distal radius. The deformity of the radius can be corrected by a closing wedge osteotomy. If the radius is fused to the humerus, the humerus frequently will have a rotational deformity; this can be relieved by a derotational osteotomy of the humerus.

In older patients with type II deformities, in whom extreme bowing of the radius and dislocation of the radial head are present, reconstructive surgery should be contemplated. With continued growth the radial head displacement will become more severe and will then interfere with elbow extension and forearm rotation. If there is enough ulna present to give the forearm stability, the radial head may be resected. If, however, there is considerable forearm instability, loss of elbow motion, and marked radial bowing, the creation of a one-bone forearm may be considered.

Surgical Technique

To construct a one-bone forearm (Fig. 116-8), approach the ulna through a posterior ulnar incision, beginning at the proximal ulna and extending to the wrist. Identify the junction of the ulna and the ulnar anlage. Osteotomize the ulna at this point and resect the anlage distally (see Fig. 116-8A). Take care to locate the ulnar artery and nerve in the distal dissection to prevent injury; these structures are closely related to the distal anlage. Resect the attachment of the fibrous extension of the anlage across the ulnar border of the distal radial epiphysis and its attachment to the carpus.

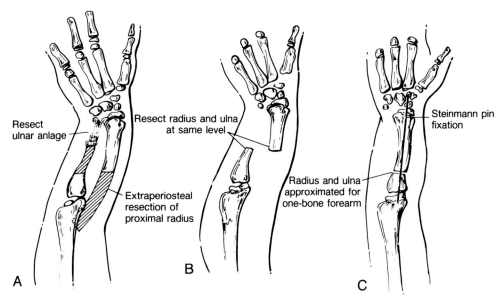

FIGURE 116-8. Technique for creation of one-bone forearm. (*A*) The distal ulnar anlage and the proximal radius (*shaded areas*) are resected. (*B*) The distal radius and proximal ulna are brought into alignment. (*C*) A Kirschner wire is used to stabilize the radial and ulnar segments and is extended to the carpals to stabilize the wrist.

When the ulnar anlage has been removed, achieve adequate exposure by dissecting across the interosseous membrane to locate the adjacent radius. The osteotomy of the radius should be made as far proximally as practical in order to maximize the length of the forearm (see Fig. 116-8*B*). Bring the distal radial shaft into alignment with the proximal ulna. Stabilize the two aligned bones by an intermedullary Kirschner wire (see Fig. 116-8*C*). If there is considerable bowing of the distal radius, a second osteotomy of the radius can be performed, and can be stabilized with the same Kirschner wire.

The radial head and proximal portion of the radius must be resected extraperiosteally to prevent recurrent growth. The resection is best performed through a separate proximal radial incision to prevent damage to the posterior interosseous nerve.

Release the tourniquet at this point, control the bleeding, and evaluate vascularity.

Postoperative Care

The extremity is placed in a well-padded long-arm splint. The dressing is changed at the end of 2 weeks. A long-arm cast is then applied and maintained until union occurs, for about 5 to 6 weeks. The Kirschner wire can then be removed and the hand and forearm supported with a removable splint until the patient regains strength and mobility in the extremity.

Complications

The complications that I have experienced have been related to the recurrence of the resected portion of the proximal radius. This resulted in loss of elbow motion that had been gained postoperatively.

ABSENT THUMB

Congenital absence of the thumb is not a common anomaly. The deformity is frequently associated with radial deficiencies. In the 100 radial deficiencies I have treated, approximately 20% had complete absence of the thumb. This anomaly is also associated with many syndromes that have much more detrimental effects on the patient's well-being.[18]

Patients with absent thumb are severely handicapped, although they may be very skillful in the use of their hands, because the thumb contributes 40% of the function of the hand. The important pulp-to-pulp pinch is missing, thus limiting their potential ability to earn a living.

Patients born without one or both thumbs are usually first evaluated shortly after birth. It is important to reassure the parents that surgical reconstruction is possible and will provide significant function and improvement.[18] However, parents are frequently reluctant to consent to surgery when it is explained that a finger or toe will have to be used in the reconstruction of the thumb. It is wise to show them pictures of, or place them in contact with, patients who have undergone this procedure. This will give the family a realistic idea of what to expect.

Principles of Treatment

The main goal of treatment is to create a thumb either from the remaining digits or from a toe. Descriptions of pollicization techniques of each of the remaining four fingers and toe transplantation are reported in the literature.[7] Pollicization of the index finger has been the most successful, through the efforts of Littler,[31] Riordan,[36] Carroll,[8] and Buck–Gramcko,[5] and is the method used by most surgeons.

Reconstruction of the thumb should begin before the patient acquires undesirable motor patterns, such as side-to-side pinch, thus allowing the child to learn proper prehension at an early age. Reconstruction should be started at 12 to 18 months of age.

Surgical Technique

There are several requirements that must be met if the index finger is to be made into a thumb.

1. It must be of the proper length, with the appropriate number of joints and phalanges.
2. The transposed digit must not be in the same plane as the fingers, so that pulp-to-pulp opposition can be accomplished.
3. A thenar eminence must be reconstructed.
4. The base must be stabilized.

Draw the skin incisions before the tourniquet is elevated. The incisions are outlined in Figure 116-9A and B. Make the incisions on the dorsum of the index finger. The longitudinal incision (see Fig. 116-9B, points F–E) begins at the middle of the proximal interphalangeal joint and extends to the level of the neck of the metacarpal. The circumferential incision of the index finger is begun on the palmar surface of the finger at the

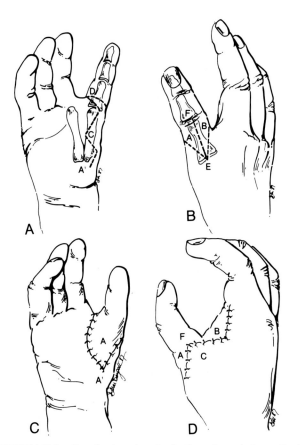

FIGURE 116-9. Drawing based on Buck–Gramcko technique of pollicization. The points along the incision labeled as A–F, and the steps in the procedure are detailed in the text.

level of the middle of the proximal phalanx (see Fig. 116-9A, point D) and continued on both sides of the finger to connect on the dorsum of the hand (see Fig. 116-9B, point E). This will create two wing flaps (see Fig. 116-9B, points A and B), which will give adequate exposure to the extensor mechanism. The radiopalmar incision (see Fig. 116-9A) starts at point D and curves proximally and dorsally, then in a palmar direction at midpalm and dorsally to the base of the second metacarpal.

Dissect the various flaps carefully, preserving the large dorsal veins to the index finger so they can be transposed with and continue to drain the index finger.

Through the palmar incision, identify the common digital artery and nerve and free them up to their bifurcation between the index and long fingers. Next, identify the index radial digital artery and nerve, and, if present, protect them.

Next, on the dorsum of the index finger expose the extensor mechanism and mobilize the lateral bands. Divide them from the central slip to the level of the proximal interphalangeal joint. Divide the dorsal fascia between the metacarpal heads, and dissect it to the transverse metacarpal ligament, which is divided with care to prevent injury to the underlying neurovascular structures.

Mobilize the flexor tendons from their sheaths and pulleys so as to free the tendons to the level of the proximal interphalangeal joint of the index finger.

Divide the first dorsal and palmar interossei at their musculotendinous attachments to the lateral bands. Carefully divide the first dorsal interosseous attachment to the proximal phalanx so as not to injure the radial collateral ligament or palmar plate. Dissect the interossei muscles proximally to the base of the metacarpal.

Identify the extensor digitorum communis and the extensor indicis proprius and divide the juncture of the communis. Free the extensor indicis proprius from the dorsal retinaculum at the metacarpal head continuing through the central slip; it thus will be free to act as the extensor pollicis longus, though it will have to be shortened later. Suture the extensor digitorum communis to the base of the proximal phalanx and capsule. This will also need to be shortened later, and will act as the abductor pollicis longus.

Again identify the common neurovascular bundle between the index and long fingers. Ligate the artery to the long finger. Gently tease the bifurcation of the common digital nerve so that the bifurcation can be split to the midmetacarpal level.

Shorten the second metacarpal by dividing it distally at its epiphyseal plate and proximally at its base and removing the shaft. This will usually provide sufficient shortening of the index ray to provide the proper length for the thumb.

The index now is completely free, except for the neurovascular bundles and the dorsal veins. The critical placement of the metacarpal head, which is to act as a new trapezium, is probably the most difficult part. The head should be placed in front of or palmar to the stump of the second metacarpal or its capsular attachment (Fig. 116-9B). This is because in the normal hand the basal joint of the thumb is not in line with, but palmar to, the line of the metacarpal bases.

Hyperextend the metacarpophalangeal joint until the palmar capsule is tight, and secure it in this position with a Kirschner wire through the base of the proximal phalanx into the hand. Then rotate the index finger 120° so that the pulp of the index finger faces the pulp of the ring finger. Pin the head of the metacarpal to the base of the second metacarpal or to the carpal bones. Place several sutures in the soft tissue surrounding the head and capsule. The Kirschner wire that is used to hold the metacarpal joint in hyperextension can then either be removed or maintained for approximately 3 weeks, at which time motion will be started.

Suture the first dorsal interosseous muscle to the radial lateral band by weaving the band through the musculotendinous junction and pulling it tight. This muscle will now function as the abductor pollicis brevis. The ulnar lateral band will be sutured in a like manner to the palmar interosseous muscle and serve as the new adductor pollicis.

Shorten the extensor tendons to further stabilize the thumb. If the extensor indicis proprius tends to rotate the thumb when it is shortened, then it will have to be pulled through above the wrist, rerouted subcutaneously, and sutured by end-to-end anastomosis. The extensor digitorum communis, having already been sutured to the base of the proximal phalangeal capsular attachment, will have to be shortened also. The flexor tendons usually will not require shortening.

Before closure it will be necessary to let the tourniquet down to determine the viability of the digit and to control excess bleeding. Use several slips of thin silastic drains in the closure. To start the closure, find the wing flap designated as point A in Figure 116-9B, and place it to the base of the palmar incision, point A' (see Fig. 116-9C). This will give you some idea how much of flap C (see Fig. 116-9D) will have to be trimmed to fit into point F. Next, close the palmar flap around the base of the finger, then along the radial side from point B distally. If after closure the finger does not continue to be pink, loosen any tight sutures or take the closure down and see if the artery is kinked or clotted. If the artery is in spasm, bathing it in lidocaine may help.

Postoperative Care

A bulky dressing with a posterior splint is applied, holding the thumb in an abducted position. The tips of the digits are left exposed to check the circulation. The dressing is changed in 1 week. The silastic drains are then removed. A short-arm thumb-spica cast is applied and then removed in 3 weeks. After immobilization is discontinued, the hand is left free and the child is encouraged to use it. Functional return is slow at first. The child is very protective of the thumb and will only start to use it when the soreness decreases. It may take several months for the flexors to the thumb to become functional. I encourage the parents to provide toys that require two-hand manipulation. Delay in the use of the pollicized thumb may be due to damage to the digital nerve during the splitting; this will delay function for 6 months or more.

Complications

There are three major causes of complications in pollicization procedures: the thumb may be too long or too short, or aseptic necrosis may occur at the head of the metacarpal. Surgical technique probably accounts for the majority of complications and failures. As the surgeon becomes more experienced, the results seem to improve.

Aseptic necrosis of the head of the metacarpal of the transposed index finger has been reported in long-term follow-up,[18] but has not decreased the function of the thumb, although the thumb may be short. If an error in thumb length is made, it is best that the thumb be short rather than too long. A short thumb is more pleasing aesthetically, and its function is not hampered.

ULNAR DIMELIA (MIRROR HAND)

Ulnar dimelia (duplication of the ulna) is an extremely rare deformity. Sixty cases have been reported in the literature.[27] The deformity has frequently been thought of as a form of duplication. However, because the defect includes failure of formation of other structures of the upper extremity, it probably should be considered as a totally separate anomaly.[44]

The deformity is characterized by duplication of the ulna and absence of the radius and thumb (Fig. 116-10). The hand has six to eight fingers, which give the appearance of a "mirror hand." The deformity is most often unilateral and involves the entire upper extremity. The shoulder is small due to defects in the scapula and pectoral muscles. The humerus has no capitellum, but two ill-formed trochleae. The proximal ulnar olecranon fossae face each other. The distal ulnae have broad carpal articular surfaces. The carpal bones are duplicated, except for the scaphoid and trapezium (see Fig. 116-10).

The occurence is sporadic and usually not inherited. However, if fibular dimelia is present, spontaneous genetic mutation should be suspected and transmission by an autosomal dominant mutant gene can occur. The most likely cause of defects in the forearm bones, with concomitant abnormality of the hand, is defective proximal–distal organization of the limb bud; this may be genetic in origin but may also be occasioned by some environmental influence at the time of morphogenesis of the limb.[24]

Principles of Treatment

The sparsity of cases treated by any one individual has hampered the development of a complete treatment plan. Many authors have published accounts of individual cases, with various methods of handling certain aspects of the deformity.[2,16,21,23,34,40] The primary concern is to create a more functional extremity and produce a better-looking hand. In order to do this it is necessary to

1. Increase elbow motion
2. Provide extension of the wrist
3. Remove excess digits
4. Reconstruct a thumb and thumb web-space

Plan your overall treatment in advance. First, observe the child at play. See how the child uses the hand in space. Determine the degree of active elbow motion and what structures activate it. Determine if lack of wrist extension interferes with hand function and what structures are present to correct the deformity. Determine which fingers are the most functional and which can be eliminated. Determine which of the digits can best be pollicized.

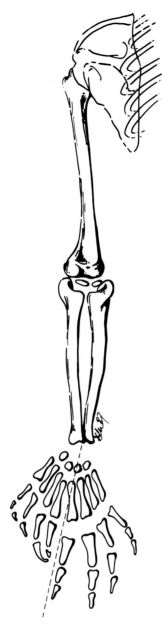

FIGURE 116-10. Ulnar dimelia, or mirror hand. At the shoulder, the clavicle is small and bowed. At the elbow, note the duplication of the ulna, with the olecranon and coracoid processes of each ulna facing the other. At the wrist, the distal ulnar articulation is broad, and double ossification centers are present for the capitate and hamate. In the hand there is duplication of four digits.

Surgical Techniques

Several operations will be necessary to reconstruct this deformity. It is best to begin with the hand because extra structures will be available following the removal of the extra digits; these structures may be used later to improve wrist function.

Hand Reconstruction

The primary goal of treatment is to reconstruct the hand so as to have four fingers and a thumb that will oppose the fingers in prehension.

I prefer the one-stage method described by Gropper,[23] based on the principles of Buck–Gramcko[6] for pollicization.

The mirror hand is usually divided by a cleft between the ulnar four digits and the radial three digits. The ulnar digits are usually the most functional and should be preserved. The middle digit or the radial duplicated digit is the most functional and is the best for pollicization.

Skin incisions are planned so that the selected digit can be isolated on its neurovascular bundles (Fig. 116-11A). In addition, a sufficient amount of skin will be available for web-space reconstruction after the digit adjacent to the ulnar side is partially filleted. The radial border of the pollicized digit can be contoured after the removal of the adjacent radial digit (Fig. 116-11B).

Careful dissection of the common neurovascular bundles to the middle digit in each web-space is necessary. Ligate the bifurcation to each adjacent digit. Tease apart the common nerves to the thenar level before division. At least two large dorsal veins should be preserved with the digit to provide adequate venous drainage.

The tendon anatomy is frequently anomalous. If the flexor tendon to the middle digit is bifurcated, sharply divide the slip to the adjacent digit even with the border of the tendon to the middle digit. The divided tendons to the radial digit can be used later to provide abductor pollicis brevis function to the pollicized digit. The extensor tendons to the excised digits can be used to provide the function of the abductor pollicis longus and extensor pollicis longus.

Shorten the metacarpal of the middle digit by dividing the shaft at its base and proximally at its physis, discarding the remaining shaft. Then align the metacarpal head with the anterior surface of the base of the middle metacarpal (see Fig. 116-11C and D). Rotate the head 120°, and hyperextend the joint. Hold the head in place in this position by two sutures. The metacarpophalangeal joint of the middle digit now becomes the carpometacarpal joint of the pollicized digit. The intrinsic muscles of the adjacent digits can then be sutured to the lateral bands of the extensor mechanism of the pollicized digit to augment adduction and abduction.

The skin flaps will have to be modified to accommodate the now-shortened digit for proper closure. Release the tourniquet after closure to evaluate the vascularity of the digits and flaps. Apply a bulky dressing with a posterior splint to hold the thumb in abduction and partial opposition. The dressing is changed in 1 week and a cast applied for 2 more weeks. Three weeks after surgery an exercise program is instituted. A removable night splint is used to hold the thumb in the opposed position to prevent overstretching for 3 months after surgery.

Wrist Reconstruction

Lack of extension and angulation of the hand to either the radial or ulnar side are the main problems. To correct the angulation, a Z-plasty and release of tight structures frequently are necessary. Release the capsule and tendons. The flexor carpi radialis or ulnaris, as the case may be, can be transferred to the extensor surface of the hand to aid in extension. Gorriz[21] recommends transferring the flexor digitorum sublimis of the pollicized digit to the extensor surface of the second metacarpal to provide extension of the wrist. Wrist extension and correction of angulation are difficult and may lead to wrist fusion at a later age.

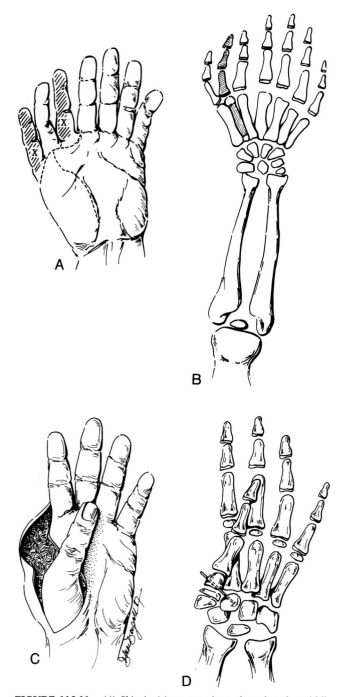

FIGURE 116-11. (*A*) Skin incisions are planned so that the middle digit (third from left) can be mobilized on its neurovascular bundles. (*B*) Adequate skin will be provided for the thumb web with the removal of the second radial ray. (*C* and *D*) The remaining head and phalanges of the third radial digit are placed anterior to the base of the third metacarpal, rotating the digit 120° and hyperextending the metacarpophalangeal joint so that the digit is in the opposed position and is out of the plane of the remaining metacarpals.

Elbow Reconstruction

Restricted elbow motion is due to weak flexor and extensor muscles and the abnormal articulations of the double ulnae with the humerus. Excision of the least-developed proximal ulna has been suggested by several authors.[24,28]

Approach the preaxial or radial ulna through a lateral incision. Expose the proximal ulna extraperiosteally, preserving a sufficient periosteal and ligamentous strip to reconstruct a collateral ligament. Excise a sufficient amount of ulna, along with its remaining periosteum, to provide adequate extension and flexion. After surgery, immobilize the limb for 3 weeks, then begin the patient on active-assistive flexion and extension exercises. A night splint is recommended to hold the elbow in 90° of flexion. It will be necessary to strengthen the flexor and extensor muscles of the elbow to maintain motion.

Complications

This is a complex problem, and proper preparation and skill are necessary to produce a satisfactory result. Infection should be minimized by use of preoperative antibiotics and sterile techniques. Skin slough should be negligible because of the excess skin available. Results will also depend on the diligence of the postoperative exercise program.

RADIOULNAR SYNOSTOSIS

Synostosis is a term that designates the failure of separation of osseous structures. Radioulnar synostosis occurs most frequently about the elbow. There are two types: type I, the pure or primary type, represents a complete fusion of the proximal portions of the radius and ulna. No radial head is present proximal to the fusion site. In type II, or secondary synostosis, the radial head is present proximal to the fusion site, but it is frequently displaced. Radioulnar synostosis is not a commonly reported deformity. However, it is probably more common than thought, because disability is somewhat minor and many patients do not seek medical attention.

Radioulnar synostosis occurs more frequently in males than females and involves the right extremity more often than the left, although it is frequently bilateral. Many cases are familial, being passed on from one generation to the next. The degree of disability depends on the position in which the forearm is fixed. A mild pronation or supination deformity can be overcome by abducting or adducting the shoulder. When pronation is severe the patient has difficulty accepting change, holding trays, and carrying heavy objects. He may have difficulty wringing water out of clothes, dealing cards, turning door knobs, or buttoning shirts, and frequently tires when writing.

Principles of Treatment

Only a small percentage of patients require surgery. Patients that should be considered for surgery are those with bilateral involvement in which one or both deformities exceeds 60° of pronation. Unilateral cases in which motion in the dominant hand is restricted by > 60° also can be considered for surgical correction.

There are two methods of treatment. One is designed to place the forearm in a more functional position by means of rotational osteotomy, and the other is designed to restore rotatory motion to the forearm.

Most mobilization techniques require extensive surgery, involving osseous as well as soft-tissue structures.[27] Dacron-reinforced silastic or soft tissue has been used to preserve the separation of the synostosis. Tendon transfers are necessary to provide motion. None of these procedures have been uniformly successful, and failure is quite common.

I prefer the method of rotational osteotomy. The osteotomy can be made at any level, but an osteotomy at the fusion site is less difficult.

The ideal position in which to place the forearm is debatable. Green and Mital[22] suggest that in bilateral cases where both hands are pronated, one forearm should be rotated in 20° to 25° of supination. Simmons[41] disputes this view, suggesting that pronation of 10° to 20° gives the best function, and citing the fact that these patients have hypermobility at the wrist of 30° to 40°, which gives them adequate supination. In bilateral cases the dominant hand should be left in 30° to 40° of pronation so as not to interfere with the patient's ability to write.

Surgical Technique

I prefer to osteotomize the forearm at the synostosis site (Fig. 116-12A). Make a longitudinal dorsal incision just to the radial side of the posterior aspect of the ulnar ridge. Subperiosteal exposure of the fusion mass is easily accomplished. Make a transverse osteotomy in the distal half of the fusion mass. I prefer to take out 1 cm of the fusion mass to shorten the osseous structures, thereby relaxing the neurovascular structures so that when the forearm is rotated they will not be twisted or stretched (see Fig. 116-12A). Place a Steinmann pin through the olecranon, across the osteotomy site, to stabilize the forearm (see Fig. 116-12B). Immobilize the forearm with an external fixator with two pins above and below the osteotomy site. Place a finger on the radial pulse as the forearm is rotated to the desired position, or until the pulse is diminished. If difficulty with circulation arises, decrease the rotation until the pulse returns. Secure the external fixator, and close the wound in the routine manner.

The patient's circulation is observed over the next few days. If full rotation was not obtained initially, the forearm can then be further rotated. Six to eight weeks is usually required for healing, at which time the external fixator is removed and the patient is started on strengthening exercises.

Complications

Simmons[41] reported eight complications in 22 operated cases. Four were due to neurovascular compromise, and three were due to loss of correction. Vascular complication is by far the most serious deterrent to correction. Shortening the fusion mass will help eliminate such complications.

MADELUNG'S DEFORMITY

Madelung's deformity is an epiphyseal abnormality characterized by dorsal and ulnar bowing of the distal radius. The hand and wrist are displaced in a palmarward and ulnar direction. The abnormality seldom becomes obvious before late childhood or adolescence.

The patient complains of pain over the ulnar aspect of the wrist. Limitation of wrist motion, especially dorsiflexion and pronation, is noted. Pain is produced by heavy work. Seldom does the patient complain of the appearance.

The radiographic findings show the radius to be short, with a marked distal medial and ulnar bow (Fig. 116-13). The distal radial epiphysis is severely sloped and triangular in shape. The medial and palmar portions of the epiphysis are fused with the radial epiphysis. The articular surface of the distal radius is ulnarly and palmarly angulated. The proximal carpal row assumes a V shape with the lunate at the apex. The lunate occupies a position between the distal radius and ulna. The distal ulna is displaced dorsally and there is a widening of the distal radioulnar joint.

The primary abnormality in this condition is failure of growth and development of the ulnar and palmar portions of the epiphyseal plate of the radius.

Principles of Treatment

The treatment of Madelung's deformity varies with the severity of the angulation. Conservative measures have not been successful. I feel that surgical intervention should not be undertaken until the distal radial epiphysis is close to closure. Pain is the primary indication for surgery.

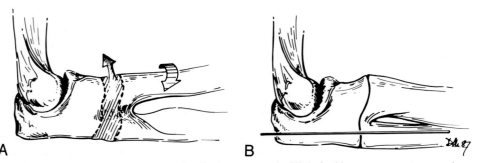

FIGURE 116-12. Surgical correction of radioulnar synostosis. (*A*) A double transverse osteotomy is made through the distal portion of the fusion mass. A 1-cm block is removed to shorten the forearm and relax the neurovascular and soft-tissue structures. (*B*) A Steinmann pin is placed through the olecranon and across the osteotomy site to stabilize the forearm while rotation is accomplished.

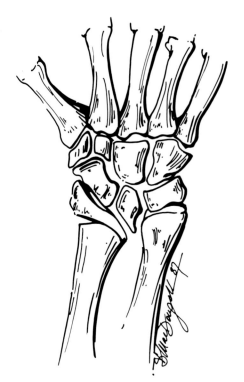

FIGURE 116-13. Schematic of Madelung's deformity. The distal radial epiphysis is wedge-shaped, and is narrow on its ulnar border. The distal radioulnar joint is wide. The lunate drops into the space between the radius and ulna.

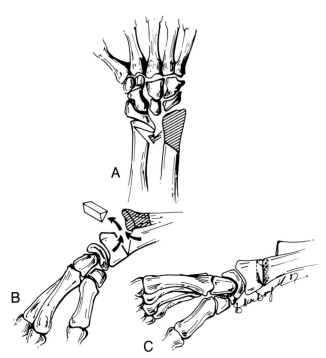

FIGURE 116-14. Technique for correction of Madelung's deformity. (*A*) The distal ulna is resected to provide adequate rotation of the forearm. (*B*) A sufficient wedge of bone is removed from the dorsal surface of the radius to correct the palmar angulation of the distal radius. (*C*) The radial osteotomy site is propped open on its ulnar surface to correct the ulnar angulation of the distal radius.

Various methods of treatment have been suggested. The Darrach[10] procedure (resection of the distal ulna) does not improve pronation or relieve pain. For the more severe deformities, Evans[17] suggests resection of the distal ulna and radiocarpal fusion, with appropriate bone wedges to correct the radial bow. Fusion is indicated only where advanced degenerative changes have occurred.

Surgical Technique

The operative treatment that I use in the more severe deformities is the method described by Ranawat.[35] Make an undulating incision over the dorsal and medial aspect of the wrist and forearm. Reflect the extensor retinaculum ulnarward. Excise the distal ulna sufficiently to allow adequate supination and pronation (Fig. 116-14*A*). Preserve the periosteal sleeve to maintain ulnar ligamentous stability. Perform a closing and opening biplane osteotomy of the radius, removing a sufficient wedge of bone from the dorsum of the radius to correct the dorsal bow (Fig. 116-14*B*). Prop the osteotomy open on the medial side of the radius to correct the medial slant of the articular surface (see Fig. 116-14*A*). Stabilize the osteotomy with crossed Kirschner wires. The osteotomies are planned to result in a 10° to 15° palmar tilt of the radial articular surface, and to correct the medial slant of the distal radial articular surface to as near to 30° as possible (Fig. 116-14*C*). The Kirschner wires are removed at 4 to 6 weeks and mobilization is begun.

Most patients obtain some pain relief and correction of the deformity. Few patients regain enough strength and tolerance

to perform heavy manual labor. Accordingly, the patient must be warned of this before surgery is decided upon.

REFERENCES

1. Albee, F.H.: Formation of Radius Congenitally Absent: Condition Seven Years After Implantation of Bone Graft. Ann. Surg. **87:**105, 1928.
2. Bayne, L.G.: Ulnar Club Hand. *In* Green, D.P. (ed.): Operative Hand Surgery. New York, Churchill Livingstone, 1982.
3. Bayne, L.G., Lovell, W.W., and Marks, T.W.: The Radial Club Hand (abstract). J. Bone Joint Surg. **52-A:**1065, 1970.
4. Bora, F.W., Jr., Nicholson, J.T., and Cheema, H.M.: Radial Meromelia: The Deformity and its Treatment. J. Bone Joint Surg. **52-A:**966, 1970.
5. Buck–Gramcko, D.: Pollicization of the Index Finger: Method and Results in Aplasia and Hypoplasia of the Thumb. J. Bone Joint Surg. **53-A:**1605, 1971.
6. Buck–Gramcko, D.: Thumb Reconstruction by Digital Transposition. Orthop. Clin. North Am. **8:**329, 1977.
7. Butler, B., Jr.: Ring Finger Pollicization with Transplantation of Nailbed and Matrix on a Volar Flap. J. Bone Joint Surg. **46-A:**1069, 1964.
8. Carroll, R.E.: Transposition of the Index Finger to Replace the Middle Finger. Clin. Orthop. **15:**27, 1959.
9. Carroll, R.E., and Bowes, W.H.: Congenital Deficiency of the Ulna. J. Hand Surg. **2:**169, 1977.
10. Darrach, W.: Derangement of the Inferior Radio-Ulnar Articulation. In Libre Jubilaire Offert au Docteur Albin Lambotte, 147, 1936.
11. Davidson, A.J., and Horwitz, M.T.: Congenital Clubhand Defor-

mity Associated with Absence of Radius, its Surgical Correction: Case Report. J. Bone Joint Surg. **21**:462, 1939.

12. Davis, R.G., and Farmer, A.W.: Mirror and Hand Anomaly: A Case Presentation. Plast. Reconstr. Surg. **21**:80, 1958.

13. Define, D.: Treatment of Congenital Radial Club Hand. Clin. Orthop. **73**:153, 1970.

14. DeLorme, T.L.: Treatment of Congenital Absence of the Radius by Transepiphyseal Fixation. J. Bone Joint Surg. **51-A**:117, 1969.

15. Dobyns, James H.: Syndactyly. *In* Green, D.P. (ed.): Operative Hand Surgery, p. 281. New York, Churchill Livingstone, 1982.

16. Entin, M.A.: Reconstruction of Congenital Abnormalities of the Upper Extremities. J. Bone Joint Surg. **41-A**:681, 1959.

17. Evans, D.C.: Wedge Arthrodesis of the Wrist. J. Bone Joint Surg. **37-B**:126, 1955.

18. Flatt, A.E.: The Care of Congenital Hand Anomalies. St. Louis, C.V. Mosby, 1977.

19. Forbes, G.: A Case of Congenital Club Hand with a Review of the Etiology of the Condition. Anat. Rec. **71**:181, 1938.

20. Goldenberg, R.R.: Congenital Bilateral Complete Absence of the Radius in Identical Twins. J. Bone Joint Surg. **30-A**:1001, 1948.

21. Gorriz, G.: Ulnar Dimelia—A Limb Without Anterioposterior Differentiation. J. Hand Surg. **7**:466, 1982.

22. Green, W.T., and Mital, M.A.: Congenital Radio-Ulnar Synostosis: Surgical Treatment. J. Bone Joint Surg. **61-A**:738, 1979.

23. Gropper, P.T.: Ulnar Dimelia. J. Hand Surg. **8**:487, 1983.

24. Harmison, R.G., Pearson, M.A., and Roaf, R.: Ulnar Dimelia. J. Bone Joint Surg. **42-B**:549, 1960.

25. Johnson, J., and Omer, G.E., Jr.: Congenital Ulnar Deficiency: Natural History and Therapeutic Implications. Hand Clin. In Smith, R.J. (ed.): Hand Clinics Symposium on Congenital Deformities of The Hand, vol 1, no. 3, p. 499. Philadelphia, W. B. Saunders, 1985.

26. Kato, K.: Congenital Absence of the Radius, with Review of the Literature and a Report of Three Cases. J. Bone Joint Surg. **6**:589, 1924.

27. Kelikian, H.: Congenital Deformities of the Hand and Forearm, p. 457. Philadelphia, W.B. Saunders, 1974.

28. Kelikian, H., and Doumanian, A.: Congenital Anomalies of the Hand. Part I. J. Bone Joint Surg. **39-A**:1002, 1957.

29. Kummel, W.: Die Missbildungen der extremitaten durch delekt. Verwachsung und uberzahl. Hefte 3. Bibliotheca Medica, Kassel, 1895.

30. Lamb, D.W.: Radial Club Hand, a Continuing Study of Sixty-Eight Patients with One Hundred and Seventeen Clubhands. J. Bone Joint Surg. **59-A**:1, 1977.

31. Littler, J.W.: The Neurovascular Pedicle Method of Digital Transposition for Reconstruction of the Thumb. Plast. Reconstr. Surg. **12**:303, 1953.

32. McKusick, V.: Mendelian Inheritance in Man, p. 133. Baltimore, Johns Hopkins Press, 1966.

33. Ogden, J.A., Watson, H.K., and Bohne, W.: Ulna Dysmelia. J. Bone Joint Surg. **58-A**:467, 1976.

34. Pintilie, D., Hatmanu, D., Olaru, I., and Ponoza, G.: Double Ulna with Symmetrical Polydactyly. J. Bone Surg. **46-B**:89, 1964.

35. Ranawat, C.S., DeFiore, J., and Straub, L.R.: Madelung's Deformity: An End-Result Study of Surgical Treatment. J. Bone Joint Surg. **57-A**:772, 1975.

36. Riordan, D.C.: *In* Crenshaw, A.H. (ed.): Campbell's Operative Orthopedics, Vol. 1, p. 277. St. Louis, C.V. Mosby, 1971.

37. Riordan, D.C.: Congenital Absence of the Radius. J. Bone Joint Surg. **37-A**:1129, 1955.

38. Riordan, D.C.: Congenital Absence of the Ulna. *In* Lovell, W.W., and Winter, R.B. (eds.): Pediatric Orthopedics, 2nd ed, vol II. Philadelphia, J.B. Lippincott, 1986.

39. Roberts, A.S.: A Case of Deformity of the Forearm and Hands with an Unusual History of Hereditary Congenital Deficiency. Ann. Surg. **3**:135, 1896.

40. Santero, N.: Dichiria con Duplicita dell Ulna e Assenza del Radio. Arch. Ital. Chir. **43**:173, 1936.

41. Simmons, B., Southmayd, W., and Roseborough, E.: Congenital Radio-Ulnar Synostosis. Presented at annual meeting of the American Society for Surgery of the Hand, New Orleans, Jan. 19, 1982.

42. Temtamy, S.A., and McKusick, V.A.: Polydactyly. Birth Defects **14**:364, 1978.

43. Temtamy, S.A., and McKusick, V.: Ulna Defects. *In* Temtamy, S., and McKusick, V.: The Genetics of Hand Malformations. Birth Defects **14**:149, 1978.

44. Wood, V.E.: Ulnar Dimelia. *In* Green, D.P. (ed.): Operative Hand Surgery, p. 404. New York, Churchill Livingstone, 1982.

BIBLIOGRAPHY

Barsky, A.J., Kahn, S., and Simon, B.E.: Congenital Anomalies of the Hand. Reconstructive Plastic Surg. Philadelphia, W.B. Saunders, 1964.

Barsky, A.J.: Congenital Anomalies of the Hand and their Surgical Treatment. Springfield, IL, Charles C. Thomas, 1958.

Bilhaur, M.: 1980 Gerison d'un Pounce Bifide per un Nouveau Procede Operatoire. Congress Française de Chirurgie, **4**:576.

Brady, L.P., and Jewett, E.L.: A New Treatment of Radio-Ulnar Synostosis. South. Med. J. **53**:507, 1960.

Brand, P.W.: The Hand, by Milford, L.I.: In Crenshaw, A.H. (ed.): Campbell's Operative Orthopedics, 4th ed. p. 229. St. Louis, C.V. Mosby.

Broudy, A.S., and Smith, R.J.: Deformities of the Hand and Wrist with Ulnar Deficiency. J. Hand Surg. **4**:304, 1979.

Burrows, H.J.: An Operation for the Correction of Madelung's Deformity and Similar Conditions. Proc. R. Soc. Med. **30**:565, 1937.

Dannenberg, M., Anton, J.I., and Spiegel, M.B.: Madelung's Deformity: Consideration of its Roentgenological Diagnostic Criteria. Am. J. Roentgenol. **42**:671, 1939.

Flynn, J.E.: Congenital Anomalies. *In* Flynn, J.E. (ed.): Hand Surgery. Baltimore, Williams & Wilkins, 1966.

Harrison, R.G., Pearson, M.A., and Rouf, R.: Ulna Dimelia. J. Bone Joint Surg. **42-B**:549, 1960.

Henry, A., and Thorburn, M.: Madelung's Deformity: A Clinical and Cytogenic Study. J. Bone Joint Surg. **49-B**:66, 1967.

Hentz, V.R., and Littler, J.W.: Abduction, Pronation, and Recession of Second Metacarpal in Thumb Agenisis. J. Hand Surg. **2**:113, 1977.

Hoover, G.H., Flatt, A.E., and Weiss, M.W.: The Hand and Apert's Syndrome. J. Bone Joint Surg. **52-A**:878, 1970.

Ireland, D.C.R., Takayama, N., and Flatt, A.E.: Poland's Syndrome: A Review of Forty-Three Cases. J. Bone Joint Surg. **58**:52, 1976.

Kelley, J.W.: Mirror Hand. Plast. Reconstr. Surg. **30**:374, 1962.

Laurin, C.A., Fevreau, J.C., and Labelle, P.: Bilateral Absence of the Radius and Tibia with Bilateral Duplication of the Ulna and Fibula. J. Bone Joint Surg. **46-A**:137, 1964.

Madelung, V.: Die spontane subluxation der hand nach vorne. Arch. Klin. Chir., **23**:395, 1979.

Marks, T.W., and Bayne, L.G.: Polydactyly of the Thumb: Abnormal Anatomy and Treatment. J. Hand Surg. **3**:107, 1978.

Mital, M.A.: Congenital Radio-Ulnar Synostosis and Congenital Dislocation of the Radial Head. Orthop. Clin. North Am. **7**:375, 1976.

Miura, T.: An Appropriate Treatment for Postoperative Z-Formed Deformity of the Duplicated Thumb. J. Hand Surg. **2**:380, 1977.

Miura, T.: Polydactyly in Japan. Hand **15**:22, 1983.

Motev, I., and Karagancheva, S.: The Madelung's Deformity. Hand **7**:152, 1975.

Riordan, D.C.: Congenital Absence of the Radius or Ulna (abstract). J. Bone Joint Surg. **54-B**:381, 1972.

Starr, D.E.: Congenital Absence of the Radius. A Method of Surgical Correction. J. Bone Joint Surg. **27**:572, 1945.

CHAPTER 117

Rheumatoid Arthritis of the Hand

JULES S. SHAPIRO

The general principles employed in planning treatment for the rheumatoid hand and wrist closely follow those described by Souter.[34] The overriding principle is to remember that the hand and wrist are attached to a rheumatoid patient. It makes little sense to undertake an involved and complicated reconstruction of the hand and wrist in a patient who is well adapted to his or her deformities, who does not have the ability to use the extremity because of severe elbow or shoulder disability, or whose functional capacity is *not* impaired by the deformities present. Whereas pain is the predominant factor in determining the need for reconstructive surgery in the lower extremities, decreasing function—usually defined by decreasing motion, development of contractures, and decreasing strength—are much more important indications for surgical intervention in the upper extremity, particularly in the hand and wrist.

A surgical procedure should not be performed if the patient's capabilities do not warrant it or no prophylactic effect is achieved by it. Prophylactic effect does not necessarily mean total eradication of the disease process, but does imply a local decrease in disease activity. The effect may be that of slowing or stopping the mechanical factors which loosen ligamentous structures, preventing musculotendinous units from producing deforming forces when applied across lax joint structures, or preventing tendon ruptures with resultant unopposed forces creating contractures. However, a procedure such as metacarpophalangeal arthroplasty, which *can* be performed on most destroyed joints, *should* be performed only when a delay in doing so would inflict limitations on the patient's ability to function. The uncooperative patient, or the patient late in life with well-developed substitution patterns is, with rare exception, not a good candidate for such surgery, no matter how "good" the results may be technically.

A second principle is that any procedure or even combination of procedures performed at one time cannot alleviate entirely the functional deficit and relieve all pain in these patients. Those areas operated upon represent but a fraction of the total number of joints and tendinous structures present in the hand and wrist; *all* structures are involved in this generalized disease process, even though only a few may be visibly involved or symptomatic. In addition, whereas surgery of the lower extremities, or even of the shoulder and elbow, involves *single* joint structures separated from each other by considerable distance, in the hand and wrist structures are often millimeters apart and successful procedures on one set of structures may be influenced by untouched disease in tendinous or joint structures lying in close proximity to the operated areas. Therefore, the surgeon must be realistic in evaluation of the procedures advocated, and more importantly, convey this realism to his or her patient. Patient expectation is often keyed to the enthusiasm of the surgeon.

INDICATIONS FOR SURGERY

General Guidelines

I have long used basic guidelines similar to those set out in 1964 by Laine and Vainio[14] as indications and contraindications for surgery in rheumatoid arthritis in general, and specifically for the hand and wrist. I divide both groups into absolute and relative as follows:

Absolute Indications
1. Imminent or manifest tendon rupture
2. Imminent or manifest nerve compression
3. Troublesome nodules
4. Imminent fractures

Relative Indications
1. Persistently painful joints
2. Persistent synovitis, tenosynovitis, or bursitis
3. Joint stiffness
4. Faulty alignment of joints and tendons

Absolute Contraindications
1. Severe cardiovascular or respiratory disease without medical clearance from an internist
2. Advanced age plus severe rheumatoid deformities
3. Lack of cooperation on the part of the patient

Relative Contraindications
1. Severe deformities if well adapted

It should be emphasized that active rheumatoid arthritis is not a contraindication for surgery; bone and wound healing are normal.

Although advances in medicine in general have altered some of these guidelines (e.g., cardiovascular and respiratory disease are no longer absolute but are still relative contraindications), in general they still comprise the fundamental indications for surgery.

Specific Indications

Synovectomy

There has been much controversy in the past regarding the efficacy of joint synovectomy in rheumatoid surgery. Much of this has come from the rheumatology community and was strengthened by several multicentered studies performed in the mid-1970s.[1,19] Other studies, usually originating in the orthopaedic community, show that there are beneficial effects from joint synovectomy, particularly if it is performed early.[10,27,28] There is a general consensus, however, that tenosynovectomy, especially of the extensor tendons at the wrist does have a prophylactic effect in preventing tendon ruptures.[12,13,37]

The rationale for synovectomy of joints of the wrist and digits revolves around the prevention of the mechanical effects of expansive synovitis on overlying joint structures. A useful analogy in understanding this concept is that of a bladder-lined ball with lacing. If the bladder is overfilled, the lacings will allow the outer casing to expand above normal size. Then, even if the internal pressure goes down, the overlying structure will remain stretched out. Translated to joint structures, once persistent synovitis is present within a joint, the structural integrity

of the joint begins to disintegrate. Ligamentous structures are stretched and no longer perform their function of guiding joint motion. Of equal importance, the overlying tendinous structures, either directly or through retinacular expansions, become deforming influences as their normal forces are applied in abnormal vectors.[33,35] Once ligamentous integrity is lost, deformities occur, often similar in appearance to those seen in degenerative arthritis; these changes are possible even without the erosive changes associated with the rheumatoid process (Fig. 117-1).

I recommend synovectomy at the wrist for

1. Persistent tenosynovitis of at least 6 months' duration despite good medical regimen
2. Persistent pain at the wrist despite such regimen

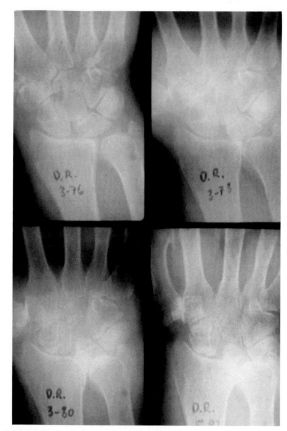

FIGURE 117-1. Example of wrist destruction in a middle-aged rheumatoid patient over a 6-year period. *Upper left,* Early scapholunate ligamentous laxity without wrist migration. *Upper right,* Two years later, advancing scapholunate ligamentous dissociation with early ulnar volar transmigration of the carpus. *Lower left,* After 2 more years, moderate subluxation at the radiolunate joint accompanies further transmigration. First evidence of sclerosis at radiolunate and distal radioulnar joints, indicating abnormal joint mechanics which produce degenerative changes. *Lower right,* Six years after initial radiograph, complete luxation of the lunate with advanced sclerotic changes at radiolunate and distal radioulnar joint. Over the entire 6-year period there have been minimal erosive changes or joint narrowing; the destruction seen is the result of ligamentous laxity leading to abnormal joint mechanics.

3. Evidence of laxity of the distal radioulnar joint on physical examination combined with a Larsen radiographic stage of less than 3.[15] (The Larsen radiographic system permits rational communication about wrist and hand deformities.

Both tenosynovectomy and radiocarpal and intercarpal synovectomy are performed at the time of repair of extensor tendon ruptures. It is always amazing how much synovitis may exist beneath the dorsal carpal capsule despite a negative physical examination and little evidence of radiographic change (see Fig. 117-4).

Metacarpophalangeal synovectomy is a relatively rare procedure in practice, and is performed primarily when the extensor apparatus has slipped into the ulnar intermetacarpal spaces. Despite severe synovitis at this level, and even in the presence of severe subluxation, hand function remains quite good for long periods of time.

Interphalangeal synovectomy is recommended in cases where persistent synovitis is creating early boutonnière deformity.

Flexor tenosynovectomy is recommended at the wrist at the time of carpal tunnel release if florid or adhesive synovitis is present. Even without signs or symptoms of median nerve compression, palmar wrist tenosynovectomy is suggested if the patient is beginning to lose ability to obtain total composite flexion actively and there is no evidence of finger tenosynovitis. In the presence of flexor tendon ruptures, tenosynovectomy at the wrist is indicated.

Flexor tenosynovectomy in the thumb or fingers is usually indicated when a persistent tenosynovitis causing either decreased range of motion or triggering of the ray is not relieved by a local steroid injection, or if the synovitis recurs within a relatively short time (i.e., 3 months).

Arthrodesis

Arthrodesis, always a staple of treatment in orthopaedic surgery, has in recent years undergone a resurgence in popularity. Some of this popularity has resulted from newer techniques and means of arthrodesis,[18,21,32] but a renewed interest in natural ankylosis patterns in the rheumatoid wrist has also developed.[6,24] Such ankylosis patterns often leave the patient with a stable, relatively painless wrist with sufficient motion to perform normal daily activities.[4] In addition, the influence of the wrist on the development of a variety of finger deformities is minimized.[26,29,30,31]

Total wrist arthrodesis is indicated in the patient with complete and painful destruction of radiocarpal and intercarpal joint surfaces, with severe bilateral wrist involvement, with evidence of rupture of all wrist extensors, and in those patients with severe deviation of the wrist secondary to carpal destruction and translation. In addition, it is the procedure of choice after failed wrist arthroplasty.

Indications for limited wrist arthrodesis have slowly expanded to include patients who previously would have undergone radiocarpal and intercarpal synovectomy alone as well as those who in the past would have been candidates for total wrist arthrodesis or arthroplasty. The choice of radiolunate versus

radioscapholunate arthrodesis depends on the amount of destruction found at surgery in the radioscaphoid articular surfaces (Fig. 117-2).

Arthrodeses in the thumb are indicated where severe joint destruction has resulted in the patterns described by Nalebuff[22] but has progressed to a point where reconstruction by means of ligament substitution or joint arthroplasty is no longer possible. In these instances, it is best to try to provide stability at one or two levels with mobility at the others—for example, metacarpophalangeal arthrodesis with synovectomy and realignment at the interphalangeal and carpometacarpal levels, or arthrodesis at both the metacarpophalangeal and interphalangeal joint levels with evidence of a good carpometacarpal joint.

In the fingers, however, arthrodeses are almost never performed at the metacarpophalangeal joint level because function is rarely improved more than can be obtained by arthroplasty, even of the resection variety. Arthrodesis at the interphalangeal joint level is indicated where there have been long-standing boutonnière deformities of greater than 60°, as in my experience it is almost impossible to regain full extension

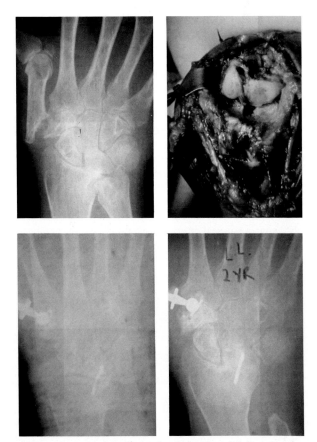

FIGURE 117-2. Radiolunate arthrodesis. *Upper left,* Preoperative radiograph, showing early ulnar translation of the carpus. *Upper right,* Intraoperative photograph showing absence of cartilage on lunate and presence of cartilage on scaphoid, an indication for radiolunate arthrodesis alone. *Lower left,* Immediate postoperative radiograph. *Lower right,* Radiograph 2 years after surgery shows radiolunate arthrodesis and no further transmigration of the carpus.

in the rheumatoid patient in this situation. Rarely is arthrodesis indicated in swan-neck deformities since useful motion can usually be obtained with either capsular or tendon releases or arthroplasty. In a mildly incapacitated patient, arthrodesis may be indicated in the proximal interphalangeal joint of the index finger to provide stability for everyday work activities.

Tendon Ruptures

By knowing the natural locations of prominent synovitis, the locations of typical tendon ruptures in the rheumatoid hand and wrist can almost be predicted.

Understanding of the pathomechanics of the distal radioulnar joint[2,38] led to an understanding of the typical patterns of extensor digiti quinti and extensor digitorum communis rupture. Radiographic evaluation may often predict the probable occurance of such ruptures.[9] The extensor pollicis longus is frequently ruptured in the third dorsal compartment at Lister's tubercle. The flexor pollicis longus often ruptures at the palmar aspect of the scaphoid tubercle,[17] followed sometimes by rupture of the flexor digitorum communis to the index finger by the same bony spicule (Fig. 117-3). Individual flexor tendons often rupture within the flexor sheaths of the digits; this is frequently preceded by progressive loss of motion from nodular entrapment[11] or severe tenosynovitis.

Swan-Neck and Boutonnière Deformities

Swan-neck deformities often remain relatively asymptomatic for many years before they interfere with function in the rheumatoid hand. Their etiology is well described by Nalebuff[23] and includes type I, flexible proximal interphalangeal joints in all positions; type II, proximal interphalangeal joint flexion limited in certain positions; type III, limited proximal interphalangeal joint flexion in all positions; and type IV, stiff proximal interphalangeal joints with poor radiographic appearance.

Type I deformity is usually well tolerated by the patient and rarely requires surgical intervention. When it does, arthrodesis of the distal interphalangeal joint will usually alleviate the most disabling segment of the deformity at the early stage of the disease. In late stages, with severe mobile swan-neck deformity, flexor tenodesis[39] will relieve hyperextension at the proximal interphalangeal joints.

Type II deformity is usually the result of intrinsic tightness, and whereas partial relief of the deforming forces created by the ulnar intrinsic tendons can be achieved at the time of metacarpophalangeal arthroplasty, any further treatment is reserved for the time when proximal interphalangeal arthroplasty is indicated.

Type III deformity is the result of long-standing deformity with resultant contracture of all tissue around the proximal interphalangeal joints. Joint manipulation and pinning, dorsal skin releases, lateral band release, and central slip release or elongation should be considered; extensive flexor tenosynovectomy may also be necessary, often extending proximally to the wrist, and distally to the insertion of the superficialis tendons.

Type IV deformity is usually amenable only to arthroplasty or arthrodesis.

Boutonnière deformity is generally insidious in the rheumatoid hand and only becomes a problem when the patient begins to develop a hyperextension deformity at the distal interphalangeal joint which inhibits ability to grasp large objects. The deformity is thought to result from expansive synovitis in the proximal interphalangeal joint interrupting the normal relationships between central slip and lateral band mechanisms. The resultant dynamic imbalance creates significantly greater flexion forces at the proximal and extension forces at the distal interphalangeal joints. Early deformity may be helped by extensor tenotomy over the middle phalanx, as here again the most disabling segment of the deformity, particularly early, may be the hyperextension of the distal interphalangeal joint. Whereas many soft-tissue reconstructions have been advocated for rheumatoid soft-tissue boutonnière deformity of moderate degree, I have never found a technique which has lasted. It is only when patients develop contractures of greater than 60° at the proximal interphalangeal joint that more aggressive treatment is recommended. This degree of contracture occurs in a relatively small number of patients.

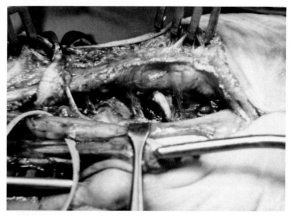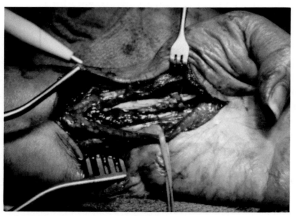

FIGURE 117-3. *Left,* Flexor pollicus longus rupture at palmar scaphoid. Synovial erosion of the scaphoid leaves a sharp bony spicule protruding into the carpal canal, which mechanically erodes the tendon. *Right,* If sufficient excursion is present, the tendon can be reattached.

SURGICAL TECHNIQUES

Synovectomy

Wrist

Dorsal Tenosynovectomy. The standard approach for most surgery on the dorsum of the rheumatoid wrist begins with a longitudinal incision, 4 to 6 inches in length, centered over the interval between the third and fourth metacarpal shafts and the distal radioulnar joint. Elevate skin and subcutaneous tissues as a single flap (to avoid skin necrosis), taking care to identify and avoid injuring the sensory branches of both the radial and ulnar nerves. Hemostasis usually involves ligation of relatively few dorsal venous cross channels.

Elevate the extensor retinaculum as a U-shaped flap, based on the radial side. Begin elevation with a scalpel over the distal ulna between the fifth and sixth dorsal compartments, followed by the use of an iris scissors to open each dorsal compartment. This protects the tendons, which can often be hard to identify due to the synovium investing them. Take particular care when approaching the extensor digiti quinti and the extensor pollicis longus, as each may be so destroyed that their fibers may blend into the surrounding soft tissues, making it easy to inadvertently cut them at the time of exposure. Once they are exposed, perform a meticulous tenosynovectomy, tendon by tendon. A small synovial rongeur is of great value in grasping the synovium and stripping it from tendons proximally and distally. Remove final remnants of synovium with a moist sponge run gently over the tendons.

Carpal and Distal Radioulnar Joint. Open the dorsal capsule of the carpus by means of a T-shaped incision, with the cross of the T lying at the distal radial articular surface. Identify the terminal sensory branch of the posterior interosseous nerve and resect it approximately 1 inch proximal to the joint in order to avoid its being entrapped during capsular closure. The ulnar limb of the T slants obliquely in a distal direction, avoiding the dorsal radiotriquetral ligament, a primary stabilizer of the carpus (Fig. 117-4).

Perform the synovectomy at both the radiocarpal and midcarpal joints using a 1-mm synovial rongeur. Traction on the hand will open the joint surfaces for better inspection and debridement. Synovium lying on the palmar sides of the carpus can often be cleared in this manner by adding flexion to the wrist in radial and ulnar deviation. Introduction of the rongeur into the recesses radial to the scaphoid and ulnar to the triquetrum usually yield significant synovium.[36] Now open the distal radioulnar joint through a straight longitudinal incision begun slightly proximal to the ulnar styloid, avoiding the dorsal elements of the triangular fibrocartilaginous complex. It is important to leave attached to the radius some capsule for closure at the end of the procedure. The distal ulna is now resected in one of two ways:

If the carpal synovectomy is to accompany a limited wrist arthrodesis, perform a classic Darrach[7] resection of the distal ulna. If however, synovectomy alone is performed, use an oblique excision[3] to maintain as much ligamentous integrity of the carpus as possible by leaving intact the styloid attachments.

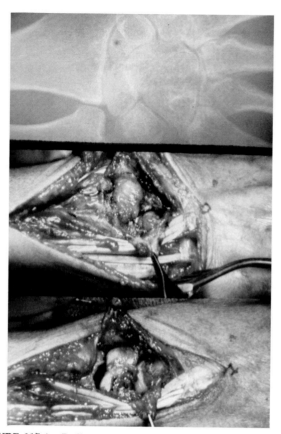

FIGURE 117-4. Radiocarpal and midcarpal synovectomy. *Top,* Radiographic appearance of the carpus before surgery. *Center,* Dorsal carpal capsule opened as described in text. The carpus is obscured by synovitis. *Bottom,* After meticulous synovectomy, carpal bones appear relatively intact.

Upon completion of the carpal and distal radioulnar joint procedure, divide the extensor retinaculum into two parts. Bring the larger portion beneath the extensor tendons and suture it over the previously closed dorsal capsule. Bring the smaller portion over the extensor tendons and suture it back to its origin. Bring the extensor carpi ulnaris dorsal on the distal ulna before such closure is made, and if sufficient retinaculum is available, create a tunnel to hold the tendon in this position, using a subportion of the retinaculum.

Metacarpophalangeal and Proximal Interphalangeal Joints

Except for the thumb, the metacarpophalangeal joints are approached through a straight dorsal transverse incision made approximately 0.5 inch proximal to the articular surface of the joint. Take care to avoid as many venous channels and sensory nerve branches as possible. Expose the extensor hood and approach each joint through a longitudinal incision in the hood at the ulnar side of the extensor tendons. Identify the ulnar intrinsic tendon together with the sagittal bands of the hood in the distal part of the incision. Elevate them from below, usually with a small hemostat, and separate them from the transverse fibers of the extensor hood. Excise a section of the tendon and sagittal bands, and flex the proximal interphalangeal joint to widen the gap between the cut ends. Now luxate the extensor tendon radially, carefully teasing the underlying capsulosynovium from it. The capsulosynovium can now be peeled out, from proximal to distal. Enter the joint just anterior to the collateral ligaments and further excise the synovium from the articular edges of the proximal phalanx. At this point, a synovial rongeur can be introduced into the distracted joint and the palmar recess cleared of synovium. Upon completion of the synovectomy, allow the extensor tendons to fall back to their normal position. While other authors advocate closure of the extensor hood, I have rarely done this and find no difference in wound healing. A reefing procedure on the radial aspect of the hood is occasionally required to centralize the tendon. Close the skin with interupted vertical mattress 4-0 nylon sutures.

Approach the thumb metacarpophalangeal joint through a curved longitudinal incision. Open the interval between the extensor pollicis longus and brevis and peel the synovium off the underside of the extensor hood. Remove the synovium in a similar fashion as described for the other finger joints. One often finds that the insertion of the extensor pollicis brevis is completely detached from its insertion. It is therefore important to elevate the capsule in continuity with the periosteum of the proximal phalanx for closure. Upon completion of the synovectomy, bring the extensor tendons together and suture them side-to-side with nonabsorbable suture, overlapping the closure to compensate for the laxity created by removal of the synovium. Close the skin with 4-0 nylon vertical interrupted sutures.

The proximal interphalangeal joints are approached through a long curved incision over the dorsum of the joint. Elevate the skin and subcutaneous tissues to expose the extensor apparatus. Elevate the edges of the lateral bands and approach the synovium anterior to the collateral ligaments. Peel the synovium from the overlying extensor apparatus, taking care where the capsule blends into the central slip at its insertion on the proximal phalanx. Clear the joint of synovium using a small rongeur, being sure to remove the hypertrophic tissue which erodes beneath the collateral ligaments. The ulnar collateral ligament may be cut and the joint opened radially for greater exposure of the inferior recesses.[25] A single suture holding the cut ends in contact is all that is necessary for closure. Allow the extensor apparatus to fall back in place and perform skin closure with 5-0 nylon suture.

Palmar Synovectomy

Wrist. Relatively little is said about the synovitis which involves the palmar aspects of the wrist and hand. However, this synovitis causes multiple symptoms in the hand. Approach the palmar wrist through a curvilinear incision extending from the distal end of the thenar crease to 2 to 3 inches proximal to the distal palmar crease. It is important to extend this incision more proximally than the standard carpal tunnel release incisions in order to give sufficient exposure for synovectomy. Take care to avoid the palmar cutaneous nerve in the radial aspect of the incision. Deepen the incision, cutting the transverse carpal ligament distally and the flexor retinaculum proximally. In the rheumatoid patient, the radial and ulnar bursae have usually hypertrophied and engulfed the flexor tendons,

often matting them together into a poorly differentiated mass. Retract the median nerve radially and ulnarward to expose the tendon sheaths, which are incised longitudinally. As normal tendon is identified, strip the synovium proximally to muscle bellies and distally to the palm. The superficialis tendons can be separated fairly easily; however, the tenosynovium encompassing the profundus tendons is much more difficult to excise. It is not possible to remove all the synovium lying between the profundi. The synovial masses surrounding the lumbrical origins should be removed.

After excising the synovium, passively move the profundi and superficialis tendons and look for independent motion between the two tendons to each finger. Strip the flexor pollicis longus of synovium, and carefully inspect the region of the scaphotrapezial joint for sharp bony spicules protruding through the palmar carpal capsule. If found, they should be smoothed off and covered over by capsular tissue.

Palm and Fingers. Flexor tenosynovitis in the fingers, presenting either as triggering or progressive loss of motion, is approached through Bruner[5] zig-zag incisions. This allows for extension of the incision proximally to the wrist if necessary, and distally to the distal portion of the middle phalanx. Care must be taken to leave important pulleys intact while performing the synovectomy. Usually an adequate synovectomy can be performed while leaving the A2 and A4 pulleys in place, if somewhat foreshortened. A pulley of 2 to 3 mm will usually suffice. After performing the synovectomy, move the profundus and superficialis tendons independently. If independent motion cannot be achieved at the time of surgery, there will not be independent postoperative excursion. Therefore, the synovectomy must proceed until such independent motion is possible. Often the last restraint is the synovial tissue lying at the A2 pulley; a small synovial rongeur introduced into the pulley area is necessary to break up the final tendon adhesions.

When the problem is one of triggering, opening the palm will usually reveal a rheumatoid nodule at the area of the A1 pulley. The nodules in this area will usually take one of two forms: discrete or diffuse. Discrete nodules lying within the tendon substance can be removed by sharp dissection with a #11 knifeblade. However, diffuse involvement in the tendon substance is almost impossible to remove. In these instances, the A1 pulley is sacrificed to allow for free motion. The incision used is still zig-zag in nature and not transverse, since sometimes the troublesome nodule is not located at the A1 pulley region, but at the bifurcation of the superficialis tendon[11] distal to the A2 pulley; in such cases, extensile exposure to this area is indicated.

The similar situation exists with the flexor pollicis longus at the region of the A1 pulley. If a discrete nodule is found, remove it by sharp dissection. If diffuse synovial infiltration is found, remove the A1 pulley.

Arthrodesis

Wrist

Total wrist arthrodesis is performed through the previously described dorsal wrist incision. If performed alone, the incision is long enough to allow reduction of the carpus in a radiodorsal direction before fixation is accomplished. Often very little is left of the carpus that is identifiable. In these instances, the third metacarpal is aligned with the distal radius. One of two methods of fixation is used. The Meuli[20] approach involves a six-hole plate and screws bridging from the radius to the third metacarpal and is useful when maximal rigidity of fixation is required. The more common approach uses a smooth Steinmann pin introduced through the third metacarpal neck and driven proximally into the radius. I use the largest pin size consistent with the size of the metacarpal shaft and prefer tapping it down the shaft of the metacarpal until the point appears in the wrist incision. Then reduce the carpal remnants as the pin is driven across the distal radius a distance of at least one-third the length of the radius. Countersink the pin in the third metacarpal (using a second pin as a punch) for at least 1 inch to allow for possible placement of an implant in the metacarpal shaft. While a pin can be placed intermetacarpally, the purchase on the amount of carpus which it traverses is relatively small and does not allow for as good fixation. Whichever method is used, two to four bone staples are used as supplemental fixation, primarily for rotational stability.

Limited wrist arthrodesis generally refers to either radiolunate or radioscapholunate arthrodesis in the rheumatoid patient. This may be indicated when there is good cartilage remaining in the midcarpal joint. The same incision is used as for dorsal synovectomy. Resect the distal ulna in either the fashion of Darrach or Bowers; the Darrach procedure allows for more bone as graft at the arthrodesis site. In opening the dorsal capsule, the ulnar side of the T-shaped incision may cut the attachment of the dorsal radiotriquetral ligament to give greater exposure. Perform a synovectomy of the radiocarpal and intercarpal joints, and flex the wrist to inspect the radiocarpal articulation. If the scaphoid surface and its corresponding radial articulation are in relatively good condition (i.e., some cartilage is still present), then perform a radiolunate arthrodesis. If eburnated bone is found in this articulation, a radioscapholunate arthrodesis is more desirable. The carpus can manually be reduced radially and dorsally to reestablish its normal relationship with the distal radius. After denuding the articular surfaces of the lunate and the radial lunate fossa (together with the scaphoid and its radial surface if radioscapholunate arthrodesis is desired), place autogenous bone between the bony surfaces and use either Kirschner wires or bone staples to hold these surfaces together. Put the wrist through a range of motion; motion should occur only at the midcarpal joints.

Metacarpophalangeal Joints

In the thumb, arthrodesis is performed through the same incision as for synovectomy. After denuding of cartilage, place the joint surfaces in 10° to 15° of flexion and hold them while placing crossed Kirschner wires or two bone staples across the joint surfaces. Carefully close the extensor hood, and reposition the extensor pollicis longus over the center of the joint.

Proximal Interphalangeal Joints

After denuding of cartilage, oppose the joint surfaces and hold them while Kirschner wires or bone staples are placed across the joint surfaces. Joints are placed from 45° to 60° of flexion

from index to little finger. In the rare instance of arthrodesis for a severe swan-neck deformity (often with ankylosis), the incision used should be shaped like a hockey stick, with the distal limb lying over the middle phalanx. Closure of skin at the end of the procedure may result in extreme tension on the suture line; in this case the distal limb of the incision may be left open to heal by secondary intent.[23]

Repair of Tendon Ruptures

Extensor Tendons

Because extensor tendons usually rupture at the dorsum of the wrist, exposure is the same as for dorsal synovectomy. At the time of dorsal synovectomy, carefully examine the extensor tendons for signs of rupture or elongation (as often happens with synovial invasion). Perform all additional procedures before the tendon reconstructions are begun (i.e., carpal synovectomy, distal ulnar resection, wrist arthrodesis). Carefully examine tendon ends for two reasons: to determine how far from the ruptured surfaces normal tendon tissue exists, and to see how much excursion still remains in the musculotendinous unit. If the rupture is recent, there may be sufficient excursion to allow for side-to-side suturing of the ruptured ends. After sharply cutting back to normal tendon substance, repair or transfer is begun.

For rupture of the extensor digiti quinti alone, I prefer transfer of the extensor indicis proprius. This muscle is used for little finger extensor transfer with rupture of the fifth extensor digitorum communis as well. Section it in the distal portion of the incision and bring it beneath the extensor digitorum communis to lie just distal to the ulnar head. Attachment is performed using side-to-side suturing with nonabsorbable suture. I prefer maximal tension for all rheumatoid tendon repairs, because one is never sure of the degree of stretching present in the sutured tendons.

Ruptures of the fourth extensor digitorum are joined with side-to-side suture to the third extensor digitorum (Fig. 117-5). If the third, fourth, and fifth or the second through fifth extensor digitorum tendons are ruptured, I prefer to use one or two flexor superficialis tendons from the ring finger and, if necessary the long finger. These may be brought around the radial border or through the interosseous membrane just proximal to the distal radioulnar joint. If the latter route is chosen (my preference), then the window must be made wide enough to allow for free excursion of the tendons. Maximal tension is particularly important in these transfers to regain finger extension.

For rupture of the extensor pollicis longus, use the extensor indicis proprius, rerouted at Lister's tubercle and joined with side-to-side nonabsorbable suture over the distal metacarpal. This may require a separate longitudinal incision in the neck region of the metacarpal.

Swan-Neck and Boutonnière Deformities

Swan-neck deformities are approached either at the time of metacarpophalangeal synovectomy (or arthroplasty) or proximal interphalangeal arthroplasty, and rarely in separate procedures. Resection of the ulnar intrinsic has been discussed, as

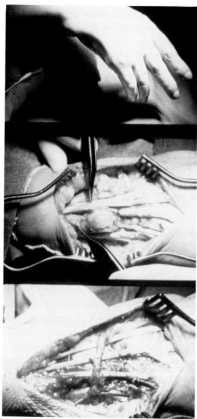

FIGURE 117-5.   Extensor tendon reconstructions. *Top,* Typical preoperative appearance of the hand with rupture of extensor tendons; note characteristic position of fourth and fifth fingers. *Center,* Appearance of ruptured tendons after tenosynovectomy. *Bottom,* Transfer of extensor indicis proprius to extensor digitorum of fifth finger and suturing of fourth extensor digitorum to third extensor digitorum. Smaller portion of extensor retinaculum is brought over the tendons to prevent bowstringing.

has flexor tenosynovectomy at the time of proximal interphalangeal arthroplasty.

Boutonnière deformities are rarely treated early. If a solitary joint is developing an early boutonnière deformity, tenotomy of the extensor tendon over the middle phalanx will give relief of the deforming force.[8] Late boutonnière deformity is best treated by arthrodesis; I have never found a reconstructive soft-tissue procedure at this level which gives uniform results in the rheumatoid patient. Boutonnière deformity in the thumb may be treated early by synovectomy of the metacarpophalangeal joint with reefing of the extensor hood mechanism. Once fixed deformity has occured (as little as 10° to 15° of flexion), reconstruction, even with tendon transfers, is of little value and arthrodesis is the procedure of choice in the symptomatic patient.

POSTOPERATIVE CARE

In general, it can be stated that postoperative care for all rheumatoid hand and wrist procedures is aimed at obtaining optimal results for whichever procedures have been performed. When multiple procedures are performed simultaneously, postoperative regimens must take into consideration the fact that both motion and stability may be desirable at different joint levels.

Postoperative dressings are voluminous and a plaster splint is used to provide rigidity. Dressings are left intact for 2 to 4 days before the first dressing change, unless temperature spikes require earlier observation of the incision. After the first dressing change, the regimen differs depending on the procedures performed.

For joint or tendon synovectomies, early motion gives the best results, within the limits imposed by the need to maintain good stability. At all joint levels, gentle passive range of motion is begun with a therapist at 2 to 4 days. At the metacarpophalangeal and interphalangeal joint levels, a dynamic extension splint is used for a minimum of 6 weeks after surgery. Patients are given a specific timetable for active range of motion exercises with the splint removed. Active-assistive motion is added at approximately 1 week. Therapy is continued for 6 to 8 weeks with emphasis on regaining motion and strength. Formal therapy is terminated when the patient has plateaued in response to treatment.

For tendon repairs or transfers, sufficient time must be permitted to allow for tendon healing to occur. The use of early passive motion[16] improves the results of flexor reconstructions and repairs; rubberband-guided flexor motion is begun at 2 to 3 days after surgery. However, immobilization with the wrist in 45° of extension and the metacarpophalangeal joints in neutral is used for 3 to 5 weeks after extensor tendon repairs.

Because of the disabilities inherent in the rheumatoid patient from generalized disease, external immobilization is kept to minimal periods of time. In performing arthrodesis, the strength of the internal fixation determines the need for and duration of external immobilization. For total wrist arthrodesis, use of plates or Steinmann pins with staples usually obviates the need for external immobilization after 1 to 2 weeks. For limited wrist arthrodesis, use of power staple fixation[32] requires immobilization for 3 weeks. Use of Kirschner wires usually requires 6 weeks immobilization before allowing unassisted activity.

In general, at the metacarpophalangeal and interphalangeal joints, both thumb and proximal interphalangeal joints are immobilized for 6 weeks after arthrodesis with Kirschner-wire fixation, or 3 weeks after power staple fixation, except in the thumb. In the thumb, mobilization is often begun several days after power staple fixation, allowing the patient to begin light resistance activities early in the postoperative period.

PITFALLS AND COMPLICATIONS

After tenosynovectomy, one must establish some form of check-rein overlying the extensor tendons. This often means using a thin, stretched-out extensor retinaculum; however, even a thin retinaculum will act as such a restraint.

If tendon repairs or transfers are performed, the duration of immobilization must be finely tuned to balance the stiffness found after immobilization for synovectomy and the danger of rupturing the tendon anastomoses. Graded mobilization is best performed with an experienced hand therapist.

Resection of the distal ulna, in my experience, is always the most painful part of any reconstructive procedure at the wrist. I always council patients that this area will be the most painful in the postoperative period, and pain will last for an average of 8 to 12 weeks. The patient should be aware that pronation/supination, being a function of both proximal and distal radioulnar joints as well as contracture of the interosseous membrane, may still be limited after distal ulnar resection. Occasionally, resection of the distal ulna will result in instability at this area. This can be avoided by *minimal* distal resection, at the neck region.

Metacarpophalangeal synovectomy, while being a good procedure for decreasing local mechanical problems, is not entirely effective. Patients should be cautioned that some joint stiffness will result after synovectomy and that recurrence of slippage of the extensor mechanism into the intermetacarpal region is possible. This is especially true if the patient has significant radial supination deformity at the wrist.

There is always a danger of nonunion at any arthrodesis site. The patient should be aware of this, and be prepared for a possible rearthrodesis, unless a stable nonunion is achieved. Often the latter provides a good, if not better, alternative than a stable arthrodesis in the rheumatoid hand.

REFERENCES

1. Arthritis Foundation Committee on Evaluation of Synovectomy: Multicenter Evaluation of Synovectomy in the Treatment of Rheumatoid Arthritis: Report of Results at the End of Three Years. Arthritis Rheum. 20:765, 1977.
2. Backdahl, M.: The Caput Ulnae Syndrome in Rheumatoid Arthritis: A Study of the Morphology, Abnormal Anatomy and Clinical Picture. Acta Rheumat. Scand. Suppl. 5:1, 1963.
3. Bowers, W.H.: Distal Radioulnar Joint Arthroplasty: The Hemiresection–Interposition Technique. J. Hand Surg. 10-A:169, 1985.
4. Brumfield, R.H., and Champoux, J.A.: A biomechanical study of normal functional wrist motion. Clin. Orthop. 187:23, 1984.
5. Bruner, J.M.: The zig-zag volar-digital incision for flexor tendon surgery. Plast. Reconstr. Surg. 40:571, 1967.
6. Chamay, A., Della Santa, D., and Vilaseca, A.: Radiolunate Arthrodesis Factor of Stability For the Rheumatoid Wrist. Ann. Chir. Main 2:5, 1983.
7. Darrach, W.: Anterior Dislocation of the Head of the Ulna. Ann. Surg. 56:802, 1912.
8. Dolphin, J.A.: Extensor Tenotomy for Chronic Boutonniere Deformity of the Finger: Report of Two Cases. J. Bone Joint Surg. 47-A:161, 1965.
9. Freiberg, R.A., and Weinstein, A.: The Scallop Sign and Spontaneous Rupture of Finger Extensor Tendons in Rheumatoid Arthritis. Clin. Orthop. 83:128, 1972.
10. Gschwend, N., Kentsch, A., Bohler, N., Lack, N., Schwagerl, W., Sollermann, C.H., Teigland, J., Thabe, H., and Tillmann, K.: Late Results of Synovectomy of Wrist, MP and PIP Joints: Multicenter Study. Clin. Rheum. Dis. 4:23, 1985.
11. Helal, B.: Profundus Entrapment in Rheumatoid Disease. Hand 2:48, 1970.
12. Kessler, I., and Vainio, K.: Posterior (Dorsal) Synovectomy for Rheumatoid Involvement of the Hand and Wrist. J. Bone Joint Surg. 48-A:1085, 1966.
13. Kulick, R.G., DeFiore, J.C., Straub, L.R., and Ranawat, C.S.: Long-term Results of Dorsal Stabilization in the Rheumatoid Wrist. J. Hand Surg. 6:272, 1981.
14. Laine, V., and Vainio, K.: Indications and Contraindications for Orthopedic Surgery in Rheumatoid Arthritis with a Special Reference to the Early Synovectomy. Rhumatismes Inflammatoires Chroniques des IV Conference Internationale des Maladies Rhumatismales, 1964.

15. Larsen, A., Dale, K., Eek, M., and Pahle, J.: Radiographic Evaluation of Rheumatoid Arthritis by Standard Reference Films. J. Hand Surg. 8:667, 1983.
16. Lister, G.D., Kleinert, H.E., Kutz, J.E., and Atasoy, E.: Primary Flexor Tendon Repair Followed by Immediate Controlled Mobilization. J. Hand Surg. 2:441, 1977.
17. Mannerfelt, L.: On Formation of Bony Spurs in the Rheumatoid Hand. With Special Reference to Attrition Ruptures of Flexor Tendons. In Tubiana, R. (ed.): La Main Rhumatoide, p. 117. Paris, L'Expansion Francaise, 1969.
18. Mannerfelt, L., and Malmsten, M.: Arthrodesis of the Wrist in Rheumatoid Arthritis. A Technique without External Fixation. Scand. J. Plast. Reconstr. Surg. 5:124, 1971.
19. McEwan, C., and O'Brian, W.B.: A Multi-center Evaluation of Early Synovectomy in the Treatment of Rheumatoid Arthritis. J. Rheumatol. Supp 1:107, 1974.
20. Meuli, H.: Reconstructive Surgery of the Wrist Joint. Hand 4:88, 1972.
21. Millender, L.H., and Nalebuff, E.A.: Arthrodesis of the Rheumatoid Wrist. J. Bone Joint Surg. 55-A:1026, 1973.
22. Nalebuff, E.A.: Restoration of Balance in the Rheumatoid Thumb. In Tubiana, R. (ed.): La Main Rhumatoide, p. 197. Paris, L'Expansion Francaise, 1969.
23. Nalebuff, E.A.: Surgical Treatment of the Swan Neck Deformity in Rheumatoid Arthritis. Orthop. Clin. North Am. 6:733, 1975.
24. Nalebuff, E.A., and Garrod, K.J.: Present Approach to the Severely Involved Rheumatoid Wrist. Orthop. Clin. North Am. 15:369, 1984.
25. Pahle, J.: Die synovektomie der proximalen interphalangealgelenke. Orthopade 2:13, 1973.
26. Pahle, J.A., and Raunio, P.: The Influence of Wrist Position on Finger Deviation in the Rheumatoid Hand: A Clinical and Radiological Study. J. Bone Joint Surg. 51-B:664, 1969.
27. Raunio, P.: Prophylactic Value of Synovectomy of the Proximal Interphalangeal Joint in Rheumatoid Arthritis. Scand. J. Rheumatol. 6(Suppl. 19):1, 1977.
28. Rodts, T.L., Payne, T., and Shapiro, J.S.: The Effects of Wrist Synovectomy on Parameters of Hand Function in Rheumatoid Arthritis. Orthop. Trans. 6:171, 1982.
29. Shapiro, J.S.: Ulnar Drift: Report of a Related Finding. Acta Orthop. Scand. 39:346, 1968.
30. Shapiro, J.S.: A New Factor in the Etiology of Ulnar Drift. Clin. Orthop. 68:32, 1970.
31. Shapiro, J.S.: Wrist Influence in Rheumatoid Swan Neck Deformity. J. Hand Surg. 7:484, 1982.
32. Shapiro, J.S.: Power Staple Fixation in Hand and Wrist Surgery: New Applications of an Old Fixation Device. J. Hand Surg. 11-A:218, 1987.
33. Smith, E.M., Juvinall, R., Bender, L., and Pearson, R.: Role of the Finger Flexors in Rheumatoid Deformities of the Metacarpal Phalangeal Joints. Arthritis Rheum. 7:467, 1964.
34. Souter, W.A.: Planning Treatment of the Rheumatoid Hand. Hand 11:3–16, 1979.
35. Swezey, R.L.: Dynamic Factors in Deformity of the Rheumatoid Arthritic Hand. Bull. Rheum. Dis. 22:649, 1971.
36. Taleisnik, J.: Rheumatoid Synovitis of the Volar Compartment of the Wrist Joint, its Radiological Signs and its Contribution to Wrist and Hand Deformity. J. Hand Surg. 4:526, 1979.
37. Thirupathi, R.G., Ferlic, D.C., and Clayton, M.L.: Dorsal Wrist Synovectomy in Rheumatoid Arthritis—a Long-term Study. J. Hand Surg. 8:848, 1983.
38. Vaughn–Jackson, O.J.: Rupture of Extensor Tendons by Attrition at the Inferior Radio-Ulnar Joint: Report of Two Cases. J. Bone Joint Surg. 30-B:528, 1948.
39. Zancolli, E.: Structural and Dynamic Bases of Hand Surgery, 2nd ed., p. 174. Philadelphia, J.B. Lippincott, 1979.

CHAPTER 118

Infections of the Hand

ROBERT M. SZABO and
JAMES D. SPIEGEL

Infection in the hand is common and can result in serious and permanent disability if appropriate management is delayed.[4,5,10,11,12,23,26,27,28,30,37,38,39,44] Loss of hand function follows an inadequately treated infection; therefore every effort should be made to achieve complete and expedient resolution. In our experience this means aggressive debridement when surgery is indicated, use of antimicrobials that cover the full spectrum of infecting agents known to be present in hand infections, and appropriate follow-up care.

Hand infection begins most often with penetration of the skin barrier and inoculation of the tissues. Tissue necrosis ensues with resultant dead space and impairment of circulation, creating an ideal environment for the bacteria to flourish. Bacterial proliferation produces the initial signs of infection: erythema, calor, swelling, and tenderness. The local tissue reaction causes edema and further impairment of local circulation, with eventual abscess formation. Clinically, an abscess is evidenced by fluctuance and induration of the surrounding tissue. One must differentiate infection from noninfectious conditions of gout, collagen vascular disease, inflammatory tenosynovitis, acute soft-tissue calcification, foreign-body reaction, and more rarely, neoplastic processes.

The goal of treatment is to arrest antimicrobial proliferation, preserve well-vascularized, pliable tissues under no tension or pressure, and remove purulent and necrotic tissue.[3,13,23] When infection presents as cellulitis, surgery is not indicated. If involvement is significant, intravenous antibiotics are required. Once the infection progresses to abscess formation, surgical drainage is necessary. In addition to incision and drainage, the abscess cavity, its walls, loculations, and all infected tissue are excised. Thorough debridement creates vascular access, enabling natural humoral and cellular antibacterial factors and antibiotics to enter the infected area. Wounds are left open to allow drainage, except in larger joints (the wrist and proximally), where closed suction is used. After surgery the hand is initially immobilized and elevated. Once the wound is nontender, nonerythematous, and not indurated, active motion is encouraged to prevent stiffness that results when edema fluid is allowed to consolidate into fibrous tissue.

Accomplishment of the surgical objectives outlined above requires a bloodless field, good lighting, skilled assistance, appropriate instruments, and anesthesia. A ''lancing'' in the emergency department is of limited use, as the extent of infection in various compartments and tissue planes may go unnoticed.[5,23,28,47] Lancing alone delays resolution of the infection and leads to unnecessary tissue destruction.[13,40] We use a tourniquet and obtain a bloodless field to adequately visualize neurovascular structures. Exsanguination is done by gravity only; an Esmarch bandage will spread the infection locally and proximally. Either a regional block or a general anesthetic is required; local anesthetics in inflamed tissues rarely give sufficient anesthesia.

Antibiotics have greatly facilitated treatment of hand infections. Their use in initial stages can often cure the infection and prevent serious sequelae. However, it is vitally important that the antibiotic be chosen based on bacteria likely to be found in hand infections. The presence of gram-positive and gram-negative anaerobic organisms has been documented in numerous hand infections[1,7,12,14–18,25,29,31,33,35] in addition to the common and well-known gram-positive aerobic organisms *Streptococcus*

TABLE 118-1. ORGANISMS CULTURED IN 175 HAND INFECTIONS IN HOSPITALIZED PATIENTS

Bacterium	Number
Gram-Positive Aerobes	
Streptococcus	111
Staphylococcus aureus	70
Staphylococcus epidermidis	29
Streptococcus faecalis	3
Bacillus spp.	1
Gram-Negative Aerobes	
Hemophilus parainfluenza	25
Hemophilus influenza	4
Hemophilus spp.	1
Branhamella catarrhalis	7
Neisseria sicca	2
Gram-Positive Anaerobes	
Corynebacterium spp.	5
Lactobacillus spp.	3
Peptococcus spp.	7
Peptostreptococcus spp.	11
Clostridium perfringens	1
Gram-Negative Anaerobes	
Eikenella corrodens	16
Bacteroides melaninogenicus	13
Bacteroides sp.	8
Veillonella spp.	3
Fusobacterium nucleatum	3
Acinetobacter wolffii	1
Acinetobacter anitratus	3
Pasteurella multocida	5
Gram-Negative Enteric Bacteria	
Enterobacter cloacae	5
Enterobacter agglomerans	1
Klebsiella oxytoca	2
Klebsiella pneumoniae	1
Escherichia coli	2
Hafnia alvei	1
Proteus mirabilis	1
Pseudomonas aeruginosa	1
	Total 346

and *Staphylococcus.* In choosing an antibiotic the following factors must be considered:

1. Penicillinase-resistant penicillins (e.g., nafcillin) are not effective against many anaerobic pathogens.[14,15,18,41]
2. Most hand infections are polymicrobial in nature (Table 118-1).[13,16,41,43]
3. Failure in initial antibiotic selection leads to a poor outcome in hand infections.[13,31,40]
4. Nonvisualization of subsequently cultured organisms on initial Gram's stain is sufficiently common[31] that this stain should not be used to exclude antibiotics (i.e., Gram's stain has too high a false-negative rate).

Therefore, we initiate treatment with two antibiotics. Effective anaerobic coverage is provided by penicillin; effective aerobic gram-positive coverage is provided by either a penicillinase-resistant penicillin (e.g., nafcillin) or by a first-generation cephalosporin such as cefazolin (Ancef, Kefzol) or cephalothin (Keflin). Anaerobic coverage in penicillin-allergic patients is provided by cefoxitin (Mefoxin).[17] Clindamycin, while effective against many anaerobes, is not effective against an important anaerobic pathogen *Eikenella corrodens*[7] and is bacteriostatic. Preferred agents are bacteriocidal.

Gram-negative enteric organisms are found in certain hand infections including those in intravenous drug abusers[33,37,43] and in mutilating injuries in "dirty environments," such as farm machinery.[12] We add an aminoglycoside antibiotic for initial treatment of these types of infections.[36]

Tetanus immunization must be current. A booster is needed if the patient has not had one in the 5 years prior to the infection or injury. History of no previous immunization requires administration of 250 to 500 units of tetanus immune globulin in addition to tetanus toxoid. A complete immunization schedule then follows.

CLASSIFICATION

Pyogenic Bacteria Infections

Aerobic

Infection within 24 to 48 hours postinjury is typical of *Streptococcus*, whereas *Staphylococcus* usually takes 4 to 6 days to make itself known. Less common but still often present are gram-negative bacteria of the Enterobacteriaceae such as *Escherichia coli, Enterobacter cloacae, Proteus,* and *Pseudomonas.*[12,40,43] The latter are more common in wounds sustained from intravenous drug abuse,[29,33,37,43] or in contaminated environments such as farms, stagnant lakes, or sewers.[12] In most hand infections multiple pathogens are isolated on culture.[40] Polymicrobial infection (see Table 118-1) demands polymicrobial antibiotic coverage from the outset if poor outcome is to be avoided.[13,31,40] Single antibiotic use rarely covers all offending organisms.[13,27,41]

Anaerobic

Anaerobic bacteria are commonly overlooked as pathogens except in special circumstances such as clostridial infection in gas gangrene. Crush injuries that result in infection create an ideal environment for anaerobes. Gram-positive anaerobic organisms, such as *Peptococcus* and *Peptostreptococcus,* are more frequently recognized; however, gram-negative anaerobic bacteria are common isolates in hand infections (see Table 118-1), either alone or with *Staphylococcus* and *Streptococcus,* especially in clenched fist and human bite injuries.[14–16,18,38,40] These anaerobes are common human mouth flora[14] and are important pathogens found in intravenous drug abuse infections,[40] because of the common practice of using saliva to lubricate the needle or to moisten cotton used to strain impurities.[33] The aerobic and anaerobic, gram-positive and gram-negative bacteria that infect hands are numerous (see Table 118-1), and we again emphasize the need to consider all pathogens when selecting an antibiotic.[5]

Nonpyogenic Infections

Herpetic infections are common in the hands of health care workers who deal with the mouth such as dentists, dental hygenists, and anesthesiologists.[24] These are self-limiting and their recognition is important to prevent overtreatment. Laboratory tests can confirm these infections, but the diagnosis is usually clinical.

The immune response to the mycobacteria,[2,9,19] fungi,[8,48] and related organisms is cell mediated rather than humeral antibody mediated, and therefore often presents as a foreign body–type reaction or nonspecific inflammation. Delay in diagnosis is common, and the diagnosis is often made only after failure of other treatment modalities. These organisms commonly infect the synovium. Once the diagnosis has been made, antibiotic treatment alone is often indicated.

TREATMENT PRINCIPLES AND TECHNIQUES

Subcutaneous Abscesses in the Hand and Forearm

In the hand venous drainage is from palmar to dorsal, and dorsal skin is not tethered to the underlying structures as it is on the palmar side of the hand. This explains the preponderance of dorsal swelling in all hand insults. Care must be taken to preserve as many of the veins as possible to reduce the deleterious effect of venous congestion. Incisions should be straight and extensile, curving only at skin creases so as to cross them at ≤60°.

Technique

1. Base the incision over the apex of the abscess. Place it in such a way that it can be extended proximally or distally in an extensile fashion (Fig. 118-1), because often the abscess proves to be larger than anticipated. Sharp angles are to be avoided because they compromise skin already suffering from the decreased perfusion produced by the edema of the infection. Skin flaps created by surgical incisions in infection are at great risk to necrose.[39]

2. Sharply enter the abscess. Open the skin along the entire subcutaneous extent to allow easy drainage.

3. Excise all infected tissue sharply; a large curette works well to remove the remains after most of the infected tissue has been sharply debrided. In infections related to intravenous drug abuse, the thrombosed, infected vein should be identified and excised along its course until uninfected tissue is found.

4. Send fluid for aerobic and anaerobic cultures. Then begin intravenous antibiotics.

5. Irrigate well with a pulsatile lavage system.

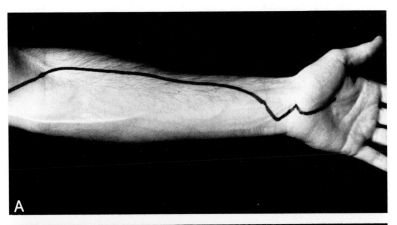

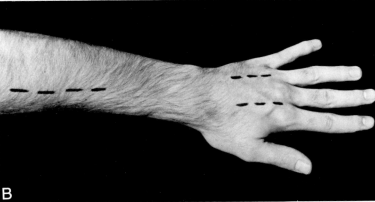

FIGURE 118-1. Incisions for drainage of subcutaneous abscesses in the hand and forearm. Incisions are extensile; only part of the incision may be necessary; however, often the extent of infection is greater than expected. (*A*) Palmar incision. (*B*) Dorsal incision.

TABLE 118-2. SPACES OF THE HAND AND THEIR INFECTIONS

Space	Corresponding Infection
Flexor tendon fibroosseous tunnel:	
Index, long, ring fingers	Flexor tenosynovitis
Thumb tendon/radial bursa	Radial bursa infection
Small finger flexors/ulnar bursa	Ulnar bursa infection
Radial and ulnar bursae	Horseshoe abscess (Hypothenar space infection)
Web space	Collar button abscess
Midpalmar space	Midpalm space infection
Anterior adductor space	Thenar space infection
Posterior adductor space	Thumb web-space infection
Parona's space	Extension anterior to the pronator quadratus

6. Let the wound close secondarily, as the vast majority will contract and epithelialize readily. For those wounds where debridement has been extensive and secondary intention healing would require a prolonged period, a meshed, split-thickness skin graft placed over a completely granulated base at a later time is recommended. Delayed closure of a wound that is not completely resolved often ends in recrudescence of the infection because unseen residual infection can no longer drain. The conditions of abscess are therefore recreated.

Necrotizing Fascitis

Necrotizing fascitis manifests itself as an overwhelming infection within a short period of time.[37,46] The population most often affected is intravenous drug abusers, who are especially at risk because of decreased effectiveness of their immune response.[32] The classic signs and symptoms are erythema, pain, advancing cellulitis, crepitance, skin necrosis, skin bullae, high fever, and other systemic signs of infection. Radiographs may demonstrate soft-tissue gas. One organ system other than the integumentary or musculoskeletal system often is in failure (e.g., delirium, shock, respiratory failure, or renal failure).

TABLE 118-3. EXTENSION OF SPACE INFECTIONS

Location of Infection	Extension
Flexor sheath infections	
Ring, middle	Midpalm space, web spaces
Index	Anterior adductor space
Thumb	Ulnar bursa (horseshoe abscess), wrist/forearm (Parona's space)
Little	Radial bursa (horseshoe abscess), wrist/forearm (Parona's space)
Midpalm	Anterior adductor space, Parona's space/forearm, web space
Anterior adductor	Midpalm, index web, index flexor sheath, wrist/forearm
Web space	Midpalm, anterior adductor, flexor digital sheaths

Group A *Streptoccoccus* is often the offending agent; however, mixed aerobic–anaerobic and gram-positive–gram-negative infections also occur.

Treatment demands immediate radical surgical debridement until healthy muscle and fascia are seen beyond the proximal limits of necrotic fascia. *All* infected tissue must be debrided radically if the infection is to be controlled.

Closed-Space Infections

The hand is compartmented by the structures that pass through it (Table 118-2). Infection in one compartment generally is manifested by pain and swelling throughout the hand, with exquisite tenderness in the confines of the involved space. Knowledge of the anatomic boundaries of these spaces is important to diagnosis and treatment.

Extension of Space Infections

Assessment of extension of infection in the hand from one compartment to the next is a necessary part of the preoperative examination, and to adequately do so one must be aware of the possible patterns of extension (Table 118-3). Visual inspection offers clues, however Kanavel states that "the most conspicuous and valuable sign is the extension of the exquisite tenderness to the area involved."[22] If there is any doubt, exploration of the space where extension may have occurred is indicated at the time of surgical drainage of the known infected space.

Web-Space Infections

In web-space infections, there is swelling and erythema over the palmar and dorsal surfaces of the involved web space, characteristically greater dorsally than palmarly because of greater suppleness of dorsal skin. A web-space infection often occurs from deep spread of a superficially infected palmar callus. The fingers bordering the web are splayed because tissue pressure holds them apart. This infection is also called a collar button abscess because it begins palmarly, then spreads dorsally through or around the transverse metacarpal ligament to the soft tissue of the dorsal web space. This creates two abscess spaces connected by a thin stalk, hence the "collar button." A neglected web-space infection can spread to the palm spaces through the lumbrical canals.[20]

Technique

1. Two incisions are needed (Fig. 118-2). Palmarly, make an oblique incision following the skin lines. Stay away from the web edge; an incision into or through the edge will cause contracture. The abscess is just below the skin, so deeper dissection is not indicated. Remember that in this area the neurovascular structures lie just beneath the skin, so great care must be exercised.
2. Spread the margins of the incision gently but sufficiently to allow adequate drainage.
3. Dorsally, make a longitudinal incision that stays at least 5 mm proximal to the web edge. Excise the dorsal abscess cavity and break up all loculations.

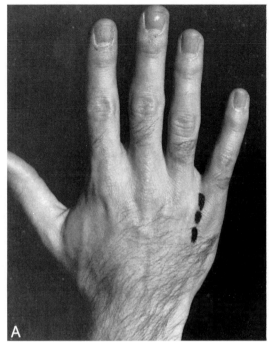
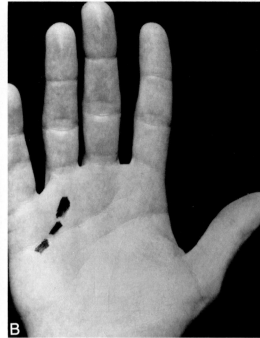

FIGURE 118-2.   Incisions for drainage of web-space infection.

4. Place drains into the incisions after irrigation. Begin intravenous antibiotics after fluid or tissue for culture is obtained. Follow with the usual aftercare.

Suppurative Flexor Tenosynovitis

Suppurative flexor tenosynovitis requires aggressive, appropriate, and prompt treatment to avoid severe disability of the digit or amputation. Kanavel[22] described the classic signs of infection of the flexor sheath as (1) exquisite tenderness over the course of the sheath, limited to the sheath; (2) semiflexed position of the finger; (3) exquisite pain on extending the finger, most marked at the proximal end where often definite swelling may be seen; and (4) symmetric, fusiform swelling of the entire finger. This type of tenosynovitis can develop from the most innocuous-appearing small abrasions and tiny punctures; do not be fooled. These minor wounds are the indication that the sheath has been inoculated with bacteria. When examining a patient with a flexor sheath infection, the other spaces of the hand must be examined as well, because extension of a sheath infection can occur into the palmar spaces, web space, carpal canal, palm bursa, and even Parona's space. Although spread to any of the hand spaces can occur, typically flexor sheath infections of the middle and ring fingers extend into the midpalmar space, and index finger infections extend into the anterior adductor space (thenar space) (see Table 118-3).

The goal of treatment is to drain the infection, allow continued drainage, yet not compromise the function and anatomy of the delicate structure that is the flexor tendon and its canal. Drainage can easily be accomplished; however the drainage procedure itself must not be detrimental to the sheath if the smooth gliding of the flexor tendon within the sheath is to occur after eradication of the infection. We believe this is best accomplished through the intermittent irrigation of the sheath using a catheter.[30]

Continuous irrigation through the catheter tube has the advantage of constant cleansing of the sheath. However, if easy egress from the distal wound does not occur, fluid can be hydraulically forced into the sheath and surrounding tissues. Intermittent irrigation requires the observation of ready egress while infusing, so this potential problem is avoided. Antibiotic irrigation within the sheath is not recommended because it has not been proven to be superior to saline irrigation alone. Also, the effect of antibiotics on the flexor sheath with respect to inducing adhesions has not been studied.

Technique

1. Two incisions are used (Fig. 118-3). Proximally make a transverse incision in the area of the A1 flexor pulley (metacarpophalangeal joint). This incision is made at the proximal palm crease in the index finger, at the distal palmar crease in the ring, and between the two for the long. Incise the skin only approximately 1 cm in length.
2. Gently dissect longitudinally in line with the palmar fascia (perpendicular to the incision), locating the digital nerves on either side of the tendon. Tag and gently retract them.
3. Identify the tendon and the A1 pulley in the base of the wound. Open the palmar synovial and fibrous covering that is the beginning of the flexor sheath; pus, or more commonly slightly cloudy fluid, will emanate. Send a sample for culture; then start intravenous antibiotics.
4. Mark the second incision along the midlateral line of the digit on the ulnar side at the distal interphalangeal joint crease. The midlateral line is that line created by con-

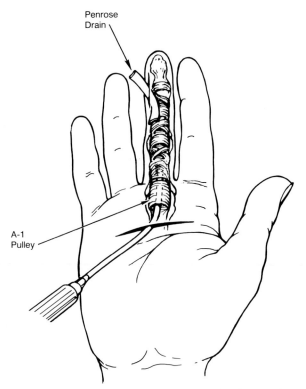

FIGURE 118-3.   Closed tendon sheath irrigation for flexor tenosynovitis.

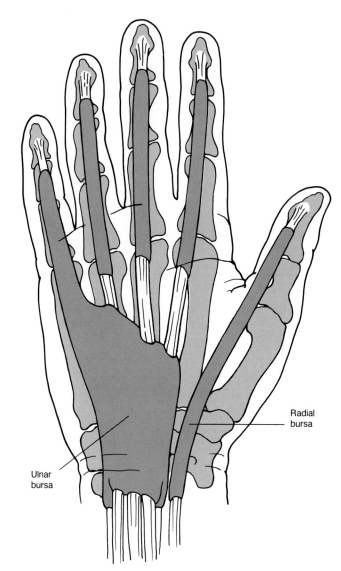

FIGURE 118-4.   Anatomy of the radial and ulnar bursae.

necting the dots that can be made at the end of the flexion creases when the finger is maximally flexed. Incise the skin. Bluntly go deeper to enter the flexor sheath.

5. Return to the proximal wound. Lift the A1 pulley, and thread a small catheter (such as a #10 pediatric feeding tube that has been fenestrated on its end) into the sheath for about 2 cm.

6. Place a syringe onto the catheter end that remains outside the wound and irrigate saline through the catheter. It should easily exit from the distal wound. If it does not, reposition the catheter, or enlarge the opening distally. Several positioning attempts may be needed to achieve the easy flow.

7. Irrigate at least 500 ml of normal saline through the sheath to thoroughly clear it.

8. Place a rubber wick made from a Penrose drain into the sheath through the distal wound to prevent closure. Secure this by a nylon suture through the skin. Nylon suture around the drain and through the skin proximally will prevent its accidental removal. Approximate the proximal wound with one or two nylon sutures.

9. Place a bulky hand dressing, allowing visualization of the distal wound but covering the palmar wound, and bring the catheter out through the dressing.

Postoperative Care

Irrigate 20 to 30 ml of room-temperature saline slowly over 30 to 60 seconds through the catheter; repeat this every 2 to 4

hours on the ward. Postoperative orders should include nursing precautions that when irrigating the catheter with saline, resistance to flow should be minimal, that egress should be seen, and that some discomfort will be experienced by the patient. However, if resistance is excessive, flow is not seen distally, and the patient experiences excessive pain, the catheter may be kinked or have moved to an inappropriate area. The catheter should be removed if easy flow cannot be regained. Continue the irrigation until the sheath is nontender (36–72 hours). Remove the catheter and wick, and apply a maceration dressing for 2 to 3 more days, continuing intravenous antibiotics. Begin active range of motion of the digit after catheter removal to prevent stiffness. Allow the wounds to close secondarily.

Radial and Ulnar Bursae Infections

Infections may occur in the flexor sheaths of the little finger and thumb flexor tendons and their bursae. The bursae are synovial sheaths surrounding these tendons that separate them from the rest of the flexors in the carpal canal (Fig. 118-4). Kanavel's signs of suppurative flexor tenosynovitis are present in the digit; in addition there is swelling, tenderness, and calor into the respective side of the palm and wrist. These are treated with catheter irrigation as described above; below are described the modifications appropriate to the anatomy of each digit and its bursa.

Technique—Radial Bursa

1. A distal thumb incision is made along the radial side at the interphalangeal joint (IPJ) crease. Stay dorsal so that the neurovascular bundle remains palmar. Identify and enter the flexor sheath.
2. Pass a probe or other blunt instrument carefully down the canal until it presses up at the palmar wrist crease. Do not push the probe if resistance is met. Gently redirect it. Make a longitudinal incision that does not cross the wrist crease.
3. Enter the space and identify your probe.
4. Pass a #10 pediatric feeding tube from proximal to distal for about 2 cm. Suture a wick distally and irrigation tube proximally as described for suppurative flexor tenosynovitis. The rest of the procedure is the same as for flexor tenosynovitis. Do not hesitate to make an additional incision in the palm if threading the catheter is difficult.

Technique—Ulnar Bursa

The technique for treating an ulnar bursa is similar to that for a radial bursa, except the distal incision on the small finger is on the *ulnar* side of the digit at the distal interphalangeal joint[21] (Fig. 118-5).

Parona's Space Infections

Parona's space is a potential space in the distal forearm between the deep flexor tendons and the pronator quadratus. It is usually only infected as a result of proximal extension of a hand space infection. Clinically it is evident by tenderness in the distal forearm and pain on pronation and supination. Drainage is accomplished by an incision at the wrist and proximal forearm that often will include communication with the proximal portion of one of the bursa or palmar space infections. Bluntly dissect deep to the flexor tendons to enter the space. Enlarge sufficiently to allow adequate drainage.

Palm-Space Infections

The palm spaces are potential spaces bounded by fascia in the central hand whose exact anatomic boundaries are not agreed upon by anatomists (Fig. 118-6). They lie dorsal to the flexor tendons, palmar to the intrinsic muscles of the hand, and

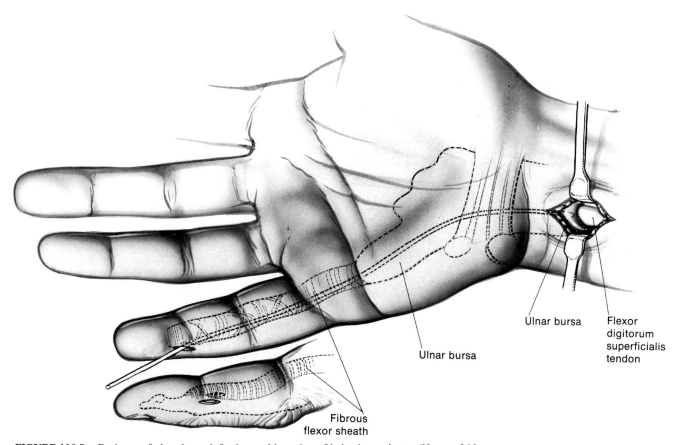

Ulnar bursa

Ulnar bursa

Flexor digitorum superficialis tendon

Fibrous flexor sheath

FIGURE 118-5. Drainage of ulnar bursa infection and insertion of irrigation catheter. (Hoppenfeld, S., and DeBoer, P.: Surgical Exposures in Orthopaedics: The Anatomic Approach. Philadelphia, J. B. Lippincott, 1984.)

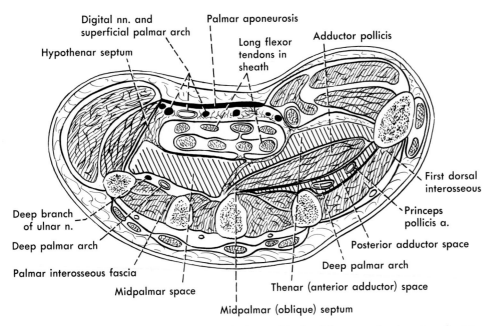

FIGURE 118-6. Cross section through the proximal part of the hand demonstrating the palmar fascial spaces. (Hollinshead, W.H., and Rosse, C.: Textbook of Anatomy, 4th ed. Philadelphia, J. B. Lippincott, 1985.)

proximally and distally merge to form potential extensions to other hand and forearm spaces. These extensions are a source of spread of infection.

Clinically a palm-space infection causes swelling, induration, pain, tenderness to palpation in that area, and tense swelling. Systemic signs of infection such as fever, chills, and malaise may or may not be present. Lymphangitis (erythematous streaking and/or proximal lymph node swelling and tenderness) may or may not be present. A puncture wound several days before is a common finding in the history. Initially dorsal swelling is the more prominent feature of a palm-space infection. Do not be fooled; the infection is palmar. If untreated, palmar swelling occurs within the confines of that compartment out of proportion to the rest of the hand. Kanavel[22] observed that the hand would look as if a balloon had been inserted into the area and blown up to its full capacity. Surgical drainage is mandatory.

Midpalmar Space Infections

The boundaries of the midpalmar space are[20]:

Anterior—flexor tendons of the ring, long, and little fingers
Posterior—second, third, and fourth palmar interossei; third dorsal interosseus; ulnar third and all of fourth metacarpal
Ulnar—hypothenar muscular septum
Radial—midpalmar septum

The midpalmar septum arises beneath the flexor tendons of the index finger, coursing obliquely posteriorly to its attachment on the third metacarpal. It divides the palm into the two main spaces of the anterior adductor (thenar) space and midpalmar space.

Technique

1. Make a transverse incision parallel and just proximal to the distal palmar crease just through the skin at the ring finger. This will be over the area of the swelling. The digital neurovascular structures lie just below the skin, so take extreme care when making the skin incision (Fig. 118-7).
2. Once through the skin, gently dissect longitudinally and identify the digital nerves. Tag these and retract them gently. Identify the deep and superficial flexor tendons to the ring finger. Since the space is dorsal to the flexors, blunt exploration radial and deep to this tendon will gain entrance into the space.
3. Spread gently and open sufficiently to allow adequate drainage. Send fluid for aerobic and anaerobic cultures, then begin intravenous antibiotics.
4. Irrigate, and leave the wound open. Place a Penrose drain within the abscess cavity.

Thenar Space Infections

What is commonly called the thenar space is more appropriately identified as either the anterior or posterior adductor spaces. Most "thenar space" infections involve the anterior adductor space. Its boundaries are[20]:

Anterior—index finger tendons, midpalmar septum
Posterior—fascial covering of the adductor pollicis
Radial—lateral (thenar) intermuscular septum
Ulnar—midpalmar septum

Clinical presentation reveals pain, tenderness to palpation, and tense swelling in the space. Distinguishing between an anterior

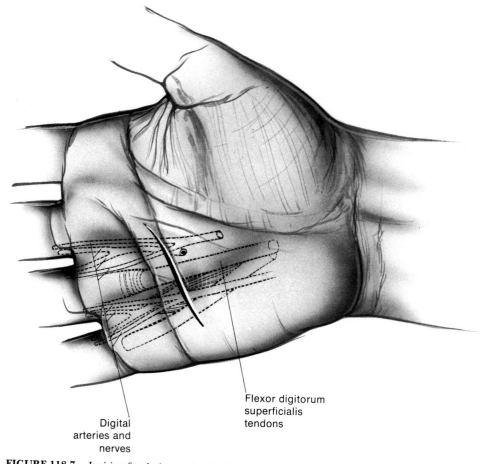

Digital
arteries and
nerves

Flexor digitorum
superficialis
tendons

FIGURE 118-7.   Incision for drainage of midpalmar space infection. (Hoppenfeld, S., and DeBoer, P.: Surgical Exposures in Orthopaedics: The Anatomic Approach. Philadelphia, J. B. Lippincott, 1984.)

adductor space infection and a posterior adductor space infection (less common, and usually in addition to an anterior adductor space infection) is done by comparison of palmar *versus* dorsal swelling, degree of tenderness, and degree of induration. If there is any doubt, open both spaces.

Technique—Anterior Adductor (Thenar) Space

1. Make a curvilinear incision in the palm parallel to the thenar crease on the ulnar side at the base of the thenar eminence (Fig. 118-8).
2. Gently spread the palmar fascia in line with the incision. Identify and tag the digital nerves and flexors to the index finger.
3. Gently retract the nerves.
4. Enter the space beneath the flexors by blunt dissection, remembering that the superficial and deep palmar arches and recurrent branch of the median nerve are in this area.
5. Open sufficiently to allow easy drainage.
6. Send fluid for aerobic and anaerobic culture, then start intravenous antibiotics.
7. Irrigate well. Place a drain within the incision to keep the space open.

Technique—Posterior Adductor Space

1. Make a longitudinal incision dorsally between the thumb and index metacarpals. Stay away from the edge of the thumb/index web to avoid web-space contractures.
2. Incise the fascia, then retract the first dorsal interosseous muscle ulnarly, and the extensor pollicis longus tendon radially. In the proximal portion of the incision is the radial artery, so take care.
3. Bluntly enter the space between the retracted muscles. Open sufficiently to allow easy drainage. Send fluid for aerobic and anaerobic cultures, then begin intravenous antibiotics.
4. Place a drain to keep the space open.

Septic Arthritis

Infection within a joint demands prompt treatment. If detected prior to fulminant proliferation of bacteria, aspiration for diagnosis and culture can be followed by antibiotic therapy alone. Medical literature documents the ability to eradicate the infection by antibiotics alone. However, the deleterious effect of pus on cartilage suggests surgical drainage is indicated if there is any doubt as to whether the infection has been detected

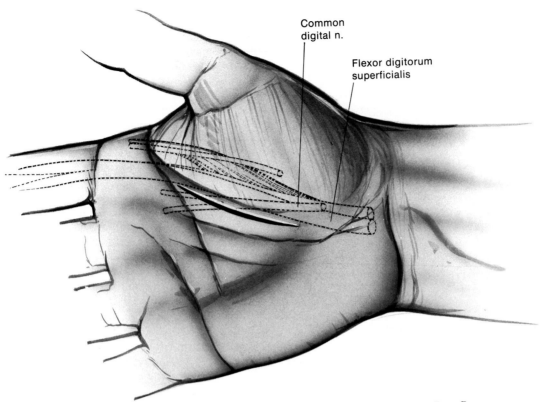

Common
digital n.

Flexor digitorum
superficialis

FIGURE 118-8. Incision for drainage of thenar space infection. (Hoppenfeld S., and DeBoer P.: *Surgical Exposures in Orthopaedics: The Anatomic Approach.* Philadelphia, J. B. Lippincott, 1984.)

and treated early. Gonococcal septic arthritis can be treated with antibiotics alone, so a sexual history is important when questioning the patient.

Usually a history of laceration, puncture wound, or systemic infection with hematogenous spread is obtained. An often-overlooked source of hematogenous spread is an oral cavity or tooth abscess. Clinical manifestations include pain, effusion, erythema, and fever. The pathognomonic sign of joint infection is exquisite pain on attempted motion of that joint. Cellulitis over a joint will cause pain on motion, but the tenderness elicited by slow, gentle, passive motion in cellulitis is much different than the severe pain caused by any attempt at motion of an infected joint. Diagnosis is confirmed by aspiration of the involved joint and the finding of frank pus or white blood cell count greater than 75,000, white blood cell differential of predominantly segmented neutrophils, or bacteria on Gram's stain of the joint fluid.

Aspiration of Phalangeal and Metacarpophalangeal Joints

Aspiration is accomplished with as large a needle as can be entered into the joint. Ideally this is 18 gauge or larger, however a 20- or 22-gauge needle usually is all that will gain entrance into smaller joints. The joint space for the metacarpophalangeal joint is easily palpated just ulnar or dorsal to the extensor hood by taking the edge of your fingernail and press-

ing. Aspirate after antiseptic prep. Local anesthetic usually causes more discomfort than the single stick of the aspirating needle; however, one cannot always convince patients of this. The interphalangeal joint spaces can be located in a similar fashion. This location just next to the extensor tendon dorsally would correspond to a 10 o'clock or 2 o'clock position if the extensor tendon (top or dorsal) is considered as 12 o'clock.

Aspiration of Wrist

The wrist joint includes the radiocarpal, radioulnar, ulnocarpal, and midcarpal joints. Septic arthritis may be found in any one or all of these joints; these spaces may or may not normally communicate. The preoperative examination should be directed toward localizing the joint(s) involved. Pronation/supination pain is indicative of involvement of the radioulnar joint. Flexion/extension pain indicates involvement of either the radiocarpal, ulnarcarpal, or midcarpal joints. Aspiration with an 18-gauge needle confirms clinical suspicions. The radial and ulnar styloids offer convenient landmarks; enter just distal to them.

Drainage of Wrist—Technique

1. The radiocarpal, radioulnar, midcarpal, and ulnarcarpal joints can be entered through either a transverse or longitudinal skin incision. A transverse incision has the ad-

vantage that if care is taken to isolate and preserve veins, a completely circumferential incision can be made so that all wrist joint spaces can be entered until the infected space can be found and drained.

2. Make the skin incision; then enter the joint space by blunt dissection between the appropriate extensor compartments. Enter between the third (extensor pollicis longus) and fourth (extensor indicis proprius, extensor digitorum communis) compartments to drain the radiocarpal, radioulnar, and midcarpal joints. Enter around the extensor carpi ulnaris or extensor digiti quinti tendons to drain the ulnocarpal joint.

3. Obtain fluid for aerobic and anaerobic cultures. Begin intravenous antibiotics.

4. Irrigate thoroughly with a pulsatile lavage system.

5. Place a closed suction system drain. Close the joint capsule and skin incision over the drain. Leave the drain in for 3 to 5 days.

6. Continue intravenous antibiotics for at least 1 week; then follow with an oral agent for several weeks after hospital discharge. Ideally the oral dose will have been determined by greater than 1:8 serum bacterocidal levels against the bacterium (bacteria) isolated. Immobilize initially, then encourage motion.

Human Bite/Clenched Fist Infections

The clenched fist injury commonly involves the metacarpophalangeal joint of the long, ring, or little fingers,[40] but any hand joint or digit can be involved. Human mouth organisms inoculated into tissue are quite virulent.[4,5,10,11,14–15,18,26,27,28,40,44] In the preantibiotic era, amputation as a means to control a human bite infection occurred in up to half of the affected patients. Death secondary to morsus humanis was reported as well. Introduction of antibiotics has not eliminated the complications associated with these infections. Even with antibiotics, 6% of human bites present needing amputation to control their infection, 4% require later amputation, and 28% develop either osteomyelitis or other causes for stiff, disabled fingers.[27]

Known history of human bite, or lacerations (especially over a joint) obtained during a fight must be treated aggressively. Treatment requires operative debridement of dead or questionably viable tissue, thorough irrigation of the subcutaneous space (especially a joint), and leaving the wound open.

Antibiotics effective against gram-positive aerobic and gram-positive and gram-negative anaerobic bacteria are mandatory.[14–18] First-generation cephalosporins such as cefazolin, cephalothin, and cephradrine, or penicillinase-resistant penicillins are effective against the common gram-positive aerobic bacteria. However, many anaerobes commonly isolated from clenched fist/human bite infections are resistant to penicillinase-resistant penicillins and clindamycin,[7,34,42] which are common first choices in treatment of "skin infections." The coverage of first-generation cephalosporins against human oral flora is variable,[17,34] so a second antibiotic is necessary. The antibiotic of choice for these anaerobes is penicillin. Cefoxitin is effective against gram-positive aerobic bacteria and the anaerobes described, so it may be used as a single agent for penicillin-allergic patients.[17]

Technique

1. Extend the traumatic laceration proximally and distally.
2. Remove the necrotic and infected tissue from the subcutaneous layer. Be aware that extension beyond the obvious site of injury commonly occurs; explore nearby potential areas of invasion such as the dorsal subcutaneous space.
3. Always open the joint if the injury is over or near a joint. One often suspects that the joint is uninvolved until arthrotomy is made and the pus wells out. Enter the joint dorsally, making a 1-cm longitudinal incision in the capsule just to the side of the extensor tendon.
4. Inspect the cartilaginous surfaces for lesions. An osteochondral defect or tooth indentation is common. Record such a finding and also the condition of the cartilage in the operative record. Divots and unhealthy-appearing cartilage are poor prognostic factors.
5. Irrigate thoroughly by pulsatile lavage. Leave the wound *open*.

Animal Bites (Dogs, Cats)

Pasturella multocida, a gram-negative anaerobic bacterium,[1,17] has been identified as an important pathogen in animal bite infections. The onset of cellulitis, lymphangitis, serous drainage, and/or pus within 12 to 24 hours of injury strongly suggests infection with this virulent organism. Penicillin is the drug of choice, with tetracycline and cephalosporins as alternative drugs. Bites seen initially should have the wound debrided of necrotic and damaged tissue; penicillin should be given prophylactically for 3 to 5 days. The wounds are left open to heal by secondary intention.

Felon

A felon is an infection in the pulp of a digit. Beneath the skin of the pulp lies fat. Numerous fibrous septae tether the skin to the bone, compartmenting the fat to make shock-absorbing spaces. Infection in the digit pulp is therefore a series of small closed-space infections, each needing incision and drainage. The patient presents with an erythematous, swollen distal phalanx on the palmar side of the digit. It is important to distinguish a felon from herpetic whitlow, because the treatment of herpetic infection of the distal phalanx is nonsurgical. When the felon has organized into an abscess, drainage is indicated.

Technique

1. Drain a felon that points palmar and midline by a midline approach (Fig. 118-9A). Drain a felon that does not point midline with a midlateral incision (Fig. 118-9B). The "fish-mouth" incision destabilizes the pulp, can cause flap necrosis, and is to be avoided.
2. Incise deeply all the way to bone and all the way across the pulp to open all compartmented spaces. Send fluid or tissue for culture. Begin antibiotics. Irrigate thoroughly.

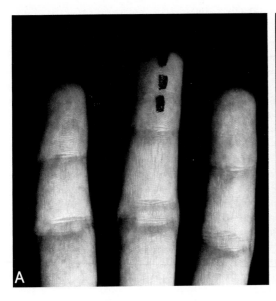
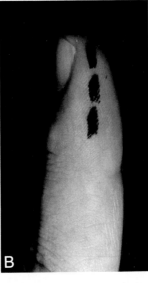

FIGURE 118-9. Incision for drainage of felon. All septae must be cut to allow appropriate drainage. (*A*) Midline incision. (*B*) Midlateral incision.

3. Leave the wound open. Place a wick into the wound; apply a bulky hand dressing to immobilize the hand for the first 24 to 48 hours.
4. Remove the wick and begin soaks four to five times a day. Apply a finger dressing incorporating damp gauze next to the wound. Active finger and hand motion is encouraged.

Nail Bed Infections—Paronychia, Eponychia, Subungual Abscess

Where the skin of the dorsal digit meets the nail is an area sensitive to the disruptive influence of daily living and nail cosmetic practices, especially in those whose work or habits cause a continually damp or wet environment. Bacteria invade the fold of skin over the nail matrix, producing the characteristic lesion of inflammation, pain, and swelling. When confined to a side of the nail, and when involving the fold of skin and not the nail, the infection is called a *paronychia;* when involving the base of the nail fold, it is an *eponychia;* when invading beneath the nail as well, it is called a *subungual abscess.* The localized superficial nail skinfold infection is not serious, but deep infection may invade bone and result in nail destruction, osteomyelitis, and amputation. The bacterium that infects is almost exclusively *Staphylococcus,* except in children where because of "thumb sucking," mouth flora can infect as well.[6]

Beware of the paronychia that is treated and then returns as a felon. Infection spreads from the nailbed to the pulp of the digit through bone; if such spread occurs, osteomyelitis of the distal phalanx is present.

Technique—Paronychia/Eponychia

1. After metacarpal block, take a Freer elevator or other blunt instrument and beginning distally to elevate a few millimeters of the nail fold from the nail as far proximally as the infection extends. A blunt instrument helps prevent scoring that can later produce nail ridging.
2. Using an 18-gauge needle, prick the infected area to

drain and break up loculations. Expect only a few drops of pus. Send these drops for culture, and begin an antibiotic effective against *Staphylococus.*
3. Cover the drained area with antibiotic-impregnated gauze and place under the nail fold. This will allow continued drainage. Begin soaks in 24 hours and continue until healed.

Technique—Subungual Abscess

1. If the nail has been elevated off the matrix by infection, a subungual abscess is present. Elevate the nail fold after incising along its borders (Fig. 118-10).
2. Remove the overlying nail plate to allow adequate drainage. If there is any question as to extent of the subungual abscess, remove the entire nail. Remember, *gently* free the nail plate from the matrix with a blunt instrument in order to avoid injury to the matrix which may result in ridging of the nail as it grows back.
3. After nail plate removal, scoop the abscess contents out with a currette, gently scraping the surface of the nail matrix.
4. Request aerobic and anaerobic culture on the fluid. Begin intravenous antibiotics.

Herpetic Infection and Herpetic Whitlow

Herpetic infection in the hand[24] most often occurs in the distal finger. Pain is the initial symptom. Vesicles 1 to 2 mm in diameter containing clear fluid occur on an erythematous base; as the infection progresses, the vesicles coalesce into bullae. The fluid may turn cloudy after being initially clear; however, it is *never* purulent. Purpuric lesions can develop beneath the nails. The pain continues for 2 to 4 weeks with decreasing erythema. The hemorrhagic areas crust, then desquamate, leaving normal tissue.

The clinical signs and symptoms found in the at-risk groups of hospital and dental personnel alert one to the diagnosis. Laboratory confirmation can be obtained by early culture of

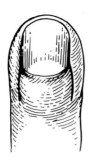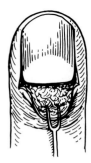

FIGURE 118-10. Incision for drainage of a subungual abscess. After folding back the eponychium, the proximal nail plate is cut with a scissor and removed.

the vesicles, which grow characteristic plaques within 1 to 3 days. Serum titers of antibody to Herpes virus over 2 to 3 weeks may rise to greater than four times normal levels.

It is important to note the self-limited nature of this illness. If incision and drainage are performed, no purulence will be expressed; an aggressive secondary bacterial infection then occurs all too often as the incision injures tissue already compromised by the edema, pressure, and unhealthy conditions the viral "cellulitis" has created. Expectant observation is the key to treatment. Antiviral agents are not indicated.

Mycobacterial Infections

Mycobacterial infections may be caused by *Mycobacterium tuberculosis*,[9] but in the hand they are more commonly caused by atypical mycobacteria such as *Mycobacterium marinum*, *M. kansasii*, *M. avium*, *M. bovis*, and *M. intracellulare*.[19] These infections typically occur in middle-aged persons with a history of puncture wound within 6 weeks of onset of symptoms. *Mycobacterium marinum*[45] is an offending organism in the setting of a seacoast environment or dock area.

With mycobacterial infections in the hand, there are usually no systemic signs of infection. Pain, limitation of motion, and fullness of the involved area are noted, but signs and symptoms are intermittent. Synovium is commonly involved. The synovitis is out of proportion to the disease initially suspected, such as collagen vascular disease, or nonspecific inflammatory synovitis. Fistulae may be present. Diagnosis is based on finding Langhans'-type giant cells in tissue and positive culture; culture results take at least 6 weeks. Diagnosis is thus typically delayed, and is made only after failure of response to initial treatment. Antibiotic treatment is the primary treatment after biopsy is obtained; complete surgical synovectomy is indicated if the synovium is heavily affected. Antituberculous therapy is recommended for 18 to 24 months with two bacterocidal antituberculous agents. Check current recommended drug therapy with an infectious disease specialist.

Fungal Infections

Fungal hand infections occur after trauma with implantation of the fungus or its spore into the skin,[8,48] or as part of systemic spread usually from a primary pulmonary infection that began with inhalation of spores. Primary cutaneous fungal infections

are found most often in gardeners, horticulturists, and others engaged in activities around soil where fungi are ubiquitous.

Cutaneous infection with one of the "systemic mycoses"— *Coccidioides immitis*, *Histoplasma capsulatum*, or *Blastomyces dermatidis*—also occurs after trauma or can actually be a systemic manifestation of a primary lesion elsewhere. After traumatic implantation and an incubation period of several days to months, a subcutaneous nodule will appear that may or may not be painful. A fistula or ulceration develops and enlarges with a raised, discolored, and verrucous border. Epithelial hyperplasia follows. Lymphatic invasion can occur; the lymph channels become cordlike. Nodules develop, ulcerate, then spontaneously resolve, only to be replaced by new lesions.

The cutaneous mycoses, sporotrichosis, chromomycosis, mycetoma, and phycomycosis, also produce hand infections. Sporotrichosis classically occurs after a prick from a rose thorn. After the *Sporothrix schenckii* organism incubates for a period of days to months, a small, nontender, moveable, subcutaneous nodule develops. Epidermal infection will ulcerate early, while a more subcutaneous nodule discolors, darkens, and then erupts through the skin. Spontaneous healing of the ulcer follows, but new lesions erupt. Lymphatic invasion occurs, raising cordlike tracks along the hand and arm. The other cutaneous mycoses present in a similar fashion.

Diagnosis of fungal infection is made by excisional biopsy of one of the lesions or by culture of drainage. Treatment varies according to the fungus isolated. The more virulent fungi require systemic therapy with amphotericin B or ketoconazole. The less virulent cutaneous mycoses may resolve spontaneously. Sporotrichosis is effectively treated by potassium iodide either orally, topically, or both.

POSTOPERATIVE CARE

Wounds are left open and covered with wet saline gauze to allow easy drainage. A plaster splint—reinforced long-arm bulky hand dressing is applied, incorporating a cord to permit continuous elevation.

The dressing is changed at 36 to 48 hours to a maceration-type dressing of 25% strength Dakin's solution. This is changed daily. Active hand motion is begun to prevent stiffness.

The patient is discharged when the wound is without erythema, tenderness, induration, or swelling.

Wet-to-dry dressings are changed three times a day at home for the open wounds; 7 days of oral penicillin, first-generation cephalosporin, or both are prescribed based on culture results. Dressing changes are continued until the wound is healed.

PITFALLS AND COMPLICATIONS

1. An undrained area of infection is a common reason for failure to improve after initial debridement. Physical examination directed toward discovering possible places of spread prior to surgery will help uncover these extensions. When in doubt, open the space at the time of surgery.
2. Keep incisions out of skin creases. If an incision for

drainage must cross the crease, angle it <60°; failure to do so results in contracture.

3. Keep out of the web spaces for the same reason.
4. Flaps in the presence of infection are prone to necrosis. Use only longitudinal or gently curved incisions.
5. Do not miss herpetic whitlow masquerading as a felon or paronychia. Incision of this already-compromised tissue may lead to secondary bacterial infection.
6. Antibiotic selection must be effective to eradicate all organisms present in a hand infection. Coverage against *Staphylococcus* and *Streptococcus*, as well as the anaerobic streptococci, is necessary. Gram-negative anaerobes are often present, especially in clenched fist, human bite, and intravenous drug abuse infections. Antibiotic selection should be based on the type of injury known or suspected.

REFERENCES

1. Arons, M.S., Fernando, L., and Polayes, I.: *Pasturella multocida:* The Major Cause of Hand Infections Following Domestic Animal Bites. J. Hand Surg. **7**:47, 1982.
2. Benkeddache, Y., and Gottesman, H.: Skeletal Tuberculosis of the Wrist and Hand: A Study of 27 Cases. J. Hand Surg. **7**:593, 1982.
3. Bingham, D.L.C.: Acute Infections of the Hand. Surg. Clin. North Am. **40**:1285, 1960.
4. Boland, F.K.: Morsus Humanus. J.A.M.A. **116**:127, 1941.
5. Boyce, F.F.: Human Bites: Analysis of 90 (Chiefly Delayed and Late) Cases From Charity Hospital of Louisiana at New Orleans. South. Med. J. **35**:631, 1942.
6. Brook, I.: Bacteriologic Study of Paronychia in Children. Am. J. Surg. **141**:703, 1981.
7. Brooks, G.F., O'Donoghue, J.M., Rissing, J.P., Soapes, K., and Smith, J.W.: *Eikenella corrodens:* A Recently Recognized Pathogen. Medicine **53**:325, 1974.
8. Bullpitt, P., and Weedon, D.: Sporotrichosis: A Review of 39 Cases. Pathology **10**:249, 1978.
9. Bush, D.C., and Schneider, L.H.: Tuberculosis of the Hand and Wrist. J. Hand Surg. **9**:391, 1984.
10. Butz, R.O.: Human Bites: A Series Treated With Antibiotics. Am. J. Surg. **9**:525, 1956.
11. Farmer, C.B., and Mann, R.J.: Human Bite Infections of the Hand. South. Med. J. **59**:515, 1966.
12. Fitzgerald, R.H., Cooney, W.P., Washington, J.A., VanScoy, R.E., Linscheid, R.L., and Dobyns, J.H.: Bacterial Colonization of Mutilating Hand Injuries and Its Treatment. J. Hand Surg. **2**:85, 1977.
13. Glass, K.D.: Factors Related to the Resolution of Treated Hand Infections. J. Hand Surg. **7**:388, 1982.
14. Goldstein, E.J.C.: Infections Following Human Bites. Infections in Surgery **000**:849, 1985.
15. Goldstein, E.J.C., Barones, M.F., and Miller, T. *Eikenella corrodens* in Hand Infections: Part 1. J. Hand Surg. **8**:563, 1983.
16. Goldstein, E.J.C., Citron, D.M., Wield, B., Blachman, U., Sutter, V.L., Miller, T.A., and Finegold, S.M.: Bacteriology of Human and Animal Bite Wounds. J. Clin. Microbiol. **8**:667, 1978.
17. Goldstein, E.J.C., Gombert, M.E., and Agyare, E.O.: Susceptibility of *Eikenella corrodens* to Newer Beta-lactam Antibiotics. Antimicrob. Agents Chemother. **18**:832, 1980.
18. Goldstein, E.J.C., Miller, T., Citron, D.M., and Finegold, S.: Infections Following Clenched Fist Injury: A New Perspective. J. Hand Surg. **3**:455, 1978.
19. Gunther, S.F., Elliott, R.C., Brand, R.L., and Adams, J.P.: Experience with Atypical Mycobacterial Infection in Deep Structures of the Hand. J. Hand Surg. **2**:90, 1977.
20. Hollinshead, H.W.: Anatomy for Surgeons, Volume 3, 2nd ed. New York, Harper & Row, 1969.
21. Hoppenfeld, S., and deBoer, P.: Surgical Exposures in Orthopaedics: The Anatomic Approach. Philadelphia, J.B. Lippincott, 1984.
22. Kanavel, A.B.: Infections of the Hand, 7th ed. London, Bailliere, Tindall, and Cox, 1939.
23. Linscheid, R.L., and Dobyns, J.H.: Common and Uncommon Infections of the Hand. Orthop. Clin. North Am. **6**:1063, 1975.
24. Louis, D.S., and Silva, J.: Herpetic Whitlow: Herpetic Infections of the Hand. J. Hand Surg. **4**:90, 1979.
25. Louria, D.B., Hensle, T., and Rose, J.: The Major Medical Complications of Heroin Addiction. Ann. Int. Med. **67**:1–21, 1967.
26. Maier, R.L.: Human Bite Infections of the Hand. Ann. Surg. **106**:423, 1937.
27. Mann, R.J., Hoffeld, T.A., and Farmer, C.B.: Human Bites of the Hand: 20 Years of Experience. J. Hand Surg. **2**:97, 1977.
28. Mason, M.L., and Koch, S.L.: Human Bite Infections of the Hand. Surg. Gynecol. Obstet. **51**:591, 1930.
29. McKay, D., Pascarelli, E.F., and Eaton, R.: Infections and Sloughs in the Hand of Drug Addicts. J. Bone Joint Surg., **55-A**:741, 1973.
30. Neviaser, R.J.: Closed Tendon Sheath Irrigation for Pyogenic Flexor Tenosynovitis. J. Hand Surg. **3**:462, 1978.
31. Nunley, D.L., Sasaki, T., Atkins, A., and Vetto, R. M.: Hand Infections in Hospitalized Patients. Am. J. Surg. **140**:374, 1980.
32. Orangio, G.R., Della Latta, P., Marino, C., Guarneri, J.J., Giron, J.A., Palmer, J., and Margolis, I.B.: Infections in Parenteral Drug Abusers: Further Immunologic Studies. Am. J. Surg. **146**:738, 1983.
33. Orangio, G.R., Pitlick, S., Della Latta, P., Mandel, L.J., Marino, C., Guarneri, J.J., Giron, J.A., and Margolis, I.B.: Soft Tissue Infections in Parenteral Drug Abusers. Ann. Surg. **199**:97, 1984.
34. Robinson, J.V.A., and James, A.L.: *In Vitro* Susceptibility of *Bacteroides corrodens* and *Eikenella corrodens* to Ten Chemotherapeutic Agents. Antimicrob. Agents Chemother. **6**:542, 1974.
35. Robson, M.C., Schmidt, D., and Hessers, J.P.: Cefamandole Therapy in Hand Infections. J. Hand Surg. **8**:560, 1983.
36. Sarubbi, F.A., and Hull, J.H.: Amikacin Serum Concentrations: Prediction of Levels and Dosage Guidelines: Part 1. Ann. Int. Med. **89**:612, 1978.
37. Schecter, W., Meyer, A., Schecter, G., Giuliano, A., Newmeyer, W., and Kilgore, E.: Necrotizing Fascitis of the Upper Extremity. J. Hand Surg. **7**:15, 1982.
38. Schmidt, D.R., and Hickman, J.D.: *Eiknella corrodens* in Human Bite Infections of the Hand. J. Trauma **23**:478, 1983.
39. Scott, J.C., and Jones, B.V.: Results of Treatment of Infections of the Hand. J. Bone Joint Surg. **34-B**:581, 1952.
40. Spiegel, J.D., and Szabo, R.M.: A Protocol for the Treatment of Infections of the Hand. J. Hand Surg., 1988, in press.
41. Stern, P.J., Staneck, J.L., McDonough, J.J., Neale, H.W., and Tyler, G.: Established Hand Infections: A Controlled, Prospective Study. J. Hand Surg. **8**:553, 1983.
42. Sutter, V.L., and Finegold, S.M.: Susceptibility of Anaerobic Bacteria to 23 Antimicrobial Agents. Antimicrob. Agents Chemother. **10**:736, 1976.
43. Webb, D., and Thadepalli, H.: Skin and Soft Tissue Polymicrobial Infection from Intravenous Abuse of Drugs. Western J. Med. **130**:200, 1979.
44. Welch, C.E.: Human Bite Infections of the Hand. N. Engl. J. Med. **215**:901, 1936.
45. Williams, C.S., and Riordan, D.C.: *Mycobacterium marinum* (Atypical Acid-Fast Bbacteria) Infections of the Hand. J. Bone Joint Surg. **55-A**:1042, 1973.
46. Wilson, B.: Necrotizing Fascitis. Am. J. Surg. **18**:416, 1952.
47. Van Niekerk, J.P.: Hand Infections: Management and Results Based on a New Classification: A Study of More Than 1,000 Cases. South African Med. J. **40**:316, 1966.
48. Zinsser: Microbiology, 17th ed. Joklik, W.K., Willett, H.P., and Amos, D.B., eds. New York, Appleton, Century, Croft, 1980.

CHAPTER 119

Tumors of the Hand

CLAYTON A. PEIMER and
JAMES S. THOMPSON

This chapter focuses on tumors that are specific to the hand and are unusual with regard to diagnosis, biologic behavior, or treatment. Tumors of the hand include soft-tissue and hard-tissue neoplasms, reactive nodules and cysts, rheumatoid proliferations, bone spurs, and foreign body reactions (Tables 119-1 and 119-2). Innocent-looking lesions may be deadly, whereas impressive-appearing ones will sometimes require minimal treatment (Fig. 119-1). Surgeons treating hand tumors must be familiar with the range of possibilities. Lesions in the hand are typically seen earlier in their course than those occurring at other sites because they are likely to be superficial (and therefore noticed). However, tumors of the hand may have a profound functional impact once treatment has begun.

Primary musculoskeletal malignancies in the upper extremity are rare, and are less common in the upper extremities than in the lower extremities.[16,18] It is unlikely that a surgeon outside a tertiary care setting will see enough difficult cases (aggressive benign and true malignant tumors) to feel truly comfortable in their management and treatment.[54] The basic principles and definitions of tumor treatment do not differ, whether applied to the hand or some other body part. Benign lesions may be latent (stage I), actively growing but limited to a small zone (stage II), or aggressive (stage III). Latent tumors of bone and soft tissue may need only observation; actively growing lesions are often controlled by intralesional or marginal excisions. Aggressive tumors require wide surgical margins or *en bloc* excision for local control and cure.

The Musculoskeletal Tumor Society (MSTS) staging system proposed by Enneking and colleagues[19,20] forms the basis for treating malignant hand sarcomas (Table 119-3). We do not yet have "standards" of safe and appropriate surgery in the hand based on objective, rigorous scientific data, owing to limited numbers and the vagaries of various reporting methods employed in the past.[8,16,51,53] What constitutes a "safe" margin and how much function need be sacrificed to save the patient have *not* been indisputably established. The MSTS staging system should make current and future treatment comparisons and definitions simpler. However, the anatomic implications of compartmentalization—based on the presence of a tissue barrier that does not permit easy extension of tumor cells—has limited application in the hand. The important issue is that a surgical margin must not be compromised if it endangers the primary goal of surgery, which is, of course, cure. In musculoskeletal tumor surgery, cure requires local control;[16] nonetheless, surgery may be supplemented and enhanced by adjunctive chemotherapy and/or radiotherapy protocols to permit retention of even small portions of the hand, and thereby allow useful function.

DIAGNOSIS

The essentials of tumor diagnosis by the combined use of history, physical examination, blood values, and diagnostic imaging studies are not included in this chapter. For information on

The authors wish to acknowledge the assistance of Frances Sherwin, M.S., in the preparation of this chapter.

TABLE 119-1. TUMORS OF SOFT TISSUE

Cystic Lesions
Ganglion cyst
Mucous cyst
Epidermal inclusion cyst

Skin Tumors
Squamous cell carcinoma
Keratoacanthoma
Malignant melanoma

Fibrous Tumors
Non-neoplastic lesions
Fibrous histiocytoma
Fibroma
Extraabdominal desmoid/desmoplastic fibroma
Fibrosarcoma

Vascular Tumors
Arteriovenous malformation
Aneurysm
Hemangioma
Glomus tumor
Hemangioendothelioma and hemangiosarcoma
Kaposi sarcoma

Nerve Tumors
Neurilemoma/schwannoma
Neurofibroma
Lipofibromatosis hamartoma of the median nerve

Lipid Tumors
Lipoma

Synovial Tumors
Giant-cell tumor of tendon sheath/
Fibrous xanthoma
Epithelioid sarcoma, synovial sarcoma,
   clear cell sarcoma

TABLE 119-2. TUMORS OF HARD TISSUE

Tumors of Cartilage
Solitary enchondroma
Multiple enchondromatosis
Osteocartilaginous exostoses (solitary and multiple)

Bone Tumors
Giant-cell tumor of bone
Aneurysmal bone cyst
Osteoid osteoma

Metastatic Tumors

inaccessible or deep tumors, lesions of the hand are best sampled by incisional or excisional biopsy technique. Biopsy is not a simple surgical procedure, and is especially crucial to the outcome of treatment of aggressive and malignant tumors.[52] If a surgeon or institution is unprepared or ill equipped to complete all diagnostic studies and proceed with definitive surgical management plus adjunctive care that might be required, the patient should be referred before biopsy is undertaken.[37] The patient and surgeon must be prepared for the unexpected, even at the time of biopsy. Sometimes incisional biopsy rather than excision may be all that is performed (Fig. 119-3).

Hand surgery is best done in a bloodless field. Tourniquet control may safely be used for performing the biopsy and treating tumors of the hand. However, unless it is certain that the lesion is benign, exsanguination of the limb with an elastic rubber wrap (Esmarch or Martin bandage) is contraindicated because it may dislodge or seed tumor cells (or bacteria from infected lesions). A bloodless field can be achieved by elevation of the arm for 2 to 4 minutes followed by inflation of the pneumatic tourniquet. Likewise, intravenous Bier block anesthesia, which also requires exsanguination, is not to be used when performing a biopsy or removing undiagnosed hand tumors.

Few pathologists are willing to make a definitive diagnosis of a bone or soft-tissue tumor on the basis of a frozen section alone. Should the lesion prove to be aggressive or malignant, then by definition the biopsy tract is contaminated with tumor cells. Biopsy incisions should be longitudinal to accommodate subsequent excision, and located to remove the lesion completely without extending the margins of dissection just to accommodate a (badly placed) biopsy site. Incisional biopsies are not likely to contaminate large areas of the hand with potentially malignant cells. Small tumors are frequently noticed early; soft-tissue lesions 1 cm or less in diameter may be biopsied by removing the entire tumor if limited to one plane or compartment. Skin lesions may be left open and/or covered with synthetic semiocclusive materials or by porcine xenograft until biopsy results are known. Questionable bone tumors are best treated by cortical incision, windowing, and *limited* curettage. Biopsy wounds are *not* drained. Postoperative care is routine for reconstructive hand surgery while awaiting definitive tissue diagnosis.

these topics, the reader is referred to Chapter 69. We would emphasize, however, that systemic studies, plain radiographs, technetium-99m and gallium-67 scintigraphy, computed tomography (CT) of the limb part and lungs, and magnetic resonance imaging (MRI) should be completed prior to surgical biopsy. The MRI and CT scan may be particularly helpful in delineating whether a lesion is contained within a bone or soft-tissue compartment, or has extended and invaded from one to the other[61] (Fig. 119-2). The data from these imaging studies may aid considerably in planning the biopsy incision (including its location) and the extent of subsequent treatment.

BIOPSY TECHNIQUE

In most cases, a specific diagnosis cannot be made without a biopsy. Although needle technique may be useful for otherwise

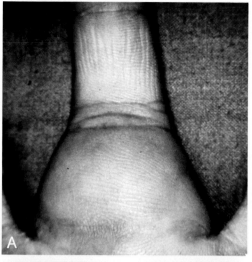

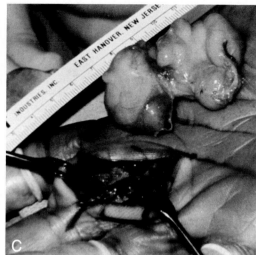

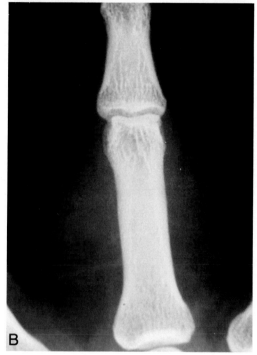

FIGURE 119-1. (*A*) A 43-year-old man with an enlarging phalangeal mass of considerable size. (*B*) Radiographs reveal the soft-tissue tumor as having a fluid density, suggestive of a lipoma. (*C*) The diagnosis was confirmed at surgery and the large lipoma removed.

TABLE 119-3. SURGICAL STAGES

Stage	Grade	Site
IA	Low (G$_1$)	Intracompartmental (T$_1$)
IB	Low (G$_1$)	Extracompartmental (T$_2$)
IIA	High (G$_2$)	Intracompartmental (T$_1$)
IIB	High (G$_2$)	Extracompartmental (T$_2$)
III	Regional or distant metastasis (M)	
	Any (G)	Any (T)

(Enneking, W.F., Spanier, S.S., and Goodman, M.A.: Current Concepts Review: The Surgical Staging of Musculoskeletal Sarcoma. J. Bone Joint Surg. **62-A**: 1027, 1980)

TREATMENT PRINCIPLES

Benign Tumors

Benign tumors of bone and soft tissue can be extirpated simply using intralesional or marginal procedures, such as shelling out of soft tissue or bone curettage. Tumors with special characteristics or presenting certain problems because of their location and biologic potential will be individually discussed later in this chapter.

Aggressive Tumors

Whether invaded locally from a primary malignancy or as a metastatic focus, the hand bones and soft tissues can be the site of many aggressive tumors. Hand anatomy and function make treatment of such lesions different from treatment of lesions occurring elsewhere. Because it is superficial, a lesion in the hand may be discovered when it is small. Yet, radical surgery in the hand limits function more severely than radical surgery performed elsewhere. Retention of even one finger may afford some useful function. Anatomic compartments and spaces in the hand communicate with those of the forearm. Strict "tumor margin" definition to effect a pure surgical cure may result in, perhaps, unnecessary debilitation when the size of a centripetal lesion is considered. For example, a tumor on or near the flexors of the little finger is contiguous with the flexor

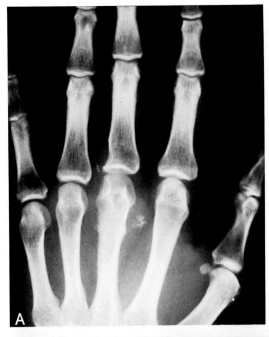

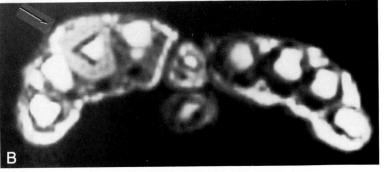

FIGURE 119-2. (A) Radiographs showing a soft-tissue mass with calcifications, plus erosion of the third metacarpal and proximal phalanx in a 27-year-old male. The findings suggest an aggressive tumor, quite possibly a (malignant) synovial sarcoma. (B) The magnetic resonance image demonstrates absence of marrow involvement by this well-defined circumferential soft-tissue tumor (*arrow*). These findings clearly support the diagnosis of benign, noninvasive neoplasm—but one which would require dorsal and palmar incisions for complete excision. Synovial chondromatosis was confirmed at surgery.

compartment, the proximal extent of which is the common flexor/pronator origin at the medial epicondyle of the humerus. Radical excision, by definition, includes removal of all tissues within a compartment; in this case, neither palmar neurovascular nor muscular structures are spared, and only the bones of the hand and forearm plus the extensor muscles are retained. The question that must be asked is whether the presence of a small, distal lesion always justifies surgery which, in effect, amputates the hand. Data to answer this question are not available, but experience suggests that aggressive tumors may often be treated by *en bloc* excision, rather than by radical resection or amputation, which would be performed for histologically similar lesions of the lower extremity. Metastatic tumors are infrequent,[3] but they may be the presenting sign of a distant primary tumor of lung or kidney (most frequently), breast, gastrointestinal, and/or hematopoietic systems (Fig. 119-4). After diagnosis by biopsy and other studies performed in conjunction with treatment of the underlying disease, the only intervention needed in those cases may be reduction by surgical, radiotherapeutic, or chemotherapeutic means.

Aggressive lesions that are frankly malignant must be distinguished from those that are only locally recurrent and invasive. Tumors in the second group can be safely and adequately addressed by *en bloc* excision as long as the cuff of normal tissue is sufficient to contain the tumor. It is usually not justifiable to include essential nerves and vessels within this normal cuff because such tumors, even if they recur, are not associated with lethal metastases. Except for skin tumors, a 2-cm to 3-cm cuff of normal tissue is usually adequate. A 4-cm to 5-cm cuff should be considered a mandatory minimum in the presence of a truly malignant tumor, because the prognosis for survival following a local recurrence is poor.[16] Ray resection or metacarpophalangeal joint disarticulation for a malignant digital lesion may be adequate surgery (Fig. 119-5). More proximal tumors would be treated by subtotal hand amputation (e.g., several contiguous rays). Definitive treatment such as *en bloc* excision or subtotal amputation, however, should not be performed until the diagnosis is clearly established by an experienced pathologist. At removal, the borders of the specimen must be carefully examined histologically for the presence of tumor and, if the lesion has not been adequately resected, the margins must be expanded. If a safe, adequate resection will destroy hand function, amputation is preferred (Fig. 119-6).

Wound closure is best effected with local tissues, local flaps, and skin grafts. Distant flaps should not be used for primary closure because tumor cells may unnecessarily contaminate the remote flap donor area. Filet flaps and local rotation flaps from portions of retained fingers are ideal for coverage in these circumstances. Complex reconstructive procedures such as vascularized flaps and digital reconstructions should be delayed and staged. If only the fourth and fifth rays are retained, rotational metacarpal osteotomy to salvage pinch is justifiable at the time of tumor resection. Index pollicization might be done in a resection that involves removal of the thumb and contiguous thenar and first web muscles.

In some institutions, these operations are most successfully performed by a team which includes a tumor surgeon and a reconstructive hand surgeon. In other situations, one person may fill both roles successfully. In all circumstances, the patient

and surgeon must weigh the lethal or destructive potential of the tumor against the value of salvaging even a small portion of the hand.[54] If preoperative studies, anatomic barriers, surgical margins, and histologic examination of the margins of resection have been adequately considered and addressed, many aggressive and malignant tumors of the hand can be cured without complete amputation. If such surgery is performed, it should be augmented by adjunctive treatment.

TUMORS OF SOFT TISSUE

Cystic Lesions

Ganglion Cyst

The ganglion cyst, the most common tumor in the hand, is seen more frequently in women than in men. The site of this lesion is most often on the dorsal carpus (scapholunate origin) or palmar wrist (scaphotrapezial and trapeziometacarpal origin).[5,38,42] Frequently the cyst arises from the palmar surface of the fibrosseous flexor sheath (retinacular cysts or sesamoid ganglia) as a small, hard, and often painful lesion at the proximal finger flexion crease.

A ganglion cyst is a mucus-filled cyst with a fibrous wall, not a neoplasm, which is typically connected to an underlying joint by an (often tortuous) stalk. The lesion may be tender as it expands or is impacted. Surgical excision is recommended for lesions which are unsightly, painful, or interfere with function and have not responded to aspiration and steroid installation. Excision is usually 95% curative if the tumor and stalk are removed with a small cuff of contiguous joint capsule (Fig. 119-7). At surgery, we prefer to aspirate the cyst and retract surrounding structures to aid visualization through the relatively small incision. No prizes are given for struggling, even if the lesion is still filled with mucus when removed; the patient wins only if there is no recurrence.

Recurrences are prevented by complete excision of the stalk, contiguous capsule, and any nearby satellite or daughter cysts. Avoid overly vigorous retraction which can endanger nearby sensory nerves, tendons, or vessels.

Mucous Cysts

Mucous cysts, nearly identical histologically to ganglion cysts, arise from arthritic distal interphalangeal joints in the fingers and thumb.[33] They often involve the nearby germinal nail matrix secondary to local pressure. As they enlarge, the overlying skin thins considerably. These lesions may be associated with a secondary, spontaneous rupture which can lead to serious complications, namely a septic infection and osteomyelitis. Like removal of the ganglion cyst, an operation to remove the mucous cyst also must include its stalk, the associated osteophytes, and the joint capsule. Protect the terminal tendon and nail matrix. Closure may require a local rotation flap or skin advancement to replace the atrophic, useless skin covering the cyst. If the underlying joint itself is significantly arthritic and symptomatic, arthrodesis is recommended (see Chap. 100).

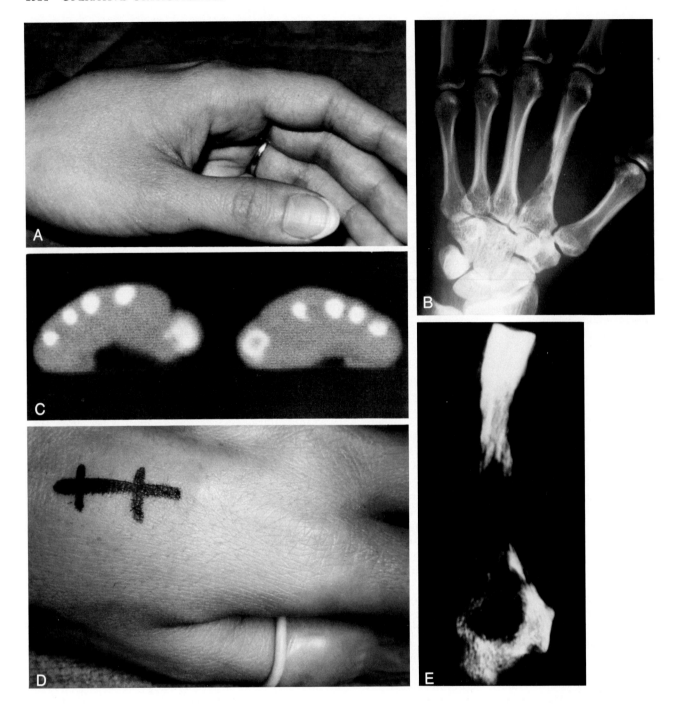

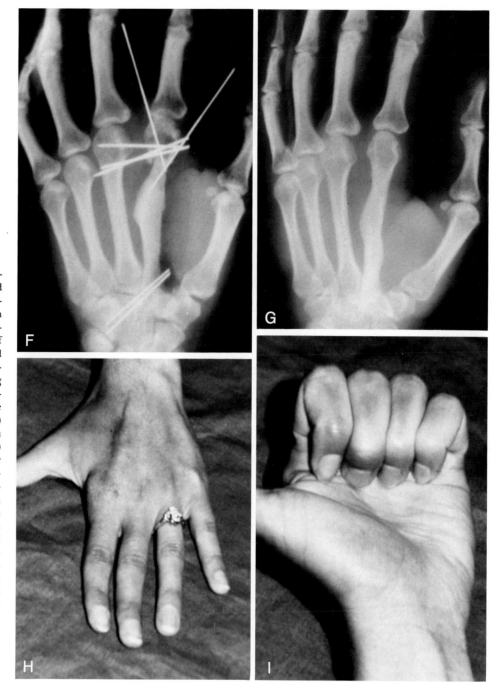

FIGURE 119-3. (*A*) Clinical appearance of the hand in a 24-year-old woman who reported a 10-week history of an enlarging, painful mass on the dorsum of the hand. (*B*) Radiographs revealed endosteal invasion of the second metacarpal diaphysis and metaphysis without new bone formation, suggestive of a rapidly growing lesion. (*C*) The CT scan revealed actual cortical destruction along the ulnar side of the metacarpal shaft. (*D*) A small dorsal longitudinal incision (located so as to be entirely excisable) was used for the incisional biopsy under tourniquet control, without exsanguination. (*E*) Radiograph of specimen. Permanent sections revealed an aneurysmal bone cyst, which was treated at a separate operation by *en bloc* second metacarpal resection and iliac graft replacement. (*F*) In order to maintain functional skeletal continuity, the second metacarpal head was transfixed to the third prior to bone resection. The Kirschner wires were left in place until union was solid. (*G*) Therapy was started 2 weeks after surgery and motion recovered rapidly. (*H* and *I*) Follow-up clinical photographs.

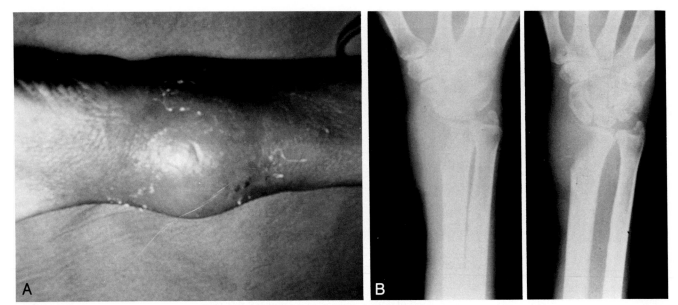

FIGURE 119-4. (*A*) Clinical and (*B*) radiographic appearance of a painful, enlarging mass and osteolysis of the radius in a 70-year-old man. Incisional biopsy disclosed bronchogenic carcinoma; the arm was irradiated.

Epidermal Inclusion Cysts

Epidermal inclusion cysts consist of buried epidermal cells which are implanted secondary to a traumatic or surgical wound.[12] The mass is attached to skin and subcutaneous tissue, contains keratin, and may enlarge to a significant size. Carefully excise these lesions, taking care to avoid spillage of the contents and damage to adjacent structures; curette intraosseous components.

Skin Tumors

Squamous Cell Carcinoma

Squamous cell carcinoma, which accounts for the vast majority of soft-tissue malignancies of the hand, is seen in older patients with a history of chronic exposure to chemicals, radiation, or the sun[10,13,48] (Fig. 119-8). The tumor is usually located on an exposed (i.e., dorsal) surface and is often accompanied by ulceration. The nailbed is a less common site. Generally, these tumors are slow growing (in contrast to keratoacanthoma). Because these primary tumors rarely metastasize, they can usually be cured by local excision, which includes a margin of 1 cm to 2 cm of normal skin (Fig. 119-9). The depth of excision required depends on the extent of the lesion. Removal of superficial tumors leaves a defect usually coverable by local advancement or skin grafting. Tumors extending into adjacent tendon or bone must be treated by *en bloc* excision or local amputation; lymph node dissection is rarely indicated unless there is nodal enlargement in the presence of a large tumor.

Keratoacanthoma

Keratoacanthoma, a benign neoplasm which resembles squamous cell carcinoma, is found in the same sites and in the same older individuals as the more serious malignant lesion but it grows more rapidly. It is usually diagnosed at excisional biopsy. Recurrences are uncommon.

Malignant Melanoma

Malignant melanoma is an aggressive and potentially lethal skin tumor. The incidence is increasing in patients with a history of chronic sun exposure.[23,34,50] Tumors may be dark, multicolored, or without pigment, and have been graded according to the level of invasion or the thickness. Most tumors can be surgically treated maintaining a 1-cm (level I or II) to 5-cm (level III through V, and nodular) margin. The adequacy of these margins is subject to some debate. Early recognition and treatment significantly increase the chance for survival if the tumor has not invaded deeper tissues and if it has not metastasized. The use of chemotherapy has not been gratifying.

Fibrous Tumors

Non-Neoplastic Lesions

The diagnoses used for these conditions include *keloid, fasciitis,* and *fibromatosis.*[2,26,46,58] Keloid is a post-traumatic phenomenon, generally occuring between the ages of 10 and 25 years, most commonly in blacks and those with a family history. Keloid may continue to grow for months or years, or involute spontaneously. Surgical excision and radiation are rarely more than temporarily successful; intradermal injection of steroids (e.g., triamcinilone) and elastic garments may be helpful. Fasciitis, also usually post-traumatic, occurs in the same age group.

The fibromatoses, frequently locally infiltrative and recurring lesions, include subdermal fibromatosis of infancy, infantile dermal fibromatosis, juvenile aponeurotic fibroma, and

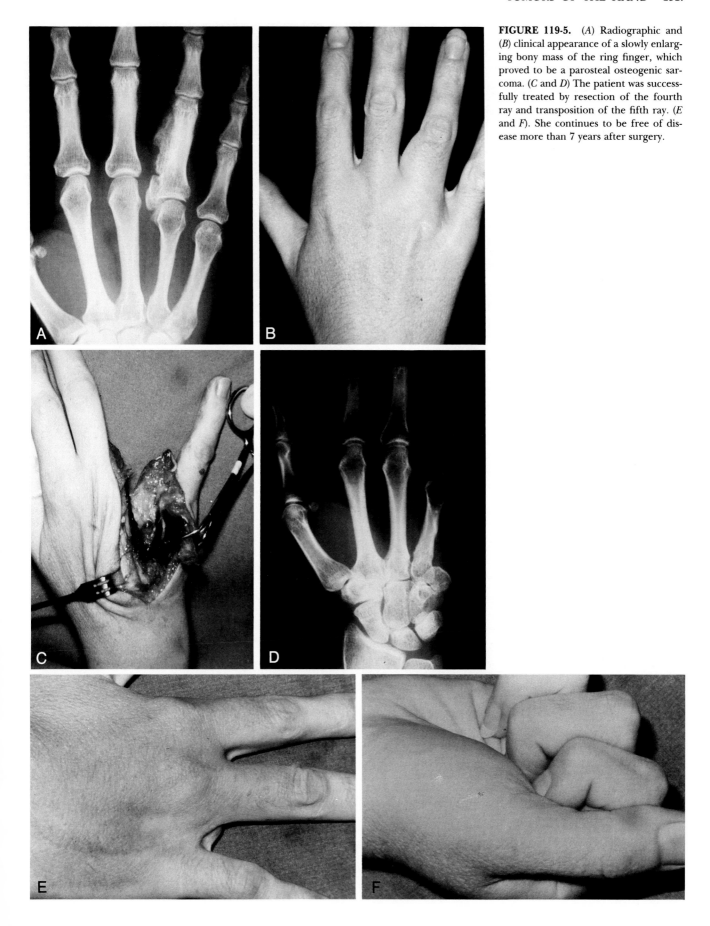

FIGURE 119-5. (*A*) Radiographic and (*B*) clinical appearance of a slowly enlarging bony mass of the ring finger, which proved to be a parosteal osteogenic sarcoma. (*C* and *D*) The patient was successfully treated by resection of the fourth ray and transposition of the fifth ray. (*E* and *F*). She continues to be free of disease more than 7 years after surgery.

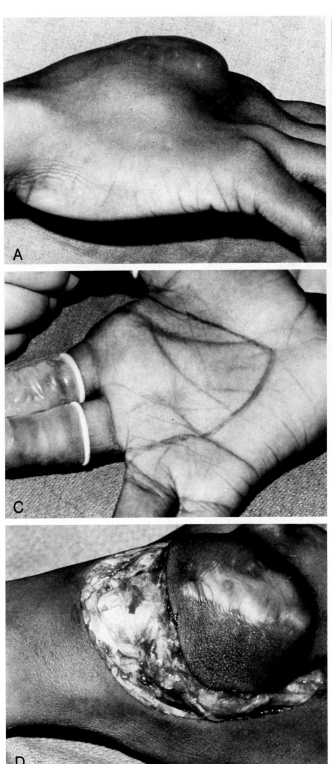

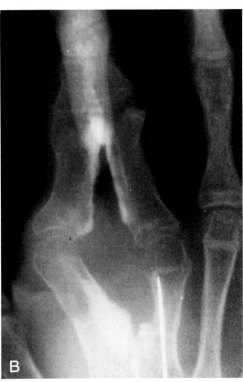

FIGURE 119-6. (*A* and *B*) After several local resections for a desmoplastic fibroma (extra-abdominal desmoid), a 14-year-old presented with an enlarging, painful, and radiographically destructive mass at the same site. The surgical plan was subtotal hand amputation with resection of the second and third rays. (*C* and *D*) At operation, the tumor was found to extend into the dorsal wrist; a below-elbow amputation was performed.

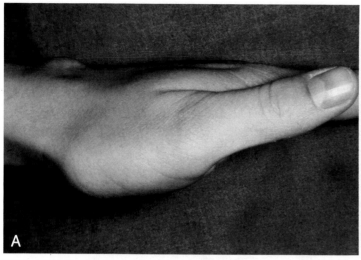 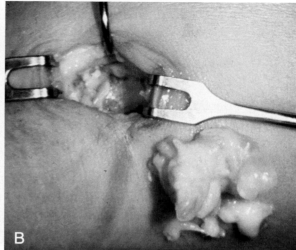

FIGURE 119-7. (A) A recurrent mass following two previous excisions of a dorsal radiocarpal ganglion cyst (performed elsewhere). (B) At operation, the cystic lesion, contiguous capsule, and satellite cysts were removed *en bloc* with the dorsal aspect of the scapholunate ligament. The lesion has not recurred.

palmar fibromatosis (Dupuytren's). These lesions must be carefully examined histologically to distinguish them from aggressive fibromatosis, fibrosarcoma, and fibrous histiocytoma. The benign forms tend to recur if incompletely excised.

Fibrous Histiocytoma

Fibrous histiocytoma—both benign and malignant—occur predominantly in males in their fourth decade.[26] The benign form has an approximate 10% to 15% recurrence rate. Marginal or wide *en bloc* excision is indicated, especially in a larger lesion. The malignant variant must be treated aggressively, often by amputation, in order to gain local control and prevent metastasis.

Fibroma

Fibroma is a benign, encapsulated lesion which, if removed completely, has a low rate of recurrence. The tumors may arise from the tendon sheath (tenosynovial) or adjacent to the fingernails (periungual).

Extra-abdominal Desmoid/Desmoplastic Fibroma

Extra-abdominal desmoid tumors are aggressive, nonmetastatic, and likely to recur. They are typically seen in young males. Effective local treatment requires a wide *en bloc* excision or amputation (see Fig. 119-6). Careful, serial observation of the site is required because of the tendency to recur locally. If the

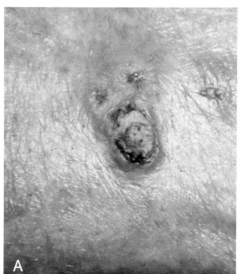 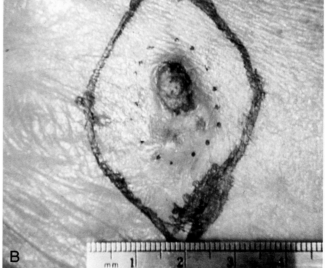

FIGURE 119-8. (A) This slowly growing skin ulcer on the hand of a 72-year-old retired construction worker was diagnosed by dermatologic punch biopsy as squamous cell carcinoma. (B) Excision included a 1.5-cm cuff of normal skin. The tumor reactive zone is marked with a dotted circle.

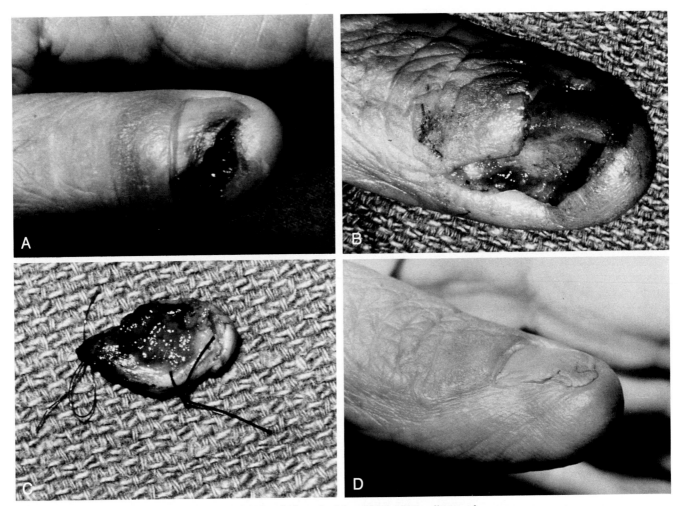

FIGURE 119-9. (*A*) A chronic ulcer beneath the thumb nail of a retired dental hygienist was diagnosed as squamous cell carcinoma by dermatologic punch biopsy. (*B*) Full-thickness excision of the radial half of the sterile and germinal nail matrix plus eponychium was performed, using suture tags (*C*) for pathologic orientation. (*D*) The frozen section confirmed tumor-free margins; a skin graft was applied to the resection zone.

lesion does recur, it should be treated promptly by repeat local excision. These lesions are notable in that they are more aggressive clinically than histologically, sometimes behaving like low-grade fibrosarcomas.

Fibrosarcoma

Fibrosarcoma is a true malignancy that may be quite aggressive. It can be found in zones that have previously been affected by trauma, burns, and scars.[15,22,28] Treatment varies with location and grade; *en bloc* excision or amputation will be necessary.

Vascular Tumors

Vascular tumors may be acquired or congenital, benign or malignant. The majority are benign, congenital lesions believed to be due to failure of differentiation of embryonic vascular channels. Acquired lesions include arteriovenous fistulae, false

and true aneurysms, pyogenic granulomata and glomus tumors.[14,49,59,65]

Arteriovenous Malformation

The true congenital arteriovenous malformation (AVM) is unusual; but whether congenital or acquired, it represents a direct shunt from arterial to venous systems.[24,43] These tumors may be difficult to excise if they are not strictly localized. They can involve bone and may require digital amputation for significant lesions not treatable by debulking. The traumatic lesion can often be treated by ligation of the feeding vessel.

Aneurysms

False aneurysms, the most common type of post-traumatic vascular injury in the hand, are seen clinically as a sometimes pulsatile but tender and enlarging mass which may bleed following minor trauma.[25,62] These lesions should be excised. If blood flow is compromised, they may require arterial reconstruction by microvein grafting. True aneurysms are rare; treatment is the same as for false aneurysms.

Hemangioma

Capillary hemangiomata are usually congenital, and most fade significantly, or disappear, by about 2 years of age. The cavernous variant, which is deep and extensive, may compress adjacent structures. Surgical treatment should be limited to enlarging or symptomatic lesions, and preoperative studies should verify the probability of distal part survival following resection of the tumor (Fig. 119-10). Tourniquet release prior to wound closure is mandatory in excising hemangiomas, because vigorous bleeding can often be encountered.

Glomus Tumor

Glomus tumor, a benign but very painful neoplasm, typically occurs beneath the fingernail. Presenting symptoms are acute and spontaneous onset of pain, marked local tenderness, and extreme cold sensitivity at the site of the lesion. Careful inspection will usually reveal a small, round nodule or bluish discoloration under the skin or nail characterized by marked localized tenderness. Patients report immediate, severe pain if an ice cube is placed on the site. A marginal excision is required. If the tumor lies beneath the nail, special care must be taken to reapproximate the sterile and germinal matrix accurately with fine, absorbable sutures. The nail or nonadherent gauze should be replaced between the nailbed and eponychium but need not be sutured in place.

Hemangioendothelioma and Hemangiosarcoma

Hemangioendothelioma and hemangiosarcoma are true malignancies that can grow rapidly and metastasize quickly. Radical excision or amputation is recommended.

Kaposi's Sarcoma

Kaposi's sarcoma was previously a rare vascular tumor, but is now seen frequently in AIDS patients.[64] The diagnosis of Kaposi's sarcoma in a reddish purple or reddish brown skin tumor nodule may be the first indication of HIV infection in an otherwise asymptomatic individual.

Nerve Tumors

Neurilemmoma / Schwannoma

Neurilemmoma/schwannoma is a common, solitary benign lesion arising from the Schwann cell usually found in the nerve trunks or branches, and most frequently occurring on the flexor surface.[18,56,60] These tumors are generally less than 4 cm in diameter; growths 4 cm to 6 cm in diameter should be viewed with suspicion. Symptoms are usually due to nerve compression from this well-defined, slow-growing tumor. Surgical removal requires microscopic dissection in order to prevent injury to compressed, secondarily atrophic, adjacent fascicles.

The malignant schwannoma is *not* a degeneration of the benign variant, but rather, a complication of neurofibromatosis. A true malignancy, the malignant schwannoma requires at

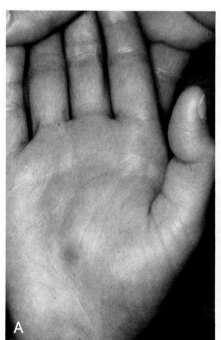 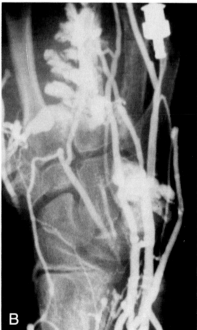 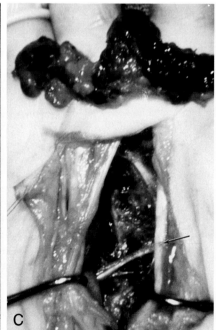

FIGURE 119-10. (A) An enlarging, painful cavernous hemangioma in a 9-year-old. (B) The venogram best demonstrated the lesion, but angiography revealed good flow to all digits. (C) Dorsal and palmar incisions were required to remove the tumor. Note preservation of the motor branch of the ulnar nerve (*arrow*).

least wide *en bloc* excision; but amputation may be necessary for aggressive and histologically poorly differentiated tumors (which carry a bad prognosis).

Neurofibroma

Neurofibroma is a diffuse growth of Schwann cells, axons, and fibrous tissue occurring as solitary or multiple lesions (von Recklinghausen's disease). The solitary variant tends not to recur following excision, but multiple plexiform neurofibromata cannot be enucleated easily from nerve trunks and require resection of segments of nerve in locally symptomatic or destructive cases. Nerve grafting is indicated for reconstruction.

Lipofibromatous Hamartoma of the Median Nerve

Lipofibromatous hamartoma of the median nerve presents as a slowly growing, painless mass, often first noticed in childhood, associated with symptoms of carpal tunnel syndrome.[36] Treatment should be limited to carpal tunnel release, occasionally with epineurotomy, and rarely, if ever, with attempted intraneural dissection. Gradual, local neurologic deterioration should be anticipated.

Lipid Tumors

Lipoma

The lipoma is a common, benign soft-tissue upper limb tumor, more often seen in women than men and typically found on the flexor surface.[35] Commonly, the patient presents with a gradually enlarging, soft, painless mass. Symptoms of a compression neuropathy (especially in the carpal canal) are usual. Local excision, including the pseudocapsule, is generally a straightforward procedure (see Fig. 119-1).

Synovial Tumors

Giant Cell Tumor of Tendon Sheath/Fibrous Xanthoma

Giant cell tumor of tendon sheath/fibrous xanthoma is not related to, and therefore should not be confused with, giant cell tumor of bone.[30,32] Most lesions are in the digits, wrist, or hand. As they slowly enlarge, they have the potential to envelop tendons, invade bones or joints, or surround neurovascular bundles. Treatment is a thorough, local excision. At surgery, avoid injury to the tendons and neurovascular structures. Up to 20% recurrence is reported, most probably from incomplete removal (Fig. 119-11).

Epithelioid Sarcoma, Synovial Sarcoma, Clear Cell Sarcoma

Epithelioid sarcoma, synovial sarcoma, and clear cell sarcoma may be among the most frequent primary malignancies of the upper extremity, especially distal to the elbow.[1,4,6,9,21,41,45,47] These lesions are aggressive in behavior, confusing in appear-

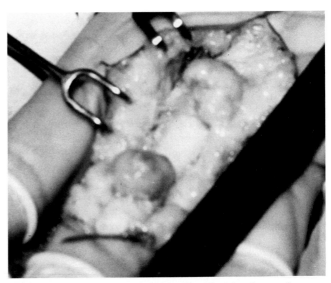

FIGURE 119-11. Giant cell tumor of tendon sheath must be completely removed to prevent recurrence, while preserving the flexor pulleys and avoiding injury to the neurovascular bundles.

ance and presentation, and capricious in their location and method of spread. The reason that an otherwise benign-appearing, solid, soft-tissue lesion of the hand and wrist should be approached with caution and suspicion when performing a biopsy is that it may be one of these tumors. Once the diagnosis is established, wide *en bloc* excision or amputation is required; axillary node dissection is advised regardless of clinical or lymphangeographic findings. Radiation and chemotherapy have been used with success in some cases, but their roles are not well defined.

TUMORS OF HARD TISSUE

Tumors of Cartilage

Solitary Enchondroma

Solitary enchondroma, probably the most common bone tumor in the hand, is frequently seen in young adults. It occurs virtually exclusively in the phalanges or metacarpals; very rarely is it reported in the carpals.[29] The tumor may be discovered incidentally on radiographs for another problem or for (pathologic) fracture; swelling may be present primarily but pain is unusual without fracture (Fig. 119-12). Very small lesions may need only periodic observation; larger tumors and those associated with fractures should be treated. Fracture through the lesion does not assure spontaneous tumor resolution during bone healing. These lesions can be cured by adequate curettage plus autogenous bone grafting to promote speedy bone reconstitution; recurrences are unusual. We prefer to treat both the lesion and the fracture simultaneously in cases of fracture through a (previously undiagnosed) lesion. In some of these patients, the addition of internal fixation (i.e., Kirschner wires) plus the bone graft may be needed to stabilize the curetted, fractured bone. Delay of surgical treatment may prolong disability, because the hand has to recover first from the fracture

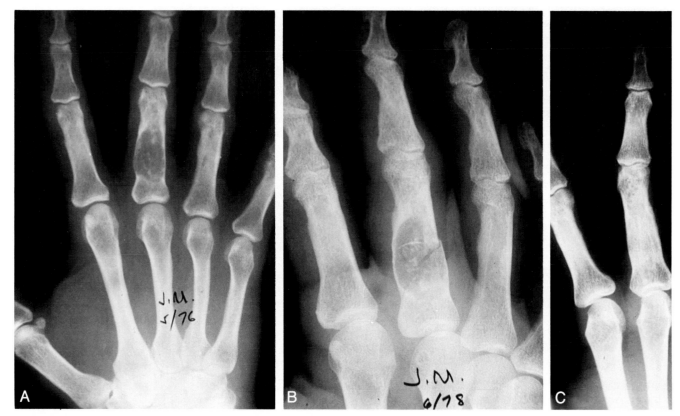

FIGURE 119-12. (A) Expansile lytic lesion of the proximal phalanx of the middle finger was found incidentally on radiographs done for a little finger injury. Speckled radiographic appearance is typical for an enchondroma. The patient declined treatment of this relatively large, albeit asymptomatic, lesion. (B) Two years later, a radiograph following a minor trauma showed a pathologic fracture through the slightly further enlarged tumor. (C) Curettage and bone grafting were performed to treat the tumor and stabilize the phalanx. Graft incorporation and remodeling occurred without incident.

and then from subsequent surgery. Furthermore, delay in treating the lesion will delay the diagnosis, should the lesion prove to be other than an enchondroma.

Approach tumors in the metacarpals longitudinally through the dorsal surface. Approach those in the phalanges through a midaxial incision so as not to disturb the dorsal or palmar tendon mechanisms. Incise the periosteum and locally strip it from the thinned, expanded cortex; remove and save a cortical window adequate to fully visualize the lesion. After complete curettage, pack cancellous bone (from the distal radius, proximal ulna, or iliac crest) into the cavity. Curette the cortical window and then pack it back into the defect. Longitudinal, smooth intramedullary Kirschner wires may be added to enhance stability in fractured bones. Resuture the periosteum to improve the tendon gliding surface. Splint the finger and protect it for 1 to 3 weeks (depending on bone stability). Start therapy as soon as practical.

Multiple Enchondromatosis

Multiple enchondromatosis is a far less frequent condition than solitary enchondromata, but the lesions tend to be larger and are associated with skeletal deformity[63] (Fig. 119-13). The risk of sarcomatous degeneration is considerably greater with these multiple lesions and should be suspected if known tumors be-

come painful, enlarge, or are associated with an acute deformity. In such circumstances, incisional biopsy is indicated. Chondrosarcomas are best treated by *en bloc* excision if purely intraosseous, or by ray resection.

Osteocartilaginous Exostoses

Multiple exostoses (solitary and multiple) are often a hereditary problem which may cause significant, generalized skeletal deformities. The hand bones are far less frequently affected than the radius and ulna. In most cases, symptoms are due to the presence of the bony mass. Treatment should remove the space-occupying lesion while preserving the nearby soft tissues. The risk of malignant transformation is extremely low for lesions of the hand. The major problem associated with these tumors may be the need for reconstructive surgery to restore proper functional hand, wrist, or forearm skeletal alignment.

Tumors of Bone

Giant Cell Tumor of Bone

Giant cell tumor of bone is relatively infrequent in the hand and wrist. When present, it is usually seen in younger patients

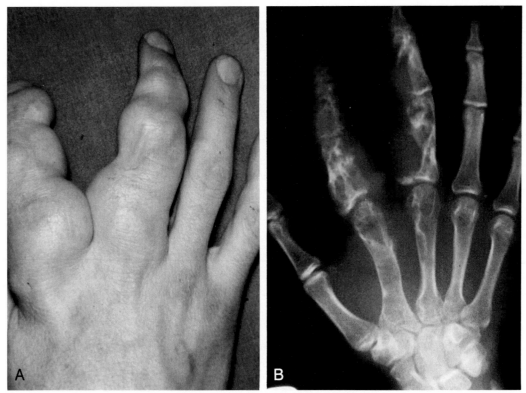

FIGURE 119-13. (*A* and *B*) Multiple enchondromatosis caused extensive deformity and dysfunction in this patient with a positive family history.

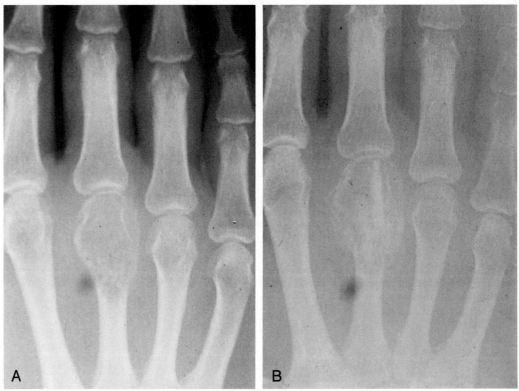

FIGURE 119-14. (*A*) Eccentric, lytic epiphyseal lesion of the third metacarpal proved to be a giant cell tumor of bone which was treated by curettage and grafting. (*B*) Tumor recurrence is seen as an enlarging zone of osteolysis, including graft destruction, nearly 4 months post-curettage. Ray resection was required.

in whom it may have multicentric foci. These lesions behave differently from those found in the larger bones.[7,39,44] For this reason, and because some smaller multicentric foci may not be easily diagnosed on routine radiographs, technetium-99m scintigraphy should be performed when this diagnosis is suspected. The lesion typically presents with pain, and is enlarged and tender, especially if it has expanded and broken through the bony cortex. Whereas giant cell tumors of bone in other locations may be amenable to treatment by curettage with or without bone grafting, giant cell tumor in bones of the hand is highly likely to recur[7] (Fig. 119-14). We believe that giant cell tumor of the bones of the hand and the distal radius and ulna should be treated by excision (ray resection or *en bloc* removal) and by replacement (as appropriate) with small autogenous bone grafts, vascularized fibular graft, or allograft.[55,57]

The precise technique of surgical approach depends on the specific lesion. The operation itself is usually performed through a dorsal or dorsolateral incision. Remove the bone extraperiosteally. If the tumor involves the articular surface (but does *not* cross it), fuse the joint or replace it with an allograft or other articular graft (e.g., toe phalanx). Fix the

bone graft to the recipient area with wires, screws, or plates. If necessary, temporarily transfix the joint to stabilize it while repaired ligaments heal. Postoperative rehabilitation is similar to other reconstructive procedures, including use of removable static or dynamic splints and supervised therapy after skeletal healing. Sometimes, the combination of early healing and rigid fixation is adequate to start mobilization quite rapidly.

Aneurysmal Bone Cyst

The aneurysmal bone cyst is a benign hemorrhagic and cystic tumor of bone with a propensity for local recurrence; it is not commonly seen in the hand.[11,31] The tumor course is usually rather rapid and clinically worrisome, and is frequently characterized by pain and swelling (see Fig. 119-3). Metaphyseal lesions are expected and often accompanied by cortical erosion. *En bloc* excision with treatment similar to that described for giant cell tumor of bone is recommended. An intercalary metacarpal resection may be stabilized by transverse intermetacarpal wires or with the addition of an external fixation device until the bone graft is solidly healed.

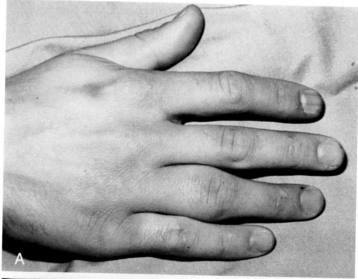

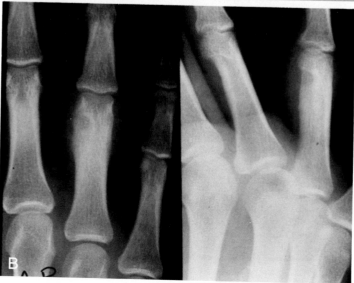

FIGURE 119-15. (*A*) Swelling and pain of 2 years' duration in a 17-year-old male whose radiographs show retrocondylar bone formation surrounding a central, lucent nidus. (*B*) At surgery, the diagnosis of osteoid osteoma was confirmed and the lesion was successfully treated by curettage.

Osteoid Osteoma

The osteoid osteoma, a benign bone-forming tumor, frequently presents as a painful and radiographically obscure lesion in a young individual. The propensity for a focus in the hand is not high but should be entertained in patients with these characteristics (Fig. 119-15). The most difficult part of treatment may be making the diagnosis. Preoperative studies may include scintigraphy, tomography, CT scans, and angiograms. Cure without recurrence is typically effected by local excision including the tumor nidus.[17,27,40]

CONCLUSIONS

The goal of this chapter is to reinforce basic principles of treatment, not to review every tumor that may occur in the hand. Specific neoplasms have been described because of their frequency, their characteristic presence in the hand, the special problems they present, or a combination of these factors.

We believe it is important to reiterate our initial statement that surgeons treating tumors of the hand must be fully prepared to examine, diagnose, biopsy, and excise these tumors appropriately. They must be concerned first with achieving a cure, but also with preserving function and with the cosmetic effects of treatment. Balancing each of these considerations is frequently not an easy task. The ultimate priority is still cure of the tumor. Surgical reconstruction after tumor excision, when needed, is an end-stage or even a separate stage, performed on a patient who is likely to survive and use his hand.

REFERENCES

1. Adeyemi–Doro, H.O., Durosimi–Etti, F.A., and Olude, O.: Primary Malignant Tumors of the Hand. J. Hand Surg. **10-A:**815, 1985.
2. Adeyemi–Doro, H.O., and Olude, O.: Juvenile Aponeurotic Fibroma. J. Hand Surg. **10-B:**127, 1985.
3. Amadio, P.C., and Lombardi, R.M.: Metastatic Tumors of the Hand. J. Hand Surg. **12-A:**311, 1987.
4. Andrew, T.A.: Clear Cell Sarcoma of the Hand. Hand **14:**200, 1982.
5. Angelides, A.C., and Wallace, P.F.: The Dorsal Ganglion of the Wrist: Its Pathogenesis, Gross and Microscopic Anatomy and Surgical Treatment. J. Hand Surg. **1:**228, 1976.
6. Archer, I.A., Brown, R.B., and Fitton, J.M.: Epithelioid Sarcoma in the Hand. J. Hand Surg. **9-B:**207, 1984.
7. Averill, R.M., Smith, R.J., and Campbell, C.J.: Giant-cell Tumors of the Bones of the Hand. J. Hand Surg. **5:**39, 1980.
8. Bowden, L., and Booher, R.J.: The Principles and Techniques of Resection of Soft Parts for Sarcoma. Surgery **44:**936, 1958.
9. Bryan, R.F., Soule, E.H., Dobyns, J.H., et al.: Primary Epithelioid Sarcoma of the Hand and Forearm: A Review of 13 Cases. J. Bone Joint Surg. **56-A:**455, 1974.
10. Butler, E.D., Hamill, J.P., Scipel, R.S., and DeLorimier, A.A.: Tumors of the Hand—A Ten-year Survey and Report of 437 Cases. Am. J. Surg. **100:**293, 1960.
11. Campanacci, M., Capanna, R., and Picci, P.: Unicameral and Aneurysmal Bone Cysts. Clin. Orthop. **204:**25, 1986.
12. Carroll, R.E.: Epidermal (Epithelial) Cyst of the Handskeleton. Am. J. Surg. **85:**327, 1953.
13. Carroll, R.E.: Squamous Cell Carcinoma of the Nailbed. J. Hand Surg. **1:**92, 1976.
14. Carroll, R.E., and Berman, A.T.: Glomus Tumors of the Hand. J. Bone Joint Surg. **54-A:**691, 1972.
15. Castro, E.B., Hajdu, S.I., and Fortner, J.G.: Surgical Therapy of Fibrosarcoma of Extremities: A Reappraisal. Arch. Surg. **107:**284, 1973.
16. Creighton, J.J., Peimer, C.A., Mindell, E.R., et al.: Primary Malignant Tumors of the Upper Extremity: Retrospective Analysis of One Hundred Twenty-six Cases. J. Hand Surg. **10-A:**805, 1985.
17. Dahlin, D.C.: Bone Tumors, 3rd ed. Springfield, Charles C. Thomas, 1967.
18. Enneking, W.F.: Musculoskeletal Tumor Surgery. New York, Churchill Livingstone, 1983.
19. Enneking, W.F., Spanier, S.S., and Goodman, M.A.: Current Concepts Review: The Surgical Staging of Musculoskeletal Sarcoma. J. Bone Joint Surg. **62-A:**1027, 1980.
20. Enneking, W.F., Spanier, S.S., and Goodman, M.A.: The Surgical Staging of Musculoskeletal Sarcoma. Clin. Orthop. **153:**106, 1982.
21. Enzinger, F.M.: Epithelioid Sarcoma: A Sarcoma Simulating a Granuloma or a Carcinoma. Cancer **26:**1029, 1970.
22. Enzinger, F.M., and Weiss, S.W.: Soft Tissue Tumors. St. Louis, C.V. Mosby, 1983.
23. Fleegler, E.J.: Skin Tumors. *In* Green, D.P. (ed.): Operative Hand Surgery, vol. 2. New York, Churchill Livingstone, 1982.
24. Gelberman, R.L., and Goldner, J.L.: Congenital Arteriovenous Fistulas of the Hand. J. Hand Surg. **3:**451, 1978.
25. Green, D.P.: True and False Traumatic Aneurysms in the Hand. J. Bone Joint Surg. **55-A:**120, 1973.
26. Hajdu, S.I.: Pathology of Soft-Tissue Tumors. Philadelphia, Lea and Febiger, 1964.
27. Huvos, A.: Bone Tumors: Diagnosis, Treatment and Prognosis. Philadelphia, W.B. Saunders, 1979.
28. Ivins, J.C., Dockerty, M.B., and Ghormley, R.K.: A Fibrosarcoma of the Soft Tissues of the Extremities: A Review of Seventy-Eight Cases. Surgery **28:**495, 1950.
29. Jaffe, H.L.: Tumors and Tumorous Conditions of Bones and Joints. Philadelphia, Lea and Febiger, 1958.
30. Jaffe, H.L.: Metabolic, Degenerative and Inflammatory Disease of Bones and Joints. Philadelphia, Lea and Febiger, 1972.
31. Johnston, A.D.: Aneurysmal Bone Cyst of the Hand. Hand Clinics **3:**299, 1987.
32. Jones, F.E., Soule, E.H., and Coventry, M.B.: Fibrous Xanthoma of Synovium (Giant-Cell Tumor of Tendon Sheath, Pigmented Nodular Synovitis). A study of One Hundred and Eighteen Cases. J. Bone Joint Surg. **51-A:**76, 1969.
33. Kleinert, H.E., Kutz, J.E., Fischman, J.H., and McGraw, L.H.: Etiology and Treatment of the So-Called Mucous Cyst of the Finger. J. Bone Joint Surg. **54-A:**1455, 1972.
34. Kopf, A.W., Bart, R.S., Rodriguez–Sains, R.S., et al.: Malignant Melanoma. New York, Masson, 1979.
35. Leffert, R.D.: Lipomas of the Upper Extremity. J. Bone Joint Surg. **54-A:**1262, 1972.
36. Louis, D., Hankin, F., Greene, T., et al.: Long-Term Follow-Up of Lipofibroma of the Median Nerve. J. Hand Surg. **10:**403, 1985.
37. Mankin, H.J., Lange, T.A., and Spannier, S.S.: The Hazards of Biopsy in Patients with Malignant Primary Bone and Soft Tissue Tumors. J. Bone Joint Surg. **64-A:**1121, 1982.
38. Matthews, P.: Ganglia of the Flexor Tendon Sheaths in the Hand. J. Bone Joint Surg. **55-B:**612, 1973.
39. McDonald, D.J., Sim, F.H., McLeod, R.A., and Dahlin, D.C.: Giant-Cell Tumor of Bone. J. Bone Joint Surg. **68-A:**235, 1986.
40. McLellan, D.I., and Wilson, F.C., Jr.: Osteoid Osteoma of the Spine. J. Bone Joint Surg. **49-A:**111, 1967.
41. Miettinen M., and Virtanen, I.: Synovial Sarcoma: A Misnomer. Am. J. Pathol. **117:**18, 1984.

42. Nelson, C.L., Sawmiller, S., and Phalen, G.S.: Ganglions of the Wrist and Hand. J. Bone Joint Surg. 54-A:1459, 1972.

43. Neviaser, R.J., and Adams, J.P.: Vascular Lesions in the Hand: Current Management. Clin. Orthop. 100:111, 1974.

44. Peimer, C.A., Schiller, A.L., Mankin, H.J., and Smith, R.J.: Multicentric Giant-Cell Tumor of Bone. J. Bone Joint Surg. 62-A:652, 1980.

45. Peimer, C.A., Smith, R.J., Sirota, R.L., et al.: Epithelioid Sarcoma of the Hand and Wrist: Patterns of Extension. J. Hand Surg. 4:275, 1977.

46. Poppen, N.K., and Niebauer, J.J.: Recurring Digital Fibrous Tumor of Childhood. J. Hand Surg. 2:253, 1977.

47. Rajpal, S., Moore, R.H., and Karakousis, C.P.: Synovial Sarcoma: A Review of Treatment and Survival in 52 Patients. N.Y. State J. Med. 84:17, 1984.

48. Rayner, C.R.W.: The Result of Treatment of 273 Carcinomas of the Hand. Hand 13:183, 1981.

49. Rettig, A.C., and Strickland, J.W.: Glomous Tumors of the Digits. J. Hand Surg. 2:261, 1971.

50. Roses, D.F., Harris, M.N., and Ackerman, A.B.: Diagnosis and Management of Cutaneous Malignant Melanoma. In Roses, D.F., Harris, M.N., and Ackerman, A.B. (eds): Major Problems in Clinical Surgery. Philadelphia, W.B. Saunders, 1983.

51. Sim, F.H.: Soft Tissue Tumors: Diagnosis and Treatment. Orthop. Surg. 1:1, 1980.

52. Simon, M.A.: Biopsy of Musculoskeletal Tumors. J. Bone Joint Surg. 64-A:1253, 1982.

53. Simon, M.A., and Enneking, W.F.: The Management of Soft Tissue Sarcomas of the Extremities. J. Bone Joint Surg. 58-A:317, 1976.

54. Smith, R.J.: Who is Best Qualified to Treat Tumors of the Hand? (editorial) J. Hand Surg. 2:251, 1977.

55. Smith, R.J., and Bushart, T.M.: Allograft Bone for Metacarpal Reconstruction. J. Hand Surg. 10-A:325, 1985.

56. Smith, R.J., and Lipke, R.W.: Surgical Treatment of Peripheral Nerve Tumors of the Upper Limb. In Omer, G.E., and Spinner, M. (eds.): Management of Peripheral Nerve Problems, Philadelphia, W.B. Saunders, 1980.

57. Smith, R.J., and Mankin, H.J.: Allograft Replacement of Distal Radius for Giant Cell Tumor. J. Hand Surg. 2:299, 1977.

58. Specht, E.E., and Staheli, L.T.: Juvenile Aponeurotic Fibroma. J. Hand Surg. 2:256, 1977.

59. Stack, H.G.: Tumors of the Hand. Br. Med. J. 1:919, 1960.

60. Strickland, J.W., and Steichen, J.B.: Nerve Tumors of the Hand and Forearm. J. Hand Surg. 2:285, 1977.

61. Sundaram, M., McGuire, M.H., Herbold, D.R., Wolverson, M.K., and Heiberg, E.: Magnetic Resonance Imaging in Planning Limb-Salvage Surgery for Primary Malignant Tumors of Bone. J. Bone Joint Surg. 68-A:809, 1986.

62. Suziki, K., Takahashi, S., and Nakagawa, T.: False Aneurysm in a Digital Artery. J. Hand Surg. 5:402, 1980.

63. Tagigawa, K.: Chondroma of the Bones of the Hand: A Review of 110 Cases. J. Bone Joint Surg. 53-A:1591, 1971.

64. Templeton, A.C.: Kaposi's Sarcoma. In Andrade, R., Gumport, S.L., Popkin, G.L., et al. (eds.): Cancer of the Skin, vol. 2. Philadelphia, W.B. Saunders, 1976.

65. Varian, J.P.W., and Cleak, T.K.: Glomus Tumors in the Hand. Hand 12:293, 1980.

CHAPTER 120

Skin Grafts

AVRON DANILLER

Skin taken from another part of the body and used to cover a wound is referred to as a *skin graft*. A graft may be described as split, full-thickness, or thick composite (Fig. 120-1).

The split-thickness skin graft is further divided into a thin split-thickness graft or a thick split-thickness graft, depending on the amount of dermis removed with the epidermis. In general the quality of a graft is entirely dependent on the amount of dermis present, with thicker grafts giving better results. (It is the dermis that makes up leather, and thus a good strong piece of leather consists of a thick dermal layer while a thin, soft piece of leather has a much thinner dermis and is less tough.) On the other hand, a thinner skin graft is more likely to survive the transfer until revascularization occurs.[59] The thicker the graft, the more hazardous is the period of devascularization and the more difficult it is to obtain an adequate result.[14,29] This is particularly true in the presence of an acute, open, nonsurgically created wound resulting from trauma, where wound conditions may not be optimal for closure with a thick skin graft.

ACUTE AND SUBACUTE TRAUMATIC WOUNDS

In principle, a fresh wound that has an adequate bed should be covered with a split-thickness skin graft and not a full-thickness one. Essential for a good "take" are absence of infection, perfect hemostasis, and a good dressing which should be left in position for a minimum of 5 to 7 days. If there are any concerns about the adequacy of the hemostasis or the infection status of the wound, the graft should be examined early, by at least the third day, as at that time it is still possible to salvage a graft with a hematoma or seroma. In the subacute situation where the wound has been open for a few days or more, no graft that is expected to survive should be placed on a wound with a bacterial count higher than 10^5/ml as shown on quantitative culture. Experience and experimentation have demonstrated that in such situations the scene changes from wound contamination to wound infection, and a very high percentage of these grafts will fail.

A second option, if one is starting off with an untidy wound, is to apply a mesh graft which allows for drainage and easily conforms to an irregular underlying bed. This method should not be used electively in a closed wound where a skin graft is placed on a fresh surgically created wound, because it not only yields an unsightly result, but by its nature is prone to even more contracture than normally occurs in a split-thickness skin graft.[20,61] For the hand this is clearly undesirable (see Fig. 120-22A).

The tendency of a split skin graft to contract must be remembered at all times. For use in the hand, such grafts must be accompanied by the placement of appropriate darts to break up the scar (Fig. 120-2). Splinting for a prolonged period of time, especially at night, should be started early. This is continued until the tendency to contract is over, which may vary from 3 to 9 months.[61] Scar and joint contracture can be prevented, but once they have commenced, they usually require reoperation.

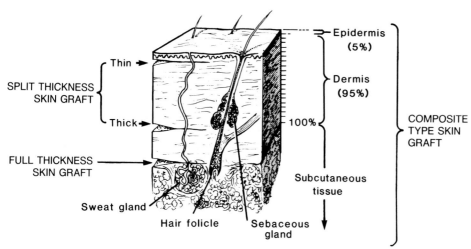

FIGURE 120-1.   Schematic showing various thicknesses of skin grafts.

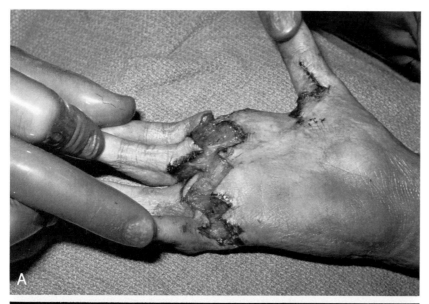

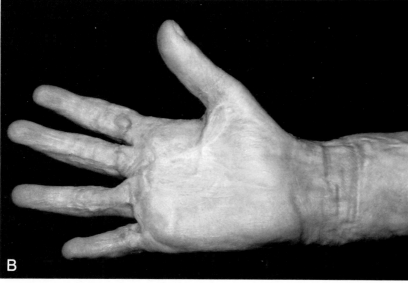

FIGURE 120-2.   (*A*) In preparing wound for placement of skin graft, darts and irregular placement of incisions in palm are used to release contractures. (*B*) Final result after maturation of wound shows no recurrence of contractures.

FIGURE 120-3. Use of composite-type graft in a heavily pigmented hand. Graft should be taken from pink skin on ulnar border of hand to replace thin, tender, split-skin graft previously placed on tip of finger.

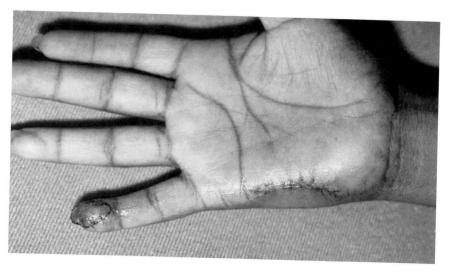

GRAFTING OF A FRESH, SURGICALLY CREATED WOUND AS AN ELECTIVE PROCEDURE

In a wound that has already healed, the surgeon can create a fresh wound under ideal conditions, making it possible to use a thick split-thickness graft or even a full-thickness graft.[40] In some situations it may be possible to place a composite-type graft. When preparing a full-thickness skin graft, all subcutaneous tissue is removed down to the white dermis. With composite-type grafts, which are much thicker, the subcutaneous tissue is minimally trimmed, leaving a thin layer of fat and loose subcutaneous areolar tissue in which much of the vascular network is still present (see Fig. 120-1). These composite-type grafts behave much like thin flaps, and are ideal for such areas as the dorsum of the hand, the palm of the hand in children, and the fingers, where they may be used to replace any thin, unstable, or scarred area (Fig. 120-3). During the period of devascularization these grafts survive with great difficulty, and

they do not heal well when placed over granulation tissue. They should be reserved only for freshly created surgical wounds. When planning such grafts, every effort should be made to break any linear scars with appropriate darts to avoid subsequent contracture, especially on the palmar surfaces. If correctly planned, this will greatly reduce the effects of contracture that occur in all grafts. It should be noted that the tendency toward contracture diminishes as the thickness of the graft or dermis increases.[29]

INSTRUMENTATION

Available for use are many varieties of dermatomes, varying from a regular scalpel, which is most commonly used in the hand, to the larger dermatomes. If a large sheet of skin is required, it is best to use a Padgett-type drum dermatome or Padgett electric dermatome, because these tend to give the most uniform thickness (Fig. 120-4). Use of a dermatome that

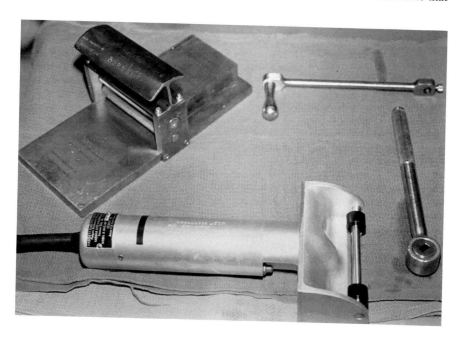

FIGURE 120-4. Dermatome and mesher are useful in skin grafts. Padgett electric dermatome is useful for obtaining grafts of uniform thickness.

produces grafts of uneven thickness will produce an inferior result.

CHOICE OF DONOR SITE

When preparing to take a skin graft, it is important to choose the site carefully. Small grafts required in young females should, for example, not be taken from conspicious areas such as the lower thigh or the forearm, but rather from well-hidden areas such as the inner arm, the panty area, or the gluteal area.

If full-thickness grafts are required for skin grafting in the hand, the most commonly used donor site is the groin. This donor site is easily hidden, and the graft can be taken under local anesthesia. Avoid use of a hair-bearing area.

In the pigmented black hand, palmar or nail bed split-thickness grafts are best harvested from the instep of the foot where the color match is better. Smaller grafts may also be harvested, in some circumstances, from the ulnar border of the hand (see Fig. 120-3). Most skin grafts become much darker with time than the surrounding tissue. However, the thicker the graft is, the less this occurs.

The wrist and elbow areas are used as donor sites by some surgeons. These may produce unsightly scars, and should not be used in the female. The inside of the upper arm is another useful hairless area where the donor site is easily hidden.

TECHNIQUES OF SKIN GRAFTING

Thoroughly clean the skin and, if necessary, remove all oils with acetone. Apply a light layer of mineral oil to allow for a smooth, steady forward movement of the dermatome. It is important to go through a mock run prior to taking the skin graft to ensure that the cord is long enough, that you are comfortable with the motion, and that there are no drapes or other objects interfering with the smooth run of the dermatome. If this is not done, one is much more likely to cut an uneven graft, or even to take full-thickness slices. With a dermatome such as the Padgett, it is not always necessary to have an absolutely flat surface, but the skin surface from which the graft is being taken should be tense and firm. This can be achieved by placing two towel clips—one proximally and one distally—and pulling them apart. This maneuver requires an assistant. A second method for obtaining adequate surface tension is the use of a tongue-blade firmly pressed at a slight angle onto the skin just in front of the dermatome, moving forward at the same pace as the dermatome. If the surface from which the graft is being taken is not kept uniformly straight, there will be a tendency to cut irregular grafts.

When setting up the dermatome it is important to choose the width setting of the blade carefully. It should not be much larger, nor should it be smaller, than what is required to cover the defect. When tightening the screws to set the blades, take care not to tighten them too much, because it is very easy to strip the threads. Before using the dermatome, set the blade reading to 0 and then gradually, one side at a time, obtain the correct opening in increments of about 1/1000 of an inch; do *not* start at 0 and go straight to 10 because this will throw a

torque into the mechanism which, if repeated too often, will lead to damage and result in uneven cuts.

Split-Thickness Grafts

For a split-thickness graft, the best thickness is in the range of .008 to .012 inch; .008 inch is a thin split-thickness graft whereas .014 of an inch is a thick split-thickness graft. If a very thick split-thickness graft is taken, causing concern about the ability of the donor site to heal appropriately without too much scarring, it is best to cover the donor site with a very thin split-thickness graft taken from a second donor site.[63]

When harvesting a skin graft for a specific defect, it is necessary to cut the graft to the exact size of the defect using a pattern. A useful trick is to place methylene blue on the skin edges of the defect, then place slightly moistened glove paper on the defect. The exact pattern will be duplicated on the moistened glove paper and the appropriate pattern can be cut. The skin graft, once taken, is then placed on the piece of paper and the exact pattern dimensions used to cut the skin graft. It has been found most useful to cut the skin with a specially designed serrated scissors (one blade of the scissors is finely serrated while the other is normal). This prevents or reduces the amount of slipping and sliding that occurs when one attempts to cut skin. When cutting skin it is important to use the "tailor technique." With each cut, the blades are not totally closed but closed only from one-half to three-quarters of the blade length. The scissors are then opened for the next cut and slid forward toward the fulcrum, followed again by a one-half to three-quarter blade-length cut. This is repeated, and reduces the likelihood of creating a jagged, irregular cut.

Defat the graft down to the white glistening dermis, and suture it into position, leaving strategically placed long ties with which to hold in position a bulky bolus-type dressing that is fashioned to exactly fit the dimensions of the graft. I use a layer of Xeroform followed by a thin layer of bacitracin ointment and a single layer of regular gauze dressing soaked with mineral oil (with the excess squeezed out), followed by a few layers of moist gauze dressing and fluffs. The pores in a single layer of Xeroform (which should never be folded into a double layer) and the mineral oil layer allow any exudate to pass through to the next layer which, when it dries, becomes firm and acts as a stent. This also reduces the accumulation of exudate and blood on the graft, and makes removal of the dressing easy and comfortable for the patient because the mineral oil does not dry out. Nonadherence reduces the likelihood of disturbing the graft at the time of dressing change.

When insetting the graft, every effort must be made to ensure that no hematoma will develop. It is well to remember that even though the bed may be perfectly dry prior to sewing in the graft, a suture needle can pierce a vessel and cause bleeding during the sewing of the graft. For this reason, make one final check for bleeding after the final suture has been placed.

Full-Thickness Grafts

Full-thickness or composite-type grafts are taken as described, but some fat and loose areolar tissue are left attached to the deep surface. This is a difficult technique and should only be used by the experienced surgeon; the failure rate can be high if all appropriate precautions are not practiced, including (1) perfect hemostasis; (2) complete immobilization for at least 5 days with a bulky bolus and dressing; (3) elevation of the part above the heart at all times; (4) no milking of the graft if a hematoma is found after 24 hours; (5) if a hematoma is present, it is removed by incision and drainage only. This principle remains a good one for all skin grafts. Milking of a hematoma from beneath a graft is only permissible in the first 24 hours. A composite-type skin graft is used only in fresh, surgically created wounds.

Use of Meshing

The use of a mesh graft, while clearly suboptimal in the hand because of its poor cosmetic appearance, can be very useful in wounds that are highly irregular and are not felt to be 100% ready for grafting. The value of the mesh is that it drapes itself extremely well around irregular surfaces. Furthermore, should there still be some infection present, drainage will occur through the fine mesh pores. Once the graft takes, contraction occurs, together with migration of epithelial cells from the graft, leading to a total sealing of the wound.

The Zimmer mesher is the most commonly used meshing instrument today. Take a regular split skin graft and place it on a special backing with the dermis facing the backing. The backings are designed to expand in various ratios; the most commonly used ratio is an expansion of 1:1.5. The backing–graft composite is then run through the mesher, which cuts the graft evenly, very much like a piece of expanded steel that is commonly used for metal lath or metal stairways. As with all dressings, it is useful to have a first layer consisting of Xeroform and bacitracin ointment, followed by a dressing soaked in mineral oil and a bulky fluff dressing.

MANAGEMENT OF THE DONOR SITE

Split-Thickness Grafts

The basic principle for management of the donor site, is that it must be kept dry and free of fluid accumulation. Failure to do so will result in secondary infection and further skin loss at the site, which then heals with a thick, unsightly, and uncomfortable scar. It also precludes the subsequent use of that site should further harvesting be required.

If Xeroform or a similar gauze-type dressing is used, it is well to remember that all of these dressings are designed to allow for appropriate drainage through the interstices of the gauze. This is destroyed if a second Xeroform or similar layer is placed, creating a dangerous occlusive dressing and thereby setting the stage for the above-mentioned series of events. After taking a graft, the oozing from the donor site can be reduced with the application of thrombin or warm, moist packs. After 10 minutes or so, these are slowly removed to prevent recurrence of bleeding. The Xeroform may then be placed, followed in my own practice by a single layer of gauze soaked in mineral oil. This is designed to allow the exudate to pass through to the next moist layer of gauze. The dressings are

removed slowly at 24 hours so as not to start bleeding. The donor site is then kept dry. The donor sites are chosen so that the patient need not lie on the area. The use of synthetic membranes ("Op-Site" or "Biobrane") is becoming more popular. Again, however, it is essential to check these areas and ensure that seromas or hematomas have not collected. If so, these must be drained and, when necessary, this must be repeated.

Full-Thickness Grafts

These are treated as any wound closed by primary closure with or without undermining.

SKIN FLAPS

When the loss of soft tissue has been so extensive as to expose vital structures that will not survive on their own intrinsic blood supply, or has produced a defect where placement of a skin graft is technically not feasible due to an inadequate bed, or a probable suboptimal functional or cosmetic result, use of a flap must be considered. To survive, the flap must include subcutaneous tissue and an intact blood supply. Where appropriate, it may also include structures such as nerve or bone (Fig. 120-5).[4,13,32,45,56]

Skin grafts, once removed from the body and hence their blood supply, lead a precarious existence in their new bed until neovascularization occurs from the bed and wound edges.[15,28] This period of devitalization clearly limits the thickness of the graft that can be used and the circumstances of its use. It is especially true when the bed of the wound consists of exposed vital tissues such as tendons with loss of paratenon, bone without periosteum, or nerves and joints. Under these circumstances it becomes necessary to cover the defect with tissue that contains within it an intact functioning blood supply with skin and subcutaneous tissue. The essence of a flap, therefore, is that its vascularity remains undisturbed and survival is thus assured. In practice this is achieved by designing the flap carefully and then making the incision down to the appropriate layer (e.g., the neurovascular layer or deep fascia) before elevation of the flap is commenced. Any elevation in the subcutaneous layer alone turns a flap into a random flap, which limits its size and safety. The distance over which the flaps may be moved is limited by the length of the vascular pedicle or base, although in the case of a free, microsurgically transferred flap, this limitation does not apply. Microsurgical flaps are discussed in Chapter 78.

Flaps may be classified according to:

Location:
  Local
  Regional
  Distant
Vascularity:
  Random
  Fasciocutaneous
  Axial and/or island
  Myocutaneous

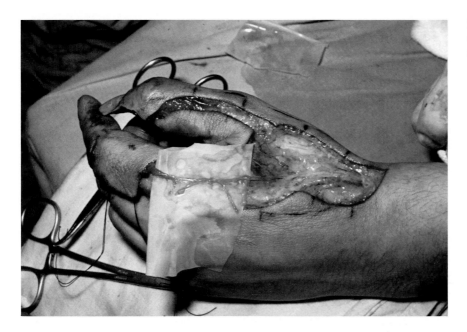

FIGURE 120-5. Elevation of sensate cross-finger flap from dorsum of index after identifying branch of radial nerve.

Physical Design:
    Transposition
    Rotation
    Bilobed
    Rhomboid or Limberg
    Z-plasty
    Advancement

Location

The flap selected to close a wound or defect depends on the availability of sufficient excess tissue. If adequate coverage can be derived from tissue adjacent to the wound, a local flap may be constructed; otherwise a regional or distant flap must be used. All flaps, when transferred in a nonmicrosurgical manner, become random once the pedicle has been divided, irrespective of their original vascular design. The most commonly designed regional flap in the hand is the cross-finger flap[19,34,37] (Fig. 120-6) or thenar flap. Distant tissue commonly comes from the groin, abdomen, chest, or opposite arm. These flaps may be tubed (Fig. 120-7) or left untubed (see Fig. 120-6B).

A distinct disadvantage of regional and distant flaps is the immobility of the hand that is required during the period of neovascularization. While this may not be significant in the younger patient, edema, immobility of the hand, and flexion contractures that result from placement of the joints in acutely flexed positions may create considerable problems in older patients. This may preclude the use of some flaps or may subject the patient to a period of prolonged postoperative rehabilitation and morbidity. In designing distant flaps, therefore, patient age and future use of the hand are factors that must be carefully considered (Fig. 120-8). For example, in a working or elderly person shortening of a digit may be preferable to a prolonged period of reconstruction that could result in an insensate or poorly sensitized finger in a stiff hand.

Vascularity

Random Flaps

Random flaps are those flaps whose survival is dependent on the subdermal plexus (Fig. 120-9).[28,53,57] No constant, identifiable vessel is present. These are probably the most commonly used flaps in hand surgery today. They were also the most commonly used flaps before current understanding of flap vascularity. However, random flaps are inherently less hardy than flaps based on an identifiable vascular pedicle. The average Z-plasty is a good example of a random flap, although it may also be designed on a fasciocutaneous principle. Certainly, all distant flaps and some regional flaps, irrespective of the nature of the original vascularity, become random flaps once the pedicle is divided at 2 to 3 weeks. Common examples in the hand are the cross-finger flap[34,37] and the thenar flap (see Fig. 120-8). If a random flap originates from areas such as the abdomen, it is usually bulky and will require defatting. This is usually done a few weeks or months after the pedicle has been divided.

Fasciocutaneous Flaps

A fasciocutaneous flap is a flap comprised of skin, subcutaneous tissue, and the deep fascia, with its deep plexus of vessels. (Fig. 120-10) It reflects one of the more recent developments in our understanding of the blood supply to skin and thus flap design.[17,60,70] It is clear that, in most instances, blood supply of the subdermal plexus arises from a deeper plexus that runs on top of the deep fascia. From this plexus, perforators run up through the subcutaneous tissue to communicate with the subdermal plexus. The plexus on the deep fascia in turn receives vessels from perforators that pass up from the underlying muscle or may receive vessels directly from segmental vessels

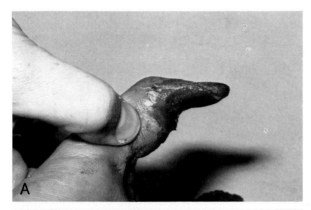

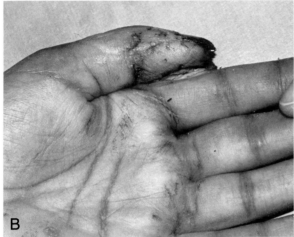

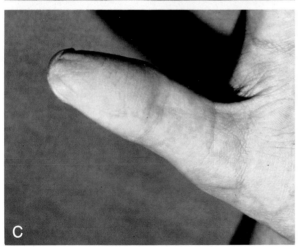

FIGURE 120-6. (*A*) Loss of soft tissue and nerves with exposed bone and tendon. (*B*) Cross-finger flap is in position after rerouting of nerve. (*C*) Final late result showing good padding with sensation.

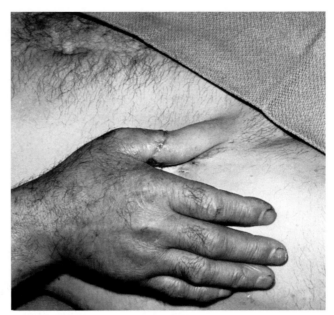

FIGURE 120-7. Salvage of avulsion injury of thumb and exposed bone with tube pedicle flap from groin.

turns it into an *island flap* (Fig. 120-11) and division of the vascular pedicle with transfer to another site in the body and microsurgical hook-up turns it into a *free microsurgical flap.* The lateral arm flap is a good example. Fasciocutaneous flaps may be designed as Z-plasties or transposition flaps (Fig. 120-12).

Myocutaneous or Muscle Flaps

It would appear that the dominant blood supply to skin is from vessels that pass up through the muscle, ramify in the plexus deep on the deep fascia, and then pass up through the subcutaneous tissue to supply the subdermal plexus (Fig. 120-13). If the entire muscle is raised with the overlying deep fascia, subcutaneous tissue, and skin, the flap thus raised is referred to as a *myocutaneous flap.* These flaps are extremely hardy and have allowed the closure and reconstruction of large defects hitherto impossible or difficult to close (Fig. 120-14). A good example is the latissimus dorsi myocutaneous flap raised with an island of skin. Muscle serves as an excellent vascular bed, thus these flaps may be raised as muscle flaps alone. A skin graft is then applied, which helps to reduce the bulky nature of most myocutaneous flaps. Muscle may also be used to restore function. There is some evidence to suggest that myocutaneous flaps may be of value in treating osteomyelitis.[11] The local delivery by the muscle of a rich vascular network, far richer than that found in a regular skin flap, appears to be the reason for this.

Axial or Island Flaps

An *axial* or *island* flap is a flap that has running within its longitudinal axis an identifiable vascular pedicle (see Fig. 120-11). The best known examples of this in the hand are the flaps based on digital vessels. Thus, we have the Moberg ad-

through the intermuscular septum. It is not surprising that most perforators come from the underlying muscle, if one recalls that an essential function of skin is to help dissipate heat generated by muscle activity.

If an identifiable vascular pedicle is seen to run in the longitudinal axis of the fasciocutaneous flap, it may also be referred to as an *axial flap.*[53,66] Skeletization of the vascular pedicle

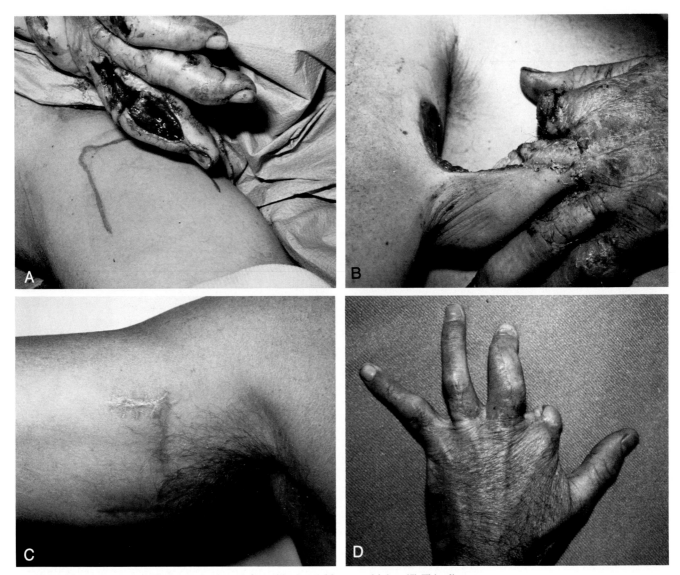

FIGURE 120-8. (*A*) Longitudinal narrow ulnar defect with exposed bone and joint. (*B*) Thin distant flap from hairless inner part of upper arm. This allows for functional use of arm during period of revascularization with injured hand in an elevated nondependent position, which greatly reduces edema. (*C*) Donor site after dividing and returning flap. Note well-hidden position of donor site. (*D*) Final result after division and inset of flap. Proximal interphalangeal joint has been fused at 35° to improve stability and function.

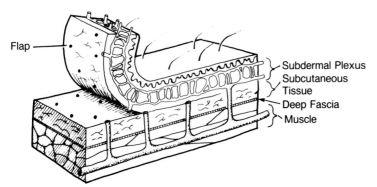

FIGURE 120-9. Random flap, in which the skin is supplied by the subdermal plexus only.

FIGURE 120-10. Fasciocutaneous flap consists of skin, subcutaneous tissue, deep fascia, and the deep vascular plexus, which is fed by a few perforators and in turn sends perforators up through subcutaneous tissue to the dermal plexus.

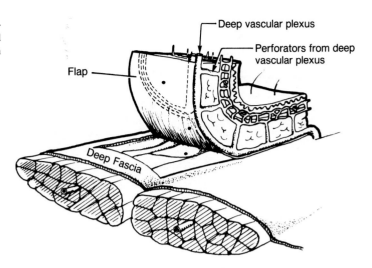

vancement flap[46] used for coverage of thumb and occasionally fingertip injuries. Isolation of the pedicle greatly increases the mobility of the flap and allows it to be transferred to almost anywhere in the hand.[12,23,41,58,62,64] The most common donor site is the ulnar or nonpinch border of a finger, used to resurface the thumb (Fig. 120-15). Many other island or axial flaps can be designed in the hand and arm. The radial forearm flap is a combination fasciocutaneous and island flap.[22,24,68,69]

In hand surgery, a commonly used axial distant flap is the groin flap,[30,48,52] although many flaps raised from the abdomen are actually myocutaneous in nature and receive their blood supply from perforators that exit the rectus abdominus muscle (see Fig. 120-14B). These flaps have a tendency to be bulky, especially in obese patients. Under these conditions, if a small flap is sufficient it may be thinned down or defatted considerably to reduce bulk. This allows for survival on the subdermal plexus but is less hardy than a flap raised on an identifiable axial vessel such as the superficial circumflex iliac in the groin or the superficial inferior epigastric in the lower abdomen. Once the flap has been set into the defect, it is allowed to sit in position for 2 to 3 weeks, at which time the pedicle is divided.[31,71]

Once divided from its pedicle, the flap immediately becomes random in nature with a less hardy blood supply; thus great

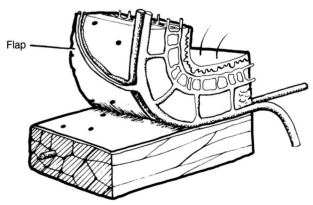

FIGURE 120-11. Axial flap, with identifiable artery running in the longitudinal axis of the flap.

care must be exercised when insetting the flap. Too much tension or undermining will result in wound edge necrosis or partial loss of the flap. If any doubt exists, delay the inset a few days or weeks. When planning the flap, it is also well to remember that every effort must be made to create darts or break straight line closure of the flap. Straight scars have a tendency to contract and may spoil the functional and even cosmetic success of the flap.

Physical Design

All flaps have a physical or mathematical design or shape, irrespective of their blood supply or location relative to the defect. This is the oldest means of classifying skin grafts, and stems from the period when the blood supply to skin (and thus the flap design) was not as clearly understood as it is today. The designs in this group are based on the surgeon's perception of how best to move local tissue from an area of relative excess to the defect requiring coverage or where the defect created by raising the flap may be easily and safely covered with a skin graft (Fig. 120-16 and see Fig. 120-12B). These flaps are therefore usually local or regional in nature.

Transposition Flaps

A transposition flap[42] is a flap that is elevated immediately adjacent to a defect and rotated about a pivot point into an immediately adjacent defect. Because the pivot point is relatively fixed, the design of the flap is such that it should be longer or must extend beyond the defect in length; otherwise it will not cover the defect (Fig. 120-17). The defect created by elevation of the flap can occasionally be closed using local tissue undermining or a skin graft (see Figs. 120-12B and 120-16).

Rotation Flaps

A rotation flap is similar to a transposition flap in that it rotates about a pivot point; however, it is semicircular in design. If too much tension exists at the pivot point and thus in the radius of the flaps, it can be relieved by making a small back cut through

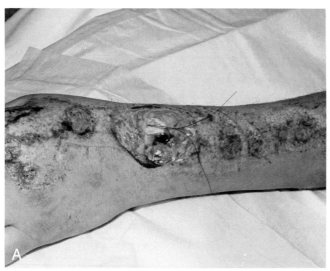
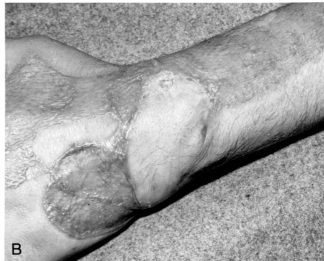

FIGURE 120-12.   (*A*) Open wound with exposed tendon and bone and joint in patient on high doses of steroid. Distant flap would have been suboptimal due to risk of infection. (*B*) Coverage of defects in one stage with fasciocutaneous-type transposition flap demonstrating relatively long narrow flap that was used safely. Donor site was covered with split-skin graft.

skin and dermis, taking great care not to disturb the underlying vascular pattern. The open triangle created is referred to as "Burow's triangle," and can usually be closed as a straight line (Fig. 120-18).

Bilobed Flaps

The principles associated with transposition flaps and the use of excess tissue near to but not immediately adjacent to a defect can be used to create a bilobed flap. The excess skin or area of greatest skin laxity is usually at right angles to the defect; thus a transposition flap is designed adjacent to the defect. The defect created by raising this flap is in turn closed by a second, somewhat smaller transposition-type flap (Fig. 120-19).

Rhomboid or Limberg Flaps

A rhomboid (Limberg) flap is a geometrically designed transposition flap (Figs. 120-20 and 120-21). The defect is made to be rhomboid in shape and thus equilateral in design to the flap.[5,16,35,40] The transverse diameter is therefore equal in length to any of the outer sides; for example, in Figure 120-20, line *ac* = line *bc*, and so forth. In designing the flap, an equal length is continued to make up the second side of the flap (see Fig. 120-20, line *ce*). The third side is a line parallel to any side of the rhomboid flap (see Fig. 120-20, line *ef*).

Z-Plasty

The Z-plasty flap is probably the most common design used in hand surgery.[21,25,65,73] It is a transposition-type flap, and is usually used to cure a scar contracture or to prevent one. Z-plasties may be single (Fig. 120-22) or multiple. The single type consists of two transposition flaps that are interchanged, effectively lengthening the scar but also breaking its length, thus reducing the likelihood of recurrence of the contracture. The sides have traditionally been of equal length but the angles may vary. The central limb or trunk that represents the con-

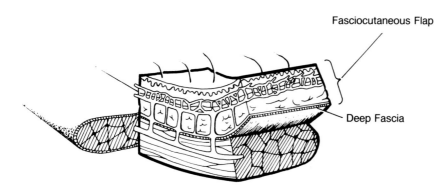

Fasciocutaneous Flap

Deep Fascia

Musculocutaneous Flap

FIGURE 120-13.   *Musculocutaneous flap* consists of muscle with overlying skin and subcutaneous tissue. Vascularity is from vessels in muscle that perforate muscle and join plexus on deep fascia. From this plexus perforators pass up through the subcutaneous tissue to join the subdermal plexus. *Fasciocutaneous flap* consists of skin and subcutaneous tissue, with the deep fascia and plexus supplied by a few dominant perforators from the underlying muscle, which itself is left undisturbed.

FIGURE 120-14. (*A*) Large defect with exposed bone, tendons, and nerves on radial side of hand and entire forearm covered with temporary dressing mesh graft. (*B*) Large, distant abdominal flap raised as myocutaneous flap based on perforators that come off the rectus abdominus muscle. External fixator in position for stabilization of associated fracture of ulna and radius. (*C*) Final result after division and inset of flap. Patient still requires reconstruction of thumb which can best be accomplished in this three-fingered, badly damaged hand with a toe-to-hand transfer.

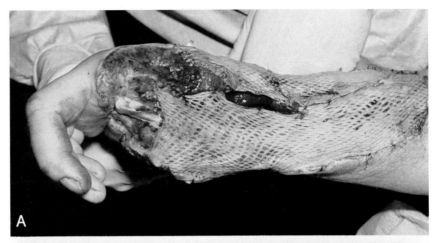

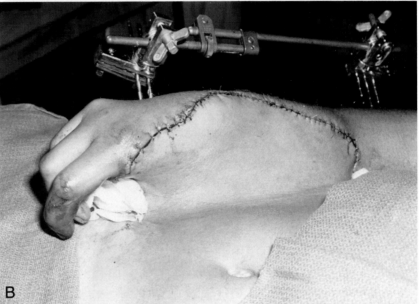

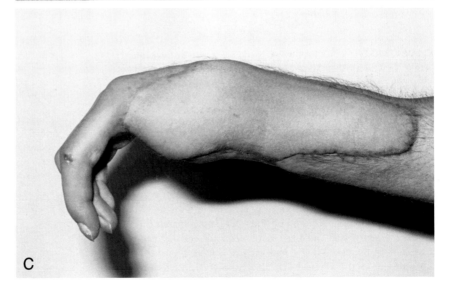

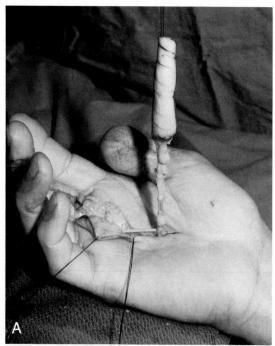

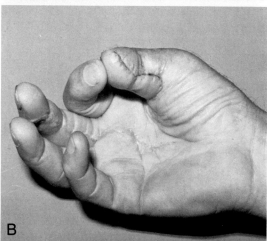

FIGURE 120-15. (A) Elevation of island sensory flap from ulnar border. Long finger flap is used to cover insensate tip of thumb, flap, and pedicle and then is rerouted subcutaneously to cover thumb. Note large island used to optimize function. (B) Final result after inset of island sensory axial-type flap and coverage of donor site with split-skin graft.

tracture should be longer than the two limbs or angle cuts.[74] In designing a Z-plasty, the scar or contracture forms the vertical component of the "Z." Choice of placement and angle of the flaps is made by first deciding on the optimal placement of the transverse scar once the flaps have been raised and repositioned or transposed. If the scar crosses a flexion crease, for example, make the vertical line along the vertical axis of the scar. Plan the crease so that it will be positioned along the midpoint of this scar. Then draw a line transecting the vertical scar and extend it laterally on each side of the scar for a dis-

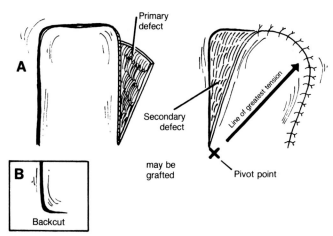

FIGURE 120-16. Classic transposition flap demonstrating transfer of locally adjacent tissue to cover a defect. Note that flap extends beyond defect to allow for shortening of flap as it rotates around the pivot point. Note also use of backcut to relieve undue tension from pivot point to apex of flap. Secondary defect is generally closed with skin graft.

tance no greater than half the length of the vertical scar. Draw a line from this point to the apex of the scar on one side and the most distal portion of the scar on the other (Fig. 120-23). The angle created is usually 60°.

Make a vertical incision down to the appropriate subcutaneous layer, making sure that the level of elevation is just above the neurovascular bundles if the dissection is being done in the finger, or down through the subcutaneous tissue, very often to the deep fascia, in other areas. If the Z-plasty is being performed to release a scar contracture, cut down deep enough to totally release or divide the scar. Then carefully elevate the flaps at exactly the same level, making sure that the subcutaneous tissue containing the diffuse vascular network is undamaged. Transpose the flaps and suture them together, using the

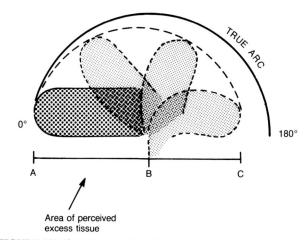

FIGURE 120-17. Transposition flap demonstrating shortening of arc of rotation and useful flap length as rotation approaches 180°. Use of a cloth pattern will aid in planning adequate length.

FIGURE 120-18. Rotation flap showing planned use of excess tissue (*A*) to cover defect. *B* and *C* illustrate techniques used to relieve excess tension from pivot point to triangular tip of flap. Cut is usually through dermis only.

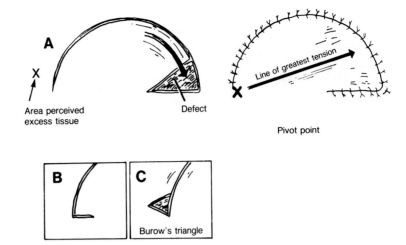

finest suture available; the minimal number of sutures required to obtain adequate approximation should be used. Ideally, the suture should never be larger than size 5-0. The needle should only pierce epidermis and dermis, leaving the underlying dermal plexis untouched. When placing a corner stitch, take great care not to damage the blood supply to the tip of the flap. This is best done by using a half-buried vertical mattress suture (Fig. 120-24).

All transposition flaps in the upper limb and hand, to ensure survival, must be raised with an intact vascular network. In practice this means that they must be raised in the hand, for example, just above the neurovascular plane. Elsewhere, they are raised just above the paratenon or the thin, loose areolar layer that invests most muscles. If the loose areolar layer over blood vessels, paratenon, or perineurium is left intact, not only is a good bed left for possible skin grafting, but flap survival with the vascular network intact is greatly increased.

Advancement Flaps

For single pedicle advancement flaps, the tip of the flap is advanced longitudinally away from its base to cover a defect.

These flaps are therefore usually rectangular in shape.[29] The advancement flap most commonly used in the hand is probably that described by Moberg to cover a tip amputation of the thumb. The volar skin elevated includes both neurovascular bundles back to the metacarpophalangeal joint. It may be necessary to flex the distal interphalangeal or metacarpophalangeal joint in order to achieve closure, and occasionally further length may be obtained by dividing the flap at its base, thereby turning it into an island flap. The defect created is closed with a skin graft. Flexion of the joint is usually corrected with time and use. More than one flap or technique may be used at any one time to optimize the result.

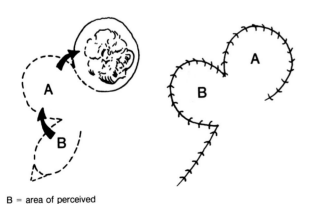

B = area of perceived tissue excess

FIGURE 120-19. Bilobed flap using transfer of perceived excess tissue from *B* to *A*, which in turn is transferred into primary defect.

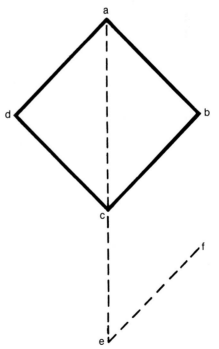

FIGURE 120-20. Diagram of rhomboid flap.

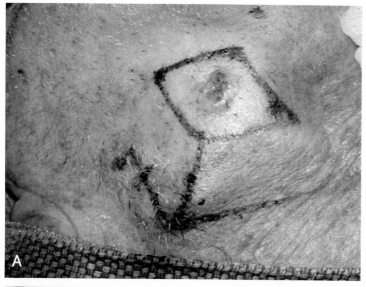

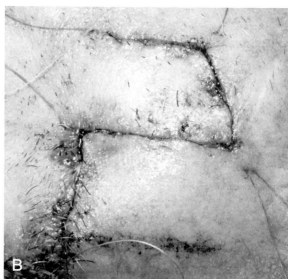

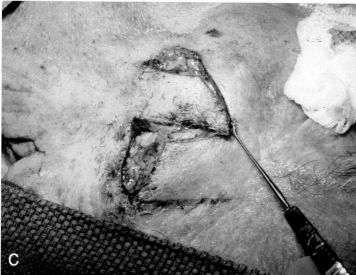

FIGURE 120-21. (*A*) Skin tumor with excision planned as rhomboid. (*B*) Elevation of transposition-type rhomboid to close defect. (*C*) Final result after closure.

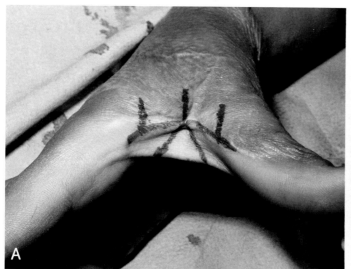

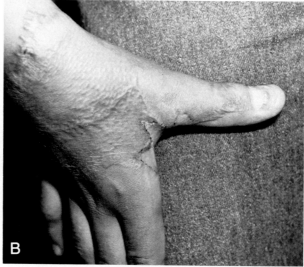

FIGURE 120-22. (*A*) Double opposing Z-plasty to release web-space conracture. Note that original use of mesh graft produced suboptimal cosmetic result on constantly exposed and visible dorsum of hand. (*B*) Final result shows good release of web space to 90° with no recurrence of contracture.

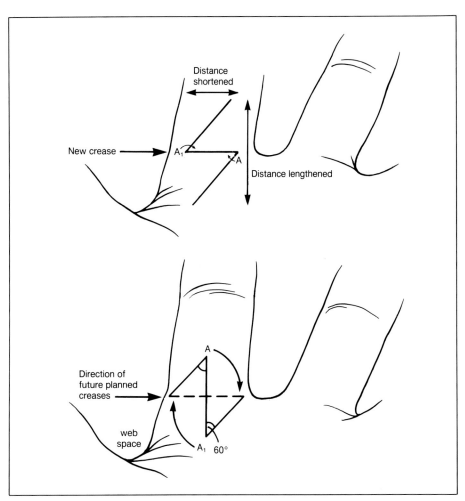

FIGURE 120-23. Technique of Z-plasty, using an angle of 60°.

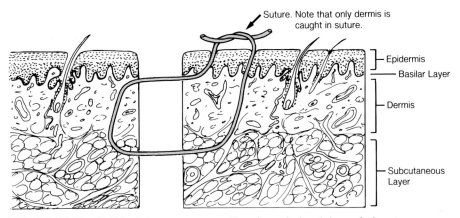

FIGURE 120-24. Half-buried mattress suture. Note that only dermis is caught in suture.

REFERENCES

1. Argamaso, R.V.: Rotation Transposition Method for Soft Tissue Replacement on the Distal Segment of the Thumb. Plast. Reconstr. Surg. **54**:366, 1974.
2. Barwick, W.J., Goodkind, D.J., et al.: The Free Scapular Flap. Plast. Reconstr. Surg. **69**:779, 1982.
3. Beasley, R.W.: Cosmetic Considerations in Surgery of the Hand. *In* Tubiana, R. (ed.): The Hand, Vol. 2. Philadelphia, W.B. Saunders, 1985.
4. Biddulph, S.L.: The Neurovascular Flap in Fingertip Injuries. Hand **11**:59, 1979.
5. Borges, A.F.: The Rhombic Flap. Plast. Reconstr. Surg. **67**:458, 1981.
6. Buncke, H.J., Buncke, C.M., and Schultz, W.P.: Immediate Nicoladoni Procedure in the Rhesus Monkey or Hallux-to-Hand Transplantation, Utilizing Microminiature Vascular Anastomoses. Br. J. Plast. Surg. **19**:332, 1966.
7. Buncke, H.J., Daniller, A.I., Schultz, W.P., et al.: The Fate of Autogenous Whole Joints. Plast. Reconstr. Surg. **39**:333, 1967.
8. Buncke, H.J., and Harris, G.D.: Skin Coverage for Challenging Hand Injuries. *In* Strickland, J.W., and Steichen, J.B. (eds.): Difficult Problems in Hand Surgery. St. Louis, C.V. Mosby, 1982.
9. Buncke, H.J., and Schulz, W.P.: Total Ear Reimplantation in the Rabbit Utilising Microminiature Vascular Anastomoses. Br. J. Plast. Surg. **19**:15, 1966.
11. Chang, N., and Mathes, S.: Comparison of the Effect of Bacterial Inoculation in Musculocutaneous and Random Pattern Flaps. Plast. Reconstr. Surg. **70**:1, 1982.
12. Chase, R.A.: Early Salvage in Acute Hand Injuries with a Primary Island Flap. Plast. Reconstr. Surg. **48**:521, 1971.
13. Chase, R.A., and Nagel, D.A.: Cosmetic Incisions and Skin, Bone, and Composite Grafts to Restore Function of the Hand. AAOS. Instr. Course Lect. **XXIII**:96, 1974.
14. Clemmesen, T.: Experimental Studies on the Healing of Free Skin Autografts. Dan. Med. Bull. **14**(Suppl. 2):1, 1967.
15. Converse, J.M.: Transplantation of Skin Grafts and Flaps. *In* Reconstructive Plastic Surgery, pp. 152–239. Philadelphia, W.B. Saunders, 1977.
16. Cormack, G.C., and Lamberty, B.G.H.: A Classification of Fasciocutaneous Flaps According to Their Patterns of Vascularization. Brit. J. Plast. Surg. **37**:80, 1984.
17. Cormack, G.C., and Lamberty, B.G.H.: Fasciocutaneous Vessels in the Upper Arm: Application to the Design of New Fasciocutaneous Flaps. Plast. Reconstr. Surg. **74**:244, 1984.
18. Cuono, C.B.: Double Z-Rhombic Repair of Both Large and Small Defects of the Upper Extremity. J. Hand Surg. **9**:197, 1984.
19. Curtis, R.M.: Cross-Finger Pedicle Flap in Hand Surgery. Ann. Surg. **145**:650, 1957.
20. Davis, J.S., and Kitlowski, E.A.: The Immediate Contraction of Cutaneous Grafts and Its Cause. Arch. Surg. **23**:954, 1931.
21. Davis, J.S., and Kitlowski, E.A.: The Theory and Practical Use of the Z Incision for the Relief of Scar Contractures. Ann. Surg. **109**:1001, 1939.
22. Fatah, M.F., and Davies, D.M.: The Radial Forearm Island Flap in Upper Limb Reconstruction. J. Hand Surg. **9B**:234, 1984.
23. Foucher, G., and Braun, J.B.: A New Island Flap Transfer from the Dorsum of the Index to the Thumb. Plast. Reconstr. Surg. **63**:344, 1979.
24. Foucher, G., van Genechten, F., Merie, N., et al.: A Compound Radial Artery Forearm Flap in Hand Surgery: An Original Modification of the Chinese Forearm Flap. Br. J. Plast. Surg. **37**:139, 1984.
25. Furnas, D.W., and Fischer, G.W.: The Z-Plasty: Biomechanics and Mathematics. Brit. J. Plast. Surg. **24**:144, 1971.
26. Gilbert, D.A.: An Overview of Flaps for Hand and Forearm Reconstruction. Clin. Plast. Surg. **7**:123, 1980.
27. Gilbert, D.A., Teot, L.: The Free Scapular Flap. Plast. Reconstr. Surg. **69**:601, 1982.
28. Grabb, W.C., and Myers, M.B. (eds.): Skin Flaps. Boston, Little, Brown, and Co., 1975.
29. Grabb, W.C., and Smith, J.W. (eds.): Plastic Surgery: A Concise Guide to Clinical Practice, 2nd ed. Boston, Little, Brown, and Co., 1973.
30. Heath, P.M., Jackson, I.T., Cooney, W.P., et al.: Simultaneous Bilateral Staged Groin Flaps for Coverage of Mutilating Injuries of the Hand. Ann. Plast. Surg. **111**:462, 1983.
31. Hoffmeister, F.S.: Studies on Timing of Tissue Transfer in Reconstructive Surgery. Plast. Reconstr. Surg. **19**: 283, 1957.
32. Hueston, J.: The Extended Neurovascular Island Flap. Brit. J. Plast. Surg. **18**:304, 1965.
33. Jacobson, J.H., and Suarez, E.L.: Microsurgery in the Anastomosis of Small Vessels. Surg. Forum **11**:243, 1960.
34. Johnson, R.K., and Iverson, R.E.: Cross-Finger Pedicle Flaps in the Hand. J. Bone Joint Surg. **53-A**:913, 1971.
35. Katsaros, J., Schusterman, M., Bepu, M., et al.: The Lateral Upper Arm Flap: Anatomy and Clinical Applications. Ann. Plast. Surg. **12**:490, 1984.
36. Ketchum, L.D.: Skin flaps. *In* Green, D.P. (ed.): Operative Hand Surgery, vol. 2. New York, Churchill Livingstone, 1982.
37. Kleinert, H.E., McAlister, C.G., MacDonald, C.J., et al.: A Critical Evaluation of Cross Finger Flaps. J. Trauma **14**:756, 1974.
38. Koss, N., and Bullock, J.D.: A Mathematical Analysis of the Rhomboid Flap. Surg. Gynecol. Obstet. **141**:439, 1975.
39. Krizek, T.J., Tani, T., Des Prez, J.D., and Kiehn, C.L.: Experimental Transplantation of Composite Grafts by Microsurgical Vascular Anastomoses. Plast. Reconstr. Surg. **36**:538, 1965.
40. Lee, K.K., Magargle, R.K., and Posch, J.L.: Free Full Thickness Skin Grafts from the Palm to Cover Defects of the Fingers. J. Bone Joint Surg. **52-A**:559, 1970.
41. Lesavoy, M.A.: The Dorsal Index Finger Neurovascular Island Flap. Orthop. Rev. **9**:91, 1980.
42. Lister, G.D.: The Theory of the Transposition Flap and its Practical Application in the Hand. Clin. Plast. Surg. **8**:115, 1981.
43. Lister, G.D., and Gibson, T.: Closure of Rhomboid Skin Defects: The Flaps of Limberg and Dufourmentel. Br. J. Plast. Surg. **25**:300, 1972.
44. Lister, G.D., McGregor, I.A., and Jackson, I.T.: The Groin Flap in Hand Injuries. Injury **4**:229, 1973.
45. Littler, J.W.: Neurovascular Pedicle Transfer of Tissue in Reconstructive Surgery of the Hand. J. Bone Joint Surg. **38-A**:917, 1956.
46. Macht, S.D., and Watson, H.K.: The Moberg Volar Advancement Flap for Digital Reconstruction. J. Hand Surg. **5**:372, 1980.
47. Mathes, S.J., and Nahai, F.: Clinical Atlas of Muscle and Musculocutaneous Flaps. St. Louis, C.V. Mosby, 1979.
48. May, J.W., and Bartlett, S.P.: Staged Groin Flap in Reconstruction of the Paediatric Hand. J. Hand Surg. **6**:163, 1981.
49. McCraw, J.B., and Dibbell, D.G.: Experimental Definition of Independent Myocutaneous Vascular Territories. Plast. Reconstr. Surg. **60**:212, 1977.
50. McCraw, J.B., Dibbell, D.G., and Carraway, J.H.: Clinical Definition of Independent Myocutaneous Vascular Territories. Plast. Reconstr. Surg. **60**:341, 1977.
51. McGregor, I.A.: Flap Reconstruction in Hand Surgery: The Evolution of Presently Used Methods. J. Hand Surg. **4**:1, 1979.
52. McGregor, I.A., and Jackson, I.T.: The Groin Flap. Brit. J. Plast. Surg. **25**:3, 1972.
53. McGregor, I.A., and Morgan, G.: Axial and Random Pattern Flaps. Br. J. Plast. Surg. **26**:202, 1973.
54. McLean, D.H., and Buncke, H.J.: Autotransplant of Omentum to

a Large Scalp Defect with Microsurgical Revascularization. Plast. Reconstr. Surg. **49:**268, 1972.

55. Miller, A.M.: Single Fingertip Injuries Treated by Thenar Flap. Hand **6:**311, 1974.

56. Murray, J.F., Ord, J.V.R., and Gavelin, G.E.: The Neurovascular Island Pedicle Flap. J. Bone Joint Surg. **49-A:**1285, 1967.

57. Myers, G., and Donovan, W.: The Location of the Blood Supply in Random Flaps. Plast. Reconstr. Surg. **58:**314, 1976.

58. Peacock, E.E.: Reconstruction of the Hand by the Local Transfer of Composite Tissue Island Flaps. Plast. Reconst. Surg. **25:**298, 1960.

59. Polk, H.C., Jr.: Adherence of Thin Skin Grafts. Surg. Forum **17:**487, 1966.

60. Ponten, B.: The Fasciocutaneous Flap. Its Use in Soft Tissue Defects on the Lower Leg. Br. J. Plast. Surg. **34:**215, 1981.

61. Ragnell, A.: The Secondary Contracting Tendency of Free Skin Grafts. Brit. J. Plast. Surg. **5:**6, 1953.

62. Rose, E.H.: Local Arterialized Island Flap Coverage of Difficult Hand Defects Preserving Donor Digit Sensibility. Plast. Reconstr. Surg. **72:**848, 1983.

63. Sawhney, C.P., and Subbaraju, G.V.: Healing of Donor Sites of Split Skin Grafts—An Experimental Study in Pigs. Brit. J. Plast. Surg. **22:**359, 1969.

64. Schlenker, J.D.: Transfer of a Neurovascular Island Pedicle Flap Based Upon the Metacarpal Artery: A Case Report. J. Hand Surg. **4:**16, 1979.

65. Shaw, D.T., Li, C.S., Richey, D.G., et al.: Interdigital Butterfly Flap in the Hand (the Double-Opposing Z-Plasty). J. Bone Joint Surg. **55-A:**1677, 1973.

66. Smith, P.J.: The Vascular Basis of Axial Pattern Flaps. Br. J. Plast. Surg. **26:**150, 1973.

67. Smith, P.J., Foley, G., McGregor, I.A., and Jackson, I.T.: The Anatomical Basis of the Groin Flap. Plast. Reconstr. Surg. **49:**41, 1972.

68. Song, R.Y., Gao, Y.Z., Song, Y.G., et al.: The Forearm Flap. Clin. Plast. Surg. **9:**21, 1982.

69. Soutar, D.S., and Tanner, S.B.: The Radial Forearm Flap in the Management of Soft Tissue Injuries of the Hand. Br. J. Plast. Surg. **37:**18, 1984.

70. Tolhurst, D.E., and Haeseker, B.: Fasciocutaneous Flaps in the Axillary Region. Br. J. Plast. Surg. **35:**430, 1982.

71. Tsur, H., Daniller, A., and Strauch, B.: Neovascularization of Skin Flaps—Route and Timing. J. Plast. Reconstr. Surg. **66:**85, 1979.

72. White, W.L.: Flap Grafts to the Upper Extremity. Surg. Clin. North Am. **40:**389, 1960.

73. Woolf, R.M., and Broadbent, T.R.: The Four-Flap Z-Plasty. Plast. Reconstr. Surg. **49:**48, 1972.

74. Yanai, A., Nagata, I., and Okabe, K.: The Z in Z-Plasty Must Have a Long Trunk. Brit. J. Surg. **39:**390, 1986.

Index

Numbers followed by *f* indicate a figure; *t* following a page number indicates tabular material.

Brachial plexus (*continued*):
  ventral approach through zig-zag incision, 1421–1422, 1421f
  injury to, 619, 742, 1393, 1425f, 2143
    causes of, 1417, 1418t
    classification of, 1419–1420, 1420t
    closed, 1417–1418
    diagnosis of, 1418–1421
    fibrosis in, 1420t
    indications for surgery in, 1421
    infraganglionic, 1418, 1418t
    lateral extension of, 1419, 1419t
    location of, 1418–1419, 1418–1419t
    open, 1417
    palliative surgery in, 1424–1426
    prognosis in, 1420t, 1421
    spinal cord lesion, 1418, 1419t
    supraganglionic, 1418, 1418t
    surgical techniques in, 1420t
    in thoracic outlet surgery, 1435
    thoracic outlet syndrome and, 1429t
    trunk, 1418, 1419t
    upper extremity amputation in, 600
  repair of:
    biceps tendon transfer in, 1424
    complications of, 1426
    epifascicular epineurotomy in, 1420t, 1423
    forearm flexor muscle transfer in, 1424
    interfascicular epineurectomy in, 1420t, 1423
    latissimus dorsi muscle transfer in, 1424
    muscle transfer in, 1424
    nerve graft in, 1420t, 1423–1424, 1425f, 1426
    nerve transfer in, 1420t, 1424
    neurolysis in, 1423–1424
    neurorrhaphy in, 1423
    pectoralis major muscle transfer in, 1424
    postoperative care in, 1424
    selection of surgical techniques in, 1424
    shoulder arthrodesis in, 1425
    surgical techniques in, 1423–1424
    tendon transfer in, 1424
    triceps tendon transfer in, 1424–1425
    wrist arthrodesis in, 1426
  surgical approach to, 1421–1423, 1421f
Brachioradialis flap, 1036
Brachioradialis muscle, 1132–1133f
  characteristics of, 1371t, 1372f
  innervation of, 1379, 1380f
  release of, in stroke, 1457, 1457f
  transfer of, in tetraplegia, 1464–1466, 1465f
Brachioradialis tendon, transfer of:
  in cerebral palsy, 1445–1446
  in high median-high ulnar palsy, 1414
  in median nerve palsy, 1398
Bracing:
  in cervical spine injury, 1903
  in fracture of tibial plateau, 430–431
Braided suture, 81
Brain stem, herniation of, 2122–2123
Brand tendon stripper, 1155, 1159–1160
Branhamella satarrhalis, 1496t
Breast, metastatic carcinoma of, 959, 968–969f, 979f, 1513
Bridge plate fixation, of fracture, of hand, 1217, 1217f
Brittain arthrodesis, of hip, 868–869
Broach, 1321, 1322f, 1325
Brodén's views, of heel, 1725, 1726f
Brooker-Wills nail, 153, 154f, 159
Brooks technique, of atlantoaxial fusion, 1888
Broomstick bar, 2166
Broomstick curl-up, 1576, 1577f
Brown-Séquard syndrome, 1895
Brucella, 2030
Brucella agglutination test, 2030
Brucellosis, 2019
  of spine, 2030–2031
Brun curette, 90f
Bruner approach, to hand. *See* Zigzag approach, to hand
Bruser approach, to knee, 55, 57f

Bucket-handle plica, 1588
Bucks-type splint, 342
Buerger's disease, 1075
Bulbocavernous reflex, 1922
Bullet, wounding characteristics of, 1328
Bunion, 69. *See also* Hallux valgus
  pain over, 1757
Bunionectomy, 1835
  chevron-type, 1759, 1762, 1762f
Bunnell drill, 94f
Bunnell's solution, 1318, 1323, 1325
Bunnell suture, 1144f
  modified, 1155, 1155f
Bunnell test, 1177t
Bunnell-type dressing, 1058
Bunnell/Williams procedure, in arthrogryposis, 2198
Bupivacaine (Marcaine), 1015, 1022–1023, 1165, 1585, 1647
Burn:
  first degree, 1117
  fourth degree, 1117–1118
  of hand, 1080
  second degree, 1117
  third degree, 1117
Burn boutonnière deformity, 1122
Burn contracture:
  axillary, 1129
  of elbow, 1128–1129, 1128f
  of hand, 1117–1129
  of index finger, 1123f
  of interphalangeal joint, 1122–1125, 1123–1124f
    Z-plasty in, 1122, 1123f
  of metacarpophalangeal joint, 1125–1128, 1127f
  of palm, 1122, 1124f
  soft tissue coverage in, 1117–1118, 1118f
  of thumb, 1118–1122, 1120–1121f
    adduction, 1119, 1120f
    adductor release in, 1119
    extension, 1119
    flexion, 1119
    opposition, 1119
    skin graft in, 1119, 1120f
    trapezial excision in, 1119
    Z-plasty in, 1119
  of wrist, 1125–1128, 1127f
Burn syndactyly, 1125, 1125–1126f
Burr, 378, 1553f, 1554
Bursitis:
  of olecranon, in tetraplegia, 1461, 1461f
  subacromial, 742
  trochanteric, 702
  tuberculous, 870, 870f
Bursography, subacromial, 742
Buttocks, heart-shaped, 2006
Button suture, 1155, 1155f, 1160–1161
Buttress plate, 139f, 140, 428–429, 429f, 431f

Cable-hook compression instrumentation, in kyphosis surgery, 2001–2003, 2003f
Cable tensioner, 1973, 1973f
Calcaneocavus foot, 2186
Calcaneocuboid joint:
  arthrodesis of, 1738, 1740f, 1743–1744, 1744f, 1747, 1811–1812, 1815–1816, 1816f
  in congenital vertical talus, 2153–2154, 2154f
  injury to, surgical techniques in, 1743–1744
  surgical approach to, 66, 66f, 1742, 1742f, 1815
Calcaneofibular ligament, 471, 472f
Calcaneonavicular joint:
  in clubfoot, 2147–2148
  surgical approach to, 65, 66f
Calcaneovalgus foot, 2161, 2199
Calcaneus:
  in clubfoot, 2148

Calcaneous (*continued*):
  fracture of, 1739f, 1811, 1813
    case studies of, 1730–1735f, 1731–1734
    with lateral fragment displaced upward, 1732–1733, 1733f
    postoperative care in, 1728
    reduction of, 1725
   joint depression-type fracture of, 1732, 1732f
    anatomy of, 1723–1725, 1724f
    classification of, 1725, 1726f
    complications of, 1734–1736
    with fragment containing entire posterior facet, 1734, 1735f
    pin fixation of, 1728–1730, 1729–1730f, 1732, 1732f
    surgical techniques in, 1725–1731, 1727–1730f
  osteomyelitis of, 841–842, 842f
    Gaenslen, 67
  osteotomy of:
    in cerebral palsy, 2161–2162, 2162f
    lateral closing wedge, 2161–2162, 2162f
    lateral opening wedge, 2162, 2162f
  surgical approach to, 1727
    lateral, 66, 67f
    medial, 66
    split heel, 67, 68f
    U approach, 66–67
  tongue-type fracture of, 1730–1731f, 1731
    anatomy of, 1723–1725, 1724f
    classification of, 1725, 1726f
    complications of, 1734–1736
    with fragment containing entire posterior facet, 1733–1734, 1734f
    pin fixation of, 1728–1730, 1729–1731f
    surgical techniques in, 1725–1731, 1727–1730f
  tuberculosis of, 862f
Calcific tendinitis, 750, 750f
Calcitonin, in fracture healing, 119
Calcium aluminate, 916
Calf, pseudohypertrophy of, 2175, 2175–2176f
Calf hypertension. *See* Compartment syndrome, acute
Calf-squeeze test, 1827
Callus, 115–117, 116–117f
  elephant's foot, 494, 494f, 498, 498–500f
  horse's foot, 494
  resorption of, 118f
Callus bone union, 118–119
Camino catheter technique, for measurement of pressure in muscle compartment, 186
Campbell triceps reflection approach, to elbow, 791
Cancellous bone graft, 97–98, 911, 1227
  chips or strips, 99
  sources of, 99, 103–104, 105f
Cancellous screw, 125–126, 127f, 1214f
Candida, 850
Cannula system:
  for arthroscopic surgery, 1555–1556, 1555–1556f, 1579, 1580f, 1592
  for needle biopsy of spine, 2133–2134, 2133f
Capillary ischemia, in compartment syndrome, 184f
Capitate, 1251, 1253f
  in capitate-lunate instability, 1299
  chondromalacia of, 1581
  displacement of, 1255, 1256f
  fracture of, 1261
Capitate-lunate joint, 1292, 1293f
  arthrodesis of, 1292
Capitellum:
  chondroplasty of, 1571
  osteochondritis of, 1574
Capsular ligament, 1669–1670, 1670f, 1673
Capsulectomy, in Dupuytren's disease, 1097, 1097f, 1103
Capsulitis, adhesive, of shoulder, 751
Capsulodesis:
  in combined nerve palsy, 1412, 1413f, 1414
  of metacarpophalangeal joint, 1210, 1445

Prostaglandin, in treatment of vascular spasm, 1007t
Prostate, metastatic carcinoma of, 959, 961f
Prosthesis:
  body-powered, 602
  immediate postoperative, 610–611
  as limb salvage procedure, 893–894
  loosening of, 376–378
  modular-design, 894, 894f
  myoelectric, 602
  upper extremity, 599, 602
Prosthetic spacer, in cervical spine, 1934, 1934f
Protection plate. See Neutralization plate fixation
Protein malnutrition, 606
Proteus mirabilis, 850, 1496, 1496t, 2017
Prothrombin time, 110
Protrusio acetabulum, 682–683, 683–685f, 690
  bipolar hip arthroplasty with, 669–670, 671f
Protrusio ring, 963
Protrusio shell, 960–962, 962–963f, 965f
Proximal intrinsic release, of intrinsic contractures
    of hand muscles, 1111–1113, 1113f
Pseudarthrosis, 500f
  in arthrodesis, of small joints of hand,
      1313–1315
  of cervical spine, 2053
  classification of, 494–495, 494t, 495f
  congenital, of tibia, 98–100
  definition of, 489, 491f
  hypertrophic, 490f
  infected, 504f, 506f
  of lumbar spine, 1947, 1954–1955, 1955f
  of proximal humerus, 532f
  in scoliosis surgery, 1988, 1993
  of spine, 2123
  synovial, 489, 491f, 500–501, 536
  of thoracolumbosacral spine, 1963–1964
Pseudogout, 847, 849
Pseudohypertrophy, of calf, 2175, 2175–2176f
Pseudomonas, 837, 1496, 2017
Pseudomonas aeruginosa, 825–826, 850, 1496t
Pseudosubluxation, of cervical spine, 1884
Pseudotendon, 1166
Psoas abscess:
  drainage of, 2034
  surgical excision of, 2038–2039
Psoas muscle, anatomy of, 1874, 1874f, 1907t
Psychological evaluation, 2046, 2055–2056,
    2056t
Pubic ramus:
  fracture of, 330
  nonunion of, 551
  surgical approach to, 37, 38f, 551
Pubis, osteomyelitis of, 843
Pulley reconstruction, 1157–1158, 1159–1160f
Pull-out wire suture, 1195, 1195f
Pulmonary atelectasis, 1954
Pulmonary complications, of cervical spine injury,
    1902–1903
Pulmonary embolism, 108–110, 692, 702, 2093,
    2107
  in cervical spine injury, 1903
  diagnosis of, 110
  in fracture of acetabulum, 330, 339
  in lumbar spine surgery, 1947
  treatment of, 110
Pulmonary function tests, 1981, 2172, 2194
Pulp approach, to hand, 33f, 35
Pulse, peripheral, in compartment syndrome,
    183, 183–184f
Pulselessness, 1635
Pulvertaft interweave suture, 1156, 1156f, 1160
Pump, Jobst, 1366
Punch:
  arthroscopic, 1581f
  Rowe glenoid, 212, 213f
Punch forceps, 1591–1592, 1591f
  upcurve, 1591, 1591f
Puncture wound, of foot, 837–839, 841f
Putti bone rasp, 92f
Pyarthrosis:
  of ankle, 852–853, 855

Pyarthrosis (*continued*):
  of carpometacarpal joint, 851
  clinical presentation in, 848–849
  complications of, 856
  diagnosis of, 849–850, 849f
  of elbow, 851–852, 855
  of finger joints, 851–852
  of foot joints, 853
  of hip, 851–852, 854–856, 855f
  of knee, 851–853, 854f, 855
  microbiology of, 850–851
  pathophysiology of, 847–848, 848f
  prognosis in, 854–855f, 855–856
  rehabilitation in, 854–855
  in rheumatoid arthritis, 847–848
  of shoulder, 851–852, 855
  of subtalar joint, 852
  of toe joint, 853
  treatment of:
    antibiotics in, 853–854
    by aspiration, 851–852
    by surgical drainage, 851–853
    by synovectomy, 852
  of wrist, 851–852, 855
Pyelogram, 293, 549, 1966
Pyrazinamide, in tuberculosis, 2032–2033

Q angle, 718, 718f, 1594–1595, 1620, 1699, 1701,
    1704–1705
Quadratus lumborum muscle, anatomy of, 1907t
Quadriceps muscle group, 413, 419, 1620, 1626
  paralysis of, 2195t
  radical compartmental excision of, in soft-tissue
      sarcoma, 988–991, 990–992f
  strengthening of, 1656, 1661, 1675, 1703,
      1703f, 1712–1713
  weakness of, 2195
Quadriceps tendon, 427
  dislocation of, 1707
Quadriga effect, 1139, 1142, 1142f, 1150, 1153,
    1162
Quadrilateral frame, 162f, 163
Quadriparesis, 1894
Quadriplegia, 1883, 1895
  interphalangeal joint arthrodesis in, 1308

Radial artery, injury to, 999, 1302
Radial collateral ligament, of index finger, 1203
Radial digital nerve, injury to, 1074–1075
Radial forearm flap, 1028, 1029f, 1037, 1037f,
    1537
Radial nerve:
  anatomy of, 1379–1380, 1380f
  compression of, 1132, 1188, 1355–1359,
      1355–1359f
  decompression of, 1134–1135
  entrapment of, 224
  fascicular topography of, 1340
  injury to, 221, 233, 536, 804, 1148, 1178,
      1193–1194, 1287, 1302
    in forearm fracture, 271
  as source of nerve graft, 1423
  surgical approach to, 20–21, 21f
Radial nerve palsy, 1182, 1375, 1379–1390. See
    also Combined nerve palsy
  Boyes transfer in, modified, 1382t, 1387–1388,
      1389–1390f
  complications of, 1389
  early tendon transfer in, 1388–1389
  flexor carpi radialis transfer in, 1382t,
      1385–1387, 1387–1388f
  flexor carpi ulnaris transfer in, 1382–1385,
      1382t, 1384–1386f
  high, 1379
  humeral fracture and, 1380
  neurolysis in, 1380

Radial nerve palsy (*continued*):
  postoperative care in, 1389
  restoration of wrist extension in, 1382, 1383f
  splinting in, 1381, 1381f
  surgical techniques in, 1381–1388, 1382t
  treatment principles in, 1380–1381
Radial tuberosity, surgical approach to, 20–21,
    21f
Radial tunnel, surgical approach to, 1358f
Radial tunnel syndrome, 1188, 1190, 1357–1359
  complications of, 1359
  postoperative care in, 1358–1359
  surgical techniques in, 1358–1359, 1358–1359f
Radial wrist extensor tendinitis, 1194
Radian, 1373, 1374f
Radiate ligament, 1252
Radical palmar fasciectomy, 1094–1095
Radical resection, in soft-tissue sarcoma, 985–986
Radicular pain symptoms, 2045–2046
Radiculopathy:
  cervical, 1428, 1429t
  in cervical disc herniation, 1929–1930
  cervical spondylosis with, 1930
Radiocapitate ligament, 1251–1252
  rupture of, 1255
Radiocarpal joint, 263
  arthrodesis of, 1295, 1299–1300
  aspiration of, 1504–1505
  fibrous nonunion of, in rheumatoid arthritis,
      1303, 1303f
  surgical approach to, 28, 29f, 30, 31f
  synovectomy of, 1487, 1489
Radiocarpal ligament, injury to, 1255, 1582
Radiohumeral joint, 263, 792
Radiolunate joint, 1292, 1293f
  arthrodesis of, 1299, 1487, 1487f
  sclerosis at, 1486f
  subluxation of, 1486f
Radioscaphocapitate ligament, rupture of, 1296
Radioscaphoid joint, 1292, 1293f, 1295, 1299
  anatomy of, 1291, 1292f
  arthrodesis of, 1299
Radioscaphoid ligament, 1251–1252
  injury to, 1252
  rupture of, 1255, 1296
Radioscaphoid-lunate ligament, injury to, 1299
Radioscapholunate joint, arthrodesis of, 1487,
    1491
Radiotriquetral ligament, 1251–1252
  rupture of, 1255
Radioulnar joint, 263, 277–278
  arthrodesis of, 1491
  aspiration of, 1504–1505
  distal:
    arthritis of, 1266
    arthrodesis of, 1272–1277, 1274f,
        1276–1277f
    in Colles' fracture, 1272–1273
    dislocation of, 1265, 1266f
    fracture of, 1265, 1266f
    hemiresection arthroplasty in, 1271–1272,
        1272f, 1277
    injury to, 1257
    repair of:
      ligamentous reconstruction in, 1267–1271,
          1268–1271f
      radial osteotomy in, 1274–1275
      resection of ulnar head in, 1265–1267
      selection of operative procedure in,
          1276–1277
      ulnar osteotomy in, 1272–1275,
          1273–1275f
    in rheumatoid arthritis, 1267–1268,
        1275–1276, 1276–1277f
    stability of, 1265–1267
    synovectomy of, 1303
  instability in, 1580–1581
  laxity of, 1487f
  proximal, 1272
  sclerosis at, 1486f
  surgical approach to, 32f, 33
  synovectomy of, 1489

CHAPMAN
Operative Orthopaedics
Volume 2

ISBN 0-397-50920-0

90000

9 780397 509201